STANDARDS FOR
CRITICAL CARE

STANDARDS FOR

CRITICAL CARE

Brenda Crispell Johanson, RN, MA, EdM, CCRN

Instructor, Staff Education, Emergency and Critical Care Specialties,
The New York Hospital–Cornell Medical Center,
New York, New York

Consuelo Urtula Dungca, RN, MA, EdM

Associate Director of Eye, Medicine, and Surgery Nursing Department,
Formerly, Medical Clinical Specialist, The Presbyterian
Hospital in the City of New York at Columbia Presbyterian Medical
Center, New York, New York

Denise Hoffmeister, RN, MA, CNRN

Administrative Nurse Clinician, Neurological Institute,
The Presbyterian Hospital in the City of New York at
Columbia Presbyterian Medical Center, New York, New York

Sara Jeanne Wells, BSN, MN

Clinical Supervisor, Critical Care Division,
The Lankenau Hospital, Philadelphia, Pennsylvania;
Clinical Instructor, Department of Baccalaureate Nursing,
Thomas Jefferson University, Philadelphia, Pennsylvania;
Formerly, Cardiovascular Clinical Specialist,
Administrative Nurse Clinician,
The Presbyterian Hospital in the City of New York at Columbia
Presbyterian Medical Center, New York, New York

SECOND EDITION

The C. V. Mosby Company

ST. LOUIS • TORONTO • PRINCETON   1985

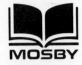

MOSBY

A TRADITION OF PUBLISHING EXCELLENCE

Editor: Barbara Ellen Norwitz
Assistant editor: Sally Adkisson
Manuscript editor: Timothy O'Brien
Book design: Jeanne Genz
Cover design: Gail Morey Hudson
Production: Kathy Teal, Judy England, Ginny Douglas

SECOND EDITION

Previous edition copyrighted 1981

Printed in The United States of America

The C.V. Mosby Company
11830 Westline Industrial Drive, St. Louis, Missouri 63146

Library of Congress Cataloging in Publication Data
Main entry under title:

Standards for critical care.

 Bibliography: p.
 Includes index.
 1. Intensive care nursing—Standards. I. Johanson,
Brenda Crispell, 1950-   . [DNLM: 1. Critical Care—
standards—nurses' instruction. WY 154 S785]
RT120.I5S7 1985   610.73′61   84-9804
ISBN 0-8016-2526-2

GW/VH/VH 9 8 7 6 5 4 3 2 1   05/A/598

Contributors

Susan C. Archbold, R.N., B.S.N.

Head Nurse, Combined Intensive Care Unit, The Lankenau Hospital, Philadelphia, Pennsylvania

Ann Aurigemma, R.N., M.A.

Inservice Instructor, Pediatrics, New York University Medical Center, New York, New York

JoAnne Bennett, R.N., M.A., C.N.A.

Administrative Assistant Director of Nursing, Long Island College Hospital, Brooklyn, New York; Adjunct Instructor, Lienhard School of Nursing, Pace University, Pleasantville, New York

Nina Eldridge Born, R.N., B.S.N.

Assistant Instructor, Staff Education, The New York Hospital–Cornell Medical Center, New York, New York

Edna Cadmus, B.S.N., M.A., CCRN

Administrative Nurse Clinician, Surgical Nursing Department, The Presbyterian Hospital in the City of New York at Columbia Presbyterian Medical Center, New York, New York

Margaret Carty, R.N., M.S.N., C.E.N., CCRN

Head Nurse, Cardiac Care Unit, The New York Hospital–Cornell Medical Center, New York, New York

Janette Cavallo-Alderman, R.N., M.A., CCRN

Instructor, New England Deaconess School of Nursing, Boston, Massachusetts

Mary K. Clark, R.N., M.A., CCRN

Research Nurse, Cardiovascular Center, The New York Hospital–Cornell Medical Center, New York, New York

Frank Costello, B.S.N., M.S.W., CCRN

Clinical Nurse Specialist, Burn Center, The New York Hospital–Cornell Medical Center, New York, New York

Mary E. Cuff, R.N., M.A., C.S.

Clinical Instructor, Medicine, New York University Medical Center, New York, New York

Joan Holter Gildea, R.N.C., M.A.

Clinical Assistant Director of Nursing, Pediatrics, New York University Medical Center, New York, New York

Barbara A. Griggs, R.N., M.A.

Associate Director, Nutritional Support Service, University Hospital, Cleveland, Ohio

Jennifer Mary Hanns, R.N., M.A., CCRN

Clinical Specialist, Eastern Region, Hewlett–Packard Co., Paramus, New Jersey; formerly Supervisor, Medical Special Care Unit, The Mount Sinai Hospital, New York, New York

Mary Fran Hazinski, R.N., M.S.N.

Pediatric Intensive Care, Vanderbilt University Hospital, Nashville, Tennessee; formerly Clinical Specialist, Cardiovascular-Thoracic Surgery, The Children's Memorial Hospital, Chicago, Illinois

Margaret A. Heenan-Chovanes, R.N., CCRN

Head Nurse, Surgical Intensive Care Unit, The Lankenau Hospital, Philadelphia, Pennsylvania

Gertrude Parker Johnson, B.S.N., CCRN

Senior Head Nurse, Cardiothoracic Intensive Care Unit, Surgical Special Care Unit, The New York Hospital–Cornell Medical Center, New York, New York

Catherine Muttart Mansell, R.N., M.A., M.S.

Consultant, Pediatric Nutritional Support and Education, New Hempstead, New York

P. Gilroy Marsella, R.N., B.A., CCRN

Senior Staff Nurse, Cardiac Care Unit, The New York Hospital–Cornell Medical Center, New York, New York

Patricia Noethling, R.N.

Supervisor, Clinical Electrophysiology Lab, The Presbyterian Hospital in the City of New York at Columbia Presbyterian Medical Center, New York, New York

Rebecca Cohen Phillips, B.S.N., M.S.

Hypertension Nurse Consultant, Bayside, New York

Laura Seche, R.N., M.S.N., CCRN

Formerly Cardiac Transplant Research Assistant, presently Staff Nurse, Surgical Cardiac Intensive Care Unit, The Presbyterian Hospital in the City of New York at Columbia Presbyterian Medical Center, New York, New York

Colette Schafran, R.N., CCRN

Nursing Care Clinician, Surgical Anesthesia Intensive Care Unit, The Presbyterian Hospital in the City of New York at Columbia Presbyterian Medical Center, New York, New York

Carol E. Shanik, R.N., M.S.

Perinatal Nursing Consultant, Chatham, New Jersey

Maryellen Sohmer, B.S.N., C.I.C.

Infection Control Coordinator, Good Samaritan Hospital, Suffern, N.Y.; Formerly Nurse Epidemiologist, The New York Hospital–Cornell Medical Center, New York, New York

Virginia P. Wahl, R.N., M.S.N., CCRN

Instructor, Staff Education, The New York Hospital–Cornell Medical Center, New York, New York

Consultants

Edna Cadmus, B.S.N., M.A., CCRN
The Presbyterian Hospital in the City of New York at Columbia Presbyterian Medical Center, New York, New York

Mary K. Clark, R.N., M.A., CCRN
The New York Hospital–Cornell Medical Center, New York, New York

Rosemary Conlon, R.N., B.S.N.
The Kontron Company, Boston, Massachusetts

Eileen Fortune Damante, R.N., M.S.N., CCRN
The New York Hospital–Cornell Medical Center, New York, New York

Ann Duckles
The New York Hospital–Cornell Medical Center, New York, New York

Antoinette Pochabet Fiorato, B.S.N.
The New York Hospital–Cornell Medical Center, New York, New York

Marianne Lichtenstein, R.N.
The Children's Memorial Hospital, Chicago, Illinois

James McCrossan, R.N.
Westchester County Medical Center, Valhalla, New York

Brent Miedema, M.D.
The New York Hospital–Cornell Medical Center, New York, New York

David Miller, M.D.
The New York Hospital–Cornell Medical Center, New York, New York

Mary Lee Warner Mohr, R.N., M.S.N.
The Lankenau Hospital, Philadelphia, Pennsylvania

Mary Moran, R.N.
The New York Hospital–Cornell Medical Center, New York, New York

Marlene Nadler-Moodie, R.N., M.S.N.
Clinical Nurse-Specialist in Psychiatric Mental Health Nursing, Carlsbad, California

Eugene Nowak, M.D.
The New York Hospital–Cornell Medical Center, New York, New York

Martha Orr, R.N., M.N.
The New York Hospital–Cornell Medical Center, New York, New York

Malcolm Perry, M.D.
The New York Hospital–Cornell Medical Center, New York, New York

Paul Stelzer, M.D.
The New York Hospital–Cornell Medical Center, New York, New York

Barbara Suchak, B.S.N., M.S., CCRN
The Presbyterian Hospital in the City of New York at Columbia Presbyterian Medical Center, New York, New York

Foreword

The first edition of *Standards for Critical Care* was published in 1981. It stands as the first publication devoted to standards for critical care nursing. Because it is written by clinicians, it has been both relevant and practical. Other critical care clinicians have applied the standards to their own patient care settings with little modification. It is for this reason that the text has been so widely accepted and used.

In the Foreword of that first edition I asked the readers to let the authors know about their experiences in implementing these standards. The response from the readers has been gratifying and has assisted the authors with the development of the second edition.

When I review the second edition of a book I want to know how it differs from the first edition. This was a very easy task with this text. In keeping with the rapid growth of critical care nursing, the number of standards has been increased by 25%. More contributors have authored sections within the text, and the pediatric standards have been expanded. This edition also separates the standards for psychosocial needs/care and infection control as well as incorporating them in other standards. Besides the extensive addition of standards, all of the previous standards have been revised. The additions as well as the revisions reflect current critical care nursing practice as well as the latest diagnostic techniques and therapeutic interventions.

The use of nursing diagnoses has been expanded in the revision of this text. As nursing diagnosis terminology is refined, its use will be extended in future editions. Because this edition is consistent with this philosophy of refining and updating, the second edition of *Standards for Critical Care* will make a significant contribution to the aggressive professional development of critical care nursing that is a goal for the 1980s.

Diane C. Adler, RN, MA, CCRN, FAAN
Clinical Director, Critical Care
Nursing, Hospital of the University
of Pennsylvania, Philadelphia

Past President, American Association
of Critical Care Nurses

Preface

Since our first edition, the formidable challenge of caring for the acutely ill patient has continued to be met by a rapidly expanding understanding of physiological and psychological interactions in multisystem diseases. Technological advancements have led to the development of more sophisticated procedures and equipment, which therefore facilitate heroic life-sustaining interventions and more subtle manipulations for altering the course of an illness. The level of sophistication necessary to carry out such large-scale intervention is indeed high.

This edition incorporates this new information into our previous standards and has grown with 15 new standards that address additional disease entities, such as hypertensive crisis, acquired immune deficiency syndrome, drug overdose, cardiomyopathies, and pleural compromise. Expanded coverage of therapeutic and/or diagnostic modalities includes the Broviac/Hickman catheter, chest tubes, transluminal coronary angioplasty, and electrophysiological testing. Separate attention to the psychological, emotional, and spiritual care of patients as well as infection control activities is provided.

The setting in which critical care occurs is unique in that continuous subjective and objective monitoring of labile parameters is essential to assure quality care. The critical care nurse therefore must integrate a knowledge of physiological principles involving multiple organ systems with a minute-by-minute monitoring of function. An accurate assessment followed by an appropriate intervention is of utmost importance.

Two primary objectives in any nursing unit are the education of new nurses and the maintenance of high standards that guarantee quality care. In critical care, the difficulties encountered in realizing these objectives are intensified by the breadth of material to be mastered and the severely compromised, often unstable, state of the patients. A comprehensive, problem-oriented manual that describes common conditions encountered in a critical care setting, along with accepted therapeutic and preventive interventions and their indications, is needed to facilitate the education process.

Nursing care standards must be in writing and must be reemphasized frequently. As before, it is our intent that this text serve as a model from which individual institutions and nurses can modify content to develop their own standards consistent with institutional policy. Standards are the basis for formulating plans for ongoing care as well as for evaluating the effectiveness with which it is delivered. They can form the basis for standard care plans. The educational value of an inclusive collection of standards is obvious. A beginning critical care nurse will be able to refer to such a source for introductory reading in an orientation program as well as when preparing a daily care plan. Moreover, instructors, clinical specialists, and head nurses are provided with a tool for evaluating the quality of care delivered and the performance of staff members in many specific situations.

Standards of care can provide the basis for prospective and concurrent audit activities, an evaluation process that helps to assure the delivery of safe, high-quality care. In this age of closer public scrutiny of health care delivery, a written policy describing established procedures at every level of hospital function is mandatory to maintain institutional accreditation and public approval.

Standards for Critical Care is designed for use in the clinical setting, in the classroom, in administrative planning, and in evaluation. This book's clinical value is its problem-oriented approach to a wide variety of conditions and its efficient delivery of essential information.

Standards for Critical Care includes more than lists of objectives and procedures. Each standard includes an introduction, assessment parameters, goals of care, and a problem-oriented chart composed of nursing activities. The introduction to each topic summarizes the salient features of pathophysiology underlying each disease state and outlines various diagnostic and therapeutic modalities that may be used. Thus the introduction provides a rationale for the sections that follow. The nurse's assessment focuses attention on a selected set of parameters that should be monitored throughout a given patient's hospital course. It serves as a guide or "organizer" of parameters to be assessed. Each assessment factor takes on more or less significance depending on the specific case as well as the staff and equipment available for monitoring. By referring to the introduction and the chart of nursing activities, the reader will be able to understand and formulate a priority for each assessment factor and integrate the information into an actual care plan. Moreover, a thorough, ongoing assessment provides for a precise definition of the patient's clinical status and permits early detection of abnormalities associated with the patient's primary health problem. For each of these "potential" problems, nursing activities that serve to prevent, identify, evaluate, and resolve the abnormality are described.

The patient and family must be adequately informed and supported during the hospital experience. Each standard outlines essential components of the teaching plan, including information about diagnostic tests, the disease process, and therapy. For surgical intervention, teaching guidelines regarding the surgery and perioperative experiences are enumerated. Special attention is given to follow-up care at the end of most standards. Finally, each standard cites comfort measures, which can make the hospital experience more pleasant.

The nursing activities in these standards form the basis for a plan of care that is tailored to the patient's illness and clinical presentation. As the nurse administers treatment to alter the patient's clinical course, nursing measures will be modified according to hospital policy and protocol in conjunction with the state nurse practice acts.

This is important to stress, because states' nurse practice acts vary, and clarification of legal activities for nursing is continuously changing, particularly in critical care nursing. Thus the activities described in these standards serve as a guide for developing a plan of care that best supports the patient at any point in an acute illness.

We would again like to thank Ms. Diane Adler for her thoughtful foreword. We would also like to thank the many clinical experts who acted as consultants and participated in reviewing our standards for this edition.

Brenda Crispell Johanson
Consuelo Urtula Dungca
Denise Hoffmeister
Sara Jeanne Wells

Contents

APPENDIXES

STANDARDS FOR
CRITICAL CARE

Respiratory

STANDARD 1

PULMONARY EDEMA OF CARDIAC ORIGIN

Acute pulmonary edema is a cardiac emergency that occurs when the hydrostatic pressure in the pulmonary capillaries (normally 7 to 10 mm Hg) exceeds the intravascular osmotic pressure (25 to 30 mm Hg), resulting in transudation of fluid into the alveoli. This reduces the amount of lung tissue available for gas exchange. It may develop suddenly or evolve slowly. The most common cause of pulmonary edema is acute left ventricular failure, usually secondary to acute myocardial infarction (AMI). Other causes include decompensating chronic heart failure, mitral valve disease, hypertension, circulatory overload, and central nervous system (CNS) injuries.

Management of pulmonary edema includes measures for decreasing venous return to the heart and, consequently, the pulmonary vasculature; improving gaseous exchange; improving cardiac output and the efficiency of left ventricular function; controlling anxiety; and treating complications that may evolve. The problems are interrelated; many of the approaches and medications used influence several of these management objectives.

For a discussion of the adult respiratory distress syndrome, or ''shock lung,'' see Standard 2, *Acute respiratory failure*.

ASSESSMENT

1. History of recent myocardial infarction (MI), left heart failure (acute or chronic), mitral valve disease, hypertension, CNS injury, and/or recent parenteral fluid administration to evaluate circulatory overload
2. Medication history, including what medications have been prescribed and level of compliance; if low level of compliance, the reason why
3. Presence of
   a. Extreme restlessness
   b. Orthopnea
   c. Tachypnea
   d. Extreme dyspnea—air hunger
   e. Bubbling rales
   f. Wheezing
   g. Coughing
   h. Nature of secretions—blood-tinged, frothy sputum
4. Level of anxiety
5. Hemodynamic status
   a. Blood pressure (BP)
   b. Pulses
   c. Heart sounds
   d. Venous pressure
   e. Fluid balance
   f. Mental status
   g. General appearance
   h. Invasive monitoring if indicated
      (1) Intraarterial pressure
      (2) Pulmonary artery pressure (PAP) and pulmonary capillary wedge pressure (PCWP)
      (3) Cardiac output
      (4) Central venous pressure (CVP)
6. Monitor electrocardiogram (ECG) for
   a. Arrhythmias
   b. Changes reflecting electrolyte imbalance, especially potassium (K^+)
   c. Changes reflecting myocardial damage, for example, AMI
   d. Drug effects
7. Lab data results of
   a. Blood gas levels
   b. Electrolytes
   c. Blood urea nitrogen (BUN)/creatinine clearance
   d. Chest radiograph for pulmonary congestion and heart size
   e. Drug levels

1

f. Any tests performed to evaluate precipitating or aggravating factors

8. Patient/family's perception of and reaction to disease process, symptoms, assessment, and treatment modalities

See Standard 15, *Heart failure (low cardiac output)*

GOALS

1. Absence of respiratory distress—adequate oxygenation and ventilation
2. Hemodynamic stability—adequate cardiac output
3. Electrophysiological stability
4. Patient verbalizes physical comfort
5. Decreased anxiety with resolution of symptoms and provision of information
6. Patient verbalizes fears and concerns
7. Maintenance goals—see Standard 15, *Heart failure (low cardiac output)*

POTENTIAL PROBLEMS	EXPECTED OUTCOMES	NURSING ACTIVITIES
■ Respiratory distress related to excessive accumulation of fluid in alveoli, resulting in abnormal ventilation/perfusion ratios	■ Normal respiratory effort	■ Ongoing assessment of patient's respiratory effort Extreme dyspnea—air hunger Orthopnea Tachypnea Wheezing Cough—often producing copious, frothy blood-tinged sputum Check for and record nature of secretions, noting amount, color, and presence of blood
	Lungs clear to auscultation	Auscultate lungs q1 hr or more frequently if indicated for presence and distribution of adventitious sounds, often described as *bubbling*
	Arterial blood gas levels within patient's normal limits	Monitor blood gas results for evidence of hypoxia and hypercapnia that is not chronically present Intraarterial line may be inserted because of frequent need for samples and to monitor BP
	Hemodynamic stability	Check BP and pulse (P) for hypertension or hypotension and tachycardia Evaluate changes in venous pressure, noting Amount of distention of neck veins Peripheral or sacral edema Engorgement of peripheral veins Hepatomegaly Ascites
	Adequate cerebral oxygenation	Assess mental status for indications of cerebral hypoxia Restlessness, extreme anxiety Confusion Stupor Coma
	Clear lung fields on radiograph	Obtain and review results of chest radiograph; radiographic changes can be delayed up to 24 hours after onset of pulmonary congestion If problem occurs, record occurrence and responses to therapy and report to physician Maintain patent IV route using microdrip or infusion pump to regulate administration of fluid and drugs Implement measures to decrease venous return, decrease pulmonary congestion, and improve gaseous exchange, as ordered Place patient in high Fowler's position with lower extremities dependent; if patient is hypotensive, this position may not be well tolerated, and feet may need to be flat and head of bed lowered somewhat until hypotension is corrected
	Absence and/or resolution of pain	Administer morphine sulfate IV as ordered to control pain, decrease anxiety, and decrease venous return and respiratory effort, thereby improving oxygen exchange Check respiration (R) for respiratory depression Check BP for hypotension Have morphine antagonist available Morphine contraindicated in presence of cardiogenic shock, history of chronic pulmonary disease, or recent cerebrovascular accident (CVA)

POTENTIAL PROBLEMS	EXPECTED OUTCOMES	NURSING ACTIVITIES

	Electrolytes within normal limits
	Urine output 30 ml/hour or more; output increases with diuretics
		Administer diuretics IV as ordered to reduce blood volume and pulmonary congestion
		Insert Foley catheter as ordered and check urine output q1 hr
		    Check specific gravity; with furosemide and ethacrynic acid, diuresis should occur within 15 to 30 minutes
		    Observe for indications of urinary tract obstruction in patients with prostatic hypertrophy
		    Check for hypotension, tachycardia, and decreased urine output, indicating circulatory intolerance
		Monitor lab report results, and observe for signs and symptoms of K^+ and sodium (Na^+) depletion
		    Administer K^+ supplements as ordered
		        Use caution and administer slowly to avoid cardiac complications
		        Never add to infusions that contain antiarrhythmics or cardiotonic agents that may be titrated
		Monitor lab report results for BUN and/or creatinine clearance
		Avoid local infiltration of IV ethacrynic acid, which is extremely irritating to tissues
		Apply rotating tourniquets if ordered
		    Connect to upper portions of three extremities (leave IV extremity free) with pressure settings midway between systolic and diastolic readings
		    Check for presence of peripheral pulses and check warmth and color of extremities; adjust pressures if necessary to maintain palpable pulse
		    Ensure that tourniquets rotate in sequence q15 min; rotate more frequently for patients with vascular insufficiency
		    Reposition tourniquet on extremity q2 hr (when rotates off)
		    Observe for edema, pain, and/or loss of function of extremity; latter two indicate prolonged constriction
		    If edema develops, elevate limb and explain to patient that condition will resolve
		    When removing, rotate off one at a time at 15-minute intervals
		    Tourniquets are contraindicated with cardiogenic shock
		Prepare for and assist with phlebotomy if ordered
		    May be indicated if initiating problem is fluid overload
		    Rarely used with concomitant left heart failure, because procedure would aggravate shock
		Administer O_2 as ordered; pressure must be high enough to exceed pressure barrier of edema fluid without excessively reducing venous return, which would result in circulatory collapse; usual airway pressure necessary is 4 to 9 cm H_2O
		Administer positive pressure as ordered; trend is to intubate more quickly and to add positive end-expiratory pressure (PEEP)
		If positive pressure mask is ordered
		    Explain to patient that it is temporary, because it may be frightening to patient who already feels suffocated
		    Adjust mask to fit snugly
		    Pad face straps for comfort if necessary
		    Set O_2 concentration at 100%
		    Begin at 0 and slowly increase sensitivity setting to patient's respiratory effort
		    When removing positive pressure mask, slowly decrease sensitivity to 0 before discontinuing
		If patient requires intubation, see Standard 6, *Mechanical ventilation;* Standard 7, *Positive end-expiratory pressure*

■ Decreased cardiac output related to left ventricular dysfunction	■ Hemodynamic stability	■ Assess for development and/or acceleration of left heart failure; early recognition allows intervention that may prevent onset of pulmonary edema See Standard 15, *Heart failure (low cardiac output)*

POTENTIAL PROBLEMS	EXPECTED OUTCOMES	NURSING ACTIVITIES
		If acute pulmonary edema has occurred Check BP q15-30 min or more frequently if indicated Initially, normotensive patient may become hypertensive secondary to extreme anxiety and activation of sympathetic nervous system; hypotension occurs as result of deteriorating left ventricular function or secondary to therapeutic maneuvers identified in Problem, Respiratory distress related to excessive accumulation of fluid in alveoli Check P q15-30 min or more frequently if indicated; decreasing tachycardia may be indication of resolution of pulmonary edema and anxiety Observe for presence and degree of Pallor Cyanosis Diaphoresis Weakness Lethargy Restlessness Auscultate or review chart for presence of S_3 gallop Participate with physician in identification and treatment of conditions known to increase myocardial O_2 consumption, such as Anxiety, fear Hypertension or hypotension Arrhythmias Tachycardia Electrolyte imbalance Hypoxia, hypercapnia Administer medications as ordered to improve cardiac function through alterations in preload, afterload, or contractility Digoxin IV commonly ordered Determine if patient has been taking digoxin Monitor lab results closely for hypoxia and hypokalemia, which promote digoxin toxicity; replace K^+ if indicated and ordered Monitor ECG continuously for development of arrhythmias Aminophylline IV Administer slowly through IV soluset or infusion pump to avoid complications of syncope or sudden death Assess effect on relieving bronchospasm and promoting diuresis in addition to inotropic effect Observe for or ascertain presence of hypotension, ventricular tachyarrhythmias, palpitations, headache, dizziness, and nausea; inform physician if any of these occur Nitroprusside or other vasodilators IV may be ordered if pulmonary edema is accompanied by hypertension and increased PCWP Maintain patent intraarterial line Administer via infusion pump Maintain patent pulmonary artery line if indicated Monitor effects of medication closely and for hypotension and arrhythmias Ensure emergency equipment is available and functional; check every shift
■ Acute anxiety related to Fear of suffocation Cerebral anoxia Treatment modalities	■ Reduction of anxiety with relief of symptoms and provision of information Patient verbalizes fears and concerns Patient cooperates with treatment regimen	■ Ongoing assessment of level of anxiety; relate findings to psychological/physiological status Remain with patient, maintaining calm, controlled appearance Provide emotional support and reassurance to patient/family that therapeutic measures will reduce symptoms Explain purpose and expectations of treatment modalities used; this is particularly important if positive pressure mask, mechanical ventilation, or rotating tourniquets are ordered; repeated explanations are necessary because of high anxiety level

POTENTIAL PROBLEMS	EXPECTED OUTCOMES	NURSING ACTIVITIES

		Make patient as comfortable as possible
		    Positioning
		    Padding face mask
		    Mouth care
		    Tourniquet suggestions as noted in Problem, Respiratory distress related to excessive accumulation of fluid in alveoli
		    Prompt relief of pain
		Reduce environmental stimuli as much as possible
		Encourage patient/family to verbalize concerns and ask questions

■ Arrhythmias related to
    Hypoxia
    Hypokalemia
    Medications
    Concomitant disease
    Anxiety
	■ Electrophysiological stability
	    Optimal cardiac rhythm
		■ Maintain continuous ECG monitoring
		    Select lead best demonstrating atrial and ventricular complexes
		    Set rate alarms; avoid use of audio component if possible without compromising patient safety
		Participate with physician in identifying cause of arrhythmias, and treat as ordered
		    Review medications patient is receiving
		    Monitor lab results for
		        Hypoxia
		        Hypokalemia
		        Acidosis/alkalosis
		    Assess alterations in level of anxiety related to onset of arrhythmia
		    Assess status of underlying disease states, particularly left heart failure, hypertension, or acute myocardial infarction
		Assess effect of arrhythmia on cardiac output and pulmonary edema
		Check emergency equipment every shift, ensuring proper function and availability
		Treat arrhythmia as ordered
		
		See STANDARD 21 *Arrhythmias*
		      STANDARD 12 *Acute myocardial infarction*
		      STANDARD 15 *Heart failure (low cardiac output)*

ACUTE RESPIRATORY FAILURE

Respiratory failure is a condition wherein the respiratory system cannot supply adequate oxygen to maintain metabolism and/or cannot eliminate sufficient carbon dioxide to prevent respiratory acidosis.

Etiological factors for the development of pulmonary failure include the following (for management of etiological factors 1 and 3 to 7, refer to the appropriate standards of care):

1. Acute primary lung disease, such as aspiration pneumonia, near drowning, hyaline membrane disease, or pneumonitis
2. Secondary lung disease caused by hypoxia, shock (adult respiratory distress syndrome, embolism, severe heart failure, or fluid overload)
3. Acute deterioration of chronic lung disease, in which some stress such as superimposed infection or heart failure precipitates decompensation in patients with chronic obstructive lung disease
4. Depression of the respiratory center related to drugs, endocrine and metabolic disorders (e.g., encephalitis), stroke, tumors, trauma
5. Neuromuscular disorders such as myasthenia gravis, Guillain-Barré syndrome, tetanus
6. Chest trauma that may cause mediastinal emphysema, flail chest, pneumothorax, etc., which may result in respiratory failure
7. Thoracic surgery produces pain and promotes hypoventilation; a pneumonectomy results in hyperperfusion of the remaining lung, which reduces capillary diffusion time and may result in perfusion of even poorly ventilated lung areas, thus promoting respiratory insufficiency and failure

Each of these etiological factors that promote pulmonary insufficiency may be associated with one or more of three pathological mechanisms.

Hypoventilation. Hypoventilation is defined as an arterial Pco_2 above 45 mm Hg, which results from reduced air reaching the alveoli with a reduced minute volume. It results in decreased Pao_2 and an increased $Paco_2$ that is inversely proportional to the alveolar ventilation. This occurs in acute airway obstruction, restrictive defects, obstructive defects, neuromuscular defect, and respiratory depression.

Intrapulmonary shunting or ventilation/perfusion mismatch. Intrapulmonary shunting refers to blood that does not participate in oxygen transfer (from alveolar air to arterial blood). The mechanism may include absence of alveolar ventilation such as occurs in atelectasis and/or bronchospasm (normal amount of shunted blood is 5% to 6%). Ventilation/perfusion mismatch refers to perfusion of unventilated alveoli (pneumonia, asthma, atelectasis, hyaline membrane disease, adult respiratory distress syndrome) or ventilation of unperfused alveoli (e.g., pulmonary embolus).

Diffusion impairment. Diffusion impairment occurs when the alveolar capillary membrane is thickened, impairing the diffusion of gases, as the result of interstitial fibrosis, interstitial pneumonia, or collagen diseases such as scleroderma or hyaline membrane disease. Hypoxemia is usually the primary effect and can often be relieved by the administration of 100% oxygen.

The clinical signs and symptoms of impending acute respiratory failure may be varied and nonspecific, resulting in delayed diagnosis and treatment. The most prominent features are related to hypoxia. Clinical manifestations usually include an altered level of consciousness (LOC), confusion, headache, asterixis, papilledema (caused by increased Pco_2), cyanosis, tachycardia, diaphoresis, and rapid shallow respirations. The onset may be either fulminant and acute or insidious in nature.

Arterial blood gas determination permits the confirmation of acute respiratory failure. Severe impairment of gas exchange and hypoxemia ($Pao_2 < 60$ mm Hg) are seen. When the patient has generally healthy lungs, compensatory hyperventilation results in lowered arterial Pco_2. When chronic lung disease or another impairment of respiratory function is present, acute respiratory failure and hypoxia are usually accompanied by hypercapnia ($Paco_2 > 75$ mm Hg). Acidosis is usually present. Once the diagnosis is established, the therapy will include treatment of the pathogenesis, maintenance of adequate oxygenation, removal of carbon dioxide, correction of acidemia, and prevention or treatment of respiratory infection.

ACUTE DETERIORATION OF CHRONIC OBSTRUCTIVE PULMONARY DISEASE

Chronic obstructive pulmonary disease (COPD) is a descriptive phrase that refers to airway obstruction, including chronic bronchitis, emphysema, and asthma.

Airway obstruction results from excessive secretions, bronchospasm, and mucosal swelling. Bronchospasm commonly occurs in patients with asthma, chronic bronchitis, and, to some extent, patients with emphysema. In patients with asthma, immune reactions produce constriction of the airway. Irritants such as fumes, dust, smoke, and cold air can also promote bronchospasm, probably via neurogenic mechanisms; chemical substances such as serotonin and histamine may constrict the airway directly. Mucosal swelling from edema and the inflammatory process in the peripheral airways may result in bronchial and peribronchial fibrosis and kinking, narrowing, and occlusion of the air passages.

Bronchitis is inflammation and production of excessive mucous secretions in the bronchial structure with a chronic cough continuing for several months and recurring annually. The principal cause of bronchitis is prolonged irritation of the bronchial mucosa due to recurrent infections, smoking (more than 20 cigarettes daily), environmental pollutants, allergy, and autoimmune diseases. It is characterized by a generalized enlargement of goblet cells lining the wall of the trachea and bronchi. There is some loss of cilia with metaplasia of the epithelium. Functional findings show increased or normal functional residual capacity (FRC), decreased vital capacity (VC), increased residual volume (RV), and decreased forced expiratory volume, or volume exhaled in first second of the forced exhalation (FEVC). Alveolar hypoventilation causes ventilation/perfusion mismatch, which may result in severe hypoxemia and hypercapnia. The alveolar-arterial oxygen difference is always increased. Chronic hypoxemia produces compensatory polycythemia (increased hematocrit [Hct]).

Emphysema is described as an anatomical alteration in the lungs characterized by overinflation of the distal air spaces beyond the terminal bronchioles with progressive destruction of the alveolar and capillary membranes. The destruction of the alveolar walls results in the loss of support of the surrounding lung and collapse of small airways during expiration. Sputum production is usually minimal. Emphysema may be caused by recurrent infections, allergy, autoimmunity, environmental pollutants, and smoking (more than 20 cigarettes daily). Functional findings include increased FRC, RV, and total lung capacity (TLC) and decreased VC and FEV. As a rule, the arterial blood gas sample shows hypoxemia from loss of alveolar surface and airway dysfunction and normal Pco_2 because of increased respiratory drive and resultant hyperventilation. The alveolar-arterial oxygen difference is always increased. A majority of patients demonstrate signs and symptoms of both chronic bronchitis (marked by thickened secretions, recurrent infections, and bronchospasm) and emphysema (marked by pulmonary hyperinflation, collapse of airways, and dyspnea).

Asthma is defined as paroxysmal dyspnea caused by spasm of the bronchial tubes, hypersecretion of mucus and edema of the mucous membrane. Because of airway compression it is often accompanied by adventitial sounds. Cough is usually the first symptom that the patient experiences; this is followed by dyspnea, tachycardia, and diaphoresis. Wheezing may or may not be present. Airway spasm results in increased work of breathing and the use of accessory muscles. Initial arterial blood gas analysis during an attack will show hypocapnia and hypoxemia as a result of increased respiratory drive and ventilation/perfusion mismatch. If the patient's respiratory status deteriorates, hypercapnia and acidosis will result. Asthma may be present in two forms. *Extrinsic* asthma usually occurs in individuals predisposed by heredity and can be induced by exogenous factors to which the patient is allergic. *Intrinsic* asthma is caused by endogenous factors such as a hypersensitivity response. Psychological factors (especially stress) play an important role in the development of asthma.

Status asthmaticus is a term used for severe asthmatic attacks that are not responsive to the patient's own maintenance regimen or parenteral sympathomimetic amines.

Prolonged, severe COPD usually leads to cardiac compromise, called *cor pulmonale*. It is characterized by degenerative, fibrotic perivascular changes with increased pulmonary vascular resistance and ultimate right heart failure. Cor pulmonale is more commonly seen in patients with chronic severe hypoxia and compensatory pulmonary vasoconstriction. The ultimate result is a permanent increase in pulmonary vascular resistance and a severe increase in right ventricular afterload. The right heart eventually fails while attempting to generate extremely high pressure.

ADULT RESPIRATORY DISTRESS SYNDROME

For reasons that are not completely understood, hypoxic, septic, or traumatic injury to the lung causes massive pulmonary edema, atelectasis, and hyaline membrane deposits. Alveolar membranes are also injured, causing further loss of fluid into the alveoli and resulting in alveolar hypoventilation; the later development of pneumonitis and interstitial fibrosis causes a decrease in diffusion capabilities.

Lung compliance and FRC are tremendously reduced. Marked alveolar hypoventilation produces ventilation/perfusion mismatch and severe hypoxemia. Hypocapnia may be present while compensatory hyperventilation occurs. Development of hypercapnia indicates severe patient deterioration. With progressive hypoxia, acidosis is unavoidable.

These patients often require mechanical ventilation with high inspiratory and end-expiratory pressures. Plasma oncotic agents are usually administered to pull fluid back into the intravascular space (although administration of these was previously controversial). Some centers advocate the administration of corticosteroids in an effort to reduce inflammation and fibrosis of alveolar surfaces. Cardiac output must be maintained at a good level to avoid further pulmonary edema and patient deterioration.

The best approach to adult respiratory distress syndrome is prevention. Individuals at risk for the development of sepsis or shock must receive careful management to avoid acute hypoxic or hypotensive episodes. Once the predisposing crises has occurred, strict fluid management with observation for early signs of respiratory distress must be performed.

ASSESSMENT

1. Baseline information regarding history, presence, and nature of
   a. Onset and length of illness
   b. Recent changes in character and amount of sputum
   c. Repeated colds
   d. Frequency of exacerbation of acute attacks and/or infections
   e. Decreased tolerance for physical activity
   f. Progressive dyspnea
   g. Chronic morning cough
   h. Complications—bronchopneumonia, pleurisy, bronchiectasis, abdominal hernia (caused by cough), pulmonary embolism
   i. Any allergies to food, drugs, or adverse reactions to changes in weather
   j. Presence of related illness
      (1) Cor pulmonale
      (2) Hypertension
      (3) Renal disease
      (4) Diabetes
      (5) Peptic ulcer
   k. Family background—members of immediate family with pulmonary illnesses
   l. Place of residence
   m. Occupation
   n. Smoking habits (past and present)
2. Presence and extent of
   a. General abnormalities indicating evidence of hypoxemia, such as
      (1) Muscle twitching, coarse tremor
      (2) Malodorous breath
      (3) Abnormalities in skin color, including pallor, cyanosis
         (a) Peripheral—note particularly appearance of extremities, tip of ears and/or nose
         (b) Central—note particularly appearance of tongue and lips
      (4) Alterations in central venous system function that may be associated with pulmonary failure, including presence of restlessness, confusion, visual defects, fatigue
   b. Pulmonary abnormalities indicating evidence of respiratory distress, including
      (1) Tachypnea, dyspnea, orthopnea, shortness of breath
      (2) Abnormal breath sounds; adventitious breath sounds, including rales, rhonchi, wheezing
      (3) Changes in voice sounds
      (4) Abnormal vocal fremitus, noting location—left and right apices, mid lung and lower lung
      (5) Abnormal resonance of underlying thoracic tissue
      (6) Pleural friction rub
      (7) Abnormalities in sputum—color, consistency, quantity, and odor
3. Signs and symptoms of chronic lung disease
   a. Abnormal posture
      (1) Short and stocky appearance
      (2) Thin and asthenic appearance
   b. Malnutrition and weight loss
   c. Abnormalities in the configuration of thorax and its movements, such as pigeon breast, funnel chest, barrel chest, scoliosis, kyphosis
   d. Use of neck muscles for quiet respirations
   e. Clubbing of fingers
   f. Abnormal rate, rhythm, and amplitude of respiratory excursions of upper, anterior, middle, and posterior lower chest
   g. Sputum—any increase in amount, color, and consistency
   h. Persistent cough; loose, rattling cough, which is usually worse in the morning and evening and worse in damp and/or cold weather
   i. Cor pulmonale, including ankle edema, evidence of pulmonary hypertension, loud pulmonic closure sound, strain and enlargement of right ventricle, right ventricular gallop
   j. Cardiovascular dysfunction, including abnormal vital signs, hypotension or hypertension, tachycardia, arrhythmias and palpitations, chest pain, abnormal location of apical pulse, jugular venous distention, peripheral edema, cool skin temperature; oliguria
4. Baseline diagnostic and lab data
   a. Serial blood count for decreased Hct and hemoglobin (Hgb); presence of polycythemia and leukocytosis
   b. Cultures
      (1) Urinalysis indicating bacteriuria
      (2) Sputum culture and sensitivity (C and S) results
   c. Electrolyte levels
   d. Sedimentation rate
   e. Arterial blood gas levels
   f. Pulmonary function tests
      (1) Lung volume

(2) Lung capacity

(3) FEV

g. Chest radiographs

  (1) Anteroposterior diameter (may be increased with COPD)

  (2) Position of trachea

  (3) Density in both lung bases

  (4) Differences in lung size

  (5) Presence of any abnormalities such as atelectasis, right ventricular hypertrophy, flattened diaphragm, hyperinflation, and bullae

h. ECG for any abnormalities, including signs and symptoms of cor pulmonale such as abnormal P wave and QRS complex

i. Lung scan for any abnormalities

j. Bronchoscopy

5. Level of anxiety related to signs and symptoms present and their effect on patient/family's behavior and life-style

6. Extent of patient/family's knowledge regarding disease process, diagnostic procedures, and planned therapy

GOALS

1. Optimal respiratory function and adequate pulmonary ventilation

2. Adequate functioning of regulatory mechanisms, that is, elimination of waste and acid-base balance within patient's normal limits

3. Absence of pneumonia and other infections

4. Absence of complications of respiratory failure—pleural effusion, pulmonary interstitial edema, pulmonary microemboli, abdominal hernia, stress ulcer, malnutrition, and anemia

5. Electrolytes and blood count results within normal limits

6. Intake of nutrients sufficient to prevent weight loss or, if needed, achieve weight gain and positive nitrogen balance

7. Reduction of patient/family's anxiety with provision of information and explanation of disease process, diagnostic procedures, and therapeutic plans

8. Before discharge patient/family is able to

  a. Explain relationship between disease process and therapy prescribed

  b. Describe dietary, medication, and activity regimen

  c. Identify signs and symptoms of respiratory infection requiring medical attention

  d. Verbalize influence of environmental factors on illness and perform necessary measures to control these factors

  e. Explain importance of follow-up

POTENTIAL PROBLEMS	EXPECTED OUTCOMES	NURSING ACTIVITIES
■ Patient/family's anxiety related to dyspnea and fear of dying	■ Patient/family demonstrates decreased level of anxiety with provision of emotional support and information Patient uses pursed lip breathing effectively	■ Assess level of anxiety Prevent physiological factors that promote restlessness, anxiety Monitor vital signs and temperature Check that O_2 delivery device is functioning properly, i.e., patent tubing Observe for signs of hypoxia Position patient with head elevated Stay with patient or reassure patient that nurse will be close at hand Encourage pursed lip breathing q1 hr Encourage verbalization of anxiety or fear related to dyspnea and course of therapy Encourage pursed lip breathing every hour Encourage participation in care as tolerated Perform treatments in unhurried manner, allowing rest periods between treatments Provide comfort measures Administer analgesics as needed if ordered
■ Patient/family's anxiety related to limited understanding of Diagnostic procedures Disease process and prognosis Therapy employed Separation from family Disruption of life-style	■ Patient/family's behavior demonstrates decreased level of anxiety with provision of information and explanations Patient/family verbalizes understanding of disease process and its relationship to therapy employed Patient/family participates actively in planning and implementing care	■ Ongoing assessment of level of anxiety Describe nature of disease process and signs and symptoms patient is experiencing Explain relationship of disease process and rationale for various therapeutic interventions at level appropriate for patient/family's comprehension and degree of anxiety present Explain anticipated procedures involved in diagnostic process/plan of care and what patient will experience Assist in preparing patient for diagnostic procedures

POTENTIAL PROBLEMS	EXPECTED OUTCOMES	NURSING ACTIVITIES
■ Obstruction to gas exchange, which may be related to Thick viscous bronchial secretions Bronchial edema Bronchospasm Fibrosis and parenchymal destruction	■ Patent airway Both lungs fully aerated as visualized on chest radiograph Clear breath sounds in all areas Absence of signs and symptoms of hypoxia	Encourage patient/family's questions and verbalization of fears and anxieties Involve patient/family in planning for care Communicate findings to physician on continuing basis ■ Prevention Employ measures to prevent respiratory infection (see Problem, Pulmonary infections) Employ measures to remove secretions as needed Frequent postural drainage for large volume of secretions Chest physiotherapy Turn and position q2 hr Cough and deep breathe Administer bronchodilators as ordered for bronchial edema and bronchospasm Encourage pursed lip breathing by having patient pursed lips or say "F" during exhalation, especially for patients with fibrosis and parenchymal destruction Provide humidification of upper airway structures by means of face mask or high-humidity tent Monitor for Tachypnea Persistent cough; syncopal episodes related to sudden fit of coughing Increasing amount of sputum with changes in color, consistency, and odor Presence of abnormal breath sounds, rales, wheezing, stridor/snorting, and use of accessory muscles (retractions, nasal flaring, jaw tugging) Fever, sore throat Altered behavior; restlessness and/or changes in obtundation Onset of urticaria and/or hay fever Deterioration in arterial blood gas levels Serial blood count for leukocytosis Decreased breath sounds Increased respiratory effort and fatigue Notify physician of any of these abnormalities If problem occurs Employ measures for removal of secretions as ordered Increase fluid intake (in absence of heart failure) Liquefy sputum by steam inhalation Administer ACORN nebulizer treatment Administer vigorous chest physiotherapy unless contraindicated; breathing exercises q1 hr Frequent change of position in accordance with therapeutic regimen q2 hr Chest physiotherapy with postural drainage q2 hr Aseptic tracheal suctioning if patient unable to cough out secretions Administer medications such as iodides, detergents, and/or enzymes Administer antibiotic therapy as ordered Check vital signs including temperature q1 hr until stable; if fever occurs, notify physician and obtain needed cultures and then administer antipyretic agent or antibiotics as ordered to decrease fever and O_2 requirements Monitor serial arterial blood gas results q1 hr until stable Monitor serial chest radiograph, sputum, C and S; look for presence of any pathogenic organisms or infiltrates Monitor for abnormalities in fluid and electrolyte balance Maintain strict intake and output; daily weights

POTENTIAL PROBLEMS	EXPECTED OUTCOMES	NURSING ACTIVITIES
		Monitor for any increase or decrease of abnormal and/or adventitious breath sounds, rales, stridor/snorting, wheezing, rhonchi, and retractions
		Observe for any marked changes in LOC such as confusion, restlessness, somnolence, and obtundation
		Observe for cyanosis and/or changes in skin color, including mucous membranes and nail beds
		Notify physician for any significant deterioration
		Allow rest periods between treatments
		Explain treatments before administration
		Provide quiet, restful environment
		Stay with patient or reassure patient that nurse will be close at hand
		Prepare patient for therapies that may be employed
		Therapeutic bronchoscopy
		Intubation with mechanical ventilation (see Standard 6, *Mechanical ventilation*)
		For COPD patients additional specific measures often include
		Monitoring for any changes in amount, color, viscosity, and odor of sputum; C and S result
		Monitoring for increasing tachypnea, dyspnea, cough, and fatigue
		Use of bronchodilators, i.e., theophylline, epinephrine, and corticosteroids; corticosteroids are specific for status asthmaticus
		Vigorous chest physiotherapy q1 hr
		Pursed lip breathing q30 min
		Postural drainage and chest physiotherapy q30 min
		Aseptic suctioning q30 min and prn; use of nebulized aerosols
		Maintain position in accordance with therapeutic regimen
		Teach breathing exercises, including pursed lip breathing
		Maintain environmental conditions to facilitate breathing
		Commonly used articles within reach
		Humidifiers in room
		Allow rest periods between treatments
		Maintain unhurried and calm demeanor when giving care

■ Pulmonary infections	■ Absence or resolution of pulmonary infection
	Chest radiograph, sputum, and C and S results show no evidence of infection
	No clinical manifestations of infection evident
		■ Prevention
		   Use strict aseptic technique in suctioning and in other nursing activities as appropriate
		   Administer prophylactic antibiotic therapy if ordered
		
		   Administer prophylactic measures such as postural drainage, inhalants, chest physiotherapy, and pursed lip breathing
		Monitor or observe for
		   Sore throat
		   Progressive dyspnea (respiratory distress)
		   Fever
		   Changes in amount, color, viscosity, and odor of sputum
		   Lab results of
		      Sputum C and S for any evidence of infection
		      Complete blood count for leukocytosis
		      Chest radiograph for atelectasis or density
		Notify physician of any abnormalities
		If problem occurs
		   Administer antibiotic therapy as ordered
		   Monitor for abnormal breath sounds or presence of rales, rhonchi, or wheezing
		   Check vital signs including temperature q1-2 hr until stable
		   Administer antipyretic as ordered to reduce fever and decrease O_2 requirements

POTENTIAL PROBLEMS	EXPECTED OUTCOMES	NURSING ACTIVITIES
		Administer vigorous chest physiotherapy as tolerated Reposition patient q1-2 hr; postural drainage if indicated Aseptic tracheal suctioning if patient is unable to cough out secretions Observe for increasing cough and changes in color, consistency, and odor of sputum Monitor result of serial sputum C and S Monitor result of serial chest radiograph

■ Acid-base disturbance, hypoxia related to alveolar hypoventilation or right to left shunting	■ Arterial blood gas levels within patient's normal limits
	Absence of signs of hypoxia including restlessness, light-headedness, dizziness, and cyanosis
		■ See problem, Obstruction to gas exchange, for prevention activities
		Monitor for
		  Arterial blood gas results indicating acidosis and/or hypoxemia
		  Symptoms of fatigue, drowsiness, headache, apathy, inattentiveness, restlessness, confusion, and somnolence
		  Signs of respiratory distress—air hunger, cyanosis, dyspnea, and tachypnea
		  Sudden changes in vital signs and temperature
		  Presence of arrhythmias
		  Increase in blood lactate level
		  Decrease in urine output
		If problem occurs
		  Careful administration of O_2 as ordered
		  Check that O_2 delivery device is functioning properly, i.e., patent
		  Monitor
		    Serial arterial blood gas levels q1-2 hr until stabilized
		    LOC
		    Serial electrolytes, specifically K^+ and chlorine (Cl^-) levels
		    Blood lactate levels
		    Temperature, P, R, and BP q2 hr
		    Heart rhythm and cardiac output
		    Chest radiograph results
		  Monitor for
		    Abnormal breath sounds, rales, rhonchi, wheezing, and stridor/snorting
		    Increase or decrease in dyspnea, tachypnea, cyanosis, restlessness, headache, and somnolence
		    Cardiac activity
		  Frequently change position for drainage of secretions q2 hr
		  Administer vigorous chest physiotherapy as tolerated; aseptic tracheal suctioning if patient is unable to cough out secretions
		  Administer antibiotics if ordered
		  Careful administration of bicarbonate to decrease lactic acid level if ordered
		  Promote effective chest expansion by positioning with pillows for comfort in accordance to therapy
		  Decrease O_2 consumption by
		    Limiting patient communication to necessary verbalization
		    Limiting patient activities
		    Providing uninterrupted rest periods
		    Providing environment conducive to rest
		    Limiting visitors
		    Reducing anxiety (see Problem, Patient/family's anxiety)
		  Notify physician for any abnormalities
		  If these measures fail, mechanical ventilation may be instituted (see Standard 6, *Mechanical ventilation*)

■ Decreased appetite related to dyspnea and weakness
Malnutrition related to prolonged debilitating lung disease
	■ Appetite improved, weight maintained, or weight gain if appropriate
	Positive nitrogen balance
	Patient consumes most of required food on meal trays
		■ Prevention
		  Gather baseline diet history data, including how dyspnea affects intake of nutrients
		  Assess patient's baseline nutritional status and plan intervention accordingly
		  Ensure intake of required fluids and nutrients
		  Frequent small meals

POTENTIAL PROBLEMS	EXPECTED OUTCOMES	NURSING ACTIVITIES

	Absence and/or resolution of any signs of malnutrition
	Regular elimination
		Monitor for
		  Signs and symptoms of malnutrition
		  Presence of swollen face with dark cheeks and circles under eyes
		  Any enlargement of parotid glands
		  Dull eyes with pale or red membranes, presence of bloodshot ring around corneas, gray spots on conjunctiva, red and fissured eyelid corners
		  Swollen lips
		  Spongy tender gums that bleed easily; presence of dental decay and missing teeth
		  Flaky, dry skin with spots or bruises
		  Brittle and split nails
		  Poor skin turgor, swollen joints, muscle atrophy, decreased subcutaneous fat
		  Altered mental status—restlessness, irritability, and confusion
		  Presence of tingling and burning of hands and feet and decreased reflexes
		  Musculoskeletal hemorrhages
		  Liver and spleen enlargement
		  Weight loss
		  Hypothermia
		  Lethargy and decreased exercise tolerance
		  Decreased albumin levels
		  Decreased lymphocyte count
		  Abnormal urea levels in 24-hour urine sample
		  Changes in anthropometric measurements
		If problem is present
		  Set required caloric and fluid intake with physician and dietitian
		  Monitor intake and output, daily weight
		  Provide required nutritional intake with meals and snacks
		  Ensure required caloric and fluid intake
		    List foods and fluids taken during meals and snacks
		    Note any abnormal eating patterns
		    Provide frequent small feedings as necessary
		    Encourage the patient to eat acidic food on meal trays first
		    Permit special food request as much as possible
		    Allow home-cooked foods within set limits
		    Have dietitian plan meals and meal substitutes with patient
		    Keep food as nearly "regular" as possible, soft rather than pureed, etc.
		  Provide conditions conducive to eating
		    Oral hygiene before and after meals and prn
		    Assist with cleaning and/or clean dentures as needed
		    Assist with eating, i.e., cutting foods, pouring liquids
		    Position patient for comfort and easy reach of foods
		    Provide equipment for eating, i.e., special device if necessary
		    Remove evidence of sputum or anything that will hinder patient's appetite
		If patient is receiving tube feedings
		  Ensure patency and proper location of tube
		  Place patient in semi-Fowler's position
		  Aspirate feeding tube before each feeding; test aspirate for heme; notify physician for abnormal amount and positive Hematest*
		  Do not feed patient if amount of aspirate is more than 100 ml or amount indicated by physician
		  Check feeding for any change in consistency and odor
		  Warm feedings before giving to patient
		  Start with small amounts of feedings at frequent intervals with gradual increase in amount and decrease in frequency as tolerated
		  Administer tube feedings at slow drip rate

*Ames Co., Elkhart, Ind.

POTENTIAL PROBLEMS	EXPECTED OUTCOMES	NURSING ACTIVITIES

		Check for bowel sounds every shift
		Monitor for
		    Abdominal cramps
		    Diarrhea and/or constipation
		    Glucosuria
		    Nausea
		    Aspiration from regurgitation
		Notify physician of any abnormalities
		Initiate bowel regimen as appropriate
		Monitor for resolution or presence of any signs and symptoms of
		    malnutrition
		Notify physician of any abnormalities

■ Emboli related to polycythemia and increased blood viscosity	■ Absence of emboli Normal pulmonary function	■ Monitor for signs and symptoms of thrombophlebitis, pulmonary emboli, and other types of emboli (see Standard 31, *Embolic phenomena*) If problem occurs, see Standard 31, *Embolic phenomena*

■ Cor pulmonale as complication of long-standing severe COPD	■ Absence of signs and symptoms of cor pulmonale
	Normal cardiac output
	Pao_2 within patient's normal limits
		■ Prevent by immediate medical therapy to alleviate problems (see
		    Problems, Obstruction to gas exchange; Pulmonary infections;
		    Acid-base disturbance, hypoxia; Decreased appetite related to dyspnea and weakness)
		Monitor for
		    Signs and symptoms of pulmonary hypertension and right ventricular strain
		        Gradual increasing edema of legs and ankles
		        Abnormal CVP, pulmonary pressures, PCWP, and cardiac output if available
		        Jugular venous distention, hepatomegaly, and puffy eyelids
		    Abnormalities in arterial blood gas levels
		    Chest radiograph evidence of cardiomegaly
		    Tachycardia and presence of gallop rhythm
		    P wave and QRS complex abnormalities/changes in ECG
		    Any alterations in LOC
		If problem occurs, see Standard 1, *Pulmonary edema of cardiac origin*

■ Gastrointestinal (GI) bleeding—ulcers and gastritis	■ Negative Hematest of emesis and/or nasogastric (NG) aspirate and stool
	Absence of abdominal pain, hematemesis, or melena
	Hct and Hgb within normal limits
	Normal GI function
		■ Prevention
		    Administer all medications with meals or when stomach is full
		    Administer antacid prophylactically as ordered
		    Minimize activities and allow for uninterrupted rest periods
		    Maintain calm and restful environment
		    Allow patient to verbalize fears and to ask questions
		    Explain all therapy before administering
		    Encourage patient to participate in care as tolerated
		    Encourage required nutrients and bland food
		Monitor for
		    Vital signs and temperature q4 hr; be aware of any sudden rise in P
		    Check all stools, emesis, and/or NG aspirate for Hematest
		    Any GI upsets—anorexia, vomiting, abdominal distention, pain, cramps, diarrhea, and/or constipation
		    Serial Hgb and Hct
		    Symptoms of sudden dizziness or syncope
		    Changes in size of abdominal girth
		Notify physician of any abnormality
		If problem occurs, see Standard 49, *Acute upper gastrointestinal bleeding*

POTENTIAL PROBLEMS	EXPECTED OUTCOMES	NURSING ACTIVITIES

■ Insufficient knowledge to comply with discharge regimen*	■ Patient/family has sufficient information to comply with discharge regimen
	Patient/family accurately describes dietary, medication, and activity regimen
	
	Patient/family identifies signs and symptoms of respiratory infection requiring medical attention
	Patient/family performs special therapeutic procedures correctly
		■ Assess patient/family's level of understanding, ability to comprehend, and any physical limitations regarding follow-up plan of care or discharge regimen
		
		Describe discharge regimen, including
		  Medications—purpose, side effects, route, dose, and schedules
		  Dietary therapy regimen
		  Activity progression—avoid overfatigue; allow for rest and relaxation
		Identify signs and symptoms that would require medical attention, especially respiratory infections such as cold, sore throat, fever, and cough irritability
		
		Describe and demonstrate to patient/family special therapeutic measures and safety precautions for specific residual pulmonary disease
		Specific therapeutic measures for patient with COPD
		  Chest drainage and chest physiotherapy
		    Assist in developing program for physical conditioning and bronchial hygiene
		    Specify positions to be assumed to facilitate drainage of lung segments
		    Emphasize that postural drainage mobilizes secretions not moved by normal air movement and brings secretions to areas where cough is effective
		    Emphasize that if patient obtains no immediate relief, he/she may cough up secretions later in the day
		  Breathing exercises
		    Emphasize that breathing exercises strengthen muscles of expiration
		    Instruct patient on breathing exercises, including diaphragmatic breathing by placing one hand on stomach just below ribs and other hand on middle of chest; breathe in slowly and deeply through nose allowing abdomen to protrude as far as possible; then breathe out through pursed lips while contracting abdominal muscles; during breathing, hands must press inward and upward on abdomen
		  Correct use of nebulizers and intermittent positive pressure breathing (IPPB) machine
		    Allow patient/family to do return demonstration of therapeutic measures
		    Encourage any questions and/or verbalization of anxiety regarding therapeutic procedures

	Patient/family verbalizes influence of environmental factors on illness and performs necessary preventive measures	Emphasize the importance of calm, safe, and comfortable environment; specific measures for patients with COPD include
		  Importance of congenial family attitude and avoidance of hostility and emotional and upsetting situations
		  Avoid exposure to crowds, people with respiratory infections, and respiratory irritants (smoke, chemicals, dust fumes, etc.)
		  Do not smoke
		  Avoid excessively dry air and extremely cold weather
		  Avoid sudden changes in temperature
		  Organize daily activity to allow work activity with least amount of effort
		  Avoid activities causing excessive dyspnea
		  Perform work and activity at slow pace
		  Allow for specific rest periods
		  Keep environment clean and free from dust
		  When using air conditioner make sure filter is clean

*If responsibility of the critical care nurse includes such follow-up care.

POTENTIAL PROBLEMS	EXPECTED OUTCOMES	NURSING ACTIVITIES
		Avoid devices in which water can stand and become stagnant
		Maintain good eating and elimination habits
		Nonflowering house plants help provide relative humidity of 50%
		Encourage fluid intake to 2000 ml daily unless contraindicated
	Patient/family accurately describes plans for follow-up care	Describe plan for follow-up visits, including purpose, when and where to come, who to see, and what specimens to bring
		Provide opportunity for and encourage patient/family's questions and verbalization of anxiety regarding discharge regimen
		Assess patient/family's potential compliance with discharge regimen
		Provide information for use of community health agencies when necessary

THORACIC SURGERY

Thoracic surgery involves entry into the chest wall or cavity for the repair or resection of abnormalities associated with the chest wall, pleura, lungs, mediastinum, esophagus, trachea, or heart.

Indications for a thoracotomy include traumatic injury in which there is evidence of extensive intrathoracic damage. Various infectious processes such as empyema and refractory bronchiectasis require surgical drainage through thoracotomy incisions. Removal of a segment, lobe, or entire lung (pneumonectomy) becomes necessary in treating malignancies that have not metastasized.

Certain nonmalignant abnormalities of the lung, such as large bullous formations, require surgical resection. A bullectomy is performed when adjacent lung tissue becomes compromised by the growing size of bullae, thus making infection and/or oxygenation problems likely.

A thoracotomy is useful for correcting various congenital or acquired deformities of the chest wall. Elevation of the sternum in pectus excavatum often improves chest wall mechanics and also provides a desirable cosmetic effect.

Postoperative goals are focused on providing adequate oxygenation and ventilation as well as hemodynamic stability. Because the integrity of the chest wall has been compromised, constant attention must be directed toward maintaining the lungs in a fully expanded state. The airway must be frequently cleared of secretions that build up quickly in the postoperative patient.

Table 3-1 lists and defines various thoracic surgeries and the indications for performing them.

ASSESSMENT

1. History, presence, nature, and severity of
   a. Pulmonary problem; previous pulmonary surgery
   b. Medical management of pulmonary problem
   c. Result of laboratory tests to date
   d. Smoking—number of packs per day, number of years
   e. Secretions—color, amount, consistency, odor
   f. Chest discomfort and, if present, the pattern (nature, duration, and severity)
   g. Altered activity levels; toleration of various activities of daily living
   h. Esophageal reflux, heartburn
   i. Pain, paresthesia, and numbness in lower arms and hand when structures in shoulder and neck are compressed by certain body movements
2. Pulmonary status, particularly
   a. Quality of respirations (e.g., rate, rhythm)
   b. Breathing pattern for presence of distress, dyspnea
   c. Presence of abnormal or adventitious breath sounds
3. Results of lab and diagnostic procedures
   a. Pulmonary function studies
   b. Arterial blood gas levels
   c. Bronchoscopy
   d. Mediastinoscopy
   e. Tomography
   f. Scalene node biopsy
   g. Pleural biopsy
   h. Open lung biopsy
   i. Radiograph—anteroposterior and/or lateral
   j. Computed tomography (CT) scan
   k. Lung scan
   l. For esophageal and esophagogastric problems
      (1) Fluoroscopic studies
      (2) Esophagoscopy
      (3) Esophageal motility studies
      (4) Other selected tests as appropriate
4. Patient/family's knowledge regarding operative therapy
   a. What they have been told
   b. Their expectations
   c. Previous experiences with surgery if any
5. Information and detail surgeon has provided about the need for surgery, the actual surgery to be done, and the expected outcomes
6. Patient/family's anxiety related to disease process, hospitalization, therapy planned, potential surgery, and expected outcome

GOALS

1. Reduction in patient/family's anxiety with provision of information and explanations
2. Patient/family complies with preoperative regimen (particularly with regard to not smoking)
3. Hemodynamic stability; absence of arrhythmias

TABLE 3-1. Thoracic surgeries

THORACIC PROCEDURE	DEFINITION	INDICATIONS
Segmental resection	Removal of segment of pulmonary lobe	Chronic, localized pyogenic lung abscess Congenital cyst or bleb Benign tumor Segment infected with pulmonary tuberculosis or bronchiectasis
Wedge resection	Excision of small peripheral section of lobe	Small masses that are close to pleural surface of lung, e.g., subpleural granulomas, small peripheral tumors (benign primary tumors)
Lobectomy	Excision of one or more lobes of lung tissue	Cancer Infections such as tuberculosis Sequestration
Pneumonectomy	Removal of entire lung	Malignant neoplasms Lung almost entirely infected with bronchiectasis Extensive chronic abscess Lung extensively infected with tuberculosis Selected unilateral lesions
Decortication of lung	Removal of fibrinous, reactive membrane covering visceral and parietal pleura	Restrictive fibrinous membrane lining visceral and parietal pleura that limits ventilatory excursion; "trapped lung"
Thoracoplasty	Surgical collapse of portion of chest wall by multiple rib resections to intentionally decrease volume in hemithorax	Closure of chronic cavitary lesions and empyema spaces Closure of recurrent air leaks Reduction of open thoracic "dead space" after large resection
Thymectomy	Removal of thymus gland	Primary thymic neoplasm; generally performed for patient with myasthenia gravis in effort to alleviate symptoms and reduce intake of medications
Correction of pectus excavatum ("funnel chest")	Depression of sternum and costal cartilage corrected by moving sternum outward and realigning cartilage-sternal junction	Cosmesis and relief of cardiopulmonary compromise that occurs most often during exercise

4. Respiratory function sufficient to maintain PaO_2 and $PaCO_2$ within normal limits; absence of atelectasis, pulmonary infection
5. Infection free, afebrile; absence of empyema
6. For specific surgery
   1. Pneumonectomy
      (1) Bronchial stump intact
      (2) Absence of pulmonary interstitial edema
      (3) Adequate cardiac output; no heart failure
   b. Esophagogastrectomy

(1) Absence of pulmonary aspiration of gastric contents
(2) Minimal to no reflux of gastric contents
(3) Food passes readily from mouth into stomach
(4) Patient complies with prescribed dietary alterations and chews food thoroughly
(5) Voice is unchanged; absence of hoarseness
   c. Lobectomy; segmental resection
      (1) Full expansion of remaining lung tissue
      (2) Absence of a pneumothorax

TABLE 3-1. Thoracic surgeries—cont'd

THORACIC PROCEDURE	DEFINITION	INDICATIONS
Repair of penetrating thoracic wounds, drainage of hemothorax	Drainage of pleural cavity and control of hemorrhage	Hemorrhage produced by injury to thoracic vessels that causes blood loss as well as compression of lung tissue and mediastinum, resulting in cardiopulmonary compromise
Excision of mediastinal masses	Removal of masses and cysts in upper anterior and posterior mediastinum	Mediastinal tumors (benign or malignant) Cysts Abscesses
Tracheal resection	Resection of portion of trachea, followed by primary end-to-end reanastomosis of trachea	Significant stenosis of tracheal orifice, usually related to mechanical pressure of cuffed tracheal tube; pressure produces tracheal wall ischemia, inflammation, and ulceration; these effects lead to formation of granulation tissue and fibrosis, which narrow tracheal orifice
Esophagogastrectomy	Resection of part of esophagus and at least cardial portion of stomach with primary anastomosis of proximal esophagus to remaining stomach	Carcinoma of esophagus anywhere from neck to esophagogastric junction Severe reflux esophagitis producing hemorrhage Extensive alkali burns of esophagus
Bullectomy	Removal by excision of cysts or pockets in lung, which result from confluence of many alveoli	Failure of medical therapy such as antibiotics and chest physiotherapy to control infection associated with such cysts or pockets Tissue adjacent to pulmonary cysts or pockets that is severely compressed
Closed thoracostomy	Insertion of chest tube through intercostal space into pleural space; chest tube is attached to water seal system, with or without suction	Provision of continuous aspiration of fluid from pleural cavity Prevention of accumulation of air in chest from leaks in lung or tracheobronchial tree
Open thoracostomy	Partial resection of selected rib or ribs, with insertion of chest tube into infected material to provide for continuous drainage	Drainage of empyemas when pleural space is fixed

  (3) Minimal air leak in immediate postoperative period, which quickly progresses to no air leak
 d. Tracheal resection
  (1) Patent airway
  (2) Breathing without distress
  (3) Tracheal anastomosis intact, without local tracheal or pulmonary infection
7. Patient has full range of motion (ROM) of arm and shoulder on the affected side

8. Coagulation studies within normal limits; absence of signs of thrombophlebitis, pulmonary embolism, or other types of emboli
9. Before discharge, patient/family verbalizes understanding of activity progression, dietary alterations, and medication regimen
10. Patient/family accurately describes signs and symptoms that require medical attention
11. Patient/family accurately describes plan for follow-up visits

POTENTIAL PROBLEMS	EXPECTED OUTCOMES	NURSING ACTIVITIES

Preoperative

■ Patient/family's anxiety related to
Disease process
Hospitalization
Medical therapy employed
Diagnostic tests planned
Impending major surgery and associated risks
Altered family roles
Separation from family members
Loss of job

■ Patient/family's behavior indicates reduction in anxiety with provision of information, explanations, and encouragement

■ Ongoing assessment of level of patient/family's anxiety
Assess knowledge and understanding of patient/family of disease process, medical therapy employed, anticipated diagnostic procedures, and anticipated surgery if planned
Explain in simple terms nature of patient's pulmonary/thoracic problem and symptoms patient is experiencing
Explain in simple terms what patient will experience during diagnostic procedures; assist in preparing patient for procedures, which may include
Radiograph, tomography
Blood samples for arterial blood gas analysis
Pulmonary function tests
Bronchoscopy, mediastinoscopy
Biopsy
Other tests specific for patient's pulmonary problem
Collaborate with physician and other members of health team on necessary teaching
When surgery is planned and physician has discussed it with patient/family, assess their understanding of information
Reinforce purpose and nature of surgery and expected outcomes
Describe perioperative experience (adjust explanation according to patient's anxiety level and desire to know), including
Preoperative
Refer to chest physiotherapist, if available, to orient patient to
Coughing and deep breathing
Incentive spirometry
Postural drainage
Prep and shave
Light dinner and NPO after midnight
Medication for sleep if needed
Morning bath/shower
Preoperative medications
Hospital gown
Care of valuables
To operating room on stretcher
Scrub suits, masks, and caps worn by operating room staff
Anesthesia
Postoperative
Regaining consciousness in recovery room/intensive care unit
Describe general environment (size of unit, room, etc.)
Nurse always nearby
Dull continuous noises
If anticipated, describe breathing tube in nose or mouth that will be in place to ease work of breathing and load on heart; explain that talking will not be possible while tube is in place but that other means of communication will be possible
NPO until "breathing tube" removed
Incision with bandage
IV, arterial lines
If anticipated, chest tubes and bloody drainage expected
ECG monitoring
Medicine for discomfort, pain
Policy for family visits
Describe responsibility of patient for achieving speedy recovery by taking active role in coughing, deep breathing, and other aspects of care
Describe process as patient progresses
Tubes, lines out
Allowed to eat
Chest physiotherapy, deep breathing, and coughing

POTENTIAL PROBLEMS	EXPECTED OUTCOMES	NURSING ACTIVITIES
		Getting stronger, ambulation Home again Provide opportunity for and encourage questions and verbalization of anxiety Reassure patient that nurse will be nearby at all times Provide calm, quiet environment Perform treatments in unhurried manner, allowing rest periods between treatments Involve patient/family in planning for care Assess reduction in level of anxiety

■ Respiratory insufficiency related to underlying disease process	■ Adequate oxygenation and ventilation with arterial blood gas levels within patient's normal limits	■ Encourage patient to stop smoking as soon as admitted to hospital with suspected pulmonary problem
		Implement chest physiotherapy as ordered to achieve optimal pulmonary function before surgery
		  Demonstrate coughing and deep breathing; have patient practice five deep slow breaths with effective cough on fifth breath
		  Demonstrate and have patient practice use of pillow
		  Teach proper diaphragmatic breathing exercises using abdominal muscles
		  Administer chest physiotherapy q2-4 hr and prn
		  Administer humidified, oxygenated air as needed, if ordered
		  Assist patient with incentive spirometry
		Monitor
		  Respirations for rate and quality; note tachypnea, dyspnea
		  Nature, amount, and consistency of sputum production
		  Breath sounds for decreased or absent breath sounds; presence of rales, rhonchi, or wheezes
		  Arterial blood gas results; note hypoxemia, hypercapnia
		  Chest radiograph results for atelectasis, fibrosis, and other abnormalities
		Notify physician of any of these abnormalities
		Administer therapy as ordered
		  Frequent chest physiotherapy to areas of atelectasis, collapse
		  Antibiotics
		  Bronchodilators
		  Expectorants, enzymes, and/or mucolytic agents
		  Incentive spirometry therapy
		Evaluate for improvement in respiratory function in response to these interventions

Postoperative
■ Hemodynamic instability related to
Pulmonary hypertension (particularly in pneumonectomy patients), resulting in heart failure
Arrhythmias that may result from hypoxia, ventricular strain, acid-base imbalance
Hemorrhage
	■ Patient hemodynamically stable
	ECG indicates absence of arrhythmias; all beats perfused
	Blood loss minimal (less than 800 ml in first 24 hours in adults)
		■ Prevent by
		  Administering fluid cautiously as ordered, particularly to pneumonectomy patient (remaining lung receives approximately twice its normal blood flow)
		  Administering therapy to prevent or to correct factors that predispose to arrhythmia formation, including acid-base imbalance and hypoxemia
		  Providing for patent chest drainage system
		Monitor
		  BP, P q½-1 hr and prn until stable; note presence of hypotension and tachycardia
		  CVP and PAP/PCWP q1 hr and prn until stable
		  Urine output with specific gravity q1 hr; note oliguria
		  Indices of adequate peripheral circulation and mentation
		  Amount and character of drainage in chest bottles (most pneumonectomy patients do not have chest tubes; if they do, suction is not continuously applied)
		  Continuous ECG reading or apical/radical pulse for arrhythmias and irregular rhythm; note concurrent signs of decreased cardiac output

POTENTIAL PROBLEMS	EXPECTED OUTCOMES	NURSING ACTIVITIES
		For signs/symptoms of heart failure, right ventricular strain and hypertrophy
		If hemodynamic instability occurs, administer therapy to correct etiological factors and to provide symptomatic relief, as ordered
		Monitor patient response to
		Fluid restriction, diuretic therapy
		Blood and blood products
		Antiarrhythmic therapy
		Inotropic agents
		O_2 supplements
		Bicarbonate, electrolyte replacement

■ Respiratory insufficiency related to improper positioning in *lobectomy and segmental resection patients;* if operated side is down, full expansion of remaining lobe(s) in affected lung is impaired	■ Respiratory function sufficient to maintain Pao_2 and $Paco_2$ within normal limits
	Respiratory rate and depth within normal limits
	Auscultation and chest radiograph reveal full expansion of remaining lung tissue, such that operative area is filled with remaining lung tissue
		■ Assess patient's respirations q½-1 hr until stable in rate and quality
		Observe for tachypnea, dyspnea
		Prevent by
		  Providing for maximal diaphragmatic excursion
		    Semi-Fowler's position
		    Frequent (q1-2 hr) repositioning
		    Support for chest around chest tube insertion site (if present) to prevent tension on tube and surrounding tissues and to give support for deep breathing and coughing
		  Positioning
		    Lobectomy and segmental resection patients—in early postoperative period many physicians preferentially position patient so that operated side is up to facilitate expansion of lobes adjacent to resected lobe; after first 1 to 2 days, patient is usually permitted to turn to either side
		    Bullectomy patients—can be turned to either side

■ Respiratory insufficiency in *pneumonectomy patient* related to compression of remaining lung by accumulation of drainage on operated side as revealed by mediastinal shift
Cardiac output may be compromised, which can contribute to respiratory insufficiency and hypoxia
	■ Mediastinum in midline position as revealed by observation, chest radiograph, and auscultation
	Full expansion of remaining lung tissue
		■ Prevent by positioning *pneumonectomy patient* on back or slightly turned to operated side; this position is usually preferred for first 1 to 2 days after surgery
		Monitor
		  Tracheal position q½-1 hr until stable; note if not in midline position, indicating mediastinal shift
		  Breath sounds q1-2 hr in remaining lung tissue
		  For arterial blood gas results indicating hypoxemia, hypercapnia
		  Results of chest radiograph, indicating mediastinal shift
		If mediastinal shift present, note concurrent signs of compromised cardiac output, hemodynamic instability
		Notify physician for abnormalities in these parameters
		If problem occurs and mediastinal shift is toward operated side, assist physician with injection of air into operated side to move mediastinum back into midline position, if necessary
		If problem occurs and the mediastinal shift occurs away from operated side
		  Assist physician with removal of drainage from operated side, or if chest tube is in place and clamped, release clamp as ordered to allow some drainage to flow out chest tube
		  Assist with insertion of chest tube if required

■ Respiratory insufficiency related to
  Inadequate chest drainage
  Hemothorax
	■ Absence or resolution of inadequate drainage and hemothorax
	Full expansion of remaining lung tissue
		■ Maintain patent draining chest tube system; "milk" or "strip" (i.e., squeeze) chest tubes as needed to move thick drainage, clots down tube
		Monitor
		  For effective suction in chest tube system
		  For thick drainage, clots that need to be mobilized
		  For fluctuation of drainage in chest tube ("tidaling"); this fluctuation will decrease gradually as space being drained decreases in size and amount of drainage subsides
		  Chest radiograph results for any collection suggesting hemothorax
		Notify physician of abnormalities in any of aforementioned

POTENTIAL PROBLEMS	EXPECTED OUTCOMES	NURSING ACTIVITIES
		If hemothorax occurs 　Assist with chest tube insertion if needed; monitor subsequent chest tube drainage 　Monitor for resolution of hemothorax by auscultation, chest radiograph results, and improved respiratory function
■ Respiratory insufficiency related to 　Atelectasis 　Hypoventilation 　Airway obstruction associated with secretions, tracheal edema (e.g., tracheal resection)	■ Absence of signs and symptoms of respiratory distress, atelectasis Adequate oxygenation and ventilation with Pao_2 and $Paco_2$ levels within patient's normal limits	■ Prevent by 　Providing for pain relief sufficient to allow for optimal pulmonary toilet while avoiding respiratory depression 　Encouraging deep breathing and coughing q½-1 hr in early postoperative period 　Supporting patient's chest 　Administering gentle chest physiotherapy q2-4 hr and prn as ordered 　Administering humidified O_2 as ordered to enhance oxygenation and to liquefy secretions (adequate systemic hydration also assists in liquefying secretions) Monitor 　Respirations q½-1 hr and prn until stable; note presence of dyspnea, tachypnea, stridorous breathing 　Breath sounds q1 hr until stable; note presence of abnormal or adventitious breath sounds in remaining lung tissue 　Arterial blood gas results; note hypoxemia, hypercapnia, or acidemia 　For signs/symptoms of hypoxia (tachypnea, tachycardia, restlessness) 　Results of sputum C and S; if sputum changes in character, send additional specimens as ordered 　Results of serial inspiratory pressures if determined 　Results of chest radiographs for presence of atelectasis and absence of full lung expansion 　BP, P q½-1 hr until stable; note presence of hypotension, tachycardia Notify physician of presence of any of these abnormalities If atelectasis occurs 　Augment chest physiotherapy to affected areas 　Assist patient with coughing and deep breathing; suction secretions if patient unable to cough 　Administer bronchodilators, mucolytic agents if ordered 　Monitor patient's response to these interventions If airway obstruction occurs 　Position head to open airway 　Augment chest physiotherapy to affected areas 　Aspirate secretions with suctioning as necessary 　Administer bronchodilators, mucolytic agents as ordered 　Assist with bronchoscopy if procedure required for diagnosis and for aspiration of a mucous plug 　Monitor patient's response to these measures
■ Respiratory insufficiency related to air leak, particularly in patients with 　*Lobectomy* 　*Segmental resection* 　*Bullectomy*	■ Absence of signs/symptoms of air collection in chest No inspired air leaks out through incision or out chest tube While chest tube(s) is in situ, drainage bottle indicates no release of air with inspiration (ventilated patient) or with expiration (extubated patient)	■ Monitor 　For air bubbling down chest tube into underwater seal bottle/chamber 　Amount of air lost in artificially ventilated patient by measuring difference between preset volume to be delivered and expired volume If air leak is present, monitor progression/resolution of by observing changes in amount of air lost Tidal volume (V_T) to be delivered by ventilator may be increased as ordered so that expired volume, or volume that does not leak out chest tube, is equal to desired V_T Monitor for inadequate drainage of air leak (signs/symptoms of pneumothorax); notify physician if this occurs

POTENTIAL PROBLEMS	EXPECTED OUTCOMES	NURSING ACTIVITIES
	While patient is intubated, amount of air expired approximates amount of air inspired	Assist with chest tube insertion if necessary
■ Respiratory insufficiency related to pulmonary interstitial edema resulting from acute increase in blood flow to remaining lung tissue in initial postoperative period (*pneumonectomy patient* is particularly susceptible to this complication)	■ Clear lungs Arterial blood gas levels within normal limits Weight remains same or decreases postoperatively (if weight gain occurred intraoperatively)	■ Prevent by administering fluids and blood products as ordered to maintain intravascular volume and hemodynamic stability, taking care to avoid administration of nonessential fluids that can contribute to pulmonary interstitial edema, ventricular strain, and/or heart failure Monitor Intake and output q1 hr Daily weights Hemodynamic parameters every hour, particularly closely in pneumonectomy patient; correlate abnormalities with presence of abnormal or adventitious breath sounds Arterial blood gas levels for hypoxemia For signs/symptoms of hypoxemia (e.g., restlessness, tachycardia) Notify physician of significant imbalance in fluid intake and output flow sheet and in daily weight pattern If pulmonary interstitial edema and associated hypoxemia occur, artificial ventilation with use of small amounts of PEEP may be ordered and instituted to achieve adequate oxygenation; see Standard 6, *Mechanical ventilation;* Standard 7, *Positive end expiratory pressure* Administer diuretics as ordered, and closely monitor response in terms of Urine output BP, P, CVP, and PAP/PCWP Weight loss or gain Arterial blood gas results; note improved PaO_2, O_2 saturation Absence or resolution of signs/symptoms of hypoxemia (e.g., restlessness, tachycardia)
■ Respiratory insufficiency related to bronchial stump leakage caused by extra tension on stump in *pneumonectomy patient*	■ Bronchial stump intact	■ Prevention When inserting suction catheter to aspirate secretions, stop before point of resistance (which may be bronchial stump suture line) When patient is intubated, V_{Ts} are reduced according to amount of lung tissue resected; pneumonectomy patient receives little more than one half of typical V_T for his/her weight (approximately 10 to 15 cc/kg) Monitor for Expectoration of old, partially clotted blood Sudden respiratory distress, including shortness of breath, with restlessness, tachycardia, hypotension If signs of bronchial stump leakage occur Notify physician at once Monitor arterial blood gas results Monitor results of emergency chest radiograph if done Prepare patient for emergency surgery to oversew bronchial stump if procedure is planned
■ Respiratory insufficiency related to breakdown of anastomosis from infection, poor healing, and bronchopleural fistula in patients with *tracheal resection*	■ Tracheal anastomosis intact	■ Prevent anastomotic breakdown in tracheal resection patient by Avoiding tension, torsion of fresh suture line by keeping patient's head flexed Avoiding rotation of patient's head by placement of suture from chin to chest or some other stabilizing measure Avoiding endotracheal intubation, which puts undue pressure against suture line Administering vigorous pulmonary toilet with modified chest physiotherapy, deep breathing, and coughing as needed q2-4 hr and prn Humidified O_2 supplements as ordered

POTENTIAL PROBLEMS	EXPECTED OUTCOMES	NURSING ACTIVITIES

		Monitor
		    For acute respiratory distress
		    For pneumothorax, subcutaneous emphysema
		    Chest radiograph results
		If problem occurs
		    Assist physician with insertion of chest tube
		    Prepare patient for surgery if planned
		    Administer antibiotics as ordered

■ Pneumothorax	■ Full lung expansion with adequate oxygenation and ventilation	■ Monitor for signs and symptoms of pneumothorax, including
		    Respiratory distress—shortness of breath, dyspnea, tachypnea
		    Anxiety, diaphoresis, pallor, vertigo
		    Asymmetrical chest movements, distant or absent breath sounds on affected side
		    Pleural pain
		    Tachycardia with weak pulse
		    Cyanosis and hypotension if severe
		Notify physician if these abnormalities occur
		If pneumothorax occurs
		    Stay with patient
		    Place patient in semi- to high Fowler's position
		    Administer O_2 therapy as ordered
		    Assist with insertion of chest tube; if done, note loss of air from patient's lung into chest tube and signs of resolution of pneumothorax with reexpansion of lung
		    Monitor q1-2 hr for continued lung expansion
		    Auscultate breath sounds q1-2 hr

■ Subcutaneous emphysema associated with collection of air and/or blood in the operative area	■ Absence of air or blood collection in operative area
	Absence of subcutaneous emphysema
	Full expansion of remaining lung tissue
		■ Monitor for
		    Subcutaneous emphysema over chest wall, which may indicate presence of additional air or blood in operative area
		    Chest radiograph results, indicating air or blood in operative area
		    Breath sounds consistent with air or blood in operative area (distant, dull)
		If subcutaneous emphysema occurs associated with air in operated area, see Problem, Pneumothorax, for nursing activities
		If subcutaneous emphysema occurs in association with collection of blood in operative area
		    Place patient in semi- to high Fowler's position
		    Assist physician with insertion of chest tube
		    Monitor patient's response, including
		      BP, P q1-2 hr
		      Nature and amount of blood lost through chest tube; notify physician of blood loss greater than 200 ml/hour in adults
		      Hct levels q1-3 hr, depending on presence of active bleeding
		    Milk chest tube q1-2 hr
		    Assist patient to cough and deep breathe q1-2 hr and prn, splinting patient's chest when patient coughs
		    Auscultate breath sounds q1-2 hr for degree of lung expansion
		    Monitor chest radiograph results for lung expansion

■ Muscle spasm of neck associated with neck flexion and shoulder immobility
Tracheal resection patient is particularly prone to this complication
	■ Absence of muscle spasm and discomfort of neck/shoulder muscles	■ Prevent muscle spasm by
		    Supporting patient's head and neck while maintaining them in flexed position, usually with aid of suture line from chin to chest
		    Massaging back and shoulder muscles frequently
		Monitor for tight neck and shoulder muscles, including patient complaints of discomfort in these muscles
		Notify physician if spasm occurs
		If neck spasm occurs
		    Continue massaging muscles and providing support of neck and shoulder
		    Administer muscle relaxant if needed, as ordered

POTENTIAL PROBLEMS	EXPECTED OUTCOMES	NURSING ACTIVITIES

■ Infection, pneumonia	■ Infection free
	Afebrile
	Arterial blood gas levels within patient's normal limits
	— Chest radiograph clear with full lung expansion
		■ Prevention
		  Administer pain medication if needed, as ordered, to avoid patient splinting and reduced respiratory excursion
		  Administer maximal chest physiotherapy, including
		    Turning q1-2 hr
		    Chest physiotherapy q2 hr with turning
		    Auscultation of breath sounds q1 hr, with suctioning as needed
		    Using pillows for support and comfort, particularly around chest tubes
		    In addition, after extubation
		      Incentive spirometry q1-2 hr
		      Deep breathing and coughing q1-2 hr
		      Assisting and supporting patient as needed
		      Ambulation as soon as possible
		Monitor
		  R q½-1 hr for rate and quality; note tachypnea, dyspnea
		  Secretions for color, amount, consistency; particularly note copious, tenacious, and/or abnormally colored sputum
		  Temperature q1-2 hr; note fever
		  For pleuritic chest pain
		  For unequal chest movements
		  Breath sounds q1 hr; note presence and nature of rales, rhonchi, and other adventitious breath sounds, or absence of breath sounds altogether
		  Color for cyanosis
		  Arterial blood gas levels; note presence of hypoxemia, hypercapnia
		  Chest radiograph results revealing infiltrates, atelectasis
		  Sputum C and S results
		  P q½-1 hr for tachycardia
		Notify physician for abnormalities in these parameters
		If pneumonia occurs
		  Administer antibiotics as ordered
		  Administer analgesics, antipyretics, and/or expectorant, if needed, as ordered
		  Liquefy tenacious secretions by administering additional systemic fluid as ordered or instilling small amounts of saline solution into endotracheal tube, followed by manual inflations

■ Embolism
Peripheral venous
Pulmonary
	■ Absence of signs/symptoms of peripheral venous embolism
	Absence of evidence of pulmonary embolus
	R, arterial blood gas levels, and cardiovascular status within patient's normal limits
		■ Monitor for evidence of peripheral venous embolism
		  Edema of lower extremity
		  Painful swelling and tenderness on palpation in area of affected vein
		  Pain when foot is forcefully dorsiflexed (Homans' sign)
		  Pain that is worse on dependency and, conversely, relieved by elevation
		  Palpable hard, cordlike vein (''cord'')
		  Cramping of extremity
		Monitor for evidence of pulmonary embolus
		  Restlessness
		  Respiratory distress, e.g., dyspnea, tachypnea, pleural or substernal pain
		  Arterial blood gas levels revealing hypoxemia, hypercapnia, or hypocapnia
		  Symptoms of hypoxia—tachypnea, air hunger, anxiety, tachycardia
		  Cardiovascular instability
		    Arrhythmias
		    Hypertension, hypotension
		    Signs/symptoms of reduced cardiac output
		  ECG changes reflecting right ventricular strain
		Notify physician if any of aforementioned occur, and administer therapy as ordered
		See STANDARD 31 *Embolic phenomena*

POTENTIAL PROBLEMS	EXPECTED OUTCOMES	NURSING ACTIVITIES
■ Infection, empyema, which may be related to bacteria introduced during surgery	■ Infection free Afebrile Absence of abnormal collection in operated area as revealed by chest radiograph, auscultation	■ Prevent by Avoiding opening closed chest drainage system (except if necessary to change system) Evacuating drainage from chest; keep drainage flowing down chest tubes by frequently "milking" (squeezing) chest tubes Monitor Temperature q1-2 hr; note fever Results of chest radiograph for results compatible with empyema CBC results for leukocytosis Erythrocyte sedimentation rate (ESR) for elevation If problem occurs Send cultures of drainage, sputum as ordered Administer antibiotics as ordered Prepare patient for surgery if necessary
■ Hoarseness related to tumor compression of laryngeal nerve or surgical damage of laryngeal nerve in *esophagogastrectomy patient*	■ Patient's speaking voice is unchanged from preoperative level Absence of hoarseness	■ Monitor For hoarseness Patient's voice if hoarseness develops For difficulty in coughing Notify physician of any of these abnormalities If problem occurs, administer therapy as ordered to facilitate patient's ability to phonate
■ Limited ROM on operated side of thoracic surgery patients related to Position used during surgery; arm is usually in very extended position taped over head or to table; occasionally this position can cause nerve damage and brachial plexus palsy Shoulder pain associated with significant amount of transsected muscle	■ Patient adequately performs breathing and body exercises Patient has full ROM of extremity on operative side	■ Prevent by Reviewing breathing, shoulder/arm and leg exercises preoperatively Instructing patient in and encouraging skeletal exercises to promote abduction and mobilization of shoulder and arm Administering pain medication, if needed, as ordered Encouraging ambulation as soon as possible, as ordered, particularly after chest tubes are removed; pneumonectomy patients are mobilized more slowly because of greater cardiopulmonary adjustments that occur Arranging for physical therapy consultation as ordered Monitor for Limited ROM of upper extremity Shoulder pain with associated decrease in movement of upper extremity Notify physician if these occur If problem occurs Administer pain medication if needed, and institute aggressive exercise program as ordered Administer physiotherapy as ordered
■ Insufficient knowledge to comply with discharge regimen*	■ Patient/family has sufficient information to comply with discharge regimen Patient/family accurately describes dietary and medication regimen and particular precautions for activities Patient/family accurately describes plan for follow-up care	■ Assess patient/family's level of understanding regarding postdischarge regimen Describe follow-up plan of care, including medications and their purpose, identification, route, dosage, frequency and timing, and potential adverse effects Instruct patient in activity progression, cautioning sternotomy or thoracotomy patient not to progress to activities faster than physician recommends; resumption of such activities as driving, vacuuming, lifting objects of prescribed weight range, or playing sports should be discussed with physician If appropriate, explain that some intercostal discomfort may normally continue for a few weeks and that it can be relieved by heat and, if necessary, mild analgesic Instruct patient/family in suture line care if appropriate; provide opportunity for practice and return demonstration

*If responsibility of critical care nurse includes this type of follow-up care.

POTENTIAL PROBLEMS	EXPECTED OUTCOMES	NURSING ACTIVITIES
		Instruct esophagogastrectomy patient not to bend over at waist but rather to bend at knees and squat to pick up items, tie shoes, and so on
		Identify signs/symptoms that require medical attention, depending on outcome of surgery and residual pulmonary dysfunction; instruct patient to seek medical attention for any untoward signs and symptoms
		Provide opportunity for and encourage patient/family questions and verbalization of anxiety regarding discharge regimen
		Describe plan for follow-up visits, including purpose of visits, when and where to go, who to see, and what specimens to bring
		Assess patient/family's potential compliance with discharge regimen

NEAR DROWNING

Drowning is the third most common cause of accidental death in the United States and one of the more common causes of death in children over 1 year of age.

Approximately 10% of all near-drowning victims do not aspirate water because of laryngospasm or forced breath holding. These individuals respond best to immediate mouth-to-mouth resuscitation and often recover spontaneous respirations within minutes. Once the patient aspirates water, however, hypoxemia, acidosis, pulmonary edema, red cell lysis, neurological injury and death can result if adequate ventilation is not quickly established and skillfully maintained.

There are theoretical differences between fresh and salt water aspiration. When the patient aspirates *fresh* water, alveolar surfactants are displaced or removed, alveolar surface tensions become high, and atelectasis can occur. Aspirated fresh water tends to be absorbed quickly into the vascular space; consequently, with greater amounts of fresh water aspiration, a mild, transient hemodilution and increase in blood volume may occur. In addition, if the fresh water was from a chlorinated swimming pool, the chlorine can destroy alveolar membranes and cause a chemical pneumonitis. *Salt* water aspiration may also interfere with alveolar surfactants; however, the predominant effect is pulmonary edema because the hypertonic salt water draws more fluid from the vascular space into the alveoli. With this fluid shift, hemoconcentration and severe hypovolemia may occur.

The end result of any significant aspiration is decreased alveolar ventilation. Aspiration causes inflammation, obstruction, and collapse of smaller airways and destruction of alveolar and capillary membranes. This produces pulmonary edema, a severe decrease in lung compliance, and alveolar hypoventilation. Arterial oxygen desaturation occurs because of the ventilation/perfusion abnormalities (perfusion of nonventilated alveoli). Healing of injured membranes can result in fibrosis and loss of intrapulmonary diffusion surface. Corticosteroid administration is thought to reduce the severity of this membrane destruction and fibrosis.

The most serious complication of near drowning is hypoxia. The patient with severe pulmonary involvement will require mechanical ventilation with high inspiratory pressures and high (up to 30 cm H_2O) PEEP to maintain adequate ventilation despite low lung compliance and pulmonary edema. Such high ventilatory pressures make the patient extremely susceptible to the development of pneumothorax and other air leaks (pneumomediastinum, subcutaneous emphysema). Acidosis may be severe and must be managed aggressively. End stage hypoxemia produces depression of cardiac, cerebral, renal, hepatic, and metabolic functions.

Beyond the second day of care, pulmonary infections can become problematic. If the patient aspirated contaminated water, severe infections can result. Many victims vomit and aspirate gastric contents during the near-drowning episode; initially, this can cause airway obstruction and later can result in severe chemical pneumonitis and pneumonia. Antibiotics will be required if evidence of pulmonary infection or lung abscess develops.

The severity of neurological sequelae following near drowning depends on the severity and duration of hypoxemia and on the temperature of the immersion water. Cold water submersion produces hypothermia before the hypoxic insult; this hypothermia may reduce tissue oxygen requirements and may result in increased patient tolerance of brief respiratory arrest. Because reports of neurological sequelae following near drowning vary considerably, aggressive management of the near-drowning victim is recommended. In the absence of associated neurological injury, if spontaneous respirations and cranial nerve reflexes do not return within hours of resuscitation (and rewarming of the patient if necessary), the prognosis for the patient is grave.

Companions or family members of the near-drowning victim may feel frustrated and guilty. Parents often will need special support, because they feel responsible for their child's condition.

ASSESSMENT

1. Circumstances of near drowning
   a. Duration of submersion
   b. Water temperature

c. Type of water—fresh, salt, or contaminated
d. Condition of patient when rescued
   (1) Presence/absence of spontaneous respirations and heart rate
   (2) LOC
   (3) Temperature
e. Evidence of associated neurological injury (concussion, skull fracture)

2. Resuscitation attempts and patient's response
   a. At scene of near drowning
   b. During transportation to the hospital
   c. On arrival in the hospital

3. Respiratory status
   a. Presence of pulmonary congestion or airway obstruction
   b. Evidence of bronchospasm, aspiration, or pulmonary edema with clinical examination or on chest radiograph
   c. Presence and efficiency of independent respiratory effort (lung aeration, use of accessory muscles)
   d. Arterial blood gas levels and acid-base balance
   e. Mechanical ventilatory assistance required (and inspiratory pressures and PEEP necessary)
   f. Chest radiograph
   g. Quantity and characteristics of respiratory secretions or sputum

4. Cardiovascular status
   a. Indirect evidence of circulating blood volume
      (1) CVP and/or left atrial pressure
      (2) PCWP
      (3) Urine output (and specific gravity)
      (4) Hct and Hgb
   b. Evidence of cardiac output
      (1) BP
      (2) Tissue perfusion
      (3) Urine output
   c. Consequences of severe hypoxemia
      (1) Progressive acidosis
      (2) Decreased myocardial function and increased irritability (and arrhythmias)
      (3) Red cell lysis and increase in serum potassium level
      (4) Decreased BP

5. Neurological status
   a. LOC
   b. Presence of cranial nerve or brainstem reflexes (gag, corneal reflex, withdrawal from pain)
   c. Seizure activity
   d. Evidence of increased intracranial pressure (caused by traumatic or hypoxic cerebral edema)
   e. Pathological posturing (decorticate or decerebrate) or flaccidity
   f. Pupil response to light and pupil size

6. Fluid and electrolyte balance
   a. Fluid balance (level of hydration, hypervolemia, hypovolemia)
   b. Electrolyte concentrations
      (1) Increased concentration indicative of hemoconcentration and hypovolemia
      (2) Decreased concentration indicative of hemodilution and hypervolemia
      (3) Increased serum potassium concentration with red cell lysis
      (4) Serum potassium concentration changes with acid-base imbalance
   c. Serum glucose level (especially important in infants, who have little glycogen storage)
   d. Renal function (especially consequences of hypoxia and acute tubular necrosis)

7. Recent history of illness
   a. Respiratory (pneumonia, emphysema, asthma)
   b. Cardiovascular (MI, coronary arteriosclerosis, congenital heart disease, arrhythmias, hypertension)

8. Current medications and allergies
9. Family members and their locations
10. Level of patient/family's anxiety

GOALS

1. Patent airway
2. Adequate ventilation
3. Adequate cardiac output
   a. Appropriate intravascular volume
   b. Effective cardiac rhythm
   c. Adequate tissue perfusion and BP
   d. Adequate Hct and Hgb
4. Normal electrolyte and acid-base balance
5. Optimal CNS function
6. Absence or resolution of pulmonary infection
7. Adequate renal function
8. Absence of nosocomial or opportunistic infection
9. Patient/family comprehends patient's health status with realistic discussion of patient's prognosis
10. Patient/family participates in hospital plan of care as appropriate
11. Patient/family demonstrates ability to provide appropriate home health care

POTENTIAL PROBLEMS	EXPECTED OUTCOMES	NURSING ACTIVITIES

■ Airway obstruction related to fluid aspiration, bronchospasm, pulmonary edema	■ Patent airway	■ Monitor for evidence of airway obstruction
		  Stridor
		  Coughing
		  Retractions (and other evidence of use of accessory muscles of respiration)
		  Nasal flaring
		  Cyanosis (or pallor if patient is anemic or an infant)
		  Excessive respiratory secretions
		  Decreased lung aeration and chest expansion
		 If aforementioned occur, suction patient's airway immediately, request that physician be called, and begin emergency resuscitation measures if patient does not respond
		 If endotracheal tube is in place, maintain tube patency with sterile suction technique, and secure tube to prevent accidental dislodgement
		 Keep suction, resuscitator bag, O_2, and appropriate sizes of prepared endotracheal tubes at bedside (tube will need to be cut to appropriate length for children)
		 Keep patient's head turned to side (unless increased ICP present) with neck slightly extended to keep upper airway as straight as possible
		 If patient is mechanically ventilated, see Standard 6, *Mechanical ventilation;* keep in mind that these patients require higher ventilatory and PEEP pressures
		  See also Standard 7, *Positive end-expiratory pressure*
		  NOTE: If patient requires high inspiratory and end-expiratory pressures, sedation will be required to ensure ventilatory control of patient (sedatives, muscle relaxants, or paralyzing agents may be used); once patient is sedated, nurse must be sure to carefully maintain adequate ventilation, because patient is totally dependent on ventilator.
		 If patient requires long-term ventilation, tracheostomy may be indicated; see Standard 5, *The patient with a tracheostomy*

■ Hypoxemia and respiratory distress related to pulmonary edema, bronchospasm, surfactant elimination, chemical pneumonitis, destruction or fibrosis of alveolar membrane, pneumonia, pneumothorax, and possible CNS depression	■ Adequate ventilation as measured by
	  Satisfactory arterial blood gas levels
	  Equal and adequate lung aeration
	  Pink nail beds and mucous membranes
	  Minimal use of accessory muscles of respiration
	  Absence of pulmonary congestion on radiograph and with clinical examination
		■ Monitor for evidence of hypoxemia
		  Altered patient LOC (patient may become more agitated or more lethargic)
		  Increased heart rate (consider patient's normal range)
		  Increased respiratory rate (consider patient's normal range)
		  Increased respiratory effort; increased use of accessory muscles of respiration and "fighting" of ventilator may be noted unless patient is sedated
		  Decreased arterial P_{O_2} and decreased pH with decreased, normal, or increased P_{CO_2} (with hypoxia, the respiratory rate is stimulated, so initial *hypocapnia* may occur)
		  Peripheral vasoconstriction
		  Cyanosis or pallor (cyanosis will appear only if hemoglobin concentration is adequate)
		 If aforementioned occur, notify physician and increase patient ventilation through hand bagging with manual resuscitator (once patent airway is assured as in Problem, Airway obstruction)
		 Monitor for evidence of increased respiratory distress
		  Aforementioned symptoms
		  Decreased lung aeration
		  Increased pulmonary congestion
		  Decreased chest excursion during inspiration
		  Arterial O_2 desaturation and/or hypercapnia
		 If aforementioned occur, ensure patent airway (as in Problem, Airway obstruction), bag patient with resuscitator bag and mask (or bag and adaptor if patient is intubated), request that physician be called, and begin emergency resuscitation measures as needed (be prepared for emergency intubation or reintubation of patient)

POTENTIAL PROBLEMS	EXPECTED OUTCOMES	NURSING ACTIVITIES
		If mechanically ventilated patient demonstrates aforementioned evidence of increased distress, the following problems should be considered

If mechanically ventilated patient demonstrates aforementioned evidence of increased distress, the following problems should be considered

Tube may be blocked; if you are unable to produce adequate ventilation by hand bagging and much resistance to ventilation is felt, tube is probably blocked; suction patient immediately; if tube remains blocked, it should be removed to allow patient to be ventilated by mask until reintubation can be accomplished

If tube is patent and patient remains severely distressed, *pneumothorax* is next consideration; physician should be notified while hand bagging is attempted and chest radiograph is obtained; nurse should have equipment assembled for emergency insertion of chest tubes

NOTE: In small infants, breath sounds are easily transmitted through thin chest wall, so adequate breath sounds may appear to be present despite pneumothorax because of transmission of breath sounds from other areas; *because pneumothorax can appear suddenly and cause rapid, severe compromise of cardiorespiratory function, health care team must be prepared to act quickly*

Maintain mechanical ventilation as ordered; see Standard 6, *Mechanical ventilation* and Standard 7, *Positive end-expiratory pressure,* but note that these patients will require high inspiratory pressures

Monitor blood gas levels and make ventilatory changes as ordered; hypercapnia, hypoxemia, and acidosis indicate increased respiratory failure

Check ventilator settings at least q1 hr if patient is mechanically ventilated

Monitor for evidence of increased pulmonary edema

Increased pulmonary congestion (by radiograph or clinical examination)

Decreased lung aeration at same ventilator inspiratory pressures, or increased ventilator inspiratory pressures at same set V_T (if patient is mechanically ventilated)

Increased respiratory effort (if patient is breathing spontaneously)

Increased respiratory secretions or sputum production

Increased PCWP

Tachycardia (increased from patient's normal range)

Tachypnea (increased from patient's previous rate, if patient is not mechanically ventilated)

Falling arterial Po_2 and pH and rising arterial Pco_2 with increasing alveolar-arterial O_2 difference

If aforementioned occur, notify physician, restrict fluid intake, and administer diuretic therapy as ordered

Colloid osmotic agents may be prescribed with diuretics to help reduce pulmonary edema; if ordered, be sure to include them as part of patient fluid intake and monitor patient response

Weaning of patient from mechanical ventilation must be performed in structured, meticulous fashion

Initially, inspiratory or PEEP pressures will be decreased; *this must be done very slowly in patients who have aspirated fresh water to make sure that they have had adequate regeneration of surfactant to tolerate weaning*

If patient tolerance permits, rate or V_T is then decreased

Only one ventilator variable should be changed at any given time, and thorough evaluation of patient response should be made before any other change is introduced

During weaning, monitor patient closely for clinical evidence of hypoxia or deterioration in arterial blood gas levels

If possible, monitor patient's end-tidal CO_2 (it should be representative of the arterial Pco_2 unless severe pulmonary disease is present)

POTENTIAL PROBLEMS	EXPECTED OUTCOMES	NURSING ACTIVITIES
		Arterial *hypocapnia* (and falling end-tidal CO_2) during weaning may indicate patient hyperventilation in response to hypoxia Arterial *hypercapnia* (and rising end-tidal CO_2) or falling arterial PaO_2 reflects respiratory insufficiency and intolerance of weaning Monitor alveolar-arterial O_2 difference; increased gradient suggests increased intrapulmonary shunting and decreased alveolar ventilation
■ Inadequate cardiac output related to inadequate circulating blood volume, peripheral and pulmonary vasoconstriction, arrhythmias, hypoxemia, acidosis, and possible pneumomediastinum	■ Stable cardiac output as measured by Effective cardiac rhythm Adequate BP Warm extremities Pink mucous membranes Brisk capillary refill Adequate urine output (0.5 to 1.0 ml/kg/hour in children; 25 to 30 ml/hour in adults) Adequate cerebral perfusion	■ Monitor for evidence of decreased cardiac output Systolic hypotension Adults—systolic BP less than 100 mm Hg (consider patient's normal range) Children—systolic BP less than 85 mm Hg (consider patient's normal range) Infants—systolic BP less than 70 mm Hg (consider patient's normal range) Tachycardia Poor peripheral perfusion (cold, clammy extremities, decreased urine output with high—greater than 1.015—specific gravity, decreased peripheral pulses) Pallor or cyanosis Increased central or pulmonary venous pressures may indicate hypervolemia, cardiac failure, or pneumomediastinum Decreased central or pulmonary venous pressures may indicate hypovolemia Arrhythmias (monitor and document any arrhythmias with rhythm strip—note BP during arrhythmias—and notify physician); be aware of electrolyte imbalance, which may precipitate arrhythmias; see Standard 21, *Arrhythmias* If symptomatic pneumomediastinum is present, it should be aspirated immediately Assess circulating blood volume Monitor Hct—notify physician and prepare to administer packed red blood cells (RBC) or whole blood if Hct is less than 30% (40% in infants) or falling rapidly Increased Hct and serum electrolyte concentrations may indicate hemoconcentration and decreased blood volume, requiring increased fluid administration Decreased serum Hct and serum electrolyte concentrations may indicate hemodilution and increased blood volume, requiring diuresis Monitor urine output—decreased urine output (less than 0.5 to 1.0 ml/kg/hour despite adequate intake) with increased specific gravity may indicate cardiac failure Administer vasopressors as ordered—note their effect on heart rate, central and pulmonary venous pressures, arterial pressure, and urine output and titrate accordingly See Standard 17, *Shock* With CNS injury, *inappropriate antidiuretic hormone (ADH) secretion* may occur; this causes increased loss of Na^+ in urine and decreased serum Na^+ concentration (H_2O intoxication); urine volume may be increased, decreased, or unchanged, but will be more concentrated (specific gravity greater than 1.015); treatment of choice is fluid restriction With CNS injury (especially following hypoxic insult), *diabetes insipidus* may occur; patient loses enormous amounts of dilute urine (specific gravity less than 1.010), and hypovolemia will result if fluid replacement is not rapid; treatment is fluid replacement and administration of vasopressin (pituitary hormone)

POTENTIAL PROBLEMS	EXPECTED OUTCOMES	NURSING ACTIVITIES
■ Cerebral edema related to hypoxemia, acidosis, fluid shifts, electrolyte imbalance, traumatic cranial injury, and extremely high ventilatory PEEP	■ Optimal CNS function as measured by Absence of seizures Absence of signs of increased intracranial pressure (ICP)	■ Monitor for evidence of increased ICP Altered LOC (increased irritability or lethargy) Increased systolic BP Decreased heart rate (although initially it may increase) Depressed respirations Decreased pupil response to light If aforementioned symptoms occur, notify physician at once and be prepared to begin emergency resuscitative measures should further deterioration and respiratory arrest occur; see also Standard 32, *Increased intracranial pressure* Perform neurological assessment q1 hr (or as indicated by patient's condition) Monitor pupil response to light and notify physician of any change in response or new pupil inequality (these findings may indicate severe cerebral edema and increased ICP) Monitor ICP if monitoring line is in place; see Standard 32, *Increased intracranial pressure* Note any pathological posturing by patient; notify physician immediately if deterioration occurs Monitor for seizure activity Ensure safety of patient environment (pad side rails, remove sharp objects, tape all tubes securely) If seizures occur, note duration, extent, and muscle involvement and notify physician Notify physician immediately if seizure activity increases in frequency or duration (additional anticonvulsants may be required) See Standard 41, *Seizures* Administer anticonvulsants as ordered (check patient's dosage and monitor patient's response) IV fluids with low salt content (e.g., 5% dextrose in water or 0.2% normal saline) may be ordered to decrease posttraumatic or posthypoxic tendency for fluid retention Diabetes insipidus or inappropriate ADH secretion may occur; see Problem, Inadequate cardiac output Osmotic diuretics may be ordered in attempt to reduce ICP by reducing cerebral edema
■ Nutritional compromise related to prolonged nasotracheal intubation, bed rest, and stress	■ Adequate nutritional status as measured by Appropriate weight gain Adequate subcutaneous tissue Moist mucous membranes Good skin turgor Adequate wound healing Normal Hgb	■ Calculate patient's daily caloric requirements; ensure adequate caloric intake via parenteral alimentation or gavage feedings if oral intake is impossible Monitor infant's serum glucose or Dextrostix* as needed; notify physician of any evidence of hypoglycemia (glycogen storage in infants is minimal) NOTE: 5% dextrose solutions provide only 200 kcal/liter and thus are inadequate for long-term nutrition If patient is given parenteral alimentation, see Standard 57, *Total parenteral nutrition* Turn patient frequently, and keep skin warm and dry to prevent skin breakdown; massage any bony prominences to improve skin circulation Monitor patient's Hct and Hgb, and notify physician of any significant changes Weigh patient daily (or twice daily if indicated), and notify physician of any significant weight gain or loss (greater than 1 kg/24 hours in adults, greater than 200 g/24 hours in children, and greater than 50 g/24 hours in infants) Monitor patient's fluid intake and output; calculate patient's daily fluid requirements, and notify physician if patient is not receiving them Monitor for evidence of dehydration; notify physician if present

*Ames Co., Elkhart, Ind.

POTENTIAL PROBLEMS	EXPECTED OUTCOMES	NURSING ACTIVITIES

■ Infection related to aspiration of contaminated water, pulmonary compromise, and multiple invasive monitoring lines	■ Absence of signs of infection, including
	Fever (or hypothermia in infant)
	Leukocytosis
	Redness, heat, or discharge at wound site
		■ If patient aspirated contaminated water obtain daily sputum cultures and notify physician of any abnormalities
		Monitor
		  For evidence of systemic infection
		    Fever (or temperature instability in infant)
		    Possible leukocytosis
		    With severe systemic infection, fall in BP and cardiac output can occur; see Standard 17, *Shock*
		  For evidence of respiratory infection
		    Increased pulmonary congestion by radiograph or physical examination
		    Increased respiratory distress (increased respiratory rate and effort, decreased lung aeration, and cyanosis or pallor)
		    Increased color, thickness, and odor of secretions (obtain specimen for C and S and gram stain)
		  For evidence of urinary tract infection
		    Fever
		    Cloudy, malodorous urine (obtain clean catch specimen for C and S and gram stain)
		    Pain with urination
		    In children, frequent voiding in small amounts is seen
		  For evidence of wound infection
		    Erythema at wound edges
		    Fluctuation of wound margins
		    Wound drainage (obtain C and S and Gram stain)
		    Heat around wound
		Administer antibiotics as ordered
		Ensure good hand washing technique by hospital personnel before and after patient contact

■ Electrolyte imbalance related to acidosis, hemodilution, hemoconcentration, red cell lysis, or fluid shifts	■ Normal serum electrolytes	■ Monitor serum electrolyte levels; notify physician if abnormal
		  K^+ shifts will occur with changes in pH; therefore before initiating any K^+ replacement, consider acid-base balance
		  With acidosis, serum K^+ rises (K^+ shifts out of cells and into serum); conversely, with correction of acidosis, serum K^+ concentration falls
		  With alkalosis, serum K^+ falls (K^+ shifts into cells and out of serum); conversely, with correction of alkalosis, serum K^+ concentration rises
		With hemodilution, serum electrolyte concentrations fall; will return to normal when diuresis occurs
		With hemoconcentration, serum electrolyte concentrations rise; will fall again with hydration
		Infants who are severely ill are particularly prone to development of hypoglycemia (they have little glycogen storage); monitor their glucose level carefully and ensure adequate source of caloric intake (5% dextrose IV solutions provide only 200 kcal/liter)
		With red cell lysis, serum K^+ will rise and hemoglobinuria will be seen; notify physician and monitor renal function

■ Hypothermia or hyperthermia related to patient submersion in cold water, CNS damage, or infection	■ Normal rectal temperature	■ Monitor patient's rectal temperature; if fever (greater than 100.5° F [38° C] is present, notify physician; note blood culture results If hyperthermia is present, this will increase patient's O_2 consumption; therefore once source of fever is established, application of hypothermia blanket may be indicated to control patient temperature; if such blanket is used, it should never be set below 72° F (22° C) and should not cool patient enough to cause shivering (or frostbite) If hypothermia is present, rewarming of patient should be accomplished gradually; rewarming should never be accomplished by application of warm object to patient's skin, as severe burns can result, particularly if cardiac output (and skin perfusion) is decreased; overbed warmers are preferred

POTENTIAL PROBLEMS	EXPECTED OUTCOMES	NURSING ACTIVITIES
■ Patient/family's anxiety related to near drowning, critical patient status, and critical care environment and equipment (in children, separation from parents will also add to child's fear)	■ Patient/family's comprehension of diagnosis and therapeutic regimen as demonstrated by their discussions and questions Patient/family's support of one another with demonstration of appropriate behavior	■ Determine concerns of patient/family Prepare family members for sight of patient with multiple IVs and many pieces of monitoring equipment Assess patient/family's understanding of condition and prognosis; elicit their opinions and comments, and attempt to clarify any misconceptions Attempt to elicit patient/family's response to patient's near drowning; provide support and reassurance during family's discussion of anger or guilt Be present when prognosis is discussed by physician, and encourage patient/family's questions, as needed Involve family in patient care as appropriate; note that family members may not have enough emotional energy to provide physical care for patient Make appropriate referrals to chaplain and to social services Assist family in anticipatory mourning and/or realistic appraisal of patient's prognosis, as appropriate
■ Patient/family may have inadequate information to provide appropriate home care for patient after discharge	■ Patient/family will possess sufficient information to enable them to demonstrate and discuss home care techniques	■ Include patient/family in discharge planning as they demonstrate readiness Keep family informed of plans for patient discharge Allow sufficient time to permit teaching at relaxed pace, with adequate time for patient/family to perform return demonstration Provide encouragement and support as needed By time of patient discharge, family should be able to discuss 　Amount, schedule, and route of administration of any medications 　Side effects of medications (if appropriate) 　What to do if medication dose is forgotten (i.e., should it be given late or omitted) 　Indications for contacting physician or primary nurse 　Follow-up appointments and telephone numbers of health care personnel Provide family and patient with written information as needed By the time of patient discharge, patient/family should be able to demonstrate 　Wound care techniques, including appropriate dressing changes 　Any required airway care (if appropriate, see Standard 5, *The patient with a tracheostomy)* Make appropriate referrals to community health services (public health nursing, visiting nurse, community groups) Assist family in obtaining needed home health care equipment If patient will be institutionalized following discharge, involve physician and social worker or chaplain in family's decision as appropriate; support patient/family in their decision, once it has been made

THE PATIENT WITH A TRACHEOSTOMY

A tracheostomy is a procedure in which an artificial opening is created between the second and fourth tracheal rings to provide an airway that bypasses upper airway structures and facilitates tracheobronchial toilet. The most common indication for a tracheostomy is upper airway obstruction (caused by congenital stricture, trauma, carcinoma, infection, hemangioma, or long-term mechanical ventilation). A tracheostomy may also be performed to enable management of respiratory secretions that cannot be removed effectively by patient cough or nasopharyngeal suction. The tracheostomy may be temporary or permanent. Generally, uncuffed tubes are used in children to avoid later tracheal stenosis. Silastic tubes are popular for this age group because they conform easily to the shape of the child's trachea; however, because they have no inner cannula, metal tubes with inner cannulas are often the choice for home-going tracheostomy intubation. Metal or cuffed tubes are more commonly used in the adult patient or the patient who requires high inspiratory pressures (cuffs prevent air leaks). The type of tube and specific methods of stomal care will depend on the experience and the preference of the physician.

Because the tracheostomy allows air to bypass the upper airway, the functions of these structures—humidification, filtration, and warming of the air—must be artificially provided until cells in the trachea can compensate. Aseptic technique is essential in all phases of tracheostomy care during hospitalization, especially because multiple caretakers will be involved in the patient's care. When the patient returns home and the caretakers are limited, a clean technique will usually be satisfactory.

Complications of the actual tracheostomy include infection, airway obstruction, hemorrhage, tracheal ulceration or stenosis, subcutaneous emphysema, tube dislodgement or displacement, increased viscosity of respiratory secretions, peristomal skin breakdown, and laryngeal injury.

ASSESSMENT

1. Purpose of tracheostomy and intended duration
2. Evidence of respiratory distress—tachypnea, increased use of accessory muscles of respiration, nasal flaring, head bobbing (in infant less than 4 months old), jaw tugging, cyanosis or pallor, copious tracheal secretions, pulmonary congestion (by radiograph or clinical examination), decreased breath sounds, decreased feeding tolerance, diaphoresis, grunting
3. Level of hydration—skin turgor, mucous membranes, fontanelle (in infants less than 18 months old), tearing (in patient more than 2 months old), urine output and specific gravity (output should be 0.5 to 1 ml/kg/hour with specific gravity less than 1.020 if fluid intake is adequate), consistency of tracheal secretions
4. Presence of stomal or pulmonary infection—pulmonary congestion, fever (or hypothermia in infants), purulent or malodorous secretions, leukocytosis, redness or fluctuance of edges of stoma
5. Appearance of stoma—retraction sutures, inflammation, size of orifice, evidence of bleeding, presence of granulomas or breakdown
6. Nutritional status—weight, wound healing, amount of subcutaneous fat, serum glucose (in infants)
7. Current medications and allergies
8. Patient/family's response to tracheostomy (and comprehension of reasons for and consequences of the tracheostomy)
9. Patient/family's concerns and fears

GOALS

1. Patent airway and adequate ventilation
2. Absence of stomal or pulmonary infection
3. Absence of tracheal stenosis or damage
4. Adequate patient hydration and nutrition
5. Patient/family's comprehension of tracheostomy procedure and necessary postoperative and home care
6. Appropriate and constructive patient/family verbalization of concerns regarding patient alterations in body image and change in life-style
7. Patient/family is able to provide home care of patient's tracheostomy as appropriate
8. Effective patient communication with health team members and family

POTENTIAL PROBLEMS	EXPECTED OUTCOMES	NURSING ACTIVITIES

■ Airway obstruction related to copious or dried tracheal secretions, pneumonia, atelectasis, hemorrhage, aspiration, or tracheostomy tube dislodgement	■ Patent airway	■ Tape spare tracheostomy tube of same size (and one a size larger and one a size smaller) to head of bed, and document size of tracheostomy tube in place
		Keep tracheal dilator with extra tube for older children and adults at bedside; tape obturator of tracheal tube that patient is wearing nearby at all times (e.g., to headboard)
		Keep suction equipment and resuscitator bag *with appropriate adaptor* at bedside
		Tape retraction sutures securely to neck or to chest wall so that they are readily accessible
		Provide humidity to inspired air as ordered; increase if secretions appear tenacious or dried
		Initially suction tracheostomy frequently, then less often as amount of mucus decreases
		  Use O_2 as needed
		  Irrigate tube with sterile saline solution (0.5 to 1.0 ml) if secretions are thick, then suction immediately
		  Once stoma is healing (after the first postoperative days) and as the patient's LOC permits, encourage patient to cough out secretions to stomal orifice so that they may be removed without suctioning or with use of only bulb syringe
		  Insert catheter *much less deeply* for tracheostomy suctioning than for endotracheal tube suctioning; irritation of carina with catheter will cause severe coughing spasm, pain, and possibly mucosal damage
		Warm inspired air for infants and young children to prevent heat loss through respiratory tract
		Restrain patient as needed to prevent removal of tube (mittens may be useful for children)
		Tie tracheostomy tube in place securely with twill or umbilical tape
		  Use square knots, and allow only one small finger-breadth of room between tape and patient's neck (tie tapes at side of child's neck to prevent loosening or dislodgement by child and development of pressure sores under knot)
		  Remember that cotton tape stretches when wet, so it may have to be changed frequently to prevent loosening
		  When changing tape, do not remove old ties until new ties are securely in place—generally two people are necessary to anchor tube and to secure new ties (especially with anxious child or combative adult)
		Remove and clean inner cannula (if present)* q2-4 hr and prn; use sterile technique and hydrogen peroxide or boiling as indicated by hospital policies
		  Use pipe cleaners to remove secretions inside of inner cannula; then rinse in sterile saline
		NOTE: Use of hydrogen peroxide may cause discoloration of silver tubes
		Change tube weekly or according to hospital policies, using sterile technique (tubes are generally changed for first time 5 to 7 days following tracheostomy)
		NOTE: Following first tracheostomy tube change, some physicians advocate *daily* tube change
		After tracheostomy is created (especially in small children), physician may gradually increase size of tube in place to provide larger patent airway; have larger tube ready as requested
		When tracheostomy is to be closed, often size of tube will be reduced slowly to allow assessment of patient tolerance and gradual reduction in size of stoma; have smaller tube ready at physician's request, but monitor patient tolerance and keep larger tubes ready to insert if patient demonstrates intolerance of smaller tube

*Silastic tubes do not have an inner cannula.

POTENTIAL PROBLEMS	EXPECTED OUTCOMES	NURSING ACTIVITIES
		Monitor for signs of respiratory distress—cyanosis, agitation, tachypnea, retractions, nasal flaring, use of accessory muscles for respiration
		Normal adult respiratory rate: 12 to 16/minute (consider patient's normal range)
		Normal pediatric respiratory rate: 18 to 30/minute (consider patient's normal range)
		Normal infant respiratory rate: 30 to 50/minute (consider patient's normal range)
		Normal newborn respiratory rate: 30 to 60/minute
		If patient demonstrates aforementioned symptoms of increased respiratory distress
		Suction tracheostomy and oropharynx with O_2 support; remove inner cannula if present
		Check position of tube and lung aeration; replace tube if needed
		Change tube if unable to suction; use caution and retraction sutures in first 5 to 7 days (as stomal tract is not yet healed)
		Notify physician and prepare for intubation of patient if these efforts are unsuccessful
		NOTE: If you are unable to replace tracheostomy tube, an endotracheal tube may even be used *only in an emergency* (and can only be inserted a *short* distance into trachea) to provide airway until proper reintubation can be accomplished; large suction catheter may also be inserted into stoma to keep it open; if this is done, catheter should be cut so that only a few inches are outside of trachea (O_2 may be administered through this catheter)
		Ventilate patient with resuscitator bag and mask *only if upper airway is intact and relatively unobstructed*
		Provide O_2 support as needed
■ Respiratory distress related to hypoventilation, pneumonia, pneumothorax, tracheostomy leakage, or perioperative sedation	■ Adequate ventilation as measured by equal and adequate lung aeration bilaterally, pink mucous membranes and nail beds, absence of pulmonary congestion, and absence of increased respiratory effort	■ Maintain patent airway as in Problem, Airway obstruction
		Monitor patient for lower airway problems
		Pneumonia
		Decreased breath sounds (indicating atelectasis)
		Increased breath sounds (indicating consolidation)
		Increase in thickness, quantity, and odor of secretions, or change in color of secretions
		Fever (or thermolability in infant)
		Increased respiratory effort (retractions or use of other accessory muscles of respiration)
		Pulmonary congestion (by radiograph or physical examination)
		Pneumothorax
		Decreased or absent breath sounds
		Cyanosis or pallor
		Increased respiratory effort
		Agitation
		Increased respiratory rate (compare to previous rate)
		Increased heart rate (compare to previous rate)
		Possible shift in mediastinum
		Hyperresonance to percussion
		If aforementioned symptoms are present, notify physician immediately, obtain chest radiograph, and prepare to assist with aspiration of pneumothorax or insertion of chest tubes if necessary
		Subcutaneous emphysema
		Swelling of neck, face, and/or trunk (results from subcutaneous air leak and is usually self-limiting, but may result in airway compression)
		Crackling with palpation
		Appearance of subcutaneous air on radiograph

POTENTIAL PROBLEMS	EXPECTED OUTCOMES	NURSING ACTIVITIES
		Administer chest physiotherapy including percussion, vibration, postural drainage (as tolerated), rib springing in infants and children, and suctioning as needed
		Provide humidity with or without O_2 continuously or during sleep
		Keep resuscitator bag *with appropriate adaptor* at bedside
■ Pneumonia related to contamination and aspiration (aspiration is much more likely if patient is neurologically impaired or if fenestrated tube is used)	■ Absence of radiographic or clinical evidence of pulmonary infection	■ Monitor for signs of pulmonary infection (congestion, fever, leukocytosis, increased respiratory distress)
		Use sterile suctioning technique
		Change humidification equipment daily; use only sterile distilled water to fill nebulizers
		Send tracheal aspirates for C and S and gram stain if infection is suspected (pulmonary tree is generally thought to be colonized with gram-negative bacteria within 48 hours of intubation)
		Administer antibiotics as ordered (double check patient dosage and allergies before administration)
		Prevent aspiration with careful attention during feedings
		If cuffed tube is in place, keep cuff inflated when patient is eating, drinking, or receiving gastrostomy feedings
		If cuffed tube is used, assess for proper amount of air in cuff, according to hospital protocol
		There should be enough air in cuff that air does not leak around it during normal tidal volume breath but when manual sigh is delivered air leaks around cuff (air is heard by placing diaphragm of stethoscope on neck over cuff site)
		Cuff pressures can be monitored using aneroid manometer or sphygmomanometer; pressures are generally kept below 20 to 25 mm Hg, but vary slightly depending on amount of air in cuff required to occlude trachea on tidal volume breath
		High-volume, low-pressure cuffs ("soft" cuffs) generate lower cuff pressures and exert less pressure on tracheal wall
		Low-volume, high-pressure cuffs ("hard" cuffs) generate higher cuff pressures and exert significantly greater pressures on tracheal wall
		If "hard" cuff tubes are used, regimen for periodic cuff deflation should be followed (per hospital protocol) to prevent tracheal wall ischemia, which can lead to necrosis, and eventual scarring and tracheal stenosis
		Administer chest physiotherapy before feedings, but no sooner than 1 hour before feeding (so patient is not coughing during feeding) or 1 hour after feeding
		If NG or gastrostomy feeding is required, check gastric tube position before each feeding, and leave gastric tube unclamped for 30 to 45 minutes following each feeding
		Have suction equipment at hand
		Keep patient in high Fowler's position or on right side during feedings and for 1 hour following feedings; do not allow patient to recline on back (flat) for 1 hour after feeding
		Avoid disturbing patient for 1 hour after feeding (no blood tests, chest physiotherapy, injections)
		Monitor for signs of aspiration
		Coughing
		Increased respiratory distress
		Cyanosis
		Vomiting
		Agitation
		If aforementioned symptoms occur, discontinue feedings immediately, gently suction oropharynx and trachea (but try not to stimulate gag reflex, which may result in further vomiting and aspiration), lower feeding tube orifice (to allow reflux), turn patient prone and slap back sharply, request that physician be notified, obtain chest radiograph (may not be positive for at least 6 to 12 hours), and prepare to institute emergency measures

POTENTIAL PROBLEMS	EXPECTED OUTCOMES	NURSING ACTIVITIES
		If patient has history of aspiration during feeding, add food coloring to feeding and notify physician if this coloring appears in tracheal secretions
▪ Stomal infection or peri-stomal skin breakdown	▪ Absence of stomal infection (no signs of inflammation of stoma, no discharge)	▪ Observe stoma for erythema, exudates, odor, and crusting lesions Notify physician and culture stoma if inflammation appears (yeast infections are most commonly detected around stoma) Cleanse stoma q8 hr and as needed with half-strength hydrogen peroxide and rinse with sterile water (use cotton-tipped applicators) Apply dressing to protect stoma during feeding and if patient has constant drooling Change tracheal tube daily, if necessary, as ordered Change tapes daily and as needed; use two people for procedure with children and uncooperative adults Do not allow secretions to pool around stoma; suction or wipe them to keep stoma as dry as possible Apply topical antifungal or antibiotic agent only if ordered; prophylactic administration may encourage growth of resistant strains of bacteria or fungi Change all humidification equipment daily and as needed Keep skin under tracheal ties as clean and dry as possible, as skin is prone to breakdown caused by abrasion and secretions
▪ Stomal bleeding related to erosion of tube through blood vessel wall or incomplete cautery of skin vessel during tracheostomy procedure	▪ No excessive stomal bleeding	▪ Monitor site for bleeding; notify physician if bleeding is occurring If bleeding is profuse, apply pressure to site to control bleeding; suction as needed to keep airway patent Change dressings as needed and weigh dressings before and after use to document amount of bleeding
▪ Tracheal erosion related to tube movement or high-pressure cuff	▪ Absence of tracheal damage and ability to resume upper airway ventilation following closure of tracheostomy	▪ Keep cuff deflated whenever possible Maintain small air leak around tracheostomy tube to prevent excessive pressure on trachea by cuff or tube Avoid movement of tube or torsion of tracheal collar when suctioning, changing tapes, and cleansing site Prevent tube dislodgement (especially in first week), as frequent tube replacement causes tracheal irritation Monitor tube shape and position; discuss with physician if tube does not conform to angle of patient's airway—a different brand of tube may be required; Silastic tubes tend to become more flexible when warmed and moistened in patient's airway, so these tubes conform most easily to angle of pediatric airway; however, these tubes are expensive and can only be used for one 2-month period (approximately); for home tracheostomy care, metal tubes with inner cannulas may be more practical Tracheostomy tube *must* be changed frequently enough to ensure its cleanliness; dirty tube will cause chronic tracheal inflammation, resulting in tracheal scarring and granulomatous tissue formation
▪ Dehydration related to inadequate humidification of inspired air or inadequate fluid intake	▪ Patent airway and adequate hydration as measured by Moist, easily suctioned secretions Moist mucous membranes Good skin turgor Adequate urine output (0.5 to 1.0 ml/kg/hour in children; 30 ml/hour in adults)	▪ Assess level of patient hydration—mucous membranes should be moist; fontanelle in infant under 18 months should be flat but not sunken; adequate eye tearing should be present in patient over 2 months of age; skin should not ''tent'' when pinched; urine output should be adequate Increase humidification of inspired air as needed Calculate patient's maintenance fluid requirements and ensure that patient receives them (through oral, IV, or gavage route); discuss requirements and route of administration with physician If secretions are dry, provide humidification via tracheal cuff Monitor fluid intake and output; discuss fluid imbalances with physician

POTENTIAL PROBLEMS	EXPECTED OUTCOMES	NURSING ACTIVITIES
■ Poor nutritional status related to prolonged hospitalization, dysphagia, anorexia, or CNS disease	■ Adequate nutritional status as measured by Appropriate weight gain Adequate subcutaneous fat Moist mucous membranes Good skin turgor Adequate wound healing Normal Hgb	■ Calculate patient's daily caloric requirements and ensure that patient receives them (discuss with physician) Monitor infant's serum glucose, and notify physician of hypoglycemia (infant glycogen stores are low) If patient is given parenteral alimentation, see Standard 57, *Total parenteral nutrition* Monitor patient's Hct and Hgb, and notify physician of abnormalities Weigh patient daily and notify physician of any significant weight loss (greater than 1.0 kg/24 hours in adults, greater than 200 g/24 hours in children, and greater than 50 g/24 hours in infants) Make food and mealtimes as appetizing for patient as possible; provide small, tasty, frequent feedings rather than large "hospital tray" ones
■ Inability of patient to communicate verbally	■ Patient can communicate his/her needs to caregivers in manner appropriate to patient's LOC and conceptual development	■ Assess patient's LOC If patient is alert Provide call bell within easy reach at all times Provide for easy observation of patient by nursing staff (and of nursing staff by patient) Provide "magic slate" or pad and pencil if patient is able to write (or communications board if unable to write) Provide communications board with illustrations if patient is preverbal or aphasic For children, nurse should be in room at all times, since child's cry or voice may not be heard In children, assess growth and developmental level and use aforementioned strategies as appropriate Provide patient with reassurance and patience; tell patient which nurses are nearby so that patient will not feel alone As appropriate, teach patient to briefly occlude airway to speak
■ Patient/family's anxiety related to patient's inability to speak, patient care required, and alterations in patient's appearance	■ Patient/family able to discuss concerns and to support one another and function appropriately	■ Explain all activities and procedures as appropriate (use play for teaching of children) Initiate appropriate referrals to social services, chaplain, and clinical specialist as needed Provide patient/family with daily reports of patient's progress (it is important to provide them with concrete daily goals and positive reinforcement) Be present when physicians discuss patient's progress with patient/family; clarify and reinforce information as needed Begin to involve patient/family in decision making and patient care as appropriate Assist patient/family in development of realistic plan for patient home health care or postdischarge care
■ Patient/family may have insufficient information to provide adequate patient home health care	■ Patient/family will be able to realistically assess their abilities to provide adequate patient home health care If patient will be discharged to home, patient/family will demonstrate adequate skills in patient health care If patient will be discharged to institution for health care, patient/family will demonstrate acceptance of this solution, while maintaining support for one another	■ Critically assess patient/family's ability to provide adequate home health care of patient with tracheostomy and to respond to any emergency situations that may arise; most families will be able to assume appropriate care; however, if both parents of an infant are blind, for example, some alternative method of care for patient may need to be explored If patient cannot be discharged to home, assist patient/family in exploring alternative forms of patient care Make appropriate referrals to community health and social service agencies If patient will be discharged to home or if patient or family will be involved in posthospital care of patient's tracheostomy, assess their readiness to learn, and begin teaching skills for home health care slowly Assessment of patient's respiratory status Maintenance of patient's airway

POTENTIAL PROBLEMS	EXPECTED OUTCOMES	NURSING ACTIVITIES
		Clean suction technique (if patient is at special risk for development of respiratory infection, sterile technique may be required—check with patient's physician)
		Stomal care
		Changing of tracheal tapes
		Changing or replacement of tracheostomy tube
		NOTE: A double-lumen metal tube is generally safest for home care
		Emergency resuscitation measures
		Medications
		Physician and nurse follow-up appointments
		Where, when, and why to contact physician, emergency personnel, nurse
		If family does not speak English, arrangements must be made to have interpreter readily available (relative, hospital personnel, etc.)
		Provide frequent and consistent reinforcement throughout teaching
		Document teaching plan and patient/family's progress
		Assist patient/family in obtaining needed home care equipment
		Ensure effective follow-up of patient following discharge; check frequently with patient/family in person and by telephone following patient's discharge
		Visiting nurse agencies may be used as part of patient home follow-up

MECHANICAL VENTILATION

Mechanical ventilation is a process by which a positive force is generated in the airway to inflate the lungs with humidified, oxygenated air. Mechanical ventilation is necessary for patients who are unable to provide enough force for their own respirations, such as patients with compromised lungs or chest wall and apneic or nearly apneic patients. Such abnormalities may result in acute respiratory failure, in which the patient is unable to maintain adequate ventilation and oxygenation and which results in hypoxemia or hypoxemia with hypercapnia.

Mechanical ventilation is necessary when conservative means cannot rectify the clinical picture of acute respiratory failure. It is employed to provide adequate exchange of blood gases in patients with a variety of abnormalities, such as the following:

Decreased CNS function (e.g., drug overdose)

Neuromuscular abnormalities, muscular weakness (as in systemic diseases associated with fibrotic, stiff lung, e.g., sarcoidosis or after cardiothoracic surgery)

Pulmonary fibrosis (e.g., Hamman-Rich syndrome)

Impaired chest wall mechanics

Flail chest

Gross obesity

Abdominal distention

Ascites

Abdominal binders

Body casts

Chest restraints

Intrinsic causes of acute respiratory failure

Asthma

Pneumonia (especially aspiration pneumonia)

Ventilation/perfusion abnormalities

Pulmonary interstitial edema

Shock lung

Fluid overload

Congestive heart failure (CHF)

Smoke inhalation

Mechanical ventilation is accomplished with the use of ventilators that inflate the lungs with a predetermined volume or preset pressure. There is a large variety of ventilators available. The volume-cycled ventilators are preferred by most clinicians because of their ability to ventilate the alveoli readily.

Volume-cycled ventilators deliver a constant tidal volume in the presence of changes in airway resistance or in compliance (distensibility) of the lungs or thorax. It terminates inspiration after a preset volume is delivered. This preset volume is delivered regardless of the pressure needed to do so. However, when excessive pressures are generated in the airway, a pressure alarm limit is activated and inspiration ends prematurely.

Examples of volume-cycled ventilators in common use include the following:

Bennett MA$_1$ and MA$_2$

Bourns Bear

Emerson

Ohio 560

There are several modes of ventilation that are available in volume-cycled ventilators. They are controlled ventilation, assist-control ventilation, intermittent mandatory ventilation, and continuous positive airway pressure/continuous positive pressure ventilation. The mode chosen depends on specific patient needs.

Controlled ventilation. With controlled ventilation, the patient is not permitted to (or cannot) initiate inspiratory efforts. The ventilator delivers a preset tidal volume at a preset rate, with the patient passive. This method is used for patients who have tachypnea and marked respiratory distress, in which the patient's breathing pattern is not in synchrony with the machine. In addition, PEEP therapy employing pressures of 5 cm H_2O or more often requires controlled ventilation. To block out the effect of patient effort, pharmacological agents such as morphine sulfate, morphine sulfate and pancuronium, or diazepam and pancuronium are generally required.

Assist-control ventilation. With assist-control ventilation, the patient can initiate each breath by creating negative pressure in the lungs through muscle contraction. The ventilator responds to this pressure by delivering a positive pressure breath called an *assisted breath*. If the patient does not initiate a breath after a preset interval, the ventilator will automatically deliver a positive pressure breath.

Intermittent mandatory ventilation (IMV). With IMV, the patient is allowed to spontaneously breathe humidified, oxygenated air from the ventilatory system at whatever rate and volume the patient chooses. Intermittent positive pressure breaths are delivered from the ventilator at preset intervals (to ensure adequate alveolar ventilation). IMV is particularly useful for patients who have been intubated for a prolonged period of time and in whom the respiratory muscles are weak. IMV allows the patient to actively contract his/her own respiratory muscles and gradually build muscle strength. This mode of ventilation is generally used for gradually weaning a patient from artificial ventilation. Special IMV valves are built into the ventilator or must be added to the inspiratory side of the ventilator tubing. Most ventilators with internal IMV valves provide synchronized IMV (SIMV), in which the ventilator senses the rhythm of the patient's breathing pattern and delivers a breath when the patient is ready for it.

Continuous positive airway pressure (CPAP) or continuous positive pressure ventilation (CPPV). With CPAP/CPPV, all patient breaths are spontaneous, with no interposed mechanical ventilator breaths. The patient breathes humidified, oxygenated air from the ventilatory system at whatever rate the patient chooses. During the expiratory phase, the patient exhales to the preset positive end-expiratory pressure level. CPAP/CPPV is useful for patients who do not require assistance in maintaining an adequate tidal volume, but who benefit from an increased end-expiratory pressure, which increases the end-expiratory volume (functional residual capacity). This effect improves gas exchange in the presence of ventilation/perfusion imbalance and other causes of impaired gas exchange.

MODES OF MECHANICAL VENTILATION

1. Controlled ventilation—patient is passive

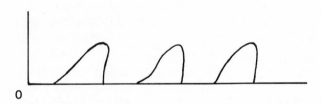

2. Assist-control ventilation—patient triggers cycle by generating inspiratory effort and negative intrapulmonary pressure (approximately 2 cm H_2O). All breaths are positive pressure

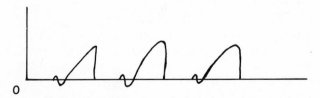

3. IMV—patient breathes spontaneously with intermittent positive pressure ventilator breaths

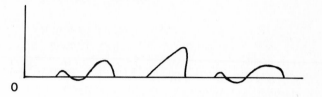

4. CPAP/CPPV—All patient breaths are spontaneous

Guidelines for effectively administering mechanical ventilation include the following:

Appropriate choice of ventilator, based on thorough assessment of the patient's needs

Serial monitoring of the arterial blood gas levels

Adjustment of ventilator settings according to the patient's response

Continuous assessment and evaluation of the patient's vital signs, color, general appearance, and other responses

Constant supervision of proper functioning of the ventilator

ASSESSMENT

1. History of underlying conditions, including
   a. Respiratory failure
   b. Renal insufficiency
   c. Cardiac disease
   d. Neurological abnormalities
2. Problem necessitating mechanical ventilation
   a. Cardiac and/or respiratory arrest
   b. Presence of apnea
   c. Acute ventilatory failure
   d. Impending acute ventilatory failure
   e. Inadequate oxygenation
   f. Severe trauma
3. Current active medical and/or respiratory problems
4. Presence, nature, and severity of abnormalities in the following systems
   a. Pulmonary
      (1) Degree of respiratory distress
      (2) Respiratory rate, quality; note tachypnea, dyspnea
      (3) Rales, wheezes, and other adventitious sounds
      (4) Ability to expectorate secretions
      (5) Amount, color, and consistency of sputum
      (6) Beside pulmonary functions; note those not within normal limits, including V_T, vital capacity, minute volume, and inspiratory force
   b. Cardiovascular
      (1) BP, heart rate, CVP, PAP, PCWP, and cardiac output for any abnormalities
      (2) ECG for arrhythmias

c. Neurological
   (1) LOC; note signs of hypoxia (e.g., restlessness, disorientation) or signs of hypercapnia (e.g., drowsiness)
   (2) Changes in pupillary size and light reflex
   (3) Abnormal motor and sensory function
d. Renal
   (1) Increase or decrease in urine output; specific gravity, pH
   (2) Presence of any drainage, e.g., ostomies
5. Patient's perception of and reaction to mechanical ventilation and intubation procedure
6. T
7. Weight
8. Results of lab and diagnostic tests
   a. Arterial blood gas values
   b. Electrolyte levels
   c. C and S of blood, tracheobronchial secretions
   d. CBC and differential
   e. Serum creatinine, BUN, total protein
   f. Chest radiograph
   g. ECG
   h. Bronchoscopy
9. Ventilation system
   a. Position of endotracheal tube
   b. Type of ventilator
   c. Settings
      (1) Mode of ventilation (e.g., assist, assist-control, control, IMV, CPAP)
      (2) Oxygen percentage
      (3) V_T
      (4) Rate
      (5) Sigh rate
      (6) Inspiratory-expiratory ratio
      (7) Sensitivity
      (8) Airway pressure
      (9) Flow rate
      (10) Humidity and temperature
      (11) PEEP (if used)
      (12) Expiratory retard (if used)
      (13) Mechanical dead space (if used)
10. Patient/family's level of anxiety and understanding of mechanical ventilation and disease process necessitating ventilation

GOALS

1. Reduction of patient/family's anxiety with provision of information, explanations, and encouragement
2. Adequate oxygenation and ventilation with PaO_2 and $PaCO_2$ levels within patient's normal limits
3. Adequate oxygenation and perfusion of organs and tissues for maximal function
4. Hemodynamic stability
   a. Adequate cardiac output
   b. Normovolemia
   c. Absence of arrhythmias
5. Infection free; absence of pneumonia
6. Electrolyte and blood count results within normal limits
7. Resolution of underlying disease condition necessitating mechanical ventilation
8. Absence of complications associated with mechanical ventilation
9. Ventilator system functioning properly
10. Synchronization of patient's breathing with ventilator

POTENTIAL PROBLEMS	EXPECTED OUTCOMES	NURSING ACTIVITIES

■ Patient/family's anxiety related to
Disease process, diagnostic tests and procedures, therapy
Mechanical ventilation
	■ Reduction of anxiety with provision of sufficient information, explanations, and encouragement	■ Ongoing assessment of level of anxiety, knowledge base, and understanding
		Collaborate with physician in providing
		  Realistic information for patient/family
		  Information relevant to level of understanding
		  Explanation of disease process, diagnostic tests and procedures, therapy
		  Explanation of need for mechanical ventilation
		Encourage verbalization of questions, fears, and anxieties
		Provide for
		  Patient decisions and participation in care
		  Periods of uninterrupted sleep
		  As much sleep as possible
		  Minimal overstimulation with meaningless noise

Inability to talk	Patient effectively communicates with alternate means	Set up alternate means of communication Relay alternate means of communication to staff, family; assist in effective use of means Reassure patient that after tube is removed, he/she will be able to talk Encourage patient to speak once tube is removed

POTENTIAL PROBLEMS	EXPECTED OUTCOMES	NURSING ACTIVITIES
		If appropriate, reassure patient that hoarseness and raspy voice will gradually subside Anticipate patient's needs Reassure and support patient/family Encourage staff/family to communicate with patient Evaluate effectiveness of alternate means of communication Provide ongoing explanation of care

■ Ventilator malfunction	■ Ventilator functioning properly
	Ventilator delivers requisite volume of humified O_2
		■ Ensure that respiratory therapist changes ventilator tubing and evaluates functioning daily
		Monitor for (q2-4 hr)
		  Correct ventilator settings (i.e., V_T, rate, O_2 percentage, sigh)
		  Delivery of correct concentration of O_2
		  Presence of any leaks (humidifier, tubing, endotracheal or tracheal cuff, nebulizer connection)
		  Patency of tubings; note condensation of H_2O in tubing or kinked, compressed, or stretched tubing
		  Functioning and setting of alarm systems (i.e., spirometer, pressure, ratio)
		  Correct temperature of H_2O vapor—95° to 100° F (35° to 37.8° C)
		  Proper needle movement on pressure gauge
		  Sufficient H_2O content in cascade
		  Secure attachment of O_2 tubing to ventilator
		  Functioning panel light indicators
		If ventilator malfunction occurs and patient is not receiving adequate V_T and/or O_2 concentrations, hand ventilate patient and ask someone to assess problem; call physiotherapist if unable to resolve problem

■ Airway obstruction related to
  Thick secretions
 	
  Improper positioning of endotracheal tube
  Bronchospasm
	■ Airway patency
	
	  Effective mobilization of secretions
	
	  Proper positioning of endotracheal tube
	  Absence or resolution of bronchospasm
		■ Prevention
		  Administer chest physiotherapy q2 hr unless contraindicated
		  Suction endotracheal/tracheal tube and mouth q1-2 hr for secretions; if secretions are thick, it may be necessary to instill normal saline solution into endotracheal/tracheal tube and infuse more parenteral fluids, as ordered
		  Auscultate lungs to ascertain bilateral expansion q2-4 hr; note decreased or absent sounds or presence of rales, rhonchi, or wheezing
		  Ensure proper positioning of endotracheal tube; monitor radiograph results for proper tube position
		  Monitor for bilateral, full expansion of lungs (by auscultation, observation, and chest radiograph)
		Provide for patency of ventilator tubings, i.e., H_2O accumulation, kinking, compression
		Monitor arterial blood gas levels q3-6 hr and prn until stable
		Increased peak inspiratory pressures (PIP) may reflect airway obstruction (e.g., secretions, mucus plugs) bronchospasm, pneumothorax, or other abnormalities that increase PIP
		Place airway or orotracheal tube if patient is biting or gumming on the tube; remind patient not to bite or gum on tube; reassure and sedate patient if necessary
		Monitor for bronchospasm: increased PIP, wheezing
		If bronchospasm occurs, hand ventilate, relax patient by reassuring and/or administering sedative; administer aminophylline, if needed, as ordered
		If bronchoscopy is necessary, assist with procedure

■ Excessive accumulation of secretions above endotracheal/tracheal cuff	■ Minimal secretion accumulation above endotracheal/tracheal cuff	■ Prevent by employing constant oral suction, using oral aspirator or intermittent oropharyngeal suctioning

POTENTIAL PROBLEMS	EXPECTED OUTCOMES	NURSING ACTIVITIES
	Absence of tracheal wall irritation	For secretions not aspirated by aforementioned methods, deflate endotracheal cuff q4-8 hr (more frequently if highpressure, hard cuffs are used); simultaneously administer vigorous manual ventilations with breathing bag, and suction oropharynx NOTE: This procedure may stimulate gag reflex in alert patients; in these patients, deflate cuff and as soon as secretions reach the trachea, suction them out
■ Accidental extubation	■ Intubation maintained	■ Reassure patient; sedate and/or restrain if necessary Position intubation tray and breathing bag nearby Keep spare tracheal tube of same size and type at bedside If extubation occurs, hand ventilate patient with mask, and call physician immediately
■ Infection related to Bypass of normal filtering system (the nose) Breach of aseptic technique for suctioning through tracheal tube Repeated, traumatic intrusive suctioning procedures	■ Infection free Afebrile	■ Prevention Employ sterile technique in suctioning Ensure that ventilator tubing is changed daily Ensure that tracheostomy tube is changed every week Change manual breathing bag at least every 3 days; keep inside plastic container Change position of patient q1-2 hr; administer chest physiotherapy when turning patient to mobilize secretions Frequent oral hygiene Monitor T, P, R, BP q2-4 hr; note elevated temperature, tachycardia or hypotension For change in secretions—color, amount, consistency, and odor Results of C and S tests of secretions every 3 days or whenever changes in color and consistency occur Notify physician of any abnormality If infection occurs Send specimen (e.g., blood, tracheal aspirate, urine) for C and S Administer fluid, antibiotic, and/or antipyretic as ordered Monitor for patient response to therapy
■ Tension pneumothorax	■ Absence or resolution of pneumothorax Full expansion of lungs	■ Prevention Avoid high volume or high pressure settings in high risk patients (COPD, emphysematous blebs) Monitor Arterial blood gas results For signs and symptoms of tension pneumothorax, including an acute increase in airway pressures, respiratory distress, unequal breath sounds, decreased or distant breath sounds, crepitant rales during inspiration and/or expiration, subcutaneous emphysema, unilateral chest expansion, tracheal deviation, decreased cardiac output and BP, tachycardia, increased CVP, and distended neck veins Chest radiograph results for pneumothorax Notify physician of any abnormality If tension pneumothorax occurs Disconnect patient from ventilator and hand ventilate with self-inflating bag Reassure and stay with patient Have someone else notify physician immediately; obtain chest tube and chest bottle/chamber setup Increase FIO_2 to 1.00 Ensure that chest radiograph is done to confirm diagnosis and after insertion of chest tube; note radiographic evidence of resolution Monitor arterial blood gas results q1-2 hr until stable

POTENTIAL PROBLEMS	EXPECTED OUTCOMES	NURSING ACTIVITIES

■ Fluid overload, weight gain from retention of inspired water vapor Pulmonary interstitial edema related to fluid overload	■ Optimal fluid balance Weight remains stable Absence of pulmonary interstitial edema; Pao_2 level within patient's normal limits	■ Prevent by
		  Administering fluids as ordered to keep fluid balance parameters within normal limits
		  Ensuring inspired air temperature controlled to 95° to 100° F
		Monitor
		  Daily weights for weight gain
		  Ankle edema
		  Intake and output q1-2 hr
		Monitor for pulmonary interstitial edema
		  Breath sounds for rales, wheezing
		  Signs/symptoms of hypoxia
		  Gradual increase in peak inspiratory pressure (observe system pressure gauge)
		  Gradual decrease in compliance or distensibility of lungs (estimated by dividing V_T by peak inspiratory pressure
		  Decrease in vital capacity
		  Chest radiograph for diffuse haziness
		Notify physician for any of these abnormalities
		Administer therapy as ordered, which may include
		  Diuretics, fluid restriction
		  CPAP or PEEP
		  Increased inspired O_2 concentrations
		  Rotating tourniquets for fulminating pulmonary edema

■ Atelectasis	■ Full lung expansion without atelectasis	■ Prevention
		  Ensure that sign mode is on 4 to 10/hour, if ordered
		  Administer vigorous chest physiotherapy q2-4 hr
		  Turn patient q1-2 hr
		Monitor
		  Arterial blood gas results q3-6 hr for any abnormality until stable
		  T, P, R, and BP q2-4 hr
		  For presence of any abnormal and/or adventitious breath sounds q2-3 hr
		  For diminished breath sounds over affected lung segment
		  For altered LOC
		If atelectasis occurs, notify physician and administer therapy, as ordered

■ O_2 toxicity related to high inspired O_2 concentrations	■ Absence and/or resolution of O_2 toxicity	■ Progressively decrease Fio_2 to below 0.5 within 24 to 48 hours of initiation of mechanical ventilation or institute other remedial measures (i.e., PEEP) to achieve adequate oxygenation, as ordered
		Keep Pao_2 level within patient's normal limits
		Monitor
		  Arterial blood gas results q2-3 hr for decreasing Pao_2 or same concentration until stable
		  Results of alveolar-arterial gradient determinations
		  For patient complaints of burning chest pain on inspiration; dry hacking cough; dyspnea
		  Actual inspired O_2 content
		  Gradual increase in PIP (observe system pressure gauge)
		  Gradual decrease in compliance or distensibility of lungs (estimated by dividing V_T by PIP)
		  Decrease in vital capacity
		  Characteristic chest radiograph changes
		  LOC
		Notify physician of any abnormality and institute therapy, as ordered

■ Hyperventilation (low $Paco_2$ levels)	■ Normal ventilatory rate with values for $Paco_2$ within patient's normal limits	■ Prevent by
		  Providing frequent reassurance and explanations
		  Administering medications for pain and/or sedation if needed, as ordered

POTENTIAL PROBLEMS	EXPECTED OUTCOMES	NURSING ACTIVITIES

		■ Monitor
		    Respiratory rate, quality for tachypnea, dyspnea
		    Arterial blood gas results q2-3 hr until stable
		  If hyperventilation occurs, notify physician; therapy is symptomatic
		    Administer sedation if needed, as ordered
		    Add dead space if patient is not breathing spontaneously
		    Decrease V_T and rate, if ordered
		    Administer medication to paralyze patient if needed, as ordered

■ Hypoventilation (high $Paco_2$ levels)	■ Ventilatory rate and $Paco_2$ levels within patient's normal limits
	  Full lung expansion by auscultation, observation, and chest radiograph
		■ Monitor
		    Respiratory rate q½-1 hr
		    Arterial blood gas results for hypercapnia
		    Breath sounds for decreased or absent sounds; presence of rales, rhonchi, or wheezes
		  If hypoventilation occurs, notify physician; therapy is symptomatic
		    Increase V_T and rate, as ordered
		    Augment chest physiotherapy, as needed

■ Transient hypotension related to
  Increased intrathoracic pressures associated with mechanical ventilation (and PEEP if used)
  Hypovolemia
	■ Hemodynamic stability
	  BP within patient's normal limits
		■ Prevention
		    Administer fluids, as ordered, to prevent hypovolemia
		  Monitor
		    BP for hypotension, CVP for elevation, and urine volume for oliguria q2 hr and prn
		    Arterial blood gas results for any abnormality q2-3 hr until stable
		  If transient hypotension occurs, notify physician
		    Administer fluids and/or inotropic agents, i.e., digoxin and/or dopamine as ordered; closely monitor patient's response; decrease PEEP, V_T or inspiratory flow rate, as ordered
		    Reassure patient

■ GI malfunction related to stress ulcers and bleeding; swallowed air with gastric distention; ileus	■ Absence of GI distress, malfunction	■ Prevent by administering antacid and/or milk as ordered, particularly to patients with NG tubes and those prone to increased anxiety
		  Encourage and support patient; sedate if needed, as ordered
		  Administer tube feeding, if ordered
		  Monitor for
		    Abdominal distention
		    Decreased Hgb and Hct daily
		    Positive Hematest results from NG aspirate and stool
		  If GI malfunction occurs, notify physician of any abnormality and administer therapy, as ordered

■ Hypoxia—inadequate oxygenation	■ Adequate oxygenation	■ Monitor
		    For signs and symptoms of hypoxia, including change in personality, decreased judgment, headache, restlessness, lack of concentration, paranoia, tachycardia, tachypnea, sudden increase in BP, cardiac arrhythmias, and cyanosis
		    For signs of respiratory distress
		    For adequate oxygenation; monitor Pao_2 levels
		    Arterial blood gas results 15 to 20 minutes after any change in ventilator settings; note concurrent signs of adequate oxygenation
		  If hypoxia occurs, notify physician and administer therapy, as ordered

■ Renal failure related to
  Decreased cardiac output associated with use of positive pressures
  Increased production of antidiuretic hormone
	■ Absence and/or resolution of renal failure	■ Ensure adequate hydration, as ordered
		  Monitor
		    Vital signs and temperature q2 hr
		    CVP, PAP q1-2 hr and prn; cardiac output measurements, if available
		    Urine output q1-2 hr; note oliguria
		    Daily weights for weight gain
		    Electrolyte levels q6-12 hr until stable
		  Notify physician of any abnormality
		  If renal failure occurs, administer therapy as ordered; see Standard 52, *Acute renal failure*

POTENTIAL PROBLEMS	EXPECTED OUTCOMES	NURSING ACTIVITIES

■ Pressure sores on side of mouth, nose, and tracheotomy site
Hyperplasia and inflammation, scarring and stenosis of trachea caused by trauma of endotracheal/ tracheal tube
	■ Minimal trauma caused by endotracheal/tracheal tube	■ Prevention
		    Change tape that secures tube daily and as necessary
		    Support tubing and maintain tracheal tube in proper alignment
		    Reposition endotracheal tube from side to side of mouth daily
		    Assist with change of tracheal tube every 7 days
		    Change tracheotomy dressings q2-4 hr and as necessary; clean skin around tube
		Monitor for presence of sores on mouth and around tracheotomy site
		If trauma occurs, reevaluate preventive measures employed and alter regimen if needed, as ordered
		Administer supportive care, as ordered

■ Tracheal esophageal fistula (TE fistula) and tracheal stenosis (ischemia, inflammation, and eventual narrowing of orifice) related to Use of high-pressure cuffs Inadequate cuff care Concurrent presence of NG tube, resulting in pressure on tracheoesophageal membrane from both sides	■ Adequate cuff care Absence of TE fistula and tracheal stenosis	■ Ensure use of low-pressure cuff on endotracheal/tracheal tube Inflate cuff to permit air leak around cuff during sigh inspirations Monitor cuff pressure q4-8 hr; cuff pressure should not exceed 30 mm Hg Maintain cuff pressure at less than 30 mm Hg, lower if possible, with minimal leak; remove NG tube as soon as feasible, as ordered Monitor contrast chest radiograph results for presence of TE fistula and tracheal stenosis Notify physician for presence of any of the aforementioned, and implement therapy as ordered

POSITIVE END-EXPIRATORY PRESSURE

Positive end-expiratory pressure (PEEP) therapy is designed as an adjunct to mechanical ventilation to maintain a prescribed amount of pressure in the patient-ventilator system at the end of each expiration. A special PEEP valve stops expiratory flow when alveolar pressure is still above atmospheric pressure. PEEP acts by reexpanding collapsed alveoli; thus recruiting additional pulmonary membranes for gas exchange. Pressure is maintained throughout the entire respiratory cycle at sufficiently high levels to prevent alveolar airway collapse, increasing both the surface area and exposure time for the diffusion of O_2.

Maintaining alveolar expansion helps to prevent shunting of blood through unventilated areas of the lungs, providing an optimal ventilation/perfusion ratio for gas exchange in an already compromised environment. Oxygenation is therefore enhanced. Improving the efficiency of oxygen diffusion provides adequate PaO_2 levels at safer concentrations of inspired oxygen (FIO_2), thereby reducing the toxic effects of inspired oxygen.

PEEP may be indicated for patients who are unable to maintain satisfactory arterial O_2 tensions (generally PaO_2 above 50 to 60 mm Hg) at reasonable levels of O_2 concentration (FIO_2 of less than 0.50 to 0.60) using conventional volume-limited mechanical ventilation.

Low levels of PEEP (3 to 5 cm H_2O) can be used prophylactically to promote alveolar patency in patients with borderline pulmonary status.

Some patients do not readily tolerate the positive pressures generated during PEEP therapy, and for this reason PEEP is generally contraindicated for patients with the following conditions:

1. COPD (bronchial asthma, bronchitis, emphysema)
2. Bullous lung disease
3. Low cardiac output states, hypotension
4. Tension pneumothorax

When low cardiac output states and hypotension are treated so that the BP and cardiac output are in the patient's normal range, PEEP therapy may be considered. Similarly, when a tension pneumothorax is resolved, cautious PEEP therapy may be considered.

PEEP levels are titrated to achieve adequate oxygenation while avoiding a diminution of venous return and subsequent decrease in cardiac output. PEEP is initiated at levels of 3 to 5 cm H_2O. The patient's arterial blood gas levels are checked, and if adequate PaO_2 levels are not achieved on a safe level of O_2 concentration (FIO_2 less than 0.50 to 0.60), the PEEP level is increased gradually in 2 to 3 cm H_2O increments until this goal is achieved. If a pulmonary artery catheter is in place, cardiac output measurements will also be performed at each level of PEEP to detect an untoward fall in cardiac output in response to augmented positive intrathoracic pressures. If cardiac output falls, the lungs receive less blood to be oxygenated. This can negate the improvement in oxygenation generated by PEEP therapy. As the physiological problems requiring PEEP therapy subside, the levels are *gradually* decreased in 2 to 3 cm H_2O increments. Arterial blood gas levels are again monitored after each change. The ventilator system pressure dial must be monitored at least hourly to determine the level of PEEP. If the pressure dial registers a PEEP level lower than that ordered, additional medication or alteration in the PEEP dial should be considered.

Weaning the patient from PEEP therapy is initiated when the PaO_2 is 60 mm Hg or more and the underlying pulmonary dysfunction is resolving. When high levels of PEEP and high levels of oxygen are being administered the FIO_2 should be reduced to a safe range first, usually 0.40 to 0.50. Then the PEEP level can be decreased gradually, 2 to 3 cm H_2O at a time, with careful assessment of PaO_2 with each decrement in PEEP. The process should be very gradual, permitting the patient's pulmonary pressures and gaseous exchange to equilibrate on the new level of FIO_2 or PEEP. A rapid reduction in PEEP levels is known to increase the amount of shunted, unoxygenated blood in the lungs.

PEEP therapy can produce some adverse effects related to the positive pressures generated. The elevated intrathoracic pressure reduces venous return to the heart, resulting in a lowered cardiac output. Patients who suffer from left ventricular dysfunction or who are hypovolemic are especially prone to this complication.

The higher intraalveolar pressure achieved in PEEP therapy promotes the formation of air leaks, permitting the escape of air into the pleural space, producing a tension pneumothorax; into the mediastinum, producing mediastinal emphysema; and into the subcutaneous tissue producing subcutaneous emphysema.

ASSESSMENT

1. History to include
   a. Presence of physiological problems commonly associated with respiratory compromise
      (1) Surgery
      (2) Heart failure
      (3) Shock
      (4) Sepsis
      (5) Pulmonary trauma
      (6) Acute pancreatitis
   b. Relative contraindications to PEEP therapy, for example
      (1) Chronic lung disease
      (2) Bullous lung disease
      (3) Hypotension
      (4) Pneumothorax
2. Respiratory function
   a. Respirations—rate, depth, quality
   b. Secretions—amount, color, consistency
   c. Breath sounds
   d. Signs of adequate oxygenation, particularly color
   e. Inspection of thorax for abnormalities
   f. Blood gas values
   g. Chest radiograph results
   h. Inflation pressures
   i. Lung compliance
   j. Alveolar-arterial oxygen gradient
3. Circulatory parameters
   a. BP, P
   b. CVP and PAP, if available
   c. Urine output
   d. Peripheral circulation
   e. Weight
4. Level of patient/family's anxiety regarding PEEP therapy and aspects of mechanical ventilation, including inability to talk

GOALS

1. Adequate oxygenation, with arterial oxygen levels within patient's normal limits
2. Delivery of prescribed levels of PEEP
3. Absence or resolution of potential complications associated with use of PEEP
4. Reduction in patient/family's anxiety with provision of information and encouragement

POTENTIAL PROBLEMS	EXPECTED OUTCOMES	NURSING ACTIVITIES
■ Patient/family's anxiety related to Hospitalization Disease process Intubation and consequent inability to talk Prolonged immobilization	■ Reduction in level of anxiety with provision of information, explanations, and encouragement	■ Ongoing assessment of level of anxiety Stay with patient or reassure patient that nurse will be close at hand Provide for alternate means of communication Explain disease process and need for intubation and use of PEEP Encourage patient/family's questions and communication of anxiety or fears related to inability to talk, course of therapy, etc. Encourage participation in care, as tolerated Perform treatments in unhurried manner, allowing rest periods between treatments Provide comfort measures
■ Inadequate oxygenation	■ Adequate oxygenation Pao_2 80 to 100 mm Hg Clear sensorium Good color Good peripheral circulation	■ Monitor Serial blood gas results for hypoxemia Color, sensorium, peripheral circulation for signs of hypoxia For signs and symptoms of hypoxia—restlessness, headache, change in personality, loss of judgment-making ability, lack of concentration, tachycardia, cardiac arrhythmias, tachypnea, and sudden elevation in BP; late signs include cyanosis, bradycardia, hypotension, and unconsciousness Select correct level of PEEP by Serial measurement of arterial O_2 levels (Pao_2) Volume of shunted blood in lungs (Qs/Qt) Capillary O_2 levels (Cao_2) Mixed venous blood O_2 levels Adequacy of cardiac output (by direct measurements and by BP, P, peripheral circulation, sensorium, urine output)
■ Inadequate oxygenation related to inadequate levels of PEEP	■ Adequate levels of PEEP	■ Monitor for Intact ventilatory-PEEP system; correct leaks if they occur Expiratory pressures on ventilator for maintenance of prescribed PEEP; adjust PEEP dial as needed Patient resistance to PEEP and patient anxiety; explain procedure and reassure patient, as needed Administer light sedation if necessary, as ordered

POTENTIAL PROBLEMS	EXPECTED OUTCOMES	NURSING ACTIVITIES
■ Inadequate oxygenation related to worsening pulmonary interstitial edema	■ Resolution of pulmonary interstitial edema FIO_2 progressively decreased to 0.4 PEEP no longer needed Extubation Clear chest radiograph *Secondary:* diminution of total body water	■ Monitor For maintenance of prescribed PEEP levels Daily weights for gain or loss For adventitious breath sounds Results of serial chest radiographs Arterial blood gas results for low PaO_2 levels Progression of inspiratory pressures (become higher as interstitial edema worsens) If problem occurs Provide for maintenance of prescribed PEEP levels; increase if needed, as ordered Administer diuretics as ordered to decrease total body H_2O
■ Patient incoordination with ventilator Positive pressure maintained throughout expiration is not natural, so patient may resist it (often called "bucking" ventilator) With higher levels of PEEP, pain is often felt in intercostal region; pain and fear cause sympathetic stimulation, which increases O_2 requirements in already hypoxic patient	■ Patient breathes in coordination with ventilator Patient is relaxed and calm	■ Prevent by Explaining procedure, what patient will experience Talking with and reassuring patient during PEEP therapy Sedating patient only if necessary, as ordered Changing sensitivity or flow rate on ventilator, if indicated Monitor For patient incoordination with ventilator system; patient breathing out of sequence with ventilator breaths For low and varying V_T (in absence of IMV system) Apparent patient resistance to ventilator breaths For factors contributing to patient restlessness, such as Hypoxia (monitor for signs and symptoms of; arterial blood gas results indicating hypoxemia) Acid-base imbalance (monitor serum electrolyte levels, arterial blood gas results for acidosis or alkalosis) Fears and anxieties (see Problem, Patient/family's anxiety) Pain Frustration because of inability to talk during intubation Notify physician of these abnormalities If patient incoordination with ventilator occurs Talk with patient; reassure and comfort him/her Reevaluate sensitivity settings and flow rates; make appropriate alterations Employ system for IMV to allow patient to breath spontaneously from reservoir of humidified, oxygenated air with addition of predetermined number of mandatory breaths per minute, if ordered Administer sedation if needed, as ordered
■ Decreased cardiac output with hypotension Hypotension may occur with initiation of or increase in level of PEEP; it reflects decreased venous return caused by additional positive intrathoracic pressure; sympathetic nervous system is stimulated, causing vasoconstriction and elevation of BP; if patient is hypovolemic, sympathetic stimulation may be insufficient to elevate BP to physiological range	■ Adequate cardiac output Hemodynamic stability Adequate venous return Adequate pulmonary blood flow Adequate blood flow to kidneys	■ Prevent by instituting PEEP in gradual increments Monitor for signs of reduced cardiac output (hypotension, tachycardia, elevated CVP, oliguria, signs of reduced peripheral circulation) when PEEP is initiated or when increments in PEEP levels are made Notify physician if any of aforementioned occur If decreased cardiac output with hypotension occurs Increase levels of PEEP in smaller increments and over longer intervals of time Administer fluid and/or cardiotonic/inotropic agent if ordered, and closely monitor patient's response

POTENTIAL PROBLEMS	EXPECTED OUTCOMES	NURSING ACTIVITIES
■ Hyperventilation, indicated by hypocapnia (low $Paco_2$); occurs as result of high inspired minute ventilation	■ Optimal $Paco_2$ and minute ventilation	■ Prevent by 　Explaining procedure to patient 　Calming and reassuring patient Monitor 　R q15-30 min for tachypnea 　Arterial blood gas levels for hypocapnia 　For patient resistance to ventilatory pressures being maintained If problem occurs 　Reassure and calm patient 　Administer light sedation if necessary 　Add ''dead space'' tubing to ventilatory system to elevate $Paco_2$ levels if necessary, as ordered
■ Atelectasis related to 　Immobility 　Primarily constant volume ventilation 　Secretions that tend to remain in periphery of lung because of high mean airway pressures	■ No atelectasis by auscultation or radiograph 　Full lung expansion as measured by pulmonary function tests	■ Prevent by administering vigorous pulmonary toilet, including 　Turn patient q1-2 hr 　Chest physiotherapy q2-4 hr Monitor 　R for tachypnea, dyspnea 　Breath sounds for localized decrease, dullness, and adventitious sounds 　Chest radiograph results for signs indicating atelectasis 　Arterial blood gas results for hypoxemia If atelectasis occurs 　Increase chest physiotherapy to affected areas 　Assist patient with coughing and deep breathing 　Administer humidified O_2 to liquefy secretions and to achieve adequate oxygenation
■ Pneumothorax related to high alveolar pressures When walls of alveoli cannot withstand positive pressure, perforation may occur; air leaks into pleural space causing pneumothorax, into mediastinum, and/or into subcutaneous spaces	■ Absence of pneumothorax 　Full lung expansion by auscultation, chest radiograph, and clinical examination	■ Prevent by 　Maintaining minimal PEEP levels necessary for adequate oxygenation 　Employing IMV system to reduce mean intrathoracic pressures, as ordered Monitor for signs and symptoms of pneumothorax 　Sudden sharp chest pain; pleuritic pain 　Anxiety, diaphoresis 　Dyspnea 　Asymmetrical chest movements 　Diminished or absent breath sounds on affected side 　Tachycardia with weak pulse 　Vertigo, pallor 　Cyanosis, hypotension 　Chest radiograph results indicating pneumothorax Notify physician if any of aforementioned occurs If pneumothorax occurs 　Monitor for resolution of small pneumothorax 　Assist with insertion of chest tube and monitor for air bubbling in drainage chamber/bottle as it is drawn from chest; monitor for resolution of pneumothorax by noting alleviation of respiratory distress and less asymmetrical chest movement on affected side; breath sounds become less resonant and distant, and chest radiograph shows resolution
■ Mediastinal emphysema	■ Absence of mediastinal emphysema or widened mediastinum on chest radiograph 　Full lung expansion by auscultation and chest radiograph	■ Monitor 　Chest radiograph results revealing widened mediastinum 　Breath sounds for decreased lung expansion 　For signs and symptoms of respiratory distress associated with decrease in lung volume 　For signs of reduced cardiac output and impaired venous return that may result from mediastinal emphysema Notify physician for any of these abnormalities

POTENTIAL PROBLEMS	EXPECTED OUTCOMES	NURSING ACTIVITIES
■ Subcutaneous emphysema	■ Absence of subcutaneous emphysema Full lung expansion by auscultation and chest radiograph	■ Monitor for air accumulation under skin, elevation of skin, "cracking" sound when skin is pressed Notify physician if any of aforementioned occur If subcutaneous emphysema occurs, air usually resorbs without treatment; if emphysema is marked, subcutaneous needles may be inserted to release some of air

CHEST PHYSIOTHERAPY

Chest physiotherapy is a coordinated series of actions consisting of manipulations designed to prevent and/or reduce respiratory complications. Chest physiotherapy also improves pulmonary function in patients with acute and chronic respiratory diseases.

This coordinated series of manipulative actions (percussion and vibration) instituted to each lung segment with the aid of gravity and coughing can mobilize secretions from a peripheral portion of the lungs into the large bronchi where they can be coughed out or removed by suctioning.

In *percussion*, cupped hands with fingers flexed and thumb against the index finger, lightly strike the chest wall in a rhythmical fashion, moving from the highest to the lowest point, with wrists alternately flexed and extended. A linen or towel is placed over the segment of the chest that is being percussed to prevent discomfort. The sudden compression of air between the hand and the chest wall during percussion produces an energy wave that is transmitted through the chest wall tissues to the lung tissue. This energy wave helps to dislodge adherent mucous plugs and moves them toward the main bronchus or trachea, where they can be easily coughed out or suctioned.

Vibration is accomplished by placing hands on the chest wall and producing a rapid vibratory motion in the arms while gently compressing the chest wall. This aids in mobilizing secretions to the main bronchus or trachea. It is performed on exhalation after a deep inhalation.

Coughing is a pulmonary defense mechanism that aids in effective mobilization of retained secretions. Cough is used after percussion and/or vibration. Instructions on effective coughing begin with proper breathing exercises followed by the mechanical components of coughing. The sequence starts with a deep breath, an inspiratory pause, and glottic closure. These actions result in increased intrathoracic pressure and expectoration of secretions when the glottis opens. Sterile suctioning is used if the patient is unable to cough.

Postural drainage is accomplished with the aid of gravity by different body positions to dislodge accumulations of mucus and other secretions from the lungs. Because of the variability and complexity of the tracheobronchial branching, practical postural drainage positions are best limited to areas of the lungs that commonly retain secretions. Precau-tions are to be considered when applying postural drainage to patients with recent myocardial infarction, postoperative neurosurgical patients, and in patients with known intracranial disease, recent spinal fusion, and/or skin graft. Techniques of postural drainage will depend on the physician's/therapist's clinical evaluation.

SEQUENCE OF THERAPY
For intubated patient

1. Auscultate to assess affected areas requiring therapy
2. Administer pain medication if needed, as ordered
3. Suction endotracheal tube and mouth
4. Position according to location of involved area and condition of patient
5. Percuss involved area for 2 minutes
6. Sigh patient two to three times
7. Vibrate on exhalation; do vibrations five times after each exhalation
8. Suction endotracheal tube
9. Auscultate lungs for evaluation of therapy

For nonintubated patient

1. Give instructions to patient on effective deep breathing and coughing exercises
2. Auscultate to assess affected areas requiring therapy
3. Administer pain medication if needed, as ordered
4. Position according to location of involved area and condition of patient
5. Percuss involved area for approximately 2 minutes
6. Instruct patient to inhale deeply, and as he/she exhales, vibrate the chest wall; do vibrations five times after each exhalation
7. Instruct patient to cough
8. If patient is unable to cough effectively, do nasotracheal suctioning
9. Auscultate lungs for evaluation of therapy

ASSESSMENT

1. Pulmonary status—quality of breath sounds, existence of full lung expansion, significance of abnormal breath sounds, and areas of pulmonary tree with abnormal or absent breath sounds

2. Presence of disease or conditions
    a. That indicate the need for chest physiotherapy, that is, COPD, pneumonia, acute atelectasis, lung abscess, bronchiectasis, cystic fibrosis, and ventilator care; postoperative patients and patients who have been on prolonged bed rest
    b. That necessitate caution in administering chest physiotherapy, that is, recent MI, increased tendency to bronchospasm, neurological conditions, spinal fusion, and/or a skin graft
    c. That contraindicate physiotherapy, that is, hypotension, unstable vital signs, dialysis, severe bleeding from esophageal varices, medical and surgical catastrophies
3. Results of lab and diagnostic tests, including
    a. Arterial blood gas levels
    b. Prothrombin time
    c. Chest radiograph
    d. ECG
4. Ability of patient to tolerate modified chest physiotherapy positions

GOALS

1. Optimal efficiency and distribution of ventilation/perfusion
2. Effective mobilization of secretions
3. Arterial blood gas and chest radiograph results within patient's normal limits
4. Hemodynamic stability; absence of arrhythmias
5. Infection free; absence of pneumonia

POTENTIAL PROBLEMS	EXPECTED OUTCOMES	NURSING ACTIVITIES
■ Anxiety related to limited understanding of therapy	■ Patient verbalizes understanding of therapy Patient's behavior indicates reduction in anxiety with provision of information, explanations, and encouragement	■ Ongoing assessment of level of anxiety and understanding Explain procedure and reassure patient Provide time for and encourage questions Administer pain medication 30 minutes before therapy if needed, as ordered Position for therapy, ensuring minimal discomfort If patient is unable to tolerate percussion, do vibration only

■ Retention of secretions	■ Effective mobilization of secretions
	Absence of atelectasis
		■ Auscultate affected areas
		Percuss affected area effectively
		    Maintain straight alignment of patient's body; support with pillows prn
		    Stand so that patient is facing you
		    Use muscle of shoulder and with cupped hands strike chest wall lightly in rhythmical fashion, flexing wrists
		    Minimize tension of muscles in forearms
		    Produce hollow sound without causing pain to patient
		Vibrate effectively
		    Place hand flat over segments that have just been percussed
		    Rhythmically tense and relax muscles of wrist and forearm (isometric movement) during exhalation
		    Instruct patient to take two to three deep breaths and cough; deliver sigh ventilation to intubated patients
		Instruct patient to cough out secretions; if patient is unable to do this, suction patient nasotracheally; suction intubated patients

■ Arrhythmias	■ Absence of arrhythmias Regular pulse rate	■ Avoid head-down position If ECG monitor is being used, increase audibility of QRS beeps and observe for arrhythmias Monitor BP and P intermittently during procedure until patient toleration is established If arterial line is in situ, set alarm limits closely and monitor BP during therapy Notify physician for significant incidence of arrhythmias Avoid percussion and emphasize vibration If problem occurs, see Standard 21, *Arrhythmias* Obtain ECG monitor if one is not already in use

PLEURAL COMPROMISE

Pleural compromise, as referred to in this standard, results when the negative pressure between the parietal and visceral pleurae is interrupted, and a foreign substance such as air or fluid enters the pleural space. This reduces or eliminates the adhesive quality of the membranes and results in a partial or total collapse of the lung and decreased oxygenation. Conditions whereby this may occur are spontaneous pneumothorax, open pneumothorax, tension pneumothorax, and hydrothorax (hemothorax, chylothorax, or pyothorax). The compromise may be slight enough to warrant simply observation or severe enough to warrant admission to an intensive care unit.

The pleural cavity, which is encased by the chest walls, the diaphragm, and the mediastinum, is lined by two smooth membranes, the parietal pleura and the visceral pleura. The parietal pleura lines the chest wall, and the visceral pleura covers the lungs. These two membranes are lubricated by approximately 2 ml of fluid that allows them to slide smoothly against each other during respiratory movement.

The term *pleural space* is a misnomer, because it infers the existence of a space between the visceral and parietal pleurae. Actually, these two membranes form an adhesive, suctionlike seal with one another, often likened to the effect of a suction cup against a smooth, moist surface. In fact, if space is formed between these two membranes, this will break the adhesive seal, and the normal functioning of the pleurae will be altered.

The adhesive quality of the visceral and parietal pleurae facilitates the synchronized movement of the lungs and chest with respiration. The lungs themselves are composed of a recoiling, sponge like tissue that is elastic because of a protein in the alveolar walls called *elastin*. If not for the seal of the pleural membranes, the lungs would naturally coil toward the bronchial tree.

The suction seal created by the two opposing pleural membranes maintains varying degrees of negative pressure during the normal respiratory cycle. The only times the intrapleural pressure becomes positive is on forced expiration or with severe lung disease or pleural compromise.

On the other hand, the inner alveolar pressures do vary during the normal respiratory cycle. On inspiration, the expansion of the chest walls causes a negative or subatmospheric pressure within the lungs, potentiating the inhalation of air. On expiration, the contraction of the chest walls causes a positive or greater-than-atmospheric pressure within the lungs, forcing the exhalation of air.

Any pleural compromise can alter normal respiratory functioning and oxygenation. Types of pleural compromise differ according to the foreign substance that enters the pleural space and its path of entry, risk of recurrence, severity, and/or potential for compromising lung and cardiac function.

Spontaneous pneumothorax. Spontaneous pneumothorax is the most common form of pleural compromise. A spontaneous pneumothorax occurs when air enters the pleural space and collapses a portion of the affected lung. The air originates from a ruptured alveolus or bulla, most commonly located at the apex of the lung. In the absence of premorbid disease, a spontaneous pneumothorax can occur in previously healthy persons of any age but is more commonly seen in adolescents during a growth spurt. The specific cause or explanation for this is still unknown.

Certain disease processes increase a person's risk of spontaneous pneumothorax because of their deleterious effects on lung tissue. These include tuberculosis; carcinoma; lung tumors, especially lymphomas; COPD; sarcoidosis; and Marfan's syndrome. Another more recent observation is the occurrence of spontaneous right-sided pneumothorax in women, usually in their 40s, during menses. This is thought to be related to catamenial pelvic endometriosis. These patients usually require medications to suppress menses or to reduce certain antigen releases from their endocrine system in addition to the more routine treatments for spontaneous pneumothorax.

There is increasing documentation of familial incidence of spontaneous pneumothorax. This occurrence has been associated with a specific HLA antigen identified in the blood.

Open pneumothorax. Also known as a "sucking wound," an open pneumothorax is usually the result of blunt trauma that penetrates the chest wall. Because the negative pressure between the pleural membranes has been broken, air will move in and out of the chest wound with every respiratory effort. This abnormal entry and exit of air into and from the pleural space results in a pendulum motion of the aorta and mediastinum. Depending on the volume of air movement in the pleural space, disruption of venous flow back to the heart can occur and subsequently decrease cardiac output.

Tension pneumothorax. A tension pneumothorax can be caused by air and/or fluid accumulation in the pleural space via an open or closed chest wound. The open chest wound was described previously. A closed chest wound is one in which the chest wall has been penetrated without leaving an open wound. When a tension pneumothorax occurs, the chest wall acts as a ball and valve, allowing air and/or fluid to continually enter the pleural space without a means for exit. Therefore the foreign substance is trapped, and a progressive process to compromise the affected lung is instituted. This characteristic of continual entrance without a mode for escape differentiates a tension pneumothorax from an open pneumothorax.

As less space is available for lung expansion and the intrapleural space becomes progressively atmospheric as opposed to subatmospheric, effective gaseous exchange is reduced. The lack of negative pressure on one side of the chest results in a mediastinal shift to the unaffected side. This shift can compress the aorta, decreasing cardiac output, and/or compress the contralateral lung. A tension pneumothorax is potentially the most dangerous type of pleural compromise because of the continuing nature of the process, and its dual effect on oxygenation and circulation.

Hemothorax. A hemothorax occurs when blood enters the pleural space. The source of the blood is usually damaged intercostal arteries, internal mammary arteries, or major hilar vessels. This damage is most commonly the result of penetrating chest wounds, chest or abdominal trauma in which the diaphragm has been lacerated, or cardiovascular surgery.

By definition, a minimal hemothorax occurs when the pleural space contains up to 350 ml of blood, a moderate hemothorax occurs when the pleural space contains 350 to 1500 ml of blood, and a massive hemothorax occurs when the pleural space contains more than 1500 ml of blood. In the presence of a massive hemothorax, the patient may be in hypovolemic shock as well as respiratory distress.

Normally, blood does not clot in the pleural space because of enzymatic action and the motion of the two membranes. However, if a hemothorax is not discovered early and evacuated, a small percentage of them will consolidate into a clot. If hemothorax is not treated after 3 to 4 weeks, infection and/or the formation of fibrous tissue may occur and require surgical intervention to restore normal lung function. The identification of a hemothorax through physical assessment is outlined in Table 9-1. Usually, more than 300 ml of blood must occupy the pleural space for a hemothorax to be diagnosed by a chest radiograph.

Chylothorax. Chyle is a milky lymphatic fluid produced in the intestines that contains digestive enzymes. It normally drains into the thoracic ducts via the left subclavian vein. Injury to this area may precipitate a chylothorax, one of the more unusual forms of pleural compromise. Most commonly, chylothorax occurs as a consequence of thoracic surgery, trauma, tuberculosis, or lymphatic tumors. Clinically, a chylothorax may not be evident for 2 to 10 days after the insult, because the chyle can accumulate in the mediastinum before entering the pleural space. IV medium chain triglycerides are usually administered to halt the formation of chyle in the lymphatic system and thereby prevent its entrance into the pleural cavity until the damaged area can heal. Medical intervention and chest tube evacuation are the preferred treatments; however, surgical evacuation may be necessary.

Pyothorax. Pyothorax occurs when pus forms in the pleural space. Pus accumulation can be associated with complications of thoracic surgery, blunt open chest trauma, or invasive lung disease. Antibiotics are a standard form of therapy. The other therapeutic measures used are more invasive and can further aggravate a preexisting infection, i.e., chest tube insertion and/or surgical evacuation. As with chylothorax, infection and recurrence are major complications.

■ ■ ■

Many procedures performed for the critically ill patient may cause a pleural compromise. Awareness of this allows the nurse to assess the patient more carefully and to take prophylactic precautions if necessary. Procedures that can cause pleural compromise include the insertion of central venous catheters or any invasive lines using neck veins, which can produce pleural compromise by accidently nicking the pleurae; the insertion of NG tubes; and maneuvers with pulmonary artery catheters.

It is not an unusual practice to ice an NG tube before inserting it. The rationale is to stiffen the tube to facilitate its passage. This can result in pleural perforation if the tube is accidentally passed into the lung, creating a pneumothorax. If a malpositioned NG tube is not identified and fluid is subsequently administered, a hydrothorax can follow.

A pulmonary artery catheter may produce a pneumothorax on insertion or if it is inadvertently wedged for any prolonged period. If the catheter is wedged in a weakened pulmonary artery of a patient with COPD, a hemothorax or pneumothorax may result. For specific information on wedging, see Standard 25, *Hemodynamic monitoring*.

Generally, the therapeutic goals for the patient with pleural compromise are related to identifying the cause, preventing occurrence when possible, treating the situation quickly to prevent further complications, and promoting

TABLE 9-1. Findings in pleural compromise

	INSPECTION	PALPATION	PERCUSSION	AUSCULTATION
PNEUMOTHORAX	May have paradoxical motion with respirations or splinting caused by pain	May have mediastinal and/or subcutaneous emphysema depending on cause	Hyperresonant	Decreased or absent breath sounds over affected area May have referred breath sounds
TENSION PNEUMOTHORAX	May have paradoxical chest motion because of mediastinal shift May exhibit splinting caused by pain	Mediastinal and or tracheal shift to unaffected side May have mediastinal and/or subcutaneous emphysema depending on cause	Hyperresonant	Decreased or absent breath sounds over entire area affected including contralateral lung May have referred breath sounds
HYDROTHORAX	Unremarkable	Unremarkable	Dull	May have decreased or absent breath sounds May have tubular breath sounds especially over consolidated areas, with "A" to "E" changes
OPEN PNEUMOTHORAX	Cover open wound to prevent more air from entering the pleural space Clean and redress when possible	Mediastinal and tracheal shift to unaffected side Mediastinal and/or subcutaneous empysema	Sucking sound	Turbulent breath sounds caused by air entering and leaving wound

patient comfort through adequate oxygenation and circulation. Interestingly, there are no clinical data suggesting that the size of the pleural compromise is in direct proportion to the presenting symptoms.

Overall, the most common treatment for any pleural compromise is the insertion of a chest tube. There are different types of pleural drainage systems that affect the patient's tolerance and nursing care. For more information on chest tubes, patient care, and management, see Standard 10, *Chest tubes*. However, several therapeutic options do exist.

A small pneumothorax, less than 20% of the affected lung, may resolve itself without treatment. In healthy, stable patients, such as an adolescent with a spontaneous pneumothorax, a simple needle aspiration via the second intercostal space can be performed in the office or ambulatory unit. This would be followed up by a chest radiograph to assess resolution.

Another alternative to hospitalization is the insertion of a one-way flutter valve, such as the McSwain dart. However, this treatment is not yet universally accepted. The dart is a polyethylene catheter with a one-way flutter valve that is attached to a four-winged flange. The flange is used to stabilize the catheter against the chest wall. The one-way flutter valve allows air to escape from the pleural space while sealing itself to prevent air from reentering the space. With proper patient education, the patient can go home with the dart in place over a period of days and be followed up in the office with chest radiographs.

Recurrent pleural compromise may require more than just acute intervention. As with most recurrent injuries, the patient with recurrent pleural compromise is more prone to develop scar tissue and adhesions in the pleural cavity, which can cause permanent damage. When this is the case, the previously mentioned treatments usually fail and further intervention is necessary. One such intervention is a pleurodesis. This is accomplished by using a sclerosing chemical over the pleural membranes to promote the uniform formation of fibrotic adhesions between them. Although many agents have been used, including silver nitrate, talc, kaolin, and olive oil, tetracycline is the most commonly used. Tetracycline causes a uniform inflammation of the pleural membranes, mimicking their natural adhesive quality. This procedure may be performed in the operating room via a thoracotomy by rubbing the pleural membranes with the sclerosing chemical, or the chemical agent may be simply injected into a pleural chest tube. This necessitates frequent changing of the patient's position to ensure that the solution gravitates to all parts of the pleural membranes. After either method, the patient will experience discomfort and will need encouragement to deep breathe and cough to prevent atelectasis.

ASSESSMENT

1. Medical and surgical history with particular attention to the presence of
   a. Catamenial pelvic endometriosis
   b. Thoracic trauma secondary to accident or surgery
   c. Underlying lung disease, such as tuberculosis, cancer, or lymphoma
   d. Other debilitating diseases, such as sarcoidosis or Marfan's syndrome
2. Presence of potential precipitating factors
   a. Adolescent growth spurt
   b. Central venous catheters or other invasive lines inserted in neck veins
   c. NG tube
   d. Pulmonary artery catheter, particularly if patient has a history of COPD
   e. Use of PEEP
3. Clinical signs and symptoms reflecting respiratory and hemodynamic status
   a. Respiratory rate
   b. Color
   c. Use of accessory muscles to breathe
   d. Dyspnea or air hunger
   e. Mental status
   f. BP
   g. P and heart rhythm
   h. Filling pressures if pressure monitoring is available
   i. Cardiac output and index, if it can be calculated
   j. General signs of decreased cardiac output, such as decreased urinary output and peripheral edema
4. Chest physical assessment; see Table 9-1
   a. Inspection
   b. Palpation
   c. Percussion
   d. Auscultation
5. Results of lab tests if indicated
   a. Arterial blood gas levels
   b. CBC
   c. Chest radiograph
   d. Cultures
6. Monitor ECG for
   a. Changes related to decreased cardiac output causing ischemia
   b. Changes related to tension pneumothorax
      (1) Rightward shift in QRS in V leads
      (2) Low-voltage QRS in V leads
      (3) Inverted T waves in V leads
      (4) Transient S-T elevations
7. Presence of other medical or surgical problems that may be secondary to or exacerbated by the pleural compromise, such as shock, pulmonary edema, or CHF
8. Presence of pain related to pleural compromise
9. Signs and symptoms of infection
   a. Elevated temperature
   b. Elevated white blood cell (WBC) count
10. Patient/family's level of anxiety
11. Patient's perception of and reaction to diagnosis and or required therapy

GOALS

1. Reduction in anxiety of patient/family in response to comfort measures, information, and explanations
2. Reduction in pain
3. Optimal respiratory function
   a. Arterial blood gas levels within premorbid baseline
   b. Full lung reexpansion by chest radiograph and assessment
   c. Afebrile without atelectasis or pneumonia
   d. Respiratory rate and quality within normal limits with absence of splinting because of pain
4. Free of infection
   a. Afebrile
   b. CBC within normal limits
   c. Absence of atelectasis or pneumonia
   d. Absence of inflamed areas around wounds or chest tubes
5. Optimal cardiac function reflected by hemodynamic stability
   a. Absence of hemorrhage
   b. Postmorbid filling pressures at patient's normal baseline
   c. Cardiac output at patient's normal baseline
   d. Absence of signs of hypovolemia and shock
6. Patient/family demonstrates understanding of pleural compromise by their reduction in anxiety and asking of pertinent questions about therapeutic treatments and outcomes
7. Before discharge patient/family is able to
   a. Describe important signs and symptoms of recurrent pleural compromise
   b. Describe factors that make patient more prone to recurrent pleural compromise
   c. Verbalize an understanding of the importance of any follow-up care necessary and when and where to obtain it

POTENTIAL PROBLEMS	EXPECTED OUTCOMES	NURSING ACTIVITIES

■ Anxiety related to
  Dyspnea
  Pain
  Insufficient knowledge
    base
  Sense of vulnerability if
    pleural compromise is
    result of trauma
	■ Patient verbalizes and
	  demonstrates reduction
	  in anxiety with provi-
	  sion of information, ex-
	  planation, and encour-
	  agement
	  Patient/family better able
	  to cooperate and retain
	  information because of
	  reduction of stress
	  Patient verbalizes decrease
	  in dyspnea and pain
		■ Promote patient comfort to reduce restlessness and pain
		  Anticipate patient needs if activity is restricted, i.e., have patient's
		    items within reach
		  Assess level of understanding regarding disease process, therapy em-
		    ployed, and diagnostic procedures planned
		  Provide information regarding disease process and therapeutic inter-
		    ventions
		  Provide support and reassurance
		  Encourage questions and verbalization of fears by patient/family
		  Use appropriate resource people if necessary—more commonly need-
		    ed if result of trauma or insult

■ Pain related to
  Respiratory distress
  Collapsed lung
  Therapeutic interven-
    tions
  Chest tube
  Needle aspiration
  McSwain dart
  Pleurodesis
	■ Patient verbalizes comfort	■ Optimize respiratory effort by placing patient in position of comfort,
		  usually semi-fowler's position
		  Provide pillow support for coughing and deep breathing exercises
		  Prevent stress at chest tube insertion site, especially while moving
		    or turning patient
		  Anticipate need for pain medication and medicate prophylactically
		    if appropriate
		  Assess for presence of pain
		  Administer O_2 therapy as ordered
		  Assess origin of pain to rule out concomitant disease processes, e.g.,
		    pulmonary embolus
		  Alleviate pain and discomfort with analgesics as ordered
		  Avoid if at all possible use of narcotics that may suppress respiratory
		    effort

■ Inadequate oxygenation re-
  lated to
  Collapsed lung
  Compression of contra-
    lateral lung
  Splinting of respirations
    because of discomfort
	■ Adequate oxygenation with
	  PaO_2 back to patient's
	  premorbid baseline
	  Acid-base balance with
	  normal limits
	  Absence of confusion
	  Patient verbalizes comfort
		■ Promote optimal positioning that will minimize patient's respiratory
		  effort
		  Promote optimal respiratory toilet by encouraging turning, deep
		    breathing, and coughing
		  Administer pain medication if needed, as ordered, to avoid patient
		    splinting, which reduces respiratory excursion
		  Assess for adequate oxygenation (see Table 9-1)
		    Physical examination
		    Sensorium
		    Color
		    Signs of inadequate tissue perfusion
		    Arterial blood gas levels
		  Administer O_2 therapy as ordered
		  Administer specific respiratory therapies as ordered, i.e., IPPB, PEEP
		  Prepare patient for and assist physician with ordered therapeutic in-
		    terventions
		    Chest tubes
		    Needle aspiration
		    McSwain dart
		    Pleurodesis
		  If patient has open chest wound, prevent further compromise by
		    covering wound to prevent more air from entering pleural space
		  If patient has or develops tension pneumothorax, prepare for *imme-*
		    diate therapeutic intervention with needle aspiration or chest tube
		    insertion

■ Hemodynamic instability
  related to
  Decreased venous return
    and reduced cardiac
    output
  Hypovolemia secondary
    to hemorrhage
	■ Hemodynamic stability
	  Absence of mediastinal
	  shift, evidenced by nor-
	  mal ECG and chest ra-
	  diograph
	  Absence of complications
	  of hemodynamic insta-
	  bility
		■ Preserve cardiac output by restricting activity if necessary
		  Monitor indices reflecting changes in cardiac status
		    Mental status
		    BP
		    Presence and/or quality of pulses
		    Respiratory rate
		    Arterial blood gas levels

POTENTIAL PROBLEMS	EXPECTED OUTCOMES	NURSING ACTIVITIES

Increased intrathoracic pressure secondary to mediastinal shift
Arrythmias secondary to hypoxia
Acid-base imbalance
		Color
		Intake and output
		Presence of peripheral edema
		Presence of hypothermia
		Trend filling pressures, including PAS, PAD, PCWP, and CVP; cardiac output; and cardiac indices if invasive monitoring lines are in place; be cautious of pressure interpretations in presence of mediastinal shifts, whereby lines themselves may be compressed, resulting in false elevations
		Monitor ECG for
		    Arrythmias secondary to hypoxia or ischemia and changes associated with a tension pneumothorax
		    S-T segment changes related to ischemia
		    Rightward shift of QRS on frontal plane
		    Decreased R wave over precordium
		    Inverted T waves in V leads related to tension pneumothorax
		Place patient in supine position to optimize blood flow during hypovolemia
		Administer volume expanders as ordered for hypovolemia
		Administer vasopressor drugs as ordered
		Administer medications as ordered for arrhythmias
		Administer O_2 therapy as ordered
		Prepare patient for and assist physician with insertion of chest tubes if indicated

■ Mediastinal emphysema	■ Absence of mediastinal emphysema or widening mediastinum on chest radiograph Full lung expansion by auscultation and chest radiograph	■ Review results of chest radiograph for presence of mediastinal emphysema or widening mediastinal border Assess for decreased breath sounds secondary to decreases in lung volumes Assess for signs and symptoms of respiratory distress associated with decrease in lung volume Assess for signs of decreased cardiac output secondary to decreased venous return resulting from compression created by mediastinal emphysema Notify physician of any of these abnormalities Prepare patient for insertion of chest tube, if necessary
■ Subcutaneous emphysema	■ Absence of subcutaneous emphysema Full lung expansion by auscultation and chest radiograph	■ Monitor for accumulation of air under skin and "crackling" sound when skin is pressed down; often found around neck Assess quantity and effect of subcutaneous emphysema; it usually causes little discomfort or compromise and should be observed for progression; usually reabsorbs without treatment Notify physician of any abnormalities Assess patient's level of anxiety about presence of subcutaneous emphysema and reassure appropriately, informing patient about normal course for this condition Prepare for chest tube insertion if indicated
■ Infection related to Traumatic wound Surgical incision Insertion of chest tube Pneumonia	■ Infection free	■ Promote good respiratory toilet to prevent atelectasis and pneumonia, including coughing, deep breathing, and suctioning Change dressings as indicated, maintaining aseptic technique Evaluate length of time any invasive line remains in patient Follow recommendations for line and equipment care identified in Standard 61, *Infection control in the critical care unit* Assess invasive line sites for redness, swelling, or drainage Assess for elevations in temperature and notify physician when appropriate Assess for signs of sepsis, including changes in vital signs, fever, chills, diaphoresis, altered LOC; notify physician if present Assess for signs of localized wound infection, including inflammation, swelling, redness, and tenderness or drainage and report to physician if present

POTENTIAL PROBLEMS	EXPECTED OUTCOMES	NURSING ACTIVITIES
		Assess for signs of pulmonary infection, including color of sputum, atelectasis, and fever, and report to physician if present Review results of lab data for elevations in WBC count Review results of cultures that have been done. Assist in good positioning for posteroanterior (PA) and lateral chest radiograph to promote early detection of lung consolidation Administer antibiotics as ordered *See* STANDARD 61 *Infection control in the critical care unit*
■ Insufficient knowledge to comply with discharge regimen	■ Patient/family will demonstrate sufficient understanding of disease process, identify potential risk factors if appropriate, and identify early presenting symptoms of pleural compromise Before discharge, patient/family Verbalizes understanding for patient's specific type of pleural compromise, risk factors, and presenting symptoms Describes medications and understands correct dosage, side effects, and complications Accurately describes activity limitation if appropriate and plans for incorporating into life-style	■ Assess patient/family's understanding of pleural compromise, follow-up care, and discharge regimen Instruct patient/family in Applicable risk factors that predispose patient to pleural compromise—COPD, lymphomas, collagen diseases, Marfan's syndrome, tuberculosis, pelvic endometriosis, adolescent growth spurt Specific therapeutic measures, such as medications Name of drug and purpose Dosage and side effects Potential complications Therapeutic interventions when necessary, such as McSwain dart, thoracentesis, pleurodesis, chest tubes Provide patient/family opportunity to ask questions and express concerns Assess patient/family's potential compliance with discharge regimen Discuss plan for follow-up visits with patient/family, including where and when to go and who to see Provide opportunity for and encourage patient/family's questions and verbalizations of anxiety regarding discharge regimen

CHEST TUBES

Chest tube placement involves the insertion of one or more tubes through the chest wall into the intrapleural space. Pleural chest tubes serve to evacuate air and/or fluid from the pleural space while also preventing their return. Chest tube insertion may be indicated for patients with pneumothorax, hemothorax, hemopneumothorax, chylothorax, pyothorax, or pleural effusion. A chest tube inserted for the removal of air will usually be inserted in the upper aspect of the anterior chest wall, because air tends to rise to the top of the pleural space. A chest tube inserted for the removal of fluid will usually be inserted in the middle to lower aspect of the lateral chest wall, because fluid tends to settle at the base of the lung. Chest tubes are often placed in both locations to remove both fluid and air.

A chest tube may also be placed within the thoracic cavity to serve as a drain, as with the mediastinal chest tubes that are commonly inserted following open heart surgery. They are usually placed outside of the pleural space and therefore are not prone to air leaks or the effects of intrapleural pressures.

The pressure between the visceral and parietal pleurae must remain below atmospheric pressure for the lungs to expand and function effectively. When this negative pressure is interrupted by trauma, surgery, or some other pathologic condition that causes a rupture in the surface of a lung, chest tube insertion serves both to prevent a tension pneumothorax and to permit the affected lung to reexpand. (See Standard 9, *Pleural compromise*.)

Air and small amounts of fluid are evacuated from the intrapleural space during exhalation, which exerts a slightly more positive pressure. To prevent the reentry of air or fluid, an underwater seal is used. The water seal functions as a barrier between the atmospheric pressure and the negative pressure within the pleural space. As air and fluid are evacuated from the intrapleural space, the pleurae are brought back into proximity with each other. The pressure in the pleural space once again becomes negative throughout the respiratory cycle.

Chest tube evacuation depends on two essential forces for proper functioning. The presence of a positive expiratory pressure helps to evacuate air and a minimal amount of fluid. The force of gravity serves to evacuate fluid and a minimal amount of air. The use of suction is an option commonly used to enhance the evacuation of both air and fluid with equal effectiveness.

The increased positive expiratory pressure created by a pleural compromise is responsible for the evacuation of air. This positive pressure will continue to expel air through the chest tube until there is no longer a significant amount of air in the intrapleural space, and the expiratory pressure returns to the normal negative pressure.

Prepare to assist the physician with the insertion of the chest tube by collecting the needed supplies. Obtain a chest tube tray and find out which type of drainage unit the physician prefers. Prepare the water seal by adding sterile water or saline solution to the water seal chamber.

Prepare the patient by explaining the procedure and its purpose. Provide the patient with as much information as needed in terms that are easily understood.

There are four drainage systems available: one-, two-, and three-bottle systems or a disposable system such as a Pleur-Evac.

The one-bottle system is the simplest and is commonly used in emergencies. In this system, the drainage goes directly into the bottle, which serves as both collection chamber and water seal. It is not recommended for the evacuation of fluid, because the drainage will raise the level of the water seal liquid, creating a resistance to drainage.

The two-bottle system provides an extra bottle for the connection of suction, which facilitates the drainage of fluid as well as air. This system also requires careful monitoring of the fluid level in the water seal/collection chamber bottle, because high levels can create resistance to drainage.

The three-bottle system provides separate bottles for collection of drainage, a water seal, and suction. Air from the pleural space passes through the collection and water seal bottles and is suctioned out. The fluid drainage remains in the collection bottle and therefore does not interfere with the water seal level.

The disposable drainage systems contain all three chambers in one unit and function the same as the three-bottle unit. They are clean and efficient and eliminate the danger of broken bottles.

Although the insertion of chest tubes has a therapeutic

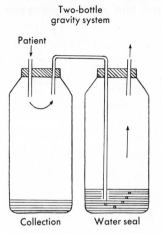

Two-bottle
gravity system

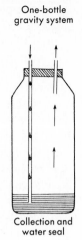

One-bottle
gravity system

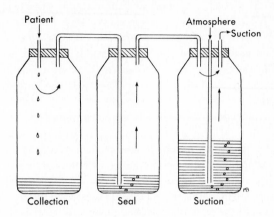

Three-bottle suction system

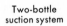

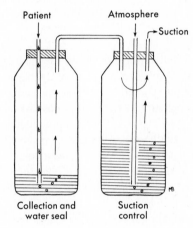

Two-bottle
suction system

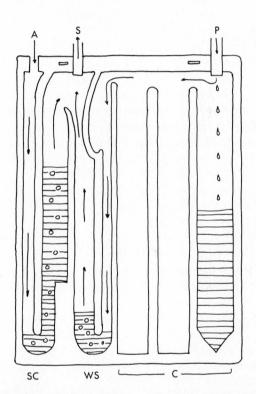

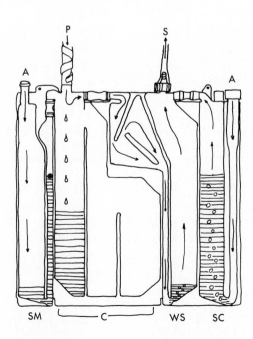

A, atmosphere. *S,* suction. *P,* patient. *SC,* suction control chamber. *C,* collection chamber. *SM,* safety seal and manometer. *WS,* water seal chamber.

purpose, there are potential complications. A new opening into the chest wall is created, and this puts the patient at risk for recurrent entry of atmospheric pressure. The integrity of the system must be monitored closely. The amount of suction used must be carefully controlled, because excessive amounts may cause the pleurae to erode and hemorrhage, while too little suction will not help the lung to reexpand.

The management of chest tubes is determined by the clinical course of the patient's condition. If the response to chest tube insertion is favorable, that is, there is a decrease in air and/or fluid accumulation along with the absence of respiratory difficulty or further air leaks, management is focused on maintaining the system. This is done by close assessment of the patient's condition along with prophylactic care to ensure the proper functioning of the equipment and to avoid the potential complications of chest tubes.

ASSESSMENT

1. History to include
   a. Presence of underlying pulmonary disease
   b. Exposure to respiratory irritants such as smoking
   c. Symptoms, onset, and duration of present illness
2. Patient's respiratory status
   a. Respiratory rate and rhythm
   b. Adequacy of oxygenation, particularly capillary refill and color of nail beds and lips
   c. Presence and quality of breath sounds
3. Patient's hemodynamic status
   a. Heart rate and rhythm
   b. BP
   c. Temperature and skin turgor
4. Type of drainage from chest tube
   a. Quantity—large, moderate, scant, or no drainage present
   b. Color—bright blood, dark blood, serosanguineous, or serous
   c. Characteristics—thin, bubbling, or clotted
5. Lab test results
   a. CBC with particular attention to Hgb for oxygen-carrying capability and WBC count for indication of an infectious state
   b. Arterial blood gas determinations
   c. Chest radiograph results for chest tube placement and degree of lung involvement
6. Chest tube insertion site for presence of an air leak, drainage, or crepitus
7. Functioning of chest tube and equipment
   a. Connections intact and absence of dependent loop
   b. Water seal bubbling sporadically
   c. Fluctuations in water seal chamber for indications of pressure changes in the pleural space and the patient's respiratory effort
8. Patient's reaction to procedure and adjustment to the environment
9. Patient/family's level of anxiety
10. Patient's threshold and response to pain

GOALS

1. Optimal respiratory function and adequate pulmonary ventilation
2. Hemodynamic stability
3. Optimal functioning of the chest tube evacuation system
   a. Respiratory status will reflect an immediate improvement with chest tube insertion
   b. Chest tube drainage will decrease to cessation
4. Absence of infection
5. Absence of atelectasis and signs or symptoms of pneumonia
6. Patient verbalizes needs
7. Reduction in patient/family's anxiety with the provision of explanations and positive reinforcement
8. Absence of pain

POTENTIAL PROBLEMS	EXPECTED OUTCOMES	NURSING ACTIVITIES
■ Patient anxiety related to Critical care environment Multiple procedures necessary for admission, workup, and treatment of patient's compromised pulmonary status Patient's past experiences with illness and hospitalizations	■ Patient is able to communicate needs and fears Patient understands and complies with procedures Patient communicates noticeable improvement in ability to breathe and thus is optimistic regarding outcome	■ Orient patient to unit environment and explain routines Explain purpose of procedures and equipment being used Reassure patient that someone is always nearby and that he/she is being observed very closely Develop care plan that is individualized to patient's needs, past experiences, and fears Assess continuously verbal and nonverbal clues of anxiety If problem occurs Stay with patient Encourage patient to verbalize concerns Ascertain by thorough assessment that anxiety is not related to hypoxia Encourage support from family members or significant others Document and report patient's level of anxiety Administer sedation ordered by physician if indicated

POTENTIAL PROBLEMS	EXPECTED OUTCOMES	NURSING ACTIVITIES
■ Family's anxiety related to Admission to critical care unit Patient's condition	■ Family feels comfortable in expressing needs and verbalizing concerns as they become evident	■ Assess level of anxiety Identify resource person to family Orient family to critical care unit, including Phone number Visiting hours Waiting area Physician's office number Encourage questions from family as they arise Supply adequate and honest answers to questions Encourage sense of hope as patient's condition improves Offer support and willingness to listen, which become even more important if patient's condition fails to improve Develop patient's care plan to include family needs
■ Acute respiratory distress	■ Patient's respirations will be easy and nonlabored Arterial blood gas levels will be adequate	■ Check chest tube functioning frequently Assess patient for presence and character of breath sounds q2 hr during acute phase of illness Obtain arterial blood gas levels as ordered Review chest radiograph for any significant changes Observe quantity, color, and characteristics of chest tube drainage as clinical status indicates Quantity may vary considerably according to clinical indication for chest tube insertion; for example, average drainage For pleural tube for pneumothorax is as little as 10 to 20 ml/hr of serosanguineous to serous fluid For pleural tube for hemopneumothorax is 50 to 100 ml/hr of bloody to serosanguineous fluid For mediastinal chest tube is 50 to 200 ml/hr of bloody to serosanguineous fluid Monitor patient's vital signs, respiratory effort, and level of anxiety Stay with and reassure patient; encourage slow deep breaths Medicate for pain if needed and as ordered Check chest tube and extension tubing for disconnection or kinking and correct as indicated Ascertain that drainage unit is below patient's chest Auscultate breath sounds for presence, quality, and any adventitious sounds Notify physician if unable to find and/or resolve cause of patient's respiratory distress
■ Atelectasis related to immobilization and splinting	■ Absence of atelectasis as evidenced by auscultation of normal breath sounds Chest radiograph will be free of atelectatic changes Patient will have effective removal of secretions	■ Assess presence and quality of breath sounds Assess patient's ability to cough and characteristics of secretions Review chest radiograph for indications of atelectasis Explain importance of coughing, deep breathing, and other treatments to patient to enhance compliance Encourage coughing and deep breathing at least q2 hr Supply patient with small pillow to splint area during treatments Splint chest tube insertion site if patient is unable to do so Turn and position q2 hr Administer chest physiotherapy q2 hr with special attention to unaffected lung Suction if necessary to induce coughing and facilitate removal of secretions Administer humidified O_2 and other respiratory therapies as ordered to help liquefy secretions
■ Decreased respiratory drive related to pain medication	■ Patient will be pain free while maintaining regular, effective respirations and strong cough	■ Assess patient's pain threshold and response to prescribed pain medication Attempt to decrease need for pain medication with comfort measures such as change in position, back rub, and pillow for splinting Avoid pain medications that tend to depress respirations and cough, such as morphine and codeine, if possible

POTENTIAL PROBLEMS	EXPECTED OUTCOMES	NURSING ACTIVITIES
		Avoid pain medications that are CNS depressants and will decrease patient's ability to assist with his/her own care
		Administer nonnarcotic analgesics, if ordered
		Assess patient's respiratory status frequently for at least 2 hours following administration of pain medication
		Notify physician if respiratory status deteriorates following pain medication
		Stay with patient, encourage patient to take regular breaths, support with O₂ therapy as ordered; prepare to administer narcotic reversal agent, such as naloxone (Narcan), as ordered
		Have intubation equipment available

▪ Recurrent or incompletely resolved pneumothorax related to ongoing air leak as evidenced by continuous bubbling in water seal chamber	▪ Bubbling in water seal chamber will become gentle and sporadic
	Full lung expansion evident by absence of adventitious breath sounds
	Improving diagnostic studies
	  Arterial blood gas levels
	  Chest radiograph
	  Respiratory parameters
		▪ Check bubbling in water seal chamber initially, then q2-4 hr thereafter for presence of increase in amount of bubbling, suggesting air leak
		Secure connections with clear tape so that disconnections can be readily identified
		Ascertain that cap is secure when using bottle system
		Assess patient's respiratory efforts for presence of dyspnea, tachypnea, or use of accessory muscles
		Observe for any increase in bubbling
		If air leak occurs
		  Check for disconnection anywhere within system
		    Clean off connection site and reconnect it; do not clamp tube, because this may put patient at risk of tension pneumothorax
		    Have patient take a deep breath and cough following reconnection; this will help expel any air that may have entered intrapleural space during disconnection
		    Clamp tubing, beginning close to insertion site and moving downward until you find source, if disconnection is not evident but air leak is present; once clamp is below leak, bubbling will stop
		  Check insertion site if unable to find air leak in tubing; exert gentle pressure on site; if bubbling stops, implying that this is source of air leak, try to seal area with petroleum gauze; chest tube may be dislodged in subcutaneous tissue and require reinsertion by physician
		  Replace drainage unit if leak cannot be found at site or in tubing; drainage unit may be cracked, which may not be evident
		Call physician if problem remains unresolved
		Prepare for possible insertion of additional chest tube

▪ Recurrent pleural compromise related to accidental removal of chest tube	▪ Patient's chest tube will remain sutured securely in place and free from tension	▪ Ascertain that chest tube is sutured securely in place on insertion
		Apply comfortably tight dressing
		Arrange tubing so that it is within sight and is kept from catching on side rails or other equipment
		Explain purpose of chest tube and warn against manipulation or handling of tubing; if patient is confused or disoriented, restrain only if necessary and as ordered
		Monitor for loosening of sutures during daily site care and bring positive finding's to physician's attention
		If problem occurs
		  Hold sterile 4 × 4 gauze securely over site until petroleum gauze can be applied
		  Assess patient for onset of respiratory distress; if respiratory distress occurs, stay with patient; provide supportive O₂ therapy as ordered and monitor vital signs; provide emotional support and reassure patient that therapeutic measures will decrease symptoms
		Notify physician and prepare for chest tube reinsertion

POTENTIAL PROBLEMS	EXPECTED OUTCOMES	NURSING ACTIVITIES

■ Delayed lung expansion or extension of pneumothorax related to loss of water seal, which can occur if
Extension tubing is disconnected
Fluid evaporates in water seal chamber
Water seal bottle breaks
	■ Full lung expansion will be maintained	■ Ascertain that water seal connection is secure
		Use appropriate stand, out of path of traffic when using bottles
		  If unavailable, tape bottles to floor, out of path of traffic
		Check water seal connections and functioning frequently
		Check fluid level in water seal chamber at least q8 hr to ensure that it is maintained at ordered level; replace as necessary
		If loss of water seal occurs
		  Reconnect tubing if indicated
		  Fill water chamber if indicated
		  Broken bottle—place water seal straw or tubing in any available container of clean fluid, such as saline bottle at bedside or even clean cup of water; this will allow time to set up new water seal bottle while minimizing any adverse effects to patient
		Assess patient for effect of loss of water seal on respiratory status
		  Dyspnea
		  Tachypnea
		  Tachycardia
		  Use of accessory muscles
		  Anxiety
		  Abnormal blood gas levels
		Loss of water seal by water evaporation may have no adverse effect, but may cause delayed lung reexpansion as seen on serial chest radiographs
		Loss of water seal by disconnection or broken bottle increases risk of extension of pneumothorax; if signs and symptoms suggest extension of pneumothorax, see Standard 9, *Pleural compromise*

■ Absence of fluctuation in water seal chamber related to
Obstruction of tubing by kink or pressure- or fluid-filled dependent loop
Lung tissue or adhesions blocking chest tube eyelets on expiration
	■ Rise and fall of fluid level will cease only when patient is free from further leaking of air into intrapleural space
	Other evidence of lung reexpansion—gradual cessation of drainage, normal breath sounds, and easy respirations—will be present
		■ Monitor chest tube functioning closely and document changes in fluid fluctuation
		Reassess breath sounds and respiratory status in conjunction with changes in fluid fluctuations
		Check for fluctuation of fluid in chest tube if drainage system is evacuating fluid
		Check for fluctuation in water seal chamber if drainage system is evacuating air
		If abnormal absence of fluctuation occurs
		  Check tubing for presence of kink and straighten as indicated
		  Reposition patient to remove pressure on tubing if necessary; this may also help if problem is caused by lung tissue obstructing eyelets
		  Coil excess tubing next to patient on bed to eliminate dependent loop; secure it with a piece of tape and a safety pin
		If normal cessation of fluctuation occurs, document observation; no other action is indicated

■ Chest tube obstruction with sudden cessation of drainage, possibly related to External pressure or kinks in tubing Presence of blood or fibrin clot on tip or within chest tube	■ Absence or resolution of obstruction	■ Check tubing for external pressure or kinks and reposition as needed Observe drainage for clot formation and strip tubing, if this procedure is advocated by institution policy Assess drainage for presence of serosanguineous or bloody fluid; air or serous fluid usually makes obstruction less likely Relieve pressure or straighten out kinks in tubing Examine tubing for presence of external clot, keeping in mind that internal clot may also be responsible If clot is present raise tubing to enhance force of gravity; gently squeeze tubing at clot between fingers to encourage slowly its movement through tubing If stripping is indicated, grip tubing close to insertion site with thumb and forefinger of one hand, and slide other hand along tubing, compressing it toward collection unit; repeat this procedure along entire length of tubing—this may generate temporarily high levels of negative pressure (See Problem, Delayed closure of pleural leaks and lung tissue damage related to excessive negative pressure) Notify physician if clot cannot be easily dislodged

POTENTIAL PROBLEMS	EXPECTED OUTCOMES	NURSING ACTIVITIES

■ Deteriorating respiratory status related to continued air leak or fluid buildup during trial clamping in preparation for removal	■ Respiratory rate will be easy and unlabored with presence of normal breath sounds	■ Explain to patient that chest tube is being clamped in preparation for removal
		Assess patient's respiratory status before clamping for presence and quality of breath sounds in all lung fields
		Clamp chest tube as ordered
		  Usually chest tube is clamped for about 24 hours before removal to ensure that normal intrapleural pressure has been restored
		Obtain chest radiograph as ordered, usually 2 hours after clamping
		Auscultate lungs and observe for signs of compromised respiratory function, initially and q½ hr after clamping
		  Tachypnea
		  Tachycardia
		  Increased respiratory effort
		  Pain
		  Decreased or absent breath sounds
		Obtain and review interpretation of chest radiograph
		If problem occurs
		  Unclamp chest tube immediately
		  Reinitiate suction, if previously in use
		  Notify physician
		  Prepare for repeat chest radiograph

■ Delayed closure of pleural leaks and lung tissue damage related to excessive negative pressure caused by stripping of chest tubes	■ Patient's chest tube will remain open and drain freely without any adverse effects of increased negative pressure	■ *Stripping is a controversial practice and should be performed only if hospital policy permits and by physician's order*
		Strip only small sections of tubing, and let tubing reexpand between squeezes; this method will produce a negative pressure of about −30 cm H₂O; pressure typically ordered is −15 to −20 cm H₂O, therefore this represents a temporary increase of only −5 to −10 cm H₂O; greater increases should be avoided
		Strip chest tubes only when necessary; if tube is for evacuation of air or even serosanguineous fluid, stripping should not be necessary; if evacuation of blood was indication for chest tube insertion, stripping should be performed carefully and not more frequently than necessary, as indicated by presence of clots or debris
		Particular caution should be taken if patient has lung disease
		Assess for indications of excessive increase in negative pressure
		  Presence of new or recurrent air leak
		  Sudden cessation of drainage, possibly caused by lung tissue trapped in eyelet of chest tube
		  Sudden increase in drainage, possibly caused by hemorrhage from damaged lung tissue
		If problem occurs
		  Notify physician
		  Refrain from further stripping until cause has been identified and resolved
		  Ascertain whether physician wants stripping to be resumed

■ Unusually large amount of drainage in a short time	■ Chest tube drainage that had initially been up to 1 to 2 liters for 24 hours will decrease to minimal or no drainage	■ Assess frequently for sudden increase in drainage in relation to previous amounts
		Monitor for changes in character of drainage, such as serous to serosanguineous or to bloody
		If problem occurs
		  Check and record amount of drainage q5-10 min
		  Check patient's BP and heart rate and for signs and symptoms of hemorrhage
		    Pale
		    Diaphoretic
		    Decreased LOC
		    Restlessness
		  If signs and symptoms of hemorrhage are present, attempt to identify source; coagulation studies may be indicated as ordered

$$\frac{}{}$$

POTENTIAL PROBLEMS	EXPECTED OUTCOMES	NURSING ACTIVITIES
		Notify physician immediately if increased drainage continues or drainage becomes increasingly bloody
		Administer volume replacement as ordered, if necessary
		Ascertain availability of blood products for replacement
		Prepare patient for surgery if it becomes necessary, as ordered
■ Infection related to presence of chest tubes	■ Absence of infection Absence of signs of local infection at insertion site	■ Provide daily site care using aseptic technique; cleanse with povidone-iodine (Betadine) and apply sterile dressing
		Replace sterile connections and tubing if disconnection occurs
		Administer pulmonary physiotherapy
		Coughing and deep breaths
		Chest physiotherapy
		Suction as indicated
		Monitor temperature at least q2-4 hr and report any elevations of 101° F (38.3° C) or above
		Observe for signs of local infection at insertion site
		Swelling
		Redness
		Warmth
		Purulent drainage
		Observe for changes in amount and/or character of sputum
		If problem occurs
		Administer prescribed antipyretics
		Administer antibiotic therapy and site care as ordered
		Notify physician

Cardiovascular

STANDARD 11

ANGINA PECTORIS

Angina is chest pain or discomfort that results from an imbalance of myocardial oxygen supply and demand. The myocardial need for oxygen may increase, as with exercise, excitement, ingestion of a heavy meal, or exposure to cold; or the supply may decrease, as with progressive atherosclerotic coronary heart disease. Angina is often the first clinical manifestation of coronary heart disease. However, the term *angina* should not imply cause, for it may also be the result of severe ventricular hypertrophy caused by aortic stenosis or regurgitation, coronary arteritis, coronary ostial stenosis, and anemia. Angina can appear abruptly or gradually. It can precede or follow an AMI. It does not always progress to MI, although specific patterns may be a warning and preinfarction angina may or may not continue following infarction.

Because myocardial metabolism is primarily aerobic and 70% to 80% of oxygen is extracted by the myocardium, increased blood flow is necessary to increase oxygen supply. Blood flow to the myocardium occurs predominantly in diastole and is determined by cardiac output, diastolic arterial pressure, coronary artery resistance, and intramyocardial pressure. The major determinants of myocardial oxygen consumption (MVO_2) are heart rate, systolic blood pressure, ventricular volume (myocardial tension), and the contractile state.

Angina that occurs with a changing pattern in terms of frequency, severity, precipitating factors, and response to rest and nitroglycerin has been given different names, including *unstable angina, crescendo angina, preinfarction angina,* and the *intermediate syndrome. Decubitus angina pectoris* is angina that occurs at rest without any identifiable precipitating cause, and *nocturnal angina* is angina that awakens a patient from sleep. *Prinzmetal's angina,* or *atypical angina,* is a variant form that may occur in the absence of exertion and may not respond promptly to rest and ni-

troglycerin. ECG changes also differ from "typical" angina.

Causes of chest discomfort from which angina needs to be differentiated include anxiety; disorders involving the bony skeleton, joints, and skeletal muscle; pulmonary problems; esophageal disorders; pericarditis; Dressler's syndrome; and AMI.

Management of angina is directed toward minimizing the imbalance between oxygen supply and demand. When the patient's condition is stable, this includes use of medications such as nitroglycerin, long-acting nitrites, beta blockers, such as propranolol, and calcium channel blocking agents, such as verapamil, nifedipine, and diltiazem; vagal stimulation; and avoidance of provoking situations and/or use of prophylactic medication. Also to be included are correction of factors known to aggravate or accelerate angina, such as smoking, obesity, hypertension, and anemia.

Management of unstable angina is more aggressive, because the course is unpredictable. This management includes hospitalization, often in a coronary care unit, ECG monitoring, drug therapy, diagnostic tests such as coronary arteriography, and procedures such as transluminal coronary angioplasty (TCA) and coronary artery bypass grafting (CABG). Indications for TCA are still evolving, but generally include good left ventricular function, adequate runoff of the distal vessels, and preferably single-vessel disease with occlusion of 50% to 95% of the involved coronary artery. A patient with multiple-vessel disease may be considered if the other criteria are present. Indications for CABG are also still evolving, but usually if coronary arteriography verifies occlusion greater than 75% of one (particularly a left main stem artery lesion) or more arteries coupled with failure of aggressive medical treatment to control pain or if the angina is significantly altering the patient's life-style, CABG is recommended.

Usually angina is seen in critical care units when it has progressed to an unstable state, when arrhythmias develop, or when it is associated with another disease that requires critical care.

ASSESSMENT

1. History of angina, hypertension, MI, left ventricular failure, aortic valve disease, or anemia
2. Patient profile, including risk factors and information regarding life-style, habits, and emotions
3. Patient's perception of and reaction to diagnosis, progression of disease, and assessment and treatment modalities
4. Precise history and description of chest pain or discomfort
   a. Location, radiation, quality
   b. Duration
   c. Frequency
   d. Precipitating factors and any recent changes
   e. Relief mechanisms and any recent changes
   f. Indicators of progression
5. Presence of other symptoms with episodes of pain
6. Evaluation of hemodynamic status
7. Monitor ECG for
   a. Changes characteristic of angina or Prinzmetal's angina
   b. Arrhythmias
8. Lab data results if indicated
   a. Chest radiograph
   b. Coronary arteriography
   c. Left ventriculography
   d. Exercise ECG test
   e. Thallium scans with or without exercise testing
9. Signs and symptoms of complications
   a. AMI
   b. Left heart failure
   c. Arrhythmias
10. Ongoing and final evaluation of effectiveness of teaching program
11. Determinants of patient compliance

GOALS

1. Absence and/or control of pain or discomfort and any associated symptoms
2. Hemodynamic stability
3. Maintenance of optimal activity level
4. Patient's behavior demonstrates reduction of anxiety with provision of information
5. Before discharge the patient/family
   a. Demonstrates comprehension of the knowledge components of the teaching program when evaluated by testing or questioning
   b. Identifies own risk factors and of those agreed on by health care team and patient, describes methods of modification
   c. Identifies own precipitating factors and/or those that frequently precipitate angina and describes appropriate action to take to avoid or treat prophylactically
   d. Lists methods for monitoring activity—demonstrates accurately skill of counting pulse, identifying own maximal heart rate
   e. Describes symptoms requiring immediate medical attention and those suggesting disease progression that should be reported to the physician within 48 to 72 hours
   f. States necessary information for compliance with discharge regimen
      (1) Medications
      (2) Follow-up

POTENTIAL PROBLEMS	EXPECTED OUTCOMES	NURSING ACTIVITIES

■ Chest pain or discomfort related to ischemic myocardium	■ Verbalizes relief and/or absence of pain
	Absence of associated symptoms
		■ Minimize discrepancy between O_2 supply and demand
		  Provide periods of rest
		  Regulate activities of patient and health care team as condition allows
		  Determine visitor preferences with patient if unit policy allows
		  Maintain comfortable, quiet environment
		  Avoid heavy meals
		  Prophylactic use of medication as ordered
		Assist patient in recognition of precipitating events and control if possible by avoidance or prophylactic use of medication; lower doses are usually required for prevention than for treatment
		Assess for verbal and nonverbal cues indicating presence of chest pain or discomfort; patient may refer to vague sensations or aches; instruct patient to inform nurse immediately when pain occurs
		Maintain patent IV line
		Administer O_2 as ordered
		If patient is admitted with unstable angina, generally treat as an AMI until ruled out; see Standard 12, *Acute myocardial infarction*

POTENTIAL PROBLEMS	EXPECTED OUTCOMES	NURSING ACTIVITIES

If problem occurs

Obtain clear description of chest pain, including

Location, radiation: most often located in retrosternal region; may radiate to neck, jaw, clavicles, shoulders, arms, and/or epigastrium; may be located only in areas of radiation without affecting retrosternal region

Quality: may be described as pressure, heaviness, squeezing, smothering, burning, or indigestion; varying intensity from mild to severe

Duration: usually lasts only 3 to 5 minutes; check carefully for change

Precipitating factors: identify and compare to prior history; note particularly if these occur at rest or at lower oxygen-expending activity

Response to relief mechanism: usually relieved by rest and/or nitrites within 15 minutes

Check heart rate and BP during episode of pain; there may be an initial rise in systolic BP in attempt to compensate

Assess for presence of associated symptoms

Dyspnea

Weakness, fatigue

Palpitations

Dizziness or near syncope

Monitor ECG for

Characteristic S-T segment depression and inversion of T waves (not always seen)

Prinzmetal's angina: S-T segments may be elevated indicative of epicardial "injury current"

Arrhythmias

Administer medications as ordered

Vasodilators and/or analgesics

Drug doses should be increased in increments as long as patient continues to have pain; response to therapy, type and dose, should be communicated to physician and recorded

Have patient in supine or semi-Fowler's position

Check BP at 1, 5, and 10 minutes after administration of medication for hypotension

Observe for and/or elicit from patient presence of headache, nausea, and vomiting, vertigo, and/or flushing of the skin; if necessary, give aspirin or acetaminophen to increase headache threshold

Beta blockers—propranolol

Determine if patient has history of heart failure, AV block, asthma, or COPD; propranolol may aggravate these conditions

Monitor closely for effectiveness of ordered dose for relief of pain without producing myocardial failure or other side effects; because a large percentage of drug is removed from portal circulation by liver before it reaches systemic circulation, effective oral doses are much larger than IV doses and vary markedly among patients

Observe for signs and symptoms of

Myocardial failure

Hypotension

Bradycardia

Bronchospasm

POTENTIAL PROBLEMS	EXPECTED OUTCOMES	NURSING ACTIVITIES

		Calcium channel blockers—verapamil, nifedipine, or diltiazem
		Verapamil
		    Determine if contraindications are present, including severe hypotension or cardiogenic shock, second- and third-degree AV heart block, sick sinus syndrome (unless pacemaker in place), CHF not secondary to supraventricular tachycardia, and concomitant beta blocker drug therapy, with which verapamil interacts
		    Administer IV ordered dose over at least 2 minutes
		    Monitor closely for indications of digoxin toxicity if patient is receiving chronic digoxin therapy; verapamil can increase serum digoxin levels
		    Assess for presence of adverse reactions including symptomatic hypotension, bradycardia, severe tachycardia, dizziness, headache, nausea and abdominal discomfort
		Nifedipine
		    Use with caution in presence of hypotension; however, nifedipine can be administered concomitantly with beta blockers
		    Administer PO or sublingually as ordered
		    Assess for presence of adverse reactions, including hypotension that is most pronounced within 20 minutes of PO dose and 5 minutes of sublingual dose; palpitations; dizziness; headache; flushing; and angina recurrence about 30 minutes after dose
		Diltiazem
		    Determine if contraindications are present, including second- and third-degree AV block and sick sinus syndrome (unless pacemaker in place)
		    Use with caution in patients with impaired renal or hepatic function and/or concomitant beta blockers or digoxin
		    Administer PO as ordered
		    Assess for presence of adverse effects, including edema, arrhythmias, flushing, CHF, bradycardia, hypotension, syncope, headache, GI symptoms, pruritus, petechiae, and urticaria
		Maintain bed rest until pain pattern resolves
		If angina persists with minimal activity or after AMI, special studies may be ordered to assess potential candidacy for TCA or CABG; see Standard 26, *Cardiac catheterization;* Standard 27, *Cardiac surgery;* Standard 13, *Transluminal coronary angioplasty*

■ Anxiety related to
    Diagnosis and awareness of being "victim of heart disease" or that disease is progressing
    Pain and limited activity tolerance
    Uncertainties about future
    Diagnostic tests
    Pending surgery
    Other
	■ Verbalizes anxiety and/or fears
	Asks questions
	Behavior demonstrates decreased anxiety with provision of information and opportunities to ventilate feelings
		■ Continuous assessment of verbal and nonverbal clues of anxiety; attempt to identify source
		Assess relationship of anxiety to pain; role of anxiety as precipitating factor
		Provide information to patient/family regarding diagnosis, pain, and diagnostic procedures
		Encourage questions from patient/family
		Provide opportunities for patient to ventilate fears and discuss future management
		Explain purpose of and expectations from invasive studies and/or therapies if indicated; remember that patients generally want to know if it will hurt, how long it will take, what to expect
		If surgery is indicated, see Standard 27, *Cardiac surgery*
		If TCA is indicated, see Standard 13, *Transluminal coronary angioplasty*
		Sedate if necessary and as ordered

POTENTIAL PROBLEMS	EXPECTED OUTCOMES	NURSING ACTIVITIES
■ Hemodynamic instability related to left heart failure—some abnormalities of left heart function may occur transiently with ischemic episodes	■ Hemodynamic stability Absence of left heart failure	■ Check BP, P, and R q2 hr and with episodes of pain Observe for signs and symptoms of heart failure Dyspnea Fatigue Rales S_3 gallop Sinus tachycardia; if present, differentiate from relationship to pain or anxiety Presence of interstitial edema on chest radiograph Inform physician of abnormalities If propranolol is being administered for angina, reevaluate its use with physician if indications of heart failure develop; may be contraindicated because of negative inotropic effect If problem occurs, see Standard 15, *Heart failure (low cardiac output)*
■ Arrhythmias	■ Absence of arrhythmias	■ Continuous monitoring of ECG for presence of arrhythmias; serious ventricular arrhythmias and AV block are common complications of Prinzmetal's angina Relate occurrence to pain Assess for presence of associated symptoms such as palpitations If problem occurs, see Standard 21, *Arrhythmias*
■ AMI	■ Absence of AMI	■ Differentiate pain of angina from that of AMI May or may not be more severe Duration longer than 20 minutes, although difficult to evaluate since pain is to be treated promptly Does not respond to nitroglycerin; requires analgesic Often accompanied by sense of impending doom or acute anxiety Associated symptoms often present Monitor daily 12 lead ECG for changes suggestive of MI If AMI is suspected, serum enzymes and isoenzymes should be evaluated for characteristic changes If problem occurs, see Standard 12, *Acute myocardial infarction*
■ Decreased activity tolerance	■ Maintenance of optimal activity level	■ Assess for indications of decreasing activity tolerance Lower levels of activity provoke onset of angina, increased pulse rate, and/or decrease in systolic BP 3 to 5 minutes before, during, and immediately after (within 1 minute) activity, check P, BP, ECG for arrhythmias and for presence of symptoms indicative of intolerance; if changes occur, have patient cease activity and immediately provide rest and/or nitroglycerin Compare pulse in early evening to that on awakening for indications of cumulative stress; increased at rest Alternate periods of rest and activity Avoid activity for 1 hour after meals; remember that activities done to patient, e.g., bathing, often result in increased activity by patient Maintain level below anginal threshold; use nitroglycerin prophylactically if indicated, as ordered Administer long-acting nitrites or calcium channel blockers as ordered; a greater workload is required to produce angina after calcium blockade When patient's condition has stabilized, gradually increase activity and record and report indices of tolerance If prolonged bed rest is required, use preventive measures to avoid complications of increased immobility Passive/active range of motion (ROM) exercises Ensure that patient deep breathes q1 hr Ensure that patient changes position at least q2 hr Apply elastic or support stockings

POTENTIAL PROBLEMS	EXPECTED OUTCOMES	NURSING ACTIVITIES

■ Insufficient knowledge and skill to comply with discharge regimen	■ Evaluation by testing or questioning demonstrates patient/family's understanding of the knowledge components of teaching program
	Asks pertinent questions regarding self-care
	Identifies own risk factors and of those agreed on by health care team and patient, describes methods of modification
	Identifies own precipitating factors and/or those that frequently precipitate angina; describes appropriate action to take to avoid or treat prophylactically
	
	Lists methods for monitoring activity; demonstrates accurately skill of counting pulse, identifying own maximal heart rate
	Describes symptoms requiring immediate medical attention and those suggesting disease progression that should be reported to physician within 48 to 72 hours
	States necessary information for compliance with discharge regimen
	Medications
	Follow-up
		■ Institute teaching program for patient/family, including
		    Nature and significance of angina
		
		    Discussion of risk factors
		        Meaning of risk factors
		        Identification of patient's own risk factors
		        Cost-benefit ratio of modification
		        Methods of modification and sources of support
		    Common precipitating factors of angina with emphasis on patient's own precipitating factors
		        Activity
		        Emotional stress
		        Ingestion of heavy meal
		        Extremes of temperature
		        Sexual activity
		    Discussion of activities or situations to avoid and/or prophylactic use of nitroglycerin
		    Importance of regulating activity to keep below threshold of angina
		        Method of counting own pulse
		        Identification of maximal heart rate
		        Work simplification techniques
		
		    Symptoms requiring immediate medical attention
		    Symptoms suggesting progression of disease to be reported to physician within 48 to 72 hours
		
		    Information regarding discharge medications
		        Name and purpose
		        Dosage
		        Frequency
		        Prophylactic use
		        Storage
		        Side effects
		        Prophylactic use of aspirin or acetaminophen to control headaches
		    Follow-up information
		Provide opportunities for patient/family to ask questions and practice palpating pulse
		Assess patient/family's potential compliance

ACUTE MYOCARDIAL INFARCTION

Myocardial infarction (MI) is death of myocardial cells resulting from impaired coronary blood flow. The impairment is most commonly the result of atherosclerosis. The area of necrosis or infarction may be small and focal or large and diffuse. Generally the infarct does not involve the cells uniformly. It is thought that there is a central area of necrosis (nonviable tissue) surrounded by injured tissue that is viable if adequate circulation is reestablished but which will otherwise become necrotic. Current therapeutic research is directed toward salvaging this tissue, thereby limiting the size of infarcts. Surrounding this injured tissue is ischemic tissue, which is viable (assuming no further infarction) but "irritable" and may be the source of some of the arrhythmias that follow the acute event.

The hemodynamic consequences of infarction range from minimal changes in left ventricular function reflected by minimal changes in the left ventricular end diastolic filling pressure and cardiac output to major elevations of left ventricular end diastolic filling pressures with low cardiac output and BP. In addition, any challenge to a compromised myocardium such as arrhythmias, hypertension, pain, and anxiety may tip the balance and result in rapid deterioration.

Healing begins immediately as the body's defense mechanisms mobilize to remove the "debris." In general, necrotic tissue is replaced with young granulation tissue between the first and second weeks after infarction; then this is replaced by fibrous tissue during the next few weeks and finally becomes a scar within 2 to 3 months.

Most key areas of the heart receive blood either from a dual arterial supply or from a coronary artery with important secondary sources. The site of infarction depends on which coronary artery is obstructed. Generally, obstruction of the left anterior descending coronary artery results in an anterior or anteroseptal MI affecting the apical portion of the anterior wall of the left ventricle and/or the contiguous portion of the ventricular septum. Obstruction of the left circumflex coronary artery produces a lateral MI affecting the lateral wall of the left ventricle, and obstruction of the right coronary artery produces an inferior MI that involves the inferior wall and contiguous septum. Infarctions of the atria and right ventricle are uncommon; therefore site classification refers to the left ventricle.

The terms *subendocardial* and *transmural* describe the amount of muscle wall involved at the site. A subendocardial infarction is one that is confined to a restricted segment of the myocardium, usually muscle in the endocardial half of the left ventricular wall. A transmural infarction is one that involves the entire (or almost entire) thickness of the muscle in the involved segment, that is, goes through the wall.

The diagnosis of MI is based on a characteristic clinical history, ECG changes, and enzyme and isoenzyme elevations. If any one of these is positive, it warrants the patient being treated for a MI unless or until it is ruled out. Technetium scans are helpful though not frequently used when the actual diagnosis of MI is questionable, because the tracer can identify areas of acute myocardial injury.

The characteristic clinical history is that of pain lasting longer than 20 to 30 minutes unrelieved by rest or nitroglycerin. Associated symptoms of dyspnea, nausea and vomiting, weakness, diaphoresis, and palpitations may or may not be present. Often the patient describes a sense of impending doom, and some degree of anxiety is present. In some cases pain is slight or absent altogether.

There are three types of characteristic ECG changes which may be seen: alterations of the QRS complexes, elevations of S-T segments, and serial T wave changes. S-T segment and T wave changes are thought to be related to the areas of injury and ischemia surrounding necrotic tissue. Alterations of the QRS complex include developing significant Q waves in leads facing the area of infarction or diminishing or disappearing R waves in one or more of the precordial leads. The exception is a true posterior infarction that usually produces broad R waves in the right precordial leads, V_1 and V_2. S-T segment elevation is temporary, occurring acutely in leads facing the area of infarction, usually with reciprocal S-T segment depression in the opposite leads. S-T segment depression that occurs for several days in all leads except aV_R suggests a subendocardial infarction. The serial T wave changes occur over several days. Initially they may be positive or biphasic, becoming negative in leads facing the infarction. The changes may not appear immediately but usually exist in some form by the fifth to seventh day. It is important to compare the ECG with a prior one if available to rule out nonspecific S-T and T wave changes.

Estimation of the site of infarction can be determined by the leads in which the ECG changes are seen. An inferior MI would be visible in leads II, III, and aV_F; an anteroseptal infarction in leads V_1, V_2, and V_3; an anterior infarction in leads V_2, V_3, and V_4; and an anterolateral MI in V_4, V_5, V_6 and leads I and aV_L. If the entire anterior wall is involved, all six V leads will reflect the changes. These are the most common sites of infarction.

Enzymes reflecting myocardial damage include creatine phosphokinase (CPK), lactate dehydrogenase (LDH), and serum glutamic-oxaloacetic transferase (SGOT). These are not specific to cardiac muscle, so isoenzymes of CPK (MB band) and LDH (LDH_1 greater than LDH_2) that are more specific are more heavily relied on. Some or all of these may increase within 24 hours after infarction and resolve within days or weeks at varying times.

Management decisions are based on limiting the size of the infarct, maintaining optimal cardiac function by maintaining adequate coronary perfusion, and decreasing myocardial oxygen demands. Electrophysiological stability is critical to both.

An intervention that is increasing in popularity is the administration of intracoronary streptokinase, ideally within the first 3 to 6 hours after infarction. It is currently thought that a transmural infarct probably has a thrombus near the plaque and that the infarct is caused by an occlusion created by both. Streptokinase administration is carried out in the catheterization laboratory for the purpose of causing fibrinolysis, which reduces coronary occlusion, with the goal of limiting the size of infarction. See Standard 13, *Transluminal coronary angioplasty.*

ASSESSMENT

1. History of angina pectoris, coronary insufficiency, MI, cardiac failure, hypertension, diabetes, arrhythmias, medications, and cardiac surgery
2. Results of special cardiac studies—past and current
   a. Coronary arteriography
   b. Left ventricular cineangiograms
   c. Exercise ECG studies; may be combined with cardiac catheterization or myocardial imaging
   d. Echocardiography
   e. Myocardial imaging with radioactive isotopes
3. Level of anxiety, depression, and denial
4. Chest pain
   a. Location, radiation, quality
   b. Duration
   c. Precipitating factors
   d. Relief mechanisms
   e. Relation to exertion, respiration, and movement
   f. Presence of associated symptoms
5. Hemodynamic status
   a. BP
   b. P

   c. Heart sounds
   d. Respiratory effort
     (1) Breath sounds
     (2) Adventitious sounds
   e. Fluid balance
   f. Venous pressure
   g. Mental status
   h. General appearance
   i. Invasive monitoring if appropriate
     (1) Intraarterial pressure
     (2) PAP and PCWP
     (3) Cardiac output
     (4) CVP

6. Continuous monitoring and daily and prn 12 lead ECG for
   a. Arrhythmias
   b. Changes characteristic of evolving MI
   c. Changes characteristic of electrolyte imbalance
   d. Changes characteristic of drugs and their toxic effects
7. Lab data results of
   a. Serial cardiac enzymes and isoenzymes
   b. Blood gases
   c. Erythrocyte sedimentation rate (ESR)
   d. WBC count
   e. BUN and/or creatinine clearance
   f. Electrolyte values
   g. Drug levels
   h. Chest radiographs
   i. Cultures to determine source of suspected infection
8. Temperature
9. Signs and symptoms of complications
   a. Arrhythmias
   b. Heart failure; pulmonary edema
   c. Cardiogenic shock
   d. Angina
   e. Extension of MI
   f. Pericarditis
   g. Infections
   h. Pulmonary/systemic emboli
   i. Rupture
      (1) Cardiac
      (2) Ventricular septum
      (3) Papillary muscle
   j. Papillary muscle dysfunction
   k. Chordae tendineae tears
   l. Ventricular aneurysm
   m. Dressler's syndrome (post-MI syndrome)
10. Information regarding patient's
   a. Risk factor profile
      (1) Family history of premature coronary heart disease
      (2) Cigarette smoking
      (3) Hypertension

(4) Elevated serum lipids

(5) Carbohydrate intolerance, diabetes

(6) Obesity—greater likelihood of hypertension, elevated blood cholesterol level, or diabetes

(7) Sedentary life-style

(8) Psychosocial factors

    (a) Type A personality

    (b) Recognition and management of stress

b. Social support systems

c. Health beliefs and perceptions

d. Perception of impact of illness; cost-benefit ratio of therapy

e. Life-style if anticipated adjustments required

11. Ongoing and final evaluation of effectiveness of teaching program

GOALS

1. Absence of chest pain—patient verbalizes comfort
2. Hemodynamic stability—absence of complications
3. Electrophysiological stability
4. Control of anxiety, denial, and/or depression
   a. Verbal and nonverbal behavior demonstrates decreased anxiety with provision of information
   b. Verbalizes understanding of disease process and purpose and expectations of equipment, procedures, and routines
   c. Asks pertinent questions regarding future; verbalizes fears and identifies sources of anxiety
   d. Uses support systems if available
5. Normal temperature after 72 hours
6. Maintains prescribed activity level
7. Performs exercises, including those to avoid deleterious effects of bed rest
8. Patient verbalizes acceptance of diagnosis and asks pertinent questions regarding future management
9. Before discharge the patient/family
   a. Demonstrates comprehension of the knowledge components of the teaching program when evaluated by testing or questioning
   b. Identifies own risk factors and of those agreed on by health care team and patient, describes methods of modification
   c. Describes home exercise program and work simplification techniques
   d. Describes parameters for monitoring own activity—symptoms and pulse; demonstrates accurately skill of counting pulse, identifying own maximal heart rate
   e. Describes symptoms requiring immediate medical attention, listing what steps to take to obtain it
   f. States necessary information for compliance with medication regimen and follow-up

POTENTIAL PROBLEMS	EXPECTED OUTCOMES	NURSING ACTIVITIES

■ Chest pain related to MI	■ Absence of chest pain and associated symptoms
	If pain occurs, patient immediately notifies staff
		■ Patient should be admitted immediately to critical care unit
		  Attach patient to cardiac monitor using lead that gives clearest tracing; note lead used and settings of rate meters
		  Ensure that patent stable IV route is obtained using indwelling venous catheter
		  Administer O_2 as ordered
		If pain is present and severe, immediately inform physician and make medication available, and/or follow standing orders for treatment
		  Check BP, P, and R before and after medication administration, at 1, 5, and 10 minutes for hypotension, tachycardia, and respiratory depression; assess response to medication
		  Obtain a full description of pain, including location, radiation, patient's description of quality, duration, precipitating factors, and relief mechanisms; determine if influenced by respiration or movement
		  Assess for presence of shortness of breath, sweating, weakness or fainting, nausea and vomiting, degree of anxiety or sense of impending doom; record and report information with the above data
		When patient's condition is stabilized, perform full admission assessment for baseline information
		  Check BP in both arms for equality and level
		  Check all pulses—carotid, brachial, radial, femoral, popliteal, dorsalis pedis, posterior tibial, and apical—for rate, rhythm, quality, and equality
		  Respiratory rate and effort
		  Neck veins for jugular venous distention
		  Weight and presence of edema
		  Mental status

POTENTIAL PROBLEMS	EXPECTED OUTCOMES	NURSING ACTIVITIES

Temperature
General appearance
Auscultate precordium for
  Quality of heart sounds
  Rate and rhythm
  Murmurs*
  Rubs*
  Gallops*
    S₄ is usually present, reflecting increased ventricular filling pressure resulting from temporary impairment of left ventricular function
Auscultate lungs for aeration and presence of rales
Palpate precordium for point of maximal impulse and abnormal precordial movements, e.g., lifts or heaves
Assess patient/family's level of anxiety
Obtain 12 lead ECG and rhythm strip from monitor noting rate, rhythm, P-R interval, QRS duration, and Q-T interval for baseline data
Ensure that blood samples are obtained and sent to lab for cardiac enzymes and isoenzymes, blood gas levels, and CBC
Obtain chest radiograph
Interview patient for information regarding past medical and surgical history and medications
Ongoing assessment and care
  Ensure that emergency equipment is functioning and readily accessible; check every shift
  Check q2 hr for 48 hours and then q4 hr, increasing frequency as needed
    BP, P (apical and radial), and R
    Auscultate precordium for normal and abnormal sounds
    Auscultate lungs for aeration and rales
    Examine neck veins
    Mental status
    General appearance
    Be alert to development of pulsus alternans and pulsus paradoxus
  Check temperature q4 hr
  Check intake and output q8 hr
  Ongoing assessment of level of anxiety, depression, denial, and readiness to learn
  Monitor lab data for results of
    Enzymes and isoenzymes
    Blood gas levels
    WBC
    ESR
    Chest radiograph
Instruct patient to inform team immediately of presence of chest pain or discomfort, emphasizing reasons why
  Relief of pain
  Importance of data collection during episode
  To prevent further muscle damage and side effects of nausea and vomiting, hypotension or hypertension
Daily 12 lead ECG for
  Changes characteristic of evolving MI
  Changes characteristic of electrolyte imbalance
  Changes characteristic of drugs and their toxicity
  Arrhythmias
When patient is stable and rested, continue admission interview to obtain items listed under 10 in Assessment; use information to determine compliance probability and tailor discharge plan

*If not nursing responsibility, review physician's notes to determine presence.

POTENTIAL PROBLEMS	EXPECTED OUTCOMES	NURSING ACTIVITIES

		Initiate measures to decrease O_2 consumption during acute phase
		  Activity regulation
		    Maintain bed rest for 24 hours
		    Patient may feed self, wash face, and brush teeth if elbows are supported on table
		    Place patient in semi-Fowler's position, which is generally most comfortable for patients and also physiologically preferable because it decreases venous return and increases lung expansion
		    If condition is stable after 24 hours, patient may be assisted to bedside commode after dangling, and men may stand to void after obtaining physician's order
		    Check BP, P, R, and ECG before activity and within 1 minute after returning to bed; always be alert to symptoms of nontolerance
		    Obtain physician's order to place patient on graded exercise program to reduce complications of physical deconditioning; refer to hospital program or literature
		    Emphasize to patient/family that activity will be progressively increased
		  Give stool softeners and laxative if necessary and ordered
		  Diet will vary according to patient's condition and danger of vomiting; for reinforcement purposes of discharge planning it is helpful to begin on low-cholesterol, low-fat diet
		    Control calories if patient is overweight and salt if patient is hypertensive
		    Avoid large meals
		    If patient is retaining fluid, limit intake of fluids
		  Maintain quiet, controlled environment; approach patient with calm, confident, reassuring manner
		Administer medications as ordered; prophylactic anticoagulation against venous thromboembolus and mural thrombi may be ordered

■ Chest pain related to angina
  Preexisting angina may or may not continue after MI; new onset of angina may develop
	■ Absence and/or control of angina sufficient for maintenance of hemodynamic stability	■ Assess hemodynamic effect of pain; check P and BP
		With physician determine cause of pain
		  Previous history of angina
		  Description of pain; may or may not be similar to that of MI in severity, location, and radiation; duration difficult to evaluate because chest pain should be treated promptly
		  Relief of pain by nitroglycerin suggests angina; however, failure of nitroglycerin to relieve pain does not confirm MI
		  Appearance of chest pain in absence of new or changing ECG, or enzyme evidence of MI suggests angina
		Treat pain as ordered, recording and reporting response; check P and BP
		Assess effect of reappearance of chest pain on patient's level of anxiety; often frightening
		
		See STANDARD 11 Angina pectoris

■ Chest pain related to extension of infarction	■ Absence and/or control of extension sufficient for maintenance of hemodynamic stability	■ Assess hemodynamic effect of pain; check P and BP Determine cause of pain with physician; continuation of pain beyond 24 hours requiring narcotic for relief and ECG or enzyme evidence of new evolution suggest extension Treat pain as ordered, recording and reporting response; check BP and P Increase frequency of observations reflecting hemodynamic instability because increased necrosis further reduces functional ventricular muscle Assist with insertion of intraaortic balloon if indicated, which it may be if pain is refractory to conventional treatment in presence of increasing hemodynamic instability; usually reserved for patient considered as candidate for CABG and cardiac catheterization (if study not recently done)

POTENTIAL PROBLEMS	EXPECTED OUTCOMES	NURSING ACTIVITIES
		Assess level of anxiety related to continuance or reappearance of chest pain
		See STANDARD 24 *Intraaortic balloon pumping (counterpulsation)* STANDARD 26 *Cardiac catheterization* STANDARD 27 *Cardiac surgery*

■ Chest pain related to pericarditis
More common with anterior or transmural infarctions
	■ Absence and/or control of pericarditis sufficient for maintenance of hemodynamic stability	■ Assess hemodynamic effect of pain; check P and BP
		Assess for following characteristics of pain and associated symptoms useful for differentiating source
		   Chest pain appearing 2 days to 1 week postinfarction that is influenced by deep inspiration or change in position (may be relieved by leaning forward); note response to narcotics; lack of response may serve as clue
		   Presence of pericardial friction rub; may not appear for 4 to 48 hours following onset of pain
		   Presence of characteristic ECG changes of pericarditis; appearance of atrial arrhythmias
		   Temperature elevation greater than 101° F (38.3° C) for more than 72 hours after MI or new appearance of fever
		Treat pain as ordered; antiinflammatory agents most commonly effective
		If patient is being treated with anticoagulants, check with physician regarding continuation; often contraindicated because of risk of cardiac tamponade but this remains controversial; usually, minimal dosages of prophylactic anticoagulants will not be discontinued
		Assess for complications of arrhythmias, heart failure, and cardiac tamponade; see Standard 18, *Pericarditis*

■ Chest pain related to Dressler's syndrome (post-MI syndrome)
Related to hypersensitivity reaction in which antigen is necrotic cardiac muscle
	■ Absence of pain and associated complications	■ Patients occasionally admitted to critical care units for diagnostic differentiation
		Determine if recent history of MI; syndrome usually develops within few weeks to months after MI
		   Assess for presence of pericardial-type pain, friction rub, and prolonged fever
		   Assess for signs and symptoms of pleuritis or pneumonitis, which are sometimes present
		   Assess for signs and symptoms of pericardial effusion or tamponade; anticoagulation usually contraindicated because of potential risk of tamponade; see Standard 18, *Pericarditis*
		If pain occurs, administer aspirin, indomethacin, or corticosteroids as ordered

■ Anxiety, depression, and denial related to
Fear and concomitant symptoms
Lack of information regarding condition, procedures and equipment, future impact of heart disease on life-style
Matters left pending at work or home
Effect of illness on others
		■ Provide a comfortable, quiet environment; avoid use of audio alarms if not necessary for safety
		Limit nursing personnel caring for patient to allow for benefit of continuity
		Orient patient/family to unit, equipment, daily routines, and expected progression of activities
		   Stress that frequent assessments are part of preventive purpose of unit and do not necessarily imply deteriorating condition
		   Explain each new procedure as it is done
		   Inform patient/family of "team qualifications"—specially trained personnel
		   Maintain confident manner
		   Repeat information as needed because of reduced attention span associated with anxiety

	Patient/family verbalizes fears, concerns, and questions	Encourage patient/family to verbalize fears, concerns, and questions
		   Provide private opportunities for both patient and family
		   Answer questions when possible; do not avoid questions
		   Remember that anxious families create anxious patients
		Allow patient as much control over environment, daily hygiene, and visitors as possible; observe effect of visitors on patient

POTENTIAL PROBLEMS	EXPECTED OUTCOMES	NURSING ACTIVITIES
		Sedate patient only if necessary and as ordered; heavy sedation makes it difficult to integrate realities of illness necessary for successful rehabilitation
		If pain occurs, treat promptly and stay with patient until resolved; narcotics also help reduce anxiety; explain source of pain
	Control or resolution of anxiety, depression, and denial with time and provision of information	Continually assess verbal and nonverbal clues of levels of anxiety, depression, and denial
		Differentiate from environmental and physiological factors, e.g., cerebral hypoxia
		Clues to *anxiety* include restlessness, sleeplessness, hostility, non-responsiveness, incessant talking, difficulty concentrating, muscular tenseness or rigidity, and watchful or frightened appearance
		Clues to *depression* include insomnia, constipation, anorexia, decreased energy drive, underresponsiveness, irritability, weeping or crying, verbalization of feelings of hopelessness about future, despondency, helplessness, depersonalization, decreased self-esteem, guilt, and general lack of interest in everything
		Clues to *denial* include explicit verbal denial; stoic or inappropriately cheerful, unrealistic statements in the face of reality; and outright refusal to comply with medical regimen
		Determine degree of denial and if it interferes with care; denial may be beneficial if it helps to reduce anxiety during acute state
		Serach for sources of anxiety; may be related to matters left pending at home or work that can be resolved
		Assess hemodynamic consequences of anxiety
	Coping mechanisms adequate to help control anxiety while not interfering with care	Participate in management of coping mechanisms
		Denial
		Accept patient's denial when it serves beneficial purpose of reducing acute anxiety, but do not reinforce it; may be inadvertently reinforced by delay of definite diagnosis pending ECG, enzyme and isoenzyme results
		Be specific when patient generalizes about, avoids, or attempts to change subject
		Identify and discuss ambiguities
		Hostility and/or sexual aggression
		Maintain calm, matter-of-fact attitude
		Avoid confrontation
		Explore causes of feelings with patient and be supportive
		Do not ignore overt behavior or overcompensate with kindness
	Acceptance of diagnosis	Begin teaching plan when patient indicates readiness
		Priority of time in unit should be to move patient toward acceptance of diagnosis
		Explain what heart attack is and healing process
		Personalize teaching to patient
		Participate in ongoing preparation of patient/family for transfer from unit
■ Arrhythmias related to Myocardial ischemia Increased sympathetic tone Abnormalities associated with reduced left ventricular function Treatment modalities	■ Electrophysiological stability Optimal cardiac rhythm	■ Continuous observation of ECG is essential
		Select best leads
		Clear QRS complexes and P waves
		Clear pacemaker artifact if present
		"Special" leads such as MCL_1 (modified V_1)
		Bundle branch blocks
		Differentiating aberrancy from intraventricular conduction problems
		Leads I and II—axis shifts
		Set rate alarms if necessary; if rate alarms are used, check rate limit indicators and alarm system regularly for accuracy and operation
		Premature beats are often warning sign of more serious arrhythmias
		Note site of origin, frequency, presence of patterns, coupling interval (relationship to preceding normal beat), and configuration (multiformed or uniformed)

POTENTIAL PROBLEMS	EXPECTED OUTCOMES	NURSING ACTIVITIES
		Check pulse to see if perfused
		Participate in management as ordered to avoid more lethal arrhythmias and negative hemodynamic consequences
		Tachyarrhythmias
		Assess effect on cardiac output resulting from decreased coronary perfusion and increased myocardial O_2 demand; significance primarily dependent on ventricular rate
		A ventricular rate of 100 to 150 is usually result of arrhythmias secondary to heart failure—sinus tachycardia, atrial flutter, and atrial fibrillation; with atrial fibrillation, assess effect of loss of atrial contraction on hemodynamic status in patients with left heart failure or mitral stenosis
		If the ventricular rate is greater than 150
		Institute treatment promptly as ordered to avoid potential circulatory collapse
		If countershock is required and time allows, assess for presence of acidosis, hypoxia, and digoxin toxicity
		If any of these are present, participate with physician in their correction, if possible, before countershock
		Bradyarrhythmias
		Assess effect on cardiac output
		May be beneficial because of increased time for diastolic coronary artery filling and decreased O_2 consumption
		Ventricular rates below 50 more likely to decrease cardiac output because of inability of left ventricle to compensate with increased stroke volume
		Observe for and treat as ordered the occurrence of premature beats
		For all arrhythmias, assess effect on cardiac output; check BP, P, and observe for changes that reflect increasing left ventricular dysfunction (see Problem, Ventricular dysfunction)
		Check emergency equipment at every shift to ensure functioning and ready availability
		Participate with physician in identification and treatment of predisposing clinical conditions or factors
		Administer antiarrhythmics as ordered; regulate IV antiarrhythmic infusions to avoid overdosing and serious side effects
		Assist with pacemaker insertion if necessary
		Relate conduction problem to site of infarction
		Anterior or anteroseptal MI—prophylactic insertion more common because of statistically higher probability of progression to complete heart block and less reliability of escape ventricular pacemaker; block is generally result of extensive septal damage
		Inferior MI—AV block generally occurs in AV node; should complete heart block develop, escape pacemaker is usually junctional (more reliable than ventricular), and block is more often transient, resolving within 14 days
		See Standard 23, *Pacemakers: temporary and permanent*
		For more detailed information, see Standard 21, *Arrhythmias*
■ Hypotension related to reflex mechanisms, probably vagal	■ Normal peripheral vascular response to compensate for hypotension, thereby maintaining BP and cardiac output	■ Assess for other indications of excessive vagal stimulation to differentiate from hypotension related to uncompensated left ventricular dysfunction
Peripheral vascular resistance remains normal or decreases in response to hypotension resulting from decreased left ventricular function rather than increasing in normal manner to maintain BP and cardiac output		Sinus bradycardia
		First-degree or Wenckebach heart block
		Nausea
		Bronchospasm
		Tracheal burning
		Assess for consequences of decreased cardiac output and increased peripheral vascular perfusion
		Monitor BP; frequency dependent on level and hemodynamic consequences

POTENTIAL PROBLEMS	EXPECTED OUTCOMES	NURSING ACTIVITIES

More commonly seen in patients with inferior or posterior MI		Administer medications as ordered
		  Parasympatholytics, e.g., atropine; often abolishes symptoms and may be given in low doses to help with differentiation
		  Vasopressors; monitor closely to avoid hypertension, tachycardia, and ventricular arrhythmias

■ Ventricular dysfunction related to heart failure, pulmonary edema
Occurs in most patients following MI to some degree during first 4 days; on continuum from asymptomatic (with minimal compensatory rise in left ventricular filling pressure) to cardiogenic shock
	■ Hemodynamic stability	■ Observe for problems known to aggravate heart failure—arrhythmias, hypotension or hypertension, acidosis, hypoxemia, pain
		  Report presence to physician
		  Treat immediately according to physician's orders
		Assess for signs and symptoms of heart failure
		  Sinus tachycardia
		  Dyspnea
		  Tachypnea
		  Orthopnea
		  Pulmonary rales
		  S_3 gallop
		  Pulsus alternans
		  Elevation of jugular venous pressure, neck vein distention
		  Hepatic enlargement
		  Positive hepatojugular reflux
		  Peripheral or sacral edema
		  Persistent hypotension continuing after relief of pain
		  Displaced or diffuse apical impulse
		Review chest radiograph for signs of pulmonary congestion or enlargement; change may follow occurrence of symptoms by as much as 24 hours
		Prepare patient for nuclear cardiology studies if ordered to differentiate whether congestive failure is caused by myocardial failure or ventricular aneurysm
		Therapy dependent on extent of failure and response to treatment; promptly inform physician of changes
		Administer O_2 as ordered, usually through nasal cannula 2 to 6 liters/minute; review results of blood gases for hypoxemia
		Administer diuretics as ordered
		  Monitor intake and output, urine specific gravity and lab results for electrolytes and BUN or creatinine clearance
		  Ensure adherence to low-sodium diet if ordered; explain purpose to patient/family, particularly when latter bring "treats" from home
		  Heart failure not responding to aforementioned will be more aggressively managed; invasive hemodynamic monitoring is recommended
		  Intraarterial lines
		  PCWP (reflecting left ventricular end diastolic filling pressure)
		  Cardiac output
		  Foley catheter
		  See Standard 25, *Hemodynamic monitoring;* Standard 15, *Heart failure (low cardiac output);* Standard 1, *Pulmonary edema of cardiac origin*

■ Ventricular dysfunction related to cardiogenic shock
Related to extensive myocardial necrosis resulting in impaired perfusion of body tissues and organs
Patients remaining in shock for over 1 hour have significantly higher mortality
	■ Absence of cardiogenic shock	■ Assess for signs and symptoms of cardiogenic shock
		  Hypotension: systolic BP less than 90 mm Hg
		  Tachycardia with poor pulse contour
		  Urine output less than 20 ml/hour
		  Mental confusion
		  Decreased peripheral perfusion
		If cardiogenic shock develops
		  Report to physician immediately
		  Participate in aggressive management to interrupt shock cycle
		In the absence of cardiogenic shock, initiate with physician invasive hemodynamic monitoring essential for determining response to therapy, thereby guiding therapy
		  Intraarterial pressures

POTENTIAL PROBLEMS	EXPECTED OUTCOMES	NURSING ACTIVITIES
		PCWP Cardiac output measurements Foley catheter for hourly urine measurements Identify and treat as ordered abnormalities such as hypoxemia, acidosis, arrhythmias, pain Institute therapy as ordered; this may include vasopressors, vasodilators, inotropic agents, fluid challenge, O_2 administration, counterpulsation and/or surgical intervention Continuous assessment required to monitor rapidly changing hemodynamic status characteristic of cardiogenic shock *See* STANDARD 16 *Cardiogenic shock* STANDARD 25 *Hemodynamic monitoring* STANDARD 24 *Intraaortic balloon pumping (counterpulsation)*
■ Ventricular dysfunction related to papillary muscle dysfunction/rupture Related to papillary muscle infarction More commonly seen with inferior, lateral, and subendocardial infarctions	■ Absence of or resolution of papillary muscle dysfunction/rupture	■ Assess for signs and symptoms of papillary muscle dysfunction, particularly during first few days after AMI Transient systolic murmur at apex indicative of mitral insufficiency Left heart failure If failure is hemodynamically significant, administer vasodilators as ordered, monitoring intraarterial pressure and PAP, urine output, etc. If mitral valve replacement is necessary because of continued heart failure, maintenance therapy with PO or IV vasodilators may be required to delay surgery for at least 6 to 10 weeks after MI to allow time for healing Onset of sudden pulmonary edema resistant to drug therapy suggests papillary muscle rupture Determine presence of Sudden onset of loud holosystolic murmur best appreciated at apex with patient lying on left side; may radiate to left axilla or back Hypotension Barely palpable pulses Signs and symptoms of severe left heart failure Electromechanical dissociation Prepare patient for cardiac catheterization and coronary arteriography to determine feasibility of surgical correction Administer vasodilators as ordered, monitoring intraarterial pressure and PAP If indicated, prepare patient for cardiac surgery; counterpulsation may be required *See* STANDARD 1 *Pulmonary edema of cardiac origin* STANDARD 25 *Hemodynamic monitoring* STANDARD 26 *Cardiac catheterization* STANDARD 27 *Cardiac surgery* STANDARD 24 *Intraaortic balloon pumping (counterpulsation)*
■ Ventricular dysfunction related to rupture of ventricular septum Rare complication, usually occurring within 2 to 10 days after infarction Seen with anterior and inferior MI	■ Absence of ventricular septal rupture	■ Determine presence of Loud holosystolic murmur near lower left sternal border with palpable thrill; may be louder at apex, which makes differentiation from papillary muscle rupture more difficult Left to right shunting Heart failure of varying degrees dependent on amount of shunting Pulmonary congestion; pulmonary edema Hypotension Prepare patient for cardiac catheterization if necessary Administer afterload reducing agents to decrease shunting as ordered, monitoring intraarterial pressure and PCWP Assist with insertion of intraaortic balloon if ordered; maintain according to protocol and physician's orders Attempts will be made to delay surgery as long as possible after MI to allow infarcted tissue to heal; development of cardiogenic shock or drug-resistant heart failure mandates earlier repair

POTENTIAL PROBLEMS	EXPECTED OUTCOMES	NURSING ACTIVITIES
		See STANDARD 15 *Heart failure (low cardiac output)* STANDARD 1 *Pulmonary edema of cardiac origin* STANDARD 26 *Cardiac catheterization* STANDARD 24 *Intraaortic balloon pumping (counterpulsation)* STANDARD 25 *Hemodynamic monitoring* STANDARD 27 *Cardiac surgery*

■ Ventricular dysfunction related to external cardiac rupture
Usually results in sudden death
	■ Absence of cardiac rupture	■ Has been noted in relation to coughing and straining at bowel movement; more common in absence of congestive heart failure
		Assess for signs and symptoms of cardiac tamponade and electromechanical dissociation
		Assist with emergency intervention
		  Pericardiocentesis
		  Constant drainage by intrapericardial catheter
		  Rapid administration of dextran and norepinephrine
		  Counterpulsation
		  Surgery to close defect

		See STANDARD 18 *Pericarditis* STANDARD 24 *Intraaortic balloon pumping (counterpulsation)* STANDARD 27 *Cardiac surgery*

■ Ventricular dysfunction related to left ventricular aneurysm
Occurs more commonly with transmural infarction from few days to 6 weeks after MI
	■ Hemodynamic stability	■ Determine presence of the following indications suggestive of aneurysm
		  Palpable prolonged outward systolic impulse medial and/or superior to point of maximal impulse
		  Persistent S-T segment elevation in precordial leads; occasionally can be produced by exercise
		  Abnormal contour of left cardiac border on posteroanterior chest radiograph
		  Paradoxical movement of left ventricle during fluoroscopy
		  Drug-resistant ventricular arrhythmias, particularly ventricular tachycardia
		  Refractory congestive heart failure
		Prepare patient for radioisotope scanning studies and/or left ventricular angiography, which may be ordered to confirm impression
		If surgery is indicated (cardiac failure and ventricular arrhythmias persist threatening hemodynamic stability; surface area involved less than 50%), it will be delayed at least 4 to 10 weeks following MI if possible
		Administer treatments directed toward controlling heart failure and arrhythmias as ordered
		Observe for signs and symptoms of systemic arterial embolization resulting from intraaneurysmal thrombosis

		See STANDARD 15 *Heart failure (low cardiac output)* STANDARD 26 *Cardiac catheterization* STANDARD 27 *Cardiac surgery* STANDARD 31 *Embolic phenomena* STANDARD 21 *Arrhythmias*

■ Thromboembolism related to deep vein thrombosis or mural thrombi from infarcted endocardium	■ Absence or resolution of thromboembolism	■ Institute preventive measures particularly for patients with severe or chronic congestive heart failure, shock, preexisting thromboembolic disease, and obesity and older (over 70) or inactive patients
		Administer anticoagulants as ordered; observe for signs of bleeding
		Assist patient with passive exercises while in bed; place footboard on bed for patient to press toes against 10 times every hour
		Instruct patient not to cross legs or ankles
		Use elastic stockings and measure calf for correct size
		  Remove twice a day
		  Make certain that stockings do not roll down, creating ''tourniquet''
		Have patient ambulate as early as possible

POTENTIAL PROBLEMS	EXPECTED OUTCOMES	NURSING ACTIVITIES

		Observe for signs of venous thrombosis
		  Positive Homans' sign
		  Change in color, temperature, or girth of extremity
		  Presence of tenderness and/or cords
		Assess for signs and symptoms of pulmonary embolus—sudden unexplained dyspnea, tachypnea, anxiety, hypotension, tachycardia, atrial arrhythmias, elevation of jugular venous pressure, elevation of PAP (if line is in place), and expiratory or fixed splitting of S_2
		Assess for signs and symptoms of pulmonary infarction—hemoptysis, pleural friction rub, dyspnea, or signs of pulmonary consolidation
		Prepare patient for lung scan if ordered
		If problem occurs
		  Inform physician
		  Administer anticoagulants as ordered
		  Observe for appearance of heart failure or pulmonary edema, which may be aggravated or precipitated by pulmonary emboli
		Assess for signs and symptoms of systemic emboli; often not recognized unless of large size or cerebral
		If systemic emboli occur
		  Inform physician
		  Administer anticoagulants as ordered
		  Treat complications
		
		See STANDARD 31 *Embolic phenomena*

■ Temperature elevation related to
  Myocardial tissue necrosis
  Pericarditis
  Infection
	■ Normal temperature after 72 hours	■ Encourage patient to cough and deep breathe every hour while on bed rest and awake
		Foley catheters should not remain in place over 2 weeks and depending on appearance may need to be changed more frequently
		Peripheral IV sites should be changed q48-72 hr
		IV tubing should be changed q48 hr
		In solutions should be changed q24 hr
		Monitoring lines should be changed as indicated in following unless detrimental to patient; employ strict aseptic technique for tubing and transducer changes
		  Pulmonary artery lines: at least every 72 hours
		  Arterial lines: at least every 7 days
		  CVP lines: at least every 7 days
		  Chamber dome and administration tubing q48 hr
		  Flush solutions at least q24 hr
		Check temperature q4 hr while patient is awake, increasing frequency as needed
		If temperature is elevated
		  Observe for associated chills and diaphoresis
		  Keep patient warm and dry
		  Administer antipyretics as ordered
		  Review lab results of WBC count and sedimentation rate
		  Inform patient that temperature elevation is expected during first 48 to 72 hours
		If temperature is elevated beyond 101° F (38.3° C) or persists beyond 48 to 72 hours, observe for other sources of infection
		  Assess for signs and symptoms of pericarditis (see Problem, Chest pain related to pericarditis)
		  Assess for other sources of infection—lungs, urine, monitoring lines
		  Obtain cultures if necessary
		  Culture tips of monitoring lines when removed if serum culture positive
		  Administer antibiotics or other medications as ordered
		
		See STANDARD 61 *Infection control in the critical care unit*

POTENTIAL PROBLEMS	EXPECTED OUTCOMES	NURSING ACTIVITIES
■ Insufficient knowledge to comply with discharge regimen	■ Evaluation by testing or questioning demonstrates patient/family's understanding of knowledge components of teaching program Asks pertinent questions about self-care	■ Institute teaching program for patient/family, including 　Normal heart function 　Explanation of what heart attack is and process of healing; relate to symptoms
	Identifies own risk factors and of those agreed on by health care team and patient, describes plans for modification	Discussion of risk factors 　Meaning and significance of 　Identification of patient's own 　Cost-benefit ratio of modification 　Methods of modification and sources of support 　　Tailor to patient 　　　Smoking 　　　Diet 　　　Recognition and management of stress 　Control of coexisting disease if present 　　Hypertension 　　Diabetes 　　Arrhythmias 　　Heart failure 　　Angina
	Describes home exercise program and work simplification techniques; demonstrates exercises Describes how own symptoms and pulse will be used to monitor activity; demonstrates accurately how to count own pulse and state maximal heart rate	Activity regulation 　Significance of activity regulation related to healing process 　Purpose of home exercise program, providing opportunity for practice 　Work simplification techniques 　Importance of avoiding or modifying activity following meals, stress, or in extremes of temperature 　Prophylactic measures if appropriate 　Method of counting pulse; meaning and significance of maximal heart rate 　Symptoms suggesting lack of tolerance and what to do if these occur 　Sexual activity: include both partners
	Describes those symptoms requiring immediate medical attention and what steps should be taken to obtain it	Symptoms requiring immediate medical attention; sources of help available to patient and how to obtain; be as specific as possible after discussion with physician
	States necessary information for compliance with medication regimen and follow-up	Information regarding discharge medications 　Name and purpose 　Dosage 　Frequency: tailor to patient's routine schedule 　Prophylactic use of and storage of nitroglycerin 　Side effects 　Group timing of medications if possible to decrease complexity of scheduling Follow-up information 　Include discussion of future tests if ordered 　　Exercise ECG 　　Cardiac catheterization 　Helpful for patient/family to be aware that periods of depression and fatigue are not uncommon, particularly during first few weeks at home
	Patient/family discusses future realistically	Provide frequent opportunities for patient/family to ask questions and express concerns or fears Provide opportunities for skills practice Assess patient's potential compliance with discharge regimen

TRANSLUMINAL CORONARY ANGIOPLASTY

The therapeutic goal for coronary artery disease (CAD) is to minimize the imbalance between oxygen supply and demand. Cardiac medications such as nitrates, beta blockers, and calcium channel blockers decrease the cardiac work load (i.e., oxygen consumption) and improve oxygen supply. In addition, risk-factor modification (reduction of weight, smoking, hypertension, and stress) is recommended to avoid progression of CAD and/or relieve symptoms. Resolution of coronary occlusion in the acute MI patient has been successfully achieved with intracoronary (IC) fibrinolytic therapy (e.g., streptokinase).

If the patient's angina is not controlled by medical management and/or interferes with the patient's life-style, CABG is generally recommended for acceptable surgical candidates. Transluminal coronary angioplasty (TCA) is an alternative mode of therapy for the patient with CAD.

Currently, TCA is performed across the country. It provides a nonoperative treatment for the relief of angina pectoris and myocardial ischemia. The physical impairment, total cost, and length of hospitalization and recovery are greatly reduced in comparison to cardiac surgery. Approximately 10% to 15% of all surgically treated patients are suitable candidates for TCA. TCA is a modification of the technique for peripheral arterial dilatations first used by Dotter and Judkins in 1964. Dilatation was accomplished by sequential passage of catheters of increasing diameters into the stenotic segment of the vessel. In Zurich in 1977, Gruntzig performed the first TCA, using a double-lumen, polyvinyl chloride, balloon-tipped catheter for dilatation. When inflated in the stenotic segment, the balloon compresses the atheromatous plaque into the arterial wall. After successful trials in Zurich, evaluation of TCA began in the United States in March, 1978.

The ideal candidate for TCA has single-vessel disease, adequate left ventricular function, and occlusion of greater than 50% but less than 95% of the proximal left anterior descending, circumflex, and/or right coronary artery. Distal stenosis is technically difficult to reach with the dilatation catheter. The atheromatous plaque should be uncalcified, discrete, short, and not eccentric (on one side). Patients with multiple-vessel disease can be considered for TCA if they have adequate runoff of the distal vessels with preserved left ventricular function.

The patient must be an acceptable surgical candidate and willing to undergo CABG if emergency coronary revascularization is required after TCA. The operating room must be on standby during the performance of TCA.

TCA can be combined with other techniques to achieve maximal myocardial blood flow. During elective CABG, myocardial perfusion may also be restored by dilatation of stenotic vessels. Alternatively, TCA may be performed after coronary recanalization with IC streptokinase. IC streptokinase restores perfusion of the coronary artery. This improved blood flow may result in reduced myocardial ischemia, improved left ventricular ejection fraction, and reduced in-hospital mortality and morbidity.

Treatment of AMI with IC streptokinase is ideally initiated in the first 3 to 6 hours after the onset of symptoms. However, successful recanalization has been accomplished up to 21 hours after infarction. Streptokinase infusion causes fibrinolysis with reduction of coronary occlusion. IC thrombolysis with streptokinase can be successfully achieved in 75% to 85% of treated patients. Complications related to IC streptokinase infusion are systemic bleeding caused by alteration of the natural clotting process, reocclusion, and/or reinfarction. Because of its effect on the clotting process, the administration of streptokinase is contraindicated in patients who are at risk for bleeding. The high-risk group for bleeding includes patients who have recently had surgery; internal bleeding; CVA; organ biopsy, thoracentesis, or paracentesis; and pregnancy or obstetrical delivery. The moderate-risk group includes patients who have severe hypertension, liver disease, or kidney disease; coagulation defects; recent cardiopulmonary resuscitation (CPR); bacterial endocarditis; and recent lumbar puncture or puncture of noncompressible vessels (e.g., the jugular vein).

The candidate for TCA is admitted 1 day before the procedure for routine preparation (ECG, chest radiograph, blood specimens). Discharge is usually 1 to 3 days after TCA. TCA is performed in the cardiac catheterization laboratory, using techniques similar to those performed during routine cardiac catheterization and angiography.

The evening before TCA, 10 grains of aspirin are administered to decrease platelet adhesion. After midnight, the patient is kept NPO except for medications to prevent ischemic symptoms (nitrates, beta blockers, and/or calcium channel blockers). Usually, a peripheral IV infusion is started and an analgesic administered before transport to the catheterization laboratory. The procedure is performed with the patient fully alert.

In the catherization laboratory, 10,000 units of heparin and dextran 40 at 50 ml/hour are infused to prevent thrombus formation and platelet aggregation. Sublinguinal nitroglycerin and oral nifedipine are administered before and during the procedure to prevent coronary spasm. IV and/or IC nitroglycerin may also be administered during the dilatation procedure to prevent spasm.

The patient is prepped, shaved, and draped for either percutaneous insertion or cutdown with the Sones arteriographic method. The rigid, guiding catheter (8.7 Fr) is introduced into the femoral or brachial artery. The flexible balloon-tipped catheter (2.0, 3.0, and 3.7 mm in diameter when inflated) is advanced through the guiding catheter. The balloon is sausage shaped when inflated and 2 cm in length.

The guiding catheter is advanced, under fluoroscopy, to the orifice of the stenotic artery. The dilatation catheter is advanced, and contrast medium is injected through the tip of the catheter to visualize the stenotic vessel. The dilatation catheter is advanced until it traverses the arterial narrowing. When the catheter tip is within the lesion, there will be a pressure gradient recorded across the stenosis. The pressure distal to the atheromatous lesion is less than the pressure proximal to the lesion (aortic root pressure).

The balloon is inflated for 5 to 15 seconds with 4 to 6 atmospheres of pressure (higher pressures have been successfully used), using a mixture of 50% saline and 50% contrast medium. Repeated inflations and deflations are performed to compress the plaque into the walls of the artery. During inflations, T waves on the ECG will peak, then return to normal on deflation. After the procedure, the pressure gradient is measured proximally and distally to the stenosis. There is a drop in the gradient with increased lumen size. The coronary flow is then revisualized with contrast medium to compare to flow before the procedure. If lumen size increases by 20% or more, the procedure is considered successful. The success rate is generally reported at 60% or greater and has been reported as high as 80%. Failure is usually associated with inability to traverse lesions that are calcific, long, and eccentric.

The most common complication of TCA is prolonged angina. Coronary spasm may occur during or after the procedure. Subintimal coronary artery dissection may occur with no early symptoms, but may later cause restenosis of the artery. Immediate dissection requires emergency CABG.

Sudden occlusion with symptoms of ischemia occurs in 6% of the patients, also requiring emergency coronary revascularization. Progression of myocardial ischemia to infarction may be averted if myocardial blood flow is restored within 60 to 90 minutes.

AMI occurs in the hospital in 6% of these patients. The in-hospital mortality is 1% for patients with single vessel disease, 2% for patients with multiple-vessel disease, and 5% for patients who have undergone previous CABG.

ASSESSMENT

1. History of cardiovascular disease
   a. Presenting symptoms (angina, shortness of breath, decreased exercise tolerance, palpitations)
   b. Previous MI
   c. Stroke, pulmonary embolism, peripheral vascular disease
   d. Risk factors for CAD—hypertension, diabetes, cigarette smoking, obesity, hyperlipidemia, sex, age, personality, stress; include family history of pertinent risk factors
2. Previous illnesses, procedures, or hospitalizations, particularly related to cardiovascular history and cardiac catheterization
3. Current medications and allergies (inquire if patient ever received radiographic contrast medium); include patient/family's comprehension of purpose and action of cardiovascular medications
4. Cardiovascular status
   a. Cardiac output and perfusion—bilateral systolic and diastolic BP, strength and presence of peripheral pulses, color and warmth of extremities, urine output, rate of capillary refill, LOC
   b. Heart rate, rhythm, and quality of pulse; presence of abnormal heart sounds—murmur, gallop, ejection clicks
   c. Blood volume—Hct, RBC count, Na^+, albumin
   d. Presence and quality of angina, shortness of breath, or palpitations
   e. Activity tolerance and relation to angina
   f. ECG—arrhythmias, evidence of past MI, hypertrophy
   g. Signs/symptoms of venous engorgement
      (1) Systemic—neck vein distention, edema (dependent or periorbital), hepatomegaly
      (2) Pulmonary—dyspnea, rales, cyanosis
   h. Cardiac isoenzymes
   i. Weight
5. Respiratory status
   a. History of COPD or other respiratory disease
   b. Rate, rhythm, quality of respirations; auscultate for rales, rhonchi, wheezing; evaluate for pulmonary edema or pulmonary venous engorgement

c. History of orthopnea
6. Renal status
    a. History of renal dysfunction or related kidney disease
    b. Adequacy of urine output
    c. Serum electrolytes; urine electrolytes and osmolality
    d. Presence of edema or weight gain
7. Temperature
8. Patient/family's knowledge related to hospitalization
    a. Comprehension of patient's cardiac disease and prognosis
    b. Comprehension of angioplasty procedure and risks involved
    c. Ability to recognize their anxiety and fears
9. Postangioplasty assessment
    a. Cardiovascular
        (1) Adequate cardiac output—BP, urine output, LOC
        (2) Heart rate and rhythm; ECG changes, noting particularly ST segment changes
        (3) Peripheral perfusion—warmth, color, pulses of extremities
        (4) Signs/symptoms of venous engorgement or heart failure
        (5) If angina occurs, note intensity and duration
        (6) Cardiac isoenzymes
    b. Respiratory—same as before procedure
    c. Renal
        (1) Urine output—osmotic diuresis may occur in response to radiographic contrast medium
        (2) Serum electrolytes—hypokalemia may potentiate ventricular ectopy
    d. Catheterization site—note amount of bleeding, hematoma formation, or presence of pain
    e. Perfusion of catheterized extremity—warmth, color, quality of pulse as compared to preangioplasty; sensation

f. Signs of prolonged clotting time/excessive bleeding related to streptokinase administration
    (1) Bleeding and excessive hematoma formation at catheterization site
    (2) Abnormal clotting profile
    (3) Bleeding around IV sites
    (4) Coffee ground emesis or black, tarry stools
    (5) Urine tests positive for RBC

GOALS

1. Reduction in patient/family's anxiety and fears resulting from verbalization opportunities and having information about own cardiac disease and procedures
2. Stable cardiovascular status
    a. Adequate cardiac output and perfusion
    b. Absence of arrhythmias
    c. Absence of bleeding—Hct and clotting profile within normal limits; absence of bleeding or thrombosis of femoral artery
    d. Absence of angina
    e. Adequate perfusion to catheterized extremity
    f. Absence of venous engorgement
    g. Cardiac isoenzymes within normal limits
3. Optimal respiratory function, with adequate oxygenation and ventilation
4. Absence of pulmonary edema or emboli
5. Adequate urine output
6. Fluid and electrolyte balance within normal limits; serum electrolytes within normal limits
7. Absence of infection
8. Absence of reaction to radiographic contrast medium
9. Patient/family demonstrates understanding of cardiac disease, prognosis, medications, and behaviors to promote health (diet, activity, stress reduction)

POTENTIAL PROBLEMS	EXPECTED OUTCOMES	NURSING ACTIVITIES

■ Patient/family's anxiety and fears related to
Cardiac disease
Hospitalization
Angioplasty
Emergency CABG
Insufficient information regarding procedure
	■ Reduction in patient/family's anxiety and fears with provision of information and encouragement
	Patient/family demonstrates understanding of risks and potential outcomes of TCA
		■ Assess patient/family's anxiety level and internal support system
		Evaluate patient/family's knowledge of cardiac disease and provide appropriate information
		Orient patient/family to preparation for procedure
		  Chest radiograph, ECG, blood specimens
		  Medications (to be given before, during, and after)
		  NPO after midnight
		Explain monitoring and nursing care after procedure
		  Frequent measurement of vital signs
		  Immobilization of catheterized extremity
		  ECG
		  Coughing and deep breathing exercises during period of bed rest
		  Medications
		Ensure that physician has explained procedure, risks, and outcomes of TCA; in some institutions, this will be done by nurse
		Assess patient/family's understanding of procedure and possible complications

POTENTIAL PROBLEMS	EXPECTED OUTCOMES	NURSING ACTIVITIES
		Encourage patient to verbalize fears related to Cardiac disease Angioplasty, which may be unsuccessful Possible emergency CABG
■ Decreased cardiac output and perfusion related to Reaction to contrast medium Heart failure MI Arrhythmias Distal coronary occlusion	■ Adequate cardiac output and perfusion Absence of angina Absence of venous engorgement	■ Prevent by maintaining adequate IV hydration during procedure; check for history of reaction to contrast medium Provide ongoing assessment before, during, and after procedure of BP Heart rate and rhythm on cardiac monitor; observe for arrhythmias and signs of myocardial ischemia (S-T segment elevation or depression, T wave changes) Respiratory rate and rhythm Monitor for evidence of decreased cardiac output Hypotension, weak peripheral pulses Tachycardia Cool, clammy skin Decreased capillary filling Decreased urine output Altered LOC Monitor for aforementioned signs continuously during procedure, then q15 min for 1 to 2 hours or until stable, then q2-4 hr and as indicated Keep epinephrine, atropine, and nitroglycerin on standby in event of reaction to contrast medium or distal coronary occlusion Notify physician immediately of Alterations in BP Arrhythmias Evidence of decreased systemic perfusion Monitor for signs and symptoms of MI Angina unrelieved by three doses of sublingual nitroglycerin Alterations in BP and P Arrhythmias, S-T segment elevation, and/or T wave changes Shortness of breath, sweating, nausea and vomiting, anxiety or sense of impending doom *See* STANDARD 12 *Acute myocardial infarction* STANDARD 15 *Heart failure (low cardiac output)* STANDARD 21 *Arrhythmias*
■ Cardiac arrhythmias related to Reaction to contrast medium Myocardial ischemia or MI Electrolyte imbalance Severe anxiety reaction	■ Absence or resolution of arrhythmias Adequate cardiac output	■ Assess for presence of predisposing factors Obtain history related to injected dye procedures (note signs and symptoms of allergic reaction) Electrolyte imbalance Anxiety related to procedure and cardiac disease Obtain 12 lead ECG before angioplasty to establish baseline rhythm for patient Monitor cardiac rhythm continuously during procedure, and at least 16 hours afterwards Assess pulses for regularity, rate, quality, and perfusion Monitor ECG for S-T segment changes Notify physician if arrhythmias or predisposing factors occur Institute therapy as ordered and monitor for response *See* STANDARD 21 *Arrhythmias* STANDARD 12 *Acute myocardial infarction*
■ Prolonged or refractory angina related to Coronary spasm MI Distal coronary occlusion	■ Absence or resolution of angina Cardiac isoenzymes within normal limits	■ Prevent by administering heparin and dextran, as ordered, to prevent thrombus formation Prevent by administering sublingual nitroglycerin and oral calcium channel blocker as ordered Maintain bed rest for 24 hours or longer after procedure, if indicated

POTENTIAL PROBLEMS	EXPECTED OUTCOMES	NURSING ACTIVITIES

		If angina occurs, monitor
		   Duration, location, radiation, and quality of chest pain
		   BP, P, R (before and after nitroglycerin administration)
		   ECG for sustained S-T segment elevations or T wave changes
		Notify physician of any anginal or hypotensive episodes
		If refractory angina occurs, see Standard 11, *Angina pectoris*
		If distal coronary occlusion occurs, patient may require emergency CABG; see Standard 27, *Cardiac surgery*
		If MI occurs, see Standard 12, *Acute myocardial infarction*

■ Inadequate perfusion of catheterized extremity	■ Adequate perfusion of extremity, with full pulses and good color	■ Monitor (before, during, and after procedure) for
		   Palpable pulses of extremity; note decreased or absent pulses
		   Warm, even color (no mottling)
		   Sensation and strength comparable to other extremity
		For care of arterial catheterization site, see Standard 26, *Cardiac catheterization*

■ Respiratory insufficiency related to
  Reaction to contrast medium
  Pulmonary edema
  Pulmonary emboli
	■ Absence of respiratory distress
	  Adequate oxygenation and ventilation
	  Absence of venous engorgement or pulmonary edema
	  Absence of pulmonary embolus
		■ Prevent by turning patient and encouraging patient to cough and deep breathe
		Monitor respiratory rate, rhythm, and quality and breath sounds before, during, and after procedure
		Note presence of signs and symptoms of dyspnea, tachypnea, hypoxia
		Monitor arterial blood gas results (note hypoxemia, hypercapnia, or hypocapnia)
		If distress occurs on dye injection, physician will discontinue injection; monitor for bronchospasm or laryngospasm; have intubation equipment available and ready for use
		Monitor for signs and symptoms of pulmonary edema
		   Rales, wheezing, dyspnea, tachypnea, hypoxemia, cough (often producing copious blood-tinged sputum)
		   Signs of venous congestion
		Notify physician of any of aforementioned abnormalities and administer therapy as ordered; monitor patient's response
		
		See STANDARD 1 *Pulmonary edema of cardiac origin*
		      STANDARD 2 *Acute respiratory failure*
		Monitor for signs and symptoms of pulmonary embolus
		   Sudden onset of chest pain
		   Dyspnea
		   Signs and symptoms of hypoxia
		
		See STANDARD 31 *Embolic phenomena*
		Notify physician of any of aforementioned abnormalities, and alter therapeutic regimen as ordered; monitor patient's response

■ Decreased renal function related to
  Contrast medium
  Decreased cardiac output
  Fluid imbalance
	■ Adequate urine output
	  Urine output greater than 30 ml/hour
		■ Prevent by administering fluids to maintain adequate cardiac output and renal perfusion/urine output, as ordered
		Monitor signs of adequate cardiac output
		   Continuously during procedure
		      BP, P, peripheral perfusion
		      Urine output
		      LOC
		   Then q1-2 hr until transfer to floor, and q2-4 hr thereafter
		Monitor for presence of renal dysfunction secondary to contrast medium
		   Urine output
		   Urine/serum electrolytes and osmolality
		   Serum creatinine and BUN
		Notify physician of abnormalities in any of aforementioned; administer therapy as ordered and monitor patient's response
		
		See STANDARD 52 *Acute renal failure*

POTENTIAL PROBLEMS	EXPECTED OUTCOMES	NURSING ACTIVITIES

▪ Bleeding related to alteration in normal clotting process if streptokinase infusion is given	▪ Absence or resolution of bleeding at arterial catheterization and IV sites
	Hct and clotting profile within normal limits
	Absence of cerebral or internal bleeding
		▪ Prevent or reduce possibility of bleeding during streptokinase therapy by
		    Immobilizing catheterized extremity to decrease hematoma formation or bleeding at catheterization site
		    Checking site q1 hr for bleeding and applying pressure if it occurs
		    Administering no injections (subcutaneously or IM), anticoagulants, or antiplatelet aggregating agents during streptokinase therapy
		Monitor BP, cardiac rhythm, and respiratory rate q1 hr
		Monitor initial and ongoing peripheral pulses, warmth, color, and sensation of extremities; monitor q1 hr during infusion, then q1 hr for 4 hours after discontinuing infusion
		Monitor baseline and ongoing lab parameters, including Hct and clotting profile; all blood specimens should be drawn through a arterial catheter or heparin lock
		Administer blood products as ordered by physician; monitor response to therapy
		Monitor for signs and symptoms of internal bleeding; test urine, emesis, and stools for blood
		Inspect IV sites and arterial catheter sites q1 hr
		Monitor for signs and symptoms of cerebral bleeding
		    Weakness, paralysis (usually unilateral) of extremities
		    Unilateral pupil changes
		    Change in LOC
		    Nuchal rigidity
		    Speech disturbance—dysphasia, aphasia
		Continue to monitor for signs and symptoms of bleeding secondary to streptokinase infusion until clotting values return to baseline
		If bleeding occurs from an intraarterial or venous catheter site, it may be necessary to apply pressure with gauze soaked in aminocaproic acid (Amicar), as ordered; if bleeding is severe, streptokinase infusion will be discontinued
		Observe for allergic reaction to streptokinase
		    Bronchospasm and dyspnea
		    Cyanosis
		    Convulsions or loss of consciousness
		If allergic reaction occurs
		    Stop infusion but maintain IV line
		    Provide ventilatory support and notify physician
		    Administer therapy as ordered

▪ Bleeding at arterial catheterization site	▪ Absence or resolution of bleeding	▪ Prevent by maintaining bed rest and extension of catheterized extremity for at least 8 hours following catheterization (or as ordered)
		Monitor for
		    Pulses, warmth, strength, and sensation of catheterized extremity
		    Bleeding or hematoma formation at catheterization site
		If bleeding or hematoma formation occurs, apply pressure and notify physician

▪ Infection of catheterization site or intracardiac structures (e.g., endocarditis)	▪ Catheterization site infection free Absence of redness, inflammation, or drainage Afebrile Absence of cardiac murmur and signs of clinical infection	▪ Prevent by changing catheterization site dressing when bleeding or drainage occurs; maintain aseptic technique when changing dressing Monitor site for redness, inflammation, or drainage Monitor temperature q4 hr Notify physician if catheterization site becomes red, inflamed, and/or develops purulent drainage; administer therapy as ordered and monitor patient's response

POTENTIAL PROBLEMS	EXPECTED OUTCOMES	NURSING ACTIVITIES
		Monitor for signs and symptoms of endocarditis
		New cardiac murmur
		Diaphoresis, fever, chills
		Anorexia, weight loss
		Malaise
		Arthralgias
		Positive blood cultures
		Notify physician of presence of new cardiac murmur and/or evidence of clinical infection
		If endocarditis occurs
		Administer antibiotic therapy as ordered
		Monitor
		BP, P, cardiac rhythm, urine output
		Heart sounds for increasing regurgitation or insufficiency
		Temperature
		See STANDARD 26 *Cardiac catheterization*
		STANDARD 61 *Infection control in the critical care unit*
		STANDARD 19 *Endocarditis*

■ Insufficient information related to
  Recommended activity level
  Diet
  Medications
  Prognosis
  Possible restenosis of treated coronary artery
	■ Identifies appropriate diet and foods to avoid
	Describes activity progression and work simplification techniques
	Accurately describes actions and side effects of medications
	Identifies risks factors and methods for reducing stress
		■ Review appropriate diet with patient/family (e.g., sodium-restricted diet)
		Discuss activity level and appropriate resumption of activities for patient
		Review all medications including name, purpose, dosage and schedule, potential side effects
		Encourage patient/family to notify physician if unrelieved episodes of angina occur; include phone number and person to call in emergency
		Provide opportunity for patient/family to discuss anxiety and fears related to resuming activities, prognosis, and discharge regimen
		Discuss modifying life-style to reduce risk factors (i.e., stress, smoking, obesity, hypertension)

		See STANDARD 27 *Cardiac surgery*
		STANDARD 12 *Acute myocardial infarction*
		STANDARD 11 *Angina pectoris*

CARDIOMYOPATHIES

Cardiomyopathy is a disease of the heart muscle. It may be classified according to etiology and pathophysiology. The cause is often unknown or obscure but may be identified with a primary or secondary process. Involvement of the heart alone is called *primary cardiomyopathy*. The cause of this primary form may be known or unknown (idiopathic). When dysfunction of other organ systems is associated with evidence of cardiomyopathy, then *secondary cardiomyopathy* is present. The pathophysiology of cardiomyopathy may be divided into three distinct groups: (1) congestive cardiomyopathy, which is considered a systolic dysfunction; (2) hypertrophic cardiomyopathy, which is considered a diastolic or obstructive process; and (3) restrictive cardiomyopathy, which is considered a diastolic dysfunction. Each group is characterized by a particular form of cardiac dysfunction, clinical picture, and appropriate therapeutic regimen.

Congestive cardiomyopathy is the most common form. It is a disease that involves the myocardium and results in a markedly dilatated left ventricle, low cardiac output, and poor systolic function. Mild to moderate regurgitation may be present. The heart is globular with poor contraction, which results in a markedly reduced ejection fraction. The myocardium is pale with areas of fibrosis but no significant hypertrophy. The endocardium may be thickened with thrombus formation. The coronary arteries are usually patent.

Toxic, infectious, and metabolic abnormalities have frequently been cited as causes of myocardial destruction resulting in congestive cardiomyopathy. Alcohol is a commonly recognized toxic agent for certain individuals. It is still unclear why some alcohol abusers develop congestive cardiomyopathy and others do not. It is believed that alcohol directly affects the heart by depressing myocardial function and thus decreasing myocardial contractility and cardiac output. The patient commonly presents with congestive heart failure, cardiomegaly, and arrhythmias.

Viruses are another cause of congestive cardiomyopathy. The relationship between viral myocarditis and congestive cardiomyopathy is being investigated. Viruses currently implicated in the development of congestive cardiomyopathy are coxsackievirus B, poliovirus, and influenzavirus. Cardiomyopathies have also been linked with endocrinopathies, electrolyte imbalances, and nutritional deficiencies. Hyperthyroidism, pheochromocytoma, beriberi, and kwashiorkor are examples of diseases associated with the development of congestive cardiomyopathy.

Another form of congestive cardiomyopathy is peripartum or postpartum cardiomyopathy. The cause is unknown, but this type of cardiomyopathy manifests itself more commonly in multiparous women over the age of 30 years, women who are delivering twins, and women who show signs of toxemia. Patients are at risk during the last month of pregnancy or the first 5 months postpartum. The patient typically presents with signs of left heart failure, including moderate respiratory distress.

Patients with congestive cardiomyopathy are usually hospitalized because of atrial and ventricular arrhythmias, conduction disturbances, mitral regurgitation, embolic phenomena, pulmonary congestion, or consequences of low cardiac output. Therapy specific for congestive cardiomyopathy includes treating the underlying factors, e.g., alcoholism, viruses, and metabolic abnormalities, and providing cardiovascular support, e.g., hemodynamic manipulation with preload and afterload adjustment, antiarrhythmic therapy, and positive inotropic support.

Hypertrophic cardiomyopathy is the second most common type of cardiomyopathy. It is characterized by muscular hypertrophy that affects the heart muscle, predominantly the ventricular septum. Left ventricular outflow tract obstruction may or may not be present. Hypertrophic cardiomyopathy with obstruction is called idiopathic hypertrophic subaortic stenosis (IHSS).

Hypertrophic cardiomyopathy does not produce dilatation as seen with the congestive form. Overall heart size is normal or nearly normal. The ventricular walls become rigid because of the overgrowth of heart muscle. In the early stage, myocardial contractility is augmented and the ejection fraction is increased. A greater percentage of blood volume is ejected earlier in systole. Cardiac output may be normal, high, or low. When cardiac output is normal or high, the patient may have no symptoms and may remain undiagnosed for years before deterioration of cardiac function is seen, and cardiac output falls.

The cause of hypertrophic cardiomyopathy is not known for certain. A familial form of inheritance and an HLA-antigen linkage has been recognized in about one third of these patients. Clinically, features of hypertrophic cardiomyopathy are variable. The disease process may be stable for a number of years or it may gradually progress after the onset of symptoms. Symptoms include dyspnea on exertion, anginal chest pain, presyncope (dizziness), and syncope. Sudden death from a cardiac arrhythmia may occur. The aim of treatment for IHSS is to decrease the obstruction. Measures to aid in this reduction include the use of beta blockers (e.g., propranolol) and calcium antagonists (e.g., verapamil), limiting or restricting physical activity, and reducing weight in obese patients.

Restrictive cardiomyopathy is the rarest form. It is characterized by abnormal ventricular compliance and increased ventricular diastolic pressures. The myocardium, endocardium, and subendocardium are infiltrated with fibroelastic tissue. This infiltration results in a rigid heart that does not distend well in diastole nor completely contract in systole. The result is a low cardiac output and eventually congestive failure.

A unique clinical presentation of restrictive cardiomyopathy is not recognized. This rare form may be easily misdiagnosed as constrictive pericarditis. Treatment of restrictive cardiomyopathy is focused on symptomatic relief. This includes the use of diuretics, digitalis, and a low-sodium diet.

The patient with a diagnosis of cardiomyopathy has a serious, lifelong condition with an overall poor prognosis. The disease may remain stable for years, it may progress slowly, or sudden death may occur. The goal of therapy is the maintenance of hemodynamic stability to control symptoms and allow an optimal quality of life. When conservative medical measures provide insufficient support of cardiac function, cardiac transplantation may be considered in appropriate surgical candidates.

ASSESSMENT

1. Chief complaint and history of present illness
2. Historical and current data necessary to rule out other conditions, such as
   a. Hypertension
   b. Congenital or valvular defects
   c. Constrictive pericarditis
   d. Ischemic heart disease
   e. Immunological disorders
   f. Toxemia
3. Historical and current data to assess other potential causes of cardiomyopathy
   a. Alcohol ingestion
   b. Viral infections
   c. Pregnancy
   d. Medications
   e. Endocrine disorders
   f. Nutritional disorders
   g. Electrolyte disorders
4. Family history of sudden death in young individuals and/or hypertrophic cardiomyopathy
5. Signs and symptoms of
   a. Dyspnea on exertion
   b. Syncope
   c. Dizziness
   d. Palpitations
   e. Chest pain
   f. Fatigue
   g. Anxiety
   h. Depression
   i. Denial
6. Parameters
   a. General appearance
   b. LOC
   c. BP
   d. P
   e. Heart sounds
   f. Jugular venous pressures
   g. Hepatojugular reflux
   h. Presence or absence and quality of arterial and peripheral pulses
   i. Presence of edema, varicosities, claudication, and thrombophlebitis
   j. Respiratory rate, dyspnea, orthopnea, paroxysmal nocturnal dyspnea, exertional dyspnea, cyanosis, clubbing, hemoptysis, cough, breath sounds, and adventitious sounds
   k. Weight, fluid balance, and urine output
   l. Temperature
7. Lab data
   a. CBC with sedimentation rate
   b. Hgb and Hct
   c. Prothrombin time and partial thromboplastin time
   d. Serial cardiac enzymes and isoenzymes
   e. Electrolyte levels
   f. Glucose
   g. BUN/creatinine clearance
   h. Lipid profile
   i. Protein and albumin levels
   j. Blood gas levels
   k. Cultures
   l. Viral titers
   m. Thyroid function tests
   n. Drug levels
   o. Urine sodium and potassium levels and routine urinalysis
8. Noninvasive methods
   a. Radiography
   b. Echocardiography
   c. Angiocardiography

d. Phonocardiography

e. Vectorcardiography

f. Multigated acquisition scanning (radioisotope)

9. Invasive methods

  a. Right heart catheterization

  b. PAP

  c. PCWP

  d. CVP

  e. Cardiac output and ejection fraction

  f. Intraarterial pressure

  g. Cardiac catheterization

  h. Coronary arteriography

  i. Ventriculography

10. Continuous ECG monitoring and daily and prn 12 lead ECG for

  a. Arrhythmias

  b. Axis deviation

  c. Drug effects

  d. Characteristic changes of biventricular hypertrophy and dilatation

  e. Changes indicative of myocardial ischemia

11. Signs and symptoms of complications

  a. Atrial and ventricular arrhythmias

  b. Emboli

  c. Infection

  d. Infective endocarditis (occurs with IHSS)

  e. Drug toxicity

  f. Risk with subsequent pregnancies

  g. Sudden death

12. Information regarding patient/family

  a. Knowledge of disease and treatment modalities

b. Perception of and reaction to diagnosis and prognosis

c. Health beliefs

d. Support systems

e. Reaction to death and dying, if appropriate

f. Presence of disturbance in body image, self-esteem, role performance, and personal identity

GOALS

1. Symptomatic stability

2. Reduction or control of anxiety, denial, and/or depression

3. Electrophysiological stability

4. Hemodynamic stability

5. Absence of complications

6. Before discharge the patient/family

  a. Verbalizes knowledge of the disease process

  b. Identifies pertinent signs/symptoms requiring medical/nursing attention

  c. Demonstrates skill in counting pulse rate and verbalizes his/her norm

  d. Verbalizes knowledge of prescribed activity limit, exercises, diet, and medications

  e. Uses appropriate other resources of the health care team (social service, home care, Meals on Wheels, occupational and/or physical therapy, and mental health counseling)

  f. Identifies the need for continued close medical/nursing follow-up

  g. Demonstrates correct CPR technique

POTENTIAL PROBLEMS	EXPECTED OUTCOMES	NURSING ACTIVITIES

■ Arrhythmias related to cardiomyopathies	■ Electrophysiological stability
	Optimal cardiac rhythm
	Adequate cardiac output
		■ Prevent by monitoring for predisposing factors and administer treatments to resolve arrhythmias or predisposing factors as ordered (e.g., hypoxia, electrolyte imbalance)
		Maintain continuous cardiac monitoring
		  Observe for clear P waves indicating atrial activity
		  Note that QRS amplitude is sufficient to trigger cardiac monitor rate meter
		  Patient's chest should be loosely covered or exposed
		  Place electrodes to allow access for defibrillation paddles if necessary
		  Place electrodes to permit monitoring of
		    MCL_1 or modified V_1—useful for distinguishing left and right bundle branch blocks; distinguishes left and right ventricular ectopic beats
		    Leads I and II—axis shifts
		  Identify and record lead selected for monitoring
		  Set rate alarms; check alarm system regularly
		Assess skin condition—skin irritation may develop in susceptible patients with prolonged use of electrodes

POTENTIAL PROBLEMS	EXPECTED OUTCOMES	NURSING ACTIVITIES

		Note rhythm changes; inform physician
		  Document with rhythm strip
		  Assess any hemodynamic changes
		  Systematically inspect rhythm strip
		  Obtain 12 lead ECG
		Administer treatments for arrhythmias as ordered
		Assess patient's response to treatment
		Have emergency equipment readily accessible
		Observe particularly for arrhythmias and ECG changes that occur with greater frequency with each form of cardiomyopathy
		  Congestive cardiomyopathy—atrial and ventricular arrhythmias, conduction disturbances, left bundle branch block
		  Hypertrophic cardiomyopathy—sudden death occurs often from lethal ventricular arrhythmias; other associated ECG abnormalities include left axis deviation, septal Q waves, and occasionally Wolff-Parkinson-White preexcitation abnormalities, conduction defects, and left atrial enlargement
		  Restrictive cardiomyopathy—ECG abnormalities include low QRS voltage, conduction abnormalities, and rhythm disturbances

■ Decreased cardiac output
  Related to decreased contractile function
  Associated with congestive cardiomyopathy
	■ Increase in cardiac output
	Decrease in afterload (decrease in impedance to ejection)
	Decrease in preload (decrease in ventricular volume)
		■ Assess for signs and symptoms of left heart failure
		  Anxiety
		  Insomnia
		  Elevated PAP and PCWP
		  Tachycardia
		  Gallop rhythm
		  Diaphoresis
		  Air hunger
		  Dyspnea
		  Basilar rales
		  Wheezing
		  Cough with frothy sputum
		  Hyperventilation
		  Respiratory acidosis
		  Cyanosis or pallor
		Assess for signs and symptoms of right heart failure
		  Oliguria
		  Dependent pitting edema
		  Elevated CVP
		  Venous distention
		  Bounding pulses
		  Arrhythmias
		  Hepatosplenomegaly
		Assess for fluid volume overload
		  Weigh daily; note increase
		  Measure intake and output hourly
		  Calculate a 24-hour fluid balance; note positive balance
		  Maintain fluid restriction as ordered
		  Monitor serum/urine electrolytes and creatinine, BUN, Hct, and specific gravity
		  Collect 24-hour urine specimens as ordered
		Assess for signs of edema
		  Measure extremities as indicated
		  Note increase in size
		Auscultate lung fields for adventitious sounds, especially rales
		Report abnormalities to physician and alter therapy as ordered
		Observe for compensatory responses—vasoconstriction caused by increased sympathetic tone and increased levels of angiotensin; salt and water retention caused by decreased glomerular filtration; and increased activity of renin-angiotensin-aldosterone system
		  Assess for signs and symptoms of edema, decreased urine output, and slight increase in BP

POTENTIAL PROBLEMS	EXPECTED OUTCOMES	NURSING ACTIVITIES

		Reduce workload on heart
		  Place patient in high Fowler's or semi-Fowler's position
		  Administer humidified O_2 as ordered
		  Administer sedatives as ordered
		  Provide environment conducive to rest
		    Dim lights at regular intervals
		    Schedule visiting hours to provide for adequate rest
		    Allow patient to rest between nursing activities
		    Anticipate and meet patient needs promptly
		    Assist with planned, graduated levels of activity
		Assess hemodynamic status
		  LOC
		  P
		  Peripheral and arterial pulses
		  PAP
		  PCWP
		  BP; Intraarterial pressure; MAP
		  Cardiac output
		  Systemic vascular resistance
		Administer therapeutic agents as ordered by physician
		  Agent such as nitroprusside, which has a direct dilating action on both arteriolar and venous beds, is usually used
		Assess for therapeutic response to nitroprusside—decreased preload reflected in decreased PCWP; decreased systemic vascular resistance results in increase in cardiac output
		Administer digitalis preparations as ordered to enhance contractility
		Following therapeutic response with IV nitroprusside administer an oral afterload reducing agent, as ordered, which promotes arteriolar dilatation
		Continue to observe hemodynamic parameters for afterload reduction and SVR reduction
		Monitor drug levels of therapeutic agents to avoid untoward effects and toxicity
		  Assess for signs of digoxin toxicity, especially in presence of hypokalemia
		
		See STANDARD 25 *Hemodynamic monitoring*
		      STANDARD 15 *Heart failure (low cardiac output)*

■ Decreased cardiac output related to left ventricular outflow tract obstruction associated with *hypertrophic cardiomyopathy*	■ Adequate cardiac output
	Absence of aggravation of obstruction
		■ Avoid conditions that increase obstruction and decrease ventricular circulation
		  Digitalis preparations
		  Beta-adrenergic stimulators (e.g., isoproterenol, dopamine)
		  Nitroglycerin
		  Blood loss
		  Diuretics
		  Nonsinus rhythms with atrial fibrillation or flutter; junctional or ventricular rhythms; tachycardia
		  Valsalva maneuvers
		  Sitting or standing suddenly
		  Exercise
		Reduce emotional stress
		Assist patient/family in identifying sources of stress
		  Identify recent life events, e.g., by use of Social Readjustment Rating Scale
		  Allow patient/family time to verbalize
		  Allow patient/family time to develop trust in nurse caring for patient by having same nurse take care of patient/family
		Encourage patient/family in importance of avoiding stress to avoid added burden to cardiovascular system
		Assist patient/family in identifying and developing coping methods

POTENTIAL PROBLEMS	EXPECTED OUTCOMES	NURSING ACTIVITIES
		Intervene with appropriate measures to lessen effects of stressors
		Promote factors that increase cardiac output by decreasing obstruction and increasing ventricular filling, as ordered
		Expansion of blood volume
		Supine or squatting position
		Beta blocking agents, e.g., propranolol
		Alpha stimulators, e.g., phenylephrine, methoxamine
		Monitor
		BP, P
		Pulses—note quality
		LOC
		Urine output
		CVP, PAP, PCWP, if available
		Cardiac output measurements, if available
		Systemic vascular resistance
		Notify physician of abnormalities in aforementioned and alter therapy as ordered
		Monitor patient's response
■ Respiratory insufficiency related to pulmonary vascular congestion associated with increased left ventricular filling pressure	■ Absence or resolution of pulmonary vascular congestion Absence of respiratory distress Adequate oxygenation and ventilation with arterial blood gas levels within patient's normal limits	■ Monitor PAP and PCWP Monitor for signs of pulmonary venous congestion
		Dyspnea
		Rales
		Cough
		S_3
		Elevated PCWP
		Determine cardiac output
		Anticipate further complications and onset of pulmonary edema
		Observe for increased dyspnea or coughing
		Note change in LOC
		Assess for increased distribution of rales
		Note presence of frothy, blood-tinged sputum
		Determine elevated PCWP—above 25 to 30 mm Hg
		Inform physician of any abnormalities
		Position for cardiac rest using Fowler's or semi-Fowler's position
		Administer digoxin as ordered and note side effects, e.g., nausea, vomiting, anorexia, headache, malaise, and arrhythmias
		Identify factors that aggravate digoxin toxicity, e.g., diuretics, renal failure, hypokalemia, and diarrhea
		Administer diuretics as ordered and monitor for side effects, e.g., weakness, muscle cramps, hypovolemia, electrolyte disturbance—especially hypokalemia
		Administer K^+ replacement as ordered
		Weigh patient daily (at same time each day)
		Maintain intake and output record with 24-hour fluid balance record
		Maintain fluid restriction as ordered
		Monitor for signs and symptoms of respiratory distress
		Monitor arterial blood gas levels for hypoxemia
		Auscultate lung fields and check for adventitious sounds
		Monitor results of chest radiograph, but remember that radiographic changes can be delayed up to 24 hours after onset of pulmonary congestion
		Administer O_2 by face mask; use low-flow rates for patient with COPD
		Anticipate need for the following therapy and administer as ordered
		Diuretics
		Digoxin
		Aminophylline
		Morphine sulfate
		Positive pressure breathing equipment

POTENTIAL PROBLEMS	EXPECTED OUTCOMES	NURSING ACTIVITIES
		Rotating tourniquets
		Advanced life support equipment
		Evaluate effectiveness of therapy and alter treatment if needed, as ordered
■ Chest pain related to left ventricular outflow tract obstruction associated with IHSS	■ Absence or resolution of chest pain	■ Assess for presence of pain
		Observe for verbal and nonverbal clues
		Encourage patient to inform health care team if pain occurs
		With occurrence of pain, assess the following (obtain clear description to assist in differentiation)
		Onset
		Quality
		Severity
		Site
		Radiation
		Influence of movement on deep inspiration
		Notify physician of pain and administer treatments as ordered for relief of pain
		Administer as ordered the following treatments to relieve or ameliorate outflow tract obstruction
		Limit or restrict physical activity
		Reduction of weight in obese patients
		Administer medications as ordered, e.g., verapamil and propranolol
		Avoid use of nitroglycerin in patient with IHSS—it worsens obstruction and may lead to syncope and sudden death
		Assess response of patient to medications and treatments
		Monitor for adverse side effects
■ Pulmonary embolism related to Immobility CHF Trauma to vessel wall associated with venipuncture Thrombus formation in heart associated with atrial fibrillation Obesity Older age groups	■ Absence or resolution of embolism	■ Assess for predisposing factors—venous stasis, hypercoagulate state, obesity, and older age
		Initiate preventive measures for high-risk patients
		Active or passive exercises as indicated for individual patients
		Apply elastic stockings—measure calf for correct size, remove q8 hr, prevent tourniquet effect with stockings
		Encourage patient to avoid straining and Valsalva maneuvers
		Provide for adequate fluid intake, as ordered
		Instruct patient to avoid crossing legs
		Demonstrate and encourage patient to perform deep breathing exercises
		Administer preventive anticoagulation as ordered
		Assist patient with early ambulation as ordered
		Assess for signs and symptoms of pulmonary embolus
		Anxiety
		Feeling of impending doom
		Tachypnea
		Diffuse chest discomfort
		Hemoptysis
		Tachycardia
		Elevation of PAP
		Fixed splitting of S_2
		Prepare patient for lung scan as ordered
		Administer O_2 supplements as ordered
		Administer anticoagulants as ordered
		Observe for signs of bleeding
		Monitor clotting profile
		Observe for complications
		Pulmonary infarction
		Pulmonary abscess
		Adult respiratory distress syndrome
		Arrhythmias
		Cerebrovascular occlusion

See STANDARD 31   *Embolic phenomena*

POTENTIAL PROBLEMS	EXPECTED OUTCOMES	NURSING ACTIVITIES
■ Systemic venous congestion related to elevated right ventricular filling pressure, right heart failure	■ Absence or resolution of symptoms of systemic venous congestion	■ Observe for symptoms of right heart failure 　Neck vein distention 　Peripheral edema 　Hepatomegaly 　Elevated CVP 　Administer diuretics as ordered 　　Monitor 　　　Intake and output 　　　Specific gravity 　　　Serum electrolytes 　　　BUN 　　　Creatinine 　　　Hct 　　　Daily weight 　Administer K$^+$ supplement for hypokalemia as ordered 　Maintain low-sodium diet and fluid restriction as ordered 　Administer O$_2$ as ordered 　Maintain bed rest to promote diuresis as ordered 　Elevate lower extremities when patient sits in chair 　Monitor CVP and cardiac output
■ Alteration in skin integrity related to 　Immobility 　Prolonged bed rest 　Nutritional deficit	■ Intact skin surface	■ Assess patient for increased risk of developing alteration in skin integrity, e.g., immobility, cachexia, bony prominences, incontinence, draining wounds, malnutrition, older age, edema, and radiation treatments 　Obtain and document baseline assessment of skin condition and assess daily 　Prevent skin alteration with high-risk patient by 　　Turning and positioning patient q2 hr and prn 　　Using appropriate skin preventive measures, but do not use as substitute for turning and positioning, e.g., air mattress, water bed, sheepskin, heel and elbow protectors, CircOlectric bed, and/or Stryker frame 　　Providing for adequate nutrition 　　　Assessing nutritional status of patient in conjunction with dietitian 　　　Using appropriate supplements as ordered, e.g., NG supplemental feedings; frequent high-calorie supplements PO as tolerated; hyperalimentation as ordered 　　　Assessing for progression to PO diet 　　Ongoing assessment and evaluation of planned diet 　　　Obtain daily weight 　　　Monitor protein, albumin, Hct, and Hgb 　　Maintain clean and dry skin 　Monitor for reddened or marked areas, or edematous areas 　Administer lotion to bony prominences q2 hr and use mild soap 　Use appropriate appliances for draining wounds/sites 　Observe for skin reactions to drugs, foods, and/or tape 　　Apply skin protector before use of adhesive tape, or use nonadhesive tape 　　Remove tape gently—do not pull 　Assess for increased activity level and progression associated with patient tolerance 　　Assist patient with passive/active ROM exercises 　　Assist patient with ambulation as early as possible, as ordered 　Evaluate interventions on daily basis 　Inform physician of any skin alteration
■ Infection related to 　Immobility 　Invasive lines 　Underlying cause of cardiomyopathy	■ Absence or resolution of infection	■ Prevent atelectasis by 　Auscultating lung fields and reporting adventitious sounds to physician 　Encouraging and assisting with coughing and deep breathing q2 hr while on bed rest and awake

POTENTIAL PROBLEMS	EXPECTED OUTCOMES	NURSING ACTIVITIES
		Turning patient q2 hr if immobile
		Providing chest physiotherapy q2 hr in selected patients
		Suctioning as needed
		Administering humidification—especially for patients with dried secretions
		Noting color, amount, and any foul odor of secretions
		Culturing as necessary for changes in sputum that suggest infection
		Obtaining radiograph as ordered by physician
		Auscultating lung fields following treatment
		Explaining importance of treatments to patient
		Prevent alteration in skin integrity
		Turn and position immobile patient q2 hr
		Apply lotion to bony prominences
		Identify patients at risk for skin alteration
		Use air mattress, sheepskin, heel protectors as necessary
		Provide adequate nutrition
		Assess for intact skin
		Prevent infection by maintaining strict aseptic technique during insertion and changing of invasive lines
		Change dressings daily and observe for signs of infection
		Change sites at least q4 days
		Change tubing and domes at least q48 hr
		Maintain closed system
		Maintain sterile technique with insertion of urinary catheter
		Administer antibiotics as ordered
		Check for drug reaction—rash, fever, bronchospasm; patient who suspects he/she is allergic to certain antibiotic may be skin tested
		Monitor for signs and symptoms suggestive of viral myocardiopathy
		Elevated coxsackie serotype B5 antibody titers
		Signs and symptoms of ischemic heart disease and rheumatic heart disease
		Monitor temperature, BP, P, and respiratory rate; report changes to physician and monitor for changes in lab data indicative of infectious process, e.g., increased WBC count with increased neutrophils
		Observe for temperature elevation, tachycardia, chills, or diaphoresis
		Keep patient warm and dry
		Institute cooling measures as ordered
		Use of hypothermia blanket requires frequent position changes and assessment for intact skin surface to avoid burns to patient's skin
		See STANDARD 61 *Infection control in the critical care unit*

■ Anxiety related to
  Fear of hospitalization
  Fear of loss of control
  Fear of death
	■ Patient identifies factors promoting fear and anxiety
	Patient identifies methods to cope with and/or resolve concerns
	Patient accepts help as needed
		■ Identify verbal and nonverbal cues of anxiety
		  Verbal cue—incessant talking, rapid speech, high-pitched voice
		  Nonverbal cue—excessive use of call bell
		Encourage patient to verbalize his/her feelings
		Assist patient to identify factors that contribute to his/her feeling of anxiety and fear
		Attempt to solve problems individually with patient
		Consult with resource individuals as necessary
		Maintain family support by allowing a family member to stay with patient when desired and/or appropriate
		Encourage development of trusting relationship between patient and nurse by having primary nurse assigned to patient
		Schedule frequent visits by nurse to diminish frequent calling by the patient
		Explain all procedures to patient/family
		Inform patient of his/her progress

POTENTIAL PROBLEMS	EXPECTED OUTCOMES	NURSING ACTIVITIES
		Keep explanations simple and brief, be prepared to offer repeated explanations Maintain calm work environment Demonstrate clinical expertise and flexibility Give sedatives and medications for sleep as ordered
■ Sleep disturbance related to fear and anxiety	■ Patient sleeps for specified periods	■ Provide environment that is conducive to sleep 　Dim lights 　Keep noise to minimum 　Maintain clean and dry environment 　Assist patient in assuming comfortable position 　Give patient a back rub 　Keep call bell within patient's reach Encourage patient to sleep by 　Alleviating pain 　Alleviating hunger 　Providing warm milk, if desired 　Administering sedative, as ordered Observe for signs of sleep deprivation 　Fatigue 　Irritability 　Time disorientation 　Behavioral changes 　Slurred speech 　Decreased muscle coordination 　Mild tremor 　Patient complains of lack of sleep Enhance sleep by 　Identifying patient's normal sleep pattern 　Establishing sense of trust and reminding patient that he/she is being monitored constantly, even while sleeping 　Attempting to identify any problems patient may have
■ Insufficient knowledge to comply with discharge regimen related to acute and chronic illness	■ Verbalizes and/or demonstrates pertinent information Verbalizes information necessary to comply with discharge regimen 　Activity 　Diet 　Medications 　Follow-up care Lists symptoms requiring medical attention Asks pertinent questions regarding self-care	■ Assess baseline level of knowledge of patient/family regarding 　Activity 　Diet 　Medications 　Follow-up care Discuss pertinent information to assist with effective discharge regimen Design teaching program to best meet needs of each individual patient/family Review with patient recommended activity regimen 　Discuss specific physical activity regimen with physician 　Discuss with patient/family significance of activity regulation related to decreasing myocardial work and increasing ventricular circulation 　Inform patient/family that patient should 　　Rest when feeling tired 　　Use work simplification techniques 　　Avoid or modify activity following stress or meals or in extremes of temperature 　　Avoid straining at stool 　　Use supine or squatting position to increase ventricular circulation and decrease obstruction with IHSS 　　Avoid sudden assumption of upright position, which would result in increase in obstruction and decrease in ventricular circulation with IHSS Discuss and distribute written material related to diet modification Discuss and distribute written materials related to medications 　Name and purpose 　Dosage

POTENTIAL PROBLEMS	EXPECTED OUTCOMES	NURSING ACTIVITIES
		Frequency—tailor to patient's routine schedule
		Side effects
		Inform patient/family that medications must not be stopped abruptly
		Inform patient/family of importance of taking medications despite possibility of feeling well
		Consult with physician before altering dose or discontinuing medications
		If appropriate, discuss pharmacologic management of IHSS
		Beta-adrenergic blocking agent commonly used is propranolol to ease ventricular obstruction
		Teach patient to count pulse before taking certain medications, and if it falls outside range set by physician, inform physician
		Inform diabetic patient that beta blocking agents may potentiate hypoglycemic effect of insulin and other oral hypoglycemic agents; in addition, beta blocking agents may mask hypoglycemic reactions by preventing symptoms of sweating and tachycardia
		Inform appropriate patients of factors related to beta blocking agents
		Asthma may worsen because of bronchial constriction
		Allergic rhinitis may be aggravated
		Discuss subacute infective endocarditis precautions before surgery, dental visits, or instrumentation—physician may order antibiotics
		Review follow-up information with patient/family
		Next scheduled appointment with physician
		Inform patient of the need for close nursing/medical follow-up
		Discuss future tests if ordered, e.g., Holter monitoring, exercise ECG, cardiac catheterization
		Encourage patient/family to ask questions and verbalize concerns
		Provide opportunities for demonstration of information given, e.g., selection of low-sodium foods, counting pulse, and family member providing CPR
		Assess potential for compliance with discharge regimen
		Provide phone number that patient/family may use to speak with nurse/physician for continued follow-up

See STANDARD 19   *Endocarditis*

HEART FAILURE
(LOW CARDIAC OUTPUT)

Heart failure occurs when the heart is unable to perform normally as a pump, which may render it unable to maintain a cardiac output sufficient to meet the body's needs at rest and/or during normal activity.

The multiple etiologies of heart failure can be organized into three major groups, depending on the way they interfere with ventricular function. These are as follows:

1. Conditions resulting in direct myocardial damage such as occurs with MI, myocarditis, myocardial fibrosis, or ventricular aneurysm.
2. Conditions resulting in ventricular overload, either by increasing the pressure against which the ventricle must work (afterload) or increasing the volume with which it must deal (preload). Increased afterload may be created by systemic or pulmonic hypertension, aortic or pulmonic stenosis, and coarctation of the aorta. Increased preload may occur with rapid infusion of IV solutions, mitral or aortic regurgitation, atrial or ventricular septal defects, and patent ductus arteriosus.
3. Conditions resulting in restriction to ventricular diastolic filling created by cardiac tamponade, constrictive pericarditis, or restrictive cardiomyopathies.

The ventricles may fail independently, but the most common cause of right heart failure is left heart failure. Right heart failure may result from pulmonary hypertension independent of left heart failure.

Failure of the ventricle results in an increase in the ventricular end diastolic filling pressure. The heart will attempt to compensate and maintain cardiac output through several mechanisms. These include increasing sympathetic nervous system activity, which results in an increase in heart rate, vascular resistance, and myocardial contractility; increasing contractility as a result of increased fiber length according to the Frank-Starling principle; and, chronically, increasing ventricular mass, resulting in ventricular hypertrophy. Hypertrophy is usually not evidenced in heart failure resulting from acute causes in critical care units unless there is preexisting heart disease.

Compensated heart failure occurs when these mechanisms are able to prevent an abnormal elevation of left ventricular end diastolic pressure and a fall in cardiac output below resting systemic requirements. Decompensation occurs as the left ventricular end diastolic filling pressure increases. If cardiac output declines with decompensation, then in addition to the pulmonary vascular congestion caused by the elevated left ventricular end diastolic pressure, there will also be a fall in renal perfusion pressure and a fall in glomerular filtration rate, which initiate renal compensatory mechanisms. The result is salt and water retention in an attempt to increase the effective intravascular volume to maintain normal renal perfusion pressure.

The early signs of cardiac failure, sinus tachycardia, S_3 gallop, dyspnea, and bibasilar rales are related to compensatory mechanisms as are many of the later complications. Recognition at this early stage with appropriate intervention may prevent complications such as arrhythmias, pulmonary edema, cardiogenic shock, and complications that occur as a result of congestion and ultimate dysfunction of organs other than the heart.

There are many degrees of heart failure, and the stage the patient is in will primarily determine the selection and aggressiveness of hemodynamic assessment and therapeutic intervention. Therapy is directed toward identifying and treating or removing precipitating or aggravating factors, reducing the work load on the heart, improving the force and efficiency of contraction, and treating the symptoms and complications resulting from congestion.

ASSESSMENT

1. History of rheumatic fever, congenital heart disease, valvular heart disease, coronary heart disease, systemic or pulmonic hypertension, myocardial disease, heart failure, endocarditis, constrictive pericarditis, infiltrative diseases, and pulmonary disease
2. Presence of factors that may precipitate or aggravate heart failure
   a. AMI
   b. Recent open heart surgery
   c. Arrhythmias
   d. Hemorrhage

e. Anemia
f. Respiratory infections
g. Pulmonary embolism
h. Thyrotoxicosis
i. Fever
j. Hypoxia
k. Excessive salt intake
l. Excessive or rapid administration of parenteral fluids
m. Emotional stress
n. Activity
o. Corticosteroid administration
p. Administration of drugs that may cause cardiac depression, such as propranolol or quinidine
3. Patient's preception of and reaction to diagnosis, progression of disease, assessment, and treatment modalities
4. Level of anxiety
5. Level of activity tolerance
6. Signs and symptoms of decreasing cardiac function
7. Signs and symptoms of pulmonary venous congestion
8. Signs and symptoms of systemic venous congestion
9. Monitor ECG for
   a. Arrhythmias
   b. P wave changes, indicating acute elevations in left atrial pressure
   c. Changes indicative of ventricular hypertrophy
   d. Changes indicative of myocardial damage, e.g., AMI or ischemia
   e. Drug effects
10. Lab data results of
    a. Electrolytes, particularly K^+
    b. BUN/creatinine clearance
    c. Blood gas levels
    d. Chest radiograph for cardiac dimensions and pulmonary congestion
    e. Cardiac catheterization
    f. Nuclear cardiac studies
    g. Echocardiography
    h. Drug levels, particularly digitalis
    i. Cultures
    j. Any other tests performed to evaluate precipitating or aggravating factors, e.g., cardiac enzymes or isoenzymes, thyroid or lung scans
11. Signs and symptoms of complications

a. Infection
b. Thromboembolism
c. Pulmonary edema
d. Cardiogenic shock
12. Ongoing and final evaluation of teaching program
13. Determinants of patient compliance with discharge regimen

GOALS

1. Hemodynamic stability
2. Absence of complications of congestion
   a. Pulmonary
   b. Systemic
   c. Renal
   d. Hepatic
   e. Intestinal
   f. Peripheral
3. Electrophysiological stability
4. Absence or resolution of complications of
   a. Infection
   b. Thromboembolic disease
   c. Pulmonary edema
   d. Cardiogenic shock
5. Patient's verbal and nonverbal behavior demonstrates reduction of anxiety with provision of information
6. Before discharge the patient/family*
   a. Demonstrates comprehension of the knowledge components of the teaching program when evaluated by testing or questioning
   b. Identifies own risk factors and/or precipitating factors, describing methods of modification or avoidance
   c. States information necessary for compliance with discharge regimen related to
      (1) Activity management
      (2) Diet
      (3) Medications
      (4) Follow-up care
   d. Accurately demonstrates skill of counting pulse, stating acceptable ranges of rate and rhythm; identifies when it is appropriate to check with physician or nurse before taking digoxin
   e. Lists symptoms requiring medical attention and appropriate actions to take to obtain it
   f. Asks pertinent questions regarding self-care

*Applies when chronic management is required.

POTENTIAL PROBLEMS	EXPECTED OUTCOMES	NURSING ACTIVITIES
■ Cardiac decompensation related to increased ventricular volume and filling pressure	■ Hemodynamic stability	■ Monitor closely for early signs and symptoms of heart failure in patient with predisposing history; early intervention and removal of aggravating factors may prevent further problems; symptom onset varies depending on ventricle involved, acute versus chronic nature, and cause
		Check BP for hypotension, pulsus alternans, and changes in pulse pressure
		Check P for compensatory tachycardia, rate and regularity, and pulsus alternans; check apical and radial pulses for deficit
		Observe for signs and symptoms of decreased perfusion
		Diaphoresis, cool skin
		Restlessness, confusion
		Cheyne-Stokes respirations
		Monitor intake and output and presence of nocturia for indication of decreased renal perfusion
		Check urine specific gravity
		Estimate diaphoretic fluid loss
		Report to physician if output is less than 30 ml/hour
		Obtain history of and observe for indications of decreasing activity tolerance and presence of fatigue (particularly significant if felt on awakening)
		Auscultate precordium or review chart for presence of S_3 and/or S_4 gallop; S_3 gallop can be normal in children and young adults
		Palpate apical impulse, noting position and quality; with ventricular hypertrophy, it becomes large and displaced to left
		Review 12 lead ECG for changes associated with ventricular hypertrophy and increased atrial filling pressure (prominent negative P waves in V_1 and V_2)
		Review chest radiograph results for evidence of ventricular hypertrophy and/or pulmonary congestion; radiographic changes can be delayed up to 24 hours after onset of pulmonary congestion
		Observe for signs and symptoms of pulmonary and systemic venous congestion listed in Problems, Pulmonary venous congestion and Systemic venous congestion
		Frequency of these observations dependent on degree of stability
		Treatment plan dependent on severity of failure
		Participate in identification and correction of aggravating factors
		AMI
		Pain
		Arrhythmias
		Hemorrhage
		Anemia
		Respiratory infections
		Pulmonary embolism
		Thyrotoxicosis
		Fever
		Hypoxia
		Excessive salt intake
		Excessive or rapid administration of parenteral fluids
		Emotional stress
		Activity
		Corticosteroid administration
		Administration of drugs that may cause cardiac depression, such as propranolol or quinidine
		If patient is receiving medications with negative inotropic effect, check with physician regarding discontinuing
		Ensure that emergency equipment is functioning and available at every shift
		If IV fluids or medications are ordered, use microdrip or infusion pump; avoid rapid or excessive hydration

POTENTIAL PROBLEMS	EXPECTED OUTCOMES	NURSING ACTIVITIES

		Institute measures to reduce work load of heart
		  Maintain bed rest; semi-Fowler or high Fowler position generally most comfortable and physiologically preferable, because venous return is decreased and lung expansion is increased
		  Organize care to allow frequent rest periods
		  Maintain quiet, controlled environment and approach patient with calm, confident, reassuring manner
		Administer medications as ordered
		  Agents to increase contractility and/or to decrease afterload or preload generally given
		  Monitor closely the effect of medication and for hypotension and arrhythmias
		  Invasive hemodynamic monitoring is essential for safe administration and therapeutic regulation with medications such as sodium nitroprusside, hydralazine, phentolamine, isoproterenol (Isuprel), or dopamine
		  Monitor pulmonary artery diastolic pressure or mean PCWP, reflecting left atrial and left ventricular diastolic filling pressures; filling pressures between 15 to 20 mm Hg are good for maintaining stroke volume; if filling pressures are above 20 mm Hg, myocardial O_2 demand probably exceeds benefit of improved stroke volume
		  Intraarterial pressure monitoring and cardiac output measurements may also be indicated
		Participate with insertion and monitoring of left ventricular assist devices, which may be indicated to prevent further deterioration until patient's condition is stabilized and/or surgical correction is undertaken
		Prepare patient for and monitor results of special studies to assess ventricular function if ordered
		
		See STANDARD 25 *Hemodynamic monitoring*
		      STANDARD 24 *Intraaortic balloon pumping (counterpulsation)*
		      STANDARD 26 *Cardiac catheterization*

■ Pulmonary venous congestion related to increased left ventricular filling pressure	■ Absence or resolution of pulmonary venous congestion and associated symptoms	■ Observe for signs and symptoms indicating pulmonary venous congestion
		  Dyspnea
		    Relate to level of activity and changing pattern; usually begins with exertion progressing to dyspnea at rest
		    Cough with dyspnea on exertion
		    Orthopnea—dyspnea occurring when patient is recumbent and relieved by patient sitting up
		    Paroxysmal nocturnal dyspnea—may or may not be associated with cough; extreme form of orthopnea; patient awakens breathless, which may be relieved in minutes by sitting or standing or may progress to pulmonary edema
		  Tachypnea
		  Auscultate lungs for presence of adventitious sounds q1-2 hr
		  Monitor results of chest radiograph for indications of pulmonary venous congestion; radiographic changes can be delayed up to 24 hours after onset of symptoms of pulmonary congestion
		  Monitor PCWP to determine left ventricular filling pressure
		Administer O_2 as ordered
		Continue measures to reduce left ventricular filling pressure identified in Problem, Cardiac decompensation

■ Systemic venous congestion related to increased right ventricular filling pressure and/or decreased renal perfusion pressure	■ Absence or resolution of systemic venous congestion and associated symptoms	■ Observe for signs and symptoms indicative of systemic venous congestion
		  Distention of neck veins
		  Peripheral or sacral edema
		  Ascites (more common with tamponade, constrictive pericarditis, or tricuspid stenosis)

POTENTIAL PROBLEMS	EXPECTED OUTCOMES	NURSING ACTIVITIES
		Hepatic congestion
		Right upper quadrant pain or tenderness
		Hepatomegaly
		Hepatic pulsation
		Jaundice
		Serum enzymes reflecting hepatic dysfunction
		Visceral congestion
		Anorexia
		Nausea
		Constipation
		Bloating
		Decreased urine output
		Increased BUN
		Proteinuria
		High urine specific gravity
		Pleural effusion (more common in right pleural space)
		Assess effect of systemic congestion on drug metabolism and excretion; adjust medication dosages as ordered
		Medications given PO may not be absorbed in presence of intestinal congestion
		Renal and hepatic congestion will interfere with metabolism and excretion
		Circulatory congestion reduces volume of distribution for medications, resulting in higher concentrations
		Administer diuretics to decrease intravascular volume as ordered
		Measure intake and output q2 hr; Foley catheter may be needed; check specific gravity
		Daily weights; notify physician if greater than 500 g/day
		Monitor lab results for BUN and electrolytes, particularly K^+ and Na^+
		Administer K^+ supplements if ordered
		If patient is receiving digoxin, observe closely for toxicity, particularly in presence of hypokalemia
		Observe for side effects of diuretic therapy; these vary with type used; loop diuretic is most potent
		Hypokalemia and hyponatremia
		Hypovolemia
		Lethargy
		Postural hypotension
		Muscle cramps
		Metabolic alkalosis
		Maintain fluid restriction if ordered (more likely if patient is hyponatremic)
		Ensure adherence to low-sodium diet if ordered
		Encourage foods high in potassium
		If patient is anorexic, do not force to eat but allow food preferences if compatible with diet; provide smaller, more frequent meals and frequent oral hygiene
		Maintain bed rest if necessary to promote diuresis
		Elevate feet when patient is up in chair
		Continue measures to improve pump efficiency indicated in Problem, Cardiac decompensation
■ Arrhythmias related to Cardiac compensatory response to decreased stroke volume Hypoxia Electrolyte disturbances Etiological condition precipitating heart failure Digoxin toxicity	■ Electrophysiological stability Optimal cardiac rhythm	■ Maintain continuous ECG monitoring
		Select lead best exhibiting atrial and ventricular complexes
		Set rate alarms
		Participate with physician in identifying cause of arrhythmia and treat as ordered
		Assess ECG changes indicating developing or progressing cardiac failure
		Sinus tachycardia as compensatory mechanism
		Atrial arrhythmias related to increased atrial pressures

POTENTIAL PROBLEMS	EXPECTED OUTCOMES	NURSING ACTIVITIES

		Monitor lab results for
		  Hypoxia
		  Electrolyte disturbances, particularly K$^+$
		  Acidosis/alkalosis
		  Serum digoxin levels
		Assess effect of arrhythmia on cardiac output and heart failure
		  Check BP and P and observe for changes reflecting increasing left ventricular dysfunction; see Problem, Cardiac decompensation
		  Bradycardias may decrease cardiac output when ventricle is not able to increase stroke volume
		  Persistent tachycardias reduce ventricular filling time, increase myocardial O$_2$ consumption, and can contribute to disordered synchrony of ventricular contraction
		  Loss of effective atrial contraction with atrial fibrillation, atrial flutter, and AV dissociation in presence of elevated left ventricular diastolic pressure can markedly reduce ventricular filling
		Check emergency equipment every shift, ensuring proper functioning and availability
		If it is necessary to treat arrhythmia, e.g., adversely compromising cardiac output and/or treatment of underlying problem not sufficient, proceed as ordered; therapy may include antiarrhythmics, cardioversion, or pacing; if cardioversion is recommended, assess for presence of digoxin toxicity; if digoxin toxicity is possibility, inform physician—cardioversion then is contraindicated; patients with long-standing atrial fibrillation may be given prophylactic anticoagulants
		
		See STANDARD 21 *Arrhythmias*

■ Decreased activity tolerance related to decreased cardiac output and/or dyspnea	■ Activity level below failure threshold
	  Absence of complications related to bed rest
	  Patient verbalizes comfort
		■ Assess level of activity tolerance; relate to fatigue or dyspnea; New York Heart Association classification helpful and may be appropriately used
		  Class I: patients with heart disease who are asymptomatic
		  Class II: slight limitation of physical activity; symptoms produced only with more than ordinary physical activity
		  Class III: marked limitation; symptoms produced with ordinary physical activity
		  Class IV: symptoms while patient is resting
		Maintain ordered activity level
		  Higher degrees of failure require bed rest during acute management; semi-Fowler's position usually most comfortable for patient and physiologically preferable, because venous return is decreased and lung expansion is increased
		  Change position q2 hr and administer skin care, particularly if edematous; observe for early indications of breakdown of skin—reddened or marked areas
		  Increase activity as ordered and as tolerated by patient; check BP, P, R, and ECG before each level increase and after activity (within 1 minute); observe for symptoms indicating poor tolerance
		Provide opportunities for patient to verbalize feelings regarding activity limitations
		Institute preventive measures to reduce thromboembolic complications of bed rest; see Problem, Thromboembolism

■ Anxiety and frustration related to
  Awareness that heart is not functioning properly, that "heart is failing"
	■ Verbalizes anxiety and fears
	  Asks questions
	  Reduction of anxiety with sufficient information, resolution of symptoms, and future planning
		■ Ongoing assessment and recording of level of anxiety
		Encourage patient/family to verbalize concerns and to ask questions
		Explain nature of heart failure relating to cause if known and to symptoms experienced
		  If probability exists that problem will be chronic, more information will be necessary as condition stabilizes and anxiety decreases

POTENTIAL PROBLEMS	EXPECTED OUTCOMES	NURSING ACTIVITIES
Resultant symptoms, particularly difficulty with breathing Lack of information regarding condition, equipment, procedures, and treatment modalities Decreased activity tolerance If heart failure is transient problem secondary to acute noncardiac problem, patient may be less aware of diagnosis		If problem is transient and not related to cardiac disease, clarify for patient If problem is recurrent, it is particularly important to identify precipitating factors with patient, allowing time for verbalization of fears and frustrations and discussion of past and future impact on life-style Explain purpose and expectations of monitoring equipment, frequency of assessments, and treatment modalities used Maintain as quiet and relaxed an environment as possible Assess hemodynamic consequences of anxiety Administer sedatives as ordered when necessary
■ Infection related to Pulmonary congestion Systemic lines Foley catheter	■ Absence or resolution of infection	■ Initiate preventive measures or precautions as appropriate Prevent atelectasis by Instituting measures or drugs as ordered to reduce pulmonary congestion Administering pain medication promptly Encouraging patient to cough and deep breathe every hour while on bed rest and awake Providing chest physiotherapy q2 hr if necessary Turning patient at least q2 hr if immobile Sterile suctioning as needed Increase level of activity as soon as possible and as ordered Maintain strict aseptic technique during insertion of hemodynamic monitoring lines and during any change of tubing or transducers Record date of insertion of each line Monitoring lines should be changed as follows unless detrimental to patient Pulmonary artery lines: at least q72 hr Arterial lines: at least every 7 days CVP lines: at least every 7 days Flush solutions should be changed at least q24 hr Chamber dome and administration tubing should be changed q48 hr IV sites for fluid administration should be changed q48-72 hr or earlier if site becomes inflamed IV solutions should be changed q24 hr IV administration tubing should be changed q48 hr Maintain sterile technique when inserting Foley catheter and apply antibiotic ointment to meatus; maintain closed system; should be removed as soon as possible and never left in place more than 14 days; bladder irrigations with antibiotic solution may be ordered; provide perineal care q8 hr; change drainage system q24 hr Check temperature q4 hr while patient is awake; increase frequency as needed; report elevation to physician If temperature is elevated, observe for associated chills or diaphoresis; keep patient warm and dry Collect data to determine source of infection Increased atelectasis on chest radiograph Increased pulmonary secretions, which may be purulent Localized signs of inflammation at IV or line insertion sites Changes in character of urine—cloudy, foul smelling, persistent hematuria, flank pain Obtain cultures and send to lab as ordered Culture tips of lines or catheters when removed if indicated Administer antipyretics and antibiotics as ordered

See STANDARD 61   *Infection control in the critical care unit*

POTENTIAL PROBLEMS	EXPECTED OUTCOMES	NURSING ACTIVITIES
■ Thromboembolism Pulmonary embolus related to Systemic venous congestion Prolonged bed rest	■ Absence or resolution of pulmonary embolus	■ Initiate preventive measures for patients assessed to be high-risk candidates for embolization Severe or chronic congestive heart failure with long-standing lower extremity edema or atrial fibrillation History of preexisting thromboembolic disease Obese Over 70 years old Prolonged bed rest anticipated Administer prophylactic anticoagulation as ordered Observe for signs of bleeding Hematest all stools, urine, and secretions Assist patient with passive/active exercises while on bed rest Place footboard on bed for patient to press toes against 10 times q1 hr Instruct patient not to cross legs or ankles Avoid use of knee gatch on bed Use elastic stockings, measuring calf for correct size Remove twice a day Make certain stockings do not roll down, causing tourniquet effect Have patient ambulate as early as possible Observe for signs of venous thrombosis Positive Homans' sign Change in color, temperature, or girth of extremity Presence of cords or tenderness Assess for signs and symptoms of pulmonary embolus—sudden unexplained dyspnea, tachypnea, anxiety, hypotension, tachycardia, atrial arrhythmias, elevation of jugular venous pressure, elevation of PAP (if line in place), and expiratory or fixed splitting of S_2 Assess for signs and symptoms of pulmonary infarction—hemoptysis, pleural friction rub, dyspnea, or signs of pulmonary consolidation Prepare patient for lung scan if ordered If problem occurs Inform physician Administer anticoagulants as ordered Assess for signs and symptoms suggesting further cardiac decompensation including pulmonary edema, which may be result of pulmonary emboli *See* STANDARD 31 *Embolic phenomena* STANDARD 1 *Pulmonary edema of cardiac origin*
■ Pulmonary edema related to pulmonary capillary pressures that exceed oncotic pressure of lungs and result in transudation of fluid into alveoli	■ Absence of pulmonary edema	■ Assess for signs and symptoms of pulmonary edema Respiratory distress Increased distribution of rales Cough and increased secretions with severe pulmonary congestion; may have blood-tinged, frothy sputum Bulging neck veins Pallor; cyanosis Diaphoresis Apprehension Restlessness Tachycardia PCWP above 25 to 30 mm Hg If problem occurs Elevate head of bed Inform physician immediately—cardiac emergency Administer medications and O_2 as ordered Apply rotating tourniquets if ordered Have someone remain with patient if at all possible *See* STANDARD 1 *Pulmonary edema of cardiac origin*

POTENTIAL PROBLEMS	EXPECTED OUTCOMES	NURSING ACTIVITIES

■ Cardiogenic shock related to left ventricular dysfunction, resulting in inadequate tissue perfusion	■ Absence of cardiogenic shock	■ Assess for signs and symptoms of cardiogenic shock
		  Hypotension: systolic BP less than 90 mm Hg
		  Tachycardia with poor pulse contour
		  Urine output less than 20 ml/hour
		  Mental confusion
		  Decreased peripheral perfusion
		If problem develops, inform physician immediately
		  Aggressive management and invasive hemodynamic monitoring must be initiated immediately to interrupt shock cycle
		  Identify and treat, as ordered, abnormalities resulting from and promoting decompensation including hypoxemia, acidosis, arrhythmias, and pain
		
		See STANDARD 16 *Cardiogenic shock*

■ Insufficient knowledge to comply with discharge regimen*	■ Evaluation by testing or questioning demonstrates patient/family's understanding of the knowledge components of the teaching program
	Identifies own risk factors and/or precipitating factors with methods for modification or avoidance
	States information necessary for compliance with discharge regimen
	  Activity
	  Diet
	  Medications
	  Follow-up care
	Accurately demonstrates skill of counting pulse
	Lists symptoms requiring medical attention
	Asks pertinent questions regarding self-care
	Patient/family discusses future realistically
		■ If heart failure requires chronic management, institute teaching program for patient/family, including
		  Explanation of normal heart function
		  Explanation of heart failure and related signs and symptoms
		  Discussion of risk factors for atherosclerotic heart disease including purpose and meaning; identification of patient's own and cost-benefit ratio of modification; if risk factor modification is indicated, discuss methods of modification and sources of support
		  Control of precipitating or aggravating factors of heart failure including diseases, e.g., hypertension or valvular heart disease
		  Activity regulation
		    Work simplification techniques
		    Importance of avoiding or modifying activity following meals, with stress, or in extremes of temperature
		    Symptoms suggesting intolerance and actions to take
		  Need for avoiding activities or clothing that promote circulatory stasis
		  Diet instruction if special diet has been ordered; give patient list of foods and beverages high in potassium if diuretic therapy is indicated, unless potassium-sparing diuretic has been ordered
		  Information regarding discharge medications
		    Name and purpose
		    Dosage
		    Frequency—tailor timing to patient's routine schedule
		    Side effects
		      Signs and symptoms of digoxin toxicity
		      Signs and symptoms of hypokalemia unless potassium-sparing diuretic has been ordered
		  Method and significance of counting pulse if patient receiving digoxin when discharged
		  Signs and symptoms of recurring heart failure and appropriate action to take; importance of daily weights
		  Information regarding follow-up
		  Provide frequent opportunities for patient/family to ask questions and express concerns
		  Provide opportunities for skills practice
		  Assess patient's potential compliance and make referrals for home follow-up if necessary

*If patient follow-up is the responsibility of the critical care unit nurse.

CARDIOGENIC SHOCK

Cardiogenic shock is a syndrome that results from inadequate tissue perfusion secondary to heart disease. It is most often the result of an AMI or cumulative infarctions in which 40% or more of the left ventricle is destroyed. It can also occur as a result of decompensating left heart failure or following cardiac surgery. In the presence of impaired left ventricular function, other factors may promote the shock syndrome including arrhythmias, drugs depressing myocardial contractility, hypoxia, acidosis, hypovolemia, and abnormalities in peripheral vascular regulation.

Cardiogenic shock consists of sustained systemic arterial hypotension with evidence of inadequate tissue perfusion of the kidneys, brain, and skin. Indications of inadequate tissue perfusion include decreased urine output (less than 20 ml/hour); changes in sensorium (restlessness, apprehension, confusion); cool, clammy skin; thready, weak brachial and radial pulses; sinus tachycardia; and hyperventilation as a compensatory mechanism for rising blood lactate levels. Most of these symptoms are caused by the redistribution of blood volume as the body attempts to maintain blood pressure in the presence of decreasing cardiac output.

Hypotension has been defined in this context by the Myocardial Infarction Research Unit Program as an arterial pressure less than 90 mm Hg for a previously normotensive person or a fall of greater than 80 mm Hg for a previously hypertensive person. Once hypotension occurs, rapid deterioration usually evolves as the "cycle" of shock begins. Coronary blood flow decreases as the blood pressure decreases, resulting in further deterioration of left ventricular function and elevation of left ventricular filling pressures. As the gradient (aortic diastolic pressure minus left ventricular diastolic pressure) diminishes, decreasing the effective coronary perfusion pressure, further impairment to coronary blood flow occurs, resulting in progressive subendocardial ischemia, progressive left ventricular dysfunction, and peripheral flow deficiencies. Hypoxemia and acidosis are established as a result and contribute to further deterioration.

Cardiogenic shock lasting more than 1 hour associated with a prior MI has a mortality greater than 80%. It is the most common cause of in-hospital death following AMI. Therefore early recognition, ideally before the cycle is established, and aggressive intervention are imperative. Invasive monitoring is essential for assessing the rapid and generally unpredictable changes in status and response to the therapeutic modalities used. Minimally this includes accurate determinations of intraarterial BP, left ventricular filling pressures (PCWP), hourly urine output, and arterial blood gas levels.

The problems and therapies employed for cardiogenic shock are interrelated and cannot be considered in isolation.

ASSESSMENT

1. Historical and current data necessary for assessing concomitant disease states and medications that contribute to or cause shock syndrome
2. Intake and output (urine via Foley catheter); urine specific gravities
3. LOC—neurological status
4. Color, temperature, and moisture of skin
5. Pulses: rate, rhythm, quality, and equality
6. R: rate, pattern, depth, and sound
7. BP and mean arterial pressure (MAP) with intraarterial line
8. Measurement of pressures
   a. Pulmonary artery diastolic pressure
   b. PCWP
   c. CVP
   d. Main aortic pressure
9. Cardiac output measurements
   a. Ejection fraction
   b. Cardiac index
10. Signs and symptoms of elevated right ventricular filling pressure
    a. Neck vein distention
    b. Positive hepatojugular reflux
    c. Increased CVP
11. Signs and symptoms of pulmonary congestion
12. Pain
13. Temperature
14. Intensity of heart sounds, presence of S_3 or S_4 gallops and murmurs
15. Lab data results for
    a. Blood gas levels
    b. Electrolytes
    c. BUN/creatinine clearance

d. Hct

e. Serial cardiac enzymes and isoenzymes

f. Chest radiographs

g. Drug levels

16. Monitor ECG for

a. Arrhythmias

b. Changes characteristic of myocardial ischemia and necrosis

c. Changes characteristic of electrolyte imbalance

d. Changes characteristic of drugs and their toxic effects

17. Results of special studies employed to determine cardiac status

a. Radioisotope scanning

b. Coronary arteriography

c. Left ventricular cineangiography

d. Two-dimensional echocardiogram

GOALS

1. Hemodynamic stability

a. Systolic BP: 90 to 110 mm Hg

b. Diastolic BP: 60 to 90 mm Hg

c. Pulse pressure: 30 to 50 mm Hg

d. Left ventricular filling pressure: 15 to 20 mm Hg

e. Cardiac output sufficient to maintain adequate tissue perfusion

2. Adequate tissue perfusion and tissue integrity

a. Urine output minimally 20 to 30 ml/hour; BUN/creatinine clearance and urine specific gravity within normal limits

b. Skin warm and dry with no pallor or cyanosis

c. Patient is oriented and able to communicate—neurological system intact

d. Adequate coronary perfusion pressure

e. Peripheral resistance sufficient to maintain BP without deleterious effects or decreased tissue perfusion

3. pH, PaO_2, and $PaCO_2$ within normal limits

4. Serum electrolytes within normal limits

5. Electrophysiological stability

6. Normal temperature

7. Absence of signs and symptoms of pulmonary congestion

8. Absence or control of pain

9. Patient/family verbalizes fears and concerns

a. Reduction of patient/family's level of anxiety with provision of information and emotional support

b. Family calmly visits with patient

c. Clergy of choice available if desired by patient/family

POTENTIAL PROBLEMS	EXPECTED OUTCOMES	NURSING ACTIVITIES

■ Inadequate tissue perfusion related to
Depressed ventricular function
Body's compensatory redistribution of blood volume
Hypoxia
Acidosis
	■ Adequate tissue perfusion and tissue integrity
	Urine output minimally 20 to 30 ml/hour
	BUN/creatinine clearance and specific gravity within normal limits
		■ Assess for signs and symptoms indicating degree of tissue perfusion and peripheral resistance
		Renal perfusion
		  Measure intake and output; include sources other than urine
		  Measure urine output q1 hr; Foley catheter required for accuracy
		    Report output less than 30 ml/hour
		    Output less than 20 ml/hour is indicative of shock; intervention is required to prevent ischemia and renal failure
		  Assess for indications of renal failure
		    Lack of response to sufficient dosages of diuretics
		    Anuria and azotemia
		    Elevated BUN or creatinine clearance
		    Decreased specific gravity
		    See Standard 52, *Acute renal failure*

	Skin warm and dry with no pallor or cyanosis	Cutaneous perfusion: check color, temperature, and hydration of skin for changes consistent with decreased perfusion—cool, pale, cyanotic, moist, or clammy
	pH within normal limits	Skeletal muscle and splanchnic perfusion: check blood gas levels for evidence of metabolic acidosis resulting from rise in blood lactate levels; may be initial isolated reduction in $PaCO_2$ in response to compensatory hyperventilation; subsequently, pH falls
	Absence of abdominal or cardiac pain	GI perfusion: check for presence of recurring abdominal pain and rigidity associated with ischemia of bowel, which may lead to necrosis and bleeding
	Patient oriented and able to communicate; neurological system intact	Cerebral and coronary perfusion are affected more by aortic perfusion pressure than by sympathetic nervous system compensatory activity; therefore signs and symptoms of inadequate perfusion more often occur with imminently pending or concurrent hypotension Cerebral perfusion

POTENTIAL PROBLEMS	EXPECTED OUTCOMES	NURSING ACTIVITIES

Observe for changes indicating altered sensorium
    Restlessness
    Confusion
    Somnolence
    Psychosis
Assess neurological status
    LOC
    Pupils and extraocular movements
    Presence of spontaneous movement of extremities
    Response to stimuli—verbal, tactile, pain
    Presence of gag reflex
    Respiratory rate and pattern; absence of spontaneous respiration

Absence or stabilization of arrhythmias and congestive heart failure

Coronary perfusion: observe for arrhythmias, signs and symptoms of CHF, and extension of MI

Adequate coronary perfusion pressure 60 to 80 mm Hg

Check pulses; poorly palpable brachial and radial pulses with bounding central pulsations may indicate intense upper extremity vasoconstriction, which may precipitate hypotension

Pao$_2$ and Paco$_2$ within normal limits

Check R for indications of hypoventilation or hyperventilation
Check blood gas results for acidosis, decreased Pao$_2$, or increased Paco$_2$; acidosis further promotes inadequate tissue perfusion

Peripheral resistance sufficient to maintain BP without deleterious effects of decreased tissue perfusion

Monitor pressures for indication of increased peripheral resistance; intraarterial line is required for accuracy
    Decreased pulse pressure; more significant finding with concurrent increased venous pressure, which helps to differentiate etiology of change from depressed myocardial function or hypovolemia
    Increased diastolic pressure (also influenced by heart rate, which determines duration of diastole)

Pulse pressure within normal limits

Increased MAP

Diastolic pressure maintained at 60 to 90 mm Hg

If measurements are available, total peripheral vascular resistance can be calculated with the following formula:

Systolic pressure maintained at 90 to 110 mm Hg

$$\frac{\text{Mean aortic pressure} - \text{Mean right atrial pressure (mm Hg)}}{\text{Cardiac output (liters/minute)}}$$

Keep physician informed of patient's status and changes indicating deterioration
Participate in management directed toward improving tissue perfusion before hypotension, acidosis, and hypoxemia become established, and toward treating complications of inadequate perfusion
Maintain patent intraarterial line; maintain patent IV line for administration of drugs; use soluset or infusion pump for control
Administer medications as ordered
    Vasodilators may be ordered when blood flow is reduced and when patient is still normotensive to decrease afterload and O$_2$ consumption
    Sodium nitroprusside most commonly used
    Nitroglycerin and long-acting nitrates more difficult to titrate
    High doses of corticosteroids may be ordered in attempt to produce same effects
    Monitor effectiveness of medication according to improvement in patient's perfusion and left ventricular performance reflected by decrease in left ventricular filling pressures and increase in cardiac output without hypotension being produced
    Titrate medication as ordered to maintain systolic BP 90 to 110 mm Hg
    Inotropic agents with vasodilator effects such as isoproterenol (Isuprel); dobutamine, and dopamine (dosage dependent); observe for side effects resulting from increased myocardial O$_2$ consumption
Initiate measures to prevent renal failure as ordered by maintaining urine output greater than 20 ml/hour
    Administer diuretics ordered by physician such as furosemide

POTENTIAL PROBLEMS	EXPECTED OUTCOMES	NURSING ACTIVITIES

Administer if ordered osmotic diuretic such as mannitol or acetazolamide (Diamox) to increase renal blood flow if output is less than 30 ml/hour in attempt to prevent renal ischemia; inform physician if this fails to induce diuresis; osmotic diuretic does not enter cells and metabolize so if it is not excreted, it may cause blood volume to overexpand and result in pulmonary edema

Dopamine or dobutamine may be ordered specifically because of ability of these drugs to increase renal blood flow

If acute renal failure develops, hemodialysis or peritoneal dialysis may be indicated

See Standard 52, *Acute renal failure*

The smallest amount of any medication that will produce desired effect should be used; inadequate renal or hepatic perfusion may interfere with metabolism and excretion of drugs and result in accumulation and toxicity

Monitor ECG for arrhythmias, a common complication of medications

Monitor PCWP to determine left ventricular filling pressure; see Problem, Depressed myocardial function

Monitor cardiac output; see Problem, Depressed myocardial function

If cerebral hypoxia results in inadequate spontaneous respiration or its absence, patient will require intubation and mechanical ventilation

If pharmacological management is not effective, counterpulsation may be instituted to decrease afterload during systole, to increase aortic pressure during diastole resulting in increased coronary perfusion, and to increase peripheral arterial blood flow

See STANDARD 25   *Hemodynamic monitoring*
     STANDARD 6   *Mechanical ventilation*
     STANDARD 24   *Intraaortic balloon pumping (counterpulsation)*

POTENTIAL PROBLEMS	EXPECTED OUTCOMES	NURSING ACTIVITIES
■ Hypotension resulting in inadequate venous return related to Depressed myocardial function Hypovolemia Vasodilator therapy Inadequate vasoconstriction—inability to compensate for decreasing cardiac output; most common with elderly or diabetic patients	■ Systolic pressure 90 to 110 mm Hg Adequate circulating blood volume Peripheral resistance sufficient to maintain BP without deleterious effects of decreased tissue perfusion Left ventricular filling pressure 15 to 20 mm Hg Absence of signs and symptoms of pulmonary edema	■ Monitor arterial BP and MAP with intraarterial pressure lines; MAP can also be calculated using the following formula:

$$\frac{\text{Diastolic pressure} \times 2 + \text{Systolic pressure}}{3}$$

Monitor CVP to determine blood volume and adequacy of central venous return

Check P for compensatory sinus tachycardia

Check for signs and symptoms of reduced cerebral or coronary blood flow, both of which are directly affected by mean aortic pressure; see Problem, Inadequate tissue perfusion

Check urine output and specific gravity q1 hr; follow lab data noted in Problem, Inadequate tissue perfusion; if tubular necrosis develops secondary to hypotension (lack of response to diuretics), urine output is less specific indicator of renal blood flow because of nephron abnormalities

Assess for presence of hypovolemia
    Review intake and output records and acute weight changes; with AMI, fluid loss can occur as result of reduced intake related to pain, nausea and vomiting, and analgesic therapy or secondary to diaphoresis, diuretic therapy, and diarrhea resulting from medications

Check for signs and symptoms indicating elevated right ventricular filling pressures
    Elevated CVP
    Neck vein distention
    Positive hepatojugular reflux
    Hepatomegaly
    Ascites
    Peripheral or sacral edema

POTENTIAL PROBLEMS	EXPECTED OUTCOMES	NURSING ACTIVITIES
		Participate in fluid challenge as ordered to help distinguish hypovolemic shock from that caused by left ventricular dysfunction
		Contraindicated if PCWP is greater than 18 to 22 mm Hg or CVP is greater than 12 cm H_2O
		Administer colloidal solution (dextran or albumin) or normal saline solution in 50 to 100 ml boluses at 5- to 10-minute intervals; challenge must be carried out rapidly to ensure vascular compartment expansion; different protocols for administering fluid challenges exist
		Check PCWP and CVP after each bolus; rise in PCWP to 20 to 22 mm Hg or increase in CVP by 2 cm H_2O is considered reasonable challenge
		Continue challenge until these pressures are reached or until flow deficiency is corrected, whichever comes first; earlier cessation is inadequate challenge
		Hypovolemia is indicated if favorable response is achieved without much increase in PCWP
		Cardiac dysfunction is indicated if PCWP increases without clinical improvement
		Participate as ordered in management directed toward maintaining an adequate circulating volume either by supplementing fluid or altering redistribution
		Maintain systolic arterial BP at 90 to 110 mm Hg; systolic pressure between 80 and 90 mm Hg is acceptable if other signs of tissue perfusion are adequate
		If problem related to hypovolemia occurs, continue fluid challenge, using guidelines described before
		Monitor
		PCWP
		CVP
		Intraarterial pressure
		Indices of perfusion noted in Problem, Inadequate tissue perfusion
		Signs and symptoms of pulmonary edema
		Administer vasoconstrictors if ordered; only indication for these drugs in patients with depressed myocardial function following AMI is hypotension; norepinephrine is usual drug of choice because it also has inotropic properties; metaraminol may also be ordered
		Monitor BP at least q15 min
		Monitor PCWP: with left ventricular dysfunction, left ventricular filling pressures at 15 to 20 mm Hg are desired to enhance contractility according to the Starling law
		Monitor ECG for arrhythmias continuously
		Monitor signs and symptoms of inadequate perfusion (see Problem, Inadequate tissue perfusion)
		Titrate to smallest dosage that raises BP and increases urine output; attempt to titrate off medication as soon as possible; if medication is necessary for prolonged period, dextran or plasma expanders may be ordered to maintain adequate left ventricular filling pressures
		Check blood gas levels for acidosis, which decreases effect of vasoconstrictor agents; adjust dosages as ordered
■ Depressed myocardial function related to Loss of functional cardiac muscle Adverse effect of medications Acidosis Hypoxemia Hyperkalemia Arrhythmias	■ Left ventricular filling pressure 15 to 20 mm Hg Cardiac output sufficient to maintain adequate tissue perfusion Cardiac index 2.5 to 4.0 liters/minute/m^2	■ Determine if patient is receiving any medications that may depress myocardial function, such as propranolol, quinidine, or procainamide (Pronestyl) Participate with physician in monitoring hemodynamic measurements essential for evaluating serial changes in left ventricular function and response to therapy PCWP reflecting left ventricular filling pressure; ideally maintained at 15 to 20 mm Hg

POTENTIAL PROBLEMS	EXPECTED OUTCOMES	NURSING ACTIVITIES
	Ejection fraction 60% to 75% of end diastolic volume Electrophysiological stability Normal temperature pH, Pao₂, and Paco₂ within normal limits Serum K⁺ within normal limits	Cardiac output measurements—several methods for determining cardiac output are available, including thermodilution, Fick principle that measures arterial-venous O₂ difference, indicator dilution method, and radioisotope scanning method if equipment is available Cardiac index is more specific determinant of adequacy of cardiac output, because body size is considered; it may be calculated using the DuBois body surface chart after measuring cardiac output, height, and weight; a normal cardiac index is 2.5 to 4.0 liters/minute/m² Ejection fraction may be calculated by the following formula:

Cardiac output measurements—several methods for determining cardiac output are available, including thermodilution, Fick principle that measures arterial-venous O_2 difference, indicator dilution method, and radioisotope scanning method if equipment is available

Cardiac index is more specific determinant of adequacy of cardiac output, because body size is considered; it may be calculated using the DuBois body surface chart after measuring cardiac output, height, and weight; a normal cardiac index is 2.5 to 4.0 liters/minute/m²

Ejection fraction may be calculated by the following formula:

$$\frac{\text{Stroke volume}}{\text{End diastolic volume}} \times 100\%$$

Normal range is 60% to 75% of end diastolic volume; decreased ejection fraction reveals inability of left ventricle to empty adequately

Intraarterial measurements of BP and mean aortic pressure; decrease in mean aortic pressure and increase in left ventricular filling pressure result in decreased coronary artery perfusion, promoting further myocardial ischemia and necrosis

Assess for indices of inadequate perfusion noted in Problem, Inadequate tissue perfusion

Assess for signs and symptoms indicative of myocardial ischemia or extension of infarction

Auscultate precordium for
  Intensity of heart sounds
  Presence of S_3 or S_4 gallops
  Murmurs

Continuously monitor ECG for
  Arrhythmias
  Changes consistent with myocardial ischemia or extension of infarction
  Drug effects

Check temperature q4 hr or as indicated; if temperature is elevated, observe for indications of increased cardiac work and myocardial O_2 demands and potential decrease in peripheral vascular resistance

Monitor blood gas levels and electrolytes for acidosis, hypoxemia, and hyperkalemia

Keep physician informed of patient's status, reporting any changes in data

Participate with physician in measures to improve myocardial function, and correct aggravating factors as ordered

Eliminate myocardial depressant drugs

Place patient in supine position; avoid Trendelenburg position

Maintain patent IV line for drug and fluid infusions

Maintain patent hemodynamic monitoring lines
  Observe for signs and symptoms of complications resulting from lines; see Standard 25, *Hemodynamic monitoring;* interpret results relating to therapeutic interventions

Administer antipyretics as ordered if temperature is elevated; keep patient warm and dry

Continue activities to correct perfusion abnormalities, acidosis, and hyperkalemia (noted in Problems, Inadequate tissue perfusion, Hypoxia-hypoxemia, and Acidosis) if present

Treat arrhythmias as ordered

Administer medications to improve myocardial function; inotropic agents with either vasoconstricting (only in presence of hypotension) or vasodilating actions will be ordered
  Monitor hemodynamic parameters indicated previously to determine response to therapy

POTENTIAL PROBLEMS	EXPECTED OUTCOMES	NURSING ACTIVITIES
		Be alert to development of arrhythmias, particularly ventricular arrhythmias, which are common side effect of medications Observe for toxic effects of all medications that patient is receiving if reduced circulation and redistribution of blood flow are present; result is decreased volume of distribution whereby smaller concentrations may be required to avoid toxicity If patient does not respond to therapy, aortic balloon counterpulsation in conjunction with medications may be employed to stabilize patient's condition for cardiac catheterization and possible emergency surgery if correctable lesions are found; see Standard 24, *Intraaortic balloon pumping (counterpulsation);* Standard 26, *Cardiac catheterization;* Standard 27, *Cardiac surgery*
■ Hypoxia-hypoxemia related to Pulmonary congestion Hypoventilation Decreased cardiac output Altered cerebral function	■ pH, PaO_2 and $PaCO_2$ within normal limits Absence of signs and symptoms of pulmonary congestion Adequate circulating blood volume to maintain cardiac output Absence of pain Serum K^+ within normal limits	■ Frequently monitor blood gas levels via intraarterial line; ensure that factors which alter blood gas results are stabilized at least 20 minutes before sampling Patient's comfort if patient is conscious Endotracheal suctioning Changes in O_2 concentration Adjustments to mechanical ventilator Administer O_2 as ordered If pulmonary congestion is present, use high flow rate and rebreathing mask If PaO_2 does not respond and remains less than 70 to 75 mm Hg, probably intubation and mechanical ventilation will be required Observe for signs and symptoms of pulmonary congestion; if present, institute measures as ordered to decrease congestion to improve oxygenation Administer diuretics as ordered following precautions noted in Problem, Inadequate tissue perfusion; hypovolemia and electrolyte imbalance augment shock state Deliver positive pressure if ordered, monitoring closely for indications of decreasing venous return, which may augment shock state Monitor respiratory effort noting rate, pattern, depth, and sound If tachypnea is present, it may indicate atelectasis, bronchospasm, pulmonary edema, or compensatory response to acidosis; if patient is being mechanically ventilated, check for increased secretions, cuff integrity, placement of tube, adequacy of ventilator settings, and patient's response Changes in patterns of respiration generally reflect cerebral perfusion problems If pain is present, treat immediately; if opiates are ordered, administer with great caution because of their respiratory depressant and hypotensive effects Review results of arterial and venous blood sampling for arterial-venous O_2 difference if performed; increase or widening of difference indicates that more O_2 is being extracted by tissues during circulation as autoregulatory response to decreased cardiac output Continue measures for improving cardiac output and perfusion noted in Problems, Inadequate tissue perfusion and Depressed myocardial function Observe for complications of hypoxia, which will promote shock cycle if they occur and are not corrected immediately Hypercapnia—always occurs with hypoventilation; results in respiratory acidosis and compensatory increase in respiration; administration of O_2 will not remove excess CO_2, so measures noted before to improve ventilation must be continued Hypotension—see Problem, Hypotension resulting in inadequate venous return Tachycardia and arrhythmias—see Problem, Arrhythmias Metabolic acidosis/hyperkalemia—see Problem, Acidosis

POTENTIAL PROBLEMS	EXPECTED OUTCOMES	NURSING ACTIVITIES
		See STANDARD 6 *Mechanical ventilation* STANDARD 7 *Positive and expiratory pressure*
■ Acidosis related to Hypercapnia Increased lactate acid production resulting from anaerobic metabolism of glucose	■ pH, Pao_2, and $Paco_2$ within normal limits Left ventricular filling pressure 15 to 20 mm Hg Absence of signs and symptoms of pulmonary congestion Electrophysiological stability Serum K^+ within normal limits	■ Monitor frequently blood gas levels via intraarterial line; initially a decrease in arterial $Paco_2$ may be seen in response to compensatory hyperventilation; if ventilation is not improved and the $Paco_2$ lowered sufficiently, the pH will fall, indicating acidosis If problem occurs, inform physician immediately and make available sodium bicarbonate IV for administration to maintain normal pH; participate with physician in correction of factors producing acidosis; check blood gas levels and pH frequently for resolution of acidosis and/or for development of metabolic alkalosis resulting from too vigorous therapy Monitor PCWP for increased left ventricular filling pressure and for signs of pulmonary congestion Observe for complications produced or aggravated by acidosis Decreased cardiac contractility Arrhythmias Hyperkalemia, which further impairs cardiac contractility and promotes arrhythmias Adjust dosages of vasoconstrictor drugs as ordered, the effect of which is lessened by acidosis Continue therapeutic modalities as ordered for improving myocardial function and tissue perfusion
■ Arrhythmias related to Inadequate tissue perfusion, particularly cardiac Hypotension Diminished myocardial function Hypoxia Acidosis Hyperkalemia Pain	■ Electrophysiological stability	■ Continuous ECG monitoring is essential Select lead best demonstrating atrial and ventricular activity Set rate alarms If arrhythmia occurs, assess effect on cardiac output; bradyarrhythmias, tachyarrhythmias, ventricular premature beats, and those resulting in loss of sequential atrial ventricular contraction may seriously alter already compromised status and promote progressive deterioration If problem occurs, inform physician immediately; continue measures to correct precipitating factor Administer antiarrhythmics as ordered through soluset or infusion pump for exact dosage control and prevention of fluid overload; remember that many antiarrhythmics further depress myocardial contractility, particularly procainamide, quinidine, and propranolol; in addition, in patient with diminished circulating volume and diminished renal or hepatic function, lower than usual doses may produce toxicity Ensure that emergency equipment is available and functioning for immediate correction of ventricular tachycardia or ventricular fibrillation *See* STANDARD 21 *Arrhythmias*
■ Pain related to decreased tissue perfusion	■ Absence or control of pain	■ Assess for verbal and nonverbal cues of pain If patient is able to communicate and is coherent, instruct patient to inform nurse immediately of presence of pain If patient is not able to communicate but is coherent, develop signals indicating presence of pain If pain is present Inform physician Determine location Cardiac Abdominal Peripheral Administer medication as ordered using as small a dose as possible

POTENTIAL PROBLEMS	EXPECTED OUTCOMES	NURSING ACTIVITIES
		If morphine is administered, monitor closely for depressive effect on cardiac and respiratory functions; it is safer to use if patient is being mechanically ventilated
■ Patient/family's anxiety related to severity of condition	■ Patient/family verbalizes fears and concerns Reduction of patient/family's level of anxiety with provision of information and emotional support Family calmly visits with patient	■ Continuous assessment of level of anxiety made difficult by altered LOC of patient and inability to speak if intubation is required Maintain quiet, controlled environment as much as possible If patient is able to speak, provide opportunities and encourage verbalization of fears, concerns, and confrontation with death but do not force communication Provide frequent explanations of who team members are and their qualifications, purpose of multiple monitoring systems and treatment modalities, and what to expect before intervention or procedure is initiated; comment on condition and presence or communications from family members Provide family with frequent information about patient; provide opportunities for family to be with patient; if desired and possible without compromising safety, provide time alone for patient and family; if possible, provide someone to whom family can talk, if not health professional, then perhaps clergy or trained volunteer; threat of death is often sudden and unexpected, and patient/family has not been allowed time for any emotional preparation
	Clergy of choice available if desired by patient/family	Determine if patient/family desires religious representative, e.g., priest, rabbi, minister

SHOCK

Shock is a clinical syndrome that is characterized by a reduction in the effective circulating blood volume and leads to a generalized inadequacy of perfusion to the vital body organs. An acceleration of circulatory impairment and progressive organ dysfunction may result in irreversible damage and death.

The common findings in all forms of shock include hypovolemia (absolute or relative) and significantly altered peripheral resistance.

Generally the patient is acutely ill and confused, restless, or stuporous, with cool extremities. The BP is low (less than 90 mm Hg) with a narrow pulse pressure. Tachycardia is often present, with weak and thready pulses. Only the larger, more central vessel pulses may be palpable. Signs of peripheral hypoperfusion and vasoconstriction may be present, including cool and clammy skin. On the other hand, septic shock may be associated with capillary dilatation and warm skin. Urine output is diminished or absent as a result of decreased renal perfusion. Metabolic acidosis is usually present. Temperature may be below normal, normal, or slightly elevated. Dyspnea may be present, with rapid and shallow respirations.

The major types of shock include the following:

1. Hypovolemic or oligemic shock with a blood volume relative to vascular space deficit; etiological factors include
   a. External fluid losses
      (1) Severe vomiting
      (2) Diarrhea
      (3) GI bleeding
   b. Internal losses; largely losses of intravascular fluid volume to the interstitial and intracellular spaces
      (1) Ileus
      (2) Intestinal obstruction
      (3) Burns
      (4) Peritonitis
2. Cardiogenic shock or inadequate cardiac output
   a. MI
   b. Acute arrhythmias
   c. Acute pericardial tamponade
   d. Severe heart valve malfunction
   e. Massive pulmonary embolus
   f. Tension pneumothorax

3. Bacteremic shock or sepsis, especially gram-negative sepsis
   a. Bowel perforation (most common)
   b. Pyelonephritis
   c. Acute cholecystitis
   d. Pneumonia in the alcoholic patient and in the patient with COPD
   e. Burn sepsis
   f. Bacterial endocarditis
   g. Nosocomial sepsis
4. Neurogenic or vasogenic shock involves the loss of neurogenic tone to vessels
   a. Spinal cord injury
   b. Anesthetic paralysis (vasodilation)
   c. Reflex vasodilation
5. Anaphylactic shock, which results from an antigen-antibody reaction that damages capillaries and results in histamine release and associated vasodilation
   a. Drugs
   b. Pollen
   c. Insect sting
   d. Foreign proteins in serum
6. Endocrine abnormalities inducing shock
   a. Diabetic ketoacidosis
   b. Adrenal crisis

Therapy for shock of any cause is directed toward improvement of arterial pressure to 90 mm Hg to restore blood flow to vital organs and management of accompanying hypoxemia, azotemia, acidosis, and other complications.

ASSESSMENT

1. History and nature of
   a. GI problem, that is, ulcers, varices, gastritis, diverticulosis, and neoplasm
   b. Severe infection with either gram-positive or gram-negative organisms, including severe respiratory infections, peritonitis, meningitis, etc.
   c. MI, cardiac failure, valvular disease, hypertension, arrhythmias, and cardiac surgery
   d. Diabetes mellitus, hypoglycemia, renal insufficiency, coagulation disorders
   e. Recent spinal cord injury

f. Severe reactions to anesthetics, drugs, diagnostic agents, vaccine, insect bites, etc.
g. Endocrine disorders
h. Nutritional status
2. Presence of signs and symptoms, including
  a. Severe hypotension
  b. Abnormally low or high CVP and PAP, if measurements are available
  c. Weak and thready or bounding pulse
  d. Cool, clammy skin
  e. Pallor, cyanosis
  f. Oliguria
  g. Acidosis and/or azotemia
  h. Restlessness, confusion, or lethargy
  i. Decreased or absent reflexes
  j. Labored, shallow respirations
  k. Chest pain
  l. Jugular venous distention
  m. Hemorrhage
  n. Severe burn injury
  o. Open wound
  p. Embolic episodes
  q. Rashes or erythema
  r. Abdominal pain and/or tenderness
3. Results of lab and diagnostic tests, including
  a. Hct level
  b. WBC count
  c. ESR
  d. BUN and/or creatinine clearance
  e. Electrolyte values
  f. Drug levels
  g. Arterial blood gas levels
  h. Cultures: sputum, blood, wound, and urine
  i. Cardiac enzymes
  j. Clotting profile
  k. Lactic acid levels
  l. Urinary electrolytes
  m. Chest and abdominal radiographs
  n. Lumbar puncture

  o. Arterial BP, CVP, PAP/PCWP
  p. Cardiac output
  q. ECG
  r. Gastroscopy or endoscopy
  s. Arteriogram
4. Patient/family's anxiety related to perception of and reaction to disease process, signs and symptoms, diagnostic procedures, therapy employed, and prognosis

GOALS

1. Patient/family's behavior indicates reduction in anxiety with provision of information and explanations
2. Hemodynamic stability; adequate cardiac output
  a. Adequate tissue perfusion of vital organs
  b. Normovolemia
3. Respiratory function sufficient to maintain
  a. Adequate oxygenation and ventilation
  b. Acid-base balance within normal limits
  c. Absence of respiratory distress syndrome
4. Serum electrolyte levels and blood count within normal limits
5. GI, neuromuscular, and integumentary function within normal limits
6. Infection free; absence of septicemia
7. Resolution and/or control of etiological factors
8. Prevention and/or resolution of accompanying complications, that is, disseminated intravascular coagulation (DIC), acute respiratory distress syndrome, etc.
9. Patient/family supplied with sufficient information for compliance with discharge regimen; before discharge the patient/family will be able to
  a. Identify factors specific to the patient that might precipitate a recurrence of shock and ways to prevent or avoid these precipitating factors
  b. Describe medications, dietary and activity regimen
  c. State signs and symptoms requiring medical intervention
  d. Describe plan for follow-up care

POTENTIAL PROBLEMS	EXPECTED OUTCOMES	NURSING ACTIVITIES
■ Anxiety related to Insufficient knowledge Monitoring equipment Diagnostic procedures	■ Reduction in level of anxiety with provision of information, explanations	■ Ongoing assessment of level of anxiety Describe nature of disease process, signs and symptoms, and therapy employed Explain anticipated diagnostic procedures, monitoring equipment, and plan of care Encourage questions and verbalization of anxieties, fears, and concerns Involve patient/family in plan of care Demonstrate concern and warmth in providing care to patient Keep patient warm (unless febrile) and comfortable Anticipate needs to minimize patient efforts and energy expenditure Position and turn patient q2 hr Encourage coughing and deep breathing

POTENTIAL PROBLEMS	EXPECTED OUTCOMES	NURSING ACTIVITIES
		Allow uninterrupted rest periods between procedures Evaluate for decrease in level of anxiety with provision of information and explanations

■ Hypovolemia related to
  External blood volume
    losses
    Wound
    GI bleeding
    Hemorrhage
  Internal losses with
    "third spacing"
    Peritonitis
    Burns
    Intestinal obstruction
	■ Normovolemia—adequate
	  volume expansion
	  Hemodynamic parameters
	  within normal limits
		■ Monitor for
		  Severe hypotension; monitor BP, P continuously in early phases of shock; thereafter note vital signs q1 hr and prn
		    Low CVP and PAP (note q½-1 until stable) and low cardiac output measurements if available
		    Oliguria; note urine output with specific gravity q1 hr
		    Signs of inadequate peripheral perfusion
		    Poor skin turgor, dry mucous membranes
		  Signs and symptoms of GI hemorrhage; see Standard 49, *Acute upper gastrointestinal bleeding*
		  Signs and symptoms of peritonitis and intestinal obstruction; see Standard 45, *Peritonitis;* Standard 50, *Gastrointestinal surgery*
		  Signs and symptoms of excessive fluid loss from burns; see Standard 64, *Burns*
		  Lab data results q6 hr
		    Electrolyte levels, particularly Na$^+$, and Hct levels
		    BUN level and creatinine clearance
		  Notify physician for any abnormality
		  If hypovolemia occurs
		    Administer volume expanders as ordered, i.e., blood, plasma, saline solution, and dextran; high-caloric solution, proteins and fats
		    Administer vasopressors as ordered (only after blood volume deficit is corrected)
		    Position patient to maximize blood flow to central organs; keep patient supine until signs of hypovolemia resolve
		    Administer corticosteroids to increase tissue perfusion if ordered (controversial)

■ Infection
  Systemic sepsis or bacteremia
  Local infection
	■ Absence of or early resolution of sepsis
	  Absence of clinical manifestations of infection
		■ Observe and monitor q½-1 hr for
		  Hyperthermia/hypothermia
		  Skin—warm and dry or cool and clammy
		  Tachycardia
		  Sudden, unexplained hypotension
		  Decreased, normal, or increased peripheral resistance, CVP, and cardiac output
		  Tachypnea, hyperventilation
		  GI symptoms, including vomiting, abdominal cramps, distention
		  Altered mental status—check LOC
		  Any swelling, redness, abnormal secretions from wounds or any part of the body
		  Abnormal bleeding indicative of DIC; see Standard 65, *Disseminated intravascular coagulation*
		  Monitor lab data daily for results of
		    C and S of organism growing in sputum, urine, blood, and/or wound
		    WBC count
		    ESR
		    Chest and abdominal radiographs
		    Clotting profile, Hct
		  Notify physician of any abnormalities
		  Maintain patent airway for efficient ventilation
		  Administer antibiotic and corticosteroid therapy as ordered
		  Administer vasoactive amine if shock persists, if ordered
		  Administer volume replacement if ordered
		  Prepare patient for surgery as ordered, if needed

POTENTIAL PROBLEMS	EXPECTED OUTCOMES	NURSING ACTIVITIES
■ Neurogenic or vasogenic shock related to spinal cord injury and/or spinal anesthesia, leading to vasodilation and hypotension	■ Absence of or resolution of vasogenic shock Adequate cardiac output Hemodynamic stability BP and peripheral perfusion within normal limits	■ Observe for 　Sudden hypotension associated with precipitating event (q½-1 hr until stable) 　Syncopal episode(s) 　Altered mental status; monitor ongoing LOC Notify physician of any abnormality Administer volume expanders if ordered Administer vasopressors if ordered (e.g., phenylephrine [Neo-Synephrine] or methamphetamine [Methedrine] to reverse reflex and depressive, vasodilating effect of anesthetic drugs)
■ Anaphylactic shock related to severe drug reaction—vaccine, serum, insect bite, etc.	■ Absence of or resolution of anaphylactic shock Hemodynamic stability	■ Delay absorption of antigen with forced emesis when appropriate or by applying tourniquet above injection site Observe for 　Severe hypotension; check vital signs, including temperature, q30 min if reaction is suspected 　Signs and symptoms of respiratory distress including choking, wheezing, and coughing 　Apprehension and restlessness 　Generalized urticaria and pruritus 　Edema and cyanosis 　Paresthesia and altered level of consciousness Notify physician of any abnormality Maintain an adequate airway—assist with intubation if needed; see Standard 6, *Mechanical ventilation* Administer epinephrine (0.5 ml—1:1000 in 10 ml saline solution as ordered, usually q5-15 min) until adequate response is elicited Administer bronchodilator as ordered to relieve bronchospasm Administer antihistamines if ordered to shorten duration of drug reaction and prevent relapses Administer hydrocortisone for prolonged reactions as ordered Administer volume expander rapidly, using saline, albumin, and/or dextran solution Treat acidosis with bicarbonate as ordered Alert health team to adverse reaction of patient to offending agent If appropriate, advise patient to avoid offending agent in future and inform future health care providers of his/her adverse reaction/allergy
■ Cardiogenic shock	■ Adequate cardiac contractility and output	■ Observe for 　Signs of decreased cardiac output (e.g., hypotension, oliguria) 　Signs of increased peripheral resistance with high CVP 　Atrial and ventricular arrhythmias 　Severe crushing pain radiating to arms and back Notify physician of any of these abnormalities If cardiogenic shock occurs, see Standard 16, *Cardiogenic shock*
■ Acute respiratory failure leading to acidosis	■ Absence of respiratory distress Respiratory function sufficient for adequate oxygenation and ventilation Arterial blood gas levels within normal limits	■ Monitor 　Arterial blood gas results q1-2 hr and prn until stable; note hypoxemia, hypercapnia, and acidemia 　Respirations q½-1 hr; note tachypnea, dyspnea 　Ongoing level of consciousness Notify physician of any of these abnormalities Maintain a patent airway Administer O_2 as ordered to maintain the arterial Pao_2 at 90 to 100 mm Hg; desirable safe Pao_2 levels are lower in patients with chronic lung disease Suction secretions as needed Administer bicarbonate as ordered Prepare for mechanical ventilation as ordered, if needed; see Standard 6, *Mechanical ventilation;* Standard 2, *Acute respiratory failure*

POTENTIAL PROBLEMS	EXPECTED OUTCOMES	NURSING ACTIVITIES

■ Renal failure related to inadequate perfusion	■ Adequate renal perfusion Indices of renal function and electrolyte levels within normal limits	■ Observe for signs and symptoms of acute renal failure
		   Note urine output q1 hr
		   If urine output is less than ½ ml/kg/hour in adults or 1 to 2 ml/kg/hour in children and infants, respectively, notify physician
		   Fixed specific gravity at or about 1.010
		   Daily weights revealing steady weight gain
		 Notify physician of any of these abnormalities
		 Monitor lab data for
		   Elevated BUN and creatinine levels
		   Acid-base imbalance
		   Electrolyte balance, Na^+ and K^+
		 Administer fluids as ordered
		 If problem occurs, see Standard 52, *Acute renal failure*

■ Insufficient knowledge to comply with discharge regimen*	■ Sufficient information to comply with discharge regimen
	 Patient/family correctly verbalizes postdischarge regimen regarding medications, diet, and activity progression
	 If appropriate, patient/family identifies etiological factors for shock, accompanying signs and symptoms, and ways to avoid or prevent recurrence
	 Patient/family correctly describes plan for follow-up care
		■ Assess patient/family's level of understanding regarding discharge regimen
		 Explain the discharge regimen, including
		   Medications—identify each medication, actions, side effects, routes, dose, schedule, and any precautionary or safety measures necessary
		   Dietary therapy
		   Activity progression—avoid overfatigue; allow for rest and relaxation
		 Describe etiological factors for patient's shock episode, if appropriate, and ways to prevent or avoid recurrence
		 Explain need for medical alert identification bracelet indicating allergy
		 Review plan for follow-up care, including purpose of visits, when to come, where to go, who to see, and what specimens to bring
		 Evaluate potential compliance of patient/family with discharge regimen

*If this type of follow-up care is the responsibility of the critical care unit nurse.

PERICARDITIS

The heart is enclosed by a pericardial sac, which is composed of two surfaces. The inner surface encasing the heart is called the *visceral pericardium,* or *epicardium.* The outer surface, which is attached to different structures in the chest including the manubrium, xiphoid process, vertebral column, and diaphragm, is called the *parietal pericardium.* Normally there is 10 to 20 ml of thin, clear pericardial fluid between the contacting surfaces of the visceral and parietal pericardium. This fluid serves as a lubricant, allowing the heart to move freely within the pericardial sac.

Pericarditis refers to an alteration of the pericardium regardless of etiology. Known causes of acute pericarditis include infection (viral, bacterial, tuberculosis, fungal), AMI, postmyocardial thoracotomy syndrome, trauma, connective tissue diseases, neoplastic disease, systemic disease such as uremia, and drugs such as procainamide, hydralazine, and phenytoin (Dilantin). Frequently the cause is not known, and the disease is labeled *idiopathic* or *nonspecific* pericarditis. Because few diseases affect the pericardium alone, the cause or associated disease must be sought.

The onset of pericarditis may be insidious or abrupt. Signs and symptoms commonly present include fever, pericardial pain, pericardial friction rub, and a typical ECG picture that will be described later. The pain must be differentiated from that of AMI, dissecting aortic aneurysm, and pulmonary embolism. Pericardial pain is classically described as sharp or knifelike; of moderate to severe intensity; precordial, often referred to the back and shoulders; and aggravated by deep inspiration or movement.

Inflammation of the pericardium may result in localized or generalized deposition of fibrin. This can produce constrictive pericarditis whereby the pericardium becomes rigid and unable to stretch. More commonly, the pericardial sac, normally a potential space with only a few drops of fluid, may fill with sufficient fluid to produce pericardial restriction (effusion or tamponade). Compression of the heart either by fibrosis or pericardial fluid results in the heart not being able to fill completely. Consequently, the systemic and pulmonary venous pressures increase and systemic BP decreases, producing a compensatory sinus tachycardia. Eventually, cardiac output will decrease.

The hemodynamic consequence of fluid accumulation in the pericardial sac is a result of the amount and speed of accumulation. The faster the accumulation, the less the volume necessary to produce hemodynamic instability and changes in intrapericardial pressure. Therefore severe tamponade can occur when a small volume of fluid rapidly enters the pericardial sac or when large volumes accumulate over time. Early identification and treatment of effusions may prevent tamponade.

Management of pericarditis is usually achieved by appropriate analgesics for pain and/or antiinflammatory agents. Some patients require steroid therapy. Treatment of the causative disease may be sufficient. Patients with frequent relapses may be considered for elective pericardiectomy. Generally, anticoagulants are contraindicated in the presence of pericarditis, because they may precipitate bleeding into the pericardial sac and tamponade if the fluid is sanguineous.

If constrictive pericarditis occurs, a pericardial resection is usually recommended. The earlier this is done, the lower the mortality and the better the prognosis.

The prognosis of pericarditis is dependent on the causative disease and/or the complications of tamponade or constriction if present.

ASSESSMENT

1. Recent history of upper respiratory tract infection
2. Presence, nature, and extent of characteristic signs and symptoms of pericarditis
   a. Temperature—diaphoresis and chills
   b. Chest pain
   c. Pericardial friction rub
   d. Respiratory status
      (1) Breath sounds
      (2) Dyspnea
      (3) Orthopnea on leaning forward
   e. Fatigue
3. Monitor ECG for
   a. Changes specific for pericarditis
   b. Tachycardia
4. Patient's perception of and reaction to the diagnosis and/or required therapy

5. Signs and symptoms and lab data changes consistent with complications
   a. Pericardial effusion
   b. Pericardial tamponade
   c. Constrictive pericarditis

GOALS

1. Absence of pain
2. Afebrile
3. Hemodynamic stability
4. Patient asks questions and verbalizes understanding of disease process and required therapy
5. Patient's behavior demonstrates decreased anxiety with provision of information

6. Absence of or resolution of complications
7. Before discharge, the patient/family
   a. Lists symptoms suggestive of recurrence to be reported to physician
   b. Asks pertinent questions regarding self-care
   c. Identifies reasons why and methods for avoiding fatigue
   d. States the information necessary for compliance with medication regimen
   e. States necessary information regarding follow-up visits to physician and/or clinic
   f. States why he/she should avoid unnecessary exposure to those with upper respiratory infections and report symptoms of colds or cough to physician

POTENTIAL PROBLEMS	EXPECTED OUTCOMES	NURSING ACTIVITIES
▪ Alterations of pericardium related to inflammation	▪ Absence of pain	▪ Assess for presence of pain Observe patient for nonverbal cues Instruct patient to inform health care team if pain is present If pain occurs Obtain clear description to assist in differentiation from AMI, dissecting aortic aneurysm, and/or pulmonary embolus; description should include Onset Quality Severity Site Radiation Influence of movement or deep inspiration Administer analgesics as ordered Administer antiinflammatory agents or steroid therapy, which may be selectively used as ordered Participate in treatment of underlying disease, e.g., uremia, which may be sufficient Position patient in high Fowler or leaning forward on padded overbed table for comfort Record and report occurrence, description of pain, and response to interventions
	Normal temperature Absence of diaphoresis and/or chills Absence of signs or symptoms of hidden infection	Check temperature q4 hr or as indicated Observe for any signs or symptoms of hidden infection If problem occurs Keep patient warm and dry Observe for diaphoresis and/or chills Administer antipyretics if indicated, and institute cooling measures if needed Maintain bed rest while chest pain, fever, and friction rub are present Assist patient to increase activity gradually after symptoms disappear while monitoring level of fatigue
▪ Alterations of pericardium related to parietal and visceral surfaces of inflamed pericardium rubbing against each other	▪ Absence of pericardial friction rub	▪ Auscultate precordium q2-4 hr for presence of friction rub; sound is similar to that produced by rubbing pieces of hair together over your ear and is described as grating or scratchy Press diaphragm of stethoscope firmly against chest Determine location of rub; usually is best appreciated along lower left sternal border to apex, but may be more diffuse Determine if rub is intermittent or continuous Determine number of components; it usually has three components related to movement of heart during atrial systole, ventricular systole, and diastole

POTENTIAL PROBLEMS	EXPECTED OUTCOMES	NURSING ACTIVITIES

		If rub is present
		  Report to physician
		  Record full description, including
		    Location
		    Number of components
		    Whether intermittent or continuous
		    Whether changing patient's position alters it

■ Alterations of pericardium related to alterations in cardiac electrophysiology	■ Resolution of ECG changes characteristic of pericarditis	■ Monitor 12 lead ECGs serially for characteristic changes of pericarditis if suspicious of presence and/or it is documented by diagnosis
		  S-T segment elevation in two or three standard leads and in some or all V leads; this occurs early in course, followed by S-T segments returning to baseline and T waves becoming flattened and then inverted in all leads except aVr
		  Absence of abnormal Q waves, loss of R wave voltage in V leads, and presence of general distribution of S-T segment changes helps differentiate pericarditis from MI; in addition, S-T segment elevation of pericarditis has concave curvature as opposed to convex curvature typical of MI
		If changes occur, save recorded strip and report to physician

■ Anxiety related to
  Limited understanding of disease and its effect on body
  Nature and degree of pain
	■ Patient verbalizes anxiety and asks questions
	Reduction of anxiety with sufficient information
	Patient notifies health care team of pain when present
		■ Ongoing assessment of level of anxiety
		Explain simply nature of disease and subsequent pain and fatigue, stressing that resolution of one will resolve other; also stress improvement in measurable parameters, indicating progress
		Explain reasons for monitoring and/or examination procedures used
		Encourage questions from patient/family

■ Collection of fluid in the pericardial sac related to pericardial effusion
Gradual accumulation of fluid in the pericardium; may be small or large in volume
	■ Absence or resolution of effusion or tamponade	■ Monitor carefully for changes in hemodynamic status; speed and amount of fluid accumulation determines onset of symptoms and frequency of observations
		Observe for the following indices of pericardial restrictions
		  Increased venous pressure*
		    Jugular vein distention
		    Elevated CVP
		    NOTE: If patient is receiving diuretic therapy, venous pressure elevation may be less obvious
		    Patient complaints of dyspnea or fullness in the chest
		  Decreased BP*
		  Narrowing pulse pressure
		  Sinus tachycardia resulting from decreased stroke volume
		  Weakening and/or absent peripheral pulse (decreased circulating blood volume)
		  Pulsus paradoxus: decrease in pulse volume and systolic BP (greater than 10 mm Hg) during normal inspiration related to changes in left ventricular filling; produced by pericardial restriction and accentuated by inspiration*
		    Palpate pulse for decrease in pulse amplitude with inspiration; check BP to confirm presence and to determine degree of pulsus paradoxus present
		    Have patient breathe normally; inflate cuff
		    Deflate cuff slowly and evenly, relating systolic reading to phase of inspiration
		    Identify and record point at which first systolic sounds are heard regardless of phase of respiration; the mm Hg difference represents millimeters of paradoxus
		  Increasing restlessness or anxiety
		  Signs of decreasing cerebral perfusion
		  Record serial 12 lead ECG to detect decreases in QRS voltages and/or development of electrical alternans (every other complex varies between two configurations)

*Indicates classic triad of tamponade.

POTENTIAL PROBLEMS	EXPECTED OUTCOMES	NURSING ACTIVITIES

		Report and record occurrence of any of aforementioned, and change timing of observations appropriately
		Prepare patient for special tests used to determine presence and amount of pericardial fluid, and monitor results if ordered
		  Echocardiography
		  Chest radiograph (enlarged heart with clear lung fields)
		  Radioisotope angiography
		  Contrast studies
		Ensure that equipment for pericardiocentesis is readily available if effusion is present and there is indication of increasing hemodynamic instability, or if presence of pus in pericardial sac is suspected
		Maintain patent IV line
		Administer steroids to treat recurrent effusions accompanied by fever and pain as ordered
		If tamponade develops
		  Place patient in low Fowler position; administer O_2 as ordered
		  Have CPR equipment and medications available for immediate use
		  Monitor venous pressure, BP, and P q15-30 min
		  Check peripheral pulses for perfusion q30 min
		  Check for changes in degree of pulsus paradoxus, q15 min
		  Monitor rhythm strips particularly for signs of tachycardia; take 12 lead ECG q30 min or as indicated
		  Observe for and record changes in mental status
		  Check for presence of Kussmaul sign resulting from restriction to diastolic filling (absence of normal fall in pressure during inspiration)
		  Assist with pericardiocentesis (removal of 100 to 200 ml usually results in dramatic improvement)
		  Administer medications and IVs as ordered for
		    Pain
		    Arrhythmias
		  Remain with patient as much as possible and provide emotional support
		  Prepare for potential surgery, which may be indicated particularly if tamponade recurs after successful pericardiocentesis

■ Constrictive pericarditis related to fibrosis of the pericardium
Usually develops slowly as a chronic disease but also may be subacute occurring in days or weeks even while effusion and/or tamponade is still present
	■ Absence or resolution of constriction	■ Determine if patient has past history of constrictive pericarditis
		Observe for
		  Fluid retention related to elevated systemic venous pressure
		  Ascites
		  Peripheral edema—may be pitting
		  Patient complaints of abdominal swelling, lassitude, and exertional dyspnea
		  Elevated jugular venous pressure
		  Decreased pulse pressure
		  Jaundice secondary to liver congestion and/or cardiac cirrhosis
		  Pulsus paradoxus (less common than in tamponade)
		  Auscultate precordium for "precordial knock," a loud third heart sound
		  Chronic, severe cachexia
		  Kussmaul sign (more common in patients with chronic pericarditis)
		Monitor ECG for
		  Atrial fibrillation—common in patients with chronic pericarditis
		  Low QRS voltage and flattened or inverted T waves
		  Conduction disturbances and pathological Q waves related to involvement of myocardium, conduction system, and/or coronary arteries
		  Notched P waves in lead II
		Prepare patient for and review results of the following, if ordered
		  Chest radiograph—useful only when pericardium is heavily calcified

POTENTIAL PROBLEMS	EXPECTED OUTCOMES	NURSING ACTIVITIES
		Liver function studies—presence of hepatic insufficiency
		Cardiac catheterization—to confirm absence of myocardial and/or valvular disease in presence of restricted ventricular filling
		If diagnosis is made, assist in preparation of patient for pericardial resection if indicated
■ Insufficient knowledge to comply with discharge regimen*	■ Evaluation by testing or questioning demonstrates patient/family's understanding of knowledge components of teaching program Patient asks pertinent questions regarding self-care	■ Institute teaching program for patient/family, including Nature of disease and effect on body; relate explanation to symptoms that patient experienced Signs and symptoms suggestive of recurrence to be reported to physician Increased fatigue without cause Elevated temperature and how to take it Chest pain Dyspnea Reasons for avoiding unnecessary exposure to people with upper respiratory infections and necessity of reporting cold or flu symptoms to physician Importance of avoiding fatigue and suggestions for doing so related to patient's pattern of activity Information regarding discharge medications, if any Follow-up information including why important, what visits involve, where to go, whom to see, and when Provide opportunities for patient/family to ask questions Assess patient/family's potential compliance

*If this type of follow-up care is the responsibility of the critical care unit nurse.

ENDOCARDITIS

Endocarditis is an infection of the endothelium and/or valves of the heart. It occurs most often in persons with structural abnormalities of the heart or great vessels but can occur in persons with normal hearts. The infection may occur on the valves or on the endocardium near congenital anatomical defects such as a ventricular septal defect. Since organisms other than bacteria, that is, fungi, viruses, and *Rickettsia,* may be responsible, it is most descriptive to use the term *endocarditis* preceded by the name of the appropriate microorganism.

The term *acute endocarditis* traditionally has been used to designate the time of fulminating onset or rapid progression of the disease. However, because even persons with subacute cases may suddenly develop serious complications, once the diagnosis is made appropriate therapy should be instituted and the differentiation loses significance.

Bacteria and other organisms can gain access to the circulation and hence the endothelium by many routes. The reason why the reticuloendothelial system, which normally handles transient bacteremia, is not successful in some people is not completely clear. People with a known predisposition to development of the disease are those with rheumatic valvular, congenital, or syphlitic cardiovascular disease. There is also a higher incidence in persons who have prosthetic valves or patches and in those who self-inject narcotics or diabetic medications. These people are particularly susceptible to bacteremia secondary to dental work, genitourinary manipulation (including catheterization), obstetrical and gynecological procedures, upper respiratory tract infections, pyoderma, and open heart surgery. Prophylactic treatment with an antibiotic should be considered. The selection of the drug is dependent on the kind of microorganisms likely to enter the bloodstream from the given site.

Endothelial vegetations develop as the bacteria multiply, initiating fibrin and platelet thrombi aggregation and deposition. If the process continues, it can lead to valvular injury or deformity. The mitral valve is most commonly involved, followed by the aortic, tricuspid, and pulmonic valves. Cardiac failure can develop or be aggravated by the resultant valvular damage or associated myocarditis. Peripheral complications may arise from endogenous im-

munological reactions to the chronic infection or from emboli released from the vegetations to various organs and tissues.

The diagnosis of endocarditis is often difficult. The disease may present itself acutely and dramatically or, more commonly, as an insidious but progressive process. The subacute form in particular may mimic almost any systemic disease, depending on the nature of the infecting organism, site of the vegetation, and the complications that have developed. Patients are often admitted to a critical care unit as a result of the complications with the diagnosis of endocarditis not yet established.

Fever, often low grade, is found in almost all cases, and cardiac murmurs are heard in the majority of patients. Once suspicion is aroused, blood cultures are drawn to confirm the diagnosis (they are not always positive) and to select the appropriate antibiotic. Cultures should be obtained before antibiotic therapy is initiated. An echocardiogram may reveal vegetations on infected valves.

Endocarditis is managed by the selection of an appropriate antibiotic for the involved microorganism. The antibiotic must be given in sufficient doses over time to eradicate the infecting organism.

Relapses may occur in a small percentage of patients following treatment; therefore follow-up cultures are obtained every 1 to 2 weeks up to 6 weeks, and the patient's temperature is monitored. The prognosis after successful treatment generally depends on the residual valvular damage.

ASSESSMENT

1. History of rheumatic, congenital, syphilitic heart disease, prosthetic cardiac valves or patches, frequent self-injections (narcotics or diabetics medication), and/or previously diagnosed endocarditis
2. Recent history of dental treatment and/or surgical procedures or instrumentation involving the upper respiratory tract, genitourinary tract, or lower GI tract
3. Signs and symptoms of infection
   a. Temperature above normal
   b. Diaphoresis and/or chills (most common at night)
   c. Anorexia; weight loss

d. Malaise
e. Arthralgias
4. New murmurs, particularly those characteristic of mitral, aortic, or tricuspid regurgitation
5. Petechiae in mucous membranes of mouth, conjunctiva, necklace area, or about wrists and ankles
6. Lab data results, including
   a. Blood culture reports
   b. Antibiotic sensitivity reports
   c. Hgb and Hct values for anemia
   d. Positive rheumatoid factor (latex agglutination titer)
   e. Echocardiograph report
7. Signs and symptoms of complications
   a. Cardiac decompensation
   b. Embolization to
      (1) Spleen
      (2) Kidneys
      (3) Brain
      (4) Coronary arteries
      (5) Peripheral arterial circulation
      (6) Lungs (right-sided endocarditis)
   c. Splenomegaly
   d. Pericarditis

8. Patient's perception of and reaction to the diagnosis and requirements of therapy

GOALS

1. Absence of infecting organism
2. Hemodynamic stability
3. Absence of or resolution of embolic complications
4. Patient asks questions and verbalizes understanding of disease, need for frequent blood samples, and therapy
5. Patient's behavior demonstrates decreased anxiety with provision of information
6. Before discharge, the patient/family
   a. Lists symptoms requiring physician notification with reasons why
   b. Asks pertinent questions regarding self-care
   c. Describes the activity regimen given him/her by the health care team
   d. Identifies methods for maintaining oral hygiene
   e. States the information regarding follow-up visits to physician and/or clinic
   g. Identifies situations or procedures for which prophylactic antibiotics may be indicated and whom to inform

POTENTIAL PROBLEMS	EXPECTED OUTCOMES	NURSING ACTIVITIES

■ Infection	■ Normal temperature
	Absence of diaphoresis and/or chills
	Absence of arthralgias related to bacteremia
	Normal appetite
	Negative blood cultures
		■ Check temperature q4 hr or as indicated
		Administer antipyretics/analgesics as ordered for elevated temperature or arthralgias; if there is little or no response, inform physician
		Institute cooling measures if needed
		Encourage fluid intake when temperature is elevated if there is no evidence of heart failure
		Avoid chills
		  Keep patient warm and dry
		  Avoid exposing body to differences in temperature
		  Change clothes and linen frequently while patient is diaphoretic
		Administer bactericidal antibiotic as ordered after checking patient's history for allergies; large doses may be required over 4 to 8 weeks
		  Maintain IV route or heparin lock; protect with armboard if necessary; check site and change dressing daily; change IV site q48 hr
		  Check for drug reaction—toxicity, rash, fever
		  Give drug on time; if patient is to be off floor unavoidably, give it early; if dose is delayed because of IV infiltration, give it promptly, inform physician, and change schedule only if necessary

■ Discomfort from IV related to phlebitis or immobilization of extremity	■ Absence of phlebitis
	Patient verbalizes comfort
		■ Observe regularly for phlebitis; if problem occurs
		  Remove IV promptly
		  Apply warm soaks
		  Culture if area is suppurating
		  Ensure that new IV is started before time of next antibiotic dose
		Alternate arms if possible when changing IV
		Provide active/passive ROM exercises
		Explore possibility of heparin lock

POTENTIAL PROBLEMS	EXPECTED OUTCOMES	NURSING ACTIVITIES
■ Malaise related to Cardiac infection Anemia Prolonged bed rest (if necessary)	■ Continuous increase in activity tolerance without fatigue	■ Evaluate extent of malaise related to immobility versus chronic infection versus anemia Maintain level of physical activity ordered during treatment as determined by the patient's situation/status If bed rest is necessary during acute phase or when evidence of heart failure is present Assist patient to turn, cough, and deep breathe q2-4 hr Assist with active or passive ROM exercises Apply elastic stockings Gradually increase activity level, monitoring cardiac tolerance Plan for rest periods between activities Avoid fatigue Provide for mobile IV stand or heparin lock, allowing greater freedom for ambulating patients Caution patient to avoid strenuous exercise (be specific) for several weeks following treatment
■ Anemia related to depressed bone marrow from chronic infection	■ Normal Hgb and Hct	■ Monitor serial Hgb and Hct values Administer blood products if ordered
■ Splenomegaly related to increased reticuloendothelial function resulting from duration of infection	■ Absence of or resolution of splenomegaly	■ Observe for indications of abdominal discomfort Spleen may be palpable 4 to 6 weeks into course of disease
■ Anxiety related to Limited understanding of disease and its effect on body Need for frequent blood samples and/or loss of blood	■ Patient verbalizes anxiety and asks questions Reduction of anxiety with sufficient information	■ Ongoing assessment of level of anxiety Encourage questions from patient/family Explain in simple terms nature of infection, relating explanation to patient's symptoms Explain purpose of frequent blood cultures and how often they will be drawn to determine organism and check response to antibiotics; note that amount drawn each time is equal to only 1 tablespoon (blood C and S tube holds 10 to 15 ml blood)
■ Valvular insufficiency related to complications of valve infection Perforation of cusp from infection eroding through leaflet Scarring may occur causing retraction/stenosis of valve Enlargement of vegetations can lead to poor closure of valve leaflets Necrosis and rupture of chordae tendineae or papillary muscles secondary to spread of infection	■ Absence of or correction of valvular insufficiency	■ Monitor for signs and symptoms suggestive of mitral, aortic, or tricuspid regurgitation; rarely are two or more valves infected simultaneously Mitral regurgitation Review chart and/or auscultate precordium for high-pitched, blowing holosystolic murmur best appreciated at apex or along lower left sternal border and which may radiate to axilla or back; turn patient to left lateral decubitus position to accentuate intensity; note also presence of S_3 and/or diminished S_1 Palpate precordium for apical impulse, which may be large, sustained, and displaced laterally Monitor for indications of left ventricular dilatation, hypertrophy, or failure, noting in particular rapid development of pulmonary congestion Aortic regurgitation Review chart and/or auscultate precordium for blowing, decrescendo diastolic murmur, that is best appreciated in third and fourth intercostal spaces along left sternal border with patient leaning forward and breath expelled and that may radiate to cardiac apex Palpate precordium for apical impulse, which may be large, forceful, sustained, and displaced downward and laterally Monitor for Wide pulse pressure Water-hammer pulse (bounding pulse with rapid rise and fall) Signs and symptoms of left ventricular failure

POTENTIAL PROBLEMS	EXPECTED OUTCOMES	NURSING ACTIVITIES

		Tricuspid regurgitation
		  Review chart and/or auscultate precordium for atrial gallop (S$_4$) and/or medium-pitched, blowing, holosystolic murmur best appreciated in fourth or fifth intercostal space close to or over sternum, accentuated by inspiration
		  Monitor for indications of right atrial enlargement and systemic venous congestion
		If problem occurs
		  Notify physician if physician is unaware of findings
		  Continue or initiate treatment as ordered for endocarditis and/or heart failure
		  Prepare patient/family for surgical replacement of artificial valve when applicable
		
		See STANDARD 15 *Heart failure (low cardiac output)*
		      STANDARD 27 *Cardiac surgery*

■ Cardiac decompensation related to altered hemodynamics from poorly functioning valves or myocarditis	■ Absence of or controlled left heart disease	■ Check BP, P, and R q4 hr or as indicated
		Auscultate chest for breath sounds at every shift
		Observe for early signs and symptoms of left heart failure
		  Sinus tachycardia
		  S$_3$ gallop
		  Bibasilar rales
		  Dyspnea
		If problem develops, see Standard 15, *Heart failure (low cardiac output)*

■ Embolic episodes	■ Absence of or resolution of embolic problem	■ Check report of echocardiogram if ordered; if vegetations are seen on valves, there is higher risk for embolization Observe for signs of embolization described in the following section at every shift and prn; report positive signs to physician immediately If embolic episode occurs; see Standard 31, *Embolic phenomena* Further diagnostic evaluation and antiembolic thrombolytic therapy may be instituted

Spleen		Observe for
		  Pain in left upper quadrant with radiation to left shoulder
		  Local tenderness, abdominal rigidity, and friction rub

Kidney		Observe for
		  Persistent hematuria
		  Oliguria
		  Costovertebral angle pain (lower back discomfort or flank pain

Brain		Observe for
		  Altered LOC
		  Paralysis; hemiplegia
		  Aphasia
		  Ptosis of eyelids, mouth droop
		  Incontinence
		  Seizures
		  Nausea and vomiting
		  Elevated BP
		  Abnormalities in respiratory pattern

Coronary arteries		Observe for signs/symptoms of MI, abscess, or pericarditis If problem occurs, see Standard 12, *Acute myocardial infarction;* Standard 18, *Pericarditis*

Peripheral arterial circulation		Observe extremities at every shift or prn for
		  Positive Homans' sign
		  Tenderness; pain
		  Swelling
		  Erythema

POTENTIAL PROBLEMS	EXPECTED OUTCOMES	NURSING ACTIVITIES
		Signs of acute arterial insufficiency to an extremity
		Decreased or absent pulse
		Coolness
		Blanching
		Decrease in capillary refilling time
		Observe acral portions of body (tip of nose, pinna of ear, fingers, and toes) for gangrenous infarctions
Lungs related to right-sided endocarditis		Observe for signs and symptoms related to hypoxia and pain
		Dyspnea
		Tachypnea
		Sudden pleuritic chest pain
		Tachycardia
		Pallor, cyanosis
		If symptoms occur
		Notify physician
		Assist with or draw arterial blood gas sample (look specifically for sudden drop in Po_2)

■ Insufficient knowledge to comply with discharge regimen*	■ Evaluation by testing or questioning demonstrates patient/family's understanding of knowledge components of teaching program
	Patient lists symptoms requiring physician notification
	Patient asks pertinent questions regarding self-care
		■ Institute teaching program for patient/family, including
		  Nature of infection and effect on heart
		  Relationship of predisposing factors to future susceptibility
		  Signs and symptoms of the disease with specific indications regarding notification of health team
		  Self-care instructions
		    Activity instructions
		    Oral hygiene
		    Suggestions for avoiding upper respiratory tract infections
		    Notification of other physicians and dentists of history
		    Situations that may require prophylactic antibiotic therapy
		  Antibiotic regimen
		    Purpose of drug
		    Dosage
		    Timing and importance of
		    Discuss importance of completing even though patient feels better
		    Side effects
		  Follow-up
		    Necessity of and timing
		    What is involved
		    Where to go and whom to see
		Provide opportunities for patient/family to ask questions
		Assess patient/family's potential compliance

*If this type of follow-up care is the responsibility of the critical care unit nurse.

HYPERTENSIVE CRISIS

Hypertension, or high blood pressure (BP), continues to be a prevalent health problem despite recent advances and increased public awareness of the condition. It is estimated that approximately 40 million Americans have hypertension, and up to an additional 25 million have borderline hypertension.

The criteria for the diagnosis of hypertension are abitrary, and several readings in various settings should be performed before the diagnosis is made. (Generally, it is recommended that BP be considered elevated if it is 140/90 mm Hg or greater for persons under age 50 years or 160/90 mm Hg or greater for persons age 50 years and older.) It is important to understand that there is no one normal BP and that readings may change within minutes in the same individual, as can easily be noted from arterial lines. Hypertension should be thought of as a continuum in which the higher the BP the greater the risk of developing the sequelae of MI, stroke, and renal failure. Because in most cases of hypertension there are no symptoms, assessing for hypertension should be an integral part of nursing care for all patients.

BP is a function of vasoconstriction (peripheral resistance) and volume (cardiac output). These two factors are regulated by both the adrenergic and renin-angiotensin systems. Hypertension occurs when one of these factors is elevated and the other is not able to compensate by a corresponding decrease or when both of these factors are elevated. The treatment is aimed at manipulating one or both of these factors.

In about 90% of hypertensive patients, no definite cause can be established. These cases are referred to as *primary* or *essential hypertension*. Primary hypertension can be controlled, but not cured. New research, however, indicates that not all cases of primary hypertension are alike physiologically. For example, one factor that may need to be considered before initiating treatment is the blood renin level.

In the remaining 10% of hypertensive patients a specific cause, most often renal or endocrine in nature, can be identified. These cases are referred to as *secondary hypertension*. It is important to identify whether or not secondary hypertension exists, because often it can be treated and cured. An example of this is renal artery stenosis, which can be treated with transluminal angioplasty, after which the hypertension is no longer present. In addition to renal artery stenosis, other causes of secondary hypertension follow:

Renal
- Renal artery stenosis
- Glomerulonephritis
- Renal failure
- Pyelonephritis

Endocrine
- Pheochromocytoma
- Cushing's syndrome
- Primary aldosteronism
- 17-Hydroxylase deficiency
- Congenital adrenal hyperplasia with virilism
- Pituitary tumor

Other
- Congenital coarctation of the aorta
- Toxemia of pregnancy
- Increased intracranial pressure (ICP)
- Oral contraceptive use

Treatment for hypertension can include both medications and nondrug therapies. Often a combination of both is used. Occasionally, nondrug therapies can eliminate the need for medication. Nondrug therapies can also make the patient feel more in control of his/her health care, an important factor in maintaining compliance. Regardless of the treatment for primary hypertension, it must be lifelong.

Antihypertensive medications can be classified into the following categories. These are listed below with examples from each group.

1. Diuretics
   a. Thiazides—hydrochlorthiazide
   b. Loop diuretics—furosemide (Lasix)
   c. Potassium-sparing diuretics—spironolactone, triamterene
2. Sympatholytics
   a. Central-acting—methyldopa, clonidine
   b. Ganglionic blockers—reserpine, guanethidine
   c. Alpha blockers—prazosin
   d. Beta blockers—propranolol, metoprolol, atenolol
3. Vasodilators
   a. Hydralazine

b. Nitroprusside
c. Minoxidil
4. Converting enzyme inhibitors—captopril
5. Calcium antagonists (not approved by FDA for hypertension)
   a. Nifedipine
   b. Verapamil

Nondrug therapies for hypertension include the following:
1. Low-sodium diet
2. Weight control
3. Exercise programs
4. Relaxation techniques
5. Cessation of smoking

Acute hypertensive crisis is aptly named, because it is sudden in onset and life threatening. Prompt treatment is imperative and includes immediate hospitalization for specialized monitoring and administration of parenteral drugs. Acute hypertensive crisis is associated with severe headache, marked elevation in arterial pressure, neurological phenomena, retinal changes, and decreased renal function. More precisely, there is a sustained diastolic pressure of at least 110 to 150 mm Hg and often higher. The neurological manifestations include nausea and vomiting, headache, visual changes, confusion, encephalopathy, convulsions, or coma. The retinal changes reflect the severity of illness and range from hemorrhage or exudate to papilledema or retinal artery spasm.

Many processes can lead to or cause hypertensive crisis. Some of the more common include history of severe hypertension (diastolic pressure >115 mm Hg); accelerated hypertension (diastolic pressure >120 mm Hg and grade III retinopathy, that is, exudates and hemorrhages on the retina); malignant hypertension (diastolic pressure >140 mm Hg and grade IV retinopathy, that is, papilledema); preeclampsia and eclampsia of pregnancy; acute or chronic glomerulonephritis; renal vascular hypertension; pheochromocytoma; and adverse reaction to concurrent intake of certain foods with monoamine oxidase (MAO) inhibitors. It is also associated, though rarely, with head injury; antihypertensive drug withdrawal; or preexisting hypertension that is further complicated by acute left ventricular hypertrophy, acute dissecting aortic aneurysm, or intracranial hemorrhage. It is important that acute anxiety states with labile hypertension be diagnosed differentially, because treatment is vastly different.

The extent and progression of hypertensive crisis vary according to the individual, the degree of hypertension, and the amount of time that has elapsed from onset to treatment.

Priorities of treatment and management of hypertensive crisis include maintenance of a patent airway and adequate pulmonary ventilation, immediate IV drug therapy to lower the arterial pressure to safe levels, treatment of any precipitating factors, prevention/control of metabolic disturbances, appropriate fluid and nutritional maintenance, and commencement and maintenance of long-term antihypertensive drug therapy once the patient's arterial pressure is sufficiently stabilized.

Complications of hypertensive crisis can be dramatically reduced by prompt treatment before their onset. Complications include widespread arteriolar necrosis, ischemic atrophy of the nephron and renal failure, left ventricular failure, MI, stroke, and coma. The most common complications are cerebral, renal, or cardiovascular problems. The usual signs of the commonly seen encephalopathy are headache, nausea, vomiting, blurred vision, drowsiness, confusion, fleeting numbness or tingling in the limbs, convulsions, and coma. It will be noted that these same signs and symptoms can also herald a cerebrovascular accident (CVA), although with a CVA the deficits are usually progressive rather than sudden and precipitous as observed in hypertensive crisis. It is important to distinguish the medical treatment of CVA from that of hypertensive crisis—a precipitous drop in arterial pressure for the patient with a CVA would be deleterious.

ASSESSMENT

1. Clinical history of
   a. New onset or current episode of hypertension, and/or any therapy
   b. Previously diagnosed hypertension or hypertension-related illness and therapy, to include any episodes of hypertensive crisis; etiological factors may include those listed on p. 144
2. Presence of risk or predisposing factors
   a. Family history
   b. Smoking—number of packs per day
   c. Obesity—self and family profile
   d. Pregnancy—full obstetrical history
   e. Dietary habits—high-sodium/high-fat diet
   f. Stressful life-style
   g. Sedentary life-style
   h. Discontinuation of medications
   i. Addition of new medications, e.g., prednisone
   j. Noncompliance with prescribed therapy
3. Patient/family's level of anxiety; reaction to illness
4. Patient assessment
   a. Appearance
   b. LOC—orientation, mental changes
   c. Findings of clinician's funduscopic examination—retinopathy
   d. Color, temperature, turgor, and moisture of skin
   e. Pain—location, type, onset, duration, any precipitating/relieving features (for example, often "anginal" type)
   f. Respirations—rate, pattern, depth, and characteristics of breath sounds, any dyspnea
   g. Temperature
   h. BP—both arms and then via intraarterial line (sys-

tolic, diastolic, MAP), any postural hypertension

i. Pulses—rate, rhythm, quality and equality; neck vein distension; heart sounds

j. Cardiac rhythm—assess for dysrhythmias, characteristic changes of myocardial ischemia, electrolyte imbalance, and drug effects

k. Nausea or vomiting

l. Fluid balance—urinary output per hour

5. Results of diagnostic studies to ascertain possible cause(s) of elevated arterial pressure and its effects

a. Urinalysis—hematuria and/or proteinuria

b. Serum electrolytes—serum K^+ low in primary aldosteronism; blood glucose

c. Serum BUN and creatinine—elevated in renal disease

d. CBC—Hct is decreased in renal failure

g. Serum uric acid—hyperuricemia is associated with hypertension

h. Urinary vanillylmandelic acid (VMA)—catecholamines are elevated

i. Blood renin levels

j. Chest radiograph

k. Abdominal radiograph

l. IV pyelogram/renal vein renins

m. CT scan

n. ECG

o. Echocardiography

6. Reaction to drug therapy

a. Hypotension—changes in mental status, urinary output, pain

b. Dysrhythmias

c. Nausea and vomiting, malaise, drowsiness

d. Impotence

e. Syncope and nightmares

7. At discharge—patient's compliance profile

a. Knowledge of condition

b. Degree of acceptance and acknowledgement of condition

c. Understanding of medical regimen—drugs, diet, rest/activity level

d. Willingness for life-style changes

e. Degree of maturity and acceptance to be responsible for level of own health and health care

f. Motivation for compliance

g. Barriers to compliance

h. Anxiety

i. Family/other support

j. Access to follow-up care

GOALS

1. Reduction of the patient's/family's anxiety by provision of information, explanation, and encouragement

2. Maintenance of arterial pressure below 140/90 mm Hg, or as individualized for the patient

3. Hemodynamic stability

4. Absence and/or resolution of any complications, including neurological, cardiac, renal, and psychological

5. Fluid balance and nutritional intake adequate and modified for positive nitrogen balance, low sodium and fat

6. CBC, acid-base balance, and electrolyte levels within normal limits

7. Absence and/or resolution of any further deterioration of associated diseases related to hypertensive crisis

8. Patient demonstrates sense of control over life and emotional stability

9. Before discharge patient/family is able to

a. Describe medication regimen

b. Describe rationale for medication regimen

c. Describe dietary regimen

d. Describe rationale for dietary regimen

e. List signs and symptoms that require medical attention

f. State necessary information with regard to clinic appointment or follow-up care

POTENTIAL PROBLEMS	EXPECTED OUTCOMES	NURSING ACTIVITIES

■ Patient's anxiety/fear related to illness and admission to hospital and critical care unit	■ Patient demonstrates decreased level of anxiety and is able to make major needs known	■ Patient's anxiety should be managed concurrent with antihypertensive therapy and other priorities of care
		Assess level of anxiety
		Develop rapport
		Demonstrate interest and concern
		  Explain critical care unit routines and environment
		  Maintain calm and competent manner to promote confidence
		  Stay with patient and reassure as indicated
		  Explain all procedures before performing them
		Maintain patient's self-esteem
		  Allow patient to have as much control and independence as possible
		  Provide comfort measures
		Encourage verbalization of any anxiety/fear/questions
		Prepare patient for and support during procedures

POTENTIAL PROBLEMS	EXPECTED OUTCOMES	NURSING ACTIVITIES
		Provide environment conducive to mental and physical rest Protect from inappropriate clinical discussions Ensure rest periods between interventions Monitor visitors according to patient's needs Monitor for sensory overload/deprivation Monitor noise pollution Ensure ordered sedation/analgesia is given with patient reaction documented and appropriate changes made to minimize/alleviate pain and discomfort

■ Family's anxiety related to
   Admission to critical
     care unit
   Threat of death
	■ Family demonstrates
	   Decreased level of anxiety
	   Sense of trust in critical
	     care team
		■ Family's anxiety should be managed concurrent with patient's therapy
		Assess level of anxiety and listen effectively to family's concerns
		Develop rapport
		Introduce key family members to key unit team members
		Give information, e.g., leaflet, concerning visiting, how to get condition reports and information, philosophy of nursing care for unit, general routines, and specialty features
		Demonstrate interest and concern in calm and competent manner to promote confidence and trust
		Encourage verbalization of anxieties/fears and any questions
		Explain purpose and encourage attendance at family group meetings, if available
		Assess for need of intervention with social worker

■ Patient/family's anxiety related to limited understanding of
   Disease process and
     prognosis
   Diagnostic procedures
     and therapy employed
   Altered family roles
   Separation from family
     members
   Loss of job
	■ Patient/family's behavior
	   demonstrates decreased
	   level of anxiety with increased understanding of
	   Disease process
	   Plan of care
	   Family relationships and
	     altered roles
	   Future possibilities
		■ Patient/family's anxiety should be managed concurrent with antihypertensive therapy and other priorities of care
		Document ongoing assessment of level of anxiety for appropriateness
		Assess inquiries for readiness of learning
		Explain nature of disease process and reasons why patient is feeling as he/she is
		Explain anticipated procedures and what patient will experience
		Assist in preparing patient for diagnostic procedures
		Explain and involve patient/family in plan of care
		Encourage patient/family's questions and verbalizations of concerns, anxieties and/or fears
		Communicate findings to physician on ongoing basis
		Support family via primary nurse and/or resource designated by primary nurse (nursing supervisor, clinician, social worker).
		Encourage patient/family's questions regarding prognosis, using primary nurse and designated resources
		Assess need for psychological evaluation of patient or need for support from primary nurse/nursing staff, using appropriate clinician(s)

■ Impaired gas exchange related to
   Decreased CNS function
   Ineffective airway clearance
   Ventilation/perfusion
     imbalance
   Pulmonary edema
	■ Adequate gas exchange
	   with adequate oxygenation and acid-base status
	   for particular patient
		■ Position patient optimally to protect airway
		Record and monitor respiratory rate, depth and characteristics of breath sounds, cough and sputum
		Report adventitious sounds and altered findings to physician
		Measure V_T and minute volume
		Monitor arterial blood gas levels and Hgb as ordered
		Give humidified O_2 as ordered
		Turn patient from side to side q2 hr to mobilize secretions, prevent atelectasis, and optimize ventilation/perfusion ratio
		Institute other respiratory nursing measures as ordered; see Standard 2, *Acute respiratory failure*
		If mechanical ventilation via artificial airway is instituted, see Standard 6, *Mechanical ventilation*
		If pulmonary edema occurs, see Standard 1, *Pulmonary edema of cardiac origin*

POTENTIAL PROBLEMS	EXPECTED OUTCOMES	NURSING ACTIVITIES
■ Elevated BP related to Severe, accelerated, or malignant hypertension Preeclampsia or eclampsia Acute or chronic glomerulonephritis Renal vascular hypertension Pheochromocytoma Adverse reaction to certain foods with MAO inhibitors	■ Return of BP to within safe limits for the particular patient	■ Maintain calm and quiet environment Record arterial pressure on both arms, in sitting and lying position if feasible, via cuff for baseline Position patient with head of bed at ordered elevation, if feasible, to increase orthostatic effect Prepare for insertion of intraarterial line immediately Monitor arterial pressure via intraarterial line continuously, setting narrow alarm limits as additional means of immediate warning of variation from current parameters Reset alarm limits as arterial pressure declines Administer antihypertensive drug(s) as ordered NOTE: For patients with *pheochromocytoma,* diagnosis is usually made by 12-hour urinary catecholamine analysis of epinephrine, norepinephrine, metanephrine, and normetanephrine, and CT scan; IV phentolamine (Regitine), an alpha-adrenergic blocking agent, is usually commenced to stabilize arterial pressure before surgical removal of tumor Institute specific measures required for antihypertensive drug used; e.g., specifics for sodium nitroprusside include: Cover container with foil, because solution is photosensitive Change solution q4 hr Obtain daily serum thiocyanate levels after first 24 hours of infusion Monitor for tolerance to drug (resistance to drug effects) Inform physician immediately of any reaction(s) to drug therapy, because drug will be titrated accordingly Monitor patient for particular side effects of antihypertensive agent used Monitor patient for dysrhythmias Monitor patient for oliguria Monitor serum electrolyte levels as ordered Observe for signs of hyperkalemia Observe for pain and report to physician, because potential change in patient's condition/diagnosis, e.g., sudden severe chest pain radiating to back, abdomen, and hips, is indicative of acute dissecting aortic aneurysm (see Standard 30, *Vascular surgery: aneurysms);* chest pain could indicate cardiac compromise Observe for and report to physician changes in LOC, visual changes, headache, nausea, and vomiting, because these changes indicate potential/actual increase in ICP and may herald seizure activity or coma
■ Hypotension related to Excessive diuretic and/ or antihypertensive therapy Hypovolemia from afterload manipulation and increased vascular space	■ Optimal arterial pressure and normovolemia	■ Monitor arterial pressure continuously and PAP if catheter is in situ, including PAWP Monitor urine output per hour Inform physician of changes in parameters Stop/decrease/titrate antihypertensive agents, as ordered Monitor intake/output balance, and weigh daily Participate in activities to restore arterial pressure as ordered, e.g., antihypertensive medication; give fluid challenge; administer vasopressor Monitor serum electrolytes, particularly serum K$^+$
■ Decrease in urinary output, related to impaired renal function as sequela of hypertension	■ Resolution of oliguria, i.e., urine output >400 to 600 ml/24 hr Normovolemia, i.e., excess body fluids removed Serum electrolytes, BUN, creatinine and bilirubin, acid-base balance within normal limits	■ Record intake and output meticulously Weigh patient daily and report to physician Evaluate need to modify nutritional intake Evaluate whether to increase concentration of IV antihypertensive therapy solutions to reduce volume and potential hypervolemia Obtain serum and urine osmolality for free water clearance Give diuretics, as ordered Monitor serum electrolytes, BUN, creatinine Observe for changes in LOC Observe for edema; see Standard 52, *Acute renal failure*

POTENTIAL PROBLEMS	EXPECTED OUTCOMES	NURSING ACTIVITIES
■ Altered LOC related to Altered arterial pressure Actual/potential increase in ICP	■ Patient returned to optimal LOC, orientation, and neurological function	■ Ensure safe environment with siderails up Document usual LOC, orientation to person, place, and time, pupillary response, and movement of extremities Note clinician's neurological examination, including funduscopic examination, and compare with physician's current examination Document and report any changes in neurological status, i.e., LOC, progressive loss of consciousness, (confusion, behavioral changes), pupillary responses, movement of extremities; also vital signs Ensure patency of IV antihypertensive drug infusion Obtain results of arterial blood gas, serum electrolytes, and glucose levels, and report to physician Assess anxiety level, reassure and remain with patient Orient patient frequently to place, person, and time Prepare patient and assist with ordered interventions and diagnostic procedures
■ Manifestations, e.g., headache, visual disturbances, nausea and vomiting, fleeting numbness/tingling of limbs, related to *Encephalopathy* as sequela of excessive arterial pressure Potential/actual increase in ICP	■ Absence/resolution of specific manifestation(s)	■ Assess patency of IV antihypertensive drug infusion Document and report manifestation(s) to physician Reassure patient and assure maximal comfort (e.g., cold compress to forehead for headache) Maintain calm, quiet milieu Document and report neurological observations q1 hr Implement physician's orders, e.g., increase/change antihypertensive therapy Perform only one intervention at a time, and allow rest period in between interventions to minimize any rise in ICP Turn patient from side to side slowly and gently, using "pull sheet"; if patient assists, instruct patient to avoid Valsalva maneuver; move patient during patient's respiratory exhalation Prepare and assist with ordered interventions/diagnostic procedures
■ Seizure activity related to Excessive arterial pressure and potential/actual increase in ICP Previous medical history	■ Absence/resolution of any seizure activity Absence of complications	■ Assess for seizure history of patient on admission; if present, note any particular aura patient experiences Instruct patient to inform nurse immediately if aura is experienced Institute seizure precautions Ensure anticipated medications are readily available Monitor for predisposing factors, i.e., hypoxia, hyperventilation, hypoglycemia, hypervolemia, electrolyte imbalance, hyperthermia, extreme fatigue/stress, and report to physician Monitor and record seizure activity, i.e., onset, progression, involvement, focus and duration, eye/head deviation, eye rolling, oral foaming, and incontinence Administer ordered medication(s) and monitor effects Maintain patent airway and prevent injury to patient's head and body Monitor postictal status *See* STANDARD 41 *Seizures*
■ Impaired cerebral perfusion, e.g., CVA, transitory ischemic events, related to Altered arterial pressure Cerebral edema and/or cerebral hemorrhage	■ Return of optimal CNS function with optimal resolution of any complications	■ Monitor and notify physician of changes in neurological status q1-2 hr; observe for Change in LOC, drowsiness and progressive loss of consciousness, confusion, and behavioral changes Pupillary reactions Speech difficulties Headache Nuchal rigidity Weakness of extremities Facial drooping Monitor hemodynamic status continuously Administer ordered antihypertensive agents

POTENTIAL PROBLEMS	EXPECTED OUTCOMES	NURSING ACTIVITIES
		NOTE: Elevated arterial pressure related to CVA should be lowered gradually rather than rapidly; precipitous drop would compromise cerebral perfusion pressure and further compromise brain function by increasing any ischemic/infarcted areas
		Protect and maintain airway patency by side-to-side positioning and judicial suctioning
		Monitor and ensure adequacy of respirations and minute volume; give O_2 as ordered.
		Turn patient from side to side q2 hr to mobilize secretions, optimize ventilation/perfusion ratio, prevent atelectasis, and preserve skin integrity
		Position limbs in correct alignment, using measures to prevent foot-drop, wrist-drop, and contractures
		Perform passive ROM exercises, and consult with physiotherapist
		Maintain adequate nutritional intake
		Monitor bowel regimen
		Monitor intake and output, and weight daily
		Monitor serum electrolyte, glucose, BUN, creatinine, Hgb, and albumin levels
		Ensure safe environment and keep siderails up
		Prepare patient and assist with diagnostic procedures, e.g., CT scan
		See STANDARD 34 *Subarachnoid hemorrhage*
■ Decreased cardiac output related to Excessive antihypertensive therapy Previous cardiac medical history Ventricular dysfunction related to Cardiac failure Increased left ventricular end diastolic pressure Myocardial ischemia MI	■ Absence or resolution of decreased cardiac output Hemodynamic stability	■ Stop/change antihypertensive agent or dose as ordered
		Monitor for diaphoresis, cool skin, tachypnea, change in LOC, decreased urinary output, rales, S_3 gallop, neck vein distention
		Monitor for factors known to compound heart failure, dysrhythmias, hypoxemia, acidosis
		Monitor LOC and urine output
		Observe and report any chest pain
		Prepare patient and equipment for insertion of PAP catheter
		Assist with insertion of PAP catheter and record right atrial and right ventricular pressures
		Monitor and record PAP systolic and diastolic and PCWP
		Participate in activities of aggressive management to prevent and/or interrupt shock cycle
		See STANDARD 16 *Cardiogenic shock* STANDARD 25 *Hemodynamic monitoring* STANDARD 12 *Acute myocardial infarction*
■ Dysrhythmias related to Electrolyte disturbance Hypoxemia Any etiological condition precipitating decreased cardiac output Compensatory mechanism for decreased stroke volume	■ Electrophysiological stability Optimal cardiac rhythm	■ Maintain continuous ECG monitoring with rate limits set appropriately
		Assess and report any ECG changes to physician
		Monitor lab results for hypoxemia, electrolyte imbalance, particularly serum K^+
		Check emergency equipment, ensuring proper functioning and/or availability of all items
		For specific arrythmias, see Standard 21, *Arrhythmias*
■ Serum electrolyte imbalance or acid-base imbalance related to Diuretic therapy Potential/actual renal disorder Respiratory compromise	■ Serum electrolytes within normal limits Acid-base balance within normal limits	■ Monitor serum electrolytes, particularly, Na^+, Cl^-, K^+, and phosphate
		Observe for ECG changes
		Monitor arterial blood gas levels; note acidosis or alkalosis
		Administer electrolyte replacements as ordered, and monitor repeat serum electrolyte values
■ Nutritional compromise related to Decreased/increased appetite	■ Normal appetite Progress toward optimal weight (gain or loss) Positive nitrogen balance	■ Assess patient's baseline nutritional status
		Obtain baseline diet history from patient and/or family, including how medical history affects intake of nutrients and patient's food preferences and dislikes
		Include data from GI assessment and history

POTENTIAL PROBLEMS	EXPECTED OUTCOMES	NURSING ACTIVITIES

Decreased/increased nutritional intake
Inability to eat
Instability of patient's condition
Stress
	Patient consumes most of required diet on food tray	Calculate patient's nutritional intake with physician, including daily caloric requirements and supplemental elements, e.g., Na^+, Cl^-, K^+, PO_4, Mg^{++}, Ca^{++}, folic acid, and vitamins
		NOTE: Elevated temperature increases caloric need
		Ensure adequate intake po, or if not possible, via NG feedings
		  Encourage even small amounts po, and give remainder via NG tube
		  If gut cannot be used, ensure adequate parenteral alimentation
		  NOTE: 5% dextrose solutions provide 200 kcal/liter and are therefore inadequate after 24 hours
		Weigh patient daily at same time and notify physician of significant weight gain/loss (>1 kg/24 hours)
		Monitor intake and output
		Provide milieu conducive to eating
		  Remove offensive or appetite-supressing items, e.g., emesis basin, syringes from bed table, etc.
		  Perform oral hygiene before and after meals and prn
		  Position patient comfortably
		  Consider distracting patient from other ongoing unit activities/procedures (e.g., with television, earphones, family member)
		  Ensure appropriate tray and utensils
		  Assist by cutting food, removing lids, opening packages
		  Prohibit interventions, e.g., blood samples
		If patient is receiving NG tube feedings
		  Assess abdomen and bowel sounds
		  Place patient in semi-Fowler position
		  Ensure proper location and patency of NG tube
		  Aspirate NG tube before feeding, and test for heme; notify physician of excessive volume of aspirate and/or positive heme result
		  Modify feedings as indicated
		  Monitor bowel regimen and intervene as indicated
		If the patient is to be given parenteral alimentation, see Standard 57, *Total parenteral nutrition*

■ Malnutrition related to
Prolonged poor nutrition
Lack of knowledge
Poor compliance to or tolerance of diet
	■ Absence or resolution of any signs of malnutrition (i.e., return to ideal body weight)
	Regular pattern of elimination
		■ Assess for signs and symptoms of malnutrition
		  Weight loss/gain
		  Presence of swollen face with dark cheeks and circles under eyes
		  Dull eyes with pale or red mucosa
		  Presence of bloodshot ring around corneas
		  Grey spots on conjunctiva, red and fissured eyelid corners
		  Swollen lips
		  Spongy, tender gums that bleed easily
		  Presence of dental decay or missing teeth; assess state of dentures
		  Any enlargement of parotid gland
		  Flaky, dry skin with spots, contusions, or ulcers
		  Brittle or split nails
		  Poor skin turgor
		  Decreased subcutaneous fat, muscle atrophy
		Request dietitian to plan meals and supplements with patient
		Ensure adequate nutritional intake
		Use appetizers as stimulants
		Provide frequent, small feedings as necessary
		List fluids and food consumed and monitor and inform dietary department of preferences and dislikes
		Note any unusual eating habits/patterns
		Permit special food requests whenever possible
		Permit, if feasible, occasional home-cooked foods
		Initiate patient teaching concerning nutritional needs, diet, purpose of weight loss/gain

POTENTIAL PROBLEMS	EXPECTED OUTCOMES	NURSING ACTIVITIES
▪ Abdominal manifestations, e.g., abdominal pain, nausea, vomiting, diarrhea, melena, related to *mesenteric ischemia,* as sequela of excessively rapid reduction of arterial pressure	▪ Absence of abdominal manifestations related to mesenteric ischemia.	▪ Monitor arterial pressure and other vital signs continuously Titrate antihypertensive agent(s) or administer as ordered Monitor response(s) to antihypertensive agent(s) continuously Observe for abdominal cramps, pain, nausea, vomiting, diarrhea, melena, and report to physician
▪ Infection related to Hospital environment (nosocomial) Invasive lines, e.g., IV, intraarterial, and/or pulmonary artery catheters; Foley catheters	▪ Absence of infection Afebrile	▪ Maintain meticulous handwashing technique before and after procedures *and in between patients* Monitor patient's temperature and report elevation Adhere to hospital and unit infection control policies Ensure that other personnel maintain standards and policy for infection control Change tubes, dressings, etc., using strict aseptic technique and according to hospital and unit policies and Centers for Disease Control recommendations Perform meticulous daily and prn care of Foley catheter Dress all puncture sites/wounds in occlusive manner Culture any suspicious foci and report to physician Perform routine cultures of urine and sputum for anergic patients Maintain clean, dry, comfortable environment for patient Report spills (blood, urine, etc.) promptly for timely cleaning; meanwhile, cover, to prevent spread and/or accident Monitor equipment for cleanliness and/or sterility on regular basis Participate in any unit audits for quality control Follow recommendations from audit(s) *See* STANDARD 61 *Infection control in the critical care unit*
▪ Insufficient knowledge to comply with discharge regimen related to* Denial of problem Anxiety Lack of knowledge Poor motivation Lack of follow-up	▪ Patient/family demonstrates or gives evidence of knowledge attained necessary for compliance with discharge regimen; by verbalization of Dietary regimen Drug regimen Rationales for drug and diet regimen Duration of regimen required, i.e., lifelong Proposed changes in life-style Signs and symptoms requiring patient to seek medical attention Information for access to follow-up care Decreased anxiety about condition	▪ Assess continuously patient's/family's understanding of disease process, discharge regimen, and follow-up care Assess any social/financial problems, and refer to social worker, if appropriate Consult with physician regarding discharge plan Assess patient/family's readiness to learn Instruct and document patient/family teaching about *Physiology,* to include Etiology, risk factors Complications Importance of regimen *Diet,* to include Types of food to avoid, (those high in saturated fat) Types of food to consume Sodium restriction Caloric requirements Encourage patient to plan his/her meals while in hospital with feedback from dietitian/nurse Obtain diet history and assist patient/family with diet plan for discharge Explain purpose of diet change simply and have patient explain to nurse to verify accuracy of information Instruct patient to regularly record weight

*If responsibility of critical care nurse includes follow-up care. Consider this an ongoing part of the care plan. Noncompliance subsequent to acute hypertensive crisis is especially common; because the patient feels better, the likelihood of denial is high.

POTENTIAL PROBLEMS	EXPECTED OUTCOMES	NURSING ACTIVITIES

Medications, to include
    Name of drug
    Dose and frequency of drug
    Purpose of drug
    Side effects and how to minimize them (e.g., postural hypotension, syncope, impotence)
        Reassure patient that if side effects do occur, they may subside over time
        Instruct patient to report side effects to physician
    Assisting patient in devising system for scheduling doses
    Refilling prescription in timely fashion
Activity level
Life-style changes, to include
    Sharing with and/or giving risk factor profile to patient/family; discussing possible life-style changes, e.g., cessation of smoking, weight reduction
    Attempting to involve patient in devising patient "contract" to be reviewed at each clinic visit to improve compliance
    Instructing patient in need to continue therapy, even in absence of symptoms

ARRHYTHMIAS

Arrhythmias are disturbances of impulse formation and/or conduction within the electrical system of the heart. To understand the pathogenesis of arrhythmias, it is necessary to review the electrophysiology of the heart.

Automaticity (diastolic depolarization) refers to the ability of cardiac cells to discharge spontaneously, not requiring an external or propagated impulse to fire. Certain specialized cells such as those in the sinus node, the conductive pathways of the atria, the AV junctional tissue, and the His-Purkinje system have this capability. This creates the potential for these cells to act as the dominant pacemaker, depolarizing the rest of the heart. Normally, the sinus node acts as the dominant pacemaker, because it spontaneously discharges faster than the other specialized cells, often called *latent* or *secondary* pacemakers. Should one of the other areas discharge more rapidly than the sinus node, it may depolarize the atria, ventricles, or both. This may occur in two ways. If the sinus node discharges at a slower rate than a latent pacemaker or if the sinus impulse is blocked before reaching the latent pacemaker site, the latent pacemaker may *passively* escape sinus domination and discharge automatically at its own intrinsic rate. These escape beats or escape rhythms will be slower than normal sinus rhythm, because the intrinsic rate of the junctional tissue is 40 to 55 times/minute and that of the His-Purkinje system is 20 to 40 times/minute. The other mechanism by which a latent pacemaker may take control is if it abnormally accelerates its discharge rate (increased automaticity) and *actively* usurps control from the sinus node. This results in a premature beat and may occur in the specialized cells of the atria, junctional tissue, or ventricles. A series of three premature beats in a row is considered a tachycardia.

For a pacemaker to depolarize the myocardium, it must be conducted from its site of origin through the heart. *Excitability* is a property of the cell receiving a stimulus that determines whether the cell will be discharged by that impulse. Many factors may influence excitability, but the most important is at what point during the recovery period following depolarization the heart is restimulated. Stages of the recovery period are related to the refractoriness of heart muscle. Immediately following depolarization is the *abso-lute refractory period,* during which excitability is zero and the tissue will not respond to a stimulus regardless of how intense it is. This is followed by the *relative refractory period,* in which excitability is improving and a strong stimulus can evoke a response. Following this period, the heart will be fully excitable, and a relatively weak stimulus could evoke a response.

The speed at which the impulse spreads through the heart is the *conduction velocity,* which varies considerably depending on the inherent properties of different portions of the specialized conduction system and the myocardium. Velocity is most rapid in Purkinje fibers and slowest in the midportion of the AV node. If conduction becomes uneven because of a difference in refractoriness, block may occur in some areas and not in others, or block may occur in a tissue but only in one direction (unidirectional). When the block is unidirectional, this uneven conduction may allow the initial impulse to reenter areas previously unexcitable that are now recovered. Should the *reentering* impulse then be able to depolarize the entire atria and/or ventricles, a corresponding extra systole (an ectopic beat, dependent on and coupled to the preceding beat) results. Maintenance of the reentrant excitation (circus phenomenon) establishes a tachycardia.

Changes in automaticity and/or conduction can conceivably occur as a result of almost any disease state or system imbalance, making them a common problem in critically ill patients, even those with normal hearts. Any form of cardiac disease may be complicated or compensated for by arrhythmias, the latter often resulting in response to decreased stroke volume or hypotension. Other conditions often implicated include alterations in body temperature; hypoxia; hypercapnia; hypovolemia; abnormal potassium and calcium concentrations; drugs, particularly digitalis; stress; and surgery, particularly cardiac.

The clinical or hemodynamic significance of an arrhythmia is ultimately dependent on its effect on the cardiac output. This is primarily determined by the patient's cardiovascular status, the duration of the arrhythmia, and the site of origin and its effect on the ventricular rate. Arrhythmias resulting in rapid ventricular rates increase myocardial oxygen consumption while decreasing the availability of oxygen to the myocardium by shortening diastole (ventricular filling time) and thereby reducing stroke volume. Those resulting in slow ventricular rates, if they are not compensated for by increased stroke volume, also result in decreased cardiac output and the consequent problems of underperfusion of vital organs and the peripheral vessels. The loss of the sequential atrial-ventricular contraction sequence can be particularly detrimental to patients with left heart failure and/or mitral valve disease who are dependent on atrial contraction for adequate ventricular filling. Finally, the electrical stability of an arrhythmia is also an important factor in determining significance, particularly in patients with AMI in whom experience has documented the incidence of one arrhythmia creating opportunities for, or resulting in, the development of other more threatening arrhythmias.

The management of an arrhythmia is dependent on its effect on the patient; accurate interpretation of the rhythm; its cause; its natural history and stability, e.g., transient or degenerative; the presence and nature of myocardial disease; the patient's electrolyte status; concomitant drug therapy; and the status of organ systems influencing drug metabolism. Based on these considerations, a number of treatment modalities may be employed. If the arrhythmia is not life-threatening, and particularly in the absence of heart disease, treatment of the underlying problem may be sufficient, such as correction of hypoxia or electrolyte imbalance. Treatment modalities include pharmacological agents; electrical intervention including pacing, cardioversion, or defibrillation; vagal maneuvers such as Valsalva or carotid sinus massage; and surgery. Combinations of modalities may be required.

One of the more significant advances in recent years in the treatment of ventricular tachycardia is clinical electrophysiological testing. This provides a method for improving the identification of the responsible mechanism, i.e., increased automaticity or reentry; for making therapeutic decisions more selectively; and for evaluating the selected therapy more objectively. See Standard 22, *The role of clinical electrophysiological testing in the treatment of ventricular tachycardia.*

Arrhythmias related to cardiac problems as opposed to those relating to acute imbalances and/or therapeutic modalities are more likely to require chronic management.

ASSESSMENT

1. History, including
   a. Preexisting arrhythmias
      (1) Precipitating factors if known
      (2) Associated symptoms
      (3) Onset, frequency, and duration
      (4) Therapeutic interventions, if any, and effectiveness
      (5) Relationship, if any, to current event
   b. Preexisting organic heart disease

   c. Medications
   d. Smoking and/or caffeine habits
2. Current medical and/or cardiovascular problems
3. Current forms of treatment, particularly pharmacological agents employed
4. Presence of factors that predispose to arrhythmias and/or influence therapy
   a. Electrolyte imbalance—K^+ and Ca^{++}
   b. Hypoxia; hypercapnia
   c. Pain
   d. Anxiety
   e. Fever
   f. Infection
   g. Hypovolemia
   h. Anemia
   i. Endocrine disorders—hypoglycemia and diabetes
   j. Hypothyroidism or hyperthyroidism
   k. Impaired organ function—liver, renal
5. Continuous monitoring and/or full ECG for accurate interpretation of arrhythmia; old tracings may be helpful
6. Results of special procedures for interpretation if required
   a. Vagal maneuvers
   b. His bundle studies
   c. Pacing studies
   d. Clinical electrophysiology testing
7. Duration and frequency of arrhythmia
8. Patient's description of associated symptoms
9. Hemodynamic consequences of arrhythmia
   a. BP changes
   b. Apical and radial pulse deficit
   c. Fatigue
   d. Changes in heart sounds
10. Patient's perception of and reaction to the diagnosis, special studies, and therapy
11. Signs and symptoms of complications
   a. Decreased cardiac output
   b. Inadequate perfusion of
      (1) Heart
      (2) Brain
      (3) Kidneys
      (4) Peripheral vascular system
   c. Electrical instability
   d. Embolic episodes

GOALS

1. Absence and/or stability of arrhythmias—optimal cardiac rhythm
2. Hemodynamic stability—adequate perfusion of brain, heart, kidneys, and peripheral system
3. Absence of or resolution of embolic complications
4. Absence of identified precipitating factors
5. Patient's behavior demonstrates reduction of anxiety with provision of information

6. Before discharge, the patient/family*
   a. Identifies factors that might precipitate arrhythmias and steps to follow to avoid

*Applies when chronic management and/or prevention is required.

b. Lists symptoms suggestive of recurrence and describes appropriate actions
c. Accurately demonstrates skill of counting pulse, stating acceptable ranges of rate and rhythm
d. States necessary information for compliance with discharge regimen
e. Asks pertinent questions

POTENTIAL PROBLEMS	EXPECTED OUTCOMES	NURSING ACTIVITIES
■ Anxiety related to Awareness of heart activity Insufficient knowledge Fear of consequences Monitoring equipment Special diagnostic procedures	■ Patient verbalizes anxiety and asks questions Reduction of anxiety with sufficient information and control of arrhythmia Absence of nonverbal responses suggestive of anxiety	■ Ongoing assessment of level of anxiety Encourage patient to verbalize fears; search for sources of anxiety; encourage questions from patient/family Maintain as quiet and relaxed an environment as possible; regulate bedside audio alarms to reduce additional stimuli without compromising patient's safety Sedate patient if necessary and as ordered Explain nature of arrhythmia to patient, stressing effectiveness of pump, i.e., difference between electrical and mechanical activity Elicit from patient indices of awareness Sensation of irregular beat Palpitations Dyspnea Feeling of fullness or throbbing in chest, neck, or head—sometimes manifested as sensation of choking Discomfort in chest because of greater than normal contractile force of postectopic beats or beats following delay Feeling that heart has stopped during long pauses Explain symptoms in relation to arrhythmia being experienced If natural history of arrhythmia suggests that it will be transient, state this to patient Explain purpose of monitoring equipment and alarm systems Explain purpose and procedure of special studies or maneuvers that may be required to identify and/or treat arrhythmia Assess effect of anxiety on patient's rhythm
■ Electrical instability related to Very rapid or very slow ventricular rates Initiation of tachycardia by premature beats Degeneration of rhythms—ventricular tachycardia to ventricular fibrillation Underlying cardiac disease	■ Electrical stability	■ Determine type of arrhythmia Select best leads Clear QRS complexes, P waves Clear pacemaker artifact if present "Special" leads such as MCL (modified V_1) Bundle branch blocks Differentiation of aberrancy from ventricular conduction problems Leads I and II—axis shifts Systematic inspection of rhythm strip—save for record Obtain 12 lead ECG if necessary, e.g., accurate interpretation of bundle branch block requires precordial leads Maintain continuous ECG monitoring for prompt recognition of changes in rhythm and for determining duration and/or frequency of arrhythmia Identify and record lead selected for monitoring Note if lead is changed Set high- and low-rate alarms Participate with physician and monitor results if special maneuvers or procedures are required for accurate interpretation Response to selected drugs, e.g., atropine, verapamil, or edrophonium (Tensilon) Response to carotid sinus massage or other vagal maneuvers Bundle of His ECG recording Atrial pacing Clinical electrophysiology testing

POTENTIAL PROBLEMS	EXPECTED OUTCOMES	NURSING ACTIVITIES

Determine cause of arrhythmia with physician
  Past and present history of medical problems and treatment modalities, particularly drugs and recent surgical intervention; instability is more common in presence of underlying heart disease
  Monitor lab data, signs and symptoms of conditions (regardless of their causes) that are commonly associated with the development and/or perpetuation of arrhythmias
    Hypotension
    Alterations in K^+ and Ca^{++} concentrations
    Alterations in body temperature
    Hypoxia
    Hypercapnia
    Hypovolemia
    Anemia
    Pain
    Anxiety
    Endocrine disorders
    Hyperthyroidism/hypothyroidism
  Relate identified cause to natural history of arrhythmia when possible
Initiate with physician progressive management to treat arrhythmia and to prevent evolution or development of new arrhythmia; selection of intervention dependent on
  Correct interpretation of arrhythmia
  Etiology
  Effect of arrhythmia on patient's clinical status
  Functional state of organs influencing drug metabolism and excretion
  Concomitant drug therapy
  Therapeutic benefit versus potential toxicity
Methods of intervention include
  Drugs
  Pacemaker—temporary or permanent
  Cardioversion
  Vagal maneuvers
    Respiratory maneuvers
    Carotid sinus massage/electrical stimulator
When administering IV medications
  Ensure that IV remains patent
  Use soluset with microdrip administration setup or IV pump
  Check q15 min to ensure adequate dosage being delivered
  Be alert to signs and symptoms of toxicity regardless of route of administration, since antiarrhythmics are potentially lethal and dosages may need to be adjusted as patient's status changes
When cardioversion is required
  Prepare patient for procedure
  If patient has been (within the last 24 to 48 hours) or is receiving digoxin, check carefully for indications of toxicity
    Check serum K^+ level if available
    If indications of toxicity are present, inform physician; procedure should be postponed for 24 to 48 hours
  If patient's status permits, explain purpose of procedure and that he/she will be given medication so that he/she will be asleep during procedure
  Ensure that IV line is in place and patent
  Have emergency equipment and drugs immediately available
If pacemaker is required, see Standard 23, *Pacemakers: temporary and permanent*

POTENTIAL PROBLEMS	EXPECTED OUTCOMES	NURSING ACTIVITIES
		Be prepared to treat lethal arrhythmia Arrest cart and defibrillator should be immediately accessible Confirm occurrence—check for presence of P, BP, and/or audible heart sounds Initiate CPR and/or defibrillate (if unit policy permits) immediately while calling for team Prepare IV medications (usually lidocaine) to maintain stable rhythm
■ Decreased cardiac output related to Persistent tachycardia and/or marked bradycardia Loss of sequential AV contraction Loss of hemodynamic benefit of atrial contraction is particularly significant in patients with left heart failure or mitral stenosis	■ Adequate cardiac output to maintain hemodynamic stability	■ Check BP q2 hr for Decrease in systolic pressure Narrowed pulse pressure reflecting reduction in effective volume If hypotension occurs, report to physician and increase frequency of observation; consider other causes, such as medications patient may be taking, MI, hypovolemia Check P q2 hr for Rate Regularity Quality—hyperkinetic or hypokinetic Pulse deficit—most common with atrial fibrillation and nonperfused premature beats Bigeminal pulse—most common with ventricular bigeminy Auscultate precordium for abnormal changes in intensity of S_1 and apical pulse Check intake and output q8 hr or more frequently if indicated Elicit description of symptoms from patient suggesting decreasing cardiac output Fatigue Dyspnea Nervousness Dizziness—relate to position Assess for early signs of left heart failure, which may be precipitated by persistent tachycardia and/or loss of atrial contribution to ventricular filling; see Standard 15, *Heart failure (low cardiac output)* If problem of diminishing output occurs Inform physician Continuous observation of ECG to determine response to therapy or effect of decreased cardiac output on electrical stability Anticipate more aggressive management of arrhythmia Increase frequency of observations noted before and in Problem, Inadequate tissue perfusion, related to decreased cardiac output Administer O_2 as ordered Ensure patent IV, and administer parenteral fluids as ordered Restrict patient's activity Give medications as ordered; in addition to those being used to treat arrhythmias, these may include drugs used to improve cardiac contractility; monitor closely to determine effectiveness on improvement of cardiac output, because increased contractility will increase myocardial O_2 consumption and therefore demand Inform patient/family of reasons for changes in observation, symptoms, and therapy
■ Inadequate tissue perfusion related to decreased cardiac output: cerebral	■ Adequate cerebral perfusion	■ Observe for signs and symptoms suggesting inadequate cerebral perfusion Yawning Mental confusion Dizziness Syncopal episodes (Stokes-Adams) Convulsions; seizures Cheyne-Stokes respirations Stroke related to transient cerebral ischemia

POTENTIAL PROBLEMS	EXPECTED OUTCOMES	NURSING ACTIVITIES
		Rule out other causes, particularly use of class II antiarrhythmics, lidocaine, and phenytoin (Dilantin), which first manifest toxicity via CNS; sensory deprivation; and organic syndrome of the aged
■ Inadequate tissue perfusion related to decreased cardiac output: myocardial	■ Adequate myocardial perfusion	■ Observe for signs and symptoms suggesting inadequate myocardial perfusion 　Angina—see Standard 11, *Angina pectoris* 　MI or extension of—see Standard 12, *Acute myocardial infarction* 　Left heart failure—see Standard 15, *Heart failure (low cardiac output)* 　Pulmonary edema—see Standard 1, *Pulmonary edema of cardiac origin* 　Cardiogenic shock—see Standard 16, *Cardiogenic shock* 　Greater electrical instability—see Problem, Electrical instability
■ Inadequate tissue perfusion related to decreased cardiac output: renal	■ Adequate renal perfusion	■ Observe for signs and symptoms of acute renal ischemia 　Check urine output q8 hr 　　If oliguria develops, check output q1-2 hr 　　If anuria develops, check output q1 hr 　　Catheterize patient if indicated and/or ordered 　　Measure specific gravity of urine 　Daily weight 　Monitor lab data for results 　　BUN 　　Creatinine clearance 　　Electrolyte balance, particularly K^+ 　　Acid-base balance 　Changes in mental status, e.g., lethargy, confusion 　Anorexia, nausea and vomiting *See* STANDARD 52, *Acute renal failure*
■ Inadequate tissue perfusion related to decreased cardiac output: peripheral system	■ Adequate peripheral perfusion	■ Observe for signs and symptoms indicative of inadequate peripheral perfusion 　Check all pulses for presence, equality, and quality 　Pallor, cyanosis, or cooling of extremities 　Sweating related to peripheral arterial constriction 　If any of the aforementioned problems occur 　　Inform physician immediately and record data 　　Increase frequency of observations and collection of aforementioned lab data 　　Prepare for specific measures to assess and improve perfusion 　　　Assist with insertion of intraarterial lines and/or pulmonary artery line 　　　See Standard 25, *Hemodynamic monitoring* 　If the problem is arrhythmia, prepare for more aggressive antiarrhythmic intervention 　Administer medications to improve cardiac function and perfusion; many pharmacological agents used for this purpose, e.g., inotropic agents and sympathomimetics, may provoke arrhythmias 　Ascertain mode of excretion of drugs, adjusting medication dosages as ordered when hepatic or renal function is altered; same amount of medication may produce toxicity if it is not metabolized and excreted because of altered hepatic or renal function
■ Embolic episodes	■ Absence or resolution of embolic complications	■ Determine if positive history of rheumatic mitral valve disease or chronic atrial fibrillation 　Initiate preventive measures for these patients and for those with previous history of thromboembolic disease or for whom prolonged bed rest is anticipated 　　Antithromboembolic stockings 　　ROM exercises, passive or active, to extremities

POTENTIAL PROBLEMS	EXPECTED OUTCOMES	NURSING ACTIVITIES
		Ambulate as soon as possible
		Patients with chronic atrial fibrillation may be anticoagulated before cardioversion
		Observe for signs of emboli routinely at every shift in high-risk patients
		Sudden onset of chest pain
		Signs and symptoms of respiratory distress
		Altered mental status
		Unexplained restlessness or anxiety
		Decreased temperature, sensation, or pulses in extremities
		If problem occurs, see Standard 31, *Embolic phenomena*

■ Insufficient knowledge to comply with discharge regimen*	■ Evaluation by testing or questioning demonstrates patient/family's understanding of knowledge components of teaching program
	Patient takes own pulse correctly and states acceptable ranges
	Patient lists symptoms requiring physician notification
	Patient asks pertinent questions regarding self-care
		■ If arrhythmia requires chronic management or if there is strong probability of recurrence, institute teaching program for patient/family, including
		Normal heart function—electrical and mechanical
		Nature of arrhythmias and potential effect on cardiovascular system
		Factors or situations that might precipitate arrhythmias and suggestions for avoiding discussed with patient/family
		Symptoms indicating recurrence and appropriate actions to take
		Medication regimen
		  Purpose
		  Dosage
		  Timing and importance of—adjust schedule to patient's lifestyle
		  Side effects and what to do about them
		Follow-up information
		Provide opportunities for patient/family to ask questions
		Assess patient/family's potential compliance

*If this type of follow-up care is the responsibility of critical care unit nurse when patient is transferred from the critical care unit.

THE ROLE OF CLINICAL ELECTROPHYSIOLOGICAL TESTING IN THE TREATMENT OF VENTRICULAR TACHYCARDIA

Ventricular tachycardia is an accelerated heart rhythm originating in either the right or left ventricle. The ventricular rate is usually between 100 and 240 beats per minute but can be as fast as 300 beats per minute (ventricular flutter). Ventricular tachycardia is a common complication of AMI and chronic ischemic heart disease. It is frequently seen in association with left ventricular aneurysms. It also may be seen in cardiomyopathy, mitral valve prolapse, drug toxicity, long Q-T syndrome, and severe electrolyte imbalance and in the absence of demonstrable heart disease. Cardiac output is usually diminished during ventricular tachycardia. This is the result of decreased diastolic filling time and the subsequent diminished stroke volume. The loss of atrioventricular sequential contraction further decreases an already compromised cardiac output by the loss of atrial systole. The clinical response to this arrhythmia varies with the underlying cardiovascular status, the hemodynamic response, and the duration and rate of the tachycardia. Symptoms can vary from none to palpitations, dizziness, diaphoresis, angina, syncope, or cardiac arrest.

Ventricular tachycardia is a remarkably common arrhythmia that has been clinically recognized for years. It accounts for approximately two thirds of the 600,000 sudden cardiac deaths that occur annually in the United States. Yet it remains a difficult rhythm disturbance to manage effectively. The diagnosis of ventricular tachycardia is not always easily made. Standard ECG observations that are suggestive of ventricular tachycardia are a wide complex tachycardia with a QRS usually exceeding 0.14 seconds, AV dissociation, fusion complexes, and often a monophasic or biphasic morphology in leads V_1 and V_6, but these observations alone may be misleading. A wide complex tachycardia may be a supraventricular tachycardia with aberrancy, Wolff-Parkinson-White syndrome using a bypass tract, or supraventricular tachycardia with preexisting bundle branch block. The symptoms noted previously are nonspecific and can have numerous etiologies. The arrhythmia is also unpredictable. There is no way of predicting when a short run of ventricular tachycardia will sustain itself, when a slow rate will accelerate, or when ventricular tachycardia will degenerate into ventricular fibrillation. The occurrences of ventricular tachycardia may be sporadic, making documentation difficult by ECG or ambulatory Holter monitoring. Without this documentation, antiarrhythmic drug therapy is carried out on an empirical basis with no objective testing of its efficacy. Even when this drug therapy is effective, the well-known side effects of these drugs makes treatment difficult and often prevents their continued use.

Over the past 20 years, a great deal of research has been done on the etiology, mechanism, and treatment of this complex arrhythmia. Perhaps one of the more significant advances in recent years in the treatment of ventricular tachycardia is clinical electrophysiological testing.

Clinical electrophysiological testing combines the use of intracardiac recording techniques and programmed electrical stimulation (pacing) to aid in the diagnosis and treatment of complex cardiac arrhythmias. Catheter stimulation techniques have assumed a major role in the treatment of ventricular tachycardia by allowing the clinician to confirm the diagnosis, to assess antiarrhythmic drug therapy, and to assess pacemaker therapy as a mode of treatment. In some cases in preparation for arrythmia surgery, endocardial mapping is performed to locate the anatomical area of the reentry circuit thought to be responsible for the tachycardia. Electrophysiological testing has been found to be most useful in treating ischemic heart disease patients with recurrent ventricular tachycardia and survivors of out-of-hospital sudden death. Patients who have symptoms of ventricular tachycardia (dizziness, syncope, etc.) but in whom no rhythm disturbance has been documented also benefit from electrophysiological testing. Patients with cardiomyopathy, mitral valve prolapse, and catecholamine-induced ventricular tachycardia are also studied. Ventricular tachycardia patients in the acute stages of MI are usually not studied for control of ventricular tachycardia but may be studied as soon as 10 to 14 days after the MI.

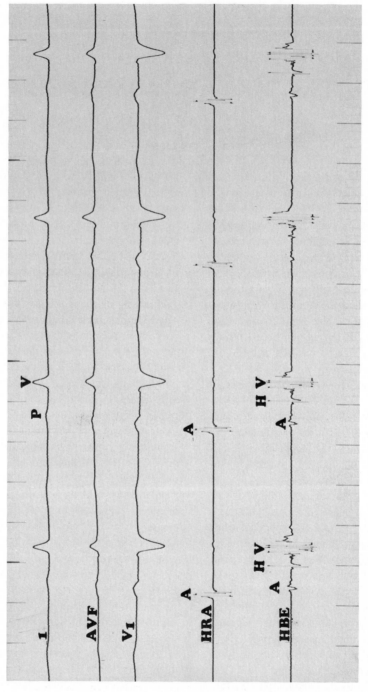

FIG. 1. His bundle ECG. From top to bottom, standard ECG leads 1, aVf, V₁, and recordings from the high right atrium and His bundle region.

Electrophysiological testing is performed by doing a right heart catheterization. Left heart catheterization may also be performed in selected cases. Two or more multipole electrode catheters are inserted into the femoral and/or antecubital veins and are guided under fluoroscopic control to the right atrium and ventricle. The catheters are then positioned for intracardiac recordings and pacing. With the catheters connected to a multichannel ECG recorder and a programmable electrical stimulator, routine measurements are made. These measurements are of intraatrial, AV nodal, and His-Purkinje conduction time. The P-A interval reflects intraatrial conduction time and is measured from the earliest deflection of the P wave in any of the surface ECG leads to the deflection of the atrial electrogram on the His bundle electrogram. The normal range is 10 to 40 milliseconds (msec). The A-H interval reflects AV nodal conduction time and is measured from the atrial deflection to the His bundle deflection on the His bundle electrogram. The normal range is 60 to 120 msec. The H-V interval measures conduction time in the His-Purkinje system and is measured from the earliest His bundle deflection in the His bundle electrogram to the earliest ventricular depolariztion in any intracardiac or body surface ECG lead. The normal range is 30 to 55 msec (Fig. 1). Sinus node, A-V node, and His-Purkinje function are then evaluated using various programmed electrical stimulation protocols. Evaluation of these areas is performed to rule out any abnormality and to assess possible contraindications to certain antiarrhythmic drug therapies. Next, the diagnosis of ventricular tachycardia is attempted by trying to induce the arrhythmia through programmed electrical stimulation. Induction is attempted by pacing the atrium and/or ventricle using impulses of 2 msec in duration at twice the diastolic current threshold. One approach of ventricular programmed stimulation is performed by pacing the ventricle at various rates (100 to 150 beats per minute) for eight consecutive beats (this pacing cycle is labeled V_1) and adding an additional premature ventricular stimulus (V_2). With a 4- to 5-second pause between each pacing cycle, this premature stimuli is programmed to enter the cycle at increasingly premature intervals, to the point of refractoriness or the induction of ventricular tachycardia. When ventricular tachycardia is not induced with V_1V_2 protocol, a second premature (V_3) and sometimes a third (V_4) is added (Fig. 2). Ventricular burst pacing of 4 to 16 beats at rates of 150 to 300 beats per minute may also be used. Stimulation protocols may vary slightly among different institutions. The pacing methods described here may be tried with the catheter in different parts of the ventricle. When patients with documented recurrent sustained ventricular tachycardia do not have their tachycardia produced in this manner, left ventricular stimulation may be attempted. Once the tachycardia has been induced and recorded, it is terminated. Termination is performed by overdrive or underdrive pacing or direct current cardioversion, or it is allowed to spontaneously terminate. The method of termination is guided by the patient's hemodynamic response to the tachycardia. When a wide complex tachycardia is initiated, dissociation of ventricular and atrial depolarization and the absence of a His bundle deflection confirms the diagnosis of ventricular tachycardia. The sensitivity of programmed stimulation in inducing ventricular tachycardia among patients who have had a spontaneous episode varies among laboratories, but generally ranges from 70% to 100%. The false-positive rate using $V_1V_2V_3$ is extremely low (3%). Protocols using different pacing methods are presently being evaluated.*

There are two basic mechanisms felt to be responsible for ventricular tachycardia: reentry and automaticity. Programmed electrical stimulation has proved to be useful in defining and differentiating these mechanisms. Reentry is felt to be the causative factor of ventricular tachycardia in chronic ischemic heart disease, which is why the sensitivity for induction is so high in this group of patients. Patients with cardiomyopathy and mitral valve prolapse do not always have the same high degree of sensitivity to arrhythmia induction, which lends to the theory that reentry may not always be the mechanism responsible for their ventricular tachycardia. The hallmark of reentry is the reproducibility, initiation, and/or termination of a tachycardia by a single or multiple extrastimuli or by rapid pacing. In contrast, automatic tachycardias are the result of enhanced diastolic depolarizations and usually can neither be initiated or terminated by programmed stimulation.†

Once the diagnosis of ventricular tachycardia has been made, antiarrhythmic drugs are evaluated on different days for efficacy and safety. The efficacy of a drug is determined by its ability to prevent the initiation of the tachycardia by programmed electrical stimulation. It has been found that if administration of an antiarrhythmic drug prevents the induction of the tachycardia, the long-term recurrence rate is extremely low (10% to 15%). When the tachycardia is still inducible on drug therapy, the long-term recurrence rate of ventricular tachycardia has been found to be as high as 80%.‡ Antiarrhythmic agents that can be administered IV are often infused during electrophysiological testing to assess this efficacy. Agents that are available in the oral form are tested only when adequate serum blood levels have been attained. When a drug is given IV, induction of ventricular

*Livelli, F., et al.: Response to programmed ventricular stimulation: sensitivity, specificity and relation to heart disease, Am. J. Cardiol. **50:**452-458, 1982.

†Josephson, M., and Seides, S.: Recurrent ventricular tachycardia in clinical cardiac electrophysiology: techniques and interpretations, Philadelphia, 1979, Lea & Febiger, pp. 247-280.

‡Horowitz, L., Josephson, M., and Kastor, J.: Intracardiac electrophysiologic studies as a method for the optimization of drug therapy in chronic ventricular arrhythmia, Prog. Cardiovasc. Dis. **23:**81-97, 1980.

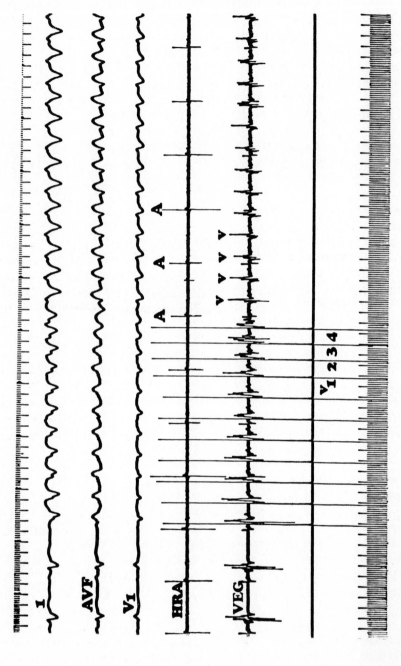

FIG. 2. Induction of ventricular tachycardia using V₁V₂V₃V₄. From top to bottom, standard ECG leads 1, aVf, V₁, and recordings from the right atrium and right ventricle. Bottom tracing represents pacing stimulus marker.

tachycardia is attempted at various dose levels. The end point of any drug infusion is (1) the inability to induce the tachycardia, (2) the achievement of the maximal dose level, or (3) an adverse effect of the drug (drug safety). Serum blood levels are drawn at every dosing level tested. When an antiarrhythmic drug given IV is successful in preventing the induction of ventricular tachycardia, the patient is re-tested with the oral form of the drug. This repeat drug study is performed when serum blood levels achieved during acute IV testing have been attained with the oral preparation. Drugs commonly used for IV testing are quinidine gluconate, procainamide, propranolol, and phenytoin. If standard antiarrhythmic drugs fail to protect the patient from inducible ventricular tachycardia, there are investigational drugs available for trial. Some commonly used investigational drugs are amiodarone, mexiletine, and flecainide The predictive accuracy of electrophsiological testing with these drugs is currently under investigation.

In addition to identifying a successful antiarrhythmic agent, electrophysiological testing documents the appropriate plasma concentration level that should be maintained orally. Another interesting fact that electrophysiological studies have shown is that higher than previously accepted levels may be required to prevent ventricular tachycardia.

Most patients undergoing electrophysiological testing for control of ventricular tachycardia are continuously monitored in the cardiac critical care unit or on a telemetry floor. The length of stay in the hospital can vary from 10 days to 8 weeks, with an average of three to six studies per patient.

Complications from electrophysiological testing are rare.

Antitachycardia pacemakers. Patients with recurrent ventricular tachycardia that is resistant to antiarrhythmic drug therapy may be candidates for pacemaker therapy. Through electrophysiological testing, a variety of pacing techniques can be explored for the prevention and termination of ventricular tachycardia. Candidates for therapy are patients who are resistant to drug therapy and patients who have had the proposed pacing method demonstrate reliability in terminating their tachycardia. Pacing techniques must be tailored to each individual patient. During electrophysiological testing, repeat induction and termination of the tachycardia must be assessed for reliability of termination and safety. Safety includes the inability of the pacing technique to cause acceleration and degeneration of ventricular tachycardia to ventricular fibrillation. This is the most catastrophic complication of antiarrhythmic pacemaker therapy. Acceleration can generally be prevented by adjustment of the rate or duration of the pacing cycle.*

Pacemaker therapy is commonly used in conjunction with drug therapy. It is not uncommon for an antiarrhythmic drug to slow the rate of the tachycardia without abolishing it. In selected cases, the use of an antiarrhythmic drug and pacemaker therapy has proved successful.

Pacing techniques for prevention and/or termination of ventricular tachycardia vary according to patient. Pacemakers are internally implanted and activate automatically or manually when ventricular tachycardia occurs. Manually activated pacemakers can be used in a selected group of patients who are subjectively aware of their tachycardia and can tolerate the arrhythmia hemodynamically. This pacemaker will fire when a radio-frequency transmitter is placed over the pacemaker. The arrhythmia should be documented by ECG before using the manually activated pacemakers. Internally controlled pacemakers will trigger automatically when ventricular tachycardia occurs.

Though still considered to be in its early stages of development, pacemaker therapy is a viable alternative for a selected group of patients.

Cardiac arrhythmia surgery. Cardiac arrhythmia surgery is yet another alternative in the treatment of ventricular tachycardia. Candidates for this type of surgery are (1) patients with ischemic heart disease in whom antiarrhythmic drug and/or pacemaker therapy has proved unsuccessful, (2) patients with a preexisting, poorly controlled ventricular tachycardia who are undergoing CABG and/or ventricular aneurysmectomy, (3) patients who can have their ventricular tachycardia induced and can tolerate it hemodynamically for mapping, and (4) patients who do not have contraindications to open heart surgery. The purpose of cardiac arrhythmia surgery is to surgically remove or interrupt the reentry circuit. In ischemic heart disease the reentry circuit felt to be responsible for ventricular tachycardia is often near a myocardial scar and/or near or in a ventricular aneurysm. It has been found that CABG and ventricular aneurysmectomy alone may not be reliable in abolishing the recurrence of ventricular tachycardia because the site of the reentry circuit may not be altered. (In blind ventricular aneurysmectomy, the aneurysm may be removed while the reentry circuit is left intact if the reentry circuit is not in the aneurysm.) The site of the reentry circuit is identified by performing ventricular mapping.

Ventricular mapping in preparation for arrhythmia surgery is best accomplished in two stages, first by preoperative endocardial mapping and then by intraoperative endocardial and epicardial mapping. Ventricular mapping requires induction of the arrhythmia. Preoperative as well as intraoperative mapping is necessary, because in some cases the tachycardia cannot be induced when the patient is under general anesthesia. Briefly, preoperative mapping is accomplished by performing a left and a right heart catheterization. Multipole electrode catheters are positioned in the right atrium and ventricle and in the left ventricle. The catheter in the right ventricle remains stationary and is the reference catheter. The catheter in the left ventricle is used for map-

*Fisher J.D., et al.: Role of implantable pacemakers in control of recurrent ventricular tachycardia, Am. J. Cardiol. **49**:194-206, 1982.

ping. While surface ECG and intracardiac recordings are simultaneously recorded, ventricular tachycardia is induced. Multiple sites are mapped and recorded. When the entire ventricle has been mapped, the data are reviewed, and the earliest site of activation is identified as the origin of the reentry circuit (this may require frequent induction and termination of the tachycardia). The entire mapping procedure can be done in 15 to 20 minutes. The second stage of mapping is performed on the day of surgery in the operating room, where direct epicardial and endocardial mapping is performed. The patient is placed under general anesthesia, and the heart is exposed. With the same recording techniques used in preoperative mapping, ventricular tachycardia is induced and direct epicardial mapping is performed. The tachycardia is then terminated, and the patient is placed on total cardiopulmonary bypass (CPB). The left ventricle is incised, ventricular tachycardia is induced, and direct endocardial mapping is performed. All three mappings are then compared, and the earliest site of activation is confirmed. This site is then surgically excised (endocardial stripping). If the reentry circuit is in an aneurysm, aneurysmectomy is performed. Commonly, CABG is performed in conjunction with arrhythmia surgery. Before discharge the patient undergoes a final electrophysiological procedure. In most cases, ventricular tachycardia cannot be induced postoperatively. In the patients whose tachycardia is still inducible and was previously drug-resistant, the ventricular tachycardia can generally be successfully treated with antiarrhythmic drug therapy.

ASSESSMENT

1. Patient/family's knowledge of arrhythmia and cardiovascular disease
2. History, including
   a. Preexisting cardiovascular disease
      (1) MI
      (2) Cardiomyopathy
      (3) Mitral valve prolapse
      (4) Angina
      (5) Other
   b. Previous cardiac surgical intervention
      (1) CABG
      (2) Valve replacement
   c. Symptoms related to arrhythmia
      (1) Palpitations
      (2) Dizziness
      (3) Near syncope or syncope
      (4) Angina
      (5) Cardiac arrest
      (6) Other
   d. Frequency of symptoms
   e. Documentation of arrhythmia
      (1) None

      (2) ECG
      (3) Ambulatory ECG
   f. Previous hospitalizations and treatment administered for arrhythmia
   g. Medications
      (1) Present drug therapy
      (2) Previous drug therapy and result
3. Patient's general condition, including
   a. BP
   b. P, temperature
   c. ECG
   d. Respiratory status
   e. Electrolyte levels
   f. Liver and renal function
   g. Emotional status
4. Patient/family's understanding of electrophysiological procedure
5. Impact of arrhythmia on patient's life-style, including physical and emotional changes
6. Assessment during electrophysiological procedure
   a. Patient's anxiety level
   b. Cardiovascular status
      (1) BP
      (2) P
      (3) ECG
      (4) Signs and/or symptoms of heart failure
   c. Patient's response to induced ventricular tachycardia
      (1) BP changes
      (2) Dizziness, syncope
      (3) Angina
   d. Patient's neurological status after cardioversion
   e. Patient's response to IV drug therapy
      (1) BP
      (2) P
      (3) ECG changes
      (4) Efficacy of drug therapy
      (5) Other
   f. Presence of symptoms of vasovagal reaction during catheter insertion and withdrawal
      (1) Pallor
      (2) Diaphoresis
      (3) Nausea, vomiting
      (4) Dizziness
      (5) Bradycardia
      (6) Hypotension
   g. Patient's emotional response to procedure
   h. Catheter insertion site for
      (1) Overt bleeding
      (2) Swelling
      (3) Perfusion of distal limb before discharge from laboratory
7. After catheterization
   a. Cardiovascular status

(1) BP

(2) P

(3) Heart rhythm

(4) LOC

b. Patient's clinical response to the procedure

(1) Inducibility of tachyarrhythmia

(2) Symptoms associated with induced tachycardia

(3) Efficacy of antiarrhythmic drug administered (control of tachycardia, side effects, etc.)

c. Catheter insertion site for

(1) Bleeding

(2) Swelling

(3) Infection

(4) Circulation to extremity

d. Patient's emotional response to procedure and repeat drug studies

8. Patient/family's understanding of antiarrhythmic drug, pacemaker therapy, and/or surgery

See Standard 23, *Pacemakers: temporary and permanent;* Standard 27, *Cardiac surgery*

GOALS

1. Absence of recurrent ventricular tachycardia through medical and/or surgical treatment

2. Hemodynamic stability

3. Patient/family demonstrates understanding of cardiovascular disease, arrhythmia, and electrophysiological procedure

4. Reduction in patient/family's anxiety regarding hospitalization, procedure, arrhythmia, and discharge from hospital

5. Absence of infection and hemorrhage at catheter insertion site

6. Reduction of physical and psychological trauma caused by multiple electrophysiological studies

7. Absence or reduction of adverse antiarrhythmic drug response

8. Before discharge patient/family is able to

a. Identify symptoms suggestive of recurrent arrhythmia

b. Provide the following information regarding prescribed antiarrhythmic drugs

(1) Name

(2) Dosage

(3) Side effects

(4) Time interval between each dose

(5) Importance of compliance to medical regimen

9. Patient/family demonstrates knowledge of how to contact members of the arrhythmia control unit

POTENTIAL PROBLEMS	EXPECTED OUTCOMES	NURSING ACTIVITIES
■ Patient/family anxiety related to disease entity	■ Reduction of patient/family anxiety with provision of information concerning arrhythmia and its treatment	■ Assess patient/family's level of anxiety and knowledge and understanding of arrhythmia and underlying disease Provide information regarding electrical conduction system of heart and its relationship to heart action and arrhythmia Elicit from patient/family subjective and objective evidence of arrhythmia Dizziness Palpitations Chest discomfort Syncope Cardiac arrest Relate symptoms to hemodynamic effect of arrhythmia Increased heart rate Decreased BP Encourage patient/family's questions regarding arrhythmia and hospitalization Maintain confident and optimistic attitude regarding treatment through electrophysiological testing
■ Patient/family's apprehension regarding electrophysiological testing	■ Reduction of anxiety with provision of information regarding procedure	■ Describe electrophysiology procedure, rationale for testing, and induction of arrhythmia Describe advantages of testing and expected results Identify symptoms that may be experienced during induction of arrhythmia Dizziness Palpitations Syncope Identify method of control and/or termination of arrhythmia Self-termination Pacing Cardioversion

POTENTIAL PROBLEMS	EXPECTED OUTCOMES	NURSING ACTIVITIES
		Describe reasons for repeat drug studies
		Because of varying properties of each individual drug
		Time is needed between administrations
		Inability to predict which drug will be effective on individual basis
		Explain potential complications of procedure and methods used to decrease possibility of occurrence
■ Symptoms related to preexisting coronary artery disease	■ Prevention and/or control of symptoms	■ Assess patient's preexisting cardiac history and initiate appropriate action if symptoms occur

See STANDARD 12   *Acute myocardial infarction*
       STANDARD 11   *Angina pectoris*
       STANDARD 15   *Heart failure (low cardiac output)*

POTENTIAL PROBLEMS	EXPECTED OUTCOMES	NURSING ACTIVITIES
■ Ventricular tachycardia	■ Electrical stability Hemodynamic stability with adequate cardiac output	■ Assess hemodynamic response to arrhythmia
		BP
		P
		Presence of angina
		LOC
		Have arrest cart and defibrillator immediately accessible
		Verify diagnosis
		Continuous ECG monitoring
		Compare rhythm with documented ventricular tachycardia if available
		Initiate with physician appropriate treatment dependent on patient's clinical response to arrhythmia
		Methods of intervention
		Drug therapy
		Cardioversion
		CPR
		Observation
		When antiarrhythmic drug therapy is administered
		Maintain patent IV route
		Have emergency IV antiarrhythmic drugs available—lidocaine, procainamide, bretyllium
		Prepare medications for administration
		Elective cardioversion may be performed if ventricular tachycardia is well tolerated, and adequate BP is maintained with no ischemic and/or cerebral symptoms
		If patient has eaten in last 8 hours, cardioversion may be contraindicated
		Explain procedure to patient
		Observe respiratory status following administration of sedative
		Maintain patent airway
		Be prepared for patient intubation
		Have Ambu bag, oxygen suction equipment, endotracheal tubes (sizes 6F and 10F), laryngoscope, and blade available
		Emergency cardioversion—nursing activities same as above
		Be prepared to initiate CPR
		When tachycardia is well tolerated, a period of observation may be warranted
		Monitor vital signs, ECG
		Be prepared to intervene with emergency procedures if tachycardia accelerates or degenerates to ventricular fibrillation
		Evaluate patient's condition after arrhythmic event
		Neurological
		LOC
		Speech
		Motor coordination
		Cardiovascular
		Vital signs
		Presence of angina
		ECG—for ischemic changes
		Respiratory status

POTENTIAL PROBLEMS	EXPECTED OUTCOMES	NURSING ACTIVITIES
▪ Patient's anxiety during electrophysiological study	▪ Reduction of anxiety with provision of information and support	▪ Evaluate patient's level of anxiety Encourage patient to verbalize fears and questions regarding procedure Reduce patient's anxiety regarding equipment by demonstrating function of equipment ECG monitor Programmable stimulator Fluoroscope, etc. Reassure patient regarding safety of procedure Inform patient of qualifications of health care team performing procedure Reiterate purpose of test Encourage patient to express any subjective symptoms experienced during procedure Explain procedure throughout testing, i.e. Discomfort from IV insertion Reproduction of symptoms Palpitations Assess patient for need of sedation Maintain relaxed, calm atmosphere
▪ Vasovagal reaction related to catheter manipulation	▪ Minimal vasovagal reaction	▪ Observe patient for signs of vasovagal reaction, especially during catheter insertion and withdrawal Pallor Diaphoresis Nausea Vomiting Dizziness Bradycardia Asystole Mild to severe hypotension Methods of intervention IV medications Pacing Observation Monitor BP P Heart rhythm LOC If vasovagal reaction occurs Assist with supportive treatment—have immediately accessible Atropine sulfate 1 to 2 mg Norepinephrine (Levophed) 4 mg diluted in 500 ml dextrose 5% in water Normal saline 0.9% 500 ml Observe response to ventricular pacing if instituted Preserve perfusion to vital ograns Place patient in Trendelenburg position if necessary Prepare infusion—normal saline and/or norepinephrine drip Be prepared for cardiac arrest Initiate CPR if necessary
▪ Induction of ventricular tachycardia during electrophysiological testing	▪ Electrical stability Hemodynamic stability	▪ Assess patient's hemodynamic response to ventricular tachycardia induction; see Problem, Ventricular tachycardia Verify diagnosis by intracardiac recordings When induction of ventricular tachycardia is accomplished, be prepared to intervene with immediate cardioversion, ventricular pacing Have immediately accessible Antiarrhythmic drugs O$_2$ Suction Defibrillator; see Problem, Ventricular tachycardia

POTENTIAL PROBLEMS	EXPECTED OUTCOMES	NURSING ACTIVITIES
		Evaluate patient's condition after ventricular tachycardia; see Problem, Ventricular tachycardia Reassure patient that induction of ventricular tachycardia is positive and expected result Diagnosis is confirmed Electrophysiological testing can be used to guide therapy High rate of success in treating ventricular tachycardia through electrophysiological testing Encourage patient verbalization of fears, anxiety
■ Cerebral emboli associated with cardioversion (extremely rare)	■ Maximal neurologic function	■ Assess patient's neurological status after cardioversion, including LOC Aphasia Dyphasia Weakness Paralysis *See* STANDARD 31 *Embolic phenomena*
■ Adverse response to antiarrhythmic drug therapy	■ Absence or resolution of adverse response	■ Monitor BP P ECG intervals P-R, QRS, Q-T Increase in ectopic activity Change in rhythm Observe for any adverse response to specific drug Notify physician of adverse responses and administer therapy as ordered
■ Infection Site of catheter insertion Endocarditis	■ Absence of infection Afebrile	■ Maintain sterile technique during electrophysiological testing Maintain cleanliness of catheter insertion site Dressing change q24 hr Apply antibiotic ointment until insertion site has healed Assess area for Swelling Inflammation, erythema Purulent exudate Assess patient for Elevated temperature Pain at catheter site *See* STANDARD 19 *Endocarditis*
■ Patient/family anxiety related to repeat electrophysiological drug studies and prolonged hospitalization	■ Reduction of anxiety with provision of information and support	■ Encourage patient to express feelings of anxiety Provide support with easy availability of supportive staff from electrophysiology lab and primary care personnel Provide opportunities for questions concerning repeat drug studies Inform patient of need for repeat studies to evaluate drug efficacy Reassure patient/family regarding high success potential of treatment Prepare for anxiety-related response to investigational drugs Provide information regarding drugs and success potential Be prepared for patient depression over prolonged hospitalization and repeated testing Maintain optimistic attitude for positive results Express understanding of depression and inform patient that this is not abnormal response Encourage activities that will minimize depression Encourage reading, television, any activity that will decrease patient/family's anxiety level Encourage frequent family hospital visits and/or verbal or written communication

POTENTIAL PROBLEMS	EXPECTED OUTCOMES	NURSING ACTIVITIES

■ Noncompliance to discharge regimen	■ Compliance
	Evaluation of patient/family's understanding of discharge regimen
		■ Instruct patient on importance of compliance, including
		    Taking medications
		    Complying with time intervals
		    Possible consequences of not taking medications—recurrence of ventricular tachycardia
		Instruct patient/family to be aware of
		    Symptoms indicating recurrence of arrhythmia
		    Side effects of medication and what to do about them
		
		See STANDARD 21 *Arrhythmias*

PACEMAKERS: TEMPORARY AND PERMANENT

A pacemaker is an electronic device that delivers an electrical stimulus to the myocardium to control or maintain heart rate when the natural pacemakers of the heart are unable to do so. The system consists of a pulse generator (energy source) and a unipolar or bipolar electrode catheter, which may be sewn on the epicardium or placed in contact with the endocardium.

When the atrium is being stimulated (paced), the pacing artifact is followed by a P wave; and when the ventricle is being paced, the pacing artifact is followed by a QRS complex.

In addition to the function of stimulation, some units also have a sensing mechanism to eliminate the problem of competition between paced and spontaneous beats, which could result in serious ventricular arrhythmias, fusion beats, or an iatrogenic parasystolic ventricular rhythm. The information that is sensed is relayed to the energy source via the same electrode that stimulates or through a second sensing electrode. The location of the electrode with this sensing capacity determines whether atrial or ventricular activity is sensed.

The several types of pacemakers available are as follows:
1. Asynchronous or fixed rate: models without a sensing mechanism
2. Demand: models with a sensing mechanism that allows the pacemaker to behave as an escape focus when the natural pacemaker does not fire during a preset escape interval and that inhibits the pacemaker when the natural pacemaker functions
3. Synchronous: models with a sensing mechanism whereby sensing in the atrium results in stimulation of the ventricle

The approach to pacemaker implantation depends in part on whether pacing is to be a temporary or permanent measure and the acuteness of the situation. Approaches include external pacing, transthoracic pacing, epicardial pacing, and transvenous endocardial pacing. For temporary pacing the energy source is external. For permanent pacing, the energy source is implanted in a pocket under the skin and connected to the heart by epicardial or endocardial electrodes. With

both methods, once the catheter is thought to be in position the stimulation threshold, the minimal current necessary to achieve one-to-one capture, is found; the sensitivity threshold is measured, if the unit has a sensing mechanism; and the rate is set.

Most permanent pacemakers implanted today can be programmed externally. This allows changes in rate, current output, sensitivity, or pulse duration to be made when there is a change in the patient's condition. This is accomplished with a pacemaker reprogrammer.

Therapeutic indications for permanent or temporary pacing include arrhythmias refractory to medication, resulting in an inadequate heart rate for the maintenance of an effective cardiac output. The rate may be too fast or too slow. The patient may be symptomatic or asymptomatic with an arrhythmia whose natural history supports pacing. "Overdrive" pacing may be employed to suppress dangerous ventricular tachyarrhythmias when medication is ineffective or when ventricular arrhythmias are related to a slow ventricular rate. Pacemaker therapy may be used in conjunction with drug therapy when independent drug therapy is not sufficient. Temporary pacing may also be employed prophylactically following open heart surgery or before permanent pacemaker implantation.

Diagnostically, temporary pacing (usually atrial) may be used to evaluate the electrophysiological response (particularly on AV conduction and sinus node function) and the hemodynamic response to increased heart rate. It also may be employed to determine the mechanism for tachyarrhythmias. A paced atrial premature beat may induce and terminate reentrant tachyarrhythmias while not affecting those resulting from enhanced automaticity. See Standard 22, *The role of clinical electrophysiological testing in the treatment of ventricular tachycardia.*

Patients being paced temporarily are considered subject to microshock hazards. The pacemaker catheter itself is insulated and electrically safe, but the exposed metal tips are not. Because the usual protective resistance provided by the skin and other tissues is bypassed, a very minimal current can potentially produce ventricular fibrillation.

Temporary pacemaker

ASSESSMENT

1. Problem necessitating pacemaker insertion
   a. Disease process
   b. ECG illustrating arrhythmia
   c. Symptoms associated with the arrhythmia
   d. Prognosis—temporary versus permanent need
2. Baseline information included in chart
   a. Date and method of insertion
   b. Location—atrial or ventricular
   c. Location of atrial and ventricular wires inserted pro-phylactically after CABG
   d. Type—asynchronous, demand, etc.
   e. Rate and threshold (MA) settings
   f. Turned on or off
   g. Frequency of use
3. Patient's perception of and reaction to pacemaker and procedure
4. Monitor rhythm strips for
   a. Frequency of need for pacing
   b. Maintenance of preset rate
   c. Paced P or QRS configuration
   d. Capture
   e. Sensing
5. Stimulation and sensing thresholds and presence of influencing factors
6. State of equipment

a. Battery
b. Connections
c. Integrity and position of catheter
7. Evaluation of hemodynamic status
8. Pulse perfusion distal to cutdown
9. Site of insertion for signs of infection, cellulitis, or phlebitis
10. Safety of electrical environment
11. Signs and symptoms of complications
    a. Aberrant pacemaker stimulation
    b. Cardiac tamponade
    c. Pulmonary embolus
    d. Pain or discomfort related to restricted mobility of extremity
    e. Cardiac arrhythmias, particularly ventricular

GOALS

1. Pacemaker unit functioning properly
2. Hemodynamic stability
3. Infection-free insertion site
4. Patient verbalizes comfort
5. Microshock-safe environment
6. Patient asks questions and verbalizes understanding of insertion procedure, reason for and function of pacemaker, and prognosis
7. Patient's behavior demonstrates decreased anxiety with provision of information
8. Absence of threatening arrhythmias

POTENTIAL PROBLEMS	EXPECTED OUTCOMES	NURSING ACTIVITIES
■ Anxiety related to Procedure Lack of physiological self-control Lack of understanding of function of pacemaker unit Unknown prognosis (permanent versus temporary need for)	■ Patient verbalizes reasonable understanding of insertion procedure, reason for and function of pacemaker, and prognosis Patient verbalizes anxiety and asks questions Reduction of anxiety with sufficient information	■ Ongoing assessment of level of anxiety Encourage questions from patient/family Explain pacemaker insertion Explain function of and need for pacing; differentiate between electrical and mechanical functions of the heart Discuss prognosis—permanent versus temporary need Ongoing explanation of care required
■ Pacemaker malfunction related to	■ Pacemaker unit functioning properly Fires at preset rate Each pacemaker stimulus produces myocardial response (capture) Senses patient's own beats (models with sensing mechanism) Hemodynamic stability	■ Continuous monitoring of ECG for Frequency of need for pacing Maintenance of preset rate Capture Paced QRS or P configuration Sensing Check initially and q8 hr Security of connections Battery Consistency between settings on pacemaker and those recorded in chart—rate, stimulation and sensitivity thresholds, and whether on or off Pulse distal to insertion site for perfusion Check threshold q24 hr or as indicated Check vital signs q4 hr or as indicated

POTENTIAL PROBLEMS	EXPECTED OUTCOMES	NURSING ACTIVITIES
		Check sense/pace needle q4 hr with vital signs
		Check for capture and sensing q4-8 hr if off
Improper care of equipment		Keep box and wires dry and a plastic cover over dials
		Clean box with water or alcohol or gas sterilize; do not autoclave
		Clean nondisposable catheters in bactericidal solution and gas sterilize
		Check to see if pacemaker must be disconnected before defibrillating
Battery failure		Check battery q8 hr
		Observe for signs of battery failure
		Complete or intermittent loss of capture
		Failure to sense
		Loss of pacing; box not discharging
		Needle on box not moving fully to sense/pace
		Alterations in discharge rate
		Ensure that fresh batteries are readily available
		Replace battery when low
Catheter displacement		Secure wire and equipment
Loss of contact between heart and electrode		Minimize motion of extremity or torso at site of insertion
		Arm: do not raise above shoulder level or lift patient under arm thereby raising shoulder
		Leg: avoid outward rotation and marked hip flexion
		Observe for signs of catheter displacement
		Change in QRS configuration
		Complete or intermittent loss of capture
		Loss of pacing artifact on ECG—box continues to discharge
		Failure to sense
		Aberrant pacemaker stimulation—spasm of chest muscle or hiccups
		If problem occurs
		Reposition patient (roll side to side)
		Increase stimulation threshold
		Inform physician of need to reposition
Improper terminal connections		Check connections q8 hr
		Observe for loss of pacing artifact on ECG—box continues to discharge
		Tighten connections if necessary
Changes in threshold		Check threshold q24 hr
		Be alert to factors that alter threshold
		Decrease threshold
		MI or ischemia
		Electrolyte abnormalities (decreased K^+)
		Frequent premature ventricular contractions
		Sympathomimetic drugs or increased catecholamine excretion
		Hypoxic states
		Increased threshold may occur 3 to 4 days after insertion because of local inflammation and fibrosis at electrode tip
		Observe for
		Complete or intermittent loss of capture
		Loss of pacing artifact on ECG—box continues to discharge
		Failure to sense
		If problem occurs
		Increase output
		Inform physician—may reposition catheter to new site
Electrode failure		Observe for complete and intermittent loss of capture
		If problem occurs, convert bipolar to unipolar
Fractured electrode—more common with epicardial electrode		Observe for complete or intermittent loss of capture
		If problem occurs, electrode will be replaced by physician
Failure to sense when catheter properly positioned and battery not failing		Observe for competition between paced and spontaneous beats
		If problem occurs
		Reposition ECG electrodes if sensing another wave as QRS
		If patient's own rhythm is adequate, turn pacemaker off and inform physician

POTENTIAL PROBLEMS	EXPECTED OUTCOMES	NURSING ACTIVITIES

		If patient's own rhythm is inadequate
		    Inform physician
		    Increase pacer rate to overdrive
		    Administer lidocaine for ectopics as ordered
		    Increase sensitivity
		    Unipolarize if bipolar system
		    If pacemaker is fixed rate, turn to demand

■ Arrhythmias	■ Absence of threatening arrhythmias	■ Observe ECG for arrhythmias, particularly ventricular
		    If premature ventricular contractions are present
		        Measure coupling interval
		        Treat with lidocaine as ordered

■ Perforation of right ventricle or septum by electrode tip	■ Electrode properly positioned	■ Observe for
		    Change in paced QRS configuration
		    Aberrant pacemaker stimulation, including hiccups
		    Complete or intermittent loss of capture
		    Loss of pacing artifact on ECG—box continues to discharge
		    Signs and symptoms of tamponade (rare)
		        Increased venous pressure
		        Decreased BP
		        Pulsus paradoxus
		        Narrow pulse pressure
		        Tachycardia
		        Restlessness, cyanosis
		        Decreased output
		    If problem occurs
		        Inform physician
		        Assist physician, who may withdraw catheter
		        Reposition patient

■ Embolization	■ Absence of emboli related to pacing	■ *See* STANDARD 31 *Embolic phenomena*

■ Infection at insertion site	■ Absence of infection at insertion site	■ Maintain sterile technique with insertion
		    Ensure clean/sterile equipment
		    Change dressing q24 hr
		        Cleanse skin with antiseptic solution
		        Apply antibiotic ointment and dry sterile dressing
		    Provide padding beneath wires to prevent ulceration of underlying tissue in predisposed patients
		    Respond to patient's complaints
		    Inspect regularly for signs of inflammation or infection
		        Tenderness
		        Redness
		        Swelling
		        Discoloration
		    Check site q4 hr or as indicated
		    Culture tip of catheter on removal if
		        Signs of infection present
		        Catheter in place over 1 week
		        Traumatic insertion

■ Pain or discomfort of affected extremity	■ Patient verbalizes comfort	■ Check pulse perfusion distal to cutdown q8 hr
		    Position extremity comfortably
		    Assist with exercises to avoid stiffness of extremity with restricted movement and edema
		    Administer medication as needed for pain

■ Tamponade related to removal of epicardial electrodes	■ Absence of tamponade	■ Closely monitor for signs and symptoms of tamponade for 3 to 4 hours following removal; note changes in
		    BP
		    Pulse pressure
		    Venous pressure

POTENTIAL PROBLEMS	EXPECTED OUTCOMES	NURSING ACTIVITIES
		Heart rate Urine output Mentation Instruct patient to avoid valsalva maneuvers after removal for at least 4 hours

■ Microshock hazard	■ Electrically safe equipment and environment	■ Insulate external metallic portions of pacing catheter
		  Safe if embedded in insulated pacemaker terminals of newer models
		  Cover with clear Scotch tape or dry surgical rubber glove
		Be certain all equipment is properly grounded with three-prong plugs only and no adaptors
		  Common ground for all equipment used on patient; avoid extension cords
		Equipment with frayed wires or other signs of disrepair *must* not be used
		If there is any question, consult hospital electrician or biomedical engineer
		Protect patient from contact with metal
		  Patient should not control line-powered equipment, e.g., television or radio
		  Staff should not touch patient or bed while simultaneously touching electrical equipment
		  Avoid electrical beds not specifically approved
		  Unplug bed lamps attached to metal beds
		  Electrical equipment should not touch bed, e.g., respirator
		  Identify patient as ''microshock precaution'' by placing sign on bed; explain to patient/family
		  Wear intact rubber or plastic gloves when handling external metallic portions of pacing catheter
		  Keep energy source and dressing dry

Permanent pacemaker

ASSESSMENT

1. Problem necessitating pacemaker insertion
   a. Disease process
   b. ECG illustrating arrhythmia
   c. Symptoms associated with the arrhythmia
2. Baseline information included in chart
   a. Date and location of implant
   b. Manufacturer's model and serial numbers for the generator and leads
   c. Set rate, ECG tracing with and without magnet held over generator
   d. Amplitude of pacemaker artifact
   e. Threshold measurements at time of implant
   f. Programmable or nonprogrammable
3. Monitor rhythm strips for
   a. Maintenance of preset rate
   b. Capture
   c. Paced QRS configuration
   d. Amplitude of pacemaker artifact
   e. Sensing
   f. Competition

4. Chest radiograph documenting location
5. Level of anxiety
6. Patient's perception of and reaction to pacemaker
7. Evaluation of hemodynamic status—signs and symptoms suggestive of pacemaker failure
8. Signs and symptoms of complications
   a. Aberrant pacemaker stimulation
   b. Discomfort at implant site and/or of affected shoulder
   c. Cardiac arrhythmias, particularly ventricular
9. Site of implantation for signs of inflammation or infection, bleeding, hematomas, and skin breakdown
10. Factors influencing learning
    a. Preexisting knowledge
    b. Level of education (formal and informal)
    c. Age
    d. Motivation
    e. State of health
    f. Level of anxiety
    g. Patient's life-style
11. Ongoing and final evaluation of effectiveness of teaching program
12. Determinants of compliance

GOALS

1. Pacemaker unit functioning properly
2. Hemodynamic stability
3. Clean, healing wound
4. Patient performs ROM exercises to affected shoulder
5. Absence of threatening arrhythmias
6. Patient verbalizes understanding of procedure, reason for and function of pacemaker
7. Patient's behavior demonstrates decreased anxiety with provision of information

8. Before discharge the patient/family
   a. Demonstrates comprehension of the knowledge components of the teaching program when evaluated by testing or questioning
   b. Takes pulse correctly, stating acceptable ranges
   c. Lists those symptoms requiring physician notification
   d. Asks pertinent questions regarding self-care
   e. Discusses future realistically, noting adjustments required
   f. States necessary information regarding follow-up visits to physician and/or clinic

POTENTIAL PROBLEMS	EXPECTED OUTCOMES	NURSING ACTIVITIES

■ Anxiety related to
   Procedure
   Lack of physiological
     self-control
   Lack of understanding
     of function of pace-
     maker unit
	■ Patient verbalizes anxiety
	   and/or fears
	   Patient asks questions
	   Patient verbalizes reason-
	    able understanding of
	    procedure, reason for
	    pacemaker, and function
	    (progression toward ac-
	    ceptance)
		■ Ongoing assessment of level of anxiety
		   Encourage questions from patient/family
		   Explain procedure, preoperative and postoperative course expecta-
		    tions
		   Explain normal conduction system and relate explanation to patient's
		    arrhythmia, which necessitates pacemaker
		   Relate patient's symptoms to arrhythmia, stressing difference pace-
		    maker will make
		   Explain function and type of pacemaker to be implanted

■ Pacemaker malfunction	■ Pacemaker unit functioning
	   properly
	   Fires at preset rate
	   Each pacemaker stimu-
	    lus produces myocar-
	    dial response (cap-
	    ture)
	   Senses patient's own
	    beat (models with
	    sensing mechanism)
	   Absence of competition
	   Hemodynamic stability
		■ Continuous monitoring of ECG for first 24 hours; then analysis of
		   ECG strip q4 hr or as indicated for
		    Maintenance of preset rate
		    Capture
		    Paced QRS configuration
		    Amplitude of pacemaker artifact
		    Sensing
		    Competition
		    Ventricular arrhythmias
		   Compare for consistency with baseline values in chart
		   Check BP, R, and temperature q4 hr or as indicated
		   Check apical and radial pulse q2 hr, then q4 hr
		    Count for *1 full minute*
		    Report rate below pacing rate or apical-radial pulse deficit
		   Observe for signs and symptoms suggestive of pacemaker failure
		    Decreased BP
		    Decreased urinary output
		    Stokes-Adams syndrome
		    Palpitations
		    Chest pains
		    Shortness of breath and fatigue
		    Light-headedness

Related to malpositioning
    of pacing catheter
		Bed rest for 24 hours and reduced activity for an additional 48 hours;
		   then increase activity as tolerated
		Arm should not be raised above the shoulder until ROM exercises
		   ordered (usually around third postoperative day)
		Observe for
		   Intermittent or complete failure to pace
		   Aberrant pacemaker stimulation

Related to generator prob-
    lems—battery depletion
    or malfunction within
    electrical circuitry
		Observe for
		   Decrease in amplitude of pacemaker artifact
		   Decrease in pulse from 5 to 10 beats/minute (rule out nonperfused
		    premature ventricular contractions as cause)
		   "Runaway" pacemaker

POTENTIAL PROBLEMS	EXPECTED OUTCOMES	NURSING ACTIVITIES
Related to malfunctioning pacing catheter Breaks in lead wire Fibrosis around site of lead tip MI in electrode area		Observe for failure to pace Notify physician if pacemaker malfunction occurs or is suspected Obtain pacemaker reprogrammer if pacemaker is programmable
■ Problems at implant site related to Incisional pain Infection Hematoma Erosion or skin breakdown caused by pressure Sterile abscesses around generator	■ Patient verbalizes sense of comfort (lack of pain) Clean, healing wound	■ Ask patient of need for pain medication; administer medication as needed Inspect site regularly (and respond to patient's complaints) for any signs of inflammation or infection, skin breakdown, or hematomas Check temperature q4 hr or as indicated If Hemovac is present, empty q8 hr or prn; report excessive bleeding When pressure dressing is removed, sterile dressings may be applied; if so, change daily Administer antibiotics as ordered for 5 to 7 days after implant procedure
■ Frozen shoulder	■ Patient performs ROM exercises to affected shoulder	■ Begin ROM exercises to affected shoulder after checking with physician, usually around third postoperative day
■ Arrhythmias	■ Absence of threatening arrhythmias	■ Observe for ventricular premature beats; note frequency, coupling interval, whether sensing or competition occurs, and whether or not they perfuse If problem occurs, notify physician and treat with lidocaine as ordered or follow standing orders
■ Insufficient knowledge and skill to comply with discharge regimen*	■ Evaluation by testing or questioning demonstrates patient/family's understanding of knowledge components of teaching program Patient takes own pulse correctly and states acceptable ranges Patient lists symptoms requiring notification of physician Patient asks pertinent questions regarding self-care Patient discusses future realistically, noting adjustments required	■ Institute teaching program for patient/family, including Normal heart function—electrical and mechanical Patient's disease process/arrhythmia, which necessitates pacemaker Pacemaker function Method of counting pulse Patient's own normal range Acceptable variations of pulse, noting specifically when to call physician Signs and symptoms indicative of pacemaker failure; relate to those patient had before pacemaker and identify when to call physician Activity instructions including work, sports, sex, and travel Necessity of identification ID card Medical alert jewelry Informing physician or dentist Electrical interference; precautions and actions to take if occurs Clothing suggestions—comfort and cosmetic Follow-up Necessity of and timing What is involved Expected battery life and procedure for generator change Provide opportunities for patient/family to ask questions and practice palpating pulse Assess patient/family's potential compliance and make referrals for home follow-up if necessary

*If this type of follow-up care is the responsibility of the critical care unit nurse when patient is transferred from critical care unit.

INTRAAORTIC BALLOON PUMPING
(COUNTERPULSATION)

The intraaortic balloon is used for patients with marginal cardiac function when augmentation of coronary blood flow and a decrease in *afterload,* or resistance to cardiac ejection, is desired. *Preload,* or the resting pressure and stretch in the left ventricle, is decreased also. These actions result in a decreased myocardial work load and oxygen consumption.

Blood supply is augmented while oxygen demand is diminished, resulting in improved myocardial efficiency and augmented stroke volume and cardiac output.

The intraaortic balloon pump is used when medical therapy is inadequate to support patients in the following clinical situations:

1. For high-risk patients requiring cardiac catheterization, particularly in the presence of unstable angina
2. Preoperatively, for patients with a recent MI and associated cardiogenic shock; mechanical defects such as mitral insufficiency, ruptured papillary muscle, septal defect; intractable angina; and arrhythmias
3. For intractable, unstable angina
4. As an adjunct to preoperative and postoperative management of surgical cardiac patients
5. When weaning from the cardiopulmonary bypass (CPB) machine is not possible using medical therapy alone; this situation occurs in patients with left ventricular failure and a low cardiac output syndrome*
6. For patients with myocardial free wall rupture following an MI to stabilize condition before and during catheterization and surgery

Intraaortic balloon pumping is avoided in patients with severe aortic insufficiency, aortic dissection, coarctation of the aorta, high-output shock, terminal noncardiac diseases, and in the presence of irreversible brain damage. Severe aortoiliac disease is a relative contraindication, although the

*Bailin, M. T.: Lectures on intra-aortic balloon pumping, 1976-1979, Cardiovascular Laboratory, College of Physicians and Surgeons, Columbia-Presbyterian Medical Center, New York; Bregman, D.: Mechanical support of the failing heart, Curr. Probl. Surg. **13**(12):1-84, 1976; Durie, M. E.: Use of an intra-aortic balloon pump following postoperative pump failure and cardiac arrest: case presentation and discussion, Heart Lung **3**:971-975, 1974.

use of guidewires for insertion reduces the risk of arterial damage, dissecting aneurysm, and emboli. In addition, femoral-to-femoral grafts can be placed to increase blood to the extremity fed by the artery into which the balloon will be placed.

The intraaortic balloon consists of a catheter with a balloon at the tip. This device can be placed in the descending aorta via an arteriotomy in the right or left femoral artery and then threaded up the descending aorta to a point 1 cm distal to the subclavian artery.

The balloon is alternately inflated and deflated with gas, such that inflation occurs during ventricular diastole when the aortic valve is closed, displacing blood into the upper torso arteries (unidirectional balloon system) or into both upper and lower torso arteries (bidirectional balloon system).

Knobs on the intraaortic balloon console are adjusted so that the balloon inflates just when the aortic valve closes. The timing is usually done using the R wave of the QRS complex as the reference point, although the arterial waveform may be used also.

Continuous BP monitoring is accomplished via a peripheral arterial catheter or via the central lumen of a double-lumen intraaortic balloon catheter. Most patients also have a pulmonary artery catheter in place to permit continuous monitoring of PAP and PCWP. Hemodynamic and circulatory monitoring activities are essential in assessing the benefit of intraaortic balloon pumping and related therapeutic interventions. Based on these observations, alterations in the therapeutic regimen may be made. Problems that arise may also require alterations in the therapeutic regimen, including hemorrhage during insertion, laceration of the aortic vessel lining, thromboemboli, and infection.

ASSESSMENT

1. Level of patient/family's anxiety
2. Patient/family's understanding of the disease process and anticipated intervention
3. Presence, nature, and severity of problem necessitating balloon insertion, including

a. Disease process
b. Hemodynamic parameters
c. Prior medical management
4. Lab and diagnostic tests, including
    a. ECG abnormalities
    b. Echocardiographic studies
    c. Radionuclide studies
    d. Electrolyte levels
    e. Cardiac isoenzymes
    f. CBC
    g. Cardiac catheterization results
    h. Chest radiograph results
5. Integrity and general function of balloon system
    a. Connector in situ; connecting tubing unkinked
    b. Lamps (lights) on console
    c. Position of balloon and catheter
        (1) External—observe for slack in balloon line and moderately tight insertion of catheter-balloon system
        (2) Internal
            (a) Chest radiograph
            (b) Note adequacy of circulation to left arm
            (c) Note adequacy of diastolic augmentation
6. Waveform and hemodynamic/circulatory status for optimal balloon pumping
    a. Proper timing
        (1) Augmented wave begins at dicrotic notch
        (2) Augmented wave reaches an optimal drop in aortic end-diastolic pressure just before next systole begins (in many patients this represents a 5 to 10 mm Hg dip below zero baseline); also called "presystolic dip"
    b. Hemodynamic parameters
        (1) Drop in height of patient's own systolic wave (indicating decreased afterload and left ventricular work); this effect may not be seen in patients with unstable angina
        (2) The pressure in the aorta at the end of diastole after the balloon deflates (end-diastolic pressure) should drop as low as possible and be accompanied be a lowering of the assisted peak systolic pressure. (in many patients this represents a "presystolic dip" of 5 to 10 mm Hg)
        (3) Presence of hypotension, tachycardia, and/or abnormal CVP and PAP/PCWP
        (4) CVP, PAP, and PCWP, and left atrial pressure, if available, in comparison with pre–balloon pumping pressures
        (5) Urine output, mental status, and adequacy of peripheral circulation in relation to pre–balloon pumping measures; note presence of oliguria, abnormal mental status, and signs of inadequate peripheral circulation

(6) Adequacy of circulation to extremities, particularly the extremities distal to the catheter insertion site and the balloon; in the left arm and affected leg note presence of
    (a) Decreased/weak pulses
    (b) Coolness, blanching, poor capillary filling
(7) Insertion site for hematoma, signs of infection, or phlebitis
(8) Signs and symptoms of complications, including
    (a) Aortic laceration
    (b) Thrombi
    (c) Microemboli
    (d) Coagulation abnormalities
(9) Respiratory insufficiency—rate, rhythm, quality of respirations—noting presence of rales, rhonchi, wheezing, shortness of breath, dyspnea, tachypnea

GOALS

1. Reduction of patient/family's anxiety with provision of information, explanations, and encouragement; patient/family asks questions and verbalizes understanding of insertion procedure and reason for and function of intraaortic balloon pumping
2. Adequate blood flow to extremity distal to site of balloon insertion
3. Absence of hematoma at site of balloon catheter insertion
4. Absence of hemorrhage from insertion site during insertion procedure
5. Absence of aortic, femoral injury
6. Signs of adequate circulation to left upper extremity and brain
7. Hemodynamic stability
8. Adequate cardiac output
9. Hemodynamic parameters and clinical signs indicate adequate perfusion of central and peripheral organs
10. Optimal function of intraaortic balloon pumping system
11. Absence or resolution of signs and symptoms of renal failure
12. Absence or resolution of a thrombus
13. Sufficient circulatory flows to affected leg, arm
14. Pulses full, extremity warm, and color good
15. Coagulation studies within desired limits
16. Infection free; absence of signs of infection at insertion site
17. Respiratory function sufficient to maintain adequate oxygenation and ventilation
18. Absence of pulmonary infection
19. Absence of signs and symptoms of a gas embolism

POTENTIAL PROBLEMS	EXPECTED OUTCOMES	NURSING ACTIVITIES
■ Anxiety related to disease process and deteriorating condition leading to need for intraaortic balloon pumping	■ Reduction in patient/family's anxiety with provision of information, explanations, and encouragement Patient/family asks questions and verbalizes understanding of disease process, purpose of hospitalization, and need for intraaortic balloon pumping	■ Assess patient/family's anxiety and understanding regarding disease process, purpose of hospitalization, deteriorating condition, anticipated balloon insertion, and diagnostic procedures (such as cardiac catheterization) Explain, in simple terms, each of aforementioned as needed Prepare patient for and provide for ongoing support and encouragement during insertion of catheter and institution of balloon pumping Prepare patient for diagnostic tests and explain them as needed Evaluate for reduction in patient/family's anxiety with provision of information, explanations, reassurance, and comfort
■ Ischemic leg, which may be related to Low blood volume Severe atherosclerosis and circulatory insufficiency Spasm of vessel at insertion site	■ Adequate blood flow to affected extremities—to leg distal to insertion site and to arm distal to balloon tip Pulses in extremities full, color good, and extremity warm	■ Prevent by Administering therapy to provide for adequate blood volume and blood flow around balloon In patient with history of severe atherosclerosis and circulatory insufficiency, prepare patient for prophylactic femoral bypass graft to augment blood flow to leg below planned insertion site, if planned During balloon catheter insertion, vessel spasm may occur; as overall hemodynamic picture improves with counterpulsation, spasm may subside; if not, assist in removal of balloon if procedure becomes necessary Monitor for ischemic leg Pulses (femoral, posterior tibial, and dorsalis pedis) before insertion of balloon, then q15-30 min (four times) and then q1-2 hr Diminished or absent pulses, which may indicate transient arterial spasm, femoral artery occlusion by catheter or thrombus, or arterial embolus to extremity; if pulses diminished or absent employ further evaluation for circulatory defects Color and temperature of extremity q30 min (four times) and then q1-2 hr Toe sensitivity and patient's ability to move toes Presence of claudication Complaints of pain and/or extreme restlessness along with signs of circulatory insufficiency to leg Monitor aforementioned indices of circulation to extremity frequently after balloon removal Notify physician of any of aforementioned abnormalities If signs and symptoms of circulatory insufficiency to extremity are marked, balloon removal may be required; assist with procedure as necessary Closely observe for continued or progressive circulatory insufficiency if pulses are weak and limb is cool; in this case reconstructive surgery may be accomplished after balloon removal to improve circulation to leg; prepare patient for surgery if planned
■ Hematoma at insertion site related to anticoagulation necessary for balloon insertion and, in some cases, operative technique	■ Absence or resolution of hematoma at site of balloon catheter insertion Coagulation profile within normal limits	■ Prevention Monitor platelet, Hct, and Hgb levels before insertion; if any or all are low, administer blood and blood products as ordered to correct the abnormalities Administer anticoagulation as ordered to achieve moderately prolonged prothrombin time (PT), activated partial thromboplastin time (APTT), and bleeding time as appropriate; be aware of pertinent baseline values Proper surgical technique (percutaneous route of insertion is most commonly used now) As soon as catheter is in place and skin incision is sutured closed, assist physician with application of pressure dressing

POTENTIAL PROBLEMS	EXPECTED OUTCOMES	NURSING ACTIVITIES

		Monitor for
		    Development of signs of hematoma at insertion site; note presence of subcutaneous swelling, bruised (black and blue) skin and subcutaneous tissue, decreased Hct, Hgb
		    Abnormally prolonged PT, APTT, and bleeding time
		If hematoma occurs
		    If large hematoma develops during balloon insertion, assist physician with removal if necessary
		    If smaller hematoma develops during and/or after insertion, maintain pressure dressing

■ Hemorrhage from insertion site
  Blood loss of more than 200 ml related to insertion of catheter into large artery
	■ Blood loss less than 200 ml
	  Restoration of normal blood volume
	  Hemodynamic stability
		■ Efforts to prevent hemorrhage include careful surgical technique during insertion procedure to reduce blood loss
		Monitor
		    For large amount of blood loss during insertion procedure
		    Serial Hct levels before, during, and after insertion procedure
		If hemorrhage occurs, administer blood replacement as ordered

■ Aortic injury: aortic rupture	■ Absence of aortic rupture	■ Prevent by
		    Assisting physician during balloon insertion
		    Avoiding head gatch of more than 30 degrees and angulation at groin when patient is turned; patients must remain in bed when balloon is in place
		Monitor
		    Vital signs throughout insertion procedure
		    For signs and symptoms of shock and cardiovascular collapse associated with aortic rupture
		If aortic rupture occurs
		    Prepare patient for emergency surgery
		    Administer blood and sympathomimetic medications if needed, as ordered

■ Aortic/femoral artery injury related to
  Dissection
  Intimal hematoma
	■ Absence of aortic/femoral artery injury	■ Prevent by
		    Assisting physicians as they employ careful technique during balloon insertion
		    Avoiding head gatch of more than 30 degrees
		    Instructing patient not to flex involved leg (leg restraints are rarely necessary)
		Monitor for
		    Difficult insertion procedure
		    Onset of patient discomfort, pain in lower back
		    Hematoma formation at or near insertion site
		    Hypotension, tachycardia, and falling Hct, with or without external bleeding, which may indicate hemorrhagic process
		Notify physician for significant abnormalities
		If aortic/femoral artery injury occurs, administer blood replacement as ordered, and carefully monitor patient's response

■ Aortic/femoral artery injury related to inadvertent partial or total removal of catheter out of artery into which it is inserted	■ Balloon and catheter remain in situ in desired location	■ Prevent by
		    Providing for slack in catheter once balloon is in place
		    Avoiding extremely tight connection of balloon-catheter system; no tape should be used
		        Risk of vessel injury and accidental dislodgement of catheter is reduced by easy disconnection of catheter from balloon when tension is applied
		    Employing comfort, support measures, and pain/sedative medication as needed to minimize patient's restlessness

POTENTIAL PROBLEMS	EXPECTED OUTCOMES	NURSING ACTIVITIES
		Monitor
		Tension/slack in intraaortic balloon catheter—safety chamber connection
		For inadvertent partial or total balloon catheter removal
		If balloon displacement is suspected, obtain radiograph
		Notify physician if displacement is noted or suspected
		If catheter removal occurs
		Apply, maintain pressure dressing as ordered
		Monitor for development of hematoma at or near insertion site
		Monitor for hemodynamic stability, stable Hct (note presence of hypotension and falling Hct; notify physician if either occurs)

■ Partial or total occlusion of subclavian and/or carotid artery; ischemic arm and/or cerebral tissue related to malposition of balloon catheter	■ Adequate circulation to left upper extremity, brain
	Upper extremity pulses full; extremities are pink in color and warm
	Patient is alert and oriented
		■ Efforts to prevent occlusion of subclavian or carotid artery include insertion of the balloon catheter using fluoroscopy or chest radiograph to achieve correct position
		Monitor
		  Pulses, circulation to left arm—note weak pulses, discomfort, pallor, and coolness of arm
		  LOC, orientation; note restlessness, confusion, irritability and other abnormalities
		Notify physician of these abnormalities
		If balloon occludes subclavian or carotid artery, assist physician to pull it out aseptically a small distance to permit better circulation to upper extremity and brain

■ Hemodynamic instability related to *inadequate diastolic augmentation*
Timing of balloon inflation/deflation inappropriate for patient's needs
Improper timing, with too short a time of inflation, allows interval of balloon deflation before next beat begins; this encourages retrograde flow of blood from arteries, including coronary arteries
	■ Diastolic augmentation properly timed such that balloon inflation begins at dicrotic notch when aortic valve closes and deflation occurs at end of diastole, just before next systole begins (during isovolumetric contraction: after mitral valve closes and before aortic valve opens)
	Pressure in aorta at end of diastole after balloon deflates drops as low as possible and is accompanied by lowering in assisted peak systolic pressure
		■ Prevention
		  Note heart rate before intraaortic balloon counterpulsation begins and set timing intervals accordingly
		  Datascope System 80, 82, 83: if heart rate changes later by more than 7 to 10 beats/minute, retiming will be necessary
		  Kontron Model 10: if heart rate changes by $\pm 20\%$, console will automatically adjust timing; if heart rate changes by more than 20%, retiming will be needed
		Objective in proper timing of balloon inflation and deflation is to time inflation to occur at dicrotic notch (or when aortic valve closes and ventricular diastole begins); try to time balloon deflation to achieve lowering of aortic end-diastolic pressure, accompanied by lowering of assisted peak systolic pressure (average drop in aortic end-diastolic pressure is 5 to 10 mm Hg; drop is affected by patient variables such as presence of heart failure (greater drop may be achieved) or unstable angina (little or no drop may be achieved)
		Initial settings may be made according to the following guidelines
		  Adjust inflation knob to inflate balloon at dicrotic notch, which represents aortic valve closure
		  Adjust deflation knob to drop aortic end-diastolic pressure as low as possible and to achieve simultaneously a lowering in assisted peak systolic pressure
		Timing can also be performed according to the following guidelines
		  Set filling time at 50 milliseconds (msec) to provide small augmented tracing while inflation and deflation interval settings are made; time for systole and balloon deflation is approximately one third of cardiac cycle + 50 msec or
		
		$$\frac{\text{R to R interval in msec}}{3} + 50^*$$
		
		Time for diastole and balloon inflation is approximately two thirds of cardiac cycle or
		
		$$\text{R-R interval} - \frac{\text{R-R interval}^*}{3}$$
		
		Check calibration and timing of balloon inflation and deflation at least q1 hr and prn

*Pastellopoulos, A.E., and Cullum, J.: Intra-aortic balloon assist for cardiogenic shock, J. Cardiovasc. Technol. **16:**21-30, 1974.

POTENTIAL PROBLEMS	EXPECTED OUTCOMES	NURSING ACTIVITIES

		Monitor
		  Appearance of augmented pressure wave for placement and timing of inflation and deflation
		    This is easily done by momentarily turning ratio of augmented beats to 1:2
		    Note whether augmented wave begins at dicrotic notch and ends just before next beat, with 5 to 10 mm Hg drop in presystolic pressure
		  For arrhythmias—mistimed balloon may be cause (balloon inflation/deflation is also slightly less accurate in presence of irregular cardiac rhythms)
		  For heart rate changes of more than 7 to 10 beats/minute (Datascope) or by 20% (Kontron)
		Notify physician of any of these abnormalities
		If inappropriate timing occurs
		  Readjust timing
		  If cause of inappropriate timing can be found, resolve problem as ordered (e.g., arrhythmias)

■ Hemodynamic instability related to *inadequate amount of gas* (CO_2, helium) in balloon
Approximately 1 to 2 cc gas lost from balloon q1 hr
	■ Sufficient diastolic augmentation to achieve BP in specified range
	When external balloon is filled, it is taut and appears smooth
	Height of augmented wave remains at maximum height achieved immediately after balloon refilling (or in systems not requiring manual inflation, augmentation wave remains at maximum height)
		■ Provide for adequate amount of gas in balloon by
		  Refilling q2-4 hr as needed (if manual refilling system)
		  After filling, note height of diastolic augmentation
		Monitor for need to refill manual refilling system
		  "Slave" balloon in external safety chamber is not taut when filled (Datascope) concurrent with
		  Decrease in height of diastolic augmented wave
		If there is inadequate amount of gas in balloon, refill if system requires manual refilling

■ Hemodynamic instability related to *kinked catheter*	■ Sufficient diastolic augmentation to maintain BP in desired range
	Catheter not kinked
	Balloon/catheter system patent
		■ Prevent kinked catheter by
		  Providing for some, but not too much, slack in external balloon catheter system
		  Keeping system visible at all times
		  Checking for unkinked line when patient is repositioned
		Monitor for alarm indicating impaired movement of gas through catheter system
		Monitor for catheter patency, presence of kinks
		If catheter kinks, straighten it

■ Problems in achieving proper diastolic augmentation related to
Difficulty in balancing/ calibration
BP monitoring system
  Faulty transducer
  "Fuzzy" or "choppy" arterial trace
  Missing arterial trace
	■ Transducer properly balanced/calibrated to console
	Appearance of crisp, normal appearing arterial tracing
		■ Prevent by
		  Recalibrating transducer to console q4 hr and prn *or*
		  Recalibrating transducer to bedside monitor and connecting jack from bedside monitor into console
		  Avoiding trauma to transducer
		  Being careful with bed rail movement so that it does not cut or damage transducer cable or balloon catheter system

POTENTIAL PROBLEMS	EXPECTED OUTCOMES	NURSING ACTIVITIES

	Console arterial BP approximates BP taken by cuff or Doppler sensor (frequently there is as much as 10 to 15 mm Hg difference)	Extra transducer should be available for immediate use
		Compare balloon console pressures with cuff BP q4-8 hr; transducer pressure is normally 10 mm Hg (5 to 15 mm Hg) higher than cuff BP
		If problem in achieving proper diastolic augmentation occurs
		  Try rebalancing, calibrating transducer
		  Transducer may need to be replaced

■ Loss of pumping capability associated with
  Leak in intraaortic balloon with rapid depletion of gas (rare)
  Gas embolism related to balloon rupture
	■ Balloon intact with adequate diastolic augmentation
	Absence of signs and symptoms of gas embolism
	Absence of leak in balloon
	If leak occurs, balloon replaced immediately
		■ Prevent by
		  Ensuring that balloon stays out of operative field during insertion procedure, thus avoiding tiny tear by surgical instruments
		  Avoiding reuse of aortic balloons; as balloon is withdrawn through Dacron graft, tiny tears may occur; autoclaving changes consistency and integrity of balloon; moreover, reuse may transmit hepatitis antigen
		Monitor for
		  Rapid depletion of gas in external (safety chamber—Datascope) balloon
		  Wrinkled appearance of external balloon instead of smooth, taut appearance (Datascope)
		  Loss of maximal diastolic augmentation capability (in comparison with postinsertion baseline augmentation)
		  Blood in catheter system
		  If inordinate loss of gas is noted, monitor for signs and symptoms of emboli to any of central organs and peripheral arterial vasculature (see Standard 31, *Embolic phenomena*)
		  Alarm on Kontron model 10 system, which sounds when there is 3 cc leak; remaining gas is automatically evacuated from balloon and catheter system, and pumping is stopped
		If balloon rupture with loss of pumping capability and/or gas embolism occurs
		  Notify physician
		  Assist with balloon and catheter removal and replacement, if procedure becomes necessary

■ Balloon catheter becomes disconnected from external balloon
This may happen if great tension is applied between internal balloon and catheter
Separation of balloon catheter from the external balloon/console when undue tension is applied is preferable to inadvertent removal of internal balloon
	■ Balloon/catheter system intact	■ Prevent by ensuring some slack in catheter; keep machine close to bed and provide for appropriate patient/catheter positioning
		Monitor for
		  Tension on external balloon line
		  Visible catheter system (so any disconnection is seen immediately)
		If balloon catheter becomes disconnected from external "slave" balloon using Datascope manual refilling system
		  Turn pump off
		  Quickly reconnect system and refill balloon (if manual method is necessary)
		  Turn pump on
		If balloon catheter disconnects from Kontron console, "high volume" alarm will sound
		  Reconnect catheter
		  Purge system
		  Press "on and auto" to refill system with gas and activate alarm system

POTENTIAL PROBLEMS	EXPECTED OUTCOMES	NURSING ACTIVITIES
■ Suboptimal pumping capability associated with *poor ECG tracing* related to Inadequate height of R wave ECG monitoring system not intact Electrode displacement	■ Intact ECG monitoring system, with crisp QRS picture; R wave of sufficient height for consistent, proper triggering of balloon inflation/deflation	■ Prevent by Providing for intact ECG monitoring system and crisp ECG picture Replacing electrodes as needed Placing electrodes to maximize R-wave height (0.5 to 1.5 millivolts) relative to other ECG waves Choosing any lead of 12 lead ECG, by adjusting lead select dial, to choose optimal lead configuration Monitor for need to replace electrodes including wide, hazy ECG baseline that may move all over screen If problem occurs and intraaortic balloon pumping console receives no ECG trigger stimulus, some units will automatically produce balloon deflation Turn pump off (until electrodes can be replaced, etc.) Switch trigger knob from "ECG" trigger to "pressure" or "pulse" trigger; turn machine on Retime inflation/deflation using this pressure/pulse mode, since the pressure spike comes later in the cycle than R wave Replace electrodes or determine any other cause for problem in ECG picture; turn pump back to "ECG" trigger; and retime intervals
■ Suboptimal pumping capability associated with *poor arterial tracing,* which may be related to occluded arterial catheter or air in system	■ Crisp arterial waveform BP via arterial catheter is within 10 to 15 mm Hg of BP by cuff or Doppler sensor	■ Provide for continuous infusion of heparin solution through arterial line to prevent occlusion Prevent/monitor for air in transducer system or kinked catheter, which can reduce accuracy of pressure readings and affect proper timing (if the arterial waveform is used to trigger balloon inflation/deflation) Prevent/eliminate kinks in transducer-flush system q4-8 hr Compare cuff/Doppler pressure against monitor pressure q4-8 hr Rebalance/recalibrate transducer system q8 hr and prn Eliminate air from system if this problem occurs Flush solution through arterial catheter periodically if necessary If clot in arterial catheter is suspected, try withdrawing clot back through arterial catheter
■ Suboptimal pumping capability associated with *suboptimal coordination of balloon inflation with source of arterial waveform*	■ Optimal pumping capability Point of inflation begins at dicrotic notch using aortic root pressure waveform *or* just before dicrotic notch using peripheral arterial waveform	■ Time inflation to occur at dicrotic notch when using aortic root arterial waveform (generated by double-lumen balloon catheter) Time inflation to occur just before (50 msec) dicrotic notch of arterial waveform generated by peripheral arterial catheter (e.g., radial) NOTE: In arterial system dicrotic notch, which represents aortic valve closure, appears later on peripheral arterial waveforms; this represents delay in waveform propagation down arterial system Monitor for Inflation (beginning of diastolic augmented wave) occurring at dicrotic notch using aortic root pressures Inflation occurring just before (50 msec) diastolic augmented wave using peripheral arterial waveforms (e.g., radial) If suboptimal pumping results from suboptimal coordination of time of balloon inflation with source of arterial waveform, reevaluate timing as described in aforementioned nursing activities

POTENTIAL PROBLEMS	EXPECTED OUTCOMES	NURSING ACTIVITIES

■ Arrhythmias
Irregular cardiac rhythm
Most intraaortic balloon pumping models automatically deflate when short coupling interval occurs
If premature beat is not very close to preceding beat, intraaortic balloon pumping system may continue to augment but at reduced efficiency on irregular beats
	■ Absence or control of arrhythmias	■ Prevent by avoiding/correcting factors that precipitate arrhythmias, such as hypoxia, acid-base imbalance, electrolyte imbalance, and anxiety
		If sympathomimetic drug is suspected offender, administer alternative medication as ordered
		Monitor
		  ECG for arrhythmias, particularly supraventricular tachycardia and ventricular arrhythmias
		  Hemodynamic response to arrhythmias if present
		Notify physician for abnormalities
		If arrhythmias occur
		  Administer antiarrhythmic therapy if ordered
		  Administer therapy to correct hypoxia, acid-abse imbalance, and electrolyte imbalance if needed, as ordered
		In patient with pacemaker, if pacing artifact is sensed as R wave, timing for balloon inflation/deflation should be appropriately altered (delay will be increased because of increased time interval between trigger [pacing spike] and dicrotic notch [aortic valve closing])
		  Kontron model 10 will ignore pacing spikes in "pattern mode" of ECG recognition, provided spike is less than 20 msec at base
		  Datascope System 83 will reject pacer spikes in "pacer reject" mode
		Until supraventricular tachycardia can be resolved using Datascope manual refill system with CO_2, frequency of augmentation may be decreased to every other beat, and 3 cc of CO_2 may be added to balloon volume as ordered
		If tachycardia develops, timing intervals will need to be decreased
		In presence of very irregular rhythm, using the Datascope system, exhaust-pressure logic may be used with arrhythmias, following procedure appropriate for console in use
		Extremely irregular rhythm may require pacing to achieve regular rhythm for proper timing of balloon counterpulsation; prepare patient for and assist with procedure

■ Cardiac arrest during counterpulsation	■ Absence or resolution of cardiac arrest	■ Prevent by administering therapy to prevent and treat arrhythmias, thus reducing the likelihood of cardiac arrest
		Monitor for
		  Arrhythmias
		  Inadequate cardiac output, hemodynamic instability
		Notify physician if these abnormalities occur
		If cardiac arrest occurs
		  Assist in institution of CPR
		  Intraaortic balloon pumping console may continue to pump in alternation with chest compressions, that is, chest is compressed as internal balloon deflates
		  A method is provided by both Kontron and Datascope consoles to enable coordination of chest compressions to balloon inflation/deflation
		    Kontron models sound each time balloon is inflated
		    Datascope systems have external "slave" balloon in a safety chamber that inflates when internal balloon is deflated; chest compressions are delivered when external balloon is inflated
		Check to see if intraaortic balloon pumping console is protected against electrical current used in cardioversion
		If cardiac arrest occurs and patient has pacemaker, balloon will continue to be triggered and filled; compress chest when internal balloon is deflated
		Intraaortic balloon pumping machine can be turned to "internal" trigger mode to trigger balloon inflation and deflation; chest compressions can be interposed with inflations of internal balloon

POTENTIAL PROBLEMS	EXPECTED OUTCOMES	NURSING ACTIVITIES
■ Continued hypotension related to low cardiac output after balloon is in place	■ Hemodynamic parameters within normal limits Hemodynamic/circulatory parameters indicate adequate cardiac output and perfusion of central and peripheral organs	■ Prevention Review chart and radiograph results to determine if balloon is placed in optimal aortic position with its tip just distal to subclavian artery Monitor P, circulation, BP to left arm, and LOC during and after catheter insertion Ensure scrupulous timing of balloon inflation and deflation; avoid delayed deflation and associated increased afterload and resistance to cardiac ejection Monitor BP, P, CVP, and PAP/PCWP, if available, jugular venous distention, urine output, peripheral circulation, and LOC q15-30 min; note signs and symptoms of low cardiac output and/or hypotension Daily weights Serial arterial blood gas results (note acidosis) Notify physician of abnormalities in these parameters If hypotension related to low cardiac output occurs Administer fluids as ordered, monitoring patient's response very closely Administer inotropic agents or inotropic/vasodilating agent combination to achieve adequate cardiac output with peak pressure of 100 to 110 mm Hg (systolic or augmented diastolic pressure, whichever is greater) and/or mean pressure of 80 to 90 mm Hg, or as ordered
■ Renal dysfunction, related to Low cardiac output Renal thromboemboli Balloon position that decreases renal artery blood flow	■ Absence or resolution of signs and symptoms of renal failure Urine output at least 0.5 ml/kg/hour for adult Indices of renal function, particularly BUN/creatinine, within normal limits	■ Prevent by maintaining adequate cardiac output and renal blood flow by administering digitalis, fluids, blood products, inotropic agents, and balloon pumping as ordered Monitor Fluid intake and output measurements q1 hr Hemodynamic measurements to determine adequacy of cardiac output q1 hr and prn Radiograph, fluoroscopy results indicating balloon position Results of daily lab studies, including BUN/creatinine levels If problem occurs, see Standard 52, *Acute renal failure*
■ Clotting abnormalities, thrombus formation, and thromboemboli, which may be related to any of several factors, including Dislodgement of atheromatous material during balloon insertion Balloon left in deflated position for more than 5 minutes Turbulence of blood flowing around balloon Hemolysis of RBC with RBC-platelet-fibrin aggregation enhanced by turbulent blood flow around balloon and by balloon acting as surface on which RBC-platelet-fibrin aggregates can adhere	■ Absence of/or resolution of thrombus or thromboembolus Adequate circulation to affected leg and arm Pulses full, extremities warm, and color good Coagulation studies within desired limits	■ Prevent by Administering prophylactic anticoagulation if ordered, which may include Continuous heparin infusion Intermittent doses of heparin Aspirin Administering dextran (10 to 20 ml/hour), if ordered, to decrease platelet aggregation Avoiding leg bending at groin or knee; when patient is turned on side, keep groin and knee straight with pillows Avoiding balloon deflation for more than 2 to 3 minutes and never for more than 30 to 60 minutes (maximum time depends on institutional policy) Manually inflate balloon if it is deflated for 5 minutes or more Monitor Circulation to affected leg, arm q½-1 hr, noting presence and quality of pulses, color, and warmth For signs of peripheral thromboembolus; arterial embolus; and embolus to kidneys, intestine, or brain, which may be followed by infarction; see Standard 31, *Embolic phenomena* Serial PT, APTT, bleeding time, and/or blood coagulation timer (e.g., Hemachron*) results

*International Technidyne Corporation, Metuchen, N.J.

POTENTIAL PROBLEMS	EXPECTED OUTCOMES	NURSING ACTIVITIES

Results of serial platelet counts done at least q24 hr
Hct and Hgb levels at least q24 hr
For signs and symptoms of bleeding—internal or external; employ anticoagulation precautions such as avoidance of bruising and so on
Record all blood loss, including blood samples
Notify physician of abnormalities in any of aforementioned and alter therapy as ordered; monitor patient response
If there are signs and symptoms of an embolus to any end organ, notify physician immediately and administer therapy as ordered; monitor for reduced function, signs of progressive ischemia of the end organ
Administer fresh blood, fresh frozen plasma, platelets as ordered
If surgical cutdown insertion procedure is performed, procure a Fogarty thromboembolectomy balloon catheter and assist physician with insertion distal to balloon insertion site to remove any thromboemboli (usually done immediately after balloon removal)
If percutaneous route of insertion is performed, use of Fogarty catheter is indicated if there is loss of distal pulse during intraaortic balloon pumping or if pulses to either leg are lost after balloon removal (secondary to dislodgement of fibrin, which collects at insertion site, during balloon removal)

■ Infection related to indwelling catheters and high frequency of invasive procedures

■ Infection free
Absence of signs of local infection at insertion site

■ Prevent by
Employing strict aseptic technique during the insertion of all lines, including balloon, and for subsequent dressing changes
Administering antibiotics as ordered
In surgical patient, generally antibiotics are instituted before balloon insertion and continued for at least 48 hours thereafter
In nonsurgical patient, a single prophylactic dose of antibiotics is generally administered at time of balloon insertion
Employing vigorous chest physiotherapy q2 hr and prn, to include turning, chest percussion and vibration, and coughing and deep breathing (if patient is extubated); if patient is intubated, see Standard 6, *Mechanical ventilation*
Monitor
For signs and symptoms of systemic and local infection, particularly of wounds or at insertion sites of invasive lines
Temperature q1-3 hr, as indicated by patient's status
Results of serial WBC counts, with differential
Culture results
If infection occurs
Continue monitoring as described before
Administer antibiotics and local care as ordered

■ Respiratory insufficiency related to
Supine position
Left ventricular power failure of any etiology leading to elevated PCWP and pulmonary edema

■ Respiratory function sufficient to maintain adequate ventilation and oxygenation
PaO_2 and $PaCO_2$ within patient's normal limits
Absence of pulmonary infection

■ Prevention
Reposition patient q1-2 hr to avoid hypostatic pneumonia
Administer chest physiotherapy q2-4 hr unless contraindicated
Administer humidified O_2 to liquefy secretions and to provide for adequate oxygenation
Monitor relationship of hemodynamic parameters with pulmonary function; particularly note PCWP, if available, in relation to signs of adequate cardiac output

POTENTIAL PROBLEMS	EXPECTED OUTCOMES	NURSING ACTIVITIES

Cardiac surgery with prolonged immobilization, minimal inflation of lungs intraoperatively, and decreased interstitial fluid/lymphatic drainage during surgery	Chest radiograph clear, indicating full lung expansion and absence of vascular congestion
	Absence of infection
		If PCWP increases concurrent with signs of falling cardiac output, notify physician
		Institute remedial measures as ordered, which may include fluids, fluid restriction, cardiotonic/vasopressor and vasodilator agents to improve cardiac output and decrease pulmonary vascular congestion
		Administer blood products as ordered to increase Hct (usually to 30%) to achieve adequate oxygen-carrying ability and sufficient intravascular colloid level
		Monitor
		  Respiratory rate, rhythm, quality
		  Breath sounds; note presence of rales, rhonchi, wheezing
		  Arterial blood gas levels, noting presence of abnormal pH levels, hypoxemia, and abnormal CO_2 levels
		  For signs and symptoms of hypoxia, hypocapnia, or hypercapnia
		  Chest radiograph results for evidence of interstitial edema, atelectasis, pleural effusion, and other abnormalities
		  Hemodynamic parameters q½-1 hr for adequacy of left ventricular function and for progress/resolution of pulmonary congestion
		  Fluid intake and output q1 hr
		  Notify physician of any significant abnormalities in these parameters
		If respiratory insufficiency occurs
		  Provide for respiratory support to achieve adequate oxygenation and ventilation, including repositioning q1-2 hr, chest physiotherapy, coughing, and deep breathing
		  Administer humidified O_2 supplement as needed and ordered
		  If these measures are insufficient, mechanical ventilation with PEEP may be instituted until precipitating cause is ameliorated (e.g., compromised myocardial function and pulmonary congestion); see Standard 6, *Mechanical ventilation;* Standard 7, *Positive end-expiratory pressure* as appropriate
		  Administer diuretic, inotropic, and vasodilatating agents as ordered to improve myocardial efficiency

HEMODYNAMIC MONITORING

Hemodynamic monitoring involves the measurement of pressures including arterial, venous, pulmonary artery, and intracranial pressures to assist in the management of the critically ill patient. This is accomplished by placing catheters in an artery, vein, heart chamber, or cerebrospinal fluid and connecting them to pressure extension lines attached to the transducer in an airtight solution-filled system. The transducer is electrically connected to a pressure monitor, scope, and recorder. Pressure transducers are electronic devices that convert mechanical pressure waves into electrical signals. The monitor/amplifier receives electrical signals through the transducer cable and processes these signals to a meaningful form, for example, a standard unit of pressure measurement, which is then displayed on the digital meters on the front panel of the amplifier.

The scope/recorder allows for continuous display and trace of waveforms processed by the monitor. An alarm system is located in the monitor, and when appropriate alarm limits are set, abnormal pressures are revealed in 3 to 4 seconds.

This direct pressure determination permits continuous patient hemodynamic monitoring, allowing for a more precise diagnosis of the patient's problems and a rapid assessment of the patient's response to therapy.

The intraarterial monitoring permits continuous BP measurements in hemodynamically unstable patients, including those receiving potent vasoactive/inotropic medications. This permits immediate detection of changes in the BP, thus guiding therapeutic alterations aimed at bringing the BP into a consistently normal range. The waveform and pressures provide information for assessment of cardiac contraction, aortic valve closure, and perfusion of ectopic beats. The arterial catheter allows for easy access to blood specimens needed for monitoring a critically ill patient. Arterial lines may be inserted into the femoral, axillary, brachial, or radial artery. Generally, the radial artery is the vessel of choice because it has been associated with fewer complications.

The CVP measures the pressure in the vena cava or right atrium. CVP/right atrial pressures reflect mean right atrial filling pressures and right ventricular end diastolic pressures (pressures at the end of the filling cycle, just before contraction). Normal CVP ranges from 1 to 6 mm Hg or 5 to 12 cm H_2O. The CVP is determined/affected by the relationship of blood volume, vascular tone, and ventricular (particularly right) function. Therapy that results in alterations in any of these three factors will alter the CVP measurement, and therefore it is a most useful guide in regulating fluid replacement and administration of diuretics as well as vasopressors and vasodilators. CVP measurement is not an accurate index of left ventricular function when the functional efficiency of the two ventricles differs. An elevated CVP may signal right ventricular failure and indirectly reflect left ventricular failure, volume overload, increased vascular tone, tricuspid valve stenosis or regurgitation, constrictive pericarditis, cardiac tamponade, or pulmonary hypertension (caused by chronic lung disease, pulmonary embolism, etc.). Other patient parameters must be assessed before diagnosis of the presence of any of these complications is made. Factors that produce low CVP/right atrial pressure include reduced blood volume and decreased venous tone.

A pulmonary artery catheter, called a *Swan-Ganz catheter,* can measure pulmonary artery diastolic pressure, pulmonary artery systolic pressure, PCWP, left atrial filling pressure, CVP, and cardiac output. It also provides information about the competency of left ventricular function, and the response of the marginal left ventricle to certain therapeutic interventions, particularly fluid administration, diuretics, inotropic agents, and vasodilators. The pulmonary artery catheter is a pliable, balloon-tipped, flow-directed catheter that is passed through a large vein, usually in the antecubital or neck area, into the right side of the heart to the pulmonary artery. There are three kinds of pulmonary artery catheters, which are as follows:

1. Double-lumen catheter: monitors pulmonary artery and wedge pressures; used for obtaining samples of mixed venous blood; used for infusion of solutions
2. Triple-lumen catheter: same capabilities as double lumen-catheter; also monitors right atrial pressure (CVP)
3. Flow-directed thermodilution catheter: same capabilities as double- and triple-lumen catheters; also monitors cardiac output via a fourth lumen connected to a cardiac output computer

Pulmonary artery systolic pressures reflect the pressures

of blood flow from the right ventricle and usually approximate the right ventricular systolic pressure in the absence of pulmonary artery stenosis. Pulmonary artery pressures (PAP) are elevated in the presence of increased pulmonary blood flow (e.g., hypervolemia), elevated pulmonary resistance, and/or left ventricular failure.

Left ventricular end diastolic pressure is reflected by the pulmonary artery diastolic and capillary wedge pressures. Left ventricular end diastolic pressure occurs at the end of the diastole when the valves on the left side of the heart open and the left ventricle, left atrium, and the pulmonary beds momentarily become a single chamber. The PCWP is obtained by inflating the balloon near the end of the catheter until the small pulmonary vessel is occluded and the catheter is said to be "wedged." The pressure reflected on the monitor is the PCWP. It reflects the resting baseline pressures in the lungs, left atrium, and left ventricle, which are nearly the same in the absence of mitral valve disease or severely increased pulmonary vascular resistance. If severe mitral valve stenosis is present, the left atrial pressures are higher and reflect a greater degree of left ventricular failure than is actually present. Serial wedge pressure measurements are useful in determining the response of the left ventricle to fluids, diuretics, and vasopressor and vasodilator drug therapy. Pulmonary wedge pressures indicating heart failure range from 18 to 20 mm Hg; for frank heart failure from 22 to 25 mm Hg; and for pulmonary edema over 30 mm Hg. For normal PAP values see Table 25-1.

Elevated PAP may occur with pulmonary embolism, which is associated with increased pulmonary vascular resistance and increased PAP. It can also be elevated in the presence of pulmonary hypertension or chronic lung disease. Pulmonary artery pressures are useful in the diagnosis of these and in the differentiation of hypovolemic shock (low PAP), cardiogenic shock (high PAP), and spinal shock (normal PAP). They also provide accurate quantification of the degree of myocardial depression after an MI, thereby permitting more precise, individualized therapy. Heart failure can be quantitated for each ventricle, and the response to therapy can be followed. Pericardial disease can be confirmed as a result of characteristic pressure changes. The presence of ventricular septal rupture can be verified with the aid of oxygen content determinations, where a step up in oxygen content between the right atrium and the pulmonary artery can be seen.

Cardiac output is the amount of blood pumped by the ventricle in 1 minute. The cardiac output of the left and right ventricles is essentially the same, since each ventricle usually pumps equal amounts of blood/minute. The two determinants of cardiac output are stroke volume (amount of blood a ventricle pumps to the body during each contraction measured in milliliters of blood/contraction) and heart rate.

Stroke volume (milliliters/beat) $\times$
Heart rate (beats/minute) $=$
Cardiac output (milliliters/minute)

The normal cardiac output ranges from 4 to 7 liters/minute in the adult, depending on body size and the effect of variables that influence the demand for cardiac output.

The determination is accomplished with the use of a pulmonary artery flow-directed thermodilution catheter connected to a cardiac output computer. An exact amount of solution of known temperature is injected into the proximal catheter lumen, which empties into the right atrium or vena cava. The change in blood temperature is detected by the thermistor at the distal end of the catheter and then transmitted to the cardiac output computer for calculation and display of the cardiac output measurement.

A left atrial catheter is used to measure the pressure in the left atrium, which is a direct reflection of the left ventricular end diastolic pressure or filling pressure. It is usually placed in patients with very marginal heart function, actual or anticipated low cardiac output, rapid blood loss, or impaired cardiac contractility and in those for whom determination of fluid administration will be partly based on the direct response of the left atrial pressures. Like the PAP, the left atrial pressure is an index to the function of the left ventricle and a guide to fluid and blood replacement. It is critical that air not enter the atrium through this catheter because an air embolus can flow directly to the brain, heart, or other organs without being filtered by the lungs.

Intracranial pressure (ICP) is the pressure exerted by the constituents of the brain, namely the brain tissue, cerebrospinal fluid (CSF), and intravascular blood. ICP normally ranges from 110 to 140 mm H_2O or 0 to 10 mm Hg. Pressures above 200 mm H_2O or 15 mm Hg are indicative of increased ICP.

Cerebral blood flow is equal to the MAP minus the ICP. Other factors such as vascular resistance and venous flow also affect the cerebral blood flow. The term *cerebral perfusion pressure* (PP) may also be used to determine the status of cerebral circulation. Under normal conditions PP in cerebral vessels is approximately equal to the MAP. Any in-

TABLE 25-1. Normal PAP values

PRESSURE	VALUE (MM HG)
Right atrial mean	− 1 to + 7
Right ventricular	
Systolic	15 to 25
End diastolic	0 to 8
Pulmonary artery	
Systolic	15 to 25
Diastolic	8 to 15
Mean	10 to 20
Pulmonary wedge mean	5 to 12

crease in ICP must be subtracted from the MAP in determining the effective PP; the resulting decrease in PP reduces cerebral blood flow. Cerebral blood flow ceases when ICP equals cerebral PP.

ICP monitoring is useful in patients who have signs and symptoms of increased ICP or potentially are at high risk for developing increased ICP. Clinical symptoms of increased ICP may not be evident until the ICP has increased well above normal levels. ICP monitoring provides for early detection of ICP elevations so that immediate interventions and therapy can be instituted to prevent irreversible cerebral damage.

There are several techniques employed to monitor ICP. These include a catheter placed in the frontal horn of a lateral ventricle; a screw, wick, or cup placed in the subdural space; and a catheter placed in the epidural space. All of the various devices are connected to a pressure transducer, and the wave forms are displayed continuously on an oscilloscope/recorder. Some devices employed can be therapeutic as well as diagnostic in providing a method for drainage of CSF when ICP elevations occur.

ASSESSMENT

1. Level of patient/family's anxiety
2. Problem necessitating hemodynamic monitoring
   a. Disease process
   b. Hemodynamic parameters
   c. Medical management employed
3. Site of insertion for pain, ecchymosis, hematoma, infection, and phlebitis
4. Signs and symptoms of complications
   a. Arterial monitoring: dissection, external hemorrhage, sepsis, plaque dislodgement, false aneurysm, local obstruction with distal ischemia, cerebral infarction (carotid artery catheter), renal dysfunction (femoral artery catheter)
   b. CVP monitoring: infection, catheter breakage, thromboembolic phenomena, air embolism, perforation of right ventricle, arrhythmias if catheter in right atrium
   c. PCWP and cardiac output monitoring: infection, pulmonary artery perforation, thromboembolic complications, pulmonary ischemic lesions, pulmonary in-

farction, pneumothorax, arrhythmias, catheter kinking, and intracardiac knotting
   d. Left atrial pressure monitoring: air embolism
   e. ICP monitoring: uncontrolled loss of CSF, infection such as meningitis and ventriculitis, CSF leakage, and cerebral trauma
5. Integrity and general function of hemodynamic monitoring system
   a. Patency of catheter
   b. Proper placement of catheter verified by chest radiograph, fluoroscopy, waveforms, characteristics on the scope, pressures
   c. Accuracy of transducer
   d. Proper balancing and calibration of the system
   e. Airtight system of pressure tubings, stopcocks, adaptors or valves; absence of bubbles
   f. Proper function of amplifier/monitor
   g. Proper function of oscilloscope and/or recorder
   h. Measurement problems, including
      (1) Overdamping of waveforms
      (2) Influence of respiratory pressures
      (3) Migration of catheter tip
      (4) Drift of electronic zero or less of calibration
      (5) Catheter whip artifact
      (6) Low pulmonary artery diastolic pressure
      (7) Faulty catheter system
6. Hemodynamic status in relation to patient's condition and therapy employed

GOALS

1. Reduction of patient/family's anxiety with provision of information and explanations
2. Hemodynamic stability—clinical signs and parameters indicate adequate central and peripheral perfusion
3. Infection free—absence of infection at insertion site or secondary sepsis
4. Absence and/or resolution of complications as stated in assessment for specific monitoring technique
5. Patient verbalizes comfort
6. Monitoring system functioning properly
7. Absence of measurement problems; waveforms correlate with patient's hemodynamic status

POTENTIAL PROBLEMS	EXPECTED OUTCOMES	NURSING ACTIVITIES
■ Patient/family's anxiety related to disease process and procedures	■ Reduction in patient/family's anxiety with provision of information and explanations Patient/family asks questions and verbalizes understanding of disease process and need for hemodynamic monitoring	■ Assess patient/family's anxiety and understanding regarding disease process, hemodynamic monitoring, and diagnostic and lab studies Explain each of aforementioned Prepare patient for and assist with diagnostic and lab studies as appropriate Prepare patient for hemodynamic monitoring and explain procedure Provide support, reassurance, and comfort for patient/family Evaluate reduction in patient/family's anxiety with provision of information and explanations

POTENTIAL PROBLEMS	EXPECTED OUTCOMES	NURSING ACTIVITIES
■ Problem during catheter insertion: pneumothorax may be associated with subclavian insertion Where air inadvertently enters pleural space Inadvertent laceration of apex of lung occurs	■ Pulmonary sufficiency Absence/resolution of pneumothorax Proper catheter placement	■ Prevention Place patient in supine or slight Trendelenburg position for catheter insertion Keep patient still during insertion Physician employs careful technique so that desired artery is entered, avoiding pleural space and lung tissue Monitor For signs and symptoms of pneumothorax, including Anxiety and diaphoresis Sudden sharp chest pain, pleural pain Dyspnea and tachycardia Absent or distant breath sounds, asymmetrical chest movement, pallor, cyanosis Hypotension Vital signs q15-30 min or more often during acute episodes Notify physician for any of these abnormalities If problem occurs Stay with patient and have someone quickly procure equipment for chest tube insertion Check vital signs and respiratory status q15-30 min and prn Reassure and try to calm patient Assist with chest tube insertion Administer O_2 therapy as ordered Place patient in semi- to high Fowler position Administer pain medication if needed, as ordered
■ Hemorrhage, which may be related to Inadvertent system disconnection Insertion technique	■ Absence/resolution of hemorrhage Flush system, including connections, tight and intact Hemodynamic stability	■ Prevention Careful tehnique is employed during insertion procedure to reduce blood loss Monitoring system alarms functioning properly with appropriate alarm limits set Set limits on monitor closely (within 20 mm Hg of patient's BP) so that staff is quickly alerted of BP drop associated with possible hemorrhage Insertion site and system should be visible at all times Ensure tight connections with no apparent leaks Tape catheter system securely All connections should be of Luer-Lok or Linden type, which are not easily disconnected Monitor for Hemorrhage from disconnected system Alarm limits and their activation, if pressure drops Blood backing up in system, caused by leak in system; tighten all connections and inspect for leaks If problem occurs If arterial line comes out, apply pressure on insertion site immediately and maintain for 10 to 15 minutes If connection comes apart, clamp tubing going to patient, ask someone to procure another system or another part of system, change contaminated portion, and reinstitute intact system If ischemia does not resolve, notify physician Catheter may be removed
■ Hematoma related to Trauma to vessel during insertion Patients with abnormal coagulation are at particularly high risk Insufficient external pressure after catheter removal	■ Absence/resolution of hematoma Atraumatic catheter insertion procedure	■ Prevention Physician avoids traumatic injury to vessel during insertion Extra precaution used for patients with abnormal clotting ability When catheter is removed, 10 to 15 minutes of direct pressure is applied to insertion site followed by placement of pressure dressing For femoral arterial puncture site; place sandbag over site for 1 to 2 hours

POTENTIAL PROBLEMS	EXPECTED OUTCOMES	NURSING ACTIVITIES

		Monitor for any
		  Signs of hematoma near insertion site—note presence of subcutaneous swelling, bruised (black and blue) appearance
		  Abnormally prolonged PT, APTT, and bleeding time; decreased Hct and Hgb
		If hematoma occurs, catheter may be removed and compresses applied to assist in resolution

■ Infection
  Endocarditis, which may be related to catheter irritation of the endocardium and associated bacterial invasion
  Septicemia
  Infection at insertion site
  Meningitis
  Ventriculitis
	■ Absence/resolution of infection
	Absence of any clinical manifestation of infection
	Intact ICP monitor system components
		■ Prevention
		  Before insertion, assist physician in adequately cleaning skin for insertion
		  Maintain aseptic technique during insertion
		  Keep patient's hands from insertion site
		  Prepare and change flush solution q24 hr, tubing system q48 hr, using sterile technique
		  Cleanse insertion site with antiseptic solution and change dressing daily, using sterile technique
		  Secure catheter well in place
		  If continuous flush system is not used, maintain sterile technique in intermittent flushing procedure
		  Arterial and CVP lines should not remain in situ for more than 3 days; pulmonary, left atrial or ICP lines should not remain in situ for more than 2 days or longer than its use is justified
		  Insertion of other lines into involved extremity should be avoided
		  Prophylactic antibiotics may be ordered in presence of known valvular abnormality
		Monitor for
		  Redness, inflammation, unusual warmth, pain, and purulent drainage at insertion site; edema, blood or CSF drainage (quality, amount)
		  Any changes in temperature
		  ECG changes consistent with endocarditis (see Standard 19, *Endocarditis*)
		  Neurological status for any abnormality/decline
		  WBC count (may be falsely elevated if patient is receiving steroids)
		  Signs/symptoms of meningitis, particularly severe headache, nuchal rigidity, altered LOC, seizures, and Kernig and Brudzinski signs
		Notify physician of occurrence of any abnormalities and/or displacement/detachment of monitoring system components
		If problem occurs
		  Monitor blood, wound, sputum culture results; CSF determinations
		  Administer medications/treatments as ordered
		  Assist physician as necessary in removal/reinsertion of catheter
		  Monitor for resolution/progression of infection
		  See Standard 42, *Meningitis/encephalitis,* or Standard 19, *Endocarditis,* if occur

■ Monitoring problems: damped waveform resulting from
Air in system
Small thrombus at catheter tip
Kinked catheter
Catheter tip against vessel wall
Compliant tubing
	■ Normal waveforms	■ Prevention
		  Of air in system
		    Ensure that all air is removed when system is assembled
		    Ensure that all connections are tight
		    Avoid vigorous flushing of line; this tends to draw some of air left in the drip chamber into line
		  Of clot in system
		    Heparin is added to crystalloid solution, infused at 3 to 6 ml/hour, and regulated by a flush flow regulator
		    Flush system with heparinized solution after every blood withdrawal
		    System is pressurized; periodically check that pressure bag gauge is at 300 mm Hg
		    Catheter is secured to skin at insertion site to prevent kinking

POTENTIAL PROBLEMS	EXPECTED OUTCOMES	NURSING ACTIVITIES

		Monitor for
		  Decreased amplitude of pressure waveform, in which systolic is usually decreased and diastolic increased with each pressure reading and prn
		  Any bleeding back to system from catheter
		If problem occurs
		  Check system and transducer connection for air
		  Check system for any kinks
		  In absence of first two problems in system, catheter may have drifted further into pulmonary artery; turn patient, have patient cough, or if he/she is intubated, manually inflate patient's lungs to encourage catheter to dislodge from small artery
		  If aforementioned activities are unsuccessful, try to gently flush solution through catheter
		  Aspirate catheter to remove suspected clot, then flush with heparinized saline solution
		  If catheter tip is suspected to be resting against vessel wall, physician may pull catheter back while observing waveforms

■ Monitoring problems: artifact or catheter whip
  May be related to long connecting line between transducer and catheter
  Related to motion of catheter caused by right ventricular contraction
	■ Pressure reading accurately reflects patient's pulmonary pressures	■ Prevention
		  Avoid excessive connecting line between transducer and the catheter
		Monitor for fuzzy, unclear pressure readings on the oscilloscope
		If catheter whip artifact occurs
		  Use pulmonary artery mean pressure reading
		  Obtain calibrated recording of pressure tracing over longer period of time to achieve most representative pressures
		  Reduce length of connecting/extension line if possible

■ Monitoring problems: inaccurate BP readings
  Arterial pressure is usually 5 to 15 mm Hg higher than cuff BP reading
  Monitor "drift"; need for recalibration
  Inaccurate PAP readings
    Movement of catheter tip to unintended location (e.g., PA → RV; PA → PCW)
    Movement of catheter tip against vessel wall
    Transducer position not at right atrial level (midchest)
	■ BP readings accurately reflect patient's actual BP
	  Accurate PAP readings
		■ Prevention
		  Use of flouroscopy and/or chest roentgenograms by physician during insertion of catheter to establish optimal catheter position
		  Suture and secure catheter near insertion site to minimize subsequent catheter movement
		  Balance and recalibrate transducer and monitor to air and to known pressure (use of sphygmomanometer), with upper part of transducer dome placed at right atrial level q8 hr
		  Check arterial monitor pressures with cuff or Doppler pressures q8 hr and prn
		  Ensure absence of air in system
		  Allow monitor-amplifier to warm up for 15 to 20 minutes before balancing/calibration and attachment to patient
		  Ensure transducer position is at midchest level to prevent inappropriately low pressure readings; subsequent measurements should be made with transducer and patient in same position
		Monitor for
		  Intraarterial pressures that are more than 5 to 15 mm Hg higher or lower than cuff BP; take cuff BP in both arms, noting any differences
		  Observe for entry of air into the system or for leaks
		If problem occurs, take action depending on cause of problem
		  Flush air out of system
		  Allow monitor, amplifier to warm up fully
		  Reposition transducer and/or patient so that transducer is at midchest level
		  Recalibrate system
		  If catheter malposition suspected, notify physician, who may reposition catheter

POTENTIAL PROBLEMS	EXPECTED OUTCOMES	NURSING ACTIVITIES
Specific for arterial lines		

■ Arterial spasm—more common with arterial catheters that have been in place 3 or more days	■ Absence/resolution of spasm	■ Prevention
		    Physician inserts arterial catheter directly, nontraumatically
		    Early removal of catheter; as soon as use is not justified
		  Monitor for complaints of severe pain at or around catheter insertion site
		  Observe circulation distal to catheter insertion site; blanching and decreased pulses may indicate spasm
		  If problem occurs, apply heat locally; if not relieved, notify physician; line may have to be removed
		    Physician may inject lidocaine hydrochloride locally around site as well as into arterial catheter (generally 10 mg)

■ Ischemia, thrombosis distal to line insertion, particularly with radial lines, related to
  Insufficient ulnar artery blood flow
  Emboli
	■ Absence of ischemic episode distal to line insertion
	  Absence of microemboli
		■ Prevention
		    Before cannulation of the radial artery, Allen test should be done to assess adequacy of blood flow through ulnar artery
		    Occlude both radial and ulnar artery
		    Have patient close hand tightly several times until hand is blanched
		    Release ulnar artery
		    Note length of time for normal color on hand to return (should be approximately 5 seconds)
		    Radial artery trauma minimized by direct, nontraumatic arterial insertion
		  Monitor
		    Circulation distal to arterial line insertion site for color, capillary filling, pulses, and sensation
		    For any complaint of severe pain at and around catheter site, with blanched appearance of limb distal to catheter
		  If ischemia occurs
		    Apply warm compress to increase blood flow to the hand
		    Increasing BP in hypotensive patient may help resolve ischemia to hand
		  If formation of clot distal to insertion site is suspected, an arterectomy and insertion of Fogarty catheter can remove clot in most patients

Specific for Swan-Ganz catheters		

■ Problem during catheter insertion: catheter curls, kinks, or knots in atrium, ventricle; more apt to occur in low-flow cardiac output states and with rapid insertion and manipulation	■ Absence/resolution of curling, kinking, or knotting of catheter
	  Uneventful catheter insertion
		■ Assist physician in partial inflation of balloon once catheter passes through tricuspid valve so that flow of blood will carry catheter into pulmonary artery
		  Catheter is advanced slowly; rapid advancement may cause curling or kinking of catheter so that further manipulation may result in knotting
		  If knotting occurs in atrium, catheter can be carefully withdrawn by physician to insertion site, and knot can be removed through small incision
		  If knotting occurs in ventricle, thoracotomy may be required to remove catheter

■ Problem during catheter insertion: perforation of pulmonary artery; may be related to insufficient air in catheter balloon such that catheter tip may injure pulmonary artery	■ Absence or resolution of pulmonary artery perforation
	  Pulmonary artery intact
		■ Prevention
		    Inflate balloon only with specified amount of air or CO_2
		    Anchor catheter firmly at insertion site
		    Observe waveform before balloon inflation; do not inflate if waveform is flattened, as this may indicate wedging
		    If wedging occurs, turn patient to side and/or stimulate coughing in attempt to dislodge the catheter from the wedged position
		  Monitor
		    For chest pain, hemoptysis, hypotension, cardiovascular collapse, and respiratory distress; notify physician immediately
		    Chest radiograph results for catheter placement

POTENTIAL PROBLEMS	EXPECTED OUTCOMES	NURSING ACTIVITIES

		If problem occurs
		  Administer medication and fluids as ordered
		  Monitor BP and P continuously
		  Prepare patient for emergency surgery if planned

■ Problem during catheter insertion: arrhythmias, which usually result from catheter irritation of the right ventricular wall	■ Absence or minimal arrhythmia occurrence
	  Absence of threatening arrhythmias
		■ Prevention
		  Monitor waveforms during insertion of catheter (or visually follow catheter under fluoroscopy)
		  Physician will partially inflate balloon as catheter is advanced to the right ventricle to blunt catheter tip and prevent irritation of endocardium
		  Physician will advance catheter slowly and cautiously
		  Administer therapy to resolve factors predisposing patient to arrhythmias including hypoxemia, acid-base imbalance, electrolyte imbalance, anxiety
		Monitor for any arrhythmia during insertion, particularly presence of premature ventricular contractions
		Have lidocaine and defibrillator available in case sudden hypotension or tachycardia develops
		If problem occurs
		  Notify physician for significant incidence of ventricular arrhythmias
		  Administer antiarrhythmic agent if needed, as ordered
		  Physician may pull catheter back slightly and wait until arrhythmia subsides before attempting to advance catheter

■ Air or CO_2 embolism, which may be related to
Balloon rupture: high incidence after 72 or more inflations
After catheter and balloon in situ for 3 or more days, lipids in blood begin decomposing balloon
Lumens of catheter, except for balloon lumen, not prefilled with flush solution before insertion
	■ Absence of air or CO_2 embolism	■ Prevention
		  Prefill all lumens of catheter except balloon with fluid solution before insertion
		  Ensure that balloon is inflated gradually until PCWP is obtained; amount of air not to exceed 0.8 to 1.5 cc
		  Allow passive inflation of balloon through stopcock by removing syringe after inflation
		  Immediate detection of balloon rupture; if no resistance is felt during balloon inflation and waveforms indicate that catheter has not wedged, balloon rupture may have occurred
		  Use CO_2 for all patients with intracardiac shunt
		  Remove catheter after 3 to 4 days in situ or with anything near 70 inflations
		  Monitor PAD readings in between PCWP determination, since PAD readings reflect PCWP readings
		If air or CO_2 embolism is suspected, notify physician and do not inject additional air or CO_2 into balloon

■ Pulmonary infarction related to occlusion of pulmonary artery by catheter as result of
Prolonged wedging of catheter
Overinflation of balloon
	■ Absence/resolution of pulmonary infarction
	  Adequate pulmonary artery blood flow as indicated by waveform and pressure reading
		■ Prevention
		  Inflate balloon for a few seconds only with 0.8 to 1.5 cc of air
		  Ensure that balloon is deflated after every wedging
		  Observe waveform frequently to detect damping (flattening) of waveform, which may indicate drift of catheter farther into artery
		  Ensure that catheter is secured at desired length and that physician sutures catheter well on skin
		  Limit frequency of wedging catheter to q2 hr if possible
		  Avoid flushing catheter vigorously while it is being wedged
		Monitor for
		  Chest pain with dyspnea, tachypnea, hemoptysis
		  Chest pain with hypertension/hypotension and tachycardia
		If problem is suspected, monitor for
		  Arterial blood gas results indicating hypoxemia (precipitous drop in Pao_2)
		  Chest pain with dyspnea, tachypnea, hemoptysis

POTENTIAL PROBLEMS	EXPECTED OUTCOMES	NURSING ACTIVITIES

		If catheter drifts in too far
		    Induce quick increase, then decrease in intrathoracic pressure by turning patient; have patient cough
		    If patient is intubated, manually inflate lungs vigorously a few times
		If pulmonary infarction occurs, administer supportive therapy as ordered, usually including humidified O_2

■ Pulmonary thromboembolism may be related to
Clot formation around the catheter
Patients with low cardiac output, hypercoagulability (e.g., with recent surgery) or other coagulation abnormalities are especially prone to this complication
	■ Normal breath sounds
	Chest radiograph clear
	Infusion fluid system working properly
		■ Prevention
		    Avoid arterial blood sampling unless necessary
		    Ensure functioning, constant, slow infusion flush system with
		        Tight connections
		        Proper tubing (high-pressure tubing) and stopcocks
		        Heparin is added to crystalloid solution, infused at 3 to 6 ml/hour, and regulated by (Sorenson) flush flow valve
		        System is pressurized—periodically check that pressure bag gauge is at 300 mm Hg
		    Anticoagulation therapy may be employed for patients at high risk for thrombus formation
		Monitor for
		    Damping of waveforms
		    Signs and symptoms of pulmonary thromboembolism, including severe substernal pain, dyspnea, tachypnea, diaphoresis, cyanosis, pallor, tachycardia, hypotension, hemoptysis, anxiety, diminished breath sounds, arrhythmias
		Notify physician for occurrence of aforementioned
		If thrombus formation at catheter tip is suspected, attempt should be made to withdraw blood and any clots through catheter

■ Monitoring problems: pulmonary wedge tracing not obtainable
Balloon rupture
Catheter not in proper position; may flip back into ventricle
	■ PCWP readings obtainable and accurately reflect patient's PCWP	■ Prevention
		    Inflate balloon with the prescribed amount of air or CO_2 to avoid rupture
		    Leave catheter in place 3 days or less; because balloon deterioration is unavoidable, balloon rupture is likely to occur after 3 days or close to 70 inflations
		    Catheter must be placed into distal pulmonary artery during initial insertions
		Monitor for
		    Absence of resistance encountered on balloon inflation and wedge pressure tracing
		    Result of chest radiograph as to position of catheter
		If signs of balloon rupture occur, leave stopcock closed to balloon and notify physician

Specific for intracranial catheter
■ Hematoma or hemorrhage related to ICP monitor insertion or maintenance
 	
Epidural hematoma
	■ Absence/resolution of hematoma/hemorrhage
	Decrease/resolution of increased ICP
	Maximal neurological functioning
		■ Establish neurological baseline and vital signs
		See Standard 32, *Increased intracranial pressure*, Problem, Progressive increased ICP, for specific activities
		Monitor ICP values and waveforms q15 min and prn
		Ongoing assessment of status-specific symptomatology ql hr and prn
		
		Monitor particularly for
		    Subtle changes in LOC
		    Frequent episodes of headaches, nausea and vomiting
		    Change in vital signs; note development of hypertension, bradycardia, altered respiratory rate and quality
		    Dilatating ipsilateral pupil that reacts sluggishly to light (from third cranial nerve dysfunction)—cardinal early sign of uncal herniation
		    Appearance/increase in contralateral hemiparesis

POTENTIAL PROBLEMS	EXPECTED OUTCOMES	NURSING ACTIVITIES
		Notify physician immediately of any change in status/vital signs; dilatating ipsilateral pupil warrants immediate surgical evacuation of clot
		Administer emergency medications and treatments as ordered
		Prepare patient for surgery as ordered
		For postoperative specifics see Standard 36, *Supratentorial craniotomy* or Standard 37, *Infratentorial craniotomy*
Subdural hematoma		Monitor particularly for
		Subtle alterations in LOC, personality, mental abilities
		Increase in restlessness, agitation, irritability
		Appearance of or increase in headache, nausea and vomiting
		Fluctuations in neurological status
		Maintain head of bed at specific degree ordered
		If ordered, assist physician with drainage of CSF to maintain ICP at specific level
		Notify physician immediately of any signs/symptoms of subdural hematoma
		See STANDARD 35 *Subdural hematoma*
Intracerebral hematoma		Monitor particularly for
		Changes in neurological status or vital signs
		Alterations of ICP values/waveforms from normal levels
		Correlation between ICP values and neurological status
		Effectiveness of therapy/medications, if ordered, for control of ICP levels
		Administer medications/treatments as ordered for elevated ICP and monitor effects on status and ICP; may include hyperventilation, osmodiuretics, narcotics, barbiturates
		If ordered, assist physician with drainage of amount of CSF sufficient to maintain ICP at predetermined level; record amount of fluid drained each time, effects on ICP value, correlation between neurological status and CSF drainage
		Notify physician immediately of any decline in neurological status or increase in ICP level above maximal limit specified

■ Brain trauma
  Blockage of ICP monitoring catheter
	■ Absence/resolution of brain trauma
	  Patent ICP monitoring catheter
		■ Employ care in intermittent flushing of ICP catheter (according to hospital protocol or as ordered; in some institutions only physicians perform this procedure)

		Monitor for
		Any abnormal secretions from insertion site
		Abnormal changes in LOC
		Notify physician if any abnormal changes occur
		If problem occurs, assist in removal of catheter/sensor/transducer

POTENTIAL PROBLEMS	EXPECTED OUTCOMES	NURSING ACTIVITIES

■ Fluid and electrolyte imbalance related to
Drainage of CSF/uncontrolled loss
Osmodiuretic administration
Increased ICP producing alterations in normal hormonal control mechanisms
	■ Fluid and electrolyte balance within normal or prescribed limits	■ Monitor for signs and symptoms of fluid and electrolyte imbalance
		Record hourly intake and output
		If CSF drainage is prescribed
		    Assist/drain specific amount ordered to maintain ICP at level specified by physician (in some institutions only physicians perform this procedure)
		    Monitor and record pre-drainage ICP level, time, CSF amount drained, and postdrainage ICP
		If continuous CSF drainage is employed
		    Monitor and record amount
		    Notify physician if CSF drainage is above usual or specified amount
		    Monitor serum electrolytes; Na+ values may decrease from loss of CSF by drainage
		    Notify physician of results and replace fluid as ordered (commonly, CSF drainage is replaced milliliter for milliliter)
		    Monitor serum and urine electrolyte/osmolality values
		    Notify physician of any fluid, electrolyte balance abnormality
		
		See STANDARD 32 *Increased intracranial pressure*

■ Abnormal intracranial pressure readings, which may be related to Loss of CSF Leakage of brain matter	■ Intracranial pressure readings are within normal limits Absence of CSF loss, leakage of brain matter, and brain trauma	■ Prevention Careful and meticulous insertion technique employed by physician Keep patient quiet and cooperative during procedures Secure catheter/sensor/transducer in place to prevent any inadvertent removal Lumen of catheter is filled with solution before insertion

CARDIAC CATHETERIZATION

Cardiac catheterization is a procedure involving insertion of a radiopaque catheter through an artery or vein into the heart using fluoroscopy. Vessels in the antecubital fossa, axilla, or inguinal region are generally used to gain intravascular access, although the umbilical vessels may be used in the neonate. Percutaneous puncture or cutdown may be performed to gain access to the artery or vein.

Pressure measurements are made and blood samples drawn via the catheter to provide information regarding hemodynamics and oxygen saturations within the heart and great vessels. Pressure measurements can demonstrate the presence of resistance to blood flow (such as that caused by valvular stenosis), and abnormal oxygen saturations confirm intracardiac or intrapulmonary shunting. Specific structures (cardiac chambers, valves, great vessels, coronary arteries) can be visualized through injection of a radiopaque contrast agent; rapid, sequential radiographs, called angiograms, record the flow of the agent through these structures. Left heart and aortic catheterization can be performed through insertion of the catheter retrograde through an artery. In children and some adults, left heart catheterization may also be accomplished by passage of the catheter from the right atrium to the left atrium through the probe-patent foramen ovale. Right heart catheterization is accomplished through insertion of the catheter through a vein and into the right atrium.

Usually catheterization with blood gas and pressure measurements is performed first. If anomalies are detected or if further visualization of structures is needed, the angiogram is then performed. Angiograms are especially useful in the diagnosis of congenital heart defects, coronary artery disease, postinfarction ventricular septal defect, valvular stenosis or insufficiency, and poor ventricular contractility.

Associated procedures may be accomplished during cardiac catheterization. His bundle mapping can be performed using an electrically sensitive catheter within the ventricles. Transvenous intracardiac pacing wires may also be inserted. Programmed electrical stimulation may be performed to assess the function of the intracardiac conduction system. (See Standard 22, *Ventricular tachycardia: treatment and clinical electrophysiology testing.*) Atrial septal defects may be created (through use of a balloon-tipped catheter) or closed (using an umbrella or plug-tipped catheter). Catheters may also be used to attempt to reduce the vessel narrowing caused by atheromas or plaques in the coronary arteries or the narrowing of surgically created shunt or repaired coarctation. (See Standard 13, *Transluminal coronary angioplasty.*) Patients may be exercised during the catheterization to monitor effects of exercise on cardiac output and coronary artery circulation. Nitrogen inhalation may also be performed; timing of nitrogen circulation can provide information regarding the presence or absence of intracardiac shunts. Medication may be administered during the catheterization to allow detailed monitoring of the patient's hemodynamic response to specific drugs.

Cardiac catheterization may be performed on an elective or an emergency basis. The patient generally receives a sedative before the procedure and local anesthetic during the catheterization.

With the increased sophistication of catheterization equipment, mortality following elective catheterization is less than 1%; risk following emergency catheterization of the sick patient, however, is somewhat higher. Risk is also increased for patients with pulmonary hypertension, arrhythmias, hypoxemia, or severe coronary arteriosclerosis and for children prone to hypercyanotic episodes (severe tetralogy of Fallot).

Morbidity is caused by intracardiac catheter manipulation (causing arrhythmias, cardiac perforation, or increased myocardial ischemia), infection, contrast agent reactions, and impaired distal perfusion of the catheterized extremity.

ASSESSMENT

1. Patient/family's comprehension of patient's cardiovascular health problem
2. Patient/family's comprehension of catheterization procedure
3. Patient/family's anxiety and concerns
4. History of cardiovascular symptoms (including unstable angina, recent MI, hypercyanotic episodes, or pulmonary hypertension)
5. Previous illness or hospitalizations and patient/family's response to them
6. Current health status

a. Current medications (especially cardiovascular medications and anticoagulants) and allergies

b. Current diseases of other body systems: renal, pulmonary, GI, neurological, musculoskeletal

7. Cardiovascular status

a. Systemic perfusion: warmth of extremities, peripheral pulses and BP, urine output, color, LOC, exercise tolerance, growth

b. Heart rate and rhythm and presence of any heart murmurs or thrills

c. Evidence of systemic venous engorgement: neck vein distention, periorbital edema, hepatomegaly, dependent edema (often not seen in children), or ascites

d. Evidence of pulmonary venous engorgement: tachypnea, increased respiratory effort, rales on auscultation (often not apparent in children until late in the clinical course), cyanosis

e. Presence and characteristics of angina or palpitations: precipitating or alleviating factors, severity, distribution

f. Presence or history of syncopal episodes, fatigue with minimal exercise

g. Cardiac isoenzyme levels (if appropriate)

h. If signs/symptoms of heart failure are present, see Standard 15, *Heart failure (low cardiac output)*

8. Fluid balance

a. Presence of edema or recent large weight gain

b. Level of hydration (mucous membranes, tearing in patients beyond 2 months, fontanelle in infants up to 18 months, skin turgor)

9. Nutritional status

a. Growth

b. Serum glucose level in infants

c. Potassium balance (particularly if patient is receiving diuretics)

10. Respiratory status

a. Evidence of pulmonary edema or pulmonary venous engorgement

b. Evidence of concurrent respiratory infection (especially in children)

c. Arterial blood gas results

11. Postcatheterization assessment

a. Cardiovascular status: heart rate and rhythm, BP and peripheral perfusion, urine output, presence of any angina, signs of pulmonary or systemic venous engorgement, LOC

b. Appearance of catheterization site: appearance of wound, presence of bleeding or hematoma, pain

c. Perfusion of catheterized extremity: warmth, color, peripheral pulses, edema, pain, sensation

d. Evidence of any infection

GOALS

1. Patient/family demonstrates comprehension of patient's condition and catheterization procedure
2. Stable cardiovascular status
3. Absence of untoward response to contrast medium
4. Adequate perfusion of catheterized extremity
5. Absence of infection
6. Patient/family demonstrates and comprehends patient's home health care routine (including wound care, medications, and health maintenance measures)
7. Appropriate fluid balance

POTENTIAL PROBLEMS	EXPECTED OUTCOMES	NURSING ACTIVITIES
■ Decrease in cardiac output related to underlying cardiac disease, hemorrhage, cardiac perforation, reaction to sedation or contrast medium, or MI (for arrhythmias, see Problem, Cardiac arrhythmia)	■ Stable cardiac output as measured by Adequate BP Good peripheral perfusion Regular cardiac rate and rhythm Minimal bleeding from catheterization site Good urine output (25 ml/hour for adults; 1 to 2 ml/kg/hour for children) Absence of systemic or pulmonary venous engorgement Absence of incapacitating angina	■ Note occurrence of any arrhythmias during catheterization procedure Monitor vital signs, LOC, and signs of peripheral perfusion frequently (q15 min initially, then q1-2 hr as appropriate) Heart rate ranges Newborn: 120 to 160/minute Toddler: 90 to 140/minute Preschooler: 80 to 110/minute School-age child: 75 to 100/minute Adolescent: 60 to 90/minute Adult: 50 to 95/minute BP ranges (systolic) Newborn: 50 to 70 mm Hg Toddler: 80 to 112 mm Hg Preschooler: 82 to 112 mm Hg School-age child: 84 to 120 mm Hg Adolescent: 94 to 140 mm Hg Adult: 105 to 145 mm Hg NOTE: Consider your patient's normal ranges when determining abnormalities If abnormalities are present, notify physician and be prepared to institute emergency measures as needed

POTENTIAL PROBLEMS	EXPECTED OUTCOMES	NURSING ACTIVITIES
		Notify physician of any arrhythmias (see problem, Cardiac arrhythmia)
		Monitor catheterization site and dressing for evidence of bleeding (dressing saturated with blood or developing hematoma); if bleeding is excessive and does not stop with application of pressure, notify physician immediately
		Obtain Hct as ordered
		Continue to apply pressure to site
		Closely monitor BP and peripheral perfusion
		Monitor for evidence of low cardiac output: cool, clammy extremities; decreased urine output; altered LOC; cyanosis, mottling, or pallor; evidence of pulmonary or systemic venous engorgement; decreasing BP; notify physician immediately if these occur
		Monitor for signs of cardiac tamponade: pallor, tachycardia, jugular venous distention, decreased BP or decreased pulse pressure, decreased heart sounds, restlessness, cool extremities, tachypnea; notify physician immediately if they occur and be prepared for emergency measures if necessary
		See STANDARD 18 *Pericarditis* STANDARD 21 *Arrhythmias* STANDARD 12 *Acute myocardial infarction* STANDARD 15 *Heart failure (low cardiac output)*
		Infants must be kept warm during and following cardiac catheterization, especially if they have low cardiac output; their O_2 consumption increases dramatically if they are subjected to heat or cold stress; small infants with little subcutaneous fat are especially prone to heat loss
		Notify physician of any complaints of angina or palpitations; check cardiac isoenzymes and ECG if angina occurs, and monitor BP
■ Cardiac arrhythmia related to preexisting cardiac ischemia, intracardiac catheter manipulation, intramyocardial contrast medium injection, or further compromise of coronary circulation with contrast medium injection	■ Appropriate cardiac rate and rhythm	■ Record patient's rhythm before cardiac catheterization and use this strip for later comparison
		Check apical and peripheral pulses frequently following catheterization procedure; if any irregularities or pulse discrepancies exist, notify physician and obtain BP and rhythm strip
		If arrhythmia exists, note its effect on systemic perfusion (note if BP drops with aberrant beat), any precipitating or alleviating factors, and response to medications
		Monitor LOC and be prepared to institute emergency measures as needed
		Assess heart rate—ascertain if it is adequate for good cardiac output; see normal ranges given before; notify physician if heart rate is excessive or insufficient
		If arrhythmia occurs, see Standard 21, *Arrhythmias*
■ Compromise of circulation to catheterized extremity	■ Perfusion of catheterized extremity remains good as measured by Warmth Pink color Good pulses Adequate movement and sensation (use opposite limb for comparison)	■ If *arterial* catheterization was performed Monitor pulses of extremity distal to catheterization site; notify physician *immediately* of any decrease in pulses (if spasm or thrombus occurs in artery, distal artery can rapidly become thrombosed and ischemia of extremity will result; this may ultimately require amputation of extremity if allowed to progress, so *prompt* attention must be given)
		Monitor color and warmth of extremity for reasons previously noted
		NOTE: When arterial circulation is compromised, extremity usually will become *pale* or *mottled*—rather than cyanotic—and cool; notify physician immediately if either occurs; heat to *contralateral* extremity may help maintain circulation to catheterized extremity (by producing reflex vasodilation), but heat should *never* be applied to *involved* extremity, because it merely increases O_2 consumption of already compromised tissue

POTENTIAL PROBLEMS	EXPECTED OUTCOMES	NURSING ACTIVITIES
		If thrombus is present, it may require surgical removal; heparin drip may be ordered to prevent further thrombus formation (monitor for bleeding if heparin is ordered) Attempt to prevent flexion of catheterized extremity at catheterization site for 6 hours or as ordered Maintain bed rest for 6 to 12 hours following catheterization (or as ordered) Administer pain medication as ordered (and needed); monitor patient's response and cardiac output Monitor for evidence of excessive edema or bleeding at catheterization site; notify physician if bleeding is not stopped by application of pressure Apply ice to catheterization site as needed If *venous* catheterization was performed Monitor pulses of extremity distal to catheterization site NOTE: When cutdown is performed, vein used for the catheterization is often tied off at end of procedure, especially in small infants; in this case, extremity distal to catheterization site would become edematous and slightly cyanotic as venous blood is trapped in extremity; collateral veins will quickly provide venous drainage, but initial discomfort should be expected If edema is present, elevate extremity to facilitate venous return; *notify physician immediately if edema causes decrease in pulses* (this would indicate compromise of arterial circulation) Monitor for evidence of bleeding at catheterization site and notify physician if it is not relieved by pressure Maintain bed rest for 4 to 6 hours following catheterization (as ordered)
■ Possible infection of Catheterization site Intracardiac structures	■ Patient will remain free of symptoms of infection Fever Leukocytosis Erythema or drainage from catheterization site Evidence of endocarditis or pericarditis	■ Monitor catheterization site for edema, erythema, heat, or discharge; notify physician if present Monitor patient's temperature; blood cultures are usually recommended if fever higher than 101.3° F (38.5° C) Monitor WBC count if infection is suspected Monitor for evidence of endocarditis (high fever, appearance of new heart murmur, hematuria) and pericarditis (cardiac friction rub, loss of heart tones, ECG changes); see Standard 18, *Pericarditis;* Standard 19, *Endocarditis*
■ Patient/family's anxiety related to patient's health status and anticipated catheterization	■ Patient/family demonstrates comprehension of preparation for procedure, catheterization itself, and postcatheterization care Patient/family's anxiety does not interfere with appropriate activity	■ Orient patient/family to nursing care unit, policies, personnel, catheterization lab (as appropriate) Orient patient/family to preparation for catheterization Chest radiograph Blood tests Appropriate medications (including withholding of anticoagulants before catheterization) Need for NPO before catheterization Premedication (include possible side effects such as dry mouth, blurred vision as appropriate) Instruct patient (as appropriate to age) and family regarding procedure itself (especially in those aspects that patient will see, hear, or feel), length of procedure, and appearance of catheterization site after procedure Discuss postcatheterization care with patient (if appropriate to age) and family Need for bed rest Postcatheterization feeding orders Required care of catheterization site (include need for immobility, ice packs, etc.) Frequency of vital sign measurements

POTENTIAL PROBLEMS	EXPECTED OUTCOMES	NURSING ACTIVITIES
		If patient is child over age of 2, toys or puppets may be used to demonstrate experiences the child will remember; in preparing any child for catheterization, nurse must be sensitive to child's cues and prepare child with only information he/she can handle; if child has little concept of time intervals, preparation just before injections and separation from parents may be most appropriate
		During and following catheterization procedure, provide support and simple explanations of catheterization results; orient patient to time and place frequently while patient is recovering from sedation
■ Possible compromise in renal function related to response to contrast medium (very concentrated contrast medium can cause oliguria, which should soon be followed by osmotic diuresis; hematuria and anuria may rarely occur)	■ Patient will demonstrate adequate urine output (25 ml/hour minimum for adults and 1 to 2 ml/kg/hour for children)	■ Monitor urine output; notify physician if urine output is inadequate *despite* sufficient fluid intake
		NOTE: Small child may become rapidly dehydrated when kept NPO for hours while awaiting catheterization; nurse must ensure that parenteral and/or oral fluid intake is adequate during period preceding and following catheterization
		If patient is anuric despite sufficient intake, fluid intake will then have to be restricted to prevent overload
		Monitor for evidence of dehydration (depressed fontanelle in infants, dry mucous membranes, decreased urine output with high specific gravity, poor skin turgor)
		Test urine for hematuria; notify physician if blood is present and monitor urine output closely
■ Possible respiratory depression related to sedation	■ Patient will demonstrate adequate respiratory function Appropriate rate Adequate and equal lung aeration bilaterally	■ Check precatheterization order against recommended dosage for patient's age and weight; notify physician if sedation order is excessive
		Monitor respiratory rate and effort and notify physician if either is insufficient or excessive
		Normal adult respiratory rate: 12 to 16 (note precatheterization range)
		Normal pediatric respiratory rate: 18 to 34 (note precatheterization range)
		Normal infant respiratory rate: 30 to 60 (note precatheterization range)
		Auscultate lungs and encourage patient to change position frequently, cough, and breathe deeply; rib-springing exercises (used only in children) or other forms of chest physiotherapy may be necessary if aeration is insufficient; notify physician immediately if respiratory effort is insufficient and begin emergency resuscitative measures if needed
■ Patient/family may have inadequate information to provide adequate home health care for patient	■ Patient/family possesses adequate information to comply with postcatheterization care regimen and general health maintenance	■ Provide patient/family with appropriate instruction regarding wound care, physician follow-up appointments, signs of infection, activity restrictions (if any), and medications
		Discuss implications of catheterization results with patient/family to obtain their perceptions of physician's recommendations and to clarify any misconceptions they may have
		Provide patient/family with appropriate telephone numbers and locations of health team members (primary nurse, cardiologist, cardiac surgeon, etc.)
		If patient is infant, discuss immunization schedule with parents; cardiologist will commonly request delay of immunizations (consult physician)

ADULT CARDIAC SURGERY

Cardiac surgery may be required for patients with congenital heart disease, coronary atherosclerosis, valvular dysfunction, great vessel abnormalities, or other degenerative or inflammatory cardiac disease.

Coronary artery bypass grafting (CABG) is a surgical technique used to shunt blood around stenotic portions of major coronary arteries. A segment of saphenous vein is usually used; the proximal end is anastomosed to the root of the aorta, and the distal end is sutured to a patent portion of coronary artery beyond the area of stenosis.

CABG is generally indicated when atherosclerotic plaques obstruct coronary artery blood flow to the point at which severe anginal symptoms occur and are unrelieved by conservative medical therapy. Placement of a bypass graft around the stenotic lesion provides additional blood flow to the myocardium fed by the artery, resulting in reduction of anginal symptoms.

The replacement or revision of heart valves is done for two major conditions: severe valvular stenosis and valvular insufficiency. In valvular stenosis the size of the valvular orifice is reduced, obstructing the forward flow of blood. In valvular insufficiency the valve cannot completely close, resulting in inappropriate regurgitation of blood.

In both valvular stenosis and valvular insufficiency cardiac output is reduced. Valvular repair or replacement can improve valvular function and dramatically improve cardiac output. Often the simple surgical division of two partially fused leaflets of the mitral valve (commissurotomy) can significantly improve valve function, but this may be only a temporary measure, because the valve will gradually restenose. Valve replacement with one of a variety of prosthetic devices may then be necessary.

Cardiac surgery is also performed for acquired defects such as ventricular aneurysms, which occur as a complication of transmural MI. A ventricular aneurysm consists of dead muscle that balloons outward during cardiac contraction rather than moving inward. This paradoxical movement of the nonviable myocardium can significantly reduce cardiac output. Resection of the dead muscle results in more effective contraction and improved cardiac output.

Cardiac surgery can be done to repair an acquired ventricular septal defect, which often occurs as a complication of an anteroseptal infarction. The septal defect permits shunting of blood from the left to the right ventricle, resulting in reduced cardiac output and pulmonary vascular congestion.

Placement of a pericardial patch or a synthetic graft over the interventricular opening restores normal intracardiac blood flows. Unfortunately, the entire septum is frequently ischemic, requiring placement of suture material into friable tissue. These sutures frequently tear postoperatively, permitting redevelopment of a septal defect.

Surgical outcome depends on preoperative cardiac function, the success of surgery, and postoperative problems that arise.

The postoperative cardiac patient is particularly prone to developing hemodynamic and fluid balance abnormalities. Continuous monitoring of the patient's volume status, serum electrolyte composition, and cardiac function is of great importance in assuring an uncomplicated course. Fluids, diuretics, vasopressors, vasodilators, and inotropic and antiarrhythmic medications are common modalities for correcting postoperative problems such as hypovolemia/hypervolemia, heart failure, angina, MI, and arrhythmias. Other conditions, such as pericardial tamponade, may require surgical intervention.

The postoperative cardiac patient remains on mechanical ventilation until it is clear that blood oxygenation and cardiac and volume status have stabilized. Pulmonary problems that must be dealt with relate to the continual production of secretions from the tracheobronchial tree. Turning the patient, chest physiotherapy, tracheal suctioning, and humidification of inspired air are all directed toward mobilizing copious secretions. After extubation, coughing and deep breathing are necessary elements in pulmonary care.

Postoperative renal problems usually arise as a result of hypoperfusion of the kidneys during or immediately after surgery. The extent of renal compromise is variable and most of the time reversible. Intravascular volume and electrolyte status must receive special attention during this period.

Psychological difficulties may be devastating in a patient who has just had cardiac surgery. Total dependency on life-support systems and the often radical change in the patient's role in his/her family often give rise to depression and a feeling of futility, which require frequent support and encouragement to counteract.

ASSESSMENT

1. History, presence, and nature of
   a. Previous hospitalization and procedures, particularly
      (1) Cardiac catheterization
      (2) Cardiac surgery
   b. Related cardiac problems
      (1) Congenital heart disease; note presence of previous palliative or corrective surgery
      (2) Valvular disease; rheumatic fever/heart disease
      (3) Coronary artery disease
      (4) Ventricular aneurysm
      (5) Septal defect
      (6) Risk factors for coronary heart disease
         (a) Hypertension
         (b) Glucose intolerance; diabetes
         (c) Hyperlipidemia
         (d) Cigarette smoking
         (e) Obesity, sedentary life-style, personality (type A), sex, age
      (7) Family history of any of the aforementioned risk factors
      (8) Past MI
      (9) Stroke, thrombophlebitis, pulmonary embolism
      (10) Angina, other signs of myocardial ischemia
      (11) Arrhythmias (palpitations)
   c. Other organ dysfunction that may be related to cardiac compromise, particularly
      (1) Pulmonary
      (2) Renal
      (3) Neurological
2. Level of cardiac function/cardiac output
   a. Activity tolerance—note level of activity restriction; presence of easy fatigability
   b. BP
   c. Pulse—note irregular rhythm, pulsus alternans, weak pulse
   d. Evaluate circulation, noting
      (1) Presence of pallor, duskiness, cyanosis
      (2) Temperature
      (3) Diaphoresis
      (4) Clubbing
   e. Heart sounds for murmurs, gallops
   f. ECG for hypertrophy, arrhythmias
   g. LOC, mentation for effects of inadequate cerebral perfusion
   h. Venous distention—sacral edema, dependent edema, distention of neck veins, ascites, hepatomegaly
   i. Signs/symptoms of cardiomegaly, pulmonary vascular congestion

   j. Presence of a syndrome such as Down or Marfan syndrome that is associated with certain types of congenital or acquired heart disease
3. Pulmonary status
   a. Rate, rhythm, quality of respirations; note presence of rales, rhonchi, wheezing, shortness of breath, tachypnea, dyspnea
   b. Inquire about presence of orthopnea
4. Weight
5. Results of lab and diagnostic tests, including
   a. ECG evidence of
      (1) Myocardial ischemia
      (2) Ventricular aneurysm
      (3) Hypertrophy
      (4) Arrhythmias
      (5) Effects of inotropic/antiarrhythmic medications
      (6) Congenital heart disease; axis and ventricular/atrial hypertrophy consistent with defect
   b. Chest radiograph for
      (1) Myocardial hypertrophy, cardiac dilatation
      (2) Pulmonary vascular congestion
      (3) Location and configuration of great vessels
   c. Myocardial catheterization for objective evidence of
      (1) Coronary artery or valvular disease
      (2) Myocardial hypertrophy; elevated intracardiac pressures
      (3) Ventricular aneurysm
      (4) Septal defect
      (5) Congenital cardiac defect
   d. Echocardiogram for evidence of
      (1) Valvular abnormalities
      (2) Hypertrophy of specific cardiac chambers
      (3) Contrast echo for intracardiac/great vessel shunts
   e. Radionuclide studies
   f. Cardiac enzymes (in adults)
   g. Electrolyte levels
6. Patient/family's level of anxiety regarding disease process, medical therapy employed, purpose of hospitalization, need for surgery, postoperative management, and general follow-up plan of care
7. Patient/family's alterations in roles, activities of daily living (ADL) associated with patient's disease process
8. Patient/family's knowledge regarding operative therapy
   a. What they have been told
   b. Their expectations
   c. Fears regarding surgery and the outcome
   d. Previous experiences with surgery
   e. Experience of other family members or friends with heart disease
9. Information and detail surgeon and/or cardiologist has provided patient/family about operative therapy, known pathology, and postoperative management

GOALS

1. a. Reduction in patient/family's anxiety with provision of information, explanations, and encouragement
   b. Patient/family demonstrates understanding of disease process, purpose of hospitalization, surgery planned, preoperative and postoperative management, and expected outcomes
2. a. Adequate cardiac output
   b. Hemodynamic stability
   c. Absence of hypotension, hemorrhage, heart failure/low cardiac output syndrome, and cardiac tamponade
   d. Absence of signs of hypervolemia, hypertension
   e. Absence of MI
   f. Absence of arrhythmias
3. a. Adequate perfusion to all vessels and end organs
   b. Absence or resolution of emboli
4. a. Respiratory sufficiency with adequate alveolar ventilation and oxygenation; arterial pH, PaO_2, $PaCO_2$ within normal limits
   b. Absence of signs and symptoms of hypoxia, pain and splinting, atelectasis
   c. Full lung expansion
   d. Absence of pneumothorax, hemothorax, or pleural effusion
   e. Absence of pulmonary edema, emboli
5. Acid-base status in balance
6. a. Absence of fluid imbalance
   b. Serum electrolyte levels within normal limits
7. Indices of renal function within normal limits
8. a. Infection free
   b. Absence or resolution of endocarditis
9. a. Absence or resolution of pericarditis
   b. Absence or resolution of postcardiotomy syndrome
10. a. Patient alert and oriented to time, place, and person according to growth and development level
    b. Patient returns to preoperative neurological status
11. Before discharge patient/family accurately describes
    a. Dietary management
    b. Plan for activity progression
    c. Medications
       (1) Identification of
       (2) Dosage/number and schedule
       (3) Potential adverse effects and precautions
    d. Care of and precautions for special devices such as the pacemaker
    e. Plan for follow-up care
12. Before discharge patient/family safely performs special procedures such as suture line care

POTENTIAL PROBLEMS	EXPECTED OUTCOMES	NURSING ACTIVITIES

Preoperative and postoperative periods

■ Patient/family's anxiety related to Disease process Hospitalization Medical therapy employed Impending major surgery and associated risks Diagnostic tests planned Altered family roles Separation from family members Loss of job	■ Reduction in patient/family's anxiety with provision of information, explanations, and encouragement Anxiety does not interfere with patient/family's functioning Patient/family demonstrates understanding of disease process, purpose of hospitalization and surgery planned, preoperative and postoperative management, and expected outcomes Patient/family actively participates in planning and implementing care	■ Ongoing assessment of level of anxiety Assess patient/family's understanding of disease process and need for surgery Describe nature of patient's cardiac problem and symptoms that patient is experiencing Provide opportunity for patient/family to discuss risks involved and the decision for open heart surgery Collaborate with physician on patient teaching to be done Explain relationship of disease process and rationale for various therapeutic interventions Explain anticipated procedures included in diagnostic process and plan of care, including what patient will experience Assist in preparing patient for diagnostic procedures Encourage patient/family's questions, verbalization of fears and anxieties Involve patient/family in planning for care Provide comfort measures for parents and/or other family members Provide opportunity to visit recovery room/critical care unit, if possible; patient/family should be acquainted with staff and visiting policies Describe preoperative experience according to patient's need to know and readiness to learn 　Preoperative 　　Chest physiotherapy 　　　Coughing and deep breathing 　　　Incentive spirometry 　　　Postural drainage 　　Shave 　　Have light dinner; then NPO after midnight

POTENTIAL PROBLEMS	EXPECTED OUTCOMES	NURSING ACTIVITIES
		Medication for sleep if needed
		Morning bath/shower
		Preoperative medications
		Hospital gown
		Care of valuables
		Ride to operating room
		Scrub suits, masks, and hats worn by operating room staff
		Anesthesia
		Postoperative
		Waking up in recovery room/critical care unit
		Describe general environment (size of unit, room, etc.)
		Nurse always nearby
		Dull, continuous noises
		Breathing tube temporarily in place to ease patient's work of breathing and load on heart; describe that speaking will not be possible while tube is in place but that other means of communication will be provided
		NPO until "breathing tube" removed
		Incision with bandage
		IV, arterial lines
		Chest tubes and bloody drainage expected
		ECG monitoring
		Medicine for discomfort, pain given as needed
		Policy on family visits
		As patient progresses
		Progression to intermediate care unit, if appropriate
		Tubes out
		Eating again
		Chest physiotherapy, deep breathing, and coughing
		Getting stronger, ambulation
		Describe responsibility of patient for achieving speedy recovery by taking active role in coughing and deep breathing to keep lungs clear, and so on
		Home again
Postoperative period		
■ Anxiety in postoperative period related to Pain Difficulty in communicating during intubation Disorientation to time and place Feelings of helplessness	■ Reduction in anxiety	■ Postoperatively, continue aforementioned measures as appropriate and, in addition Provide for pain relief, sedation if needed, as ordered Frequently orient patient to time and place Remind patient that operation is over Develop mode for patient communication during intubation period Encourage and provide opportunity for patient/family's participation in care

■ Hypovolemia related to
Inadequate fluid replacement
Use of deep hypothermia, which produces high peripheral resistance; with warming, peripheral vasodilatation occurs, which may result in inadequate circulating blood volume relative to vascular space
	■ Hemodynamic stability, adequate cardiac output
	BP, P, CVP, and PAP/PCWP within patient's normal limits
	Adequate peripheral perfusion
	  Warm, dry skin
	  Full peripheral pulses
	  Alert and oriented
	  Urine output at least 0.5 ml/kg/hour
		■ Prevent by
		Scrupulous monitoring of hemodynamic parameters (q5 min while patient is warming, then q15 min until stable, then q½-1 hr), including
		BP, P, PAP/PCWP, and CVP
		Peripheral perfusion—skin temperature, color, peripheral pulses
		Urine output (q1 hr)
		Chest tube drainage (q½-1 hr)
		Note above-normal amount of blood loss
		Notify physician for blood loss of more than 100 ml/hour in 2 or more consecutive hours or more than 150 ml in any 1 hour

POTENTIAL PROBLEMS	EXPECTED OUTCOMES	NURSING ACTIVITIES

	Chest drainage less than 100 ml/hour for first few postoperative hours in adults
	Absence of bloody urine or secretions, or above-normal amounts of wound drainage
	Hct above 30%
		Monitor for signs and symptoms of hypovolemia
		  Hypotension, tachycardia
		  Low CVP, PAP, and PCWP relative to patient's norm
		  Signs of peripheral hypoperfusion
		  Oliguria
		Notify physician of abnormalities
		If hypovolemia occurs
		  Administer fluids, blood, blood products as ordered, closely monitoring patient's response
		  If patient is hypovolemic in presence of very marginal heart function, administer inotropic and/or vasodilator medications with concurrent fluid administration as ordered
		  Keep patient in supine position until hemodynamic parameters are within patient's normal limits

■ Hemorrhage/low Hct related to
  Inadequate blood replacement
  Platelet destruction in cardiopulmonary bypass (CPB) machine
  Blood replacement with old blood—deficient in platelet and clotting factors
  Inadequate reversal of heparin
  Liver congestion and deficient production of clotting factors in patient with right-sided congestion (heart failure)
  A missed bleeding artery and/or diffuse intrathoracic ooze, especially if chest has been entered before
	■ Adequate cardiac output
	  Hemodynamic parameters within patient's normal range
	  Absence of inordinate blood loss, hemorrhage
	  Chest drainage less than 100 ml/hour for first few postoperative hours
	  Absence of bloody urine or secretions, or above-normal amounts of wound drainage
	  Hct above 30%
		■ Monitor coagulation profile
		  Note dosage of protamine given to reverse heparin effects after CPB; administer additional protamine if needed, as ordered
		  Administer fresh blood, fresh frozen plasma, appropriate clotting factors if ordered
		Monitor for signs and symptoms of hemorrhage
		  Brisk, large amounts of bright red drainage through chest tubes
		  Falling Hct (check q½-1 hr until stable)
		  Signs of hypovolemia (see Problem, Hypovolemia)
		Monitor for signs of coagulopathy, including
		  Blood oozing from incision site
		  Bloody secretions from endotracheal tube
		  Hematuria
		  Heme-positive NG aspirates and stool
		Notify physician for presence of these abnormalities
		Administer blood and blood products as ordered, closely monitoring patient's response

■ Cardiac tamponade related to
  Inordinate blood loss
  Malposition of chest tube
  Blood that cannot be readily drained by chest tubes (e.g., formation of clot around internal orifice of tube)
	■ Adequate cardiac output, peripheral perfusion
	  Absence of cardiac tamponade
		■ Prevent by milking (stripping) chest tubes frequently to ensure patency and prevent clot formation around internal orifice of tube
		Monitor for signs/symptoms of cardiac tamponade, including
		  Sudden, marked orthopnea
		  Hypotension
		  Narrowing pulse pressure
		  Weakening and/or absent peripheral pulse from decreased circulating blood volume
		  Tachycardia
		  Increased venous pressure, venous congestion, which may be manifested by
		    Jugular venous distention
		    Increased CVP
		    Patient complaints of dyspnea or fullness in chest
		  Pulsus paradoxus—decrease in pulse volume and systolic BP (greater than 10 mm Hg) during normal inspiration related to changes in left ventricular filling; produced by pericardial restriction and accentuated by inspiration (For technique to elicit this sign, see Standard 18, *Pericarditis*)
		  Distant heart sounds
		  Decreased size (voltage) of QRS complex and/or development of electrical alternans (every other complex varies between two configurations)

POTENTIAL PROBLEMS	EXPECTED OUTCOMES	NURSING ACTIVITIES

		Abrupt decrease in chest tube drainage (may occur if chest tubes are clotted)
		Signs of decreasing cerebral perfusion
		  Increasing restlessness, anxiety
		  Altered LOC
		Prepare patient for special tests used to determine presence and amount of pericardial fluid and monitor results if ordered
		  Chest radiograph—increased heart size
		  Echocardiography
		  Radioisotope angiography
		  Contrast studies
		If signs and symptoms of cardiac tamponade occur, notify physician immediately
		If chest tube losses abruptly decrease, milk tubes vigorously to remove clot
		Assist with pericardiocentesis if procedure is necessary
		Institute other remedial measures as ordered, including preparing patient for thoracotomy and return to operating room
		
		See STANDARD 18 *Pericarditis (includes cardiac tamponade)*

■ Myocardial failure, which may be associated with
Ventriculotomy
Cardiomyopathy (preexisting)
Intraoperative myocardial ischemia
Recent or perioperative infarction
Tachyarrhythmias, bradyarrhythmias
Hemopericardium with tamponade
Residual cardiac depressant effects of anesthesia
Metabolic abnormalities, including acid-base imbalance
Pulmonary embolus
	■ Adequate cardiac output	■ Reduce myocardial O_2 consumption by
		  Bed rest in early postoperative period
		  Providing for quiet, calm environment
		  Comfort measures
		  Administering pain medication
		  Administering medications that directly reduce myocardial O_2 requirements (e.g., beta blockers) if ordered
		  Administering therapy to reduce incidence of or resolve arrhythmias
		Monitor for signs/symptoms of heart failure, including
		  Hypotension, tachycardia
		  Elevated CVP and PCWP, venous congestion
		  Pulmonary vascular congestion, pulmonary edema
		  Rales
		  Tachypnea
		  Peripheral hypoperfusion
		  Lethargy, easy fatigability
		  ECG changes associated with myocardial ischemia and/or infarction
		Notify physician of significant abnormalities
		Administer therapy as ordered to achieve adequate cardiac output
		  Inotropic, vasopressor agents
		  Vasodilator agents
		  Diuretics
		  Intraaortic balloon pumping
		Monitor patient's response closely
		
		See STANDARD 15 *Heart failure (low cardiac output)*

■ Hypertension, which may be related to
Hypervolemia, fluid overload
Delayed action of catecholamines stored in capillaries during deep hypothermia
Continuing preoperative hypertension
	■ BP within patient's normal limits
	Normovolemia
	Blood volume within patient's normal limits
		■ Monitor hemodynamic parameters q5 min in early postoperative period (continuous monitoring via arterial, venous catheters whenever possible)
		Notify physician for presence of hypertension and administer therapy as ordered, including continuous IV infusion of antihypertensive agent
		Monitor for signs and symptoms of hypervolemia
		  Hypertension, tachycardia
		  Elevated CVP and PAP
		  Elevated urine output (if heart function is adequate)
		  Dramatic weight gain over preoperative weight (measure at least q24 hr)

POTENTIAL PROBLEMS	EXPECTED OUTCOMES	NURSING ACTIVITIES
		Notify physician for these abnormalities If hypertension occurs administer diuretic and/or vasodilator medication if needed, as ordered; institute fluid restriction if ordered

■ MI	■ Absence of signs and symptoms of myocardial ischemia or MI	■ Prevent by administering therapy as ordered to maintain adequate cardiac output/coronary artery blood flow and to maintain Hct at prescribed level (usually above 30%)
		Monitor for
		  ECG changes indicating myocardial ischemia/MI
		  Restlessness, anxiety associated with signs/symptoms of low cardiac output, severe anginal pain, dyspnea, shortness of breath, wheezing, cough, rales
		  Results of serum cardiac enzyme levels
		    Presence of CPK (MB band)
		    Elevated LDH (LHD_1 and LDH_2) isoenzyme levels
		If any of these abnormalities occur, notify physician
		If MI is suspected, see Standard 12, *Acute myocardial infarction*

■ Arrhythmias, which may be related to
Cellular metabolic abnormalities
Acid-base imbalance
Hypoxia
Intracellular shifts in K^+, Na^+, Ca^{++}
Circulating catecholamines and cardiotonic drugs
Dilatation of cardiac chambers
Surgical injury of conduction system
Preoperative or postoperative atrial fibrillation, often associated with pericarditis, heart failure, and myocardial hypertrophy
Sinus node injury, atrial ischemia, or infarction
Pulmonary emboli
	■ Absence or resolution of arrhythmias, with adequate cardiac output	■ Prevent by monitoring for and administering therapy to correct factors that predispose patient to arrhythmias, including
		Acid-base imbalance
		Hypoxia
		  Administer humidified O_2 if needed, as ordered
		  Monitor Hct and Hgb for adequate oxygen-carrying capacity
		  Administer blood if needed, as ordered
		Electrolyte imbalance
		Psychosocial stress
		Monitor
		  ECG continuously, with high- and low-rate alarms set at all times
		  Notify physician of any significant changes in rate and/or rhythm and of associated changes in cardiac output (BP, P, and/or peripheral perfusion)
		  NOTE: Patients with marginal heart function have limited cardiac reserve and are less able to maintain stroke volumes in presence of bradyarrhythmias or tachyarrhythmias; thus heart rate must be kept within patient's physiological range
		If arrhythmias occur
		Document arrhythmias with rhythm strip in chart; compare ECG with baseline serial lab (12 or 15 lead) ECGs in chart
		Administer therapy as ordered, which may include:
		  Antiarrhythmic agent
		  Correction of factors predisposing patient to arrhythmias
		Document therapy given and patient's response
		Make appropriate entries in nursing care plan
		Assist with insertion of pacemaker, if necessary, for patients with complete heart block and/or unstable rhythms with poor cardiac output; for patients who have pacing wires in place for standby use, keep pacemaker at bedside
		See Standard 23, *Pacemakers: temporary and permanent*

■ Respiratory insufficiency related to *hypoventilation* and *atelectasis*, resulting from
Discomfort, pain, and splinting, with difficulty deep breathing and coughing
Thoracotomy with direct trauma to chest wall
Interstitial edema
	■ Adequate oxygenation and ventilation, with arterial pH, PaO_2 and $PaCO_2$ levels within normal limits
	Absence of signs and symptoms of hypoxia, tachypnea, dyspnea, pain and splinting, and/or atelectasis
	Lungs clear by auscultation and chest radiograph
		■ Prevention
		Administer pain medication, particularly in first few postoperative days (administer sufficient medication to reduce pain, but not so much that respirations are depressed and shallow and cough effort is weak)
		Maintain patent airway by
		  Turning q1-2 hr
		  Chest physiotherapy q2 hr with turning
		  Auscultation of breath sounds q1 hr
		  Suctioning as needed

POTENTIAL PROBLEMS	EXPECTED OUTCOMES	NURSING ACTIVITIES

Decreased compliance associated with interstitial edema and fibrosis	Aeration equal and adequate bilaterally	After extubation, also
		  Incentive spirometry q½ hr
		  Deep breathing and coughing q1-2 hr and prn
		  Promote optimal chest expansion by positioning patient in semi-Fowler position
		  Maintain NG tube to prevent gastric distention with air and diaphragmatic elevation if needed, as ordered
		Use pillows for support, comfort (considering placement of chest tubes)

■ Respiratory insufficiency related to *ventilation/perfusion abnormality,* which may result from
  Postperfusion syndrome
  Atelectasis
  Microemboli
  Residual intracardiac shunting
Respiratory insufficiency related to *impaired gas diffusion* in lung, resulting from pulmonary edema
	■ Adequate oxygenation and ventilation, with PaO_2 and $PaCO_2$ within patient's normal limits	■ Monitor
		Respiratory status q1 hr and prn, including
		  Presence of spontaneous respirations
		  Respiratory rate—note presence of tachypnea
		  Quality of respirations—note presence of dyspnea, shallow breathing
		  Respiratory effort
		  Breath sounds—note presence of rales, rhonchi, wheezing
		  Color (note cyanosis cannot be detected if patient is anemic)
		Serial arterial blood gas levels q1-2 hr until stable and q15 min after any change in ventilator settings or O_2 concentration is made; note levels not within patient's normal limits and notify physician
		For signs and symptoms of hypoxia, including tachypnea, tachycardia, and restlessness and confusion
		Verify and document ventilator settings q1-2 hr
		Monitor chest radiograph results for presence of
		  Infiltrates indicating atelectasis
		  Diffuse haziness indicating pulmonary interstitial edema
		Monitor for increased pulmonary interstitial edema and alveolar water by noting presence of
		  Rales
		  Increased CVP, left atrial pressure, and/or PCWP
		  Hypoxemia
		  Increased respiratory rate
		Notify physician of these abnormalities
		If pulmonary interstitial edema occurs
		  Administer diuretics and CPAP or PEEP and increase O_2 concentration as ordered
		  Monitor patient for response to therapy; notify physician if there is no response or poor response
		  See Standard 1, *Pulmonary edema of cardiac origin;* Standard 7, *Positive end-expiratory pressure* as appropriate
		If intubation and mechanical ventilation are necessary, see Standard 6, *Mechanical ventilation*

■ Respiratory insufficiency related to *pneumothorax, hemothorax,* or *pleural effusion*	■ Fully expanded lungs	■ Monitor for decreased breath sounds, decrease in chest tube drainage, bubbles in chest bottle, and signs/symptoms of hypoxia; notify physician of these abnormalities
		Maintain patent chest drainage system
		  Chest tubes to water seal drainage and suction as per physician's order
		  Milk chest tubes q1 hr and prn while tubes are in place to facilitate drainage
		Monitor for evidence of pleural effusion or hemothorax
		  Localized chest discomfort, pain
		  Respiratory distress: shortness of breath, tachypnea, dyspnea
		  Distant, decreased, or absent breath sounds over affected area
		  Pleural friction rub
		  Asymmetrical chest movements
		  Tachycardia; hypotension may occur with large hemothorax

POTENTIAL PROBLEMS	EXPECTED OUTCOMES	NURSING ACTIVITIES
		Restlessness
		Elevated temperature
		Tension pneumothorax
		Monitor for evidence of tension pneumothorax
		If chest tube in place, air bubbles in drainage compartment/bottle
		Chest discomfort, pain
		Respiratory distress: tachypnea, dyspnea
		Distant, decreased breath sounds over affected area
		Pallor
		Restlessness
		Tachycardia, weak pulse
		If more severe
		Vertigo
		Tracheal deviation
		Asymmetrical chest movements
		Cyanosis
		Increased CVP
		Distended neck veins
		Be aware of chest radiograph results compatible with pneumothorax, hemothorax, or pleural effusion
		Notify physician of abnormalities in aforementioned signs and symptoms
		If problem occurs
		Have chest tube and drainage system available
		Prepare patient for and assist with chest tube insertion or needle aspiration of fluid/blood; if chest tube inserted, aseptically attach tube to drainage system
		Monitor for resolution of signs and symptoms
		When chest tubes are removed
		Assist physician in suturing insertion site closed to prevent air entry through site
		Apply air-occlusive dressing to site
		Assist with chest radiograph if ordered
		Auscultate chest for equality of aeration
		Notify physician of any changes
■ Respiratory insufficiency related to *thromboemboli*	■ Absence of pulmonary embolus and peripheral thromboembolus	■ Prevent by
		Providing for early, gradual ambulation as tolerated and as ordered
		Passive and active leg exercises
		Antithromboembolic stockings or Ace bandages
		Changing IV sites before they become inflamed and/or swollen (q48 hr)
		Monitor for
		Evidence of thrombus formation in deep leg veins
		Edema of extremity
		Painful swelling and tenderness in affected area
		Pain that is worse on dependency and, conversely, relieved by elevation
		Palpable, hard, cordlike vein ("cord")
		Evidence of pulmonary embolus
		Respiratory distress: tachypnea, dyspnea
		Chest discomfort, pain
		Restlessness
		Diaphoresis
		Arterial blood gas results indicating hypoxemia
		Cyanosis
		Notify physician immediately of aforementioned signs/symptoms of peripheral thromboembolus and pulmonary embolus
		If thromboemboli occur, see Standard 31, *Embolic phenomena*

POTENTIAL PROBLEMS	EXPECTED OUTCOMES	NURSING ACTIVITIES
▪ Acid-base imbalance, which may be related to Metabolic acidosis associated with poor perfusion, tissue hypoxia, increased lactic acid production during CPB (elevated levels are present in early postoperative period) Metabolic alkalosis associated with many transfusions (citrate metabolized to bicarbonate), use of certain diuretics	▪ Acid-base balance within normal limits Blood gas levels within patient's normal limits, including pH Pao_2 $Paco_2$ Base excess Total CO_2 Bicarbonate Other anions, cations that help to determine acid-base status within normal limits	▪ Prevent by Administering fluids and electrolytes to keep fluid balance and serum electrolyte levels within normal limits Administering therapy to support cardiac output to achieve adequate peripheral perfusion, thereby minimizing anaerobic metabolism and acidosis Monitor serial arterial blood gas results for pH, Pao_2, $Paco_2$, and bicarbonate levels Monitor lactic acid levels if appropriate Note results not within normal limits and notify physician If problem occurs Administer therapy as ordered to correct acid-base imbalance (e.g., bicarbonate, electrolytes) Administer therapy to correct etiological factors for acid-base imbalance present (e.g., alter diuretic therapy) Administer therapy as ordered to provide for adequate oxygenation
▪ Fluid imbalance	▪ Fluid output is approximately two thirds of fluid intake Weight gain per day is less than 0.5 to 1 kg Urine output is at least 0.5 ml/kg/hour Adequate cardiac output with hemodynamic parameters within patient's normal limits	▪ Prevent by Monitoring fluid intake and output q1 hr in the early postoperative period; particularly note the following IV intake Urine output for oliguria Chest tube drainage for hemorrhage NG tube drainage Monitor hemodynamic parameters continuously—correlate systemic arterial BP, PAP, PCWP, CVP, P, peripheral perfusion, urine output and daily weight and note clinical signs of dehydration to determine adequacy of hydration and cardiac output Notify physician of significant abnormalities If fluid imbalance occurs Administer fluids, institute fluid restriction, and/or administer diuretics as ordered Note patient's response to therapy employed, particularly in terms of fluid and hemodynamic parameters
▪ Electrolyte imbalance, which may include Hypokalemia associated with use of Diuretics CPB machine Deep hypothermia Diuretic phase of renal failure K^+ shifts with acidosis/alkalosis NOTE: Significant total body depletion may exist in the presence of a normal serum K^+ level Hyperkalemia associated with decreased renal function Hypocalcemia related to multiple blood transfusions	▪ Serum electrolyte levels within normal limits Absence of signs and symptoms of electrolyte imbalance	▪ Monitor lab reports for serum K^+, Na^+, Cl^-, and Ca^{++} levels Monitor for evidence of hyperkalemia Nausea, diarrhea Hypotension ECG changes Wide to absent P wave Depressed S-T segment Tall, peaked T wave Prolonged Q-T interval Irritability, restlessness Paresthesias, difficult speech Spastic to flaccid muscle tone Monitor for evidence of hypokalemia Weak, faint pulses ECG changes Elevated P wave Flattened or inverted T wave Prolonged Q-T interval Flabby to flaccid muscle tone; paralysis; absent reflexes Apathy, depression; lethargy Monitor for evidence of hypocalcemia Palpitations ECG changes: prolonged S-T segment Abdominal cramps; constipation Positive Chvostek and Trousseau signs

POTENTIAL PROBLEMS	EXPECTED OUTCOMES	NURSING ACTIVITIES
		Spastic muscle tone Numb, tingling sensation Seizures Malaise, weakness Notify physician of any of aforementioned and administer therapy as ordered, which may include 　Electrolyte replacement for hypokalemia, hypocalcemia* 　　K^+ should never be added to infusions that contain antiarrhythmic or cardiotonic agents, since increasing rate of these medications would result in patient receiving too much K^+, resulting in arrhythmias and possibly cardiac arrest 　　High concentrations of K^+ should be avoided 　Therapy to decrease K^+ levels in hyperkalemia 　　Peritoneal dialysis 　　Potassium-binding resins (e.g., sodium polystyrene sulfonate [Kayexalate]) 　　Insulin and glucose
■ Renal dysfunction, which may be related to Inadequate cardiac output and renal blood flow Renal capillary occlusion with microemboli	■ Indices of renal function within normal limits Urine output at least 0.5 ml/kg/hour After early postoperative period, specific gravity indicates renal ability to concentrate Serum and urine electrolyte and creatinine levels within normal limits BUN levels within normal limits Urine pH, glucose, ketone, and protein levels within normal limits	■ Prevent by administering therapy to maintain adequate cardiac output and renal blood flow, including blood products, fluids, and cardiotonic agents Monitor 　Indices of cardiac output; note signs of decreased cardiac output 　　Hypotension, tachycardia 　　Restlessness 　　Evidence of peripheral hypoperfusion, oliguria 　Fluid intake and output q1 hr, noting imbalances 　Lab reports serially for 　　BUN and urine and serum creatinine levels 　　Urine glucose, ketones, protein, electrolyte and pH levels 　For adequate cardiac output Notify physician for any of these abnormalities If renal dysfunction/failure occurs, see Standard 52, *Acute renal failure*
■ Emboli, which may result from Thromboemboli related to 　Imperfections in CPB machine gas exchange membrane, causing release of lipids, hemolysis of RBC 　Direct contact of RBC with O_2 　Increased incidence in patients with cyanotic heart disease, particularly in presence of high Hct Calcium from resected valve	■ Adequate tissue perfusion Absence or resolution of emboli formation Absence of emboli in microcirculation	■ Prevention 　Heparin while patient is on CPB machine 　Hemodilution while patient is on CPB machine 　Maintenance of adequate systemic blood flow and perfusion with fluids and blood products, and inotropic/vasodilator medications as ordered 　Prevent thromboemboli from occurring in lower extremities with 　　Antithromboembolic stockings 　　Passive or active ROM exercises 　　Early ambulation 　　Anticoagulation in patients with valve replacements as ordered 　　　Mechanical valves—generally long-term anticoagulation with warfarin compound 　　　Tissue valves—generally short-term anticoagulation with acetylsalicylic acid 　　　Anticoagulation is often continued longer if atrial fibrillation, mitral valve disease with enlarged atria, or certain other complicating factors are present; in these patients, a warfarin compound (e.g., Coumadin) may be drug of choice

*K^+ solutions should be clearly labeled to prevent accidental bolus administration.

POTENTIAL PROBLEMS	EXPECTED OUTCOMES	NURSING ACTIVITIES

Vegetations from resected valve
Fat from sternotomy
Air
Disintegration of ball in ball-cage prosthetic valve, releasing fragments into circulation
Disintegration of tissue valves (porcine and cadaver)
		In presence of abnormalities with which patient is at high risk for bleeding (e.g., GI bleeding, lupus erythematosus, conditions causing low platelet levels), no anticoagulation may be employed
		Monitor for evidence of pulmonary embolus
		  Restlessness
		  Respiratory distress, e.g., dyspnea, tachypnea, pleural or substernal pain
		  Arterial blood gas levels revealing hypoxemia, hypercapnia, or hypocapnia
		  Symptoms of hypoxia: tachypnea, air hunger, anxiety, tachycardia
		  Cardiovascular instability
		    Arrhythmias
		    Hypertension, hypotension
		    Signs/symptoms of reduced cardiac output
		  ECG changes reflecting right ventricular strain
		Notify physician if any of aforementioned occur and administer therapy as ordered
		
		See STANDARD 31 *Embolic phenomena*
		
		Monitor for evidence of a coronary embolus and MI
		  Severe, crushing precordial or substernal chest pain (unrelated to movement)
		  ECG changes
		    S-T segment elevation
		    T wave inversion
		    Q waves (later)
		  Arrhythmias
		  Hypotension, tachycardia
		  Diaphoresis
		  Cold, clammy skin
		  Restlessness, anxiety
		  Elevated cardiac enzyme levels
		Notify physician if any of aforementioned abnormalities occur and administer therapy as ordered; monitor patient response
		
		See STANDARD 12 *Acute myocardial infarction*
		
		Monitor for evidence of cerebral vascular embolus and infarct
		  Sudden dizziness
		  Altered LOC
		  Aphasia, dysphagia
		  Seizures
		  Unilateral weakness
		  Paralysis
		  Ptosis of eyelids, mouth
		Notify physician of any of aforementioned and administer therapy as ordered; monitor patient response
		
		See STANDARD 39 *Carotid endarterectomy*
		
		Monitor for other types of emboli, particularly mesenteric, renal, splenic, and others; see Standard 31, *Embolic phenomena,* for specific signs and symptoms
		If problem occurs
		  Administer heparin continuously or intermittently as ordered
		  Administer long-term warfarin if appropriate, as ordered (e.g., in patients with metal valve replacements)
		  Administer fibrinolytic/enzyme therapy if ordered
		
		See STANDARD 31 *Embolic phenomena*

POTENTIAL PROBLEMS	EXPECTED OUTCOMES	NURSING ACTIVITIES
■ Altered LOC related to Cerebral hypoxia and edema from decreased cardiac output and/or hypoxemia Cerebral microemboli (more common in children with cyanotic heart disease and high Hct) Metabolic alterations from renal and/or he- patic damage CNS depressant medica- tions Sleep deprivation, noise, sensory monotony of environment Anxiety and fear	■ Patient is alert and ori- ented and has normal neuromuscular function	■ Assess neurological status with vital signs, noting Pupillary response Spontaneous, purposeful movement of all extremities LOC; note restlessness, disorientation Response to commands Response to touch (to painful stimuli if appropriate) Spontaneous respiration Notify physician for abnormalities in these parameters If basic neurological examination is abnormal, perform further testing as appropriate Response to pain Reflexes Extremity Pupillary Corneal Visual and auditory function Note signs of cerebral embolus, including Unilateral weakness Dysarthria Aphasia Monitor for physiological abnormalities that predispose patient to altered LOC, including Infection Acid-base imbalance Hypoxia Cerebral emboli Medications Alcohol withdrawal Notify physician if these abnormalities occur Monitor for complications of cardiac surgery that predispose patient to abnormal psychological responses, including cardiac, respira- tory, and/or renal failure Notify physician of abnormalities, and administer corrective/sup- portive therapy as ordered Administer therapy to minimize incidence of predisposing factors for altered LOC Administer therapy to augment cardiac output and cerebral blood flow if needed, as ordered (e.g., inotropic agents) Administer therapy to alleviate cerebral edema (e.g., restriction of Na^+ and fluid intake, administration of steroids and/or osmotic diuretics, as ordered) Correct metabolic abnormalities Avoid or reduce dosage of drugs that produce CNS depression Provide for rest periods and as much sleep as possible Provide for meaningful sensory stimuli; reduce meaningless stimuli Provide for psychological support and appropriate encouragement (see Problem, Patient/family's anxiety) Establish trusting confident relationship between physician, nurse, and patient Spend time with, reassure, and comfort patient Explain procedures and what patient will experience in simple terms Provide for and encourage increasing amounts of patient decision making and control in his/her care Monitor for more pronounced abnormalities such as visual and au- ditory hallucinations, paranoid delusions; notify physician if these occur Limit or reduce extraneous, monotonous noise in patient's environ- ment as much as possible Provide for objects in environment that assist in reorientation of patient to surroundings; clock should be within patient's vision

POTENTIAL PROBLEMS	EXPECTED OUTCOMES	NURSING ACTIVITIES
		Administer medication to patient for pain regularly in early postoperative period; administer sedatives if needed, as ordered (NOTE: Metabolism of narcotics may be decreased in presence of chronic liver engorgement; reduced dosages may be necessary)
		Build supportive relationship with family; mobilize their resources to encourage and assist patient during the recovery period
■ Infection related to Sternotomy IV cutdown sites Prosthetic materials CPB Decreased lung compliance with atelectasis Mechanical ventilation Urinary tract infection related to urethral catheter Certain types of prosthetic valves Damage to protein antibodies Early postoperative decrease in number and phagocytic activity of WBC	■ Infection free Afebrile	■ Prevent by Being aware of length of time IV or arterial lines have been in place; remind physician if line has been in place longer than recommended time interval IV lines—2 days (48 hours); *maximum* 3 days Arterial lines—4 days Central, Swan-Ganz catheters—3 to 4 days Observing site daily for signs of inflammation; notify physician, and assist with line removal (earlier than maximal recommended time) if this occurs Maintaining appropriate aseptic technique when administering IV fluids, changing IV bottles, giving medications, etc. Administering antibiotics as ordered Applying povidone-iodine (Betadine) solution to sternotomy and chest tube site daily after dressing is removed, as ordered Maintaining aseptic technique in handling urethral catheter; should be removed as soon as possible Administering respiratory care as in Problem, Respiratory insufficiency, to decrease potential for atelectasis, pneumonia Monitor Vital signs q½-2 hr until stable, with special attention to unusual fever spikes or hypothermia (in infants); notify physician for temperature over 101° F or less than 97° F (over 38.4° C or less than 36.2° C) For signs of sepsis: fever, chills, diaphoresis, altered LOC For signs of localized wound infection; check sternotomy, chest tube sites, and all IV sites for redness, warmth, pain, edema, and drainage For pulmonary infection, especially changes in character of sputum (note amount, color, consistency), fever, atelectasis For signs of urinary tract infection: cloudy urine, dysuria, flank pain, persistent hematuria, foul smelling urine Notify physician of aforementioned abnormalities and alter therapy as ordered If problem occurs Administer antipyretics as ordered for elevated temperature (as fever increases, so does cardiac work); if patient is hypothermic warm him/her using warm blankets Administer antibiotics as ordered Administer specific therapies as ordered to hasten resolution of infection, according to site/organ system involved
■ Endocarditis, which may be related to secondary infection associated with multiple invasive lines, particularly in early postoperative period	■ Absence or resolution of endocarditis	■ Prevent by Removing lines, catheters as soon as possible Administering prophylactic antibiotics as ordered in perioperative period Monitor for ECG abnormalities, including S-T segment elevation or depression Fever, diaphoresis Petechiae on skin, mucous membranes Splinter hemorrhages under nails Anorexia, weight loss Malaise, arthralgias

POTENTIAL PROBLEMS	EXPECTED OUTCOMES	NURSING ACTIVITIES

		Monitor laboratory results for
		  Positive blood cultures
		  Anemia
		If severe endocarditis is suspected or occurs, monitor for signs of
		  Valvular dysfunction
		  Low cardiac output
		If endocarditis occurs, see Standard 19, *Endocarditis*

■ Pericarditis, which is related to direct surgical manipulation, trauma	■ Absence or resolution of postoperative pericarditis	■ Monitor for
		  ECG changes including S-T segment elevation and T wave abnormalities
		  Pericardial friction rub
		  Persistent chest discomfort, pain
		  Persistent fever
		If pericarditis occurs, see Standard 18, *Pericarditis*

■ Postcardiotomy syndrome, which may be related to Hypersensitivity, immune response to pericardial injury
Signs and symptoms usually begin about 7 days postoperatively, although syndrome may begin as early as 3 days postoperatively and as late as many months postoperatively
	■ Absence or resolution of postcardiotomy syndrome	■ Monitor for
		  Signs and symptoms of pericarditis, which may include ECG changes such as T wave abnormalities and/or S-T segment elevation (see Standard 18, *Pericarditis*)
		  Pericardial friction rub
		  Persistence of chest discomfort, pain
		  Persistent fever or recurrent fever continuing after first few postoperative days
		  General malaise
		  Arthralgia, joint pains
		  Pleurisy, pleural effusion, hemoptysis
		  Leukocytosis
		  Increased ESR
		Notify physician for any of these signs and symptoms
		If postcardiotomy syndrome occurs
		  Administer antipyretics and analgesics as ordered, usually aspirin
		  Administer steroids if ordered

■ Insufficient information for compliance with discharge regimen*	■ Patient/family has sufficient information to comply with discharge regimen
	Before discharge, patient/family
	  Verbalizes dietary management
	  Describes activity progression; identifies activities to avoid in first few weeks at home
	  Accurately performs specific procedures; describes precautions regarding special devices such as pacemaker
	  Accurately identifies medications and pertinent information
		■ Assess patient/family's understanding of disease process, follow-up plan of care, and discharge regimen
		Consult with physician regarding rehabilitation plan
		Discuss modification of risk factors present
		  Atherosclerosis
		  Hyperlipidemia
		  Glucose intolerance, diabetes
		  Hypertension
		  Type A personality (method of relaxation)
		  Amelioration of job, home stress
		  Smoking
		  Obesity
		Discuss ways to prevent thromboemboli
		Instruct patient/family in (as ordered, when appropriate)
		  Diet
		    Type of food to consume; foods to avoid (e.g., those high in cholesterol, saturated fat, sodium)
		    Sodium/salt restriction
		    Calorie restriction
		    After instruction, permit and encourage patient to do his/her own meal planning, selecting proper foods from hospital menu, if possible
		  Fluid intake (restriction if appropriate)
		    Monitor for swelling of lower legs, with limitation of fluid intake if this occurs; notify physician if inordinate swelling occurs

*If responsibility of critical care unit nurse includes follow-up care.

POTENTIAL PROBLEMS	EXPECTED OUTCOMES	NURSING ACTIVITIES
		Daily weight; notification of physician if weight gain is more than 4 to 5 pounds in 1 week or if marked ankle swelling is present
		Avoidance of excessive eating and drinking of alcoholic beverages
		Medications
		Name of drug and purpose
		Indications for use if drug is to be taken prn
		Identification of
		Dosage/number of pills and schedules
		Potential adverse side effects and how to minimize
		Avoidance of over-the-counter medications that can change activity of medications prescribed
		Other precautions for each medication
		Assist patient in keeping chart on which medications taken can be recorded
		If chest pain (anginal pain) does not respond to antianginal medication, physician should be notified
		Avoidance of situations at home or work that elicit tense or angry feelings or marked fatigue
		Activity levels; patient should
		Consult physician before resuming more vigorous activities such as driving a car, lifting stuck windows, vacuuming
		Get plenty of rest, with 8 hours or so of sleep at night and spaced activities during day, with rest periods in between
		Exercise on regular, moderate basis
		Avoid prolonged periods of activity in very hot or cold temperatures
		Avoid undue straining with bowel movements; if this occurs, patient may be instructed to add fiber and certain fruits to his/her diet; if straining is pronounced, physician should be notified; stool softener and/or increase in fluid intake may be ordered
		Encourage patient that chest movements associated with coughing, housework, driving a car may cause some discomfort for several weeks; in first few weeks at home, mild analgesic may be ordered (to be taken as needed)
		Special care activities, followed by return demonstration
		Suture line care
		Precautions with pacemaker if in situ (see Standard 23, *Pacemakers: temporary and permanent*)
		Other activities
	Indicates understanding of untoward signs and symptoms, including those which require medical attention	Describe indications for notification of physician (e.g., chest pain, fever, malaise, and other difficulties); include phone number and person to call in emergency
	Accurately describes plan for follow-up care, including procedure for clinic visits	Describe plan for follow-up with cardiologist and, if needed, visiting nurse, physiotherapist and/or occupational therapist, as ordered
		Provide opportunity for patient/family to ask questions and verbalize anxieties, fears regarding discharge regimen
		Assess patient/family's potential compliance with discharge regimen
		Provide information about and assistance in obtaining referral services for available community resources as appropriate

PEDIATRIC CARDIAC SURGERY

Children most commonly require cardiovascular surgery because of congenital heart defects. Since the child may be emotionally and physically immature, the critical care nurse should modify assessment techniques and interventions to suit the psychosocial and physical levels of maturity of the child. Throughout the child's hospitalization, it is important to treat the child and family as a unit, because the response of the family will usually influence the child's responses to situations and therapy. Preparation of the child for procedures or surgery should be planned only after careful assessment of the child's cognitive and psychosocial developmental levels and the child's concepts of time intervals. Use of therapeutic play or art can be extremely valuable in assessing the level and source of the child's anxiety and in providing a mechanism for reducing anxiety. The surgery and postoperative critical care experience can be terrifying for the child and family; as a result, the support and care provided by the nurse will play a vital role in the child's recovery.

The most common preoperative problems occurring as a result of congenital heart disease are CHF and hypoxemia.

When CHF is a problem in children, the following symptoms may be noted:

Tachycardia

Tachypnea

Increased respiratory effort (retractions, jaw tugging, head bobbing, grunting)

Diaphoresis

Decreased urine volume

Peripheral vasoconstriction

Poor feeding, slow weight gain

Decreased exercise tolerance

Rales, ascites, and dependent edema may be only very *late* signs of CHF in children. If rales are present, a concurrent respiratory infection should be suspected. Rales will be evident, however, if severe left heart obstruction (mitral or aortic stenosis) exists.

The child who has *cyanotic heart disease* with resultant hypoxemia and compensatory polycythemia has possible systemic complications. He/she is at increased risk for thromboembolus formation, particularly when the Hct level is above 60%. Dehydration can cause hemoconcentration and increased blood viscosity, so care should be taken to prevent dehydration in these children. No air should be allowed in the IV line, because it could be shunted right to left and into arterial circulation, causing a cerebral embolus. These children are also at increased risk for the development of brain abscesses (especially beyond the age of 2 years). Their platelets are often decreased in number and/or function, so these patients are prone to bleeding postoperatively.

Surgical palliation of a congenital heart defect may be performed to *reduce* the volume and pressure of pulmonary blood flow by placement of a pulmonary artery band when the child has complex heart disease and increased pulmonary blood flow. Palliative surgery may also be performed to *increase* the amount of pulmonary blood flow by creation of a systemic to pulmonary artery shunt when the child has cyanotic heart disease. When palliative surgery is performed, the nurse must monitor for postoperative complications of the palliative procedure as well as for continued problems caused by the child's underlying defect.

When corrective surgery is performed, an atrial or ventricular septal defect may be closed, a conduit or valve may be inserted, or areas of stenosis may be resected or enlarged. Since these procedures may result in alteration of ventricular preload, contractility, and afterload, it is necessary to monitor for postoperative signs of low cardiac output and CHF. If sutures are placed near the intracardiac conduction system or if cardiac exposure requires a ventriculotomy, the nurse should expecially monitor for evidence of postoperative arrhythmias. The nurse who cares for any patient after cardiovascular surgery should monitor for evidence of hemorrhage and complications such as hypovolemia, hemothorax, and tamponade. Because the child's circulating blood volume is quantitatively smaller than an adult's, it is imperative that significant blood loss be replaced and sources of bleeding promptly identified and remedied.

If the child's spontaneous respiratory effort is inadequate after the surgery or if the child required lengthy and complex surgery, mechanical ventilatory support will be required postoperatively. If the child has pulmonary hypertension with an elevation in pulmonary vascular resistance preoperatively, metabolic acidosis, hypothermia, and alveolar hypoxia must be avoided, because these will enhance pulmonary vasoconstriction and may result in a fall in cardiac output. In these children, weaning from mechanical ventilatory support and oxygen therapy must be performed slowly. Following any cardiovascular surgery, the nurse should perform frequent assessment for evidence of atelectasis, pneumothorax, hemothorax, and pleural effusion. Throughout the child's postoperative care, the nurse is responsible for maintaining adequate ventilatory support (if needed), ensuring acceptable pulmonary function, and providing vigorous chest physiotherapy and pulmonary toilet.

Fluid and electrolyte imbalances commonly develop after cardiovascular surgery and use of CPB. The electrolyte imbalances most commonly seen in children after cardiovascular surgery include metabolic acidosis, hyperglycemia, hypocalcemia, hypokalemia, and hyperkalemia. These imbalances should be promptly detected and treated, because they can depress cardiovascular function. Renal failure can also complicate the child's postoperative course, though it is unusual unless the child develops poor systemic perfusion.

Neurological complications can occur throughout the postoperative course. They are more likely to occur during the immediate postoperative period if the child had preoperative cyanotic heart disease with significant polycythemia (Hct greater than 60%) and a microcytic anemia. Seizures or hypoxic encephalopathy can result from postoperative acidosis, hypotension, hypoxemia, and electrolyte imbalance.

Because postoperative care requires the use of multiple invasive monitoring lines and other invasive equipment, the child is at risk for the development of infection. If the child's surgical repair requires insertion of prosthetic material (e.g., valves, arterial patches), the development of infection and bacteremia can quickly progress to endocarditis, because bacteria will adhere to areas of turbulent intracardiac or intraarterial blood flow. The nurse is responsible for maintenance of clean IV access sites and incisions, and must often monitor the hand-washing techniques of other members of the health care team to ensure hand washing before and after every patient contact.

When the child's condition stabilizes, the child, family, and health care team can begin to focus on planning for the child's return home, and discharge teaching can begin. Any teaching provided should be carefully documented in the child's nursing care plan so that the information can be consistently reinforced. The critical care nurse should help to ensure that the child's transitions from the critical care unit to the pediatric floor and from the hospital to home are smooth ones.

Because there are many common forms of congenital heart defects that require surgical intervention, Table 28-1 provides a brief summary of several types of congenital defects, their hemodynamic consequences, surgical repair, and postoperative complications. For additional information about postoperative complications and nursing interventions, please refer to the more detailed nursing care plan that follows. Text continued on p. 231.

TABLE 28-1. Congenital heart defects

LESION	PREOPERATIVE PROBLEMS	SURGICAL REPAIR	POSTOPERATIVE PROBLEMS
Patent ductus arteriosus (PDA)	Increased pulmonary blood flow (from aorta into pulmonary artery) CHF may be a problem in infants, particularly premature infants Older children may be asymptomatic with murmur and waterhammer pulses PDA may be *lifesaving* in infants with cyanotic heart disease and compromised pulmonary blood flow	Ligation and/or division of ductus may be performed using a left thoracotomy incision (closed heart procedure) Indomethacin (a prostaglandin inhibitor) may be administered to neonates to promote ductus closure without surgery Prostaglandin E₁ may be administered to *maintain* ductal potency in infant who is dependent on ductus	CHF may be present (if it was present preoperatively) Other complications are those associated with thoracotomy incision (possible chylothorax, phrenic nerve paralysis, bleeding, etc.)
Atrial septal defect (ASD)	Usually children are asymptomatic, although CHF may occur if right ventricular dysfunction or small left ventricle is present Left to right shunt will cause increased pulmonary blood flow under low pressure	Stitch or patch closure of ASD using CPB (open heart surgery) Experimental closure of ASDs has been performed during cardiac catheterization	Conduction disturbances (especially heart block) Complications of CPB (postcardiotomy syndrome, bleeding, tamponade, etc.)

Modified from Hazinski, M.F.: Nursing care of the critically ill child, St. Louis, 1984, The C.V. Mosby Co.

TABLE 28-1. Congenital heart defects—cont'd

LESION	PREOPERATIVE PROBLEMS	SURGICAL REPAIR	POSTOPERATIVE PROBLEMS
	Atrial arrhythmias, CHF, and pulmonary hypertension may occur in middle adulthood		CHF is a rare complication but is more likely if it was present preoperatively or if pulmonary hypertension or small left ventricle is present
Ventricular septal defect (VSD)	If VSD is small, child may be asymptomatic and defect may close spontaneously If VSD is large, increased pulmonary blood flow under high pressure and CHF will result once pulmonary vascular resistance has fallen (at approximately 4 to 9 weeks of age); CHF may be present earlier if additional defect (such as PDA) is present Pulmonary hypertension may result from large shunt	Pulmonary artery banding may be performed as palliative procedure (closed heart procedure) to reduce volume and pressure of pulmonary blood flow and alleviate CHF; later debanding and closure of VSD are required Open heart patch or suture closure of VSD is definitive open heart repair Atrial or ventricular cardiac incision may be used for definitive repair	CHF is more likely if it was present preoperatively, if ventriculotomy cardiac incision was used for repair, or if pulmonary hypertension is present Conduction disturbances, especially heart block, may occur; right bundle branch block will result if right ventriculotomy incision was used Respiratory insufficiency may be present, particularly if CHF or pulmonary hypertension was present preoperatively
Endocardial cushion defect (partial or complete AV canal may be present), consisting of 1. Primum ASD (low in atrial septum) 2. Cleft in anterior leaflet of mitral valve 3. Possible common AV valve 4. Possible membranous ventricular septal defect 5. Left ventricle to right atrial shunt may be present in addition to ASD and VSD shunting	If simple primum ASD and small mitral valve cleft are present, child may be asymptomatic With larger left to right shunt and mitral insufficiency (from cleft in mitral valve), greater increase in pulmonary blood flow and CHF may result With large VSD component, CHF can be severe Right bundle branch block and left axis deviation are common ECG findings Children with AV canal are generally small for age with frequent upper respiratory infections This defect is most common cardiac defect associated with children with Down's syndrome	Pulmonary artery banding may be performed as palliative procedure if large VSD has caused CHF; banding will *not* be performed if left ventricle to right atrial shunt or severe mitral insufficiency is present Definitive repair requires division of common AV valve (if present), patch closure of ASD and VSD (if present), and repair of mitral insufficiency (using suture closure of valve cleft), using CPB (and possible hypothermia and circulatory arrest in infants, if necessary)	CHF is common complication NOTE: With closure of ASD, severe residual mitral regurgitation can cause pulmonary edema and left ventricular failure Heart block may occur, since conduction system (including AV node and His bundle) is located along margin of defect Respiratory insufficiency may complicate CHF and pulmonary edema Preoperative pulmonary hypertension will make postoperative right ventricular failure and respiratory insufficiency more likely
Pulmonary valvular stenosis or atresia without VSD	With pulmonary valvular atresia, there is no continuity between right ventricle and pulmonary artery, so blood must pass into left heart (via a patent, or "stretched," foramen ovale) and then back into the pulmonary artery via the ductus arteriosus; signs of systemic venous engorgement may be present; severe cyanosis and sudden deterioration may occur if ductus closes Right ventricle may be rudimentary	Prostaglandin E₁ is usually administered to maintain patency of ductus arteriosus until diagnostic studies and surgery can be performed in the neonate Emergency pulmonary valvulotomy in neonatal period is called *Brock procedure;* no bypass is used, and curved blade is inserted in right ventricle (surrounded by pursestring sutures) to cut open atretic pulmonary valve	CHF may develop If child has cyanosis and compensatory polycythemia preoperatively, bleeding and embolus formation may develop postoperatively Respiratory insufficiency may occur if severe cyanosis is present preoperatively (pulmonary microthrombi may occur, and pulmonary vessels will react to increased flow) or if CHF is present postoperatively

Continued.

TABLE 28-1. Congenital heart defects—cont'd

LESION	PREOPERATIVE PROBLEMS	SURGICAL REPAIR	POSTOPERATIVE PROBLEMS
	With pulmonary stenosis, pulmonary blood flow may be normal or decreased	Hypothermia and circulatory arrest may be used to perform emergency valvulotomy under direct visualization Open heart surgery allows pulmonary valvulotomy with direct visualization NOTE: If pulmonary atresia is present and neonate is rapidly decompensating as ductus is closing, prostaglandin E_1 may be administered by continuous IV infusion to keep ductus open until neonate can be brought to surgery	
Tetralogy of Fallot consists of four associated defects: 1. VSD 2. Pulmonary infundibular stenosis 3. Overriding aorta (overrides VSD) 4. Right ventricular hypertrophy	Severity of cyanosis (and decrease in pulmonary blood flow) is related to severity of infundibular pulmonic stenosis Generally infants are mildly cyanotic at birth and become progressively more cyanotic during first months of life as ductus closes and infundibular stenosis becomes relatively more severe Spasm of infundibulum and resultant severe decrease in pulmonary blood flow can cause severe cyanosis, hypoxia, and loss of consciousness; placing child in knee-chest position may promote increased pulmonary blood flow and alleviate spell (morphine sulfate or propranolol may also be given) Compensatory polycythemia and right to left intracardiac shunting (allowing some venous blood to bypass filtration of pulmonary macrophages) makes these children more prone to thromboembolus formation and brain abscess These children may instinctively squat during play to increase pulmonary blood flow Clubbing of fingertips and toes will occur with severe cyanosis	Waterston shunt (ascending aorta to pulmonary artery shunt, as side to side anastomosis) or Blalock-Taussig shunt (subclavian artery to pulmonary artery shunt, as end to side anastomosis) may be created as palliative (closed heart) surgery to increase pulmonary blood flow; Gortex shunt may also be inserted between subclavian artery and pulmonary artery Definitive (open heart) repair involves patch closure of VSD, resection of infundibular stenosis, and widening of pulmonary outflow tract (gusset or conduit may be required to produce a large enough pulmonary outflow tract); right atrial or ventriculotomy incision is used for repair NOTE: If neonate's condition is rapidly deteriorating as ductus closes, continuous IV infusion of prostaglandin E_1 may be given to keep ductus open until neonate can be brought to surgery	CHF will occur postoperatively NOTE: If CHF is *severe* following surgery, residual VSD should be suspected Arrhythmias, especially heart block, may be present Respiratory insufficiency may be present NOTE: Pulmonary vasoconstriction from alveolar hypoxia can produce increased right ventricular afterload (and increased right ventricular failure); pulmonary microthrombi can cause ventilation/perfusion abnormalities; CHF will increase work of breathing; thus respiratory support must be skilled Bleeding is more likely postoperatively as a result of preoperative cyanosis and compensatory polycythemia (these cause platelets to be decreased in number and function) Increased risk of postoperative thromboembolism is present

TABLE 28-1. Congenital heart defects—cont'd

LESION	PREOPERATIVE PROBLEMS	SURGICAL REPAIR	POSTOPERATIVE PROBLEMS
Truncus arteriosus (types I, II, and III) A single great vessel (the aorta) gives rise to systemic pulmonary and coronary circulations; the single great vessel straddles a large VSD, so it receives blood from both ventricles	Most infants are cyanotic as the result of mixing of systemic and pulmonary venous blood in trunk and as the result of decreased pulmonary blood flow (caused by pulmonary stenosis); if pulmonary blood flow is severely reduced, neonate may become profoundly hypoxemic when ductus begins to close In some infants, CHF and pulmonary hypertension can result from increased pulmonary blood flow under high pressure	Prostaglandin E₁ may be administered during neonatal period if cyanosis and profound hypoxemia develop when neonate's ductus arteriosis begins to close A systemic to pulmonary artery shunt may be surgically created to increase pulmonary blood flow (see discussion under tetralogy of Fallot) Pulmonary artery banding may be performed as palliative measure to reduce volume and pressure of pulmonary blood flow if CHF develops (later debanding and repair will be necessary) Open heart repair involves closure of VSD to allow left ventricular and aortic continuity; right ventricular to pulmonary artery continuity is established through insertion of valved conduit; ventriculotomy cardiac incision is used Deep hypothermia and circulatory arrest may be used in infants	CHF or low cardiac output is present postoperatively Arrhythmias (especially heart block) may occur; right bundle branch block will be present because of ventriculotomy incision Respiratory insufficiency may be present (especially if severe CHF and pulmonary hypertension are present preoperatively) Preoperative cyanosis and compensatory polycythemia will make child more prone to bleeding and thromboembolus perioperatively
Truncus type IV or pseudotruncus (pulmonary atresia); only aorta arises from ventricles, and distal pulmonary vessels are perfused only through collateral circulation—a VSD is also present	Pulmonary blood flow is accomplished only through PDA and collateral circulation, so pulmonary blood flow is *decreased* Cyanosis is present and may become profound when ductus arteriosus closes after birth	Prostaglandin E₁ may be administered during neonatal period to keep ductus arteriosus patent Palliative procedure may be performed to increase pulmonary blood flow (Waterston or Blalock-Taussig shunt) Repair involves closure of any associated septal defects and/or PDA, and establishment of right ventricle to pulmonary artery blood flow through use of valved conduit	CHF or low cardiac output is often present Arrhythmias may be present particularly as a result of a ventriculotomy cardiac incision and closure of septal defects Cyanosis and compensatory polycythemia will make child prone to bleeding (decreased platelet function) and thrombus formation perioperatively Respiratory insufficiency may be increased by presence of severe cyanosis preoperatively (causing pulmonary microthrombi), by CHF postoperatively, and/or by low cardiac output postoperatively NOTE: Alveolar hypoxia may cause pulmonary arterial vasoconstriction and increased right ventricular afterload, so these children should be weaned from mechanical ventilation carefully

Continued.

TABLE 28-1. Congenital heart defects—cont'd

LESION	PREOPERATIVE PROBLEMS	SURGICAL REPAIR	POSTOPERATIVE PROBLEMS
Tricuspid atresia NOTE: ASD and/or VSD will be present; other lesions (such as PDA, pulmonary stenosis, or transposition of great vessels) may be present and complicate the clinical presentation and repair	Systemic venous return shunts from right atrium to left atrium; pulmonary blood flow depends on left to right shunt through VSD, PDA, or surgical shunt; thus, pulmonary blood flow is usually decreased (but *may* be increased if another large shunt is present) Cyanosis is present to variable degree (depending on amount of pulmonary blood flow); severe hypoxemia may be present CHF may be present if large left to right shunt is present through VSD Clubbing will be present in older cyanotic child Compensatory polycythemia and right to left intracardiac shunt will make child more susceptible to spontaneous thromboembolus formation (especially if child is under 2 years old and anemic) and brain abscess Signs of systemic venous engorgement will be present if ASD (patent foramen ovale) is restrictive	Palliative shunt may be performed to increase pulmonary blood flow—Waterston shunt is side to side anastomosis between aorta and pulmonary artery; (this is performed infrequently because it can be associated with significant late complications including pulmonary hypertension); Blalock-Taussig shunt is made by end to side anastomosis between subclavian and pulmonary artery; modified Blalock-Taussig shunt is created by anastomosis of Gortex between subclavian artery and pulmonary artery; Glenn procedure is side to side anastomosis between superior vena cava and right pulmonary artery If CHF caused by large VSD is occurring, pulmonary artery banding may be performed as palliative procedure If patent foramen ovale is too small to allow free right to left atrial shunting, Rashkind balloon septostomy may be performed in cardiac catheterization lab, or Blalock-Hanlon septectomy may be performed (through mediastinal incision but without use of CPB) Corrective procedure is known as *Fontan procedure* and consists of placement of a valved or valveless conduit between right atrium and main pulmonary artery; other existing shunts (ASD, VSD, Waterston, etc.) would be closed; surgical correction is ideally performed when child is old enough to allow insertion of large conduit; Glenn procedure may be left in place after the Fontan procedure	CHF is likely, so CVP will need to be high, but watched carefully; fluid management must be judicious; development of ascites, pleural effusions, and other signs of systemic venous engorgement will probably occur Preoperative cyanosis and compensatory polycythemia will make child more prone to development of postoperative bleeding and perioperative thromboembolism formation Arrhythmias are likely, especially if VSD closure was performed Atrial arrhythmias are common Respiratory insufficiency can occur (related to CHF, pulmonary microthrombi, preoperative pulmonary hypertension, etc.)

TABLE 28-1. Congenital heart defects—cont'd

LESION	PREOPERATIVE PROBLEMS	SURGICAL REPAIR	POSTOPERATIVE PROBLEMS
Transposition of great vessels (TGV) Other possible associated lesions (VSD, aortic or pulmonic stenosis, or coarctation of aorta) will complicate clinical picture and surgical repair	Since aorta arises from right ventricle and pulmonary artery arises from left ventricle, two "closed loops" (right heart with systemic circulation and left heart with pulmonary circulation) are present, communication must exist between two circuits to allow survival; often PDA and ASD provide communication, and child may decompensate rapidly once PDA begins to close Cyanosis is generally present within hours of birth and can be severe, depending on degree of mixing between arterial and venous blood Clubbing will be present in older children Compensatory polycythemia and intracardiac shunting will make child more susceptible to spontaneous thromboembolus formation (especially before age 2 and in patients with microcytic anemia) and brain abscess formation	Prostaglandin E_1 is usually administered during neonatal period to maintain patency of ductus arteriosus Rashkind balloon septostomy is usually performed in catheterization lab to facilitate intraatrial mixing of arterial and venous blood Blalock-Hanlon septectomy may be performed as palliative surgery (via mediastinal incision but without use of CPB) to facilitate mixing between arterial and venous blood Corrective surgery will be performed by switching venous return or arterial circulation; Mustard, Senning, or arterial switch (Jatene) operation 1. Mustard procedure involves excision of atrial septum and use of pericardial baffle to redirect venous return; right ventricle remains systemic ventricle and left ventricle remains pulmonary ventricle; end result of Senning procedure is similar, though parts of atrial septum are used for baffle 2. Arterial switch operation involves closure of existing septal defects, great vessels are divided immediately above their semilunar valves, and coronary arteries are removed from aorta; great vessels are "switched" and resewn to their proper locations, and coronary arteries are anastomosed to aorta (in its new position); this procedure is performed early in life or after pulmonary band has been placed during neonatal period, or it may be performed in later infancy if large VSD is present	CHF is likely because of intraatrial manipulation or ventriculotomy incision Arrhythmias are extremely common with any of these corrective procedures; atrial arrhythmias and heart block are particularly likely following Mustard procedure; heart block and ventricular irritability are more common following arterial repair or Rastelli procedure; right bundle branch block will be present if ventriculotomy incision was made (as in Rastelli procedure) Preoperative compensatory polycythemia makes child more prone to postoperative bleeding and perioperative thromboembolus formation If intraatrial baffle is too restrictive following Mustard or Senning repair, systemic venous engorgement and pulmonary venous engorgement can occur (will require reoperation) Respiratory insufficiency will be likely and will be worsened by pulmonary microthrombi and CHF; weaning from mechanical ventilation must be gradual (since pulmonary vasoconstriction caused by hypoxia may increase ventricular afterload)

Continued.

TABLE 28-1. Congenital heart defects—cont'd

LESION	PREOPERATIVE PROBLEMS	SURGICAL REPAIR	POSTOPERATIVE PROBLEMS
		If pulmonary stenosis or atresia is present, Rastelli procedure may be employed for correction of TGV; VSD would be closed with baffle, which allows left ventricular output to flow through VSD and into aorta; pulmonary valve is sewn closed, and conduit connects right ventricle to main pulmonary artery Repair may be accomplished in infancy with use of deep hypothermia and circulatory arrest	
Total anomalous pulmonary venous return (TAPVR) NOTE: TAPVR may be to vessel *above* diaphragm or *below* diaphragm; infradiaphragmatic type is most frequently associated with obstructive pulmonary edema	Since all venous return flows into right atrium and then passes into left heart only through ASD or VSD, right heart failure and evidence of systemic venous engorgement will often be present Cyanosis is often present (since systemic and pulmonary venous return mix) If pulmonary venous drainage is *obstructed* (as in TAPVR *below* diaphragm into portal venous system) severe pulmonary edema will result within weeks of birth	Rashkind balloon septostomy may be performed in catheterization lab to allow greater intraatrial mixing (and more flow to left side of heart) Pulmonary veins must ultimately be anastomosed to left atrium (open heart surgery) Repair is often accomplished through use of deep hypothermia and circulatory arrest in infants	CHF or low cardiac output is often present postoperatively; left atrium and ventricle generally are small and will need to adjust to normal pulmonary venous return Respiratory failure will be most troublesome complication for infants who have had repair of obstructed TAPVR, such as TAPVR below diaphragm; these infants should be monitored closely for pulmonary edema, atelectasis, and consolidation, and they require excellent pulmonary toilet and gradual weaning from ventilatory support Arrhythmias may occur (particularly atrial arrhythmias and evidence of ventricular irritability) Since infant often demonstrates cyanosis and compensatory polycythemia preoperatively, he/she will have increased risk of postoperative bleeding and perioperative thromboembolus formation
Coarctation of aorta (preductal type); this defect may be associated with other left heart anomalies	If aortic arch is small, symptoms of severe CHF may be apparent within hours or days of birth If hypoplastic left heart is present, condition will deteriorate rapidly If narrowing is located in arch of the aorta, difference in BP between right and left arms may be present	Narrowed aortic segment must be increased during thoracotomy with aortic cross-clamping (closed heart surgery); aorta is then closed using patch (the newborn's proximal left subclavian artery may be used as a patch) If aortic arch must be extensively reconstructed, hypothermia and circulatory arrest may be used	CHF may be severe in postoperative period Transient upper extremity hypertension may be present Mesenteric arteritis may occur following restoration of strong, pulsatile blood flow to distal aorta Renal failure may occur Chylothorax may develop

TABLE 28-1. Congenital heart defects—cont'd

LESION	PREOPERATIVE PROBLEMS	SURGICAL REPAIR	POSTOPERATIVE PROBLEMS
	Lower extremities may be cyanotic (they will receive blood flow from right ventricle through ductus)		
Coarctation of aorta (postductal type) NOTE: Bicuspid aortic valve is present in majority of these patients and may become calcified and/or stenotic	CHF may occur in infancy if coarctation is severe or associated with another defect (PDA, VSD, etc.) Decreased BP in lower extremities will cause decreased pulses and may cause claudication Increased BP (hypertension) in upper extremities will be present Development of large collateral circulation will cause "rib notching" on radiograph in older children	Narrowed segment of aorta must be incised and aorta patched during left thoracotomy incision and aortic cross-clamping (closed heart surgery) Patch may be necessary to achieve reanastomosis of aorta without stenosis	CHF (if present preoperatively) Tachycardia and transient upper extremity hypertension may be present for days postoperatively Mesenteric arteritis may occur following restoration of strong, pulsatile blood flow to descending aorta (monitor for ileus and begin feedings slowly) Movement of or sensation in lower extremities may be impaired if spinal cord circulation is decreased during aortic cross-clamping Renal failure may occur Chylothorax may develop
Aortic stenosis/insufficiency	←————————————————— See adult open heart surgery —————————————————→		
Mitral stenosis/insufficiency	←————————————————— See adult open heart surgery —————————————————→		
Anomalous left coronary artery (left coronary artery arises from pulmonary artery, so venous blood is provided to left ventricle coronary artery supply)	Angina and infarction can occur in early childhood because of left ventricular ischemia Ventricular arrhythmias or S-T segment changes also indicate ischemia	Coronary artery must be detached from pulmonary artery and reimplanted into aorta; graft may be used CPB may be used if coronary artery is difficult to reanastomose to aorta	Myocardial ischemia and/or infarction Left ventricular failure requiring vasopressor support Arrhythmias (particularly those indicating ventricular irritability) may develop

ASSESSMENT

1. History, presence, and nature of
   a. Previous hospitalizations and procedures, particularly
      (1) Cardiac catheterization
      (2) Palliative or "corrective" cardiac surgery
   b. Related cardiac problems
      (1) CHF
      (2) Cyanosis, hypercyanotic episodes, chronic hypoxemia
      (3) Rheumatic heart disease
      (4) Subacute bacterial endocarditis (or risk for, caused by the presence of areas of turbulent blood flow within the heart or great vessels)
      (5) Arrhythmias
      (6) History of syncope
   c. Nonspecific signs of cardiorespiratory distress
      (1) Delayed motor milestones (may be noted in the presence of normal intellectual and social development)
      (2) Feeding difficulties (the infant often takes longer to feed, then may take very little formula or vomit after feeding)
      (3) Poor weight gain during infancy or "failure to thrive"
      (4) Decreased exercise tolerance
      (5) Increased irritability or lethargy
   d. Other organ dysfunctions which may be related to the cardiovascular problems, particularly
      (1) Pulmonary
      (2) Renal

(3) Neurological (monitor especially for history of cerebral thromboembolic events in the infant with cyanotic heart disease under the age of 2 years, and history of brain abscess in the child over the age of 2 years with cyanotic heart disease)

e. Malformations or disorders of other systems (e.g., skeletal or GI anomalies), which affect approximately one third of children with congenital heart disease

2. Level of systemic perfusion

a. Activity tolerance—note level of activity restriction; differentiate between activity restrictions imposed by parents and those self-imposed by child; note the presence of easy fatigability or lethargy or squatting during play (particularly in the child with cyanotic heart disease)

b. BP should be appropriate for age (consider patient's normal BP)

c. Heart rate should be appropriate for age and clinical status

d. Peripheral pulses should all be strong and equal

e. Extremities should be warm and well perfused; nail beds should be pink, and capillary refill should be brisk

f. Urine output should equal 0.5 to 1.0 ml/kg/hour if fluid intake is adequate

g. Signs of CHF

(1) Evidence of adrenergic stimulation: tachycardia, diaphoresis, peripheral vasoconstriction, decreased urine output

(2) Evidence of systemic venous engorgement: high measured CVP or right atrial pressure, hepatomegaly, periorbital edema, ascites (rare in children)

(3) Evidence of pulmonary venous engorgement: tachypnea, increased respiratory effort, rales (often not present, unless the child has a concurrent upper respiratory infection)

h. A gallop rhythm may be present when the infant or child has CHF, and murmurs noted may be characteristic of specific congenital heart defects

i. Review ECG for signs of arrhythmias that may be compromising the child's cardiac output

j. Evaluate the child's fluid balance

(1) Mucous membranes should be moist

(2) The fontanelle should be flat in infants less than 16 to 18 months of age (before the sutures close); the fontanelle may be sunken if the infant is hypovolemic, and full and tense if the infant is hypervolemic

(3) Urine output should total approximately 0.5 to 1.0 ml/kg/hour if fluid intake is adequate; urine should be appropriately concentrated if urine volume is small

(4) Skin turgor should be good; with dehydration the skin may remain ''tented'' after it is pinched, and with hypervolemia the skin may be tense and shiny over edematous areas

(5) Tearing should be present during vigorous cry in infants older than 6 weeks if hydration is adequate

(6) Evaluate daily weight; weight gain should be consistent and steady; rapid weight gain may indicate fluid retention; weight loss can occur as the result of vigorous diuresis and poor fluid intake

(7) Total all recent sources of fluid intake and output

k. Note the child's position of comfort; the child with cardiorespiratory distress usually prefers the upright position

3. Pulmonary status

a. Rate, rhythm, and quality of respirations; note presence of rales, rhonchi, wheezing, stridor, grunting, retractions, or nasal flaring

b. Presence of pulmonary problems (e.g., pleural effusion) secondary to either cardiovascular or pulmonary problems (e.g., atelectasis) that may complicate cardiovascular recovery

4. Results of laboratory and diagnostic tests, including

a. ECG evidence of

(1) Arrhythmias

(2) Signs of abnormal axis or chamber hypertrophy, which may be consistent with specific forms of congenital heart defects

(3) Effects of chronotropic or inotropic medications

(4) Myocardial ischemia (may be noted in children with severe aortic stenosis)

b. Chest radiograph for signs of

(1) Cardiac enlargement (NOTE: Heart size will not increase when hypertrophy is present—it can increase when one or more chambers dilatate)

(2) Pulmonary vascular markings

(3) Location of great vessels

c. Cardiac catheterization for evidence of

(1) Abnormal oxygen saturation in chambers of the heart or in the great vessels indicating the presence of a shunt

(2) Abnormal pressure measurements within the heart or great vessels, indicating the presence of areas of stenosis or pulmonary hypertension

(3) Abnormal blood flow patterns depicted by the angiocardiogram, indicating specific areas of intracardiac shunts or areas of obstruction

d. Echocardiogram for evidence of

(1) Structural abnormalities within the heart or great vessels

(2) Secondary evidence of chamber hypertrophy or decreased chamber or valvular size

e. Radionuclide studies

f. Exercise testing

g. His bundle mapping or other studies of intracardiac conduction

h. Electrolyte and acid-base balance

i. CBC (monitor for evidence of severe polycythemia and microcytic anemia in the child with cyanotic heart disease, as this increases the child's risk of spontaneous thromboembolic events)

5. Patient/family's level of anxiety regarding disease process, medical therapy employed, purpose of hospitalization, need for surgery, postoperative management, and general follow-up plan of care

6. Patient/family's past alterations in roles, ADL, associated with patient's disease process

7. Parent's fears and concerns about their child's congenital heart disease

8. Patient/family's knowledge regarding operative therapy

a. What they have been told

b. Their expectations

c. Fears regarding surgery and the outcome

d. Previous experiences with surgery

e. Experience of other family members or friends with heart disease

9. Information and detail surgeon has provided patient/family about operative therapy, known pathology, and postoperative management

GOALS

1. Reduction of patient/family's anxiety with provision of information and support

a. Patient/family demonstrates understanding of the disease process, the purpose of the child's hospitalization, the plan of surgery, the preoperative and postoperative treatment plans, and the expected outcomes

b. Patient/family participates in planning and implementing the child's care, as appropriate

2. Adequate systemic perfusion, without evidence of

a. Hypovolemia

b. Hemorrhage

c. Tamponade

d. Electrolyte or acid-base imbalance

e. Poor cardiac contractility

f. Increased systemic or pulmonary vascular resistance

g. Arrhythmias

h. Hypothermia

3. Absence of CHF

4. Adequate pulmonary function

a. Arterial blood gas levels will reflect good alveolar ventilation with appropriate pH and oxygen and carbon dioxide tension

b. Absence of auscultatory or radiographic evidence of atelectasis, pneumothorax, hemothorax, pleural effusion, chylothorax, or inadequate inspiratory effort as a result of pain or "splinting" of incision

5. Serum electrolyte levels within normal limits

6. Parameters of renal function within normal limits

a. Urine output adequate with average of 0.5 to 1.0 ml/kg/hour

b. Urine concentration will be appropriate

c. Serum creatinine and BUN will be normal

7. Neurological function within normal limits, with no evidence of seizures or impairment (or will demonstrate same neurological function as preoperatively)

8. Wound heals completely without evidence of systemic or local infection

9. Patient/family demonstrates knowledge of and proficiency in techniques needed to provide postdischarge care for the child

POTENTIAL PROBLEMS	EXPECTED OUTCOMES	NURSING ACTIVITIES

■ Patient/family's anxiety related to
Child's cardiovascular disease
Surgery
Prognosis and/or hospitalization
	■ Absence of behavior that interferes with medical care
	Patient (if appropriate) and family discuss child's disease, purpose of hospitalization, goals and potential complications of surgery, planned postoperative management, and prognosis
	Patient/family involved in care as appropriate
		■ Orient child and significant family members to nursing care unit (including preoperative unit and critical care unit)
		Assess child's preparation for surgery
		  Ascertain what child has been told about his/her hospitalization and surgery
		  Ask parents how they think child can best be prepared for surgery
		  Assess child's level of cognitive and psychosocial development
		Plan preoperative teaching approach based on child's prior preparation and individual level of comprehension; collaborate with other members of health care team
		Provide general information and repeated assurances that parents will be waiting after surgery (if this is true), and that child will be returning home soon; most children under 2 to 3 years of age do not have sufficient conceptual ability to grasp details about surgery or postoperative care

POTENTIAL PROBLEMS	EXPECTED OUTCOMES	NURSING ACTIVITIES

Plan unstructured sessions to assess child's understanding of hospital procedure and his/her fears and concerns; structured sessions may then be planned for child older than approximately 2 years of age to teach about planned treatment or clarify serious misconceptions; it is important that child not be given more detailed information than he/she can handle—take cues from child about tolerance and acceptance of information

Children may enjoy and benefit from use of dolls or other play equipment preoperatively and postoperatively

Describe postoperative experience according to child's (and family's) *need to know* and *readiness to learn;* do not overwhelm child with threatening details about events that will occur while he/she is asleep or about things child will not see, hear, or feel

Take cues from child and family and do not give child more information than he/she is able to handle; it may be necessary to provide child with small amounts of information at a time, with frequent reinforcement of important points

Use human figure drawings during explanation or child's preoperative and postoperative care for school-age child

Plan timing of child's teaching carefully; if child does not have well-developed sense of time intervals, explanations may be given evening before surgery and should not be complex; if child has well-developed concept of time intervals, preparation may be accomplished gradually, focusing on different aspects of postoperative care at different sessions

Teach child those things that *he/she* can do that will hasten recovery (e.g., deep breathing and coughing)

Avoid telling child that surgery will make him/her feel better (if child is asymptomatic) since child will actually feel worse in early postoperative period; it may be more accurate to tell child that noise in his/her heart will be fixed (child may be frightened to hear that he/she has a "leaky" heart or a "hole" in his/her heart, so these terms should probably be avoided)

Provide child (as appropriate) and family with opportunity to visit critical care unit and to meet with nursing staff; very young children, however, may be more frightened by sight of critically ill children, so preoperative visit to critical care unit should be carefully planned and supervised

Discuss general activity schedule (preoperative and postoperative) with child (as appropriate) and family

Time of surgery

Need for preoperative NPO orders

Approximate length of surgery (overestimations are usually better than underestimations)

Anticipated length of stay in critical care unit (overestimations are usually better than underestimations)

Anticipated postoperative and postdischarge activity

Encourage child/family to ask questions and discuss concerns; it may be helpful to ask child to "name the one scariest thing" to obtain concrete examples of child's fears

Assist in preparing the child for diagnostic procedures

Assess continuously child/family's level of anxiety and be prepared to provide more information, reassurance, or comfort as needed; occasionally, anxious parent continues to ask many questions, when in fact reassurance or comfort is really needed; in this case, nurse should avoid providing more and more information and should attempt to determine what parent *really* wants to know

Record specific teaching information (including specific terminology used to describe procedures or equipment) in child's chart or care plan so health care team can reinforce same information consistently

POTENTIAL PROBLEMS	EXPECTED OUTCOMES	NURSING ACTIVITIES

Provide further teaching as new problems arise

Provide child with postoperative opportunities to discuss surgical or critical care experience through use of play, art, or games

Encourage child's expression of feelings and emphasize acceptability of such expression (e.g., it is "okay to cry" if it hurts); if some of child's expressions of anger are harmful (e.g., if child pulls out an IV line), consistent limits should be placed on this form of expression, and this should be discussed with child

Assess and document family strengths and family stresses, since these may influence family's response to stress

Assess family's need for financial assistance or other additional support, and refer them to appropriate hospital support personnel, including social worker, hospital financial advisor, or state or local agencies, as indicated

■ Postoperative inadequate systemic perfusion and low cardiac output related to

Hypovolemia (as result of hemorrhage, diuresis, or inadequate fluid administration)

Tamponade

Decreased cardiac contractility (related to hypervolemia, electrolyte or acid-base imbalance, or cardiac dysfunction)

Increased systemic or pulmonary vascular resistance

Arrhythmias

Hypothermia

NOTE: Each of these problems will be discussed separately

■ Adequate systemic perfusion as demonstrated by

Warm extremities

Pink mucous membranes and nail beds

Strong peripheral pulses

Good capillary refill

Urine output of 0.5 to 1.0 ml/kg/hour

Arterial BP within patient's normal range ("normal" range for each patient to be determined after consideration of normal range for patient's age and patient's preoperative BP)

Arterial blood gas levels within normal limits (pH of 7.35 to 7.45; Po_2 80 to 100 mm Hg in child or 60 to 80 mm Hg in neonate; Pco_2 of 35 to 45 mm Hg)

■ Assess indirect evidence of child's systemic perfusion, including

Temperature of extremities (should be warm)

Color of mucous membranes and nail beds (should be pink)

Quality and intensity of peripheral pulses

Capillary refill time (should be brisk)

Notify physician of signs of poor systemic perfusion

Measure and record hourly urine output; report output of less than 0.5 to 1.0 ml/kg/hour to physician; measure urine specific gravity q4-8 hr and correlate with urine volume; if urine volume is low and specific gravity is low, renal dysfunction may be present

Measure patient's arterial blood pressure. Notify physician of arterial hypotension or hypertension (see normal arterial systolic pressures below)

Age	Normal systolic arterial BP ranges (mm Hg)
Neonate	50 to 70
Infant	74 to 100
Toddler	80 to 112
Preschooler	82 to 110
School-age child	84 to 120
Adolescent	94 to 140

If cardiac output thermistor probe is in place, measure child's cardiac output as ordered or as indicated by patient's condition; include amounts of fluid injected as part of patient's fluid intake; convert any cardiac output measurements to *cardiac index*

$$\text{Cardiac index} = \frac{\text{Cardiac output}}{\text{m}^2 \text{ body surface area}}$$

Report cardiac index of less than 2.5 liter/min/m² body surface area to physician immediately

Determine simultaneous arterial and venous O_2 saturation measurements which may be made and used to calculate arterial and mixed venous O_2 content, if Swan-Ganz catheter is in place

NOTE: If difference between child's arterial and mixed venous O_2 content is increasing, child's cardiac output is probably falling; if difference is decreasing, child's cardiac output is probably increasing

Monitor child's arterial blood gas levels and report any metabolic acidosis, hypoxemia, or hypercapnia to physician

Total all fluid intake patient is receiving and discuss with physician if total fluid intake greatly exceeds total fluid output

See STANDARD 16   *Cardiogenic shock*

POTENTIAL PROBLEMS	EXPECTED OUTCOMES	NURSING ACTIVITIES
■ Postoperative hypovolemia related to 　Hemorrhage 　Diuresis 　Inadequate fluid administration	■ Minimal chest tube drainage (less than 3 ml/kg/hour or less than 5% to 7% of total circulating blood volume during first 6 hours postoperatively) Hct within normal limits determined by health care team—approximate ranges are 　40% minimum for infants 　30% minimum for children Adequate CVP or right atrial pressure Adequate PAWP or left atrial pressure Moist mucous membranes Good skin turgor Urine output of 0.5 to 1 ml/kg/hour with appropriate specific gravity	■ Calculate child's circulating blood volume (see below) and consider all blood loss in terms of that blood volume; notify physician if unreplaced blood loss totals 7% to 10% of child's circulating blood volume; transfusion may then be ordered

<table>
<tr><th>Age</th><th>Circulating blood volume (ml/kg)</th></tr>
<tr><td>Neonate</td><td>85 to 90</td></tr>
<tr><td>Infant</td><td>75 to 80</td></tr>
<tr><td>Child</td><td>70 to 75</td></tr>
</table>

Record running total of unreplaced blood drawn for laboratory analysis for any patient under 1 year of age; discuss replacement of this blood with physician once it totals 7% to 10% of infant's circulating blood volume

Strip chest tubes gently but firmly enough to keep them free of clots; Notify physician if chest tube output totals ≥3 ml/kg/hour for 3 or more hours, or 5 ml/kg/hour in any 1 hour

NOTE: *Bleeding totaling 3 ml/kg/hour for 3 hours usually constitutes a 12% to 15% hemorrhage*

Draw blood sample for Hct determination immediately after surgery (as ordered), and repeat sample as patient's condition or physician's order indicates; if Hct is low or has fallen suddenly, report this to physician immediately

Draw blood samples for coagulation studies (as ordered by physician or per unit policy) if excessive chest tube output is present; discuss abnormal results with physician, so appropriate blood component therapy may be administered

Discuss possibility of surgical bleeding with physician if excessive chest tube output is present in absence of any coagulopathy

NOTE: Patient may require reoperation to locate and repair site of bleeding; surgical bleeding should be suspected when any patient demonstrates excessive chest tube output with evidence of good clot formation in tube; these patients are most at risk for clot obstruction of chest tubes and resultant tamponade

Total all fluid intake and output and report patient's fluid balance to physician

Measure patient's CVP and/or right atrial pressure, PAWP and/or left atrial pressure; maintain these cardiac filling pressures at level where systemic perfusion is best, as ordered

Postoperative filling pressures are usually maintained at 5 to 15 mm Hg, but specific ideal pressures should be determined by surgeon and other members of health care team; these filling pressures are usually maintained with infusions of blood components or crystalloid or colloid solutions

Whole blood or packed cells are usually administered if additional fluid administration is required and child's Hct is low; fresh frozen plasma, albumin, or other colloid or crystalloid solutions are usually administered if additional fluid is required and child's Hct is satisfactory

If high filling pressures are required to maintain satisfactory systemic perfusion, child's cardiac contractility is probably low, and correction of acid-base or electrolyte balance or administration of inotropic medications may be required (per physician's order); see also Problem, Decreased cardiac contractility

If child's filling pressures rise rapidly with administration of only small volumes of fluid, child's ventricular compliance is reduced, and fluid administration should be accomplished very slowly

Assess patient's level of hydration

Mucous membranes should be moist

Infant's fontanelle should be level (not sunken)

Tearing should be present with cry beyond 4 to 8 weeks of age

POTENTIAL PROBLEMS	EXPECTED OUTCOMES	NURSING ACTIVITIES
		Skin turgor should be good (skin should not remain tented after pinching)
		Urine output should be 0.5 to 1.0 ml/kg/hour if fluid intake is adequate; urine specific gravity should be <1.020
		Report signs of inadequate hydration to physician
■ Tamponade and resultant low cardiac output caused by mediastinal bleeding and inadequate mediastinal drainage	■ Absence of the following signs of cardiac tamponade High CVP (or right atrial pressure) and left atrial (or PAWP) with falling systemic arterial pressure and decreasing systemic perfusion Pulsus paradoxus Decreased intensity of heart sounds (late) others; see nursing activities	■ Assess patient continuously for signs of *cardiac tamponade* Elevated venous and atrial pressures (NOTE: Isolated right or left atrial tamponade can produce isolated elevation in right or left atrial pressure) Poor systemic perfusion Pulsus paradoxus (fall in systolic arterial pressure by more than 8 to 10 mmHg with spontaneous inspiration) NOTE: Pulsus paradoxus will not be observed if patient is receiving positive pressure assisted ventilation Monitor for late signs of tamponade, including Distant heart sounds Bradycardia Hypotension Widening of mediastinum on chest radiogram Report any of these findings to physician and be prepared to institute emergency measures, as needed Keep chest tubes patent with gentle stripping NOTE: Tamponade as result of clotted chest tubes is especially likely in patient demonstrating evidence of clotting and a history of chest tube output that ceases abruptly with concurrent deterioration in patient's clinical appearance; ''back-stripping'' of mediastinal tubes or direct suctioning of mediastinal tubes may be necessary (with physician's order) if tamponade is suspected If tamponade develops, notify physician; prepare thoracotomy tray for emergency thoracotomy (or prepare for patient return to operating room, as hospital policy dictates)
■ Decreased cardiac contractility related to hypervolemia, acid-base or electrolyte imbalance, or cardiac dysfunction	■ Absence of signs of systemic or pulmonary venous engorgement (see Problem, Congestive heart failure) Arterial blood gas levels within normal limits, with pH of 7.35 to 7.45, an arterial oxygen tension of 80 to 100 mm Hg (60 to 80 mm Hg in neonates), and arterial carbon dioxide tension of 35 to 45 mm Hg Serum electrolyte concentrations within normal limits (particularly glucose, Ca^{++}, and K^+) Minimal fluid weight gain ≤50 g/24 hours in infants ≤200 g/24 hours in children ≤500 g/24 hours in adolescents	■ Monitor for signs of *systemic venous engorgement* High measured CVP or right atrial pressure Hepatomegaly Jugular venous distention (useful only in older child) Periorbital edema Pleural effusion Ascites Discuss these findings with physician; patient may require diuresis (per physician's order) Monitor for signs of *pulmonary venous engorgement* Tachypnea (if patient breathing spontaneously) Increased respiratory effort (if patient is breathing spontaneously) Increased peak inspiratory pressures or decreased lung compliance (as assessed during hand ventilation with manual resuscitator when patient is intubated), or increased pulmonary secretions (if patient is intubated and mechanically ventilated) Increased pulmonary vascular markings on chest radiograph NOTE: Child's heart size may be increased, and pleural effusion may be present when child has cardiac dysfunction Monitor patient's arterial blood gas values and report development of acidosis, hypoxemia, or hypercapnia to physician; initiation of or adjustment in ventilatory support may be required (see Problem, Respiratory distress) Monitor child's serum electrolyte concentration, and report any abnormalities to physician so treatment can be instituted, as indicated Administer sodium bicarbonate, as ordered, if *metabolic acidosis* is present

POTENTIAL PROBLEMS	EXPECTED OUTCOMES	NURSING ACTIVITIES

NOTE: Since administration of sodium bicarbonate results in formation of CO_2, it is imperative that ventilatory function and/or ventilatory support be adequate to prevent development of secondary hypercarbia and respiratory acidosis

Administer hypertonic glucose solution as ordered if *hypoglycemia* is present

Administer calcium solutions as ordered if *hypocalcemia* is present

Administer any calcium infusion through large-bore venous catheter, and administer slowly to prevent bradycardia (administration rate should not exceed 100 mg/min)

Administer potassium chloride as ordered if *hypokalemia* is present

Administer IV potassium chloride through large-bore or central venous catheter; if peripheral administration of potassium chloride is required, solution should be sufficiently diluted so vascular irritation is prevented; inadvertent bolus administration of drug can be prevented if IV tubing is carefully labeled during potassium chloride infusion

Administer calcium, sodium polystyrene sulfonate (Kayexalate) enema, or glucose and insulin, as ordered, if *hyperkalemia* is present

Discuss with physician initiation of inotropic cardiac support or afterload reduction, as needed

If poor systemic perfusion persists despite presence of adequate (or even high) cardiac filling pressures and correction of acidosis, hypoxemia, or electrolyte imbalances, administer dopamine by continuous IV infusion as ordered; desired dose of dopamine should be titrated according to desired clinical effect, as ordered (see Appendix D for dosages); lower dosages of dopamine produce dopaminergic renal artery dilatation and beta-1 adrenergic effects; higher dosages produce alpha-adrenergic effects (these are usually undesirable)

Administer dobutamine by continuous IV infusion as ordered (see Appendix D); dobutamine provides primarily beta-1 adrenergic effects, including increased cardiac contractility and increased cardiac output; *dobutamine produces no selective renal artery dilatation*

Administer medication through separate IV line if any continuous infusion medication is ordered so that infusion will not have to be interrupted for administration of other medications or fluid therapy

Refer to Appendix D for a complete description of guidelines for administering medications to children

---

POTENTIAL PROBLEMS	EXPECTED OUTCOMES	NURSING ACTIVITIES
■ Decreased cardiac output related to increase in systemic or pulmonary vascular resistance	■ Adequate peripheral perfusion as indicated by Warm extremities Pink mucous membranes and nail beds Strong peripheral pulses Good capillary refill Urine output of 0.5 to 1.0 ml/kg/hour Systemic vascular resistance within normal limits 10 to 15 units/m² body surface area in neonate 15 to 20 units/m² body surface area in toddler 20 to 30 units/m² body surface area in child	■ Assess child's indirect evidence of systemic perfusion (see Problem, Postoperative inadequate systemic perfusion), and notify physician if patient demonstrates evidence of poor systemic perfusion Calculate child's systemic vascular resistance (SVR) if necessary parameters can be measured, as follows

$$\text{SVR in units} = \frac{\text{MAP (mm Hg)} - \text{Mean right atrial pressure (mm Hg)}}{\text{Cardiac index}}$$

Unit computers may perform this calculation

NOTE: Even ''normal'' systemic vascular resistance may be too high if child's cardiac contractility is significantly reduced; therefore *trends* in child's calculated SVR and child's clinical status are usually considered more important than any single SVR calculation

Administer an afterload-reducing agent, as ordered, if high systemic vascular resistance is thought to be producing increased left ventricular afterload and decreased cardiac output; afterload reduction may be attempted with any of the following IV medications

POTENTIAL PROBLEMS	EXPECTED OUTCOMES	NURSING ACTIVITIES

	Pulmonary vascular resistance within normal limits
	8 to 10 units/m² body surface area in neonate
	1 to 3 units/m² body surface area in infant and child
		Nitroglycerine (ointment form of medication may be given instead of IV form)
		Sodium nitroprusside
		Dobutamine
		Isoproterenol
		NOTE: These drugs may be administered alone or in combination with other vasopressors or vasodilators
		If continuous-infusion systemic vasodilators are used
		  Administer vasodilator through separate IV line, and label line carefully; prevent interruption in or acceleration of rate of vasodilator infusion, and prevent inadvertent bolus administration of medication when IV tubing is changed
		  Administer fluids if needed, as ordered, to maintain stable right or left atrial pressure during vasodilator therapy
		  NOTE: *Hypotension is more likely to occur during vasodilator therapy if hypovolemia is present*
		  Monitor indirect evidence of child's systemic perfusion throughout vasodilator therapy and notify physician of signs of inadequate systemic perfusion
		Calculate child's pulmonary vascular resistance (PVR) if necessary parameters are available, as follows

$$\text{PVR in units} = \frac{\text{Mean pulmonary artery pressure (mm Hg)} - \text{Mean left atrial pressure (mm Hg)}}{\text{Cardiac index}}$$

Unit computer may perform this calculation

If child's calculated pulmonary vascular resistance is high, or if child is known to have increased pulmonary vascular resistance from preoperative catheterization studies

  Ensure that child's alveolar ventilation is adequate, since alveolar hypoxia can produce pulmonary arterial vasoconstriction and increased pulmonary vascular resistance; as a result, child with high pulmonary vascular resistance or reactive pulmonary vascularity should be weaned *very slowly* from ventilatory support

  Prevent hypothermia, since it may contribute to development of pulmonary vasoconstriction and increased pulmonary vascular resistance

  Prevent or ensure prompt treatment of hypoxemia or acidosis, since they can also produce pulmonary arterial vasoconstriction

  NOTE: Postoperative care of child with pulmonary hypertension requires excellent respiratory support, since inadequate ventilation will enhance pulmonary arterial vasoconstriction, and can quickly produce fall in cardiac output

If pulmonary vascular resistance is high, administration of systemic vasodilator, particularly nitroglycerine or sodium nitroprusside, is usually ordered (see Appendix D for dosages); additional pulmonary vasodilators may also be prescribed

  Tolazoline—*watch for signs of systemic hypotension*

  Isoproterenol

Check child's platelet concentration, if child receives sodium nitroprusside therapy for 48 hours or more, since sodium nitroprusside administration can produce thrombocytopenia; in addition, check child's serum thiocyanate level, since metabolism of nitroprusside produces thiocyanate and cyanide

Change only one medication dose at a time when patient is weaned from vasodilator or inotropic support to facilitate evaluation of child's response to change

POTENTIAL PROBLEMS	EXPECTED OUTCOMES	NURSING ACTIVITIES

■ Decreased cardiac output as result of arrhythmia	■ Electrophysiologic stability
	Adequate cardiac output
	Hemodynamic stability
		■ Monitor patient ECG continuously; ensure display of clear tracing with proper lead placement and good skin preparation
		Assess (immediately) effect of any arrhythmias on child's systemic perfusion
		  Assess indirect evidence of child's systemic perfusion (warmth of extremities, color of mucous membranes and nail beds, strength of peripheral pulses, quantity of urine output); notify physician immediately of any arrhythmias associated with decreased systemic perfusion
		  Initiate CPR as needed if arrhythmia causes inadequate systemic perfusion
		Obtain rhythm strip to document any arrhythmia (include at least 10 to 12 ventricular complexes)
		Attempt to determine potential contributing factors when any arrhythmia develops
		  Changes in intravascular K^+ and Ca^{++} concentration
		  Acidosis
		  Hypoxemia
		  Digitalis toxicity
		  Monitor arterial blood gas and/or serum electrolyte concentrations (as ordered or per unit policy)
		  Check with physician before administering digoxin, and obtain blood sample for digoxin level as ordered
		If temporary pacing wires are in place, and are connected to external pacemaker, check function of wires and pacemaker
		
		See STANDARD 23 *Pacemakers: temporary and permanent*
		      STANDARD 21 *Arrhythmias*
		
		Administer electrolyte supplements, sodium bicarbonate, or antiarrhythmic medications as ordered, and assess patient response
		
		See STANDARD 21 *Arrhythmias*

■ Low cardiac output in young infant as result of hypothermia	■ Rectal temperature of approximately 37° C (98.6° F), and skin temperature of approximately 36° to 36.5° (96.8° to 97.7° F) Evidence of good systemic perfusion (including warm extremities, pink mucous membranes and nail beds, strong peripheral pulses, good capillary refill, and urine output of 0.5 to 1.0 ml/kg/hour)	■ Monitor patient's rectal and skin temperature q1 hr, and more often as needed postoperatively Use overbed warmer or Isolette to provide infant with neutral thermal environment (that environmental temperature at which infant can maintain normal rectal temperature with lowest O_2 consumption—these temperature ranges can be found in the form of Scope charts, and should be posted in every critical care unit caring for neonates) Notify physician if infant has a rectal temperature below 36° to 36.5° C despite warming measures Notify physician if patient's rectal temperature *exceeds* 37° C in presence of low skin temperature or poor systemic perfusion, since this may indicate presence of low cardiac output

■ CHF related to
  Uncorrected congenital heart defect (e.g., after palliative surgery)
  Correction of congenital heart defect (and alteration in ventricular preload, contractility, and afterload)
  Postoperative hypervolemia
  Electrolyte imbalance
	■ Adequate systemic perfusion
	Absence of evidence of systemic venous engorgement, including
	  High CVP or right atrial pressure
	  Hepatomegaly
	  Periorbital edema
	  Ascites
		■ Monitor child's heart rate and evidence of systemic perfusion (including warmth of extremities, color of mucous membranes and nail beds, strength of peripheral pulses, speed of capillary refill, and urine output); notify physician if evidence of poor systemic perfusion is present
		Measure urine output hourly, and notify physician if total is less than 0.5 to 1.0 ml/kg/hour
		  If decreased urine output is accompanied by increased urine specific gravity and fluid intake is thought to be inadequate administer additional fluids as ordered
		  If child's CVP is high and periorbital edema, hepatomegaly, or ascites is present, decreased urine output is probably caused by CHF; administer diuretics as ordered

POTENTIAL PROBLEMS	EXPECTED OUTCOMES	NURSING ACTIVITIES
	Absence of pulmonary venous engorgement, including Tachypnea (if breathing spontaneously) Increased respiratory effort, including retractions, nasal flaring, and grunting (if breathing spontaneously) Increased left atrial pressure or PAWP Increased peak inspiratory pressure or decreased lung compliance (if patient receiving mechanical ventilation) Minimal fluid weight gain ≤50 g/24 hours in infants ≤200 g/24 hours in children ≤500 g/24 hours in adolescents	Monitor for evidence of *systemic venous engorgement* High CVP or right atrial pressure Hepatomegaly Periorbital edema Ascites or pleural effusion Discuss these findings with physician as soon as they are observed Monitor for signs of *pulmonary venous engorgement*, including Tachypnea (if patient is breathing spontaneously) Increased respiratory effort, as indicated by nasal flaring, retractions, and grunting (if patient is breathing spontaneously) Increased left atrial pressure or PAWP Increased peak inspiratory pressure or decreased lung compliance (as assessed during hand ventilation of intubated patient), or increased volume of respiratory secretions in patient receiving mechanical ventilatory assistance Pleural effusion Monitor patient fluid intake and output and discuss positive fluid balance with physician Administer digitalis derivative as ordered; check dosage before administration, and monitor for arrhythmias or other signs of toxicity (see Appendix D for dosages) Administer diuretic therapy as ordered Check dosage and possible urinary electrolyte losses Assess patient urinary response to diuretic and notify physician if this response is inadequate Check patient electrolyte concentration (per physician's order or unit policy) and administer electrolyte supplement as ordered Measure child's weight daily or twice daily on same scale at same time of day; notify physician of significant weight gain *See* STANDARD 15 *Heart failure (low cardiac output)*
■ Respiratory distress related to Atelectasis Pneumothorax Hemothorax Pleural effusion Chylothorax CHF Low cardiac output Pulmonary hypertension Inadequate ventilatory support Malfunctioning chest drainage system Pain and splinting of incision and resultant hypoventilation	■ "Normal" respiratory rate—range to be determined by consideration of child's age, clinical condition, and preoperative respiratory rate Minimal evidence of increased respiratory effort (including nasal flaring, retractions, and grunting) Adequate and equal lung aeration bilaterally, with no evidence of congestion on auscultation	■ Assess child's chest expansion, lung aeration, respiratory rate, respiratory effort (if patient breathing spontaneously), and evidence of lung compliance (e.g., pressure required to inflate lungs or by ease of hand ventilation of intubated patient); report abnormal findings to physician Monitor for evidence of *atelectasis* (especially of right upper lobe) Decreased breath sounds Change in quality or pitch of breath sounds Dullness to percussion Decreased chest movement with respiration Tachypnea (if patient breathing spontaneously) Evidence of atelectasis on chest radiograph NOTE: Since breath sounds are easily transmitted through thin chest wall of infant, significant atelectasis can be present without appreciable decrease in intensity of associated breath sounds; as result, assess for changes in quality or pitch of breath sounds Monitor for evidence of *pneumothorax* Decreased breath sounds Change in pitch of breath sounds Hyperresonance of chest to percussion Decreased chest movement during inspiration Increased respiratory rate, effort, or dyspnea (if child is breathing spontaneously) Increased peak inspiratory pressures and increased resistance to hand ventilation (if patient is intubated and mechanically ventilated) Evidence of pneumothorax on chest radiograph Notify physician if any of these signs develop, and prepare for chest tube insertion or tap, as ordered

POTENTIAL PROBLEMS	EXPECTED OUTCOMES	NURSING ACTIVITIES
		Monitor for signs of development of *tension pneumothorax*
		Marked respiratory distress
		Restlessness or agitation with significant respiratory distress
		Mediastinal shift away from side of pneumothorax (heart sounds will be heard better on side of chest opposite pneumothorax)
		Hypotension (caused by decreased venous return and decreased ventricular diastolic filling)
		High peak inspiratory pressures and extreme difficulty in providing hand ventilation (if patient is intubated and receiving mechanical ventilatory support)
		Decreased arterial oxygen tension and possible cyanosis
		Notify physician immediately of these findings; emergency decompression of pneumothorax is essential; prepare for emergency needle aspiration of pneumothorax or chest tube insertion
		Monitor for signs of development of *hemothorax* or *pleural effusion*
		Increased respiratory rate and effort (if patient is breathing spontaneously)
		Decreased intensity or change in quality of breath sounds
		Dullness to percussion of chest
		Increased peak inspiratory pressures or resistance to hand ventilation (if patient is intubated and receiving mechanical ventilatory assistance)
		Evidence of free pleural fluid on chest radiograph (this will be especially apparent if lateral decubitus film is obtained)
		If significant hemothorax develops, patient may develop signs of circulatory compromise caused by hypovolemia (see Problem, Postoperative hypovolemia)
		Notify physician if any of these signs develop and prepare for thoracentesis and/or chest tube insertion
		Check patient chest radiograph as ordered or per unit policy
		Observe appearance of chest tube drainage (if pleural tube is in place); if lymph is present or if large amounts of serosanguineous fluid are draining continuously, notify physician; chest tube is usually left in place until such drainage ceases
		If *chylothorax* is present, chest drainage often becomes milky after patient ingests food or liquid containing fat
		If *chylothorax* is present, chest tube may be left in place to prevent development of respiratory insufficiency; child may be placed on special (medium-chain triglyceride) diet to reduce quantity of drainage; child usually also requires administration of supplemental fat-soluble vitamins (A, D, and E)
		See Problems, CHF; Low cardiac output; Pulmonary hypertension
		Ensure provision of adequate ventilatory support if child is intubated
		Monitor chest expansion and aeration; child's chest is soft and compliant, and therefore will move if adequate inspiratory volume is provided—*if child's chest is not expanding with inspiration, ventilatory support is not adequate*
		Notify physician and check endotracheal tube patency, position, and effectiveness of ventilation; if child appears restless, irritable, or cyanotic, suction and provide hand ventilation as necessary
		Provide effective tidal volume (7 to 20 ml/kg—specific volume is determined by patient's problem, manufacturer's recommendations, ventilator dead space and tubing compliance, and unit policy) and PEEP (2 to 4 cm H_2O is considered physiological), as ordered
		Verify ventilator settings and measure vital signs at least q1 hr and more often if patient's condition changes; ensure that humidification of inspired air is adequate
		Check patient's arterial blood gas levels per hospital policy or physician's order; notify physician of abnormal results

POTENTIAL PROBLEMS	EXPECTED OUTCOMES	NURSING ACTIVITIES
		Frequently verify tube patency and proper endotracheal tube position through frequent auscultation of breath sounds and provision of pulmonary toilet
		Hand-ventilate patient and suction as needed to keep endotracheal tube clear and lungs clear to auscultation
		Turn patient frequently (if condition is stable), and provide percussion, vibration, and rib-springing, as needed
		Provide postural drainage if needed, as ordered (per patient condition or unit policy)
		If problems arise
		Hand-ventilate patient while ventilator is checked
		Assure tube patency and adequate lung aeration
		Notify physician if hand-ventilation is difficult or unsuccessful
		If tube is obstructed, it may be necessary to remove tube and hand-ventilate child with bag and mask until tube can be replaced
		NOTE: If child "fights" ventilator and hypoxemia is not present it may be necessary to paralyze child to provide effective ventilation; if child will be paralyzed, it is important to tell child that he/she will not be able to move, and it is also imperative that child continue to receive analgesics; see Standard 6, *Mechanical ventilation*
		Monitor child's arterial blood gas levels (as ordered and per unit policy) and discuss results with physician
		When the child is extubated
		Elevate head of bed (to allow maximal diaphragmatic excursion) and place small linen roll under child's shoulders (to extend airway)
		Monitor for signs of upper airway obstruction (stridor, decreased air movement, increased respiratory effort) as result of subglottic edema
		Monitor effectiveness of child's spontaneous ventilation
		Provide bronchial (postural) drainage, chest percussion and vibration, rib-springing, and deep-breathing exercises as needed; see Standard 8, *Chest physiotherapy*
		Ensure proper function of chest drainage system (if present)
		Provide adequate pain medication per physician's order; if child is breathing spontaneously, be alert for signs of respiratory depression if narcotics are administered
		Assist child in splinting chest incision to minimize discomfort and maximize inspiratory effort when child attempts to cough or take deep breaths
■ Electrolyte imbalance related to Use of CPB Use of diuretics Stress response Fluid and blood component administration	■ Serum electrolyte concentrations within normal limits Absence of any secondary signs or complications of electrolyte imbalance	■ Monitor serum electrolytes; in young infants, serum glucose, calcium, and K$^+$ balance should be monitored closely during periods of illness or stress Refer to problem, Decreased cardiac contractility, for guidelines for administration of sodium bicarbonate and electrolyte supplements If metabolic acidosis, hypoglycemia, hypocalcemia, hypokalemia, or hyperkalemia develop, monitor patient closely for evidence of depressed cardiovascular function or arrhythmias or for other systemic signs of electrolyte imbalance (such as decrease in muscle tone or neuromuscular irritability)
■ Renal dysfunction related to Poor systemic perfusion Intravascular hemolysis Thromboembolus Complications of medications	■ Urine output of 0.5 to 1.0 ml/kg/hour when fluid intake is adequate Appropriate urine concentration when urine volume is reduced Serum creatinine and BUN within normal limits	■ Measure urine output, and discuss with physician if output totals less than 0.5 to 1.0 ml/kg/hour Test urine for presence of blood and protein; monitor specific gravity q4 hr postoperatively

POTENTIAL PROBLEMS	EXPECTED OUTCOMES	NURSING ACTIVITIES

		If problem occurs
		   Administer fluid bolus totalling 5 to 10 ml/kg and diuretic (e.g., furosemide) if child's urine output is inadequate and CVP is low
		   Initiate fluid restriction as ordered if urine output remains inadequate despite presence of adequate circulating blood volume (CVP or right or left atrial pressure of 5 to 10 mm Hg) and administration of diuretics
		
		See STANDARD 52 *Acute renal failure*
		        STANDARD 53 *Peritoneal dialysis*
		        STANDARD 54 *Hemodialysis*
		
		Urine sample should be spun down in centrifuge if red urine is observed; if blood precipitates after spinning, this suggests that whole RBCs are present in urine, and bleeding is probably from bladder trauma; if, despite centrifuge spinning, urine remains rusty in color, this suggests that urine contains RBC fragments as result of intravascular hemolysis
		   NOTE: If intravascular hemolysis is present, it is important that adequate urine flow be maintained to "flush" RBC fragments from kidneys (especially glomeruli); adequate urine flow may be maintained through judicious use of fluid and diuretic administration (per physician's order)
		Restrict child's fluid intake to equal urine output plus child's insensible fluid losses (if this is possible without compromising systemic perfusion) if acute tubular necrosis or renal failure is suspected, closely monitor child's serum creatinine, BUN, and K$^+$
		If renal dysfunction is suspected and urine output is present, simultaneous sample of urine and serum for creatinine measurement will probably be requested to attempt to determine child's urine creatinine clearance
		Prepare patient for peritoneal dialysis or hemodialysis, as ordered, if child becomes severely hypervolemic, hyperkalemic, uremic, or acidotic
		Reevaluate drug dosages for any drug that requires renal excretion if urine output falls
		Administer calcium, glucose and insulin, or sodium polystyrene sulfonate (Kayexalate) enema as ordered if hyperkalemia develops (see Appendix D for dosage)

■ Neurological impairment related to
  Hypoxia
  Acidosis
  Poor systemic perfusion
  Thromboembolism
  Electrolyte imbalance
  Prolonged undetected seizure activity
	■ Maximal neurological functioning with no abnormal posturing, clonus, or flaccidity
	Age-appropriate response to stimulation and questions
	Brisk, equal pupil constriction in response to light
		■ Assess child's neurological function as soon as possible after surgery
		  Check pupil size, equality, and response to light
		    If child is awake, check movement and strength of all extremities
		    If child is asleep, note muscle tone and withdrawal from mildly noxious stimuli
		Report any abnormal findings to physician immediately
		  NOTE: Pupil dilatation is normally present when patient is receiving sympathomimetic agents (e.g., dopamine)
		Assist in correction of hypotension, hypoxemia, or acidosis (per physician's order) as quickly as possible to prevent neurological sequelae
		  Assess child's neurological status if any of these problems arise
		If neurological impairment is suspected, discuss plan of care with physician immediately, and document *all* information that is given to parents in nursing care plan so that consistent information can be provided
		If neurological impairment is present, begin to provide passive ROM exercises to prevent development of contractures
		  Obtain order for physiotherapy or occupational therapy consultation
		  Develop rehabilitative care plan and share this with all members of health care team

POTENTIAL PROBLEMS	EXPECTED OUTCOMES	NURSING ACTIVITIES
		Monitor for evidence of seizure activity; if child requires paralyzing agents postoperatively, clinical diagnosis of seizure activity becomes very difficult; suspect seizures if child demonstrates wide fluctuations in BP in absence of any cardiovascular problem or changes in pupil size and reactivity; electroencephalogram (EEG) is often required to determine if seizures are present in these children
		If seizures develop, notify physician immediately and position patient for maximal safety—*do not stick anything in patient's mouth* once patient is in clonic state (unless airway obstruction develops)
		Check blood gas and serum electrolyte concentrations (as ordered or per unit policy), particularly if metabolic imbalance is thought to be cause of seizures
		Report any abnormal results to physician
		Administer anticonvulsant medications as ordered; check dosage and monitor for therapeutic effect, side effects, and anticonvulsant drug levels
		See STANDARD 41 *Seizures*
		Provide for periods of rest, and attempt to reduce visual and auditory stimulation
		Provide meaningful stimulation between periods of rest; orient child to time and place, and reinforce information that surgery is over and that parents are nearby
		Administer pain medications as needed
		Monitor for signs of increased ICP if hypoxic encephalopathy is present
		Increased irritability or lethargy
		Pupillary dilatation or constriction and decreased response to light
		Bradycardia
		Changes in respiratory pattern (if patient is breathing spontaneously)
		Increased systolic BP with widening of pulse pressure (this is a very *late* sign)
		Report signs of increased ICP to physician immediately; attempt to hyperventilate patient, if ordered, since this can produce immediate temporary reduction in cerebral blood volume and ICP
		See STANDARD 32 *Increased intracranial pressure*
		If increased ICP is present
		Administer osmotic diuretics (e.g., mannitol) and/or steroids (e.g., dexamathasone) as ordered
		Administer antipyretics (with physician's order) if rectal temperature exceeds 39° C (102.2° F)
■ Infection or inflammation as result of Cardiovascular surgery Insertion of prosthetic material Invasive monitoring techniques Compromised nutritional status Postcardiotomy syndrome	■ Infection free Absence of: Fever above 38.5° C (101.3° F) Chills Leukocytosis Local wound infection or inflammation (including erythema, wound exudate, or wound fluctuation) Positive wound cultures Positive blood cultures	■ Keep all incisions and venous and arterial entrance sites clean and dry
		Change all dressings according to hospital policy; apply occlusive dressings and iodophor ointment (per physician's order and unit policy) to all central venous lines
		Observe all skin puncture sites for signs of erythema, drainage, or fluctuation; notify physician of any signs of inflammation
		Maintain strict aseptic technique when handling invasive equipment; ensure that all staff members wash hands before and after each patient contact
		Calculate child's maintenance caloric requirements
		If child is unable to take oral maintenance calories within 24 to 48 hours after surgery, discuss alternative methods of alimentation with physician (e.g., NG feeding or parenteral alimentation); see Standard 57, *Total parenteral nutrition through central venous catheter*

POTENTIAL PROBLEMS	EXPECTED OUTCOMES	NURSING ACTIVITIES

	Absence or resolution of postcardiotomy syndrome; absence of
	Low-grade fever approximately 10 days postoperatively
	Leukocytosis
	Pleural or pericardial effusions
	Elevation of ESR
	Serologic evidence of antiheart antibodies
	Rise in viral titers
	If postcardiotomy syndrome develops, cardiovascular compromise will be prevented
		Monitor child's temperature; notify physician if fever over 101.3° F (38.5° C) develops; physician may order blood cultures (particularly if child's surgical repair required insertion of prosthetic material)
		NOTE: Neonates may become *hypothermic* when serious infection develops, and infants and children may develop acidosis and thrombocytopenia when sepsis develops
		Assess for evidence of overt infection
		Monitor for evidence of urinary tract infection, including
		  Burning sensation with urination (or other signs of patient discomfort with voiding)
		  Cloudy or odorous urine
		  Hematuria
		NOTE: Glucosuria may be sign of infection in children
		Monitor for signs of postcardiotomy syndrome approximately 7 to 10 days after surgery, including
		  Fever over 101.3° F (38.5° C)
		  Substernal or pericardial chest pain, which is exacerbated by respiration and may radiate to shoulder
		  Pericardial friction rub
		  Pericardial effusion (may be apparent on echocardiogram)
		  Pleural effusion (may be evident on clinical examination and chest radiograph)
		  Leukocytosis
		  Malaise or arthralgia
		  Elevation in ESR
		  Serologic evidence of antiheart antibodies
		  Rise in viral titers
		  Serial electrocardiographic evidence of pericarditis
		Report these findings to physician
		If postcardiotomy syndrome develops, administer aspirin and/or steroids, as ordered
		Administer antibiotics as ordered; check dosage and monitor for side effects

■ Insufficient knowledge to comply with discharge regimen	■ Patient (as appropriate) and family demonstrate knowledge of medications and care techniques necessary for child's care at home	■ Provide child (as age-appropriate) and parents with information necessary to manage child's care at home when patient's condition is stable, including
		  Dosage, route, effects, and side effects of all medications that child will receive
		  Times and intervals of child's follow-up appointments
		  Indications for contacting physician
		  Telephone numbers of child's primary nurse and physician
		  Techniques for any special care techniques (e.g., postural drainage)
		Initiate appropriate referral to supportive services, including
		  Social services
		  Visiting nurse or home care nurse
		  Outpatient physiotherapy
		  Outpatient physician contacts
		Document all teaching in child's care plan so that all information is reinforced consistently

VASCULAR DISEASE:
MEDICAL AND SURGICAL MANAGEMENT

Peripheral vascular diseases are a distinct group of diseases and syndromes that involve the arterial, venous, or lymphatic system and have well-defined clinical features. The term *peripheral vascular disease* in its broadest sense applies to disease of any of the blood vessels outside the heart and to diseases of the lymph vessels.

Arterial insufficiency and *ischemia* are the terms used to indicate inadequate arterial circulation. This condition is acute in arterial embolism and spasm and is chronic in arteriosclerosis obliterans and thromboangiitis obliterans. It is usually characterized by pain (intermittent claudication, neuropathy, or pain at rest), by absent or diminished arterial pulsation, and by color changes that are dependent on the position of the affected limb. Inadequate arterial circulation may also be manifested by ulceration, gangrene, coldness, and pallor of the skin.

Venous insufficiency indicates inadequate venous circulation. It is severe in acute ileofemoral thrombophlebitis and may be chronic in varicose vein disease. Acute venous insufficiency is usually characterized by swelling of the limb and prominent superficial veins. In chronic venous insufficiency, stasis dermatitis, pigmentation, and ulceration may also be present.

Arteries normally undergo an aging process characterized by an increase in the thickness of the intimal area, a loss of elasticity, an increase in calcium content, and a decrease in luminal diameter. These changes are thought to occur generally throughout the major arterial system and have been referred to as *arteriosclerosis*.

In contrast, *atherosclerosis* is characterized by the focal accumulation of lipids, carbohydrates, blood products, fibrous tissue, and calcium deposits, seen first in the intima of the arteries. The pathogenesis of atherosclerosis depends on a precise sequence of critical events occurring in the interaction of blood elements with the arterial wall. Risk factors may potentiate the critical events leading to atherosclerosis.

Evidence indicates that both lipid transport and platelet interaction with the arterial wall play important roles in the formation of atherosclerotic plaques. The characteristic localization of early lesions in the arterial tree may be a result of the anatomic presence of intimal cushions in these areas at the time of birth. The extent of intimal thickening increases with age, presumably because of stressors on the arterial wall, and this contributes to the development of atherosclerosis.

The major "critical events" in the development of atherosclerosis seem to be as follows:
1. Hemodynamic stress, endothelial injury, and arterial wall–platelet interaction
2. Smooth muscle cell proliferation
3. Lipid and lipoprotein entry and accumulation
4. Altered mechanisms of lipid removal
5. Fibrosis and development of thrombi
6. Ulceration, calcification, and formation of aneurysms

Chronic atherosclerotic occlusive disease of the extremities involves the aorta, its major branches to the limbs, and the arteries of the extremities. The great majority of cases affect the lower extremities and are caused by atherosclerosis of the terminal portion of the abdominal aorta, the ileofemoral and popliteal arteries, and the medium-sized arteries below the knee. The clinical disease is usually designated by a term such as *arteriosclerosis obliterans* or *atherosclerosis obliterans* and is often abbreviated ASO.

The diagnosis of arterial obstruction should be made by clinical assessment backed by lab data. In the majority of patients with occlusion or narrowing of the arterial supply to the extremities, clinical assessment is adequate to detect even mild degrees of narrowing. Intermittent claudication is strongly suggestive of occlusive arterial disease, but to diagnose atherosclerosis of the extremities definitely, one must establish the presence of occlusive arterial disease by objective examination. Pulsations may be absent or impaired. Postural color changes, particularly when they are unequal in the two limbs, are valuable but nonessential confirmatory evidence of occlusive arterial disease. Ischemic ulcers or gangrene of the digits is strongly suggestive of occlusive arterial disease.

Radiographic studies for the purpose of detecting arterial calcification may be of value in distinguishing atherosclerotic disease from other types of occlusive arterial disease. Calcification may be noted in the abdominal aorta and iliac, femoral, and anterior and posterior tibial arteries.

Arteriograms are rarely necessary to establish the diagnosis of occlusive arterial disease, and arteriography is not recommended as a routine diagnostic procedure. Arteriography *is* indicated in every case of atherosclerosis of the extremities in which arterial bypass surgery is being contemplated. Although the proximal sites of arterial occlusion can often be delineated by means of the history and physical examination, the surgeon requires more precise knowledge of the arterial inflow and outflow to assess operability and to plan the operation itself.

Noninvasive detection of blood flow using a commercially available ultrasound transducer is based on the *Doppler effect*. Sound waves reflected from a moving column of blood are changed in frequency to a degree that is proportional to the velocity of flow. The back-scattered sound is converted into an audible signal, which indicates that flow is present. Transcutaneous Doppler signals may be processed to produce analog recordings of flow velocity, and directional flow instruments are available for assessment of normal and pathologic directional flow changes.

Systolic ankle pressures measured at intervals after treadmill exercise are most useful in assessing the degree of lower limb ischemia. The pressures are obtained with the Doppler probe at either the posterior tibial or the dorsalis pedis position and a standard inflatable BP cuff just above the ankle. Systolic ankle pressures obtained at 1, 3, 5, and 10 minutes after exercise are compared with the simultaneously obtained brachial pressures, and the result may be expressed as an index. The more severe the ischemia, the lower the postexercise systolic ankle pressure becomes, and the longer it takes to return to preexercise levels.

The basic principles of *medical treatment* of atherosclerosis of the extremities include procedures designed to arrest progression of the disease, improve blood flow, relieve pain, and treat ulcers and gangrene.

Hyperlipidemia is generally accepted as a factor in the pathogenesis of atherosclerosis. Primary hyperlipidemia is often familial. Dietary measures are fundamental to most efforts to reduce abnormally high blood lipid levels. For primary hypercholesterolemia, the diet is restricted in cholesterol and saturated fats, which usually occur together in foods. For a mild disorder, the so-called prudent diet is often recommended. This diet is limited in egg yolks, shellfish, butterfat-containing dairy products, and fatty meats.

Bile acid sequestrants are anion-exchange resins that bind bile acids in the intestine, and the resulting complex is then excreted in the feces. This increased fecal loss leads to a decline in the concentration of cholesterol, the precursor of the bile acids. Bile acid sequestrants are generally well tolerated and are moderately effective in patients who have hypercholesterolemia.

Large doses of niacin are used for patients with hypercholesterolemia that is refractory to diet and other medication. Although large doses of niacin may control hyperlipidemia for long periods, the patients should be assessed cautiously, because serious side effects may occur. These include abnormal liver function tests and even jaundice, abnormal glucose tolerance, hyperuricemia, and, rarely, acute gouty arthritis. Some patients have also experienced symptoms of peptic ulceration while receiving long-term niacin therapy.

Diabetic patients with atherosclerosis should have optimal control of their diabetes, because diabetes increases the prevelance and severity of ASO. There is evidence to suggest that diabetes mellitus increases the incidence and severity of peripheral vascular disease. Reports have shown that arteriosclerotic gangrene of the extremities occurred about 40 times more commonly in diabetic patients than in nondiabetic patients over 50 years of age.

Nicotine produces peripheral vasoconstriction in almost all persons. For this reason alone, tobacco smoking has an unfavorable effect on patients with ASO and should be discontinued.

It is generally conceded that hypertension increases the rate of development of atherosclerosis in coronary arteries. However, evidence that hypertension is an important factor in the pathogenesis of atherosclerosis of the extremities is not well documented.

Patients with ASO who receive anticoagulants are less likely to have complete occlusions, and they have less of a tendency for propagation of occlusive thrombi than similar patients not treated with anticoagulants.

The use of vasodilators in patients with chronic arterial occlusive disease is controversial. It has been demonstrated, for instance, that vasodilator drugs will dilatate vessels in normal vascular beds, divert flow to these beds, and actually further reduce flow to an ischemic limb.

Destruction of sympathetic ganglia may be accomplished by the careful injection of small amounts of absolute ethyl alcohol into the region of the second or third lumbar sympathetic ganglion. The effect is frequently not permanent, and sympathetic function may return in 6 to 12 months. Arterial flow can be improved by the vasodilatation produced by a sympathectomy.

The factors that produce atherosclerosis of the lower extremities are likely to lead to similar lesions in other arteries of the body. The coronary and cerebral arteries are of particular interest in this respect, because occlusive lesions of these arteries have serious prognostic implications. Symptomatic coronary or cerebral artery disease may precede or follow the clinical manifestations of lower extremity disease. Most patients who have atherosclerosis of the lower extremities die of coronary heart disease or in a manner highly suggestive of it.

Patients with atherosclerosis of the extremities have a

shortened life expectancy. The 5-year survival rate of non-diabetic patients in whom aortoiliac occlusive disease develops before the age of 60 years is approximately 73%.

The goal of vascular *surgical treatment* of atherosclerosis is the restoration of circulation to the affected extremities. Patients presenting with far advanced occlusive disease usually have more severe atherosclerotic disease than those whose only presenting symptom is claudication. The success rate is directly related to the degree of underlying disease, collateral circulation, age, and BP control/abnormalities.

The surgeries described in Table 29-1 are the most common ones performed to relieve occlusive disease of the lower extremities.

TABLE 29-1. Common vascular surgeries

SURGERY	DEFINITION AND RATIONALE	REPRESENTATION
Femoral-femoral bypass	Performed in poor-risk patients who present with unilateral claudication or ischemia; this surgery is performed only if donor artery has no marked proximal stenosis.	
Femoropopliteal bypass	Remains the standard operation for relieving ischemic symptoms secondary to femoropopliteal occlusive disease; patients presenting with this disease process usually have involvement of distal popliteal artery and its tibial branches as well	
Aortoiliac bypass	Limb-threatening ischemia is not usually seen with aortoiliac occlusions unless femoropopliteal disease is also present; aortoiliac occlusive disease is that in which distal aorta, including iliac arteries, is affected	
Aortobifemoral bypass	Same as aortoiliac	
Sympathectomy	Infrequently performed in addition to arterial bypass surgery; its use is said to improve early patency of new grafts by increasing total limb blood flow during early postoperative period	
Amputations	Performed only when extensive destruction of tissues that cannot be treated conservatively is present; degree of amputation depends solely on extent of disease present; immediate amputation of limb is indicated when uncontrolled sepsis, associated with abscesses, and severe cellulitis are encountered	

ASSESSMENT

1. History—nature, presence and severity of
   a. MI and/or angina (plaques within the coronary arteries)
   b. Cerebrovascular disease (plaques within the carotid arteries)
   c. Intermittent claudication (include frequency and distance required to elicit symptoms)
   d. Asymmetrical coldness of extremities
   e. Limb pain while patient is supine (sign of ischemic pain)
2. Previous and current medical therapy and prior surgery
3. Clinical signs and symptoms, including
   a. Decreased or absent pulses unilaterally
      (1) Temporal arteries
      (2) Carotid arteries
      (3) Subclavian arteries
      (4) Axillary arteries
      (5) Brachial arteries
      (6) Radial and ulnar arteries
      (7) Iliac arteries
      (8) Femoral arteries
      (9) Popliteal arteries
      (10) Dorsalis Pedis artery
      (11) Posterior tibial artery
   b. Disappearance of pulses after exercise
   c. Abnormal skin temperature of affected limb
   d. Auscultation—murmurs or bruits may be produced by arteriovenous fistulae, aneurysms, or vascular tumors
   e. Topical inspection
      (1) Persistent cyanosis
      (2) Chronic ulcers or gangrenous lesions
      (3) Pallor of the skin
      (4) Stasis dermatitis
      (5) Increased pigmentation
      (6) Decreased capillary refill
   f. Impairment of nerve function secondary to ischemia of affected extremity
   g. Cerebral status
      (1) LOC, noting abnormalities
      (2) Episodes of syncope (decreased carotid blood flow)
4. Weight
5. ECG, BP, (record BP on both arms), and P: note abnormalities
6. Results of lab tests, including
   a. Arteriogram
   b. Doppler studies
   c. Systolic ankle pressures
   d. Hgb, Hct, and platelet counts
   e. Coagulation studies
   f. Kidney function tests
   g. Liver function tests
   h. Blood lipid levels
7. Patient/family's knowledge regarding disease condition
   a. Family roles regarding illness
   b. What they have been told
   c. Their expectations
   d. Fears and previous experiences
   e. If surgery is being considered and patient/family has been told
      (1) Reactions to surgery
      (2) Knowledge of surgical procedure and teaching if appropriate

GOALS

1. Reduction of patient/family's anxiety with provision of information and encouragement
2. Patient uses available support systems
3. Patient verbalizes acceptance of diagnosis and asks pertinent questions regarding future management
4. Absence of pain; patient verbalizes comfort
5. Patent graft postoperatively
6. Hemodynamic stability; absence of complications
7. Absence of embolic complications
8. Absence of infection
9. Nutrition adequate to maintain a positive nitrogen balance and prevent loss of weight
10. Maintenance of preoperative pulmonary function
    a. Arterial blood gas levels within patient's normal limits
    b. Clear lungs on auscultation
    c. Full lung expansion
11. Maintenance of preoperative renal function
    a. Urine output greater than 30 ml/hour
    b. Normovolemia
    c. Lab indices within normal (or preoperative) limits
12. Before discharge, the patient/family
    a. Describes the follow-up regimen
    b. Describes the plan for follow-up visits
    c. Describes the activity regimen
    d. Describes the rationale, dosage, frequency of administration, and potential adverse effects of any medications
    e. Describes the symptoms requiring immediate medical attention and the steps to take to obtain it

POTENTIAL PROBLEMS	EXPECTED OUTCOMES	NURSING ACTIVITIES
Medical management		
■ Patient/family's anxiety related to insufficient information regarding Disease process Hospitalization Diagnostic procedures Altered life-style Therapeutic regimen	■ Reduction in patient/family's anxiety with provision of information and encouragement	■ Ongoing assessment of patient/family's anxiety Ongoing assessment of patient/family's knowledge of disease process, planned diagnostic tests, therapeutic regimen, possible surgery, and anticipated dependency/altered life-style Collaborate with other health care team members concerning teaching to be done Discuss disease process with patient/family, including any symptoms patient may be experiencing Thoroughly explain all planned diagnostic tests Provide opportunity for patient/family verbalization of anxiety, questions, and fears
■ Discomfort/pain related to ischemia	■ Absence or resolution of pain/discomfort	■ Assess patient for presence and nature of pain; note quality, site and severity of pain Assess influence of pain on ADL Assess level of activity at which discomfort or pain occurs Administer Analgesics as ordered Vasodilatory agents as ordered; monitor for increase/decrease in perfusion Monitor for relief of pain Assist patient in altering ADL to compensate for altered life-style/dependency
■ Tissue ischemia in affected limbs	■ Absence of tissue ischemia Adequate arterial blood flow	■ Assess extent of tissue ischemia and arterial flow to affected areas Quality of pulses Limb color Level of discomfort Temperature Immobility Doppler-flow studies Explain noninvasive and invasive vascular studies, such as Arteriograms Doppler studies Systolic ankle BP measurements Monitor test results Notify physician of abnormal signs and symptoms If problem occurs, administer the following as ordered Analgesics Vasodilatory agents; monitor for increase/decrease in perfusion Prepare patient for possible surgery, if planned
■ Insufficient information to comply with discharge regimen	■ Sufficient information to comply with regimen	■ Assess patient/family's understanding of discharge regimen Instruct patient/family About medications, including name, route, dosage, and potential side effects To report any increase in pain To report any limb discoloration To report any temperature difference in limb To keep affected limb warm To avoid massaging affected limb In ways to avoid smoking To avoid remaining in one position for lengthy periods of time Describe follow-up plan of care with frequent visits and monitoring of disease process Provide opportunity for patient/family verbalization of questions and fears Reassess potential compliance to discharge regimen

POTENTIAL PROBLEMS	EXPECTED OUTCOMES	NURSING ACTIVITIES

Surgical management

■ Patient/family anxiety related to insufficient information regarding

   Diagnostic and preparatory tests before surgery

   Surgery, its expected outcomes, and potential problems

■ Reduction in patient/family anxiety with provision of information and encouragement

■ Ongoing assessment of patient/family's anxiety

   Assess patient/family's knowledge and understanding of certain diagnostic tests, rationales for these tests, and what patient will experience

   Explain, in simple terms, disease process, need for surgery, expected outcomes (and associated benefits), and potential problems

   Explain purpose of diagnostic tests and what patient will experience

   Encourage patient/family to verbalize fears and ask questions

   Assess reduction in level of anxiety with provision of information, explanations, and encouragement

■ Hemodynamic instability related to

   Hypotension secondary to

      Hypovolemia

      Hemorrhage

   Hypertension

■ Hemodynamic stability, BP, P, CVP, PAP/PCWP, urine output, and Hgb/Hct within patient's normal limits

   Absence of postoperative hemorrhage

■ Prevent by administering ordered fluid and blood products to maintain adequate intravascular volume

   Monitor BP and P q15 min and prn until stable, then q½ hr for 2 hours, then q1 hr

   Monitor for evidence of hypovolemia, hemorrhage

      Hypotension

      Tachycardia

      Weak, thready pulses

      Decreased CVP/PAP if available

      Decreased urine output

      Decreased Hct/Hgb

      Cool, mottled extremities

      Altered LOC

   Monitor abdominal girth q2 hr for 24 hours or until stable, if appropriate for surgery performed

   Monitor affected limb girth q2 hr for 24 hours or until stable, if appropriate for surgery performed

   Notify physician of abnormalities in the aforementioned

   If hemorrhage occurs

      Administer fluid and/or blood products as ordered

      Frequently assess hemodynamic profile as previously stated

   If hypovolemia occurs as result of hemorrhage

      Administer fluids, blood, and blood products as ordered

      Continually assess hemodynamic profile as previously stated

   If hypertension occurs

      Administer antihypertensive and/or diuretic medications as ordered

      Closely monitor hemodynamic profile as previously stated

      All potent antihypertensive medications should *only* be administered via infusion pump, and monitoring of BP should be accomplished by use of intraarterial catheter

■ Graft occlusion

■ Patent graft

■ Prevention

   Turn patient maintaining straight legs and support legs with pillows

   Avoid turning axillobifemoral bypass patient onto grafted side

   Monitor all circulatory parameters distal to graft

      Pulses

      Color

      Temperature

      Sensation

   Notify physician of abnormalities in aforementioned

   Administer therapy as ordered and monitor patient's response

■ Embolic formation related to possible dislodgement of atherosclerotic plaque or thrombus

■ Absence of emboli

■ Prevention

   Apply antithromboembolic stockings where indicated and ordered

   Administer anticoagulants if ordered

   Assist patient with ROM exercises

   Monitor for signs and symptoms of

      Pulmonary emboli and infarction

      Cerebrovascular emboli and infarction

      Renal emboli and infarction

   Notify physician of abnormalities in aforementioned

   If embolism/infarction occurs, administer therapy as ordered

See STANDARD 31 *Embolic phenomena*

POTENTIAL PROBLEMS	EXPECTED OUTCOMES	NURSING ACTIVITIES

■ Infection
  Wound
  Vascular graft
  Blood
	■ Infection free
	  Afebrile
		■ Prevention
		    Use aseptic technique for wound care
		    Administer prophylactic antibiotics, if ordered
		  Monitor for
		    Elevated temperature
		    Erythematous, inflamed wound
		    Purulent wound drainage
		    Diaphoresis, shaking, chills
		    Tachycardia
		    Altered LOC
		    Elevated WBC count
		    Positive blood culture
		  Notify physician of any abnormalities
		  Administer therapy as ordered (e.g., antibiotics) and monitor patient's response
		
		  See STANDARD 61 *Infection control in the critical care unit*

■ Respiratory insufficiency	■ Adequate respiratory function	■ Prevention
		    Administer chest physiotherapy q2-4 hr and prn
		    Encourage deep breathing and coughing
		    Administer humidified, oxygenated air, as ordered
		    Assist patient with incentive spirometry as ordered
		    Employ tracheal suctioning as necessary
		  Monitor
		    Rate and quality of respirations q1 hr
		    For decreased or absent breath sounds and/or rales or rhonchi
		    For signs and symptoms of hypoxia
		    Chest radiographic results
		    Arterial blood gas results
		  Notify physician of abnormalities and alter therapeutic regimen as ordered
		
		  See STANDARD 2 *Acute respiratory failure*

■ Renal insufficiency	■ Indices of renal function within normal limits	■ Prevention
		    Administer fluids, blood, and blood products as ordered to maintain adequate cardiac output and kidney perfusion
		    Administer inotropic agents, if ordered, to increase renal blood flow and urine output
		    Administer diuretics as ordered, monitoring patient's response
		  Monitor
		    For signs of inadequate cardiac output: hypovolemia; hypotension, tachycardia, low CVP, PAP (if available); oliguria
		    Lab indices of renal function, including BUN, uric acid; serum and urine creatinine and electrolyte levels
		    Arterial blood gas results for acid-base imbalance
		  Notify physician of any abnormalities and administer therapy as ordered
		  If kidney dysfunction or failure occurs, see Standard 52, *Acute renal failure*

■ Myocardial ischemia	■ Absence or early resolution of myocardial ischemia	■ Monitor for
		    Chest pain
		    ECG changes indicating ischemia
		    BP, P, PAP, CVP (if available) during episode of chest pain
		  Notify physician of any abnormalities
		  If angina occurs
		    Administer antianginal medications as ordered and monitor patient response
		    Monitor BP, P, q15 min and prn until anginal chest pain resolves
		
		  See STANDARD 11 *Angina pectoris*

- Insufficient knowledge for compliance with discharge regimen*

- Before discharge
  Patient/family verbalizes knowledge of discharge regimen, including precautions, medications, diet, and activity
  Patient/family is able to describe follow-up plan, including where and when to go, who to see, and what specimens to bring
  Patient/family accurately describes signs and symptoms requiring medical attention

- Assess patient/family's understanding of discharge regimen, including dietary regimen, medications, activity modifications, and special precautionary measures
  Describe discharge regimen, including
    Medications—purpose, identification of, route, dosage, timing, frequency, and potential adverse effects
    Dietary regimen
    Activity progression; position modifications
    Avoidance of constricting clothing
    Avoidance of one position being maintained for more than 1 hour
    Monitoring circulation to affected extremity
  Instruct patient/family in specific measures according to residual impaired organ circulation and associated dysfunction
  Describe signs and symptoms requiring medical attention, depending on site of vascular disease and outcome of surgery
  Discuss plan for follow-up visits with patient/family, including where and when to go, who to see, and what specimens to bring
  Provide opportunity for and encourage patient/family's questions and verbalization of anxiety regarding discharge regimen

*If critical care nurse is responsible for this type of follow-up care.

VASCULAR SURGERY: ANEURYSMS

An aneurysm is a local dilatation of a weakened vessel wall. A true aneurysm involves a ballooning of the entire wall, whereas a false aneurysm involves a tear in the vessel lining that allows blood to collect outside the artery. Bleeding is contained by the surrounding tissues, producing a cavity that is surrounded by a clot but that connects with the arterial lumen.

Aneurysms most commonly occur in the aorta, although they are also found in the cerebral arteries, in the ventricle of the heart after a MI, and in other central and peripheral vessels.

The etiology of aneurysms may be classified as hereditary (e.g., congenital abnormalities, connective tissue abnormalities of the vessels, arteriovenous communications) or acquired (e.g., mycotic, syphilitic, traumatic, atherosclerotic, or dissecting lesions).

The atherosclerotic lesions involve intimal degeneration, subintimal proliferation, fibrosis and atrophy of the underlying media and associated weakening of the vessel wall. Calcification of the lining often develops as the fibrotic process continues. These lesions are often precursors of atherosclerotic aneurysms, which occur most often in the abdominal aorta between the origin of the renal arteries and the aortic bifurcation. Occasionally, the thoracic aorta and other vessels are involved.

A predisposing factor for aneurysm formation is hypertension. Hypertension adds to the mechanical pressure and force of turbulent blood flow against a weakened vessel wall and is thus associated with a greater tendency for aneurysm rupture and dissection.

Aortic aneurysms are classified into five major types according to location: thoracic-ascending, transverse, descending; thoracoabdominal, and abdominal.

Ascending thoracic aneurysms are located in the ascending portion of the thoracic aorta, which is the portion of the aorta closest to the heart.

Aneurysms of the transverse aortic arch involve the carotid, subclavian, and upper vertebral arteries. Aneurysms of the descending thoracic aorta are located in the proximal portion of the descending aorta.

Thoracoabdominal aneurysms extend from immediately above the diaphragm to the subdiaphragmatic aorta. This type is occasionally associated with reduced blood flow to the celiac, superior mesenteric, and renal arteries. Abdominal aneurysms are located below the renal arteries and extend to the iliac artery, which is commonly involved to some extent.

Dissecting aneurysms involve progressive longtitudinal tearing of the media from the intima. If a rapid aortic dissection occurs, serious hemodynamic compromise results and may lead to cardiovascular collapse.

Most aneurysms are asymptomatic until they begin to leak, rapidly enlarge, or dissect. When any of these occur, the primary symptom is pain. Pain may develop as a result of the direct expansile process or as a result of hypoperfusion of an organ or an extremity (i.e., bowel ischemia).

Physical signs of aneurysms include a palpable pulsatile mass, pulse differences in the extremities, and evidence consistent with an intracranial, intrathoracic, or intraabdominal mass.

Aneurysms may first be observed as masses on a radiograph if the walls are calcified. Conclusive diagnosis can be reached by ultrasonography and arteriography.

Medical management is employed when the patient is admitted with a dissecting aneurysm. Hypertensive patients are treated with potent vasodilators to immediately lower the BP. If possible, continuous pressure monitoring should be provided for such patients.

Other types of aneurysms of the ascending thoracic aorta and abdominal aorta may be treated surgically. Surgery is performed if the aneurysm is compromising blood flow to distal or adjacent organs or is large enough to suggest that the risk of rupture is significant. Surgical repair can prevent extension of the aneurysm and reduce ischemic injury and the risk of rupture. Restoration of circulation to arteries and organs adjacent and distal to the aneurysm improves organ function. The aneurysm is either excised with a primary anastomosis or an interposition graft, or bypassed using a synthetic graft.

Hazards of surgery include hemorrhage and ischemic injury to the involved end organs during the surgical repair. Severe intraoperative ischemia can occasionally produce visceral organ ischemia (e.g., kidney or liver with thoracoabdominal aneurysms) or spinal cord ischemia.

Each type of aneurysm has unique potential preoperative and postoperative complications depending on the nature, location, and extent of the aneurysm and the difficulty of operative repair.

Mortality varies according to the location of the aneurysm. The lowest mortalities are reported for abdominal aortic and peripheral aneurysms in the lower extremities (less than 2%). The risk increases for aneurysms of the ascending or transverse thoracic aorta where the carotid and coronary arteries and aortic valve are commonly involved. Surgical outcome is also determined by the patient's age, BP abnormalities, and the degree of atherosclerosis present.

Postoperative nursing care is focused on achieving optimal hemodynamic stability. Therapy is directed toward preventing, monitoring for, and, if necessary, resolving problems associated with ischemic injury.

ASSESSMENT

1. If patient is known to have an aneurysm and presents with cardiovascular collapse, the aneurysm may be dissecting or have ruptured; obtain a brief history from patient or family while patient is prepared for emergency surgery
2. History, nature, presence, and severity of
   a. Palpitations, angina (aortic valve insufficiency, decreased coronary blood flow)
   b. Syncope (decreased carotid artery blood flow)
   c. Dyspnea (aneurysm compression of trachea, bronchus)
   d. Hoarseness (compression of recurrent laryngeal nerve)
   e. Abdominal pain (decreased mesenteric blood flow, aneurysm compression of abdominal organs)
   f. Bloody diarrhea (ischemic bowel)
   g. Hematuria (ischemic bowel)
   g. Hematuria (ischemic kidney)
   h. Painful, weak extremities (ischemia)
3. Previous and current medical therapy and prior surgery
4. Clinical signs and symptoms, including
   a. Deficits in circulation to extremities
      (1) Painful, weak extremities; presence of ischemic pain in one arm that is constant and nagging in character; pulsating mass present with decreased circulation distal to mass
      (2) Quality of pulses distal to aneurysm, noting fullness, pattern of filling, and occlusion pressure; note presence of edema
      (3) Capillary circulation of extremity distal to vascular problem—note color, relative temperature (warmth versus coolness), sympathetic discharge (clamminess versus dryness)
      (4) Impairment of nerve function secondary to ischemia of affected extremity

   b. Cardiac status
      (1) Note abnormalities in BP, P, and heart sounds and, if available, CVP and PAP/PCWP; ECG and presence of arrhythmias
      (2) Note signs of insufficient blood flow—angina, palpitations (may also indicate aortic valve insufficiency)
   c. Pulmonary status, including
      (1) Rate and quality of respirations
      (2) Breath sounds
      (3) Arterial blood gas levels
      (4) Signs of distress; dyspnea; paroxysmal cough (aneurysm may compress trachea, bronchus); hoarseness (compression of recurrent laryngeal nerve)
   d. Renal status
      (1) Presence of flank pain
      (2) Hematuria
      (3) Note abnormalities in volume of urine and specific gravity
   e. GI status, including presence of
      (1) Abdominal pain (decreased mesenteric blood flow or compression of abdominial organs by aneurysm)
      (2) Bloody diarrhea (ischemic bowel)
      (3) Dysphagia (impingement of esophagus)
   f. Cerebral status
      (1) LOC, noting any abnormalities
      (2) Any episode of syncope (decreased carotid blood flow)
      (3) Presence of unequal pupils (compression of cervical sympathetic chain)
5. Weight
6. Results of lab and diagnostic tests, including
   a. Hgb, Hct, and platelet levels
   b. Coagulation studies
   c. WBC count
   d. Kidney function tests
   e. Liver function tests
   f. ECG
   g. Radiographs
   h. Arteriography
   i. Aortograpy
   j. Cardiac catheterization
   k. Ultrasound studies, as appropriate
7. Patient/family's knowledge regarding operative therapy
   a. What they have been told
   b. Their expectations
   c. Fears regarding surgery and the outcome
   d. Previous experiences with surgery, if any
8. Information and detail surgeon has provided patient/family about the need for surgery, the actual surgery to be done, and the expected outcomes

9. Patient/family's level of anxiety related to disease condition, accompanying signs and symptoms of circulatory insufficiency, hospitalization, and family role alterations associated with illness

GOALS

1. Reduction in patient/family's anxiety with provision of information, explanations, and encouragement
2. Hemodynamic stability—absence of hemorrhage; minimal postoperative bleeding; aneurysm repaired with no recurrence; adequate circulation distal to vascular repair
3. Patent vessel, graft
4. Respiratory function within normal limits
   a. Arterial blood gas levels within normal limits
   b. Full lung expansion with no atelectasis, pulmonary interstitial edema, or compressed bronchus
   c. Afebrile without atelectasis or pneumonia
5. Acid-base balance and electrolyte levels within normal limits
6. Absence of signs of mesenteric ischemia, infarction
7. Kidney function adequate for removal of body's nitrogenous waste products and maintenance of body fluid volume
8. Nervous system function within normal limits; no evidence of cerebral embolus, infarction
9. Spinal function and associated neuromuscular, autonomic, genitourinary function within normal limits; absence of paralysis
10. Coagulation studies within normal limits; absence of emboli formation
11. Patient/family verbalizes knowledge of discharge regimen, including special precautionary measures, medications, diet, and activity modifications; patient/family able to describe follow-up plan of care including where and when to go, who to see, and what specimens to bring

POTENTIAL PROBLEMS	EXPECTED OUTCOMES	NURSING ACTIVITIES
Preoperative		

■ Patient/family's anxiety related to
Disease process
Hospitalization
Therapeutic regimen
Diagnostic tests planned
Impending major surgery and associated risks
Altered family roles
Separation from family members
Loss of job
	■ Reduction in patient/family's anxiety with provision of information, explanations, and encouragement	■ Ongoing assessment of level of patient/family's anxiety
		Assess patient/family's knowledge and understanding of disease process, therapeutic regimen, anticipated diagnostic procedures, and anticipated surgery, if planned
		Explain nature of patient's circulatory problem and symptoms patient is experiencing in simple terms
		Explain in simple terms what patient will experience during certain diagnostic procedures
		Assist in preparing patient for procedures, which may include radiographs, ECG, cardiac catheterization with angiography and ultrasonography as appropriate, if ordered
		Collaborate with physician and other health team members on teaching to be done
		When surgery is planned and physician has discussed it with patient/family, assess their understanding of information
		Reinforce purpose and nature of surgery and expected outcomes
		Describe perioperative experiences (adjust explanation according to patient's anxiety level and desire to know), including
		Preoperative
		    Orient patient to (call chest physiotherapist, if available)
		      Coughing and deep breathing
		      Incentive spirometry
		      Chest physiotherapy
		    Shave and light dinner
		    NPO after midnight
		    Medication for sleep if needed
		    Morning bath/shower
		    Preoperative medications
		    Hospital gowns
		    Care of valuables
		    Ride to operating room
		    Scrub suits, masks, and caps worn by operating room staff
		    Anesthesia

POTENTIAL PROBLEMS	EXPECTED OUTCOMES	NURSING ACTIVITIES
		Postoperative
		Waking up in recovery room/critical care unit
		Describe general environment (size of unit, room, etc.)
		Nurse always nearby
		Dull, continuous noises
		If anticipated, describe breathing tube that may be in place to ease patient's work of breathing and load on heart; explain that talking will not be possible while tube in place but that other means of communication will be possible
		NPO until breathing tube is removed
		Incision with bandage
		IV, arterial lines
		If anticipated, chest tubes, bloody drainage expected
		ECG monitoring
		Medicine for discomfort, pain
		Policy for family visits
		Describe responsibility of patient for achieving speedy recovery by taking active role in coughing and deep breathing to keep lungs clear and so on
		As patient progresses
		Tubes, lines out
		Eating again
		Chest physiotherapy, deep breathing, and coughing
		Getting stronger, ambulation
		Home again
		Provide opportunity for and encourage questions and verbalization of fears, anxieties
		Reassure patient that nurse will be nearby at all times
		Provide calm, quiet environment
		Perform treatments in unhurried manner, allowing rest periods between treatments
		Involve patient/family in planning for care
		Assess for reduction in level of patient/family's anxiety
■ Hemodynamic instability related to involvement of aortic valve *(ascending aortic aneurysm)*	■ Hemodynamic stability BP, P, CVP, PAP/PCWP, urine output, peripheral circulation, and mentation are within patient's normal limits	■ Evaluate nature of pain, particularly location and severity
		Assess cardiovascular status at least q½-1 hr until stable, and monitor
		For changes in BP
		Pulses: palpate and auscultate, noting peripheral perfusion
		Heart sounds, noting murmurs
		CVP and PAP if available
		ECG, noting presence of arrhythmias, signs of left ventricular hypertrophy, myocardial ischemia
		For symptoms of ischemia; complaints of angina, palpitations
		Assess circulation to extremities and monitor for changes; note
		Presence of pain, particularly pain that is constant and nagging in character
		Presence of pulsating mass with decreased circulation distal to mass
		Evaluate pulses distal to pulsating mass, noting fullness, pattern of filling, occlusion pressure
		Evaluate capillary circulation of extremities distal to vascular problem; note color, relative temperature (warmth versus coolness), sympathetic discharge (clamminess versus dryness)
		Monitor
		For impairment of nerve function secondary to ischemia of spinal cord and/or extremities
		For paralysis of nerves originating in spine, which may result from compression of aneurysm on arteries that feed spinal cord

POTENTIAL PROBLEMS	EXPECTED OUTCOMES	NURSING ACTIVITIES
		Assess signs/symptoms of impaired circulation to or compression of organs located along or distal to aneurysm and monitor for progression; evaluate
		Lungs
		Respiratory rate, quality of respirations, breath sounds; note decreased or absent sounds, presence of rales, rhonchi, or wheezing
		For signs of hemothorax
		For signs/symptoms of hypoxia
		For dyspnea, paroxysmal cough, hoarseness, hemoptysis
		Arterial blood gas results
		Chest radiograph results for upper airway compression
		Kidney
		For presence of flank pain, hematuria
		Volume of urine, specific gravity
		Lab data
		BUN
		Serum and urine electrolyte and creatinine levels, osmolality
		GI
		For abdominal pain
		For presence of bloody diarrhea
		Dysphagia
		Neurological
		LOC, mentation
		For presence of syncope, unequal pupil size
		For neurological abnormalities and weakness in upper spine and upper extremity region
		Liver
		For jaundice, icteric selera
		For anorexia, nausea, vomiting; malaise
		Lab data
		Enzymes: SGPT; SGOT
		Bilirubin (total; indirect, direct)
		Serum proteins, including total protein, albumin levels; albumin-globulin rate
		Coagulation studies, including clotting factors and platelets
		Monitor lab results, noting abnormalities in
		Hgb, Hct, platelet levels, coagulation studies
		WBC counts
■ Hemodynamic instability related to *dissecting aneurysm*	■ Aneurysm does not extend; remains stable in size Hemodynamic stability	■ Prevent progression of dissecting aneurysm by
		Administering IV vasodilators if ordered to lower BP; provide for continuous BP monitoring via an intraarterial line
		Administering diuretics and sedatives as ordered
		Maintaining quiet, peaceful environment
		Monitor for
		Abrupt onset of severe pain, with localization depending on organs involved
		Aortic diastolic murmur, which occurs with detachment of aortic valve cusp
		Neurological symptoms, including syncope
		Chest radiograph results indicating widened aortic silhouette and mediastinum and, occasionally, hemothorax
		ECG and cardiac enzymes to rule out MI
		Signs of left ventricular hypertrophy, particularly if patient is hypertensive
		Circulatory insufficiency of organs involved (see Problem, Hemodynamic instability)

POTENTIAL PROBLEMS	EXPECTED OUTCOMES	NURSING ACTIVITIES
		Monitor for *acute extension* of dissecting aneurysm, including sudden hypotension, extension of area of pain, signs of aortic regurgitation, sudden drop in urine output, reduced peripheral circulation, sudden weakening or disappearance of peripheral pulses, altered LOC with sudden confusion, restlessness Notify physician of appearance of any of these abnormalities and administer therapy as ordered; monitor patient's response

Postoperative
■ Hemodynamic instability related to
  Hypotension associated with hypovolemia from hemorrhage
  Hypertension
	■ Hemodynamic stability
	  BP, P, CVP, PAP/PCWP, urine output, peripheral circulation, and mentation are within patient's normal limits
	  Absence of postoperative hemorrhage
	  Hct and Hgb levels remain stable
		■ Prevent by
		  Administering fluids, blood products as ordered to maintain adequate intravascular volume and Hct
		  Closely monitoring patient's hemodynamic response and Hct levels
		  Administering antihypertensive medication to lower BP in the hypertensive patient, as ordered
		Monitor
		  BP, P q½-1 hr until stable; note hypotension or hypertension, tachycardia
		  For signs and symptoms of hemorrhage
		    Hypotension, tachycardia
		    Oliguria
		    Falling CVP, PAP/PCWP
		    Cool, clammy, blanched extremities
		    Altered mentation—restlessness, confusion
		    Falling Hct levels
		  Abdominal girth q2-4 hr until stable; note increasing size
		  For tenseness of abdomen q2-4 hr until stable, then q4-8 hr
		Notify physician of these clinical abnormalities
		If hemorrhage occurs
		  Administer blood and blood products as ordered, closely monitoring patient's vital signs, CVP, PAP, urine output and Hct levels
		  If hypovolemia occurs, administer fluids as ordered, closely monitoring patient's hemodynamic response as before
		  If hypertension occurs, administer diuretics, antihypertensives as ordered; potent IV antihypertensive medications should be given via infusion pump with continuous monitoring of arterial BP via intraarterial line

■ Myocardial ischemia with angina related to hypotension and/or decreased coronary artery blood flow	■ Absence or early resolution of myocardial ischemia	■ Monitor for
		  Chest pain
		  ECG changes indicating ischemia—S-T segment elevation or depression, T wave inversion
		Notify physician if these abnormalities occur
		If angina occurs
		  Administer antianginal medication as ordered, and monitor patient's response
		  Monitor BP, P q15 min and prn during and immediately after acute anginal episode
		
		See STANDARD 11 *Angina pectoris*

■ MI	■ Absence of MI	■ Monitor for
		  Chest pain unrelieved by antianginal medications
		  Other signs/symptoms of MI
		    Indigestion
		    Shoulder, arm, or jaw pain
		  ECG changes including S-T segment elevation, T wave inversion and diagnostic Q waves
		  Hemodynamic response to severe, unrelenting chest pain
		Notify physician of these abnormalities
		If problem occurs, monitor vital signs q¼-½ hr and prn until stable
		Administer supportive therapy as ordered (e.g., O₂, pain medication)
		
		See STANDARD 12 *Acute myocardial infarction*

POTENTIAL PROBLEMS	EXPECTED OUTCOMES	NURSING ACTIVITIES

■ Vascular defect (aneurysm) recurs	■ Aneurysm does not recur Abdominal girth remains stable postoperatively Adequate circulation to arteries distal to vascular repair	■ Monitor
		  Circulation distal to aneurysm repair, including pulses, color, capillary filling
		  For occurrence of pain distal to repair
		  Abdominal girths after repair of thoracoabdominal, abdominal aneurysms
		  For compression of organs adjacent to aneurysm
		  Results of serial chest, abdominal radiographs
		Notify physician of abnormalities in any of aforementioned
		If vascular defect recurs, administer therapy as ordered
		To enhance circulation to lower extremities place patient in reverse Trendelenburg position if ordered

■ Occlusion of peripheral vessel repair/graft, which may result from low BP and blood flow with circulatory stasis, clotting, and vessel occlusion	■ Patent vessel or graft Circulation distal to aneurysm is sufficient with full pulses, good color, and warmth in extremities	■ Prevent by
		  Avoiding constricting clothing or apparatus and angulation at groin or knee; avoid high Fowler position
		  Turning patient (or he/she turns) with leg straight and supported with pillows
		  Applying antithromboembolic stockings as ordered in patients without severe peripheral circulatory insufficiency
		  Assist with ROM, passive-assistive, and active-assistive exercises
		  Assist in early ambulation as ordered
		Monitor
		  Pulses distal to repair; ultrasound device (Doppler) may be needed for weak pulses
		  Other circulatory parameters distal to repair, including color, temperature, and sensation
		Notify physician if abnormalities in aforementioned occur, and alter therapy as ordered; monitor patient's response
		Prepare patient for surgery if planned, as ordered

■ Respiratory insufficiency related to
  Pulmonary interstitial edema as result of vigorous fluid administration
  Atelectasis
  Pneumonia
  Elevated diaphragm from abdominal surgery and associated distention, ileus
  Dyspnea caused by compression of upper airway by aneurysm
  Respiratory acidosis, alkalosis
	■ Respiratory function within normal limits Arterial blood gas levels within patient's normal limits Clear lungs; no adventitious sounds Auscultation and chest radiograph reveal full lung expansion without atelectasis, pulmonary interstitial edema, or compressed bronchus Afebrile, without pneumonia	■ Prevent by providing frequent chest physiotherapy
		  While patient is on bed rest, turn at least q2 hr
		  Encourage deep breathing and coughing
		  Administer humidified, oxygenated air as ordered
		  Employ incentive spirometry as ordered according to patient's clinical picture
		  Employ tracheal suctioning as necessary
		Monitor
		  Rate and quality of respirations q1-2 hr
		  Secretions for amount, color, and consistency
		  For decreased or absent breath sounds, rales, rhonchi, or wheezing
		  For respiratory distress and hypoxia, e.g., tachycardia, restlessness, tachypnea, dyspnea
		  Temperature q1-2 hr for fever
		  Arterial blood gas levels; note hypoxemia, hypercapnia, or hypocapnia
		  Chest radiograph results
		If respiratory insufficiency occurs
		  Emphasize direct chest physiotherapy to atelectatic areas
		  Emphasize gravity drainage of involved pulmonary lobe(s)
		  Assist with intubation if procedure becomes necessary
		  Manage mechanical ventilation and PEEP if needed to maintain adequate gas exchange
		
		See STANDARD 6 *Mechanical ventilation*
		      STANDARD 7 *Positive end-expiratory pressure*
		
		If respiratory acidosis occurs
		  Administer therapy as ordered to increase alveolar ventilation
		  Monitor arterial blood gas results q1-2 hr until stable for decrease in $Paco_2$ levels to within patient's normal limits

POTENTIAL PROBLEMS	EXPECTED OUTCOMES	NURSING ACTIVITIES
		If respiratory alkalosis occurs
		Administer therapy to correct etiological factors (e.g., pain) as ordered
		Monitor arterial blood gas results q1-2 hr until stable for increase in $Paco_2$ levels to within patient's normal limits

■ Kidney dysfunction related to
  Preoperative renal ischemia in presence of renal artery aneurysm
  Intraoperative renal ischemia associated with repair of renal artery aneurysm
	■ Kidney function within normal limits and adequate to maintain BUN, creatinine, electrolyte levels, body fluid volume, and acid-base balance within normal limits	■ Prevent by
		  Administering fluids, blood, and blood products as ordered to maintain adequate cardiac output and kidney perfusion
		  Administering inotropic agents, if ordered, to increase renal blood flow and urine output
		  Administering diuretics, as ordered, closely monitoring urine output response
		Monitor
		  For signs of inadequate cardiac output, hypovolemia
		  Hypotension, tachycardia
		  Low CVP and PAP
		  Oliguria
		  Inadequate periperal circulation
		  For hematuria
		  Urine volumes and specific gravity q1 hr; note oliguria, high specific gravity
		  Daily weight for gain or loss
		  Arterial blood gas results for acid-base imbalance
		  Lab indices of renal function, including level of BUN, uric acid, serum and urine osmolality, creatinine, and electrolytes
		Notify physician for abnormalities
		If kidney dysfunction or failure occurs, see Standard 52, *Acute renal failure*

■ GI dysfunction, ileus related to
  Mesenteric infarction
  Recurrence of abdominal aneurysm
	■ GI function within normal limits
	  Bowel sounds within normal limits
	  Absence of abdominal distention, rigidity, or other signs of mesenteric ischemia, infarction, or abdominal aneurysm
		■ Monitor
		  Abdominal girths q2-4 hr for increasing abdominal distention
		  Abdominal tenseness for increasing rigidity q2-4 hr
		  Bowel sounds q4 hr for decreased or absent bowel sounds
		  For signs/symptoms of mesenteric infarction, including
		    Patient's complaints of discomfort, malaise
		    Temperature elevation
		    Bloody diarrhea (test for heme-positive results)
		    Elevated WBC count
		Notify physician of these clinical abnormalities
		If mesenteric infarction, recurrence of abdominal aneurysm, or ileus occurs
		  Administer therapy as ordered, closely monitoring patient's response
		  Prepare patient for surgery if planned

■ CNS dysfunction related to
  Ascending and *transverse thoracic aortic aneurysm* associated with deficient carotid artery blood flow
  Arterial embolism associated with atherosclerosis, cholesterol plaques
	■ CNS function within normal limits
	  Absence of confusion, disorientation, restlessness
	  No evidence of cerebral embolus, infarction
		■ Monitor
		  Neurological status, LOC on admission and serially thereafter
		  For signs of general cerebral ischemia, headache, confusion, disorientation, particularly in patients with thoracic aneurysm
		  For delayed regaining of consciousness after anesthesia
		  For signs of cerebral embolism, infarction, particularly unilateral neurological deficiency, including weak limbs, ptosis of eyelid and/or side of mouth
		  Neurological function to extremities for abnormalities in sensation, movement, strength
		Notify physician of any of these abnormalities
		Alter therapeutic regimen as ordered, and monitor patient's response

POTENTIAL PROBLEMS	EXPECTED OUTCOMES	NURSING ACTIVITIES

■ Emboli formation related to
  Frequent association of aneurysm with atherosclerosis
  Dislodgement of thrombus during surgery
	■ Coagulation studies within normal limits
	  Absence of emboli formation
		■ Prevent by
		  Assisting patient with ROM exercises and ambulation as ordered
		  Applying antithromboembolic stockings as ordered
		Monitor for evidence of pulmonary embolus
		  Restlessness
		  Respiratory distress, e.g., dyspnea, tachypnea, or pleural or substernal pain
		  Arterial blood gas levels revealing hypoxemia, hypercapnia, or hypocapnia
		  Symptoms of hypoxia; tachypnea, air hunger, anxiety, tachycardia
		  Cardiovascular instability
		    Arrhythmias
		    Hypertension, hypotension
		    Signs/symptoms of reduced cardiac output
		  ECG changes reflecting right ventricular strain
		Notify physician if any of aforementioned occur, and administer therapy as ordered
		
		See STANDARD 31 *Embolic phenomena*
		
		Monitor for evidence of coronary embolus and MI, e.g.
		  Severe, crushing precordial or substernal chest pain (unrelated to movement)
		  ECG changes
		    S-T segment elevation
		    T wave inversion
		    Q waves (later)
		  Arrhythmias
		  Hypotension, tachycardia
		  Diaphoresis
		  Cold, clammy skin
		  Restlessness, anxiety
		  Elevated cardiac enzyme levels
		Notify physician if any of aforementioned abnormalities occur and administer therapy as ordered; monitor patient response
		
		See STANDARD 12 *Acute myocardial infarction*
		
		Monitor for evidence of cerebral vascular embolus and infarct, e.g.
		  Sudden dizziness
		  Altered LOC
		  Aphasia, dysphagia
		  Seizures
		  Unilateral weakness
		  Paralysis
		  Ptosis of eyelids, mouth
		Notify physician of any of aforementioned and administer therapy as ordered; monitor patient response
		
		See STANDARD 39 *Carotid endarterectomy*
		
		Monitor for renal emboli and infarction
		  Costovertebral angle back pain, lower back pain
		  Persistent hematuria, pyuria, and/or oliguria
		  Edema
		  Abnormal renal function tests
		    Urine volume, specific gravity
		    Serum, urine creatinine, electrolytes, osmolality
		    BUN, serum uric acid
		Notify physician of any of aforementioned and administer therapy as ordered; monitor patient response

POTENTIAL PROBLEMS	EXPECTED OUTCOMES	NURSING ACTIVITIES
		Monitor for evidence of mesenteric artery embolus, infarction of intestine Fever Lower abdominal discomfort, pain Bloody diarrhea Shock—pallor, diaphoresis, cold and clammy extremities, tachycardia, hypotension Lab results indicating elevated WBC count, ESR, and LDH Notify physician of any of aforementioned abnormalities and administer therapy as ordered; monitor patient response ***See*** STANDARD 31 *Embolic phenomena* If embolism and infarction occur, administer anticoagulation therapy as ordered
■ Ischemic injury to spinal cord may occur, particularly during repair of *transverse, descending thoracic aneurysms* and *dissecting thoracic aneurysms*	■ Spinal function and associated neuromuscular, autonomic, genitourinary function within normal limits Absence of paralysis	■ Monitor for Impaired sensation, motor responses Weakness Neuromuscular abnormalities Decrease or loss of deep tendon and cutaneous reflexes Bladder/bowel disturbance Hemiplegia, paraplegia If problem occurs Evaluate for neuromuscular abnormalities, alterations in sensation q1-2 hr Reposition patient at least q2 hr Assist patient with exercises (e.g., ROM) Administer therapy to support bowel and/or bladder function if impaired, as ordered Provide for skin care q2-4 hr Provide for adequate nutrition, as ordered
■ Acid-base, electrolyte imbalances, including Metabolic alkalosis related to Upper GI tract fluid losses (NG tube) Hyperaldosteronism associated with Use of diuretics Hypovolemia Hyponatremia (use of IV fluids low in Na^+) Hypokalemia Hypochloremia Blood administration Citrate metabolized to bicarbonate, appearing several hours after administration Electrolyte imbalance, particularly hyponatremia, hypokalemia	■ Acid-base balance within normal limits Electrolyte levels within normal limits	■ Prevent by Administering fluids, as ordered, based on fluid losses and consideration for variables that increase or decrease fluid requirements Administering electrolyte supplements as ordered based on losses in urine, stool, and drainage and on serum electrolyte levels Avoiding vigorous diuretic administration; if brisk diuresis is necessary, administer careful electrolyte replacement as ordered Monitor Intake and output records for imbalances Serum and urine electrolyte levels For symptoms of fatigue, drowsiness, headaches, apathy, inattentiveness, restlessness, confusion, weakness Serial arterial blood gas levels for acid-base imbalance Vital signs q1-2 hr until stable Notify physician for abnormalities If problem occurs Monitor arterial blood gas levels q1-2 hr until stable Vital signs q1-2 hr until stable If electrolyte imbalance occurs Administer electrolytes as ordered Monitor for alleviation of signs/symptoms of electrolyte imbalance If acid-base imbalance occurs and is related to use of a certain diuretic, alter diuretic regimen as ordered

POTENTIAL PROBLEMS	EXPECTED OUTCOMES	NURSING ACTIVITIES

■ Insufficient knowledge for compliance with discharge regimen*	■ Before discharge
	Patient/family verbalizes knowledge of discharge regimen, including precautions, medications, diet, and acitivty
	Patient/family is able to describe follow-up plan, including where and when to go, who to see, and what specimens to bring
	Patient/family accurately describes signs and symptoms requiring medical attention
		■ Assess patient/family's understanding of discharge regimen, including dietary regimen, medications, activity modifications, and special precautionary measures
		Describe discharge regimen, including
		  Medications—purpose, identification of, route, dosage, timing, frequency, and potential adverse effects
		  Dietary regimen
		  Activity progression; position modifications
		  Avoidance of constricting clothing
		  Avoidance of maintaining one position for more than 1 hour
		  Monitoring circulation to affected extremity
		Instruct patient/family in specific measures according to residual impaired organ circulation and associated dysfunction
		Describe signs and symptoms requiring medical attention, depending on site of original aneurysm and outcome of surgery
		Discuss plan for follow-up visits with patient/family, including where and when to go, who to see, and what specimens to bring
		Provide opportunity for and encourage patient/family's questions and verbalization of anxiety regarding discharge regimen

*If critical care nurse is responsible for this type of follow-up care.

EMBOLIC PHENOMENA

An embolus has been defined as "a detached intravascular mass (solid or gaseous) that is carried by the blood to a site distant from its point of origin. Inevitably these lodge in vessels too small to permit their further passage, resulting in partial or complete occlusion of the vessel."*

An embolus may travel in either the venous or the arterial system. In rare cases an embolus may originate on the venous side but pass through a septal defect in the heart and become arterial (paradoxical embolus). Usually venous emboli that become clinically significant are lodged in the pulmonary circulation, causing varying degrees of respiratory compromise. Arterial emboli are more unpredictable in their ultimate destination, and because they potentially can obstruct a significant percentage of blood flow to one of several end organs (brain, kidney, bowel), their effects are usually more devastating.

Emboli may be composed of blood clots (thrombi), fat, air, calcium, amniotic fluid, fragments of tumors, and infected and foreign materials that enter the bloodstream and lodge in various end organs.

Thrombi are formed intravascularly by blood cells, platelets, and fibrin. They are the most common source of embolic phenomena. Factors predisposing to the formation of thrombi include stasis of blood flow, injury to a blood vessel lining (e.g., sepsis, trauma), and a hypercoagulable state. The latter occurs in cancer patients, postoperative patients, and patients suffering from chronic, debilitating diseases. Other high-risk patients include those with conditions such as varicosities, obesity, polycythemia vera, collagen vascular disease, vasculitis, pregnancy, and older age. The intake of certain medications (e.g., progestational agents such as oral contraceptives) also predisposes to the formation of thromboemboli.

Fat emboli result from the release of fatty aggregates into the vascular system, the most common source of these being bone marrow in the setting of a fracture or operative procedure. Fat emboli travel until they reach a capillary bed, frequently in the lungs, where a reactive inflammatory process causes interstitial edema. A large embolus or shower of microemboli is capable of causing severe respiratory insufficiency.

Air emboli are usually introduced into the vascular system through catheters that have been inadvertently left open to air. Large amounts of air (1 cc/kg) are required intravenously before significant clinical findings become evident. A situation capable of producing such an effect is that in which a deep inspiration takes place in the presence of a large-bore central venous catheter left open to air. The negative intrathoracic pressure may pull a bolus of air into the line, which can enter the venous circulation, flow to the lungs, and compromise pulmonary circulation in that area.

Arterial air emboli, on the other hand, require much less volume for disastrous effects. Air may be delivered into the arterial system at the beginning or end of CPB or hemodialysis or through various arterial monitoring lines.

Other, less common sources of emboli include calcium from damaged heart valves, which may be released during surgical resection. Septic emboli originate from a nidus of intravascular infection such as a vegetation on a heart valve or an infected thrombus.

Amniotic emboli are contents of the amniotic sac that are forced into the systemic circulation by contractions during abortion or normal delivery. This sort of embolus is especially dangerous because of the intense systemic reaction that may result (i.e., shock, disseminated intravascular coagulation [DIC]).

Consideration of predisposing factors and careful attention to historical detail are important in formulating a diagnosis of embolic phenomena. Physical findings will vary, depending on the arterial or venous origin of the embolus and the organ systems involved. The significance of lab tests will likewise be determined by the location of the presumed embolus.

Therapeutic goals for embolic phenomena are the restoration of blood flow to affected systems and the prevention of further embolic events by removing or suppressing the source. In the case of thromboemboli, anticoagulation has been shown to effectively control the recurrence of such problems. Arterial emboli and large pulmonary emboli are often surgically removed in addition to their source being located and dealt with appropriately.

*From Robbins, S.L.: Pathologic basis of disease, Philadelphia, 1974, W.B. Saunders Co., pp. 334-335.

ASSESSMENT

1. History, presence, and nature of
   a. Physiological factors that predispose patient to the formation of blood clots, including
      (1) Stasis of blood flow as in prolonged immobility
      (2) Injury to a vessel lining as in trauma or sepsis
      (3) Hypercoagulable state as in some cancers and in the immediate postoperative period following major surgery
      (4) Obesity
   b. Physiological factors that predispose patient to the formation of fat emboli
      (1) Recent trauma to long bones, ribs (e.g., thoracic surgery, fracture), sternum (e.g., thoracic surgery)
      (2) Metabolic/hematological abnormalities such as
         (a) Diabetes, pancreatitis
         (b) Severe infections, burns
         (c) Carcinoma
         (d) Leukemia, blood dyscrasias, sickle cell disease
   c. Physiological factors that predispose patient to the formation of an air embolism
      (1) Atrial, pulmonary artery, and/or central venous lines
      (2) Hemodialysis therapy
      (3) Recent cardiac surgery
   d. Physiological factors that predispose patient to the formation of calcium emboli, including
      (1) Recent cardiac surgery for valvular replacement
      (2) Fracture or trauma of long bones, sternum, ribs
   e. Physiological factors that predispose patient to the formation of septic emboli, including
      (1) Any kind of infection, particularly systemic infection
      (2) Local infections such as vegetations on heart valves
   f. Physiological factors that predispose patient to the formation of amniotic fluid emboli, including
      (1) Pregnancy, delivery
      (2) Recent abortion
   g. Presence of any kind of tumor that predisposes patient to emboli made of tumor fragments and also to hypercoagulability

2. Presence, nature, and extent of characteristic signs and symptoms of emboli (see more specific description in standard that follows) according to type and location
   a. General restlessness, anxiety, dizziness
   b. Fever
   c. Respiratory distress
   d. Signs and symptoms of hypoxia
   e. Hemodynamic instability
   f. Altered mental status concurrent with unilateral weakness, aphasia, fainting, and/or incontinence
   g. Lower back pain with hematuria; note oliguria and/or pyuria
   h. Lower abdominal discomfort; pain with bloody diarrhea
   i. Pain in left upper quadrant of abdomen radiating to left shoulder; pleural friction rub

3. Results of lab and diagnostic tests, including
   a. Doppler ultrasound
   b. Impedance plethysmography
   c. Iodine-labeled fibrinogen uptake test
   d. Venograms, arteriograms
   e. Scans (e.g., ventilation/perfusion scan)
   f. WBC count; ESR
   g. Renal function tests
   h. Myocardial enzyme levels
   i. ECG
   j. Arterial blood gas levels
   k. Radiograph (e.g., chest)

4. Level of anxiety related to disease process, hospitalization, anticipated therapy, anticipated diagnostic procedures, altered family roles, and other factors

5. Patient/family's understanding of purpose of hospitalization, therapy planned, and, if appropriate, anticipated surgery, expected outcome, and perioperative experiences

GOALS

1. Reduction in patient/family's anxiety with provision of information, explanations, and encouragement
2. Absence or resolution of emboli
3. Resolution of organ dysfunction manifested by indices of organ function within normal limits
4. Hemodynamic stability
5. Absence or resolution of arrhythmias
6. Before discharge patient/family is able to
   a. Accurately describe activity, dietary, and medication regimen
   b. Identify signs and symptoms requiring medical attention
   c. Accurately describe plan for follow-up care

POTENTIAL PROBLEMS	EXPECTED OUTCOMES	NURSING ACTIVITIES
■ Patient/family's anxiety related to Hospitalization Disease process Therapeutic regimen Diagnostic procedures	■ Reduction in anxiety with provision of information, explanations, and encouragement	■ Assess level of patient/family's anxiety Assess level of understanding regarding disease process, therapy employed, and diagnostic procedures planned Explain relationship of disease process and rationale for various therapeutic interventions Explain in simple terms the diagnostic procedures anticipated and what patient will experience Assist in preparation of patient for diagnostic procedures Provide opportunity for and encourage questions, verbalization of fears Assess reduction in patient/family's level of anxiety
■ Thromboemboli formation	■ Absence of/or resolution of embolus	■ Prevent thromboembolism Apply antithromboembolic stockings without wrinkles or any tight areas that can cause hemostasis and clot formation; prevent constriction at joint areas by keeping lower leg stockings 2 inches from knee joint and ending stocking or elastic bandage extending to upper leg 2 inches below groin Remove stockings/elastic bandage for 10 to 15 minutes q8 hr to allow for better superficial capillary filling, thereby preventing skin breakdown, and to correct any uneven pressure areas Enhance lower extremity circulation with passive and active ROM exercises Reposition patient at least q2 hr Elevate patient's legs with knees straight while patient is out of bed Position patient to avoid marked angulation at groin or knee Provide for early ambulation as tolerated, as ordered Prevent injury to vessel lining by preventing local trauma, infection, or sepsis Do not massage or hold leg muscles tightly Avoid prolonged bed rest Instruct patient not to cross feet at ankles Ambulate patient q1-2 hr unless contraindicated Minimize/prevent hypercoagulability Discontinue oral contraceptives and any medication that may cause hypercoagulability as ordered, particularly if surgery is planned Administer prophylactic low-dose heparin, if ordered, in certain high-risk patients, particularly if surgery is planned (persons over 60 years old, those in heart failure, persons with carcinoma or history of thrombophlebitis and/or embolization) Administer adequate fluid intake as ordered Administer stool softeners if ordered to limit straining that could dislodge thromboemboli Encourage patient to avoid straining—valsalva maneuvers
■ Peripheral venous embolism	■ Absence of peripheral venous embolism Adequate peripheral blood flow	■ Monitor for Edema of lower extremity by comparing differences in circumferential measurements of leg at several levels Painful swelling and tenderness on palpation in area of affected vein Pain when foot forcefully dorsiflexed (Homans sign) Pain that is worst on dependency and, conversely, relieved by elevation Palpable hard cordlike vein (cord) Severe cramping of extremity Local warmth around clot Fever Results of venogram, Doppler ultrasound, impedance plethysmography, iodine-labeled fibrinogen uptake test, if performed If any of these abnormalities occurs, notify physician

POTENTIAL PROBLEMS	EXPECTED OUTCOMES	NURSING ACTIVITIES

		If peripheral venous embolism occurs
		  Administer anticoagulation, using continuous or intermittent doses of sodium heparin during acute period followed by sodium warfarin compound in subacute period as ordered
		  Monitor for
		    Serial PT/APTT levels during heparin therapy (therapeutically prolonged to 1½ to 2 times normal or 90 to 100 seconds)
		    Signs of bleeding (e.g., easy bruising)
		    Guaiac test results on all stools and NG drainage
		  Administer antacids if ordered
		  Monitor neurological status for signs of intracranial bleeding
		  Avoid IM injections
		  Administer analgesic if needed, as ordered
		  Maintain patient on bed rest during acute period
		  Keep edematous extremity elevated during acute period
		  Avoid squeezing, massaging, or pressure against extremity where peripheral thrombus resides
		  Avoid use of pillows
		  Avoid gatching knees
		  Instruct patient not to cross legs
		  Reposition patient q1-2 hr
		  Apply moist heat to affected area if ordered
		  Use bed cradle over affected extremity
		  Administer active and passive ROM exercises to *unaffected* extremities
		  Apply antithromboembolic stockings to unaffected extremity if ordered
		Monitor for mobilization of peripheral venous embolus; particularly note signs/symptoms of pulmonary embolus (see Problem, Pulmonary emboli)

▪ Peripheral arterial embolism	▪ Absence of peripheral arterial emboli
	Adequate circulation to extremities; color, pulses, skin temperature within normal limits
		▪ Monitor for
		  Signs and symptoms of arterial embolus and concurrent circulatory insufficiency to extremities, particularly noting tenderness, pain, blanching, decreased capillary filling, coolness, decreased to absent pulses in affected area, q½-2 hr as needed
		  Numbness and tingling
		  Circulation to tip of nose, pinnae of ears, fingers, and toes for infarction of tissue, which can become gangrenous
		  Pulses that cannot be easily palpated
		  Results of ultrasound (or Doppler) testing or noninvasive electrical impedance plethysmography
		  Results of arteriogram, if performed
		  Scaling and dryness of skin
		If any of these signs and symptoms occur, notify physician
		If peripheral arterial embolism occurs
		  Administer anticoagulation with continuous or intermittent doses of heparin sodium as ordered
		    Monitor for
		      Serial PT/APTT levels during heparin therapy (therapeutically prolonged to 1½ to 2 times normal or 90 to 100 seconds)
		      Sign of bleeding (e.g., easy bruising)
		      Guaiac test results on all stools and NG drainage
		    Administer antacids if ordered
		    Monitor neurological status for signs of intracranial bleeding
		    Avoid IM injections
		  Administer vasodilator medications if ordered
		  Keep patient on bed rest during acute period; use of bed cradle; cotton blankets next to patient
		  Avoid heating devices to or chilling of lower extremities
		  Reposition patient q½-1 hr

POTENTIAL PROBLEMS	EXPECTED OUTCOMES	NURSING ACTIVITIES
		Avoid any one position for long periods of time
		Avoid raising lower extremity above level of heart
		Administer active and/or passive ROM exercises to extremities q2-4 hr unless contraindicated
		Apply antithromboembolic stockings to unaffected extremity, if ordered
		Prepare patient for surgical removal of embolism, if planned
		For cleansing use small amount of mild soap, rinse well, and dry gently but thoroughly; avoid vigorous rubbing; apply lanolin-base lotions; do not permit skin to remain wet
		Administer analgesic if needed, as ordered
		In subacute period for both peripheral venous and arterial embolism
		Ambulation should start gradually, such as with short walks q1-2 hr
		Legs should be elevated periodically throughout day, such as for 10 minutes q1-2 hr
		Remaining in one position for long periods (more than 1 to 2 hours) should be avoided
		Calf muscles should be periodically flexed when patient is sitting
		Apply antithromboembolic stockings
		Avoid extremes of temperature; keep extremities comfortably warm
		Patient should avoid
		Constricting clothing, including girdles, garter belts
		Leg crossing
		Smoking
		Rubbing, massaging legs
■ Pulmonary emboli associated with Respiratory insufficiency Hypoxia resulting from Significant intrapulmonary shunting Dyspnea associated with bronchoconstriction resulting from regional ischemia, pain, and anxiety Signs and symptoms vary according to size of embolism and patient's unique response Small embolism may cause mild tachycardia, mild dyspnea, unexplained wheezing, cough, tachypnea, and mild temperature elevation	■ Absence of or resolution of signs, symptoms of pulmonary embolus Adequate oxygenation and ventilation with Pao_2 and $Paco_2$ levels within normal limits Respirations without distress; respiratory rate within normal limits Clear chest radiograph without atelectasis, pleural effusion, cardiac enlargement Cardiopulmonary stability	■ Prevent by employing prophylactic measures to prevent emboli formation (see Problem, Peripheral venous embolism) Monitor for Restlessness, anxiety, fever, dizziness, faintness, or any unusual sensation in chest Respiratory distress: dyspnea, tachypnea, pleural and/or substernal pain that may be sharp or stabbing in nature; auscultation may reveal pleural rub over infarcted tissue, rales, wheezing with bronchoconstriction, pleural effusion, accentuation of pulmonary component of second heart sound Arterial blood gas levels indicating hypoxemia, hypercapnia, or hypocapnia Signs of hypoxia: tachypnea, air hunger, anxiety, dyspnea, tachycardia, hypertension or hypotension Cardiovascular instability Arrhythmias Hypertension Signs of reduced cardiac output—hypotension, tachycardia, angina, oliguria, peripheral vasoconstriction—and signs of venous congestion—jugular venous distention, elevated CVP measurements, presacral and peripheral edema Increased loudness of pulmonic component of second heart sound ($\uparrow S_2 P$) (closure of pulmonic valve is accentuated by pulmonary hypertension) ECG changes, including tall peaked P waves in leads II, III, and right atrial and ventricular strain pattern, right QRS axis shift, RBBB pattern, S-T segment and T wave changes in massive pulmonary embolism; auscultation may reveal right ventricular gallop rhythm, S_3, S_4, systolic murmur, and widely split S_2; atrial fibrillation may develop secondary to pulmonary emboli LDH, transaminase, and bilirubin levels; note elevation without concurrent SGOT elevation

POTENTIAL PROBLEMS	EXPECTED OUTCOMES	NURSING ACTIVITIES

Moderate-sized embolism often presents with pleuritic chest pain, anxiety, restlessness, dyspnea, cough, tachypnea; arterial blood gas analysis reveals hypoxemia and hypocapnia; cardiac compromise may result from sympathetically induced tachycardia and from pulmonary hypertension (associated with local pulmonary vasoconstriction)
 	
Massive embolism may produce tachypnea, marked dyspnea, air hunger, a feeling of impending doom, anxiety, mental clouding, and occasionally hemoptysis, cyanosis, a marked tachycardia, and hypotension and may progress to cardiovascular collapse
		Fibrinogen degradation product (FDP) levels, which are elevated as result of fibrinolysis of clot (normal levels <5 mg/ml); FDP is less reliable in presence of liver disease, DIC, or other coagulation abnormalities
		Serial chest radiograph results, particularly noting consolidation, atelectasis, dilated central pulmonary arteries with decreased distal vascular markings, pleural effusions, elevated diaphragm on affected side, cardiac enlargement with prominent right atrial border and/or right ventricular dilatation, dilatated superior vena cava
		Results of arteriogram, ventilation/perfusion lung scan, radioactive fibrinogen test, if performed; prepare patient for these tests
		Notify physician of any clinical abnormality
		If pulmonary embolism occurs
		  Assess nature, severity of signs and symptoms
		  Administer therapy to attenuate signs and symptoms (particularly chest pain, hypoxia) as ordered
		    Pain medication (e.g., morphine sulfate)
		    O_2 supplements
		    Chest physiotherapy
		      Monitor breath sounds q1-2 hr, noting decreased or absent sounds or presence of rales, rhonchi, or wheezing
		      Monitor chest radiograph results for areas of consolidation; emphasize gentle chest physiotherapy to affected areas
		    Bronchodilator if ordered
		    Mechanical ventilation with PEEP, which may be necessary for adequate gas exchange
		  Position patient for comfort and to ensure optimal diaphragmatic excursion
		  Provide for psychological support
		  Monitor patient's progress, and institute therapy as ordered
		    Monitor
		      Serial chest radiograph results for resolution
		      Serial arterial blood gas results for adequate oxygenation, ventilation
		      For arrhythmias associated with pulmonary embolism; if significant incidence occurs, notify physician; provide for continuous monitoring of ECG using cardiac monitor
		      For signs of cor pulmonale and right ventricular strain; administer fluids and vasoactive agents cautiously to maintain cardiac output
		    Monitor for amelioration of dyspnea, pain, and anxiety with therapy
		  Administer thrombolytic agents to lyse clots if ordered; because this therapy is associated with considerable risk, particularly untoward bleeding, it is reserved for patients with massive pulmonary embolism and shock; agents used include streptokinase and urokinase
		  Administer anticoagulation therapy if ordered
		    Monitor for
		      Serial PT/APTT levels during heparin therapy (therapeutically prolonged to 1½ to 2 times normal or 90 to 100 seconds)
		      Signs or bleeding (e.g., easy bruising)
		      Guaiac test results on all stools and NG drainage
		      Administer antacids if ordered
		      Monitor neurological status for signs of intracranial bleeding
		      Avoid IM injections

POTENTIAL PROBLEMS	EXPECTED OUTCOMES	NURSING ACTIVITIES
		Prepare patient for surgery if ordered; surgery is considered for patients in whom anticoagulation therapy has failed to prevent recurrent emboli or for whom anticoagulation is contraindicated, (e.g., GI bleeding, thrombocytopenia); surgeries include Surgical embolectomy, which is reserved for patients who achieve inadequate relief of signs and symptoms with medical therapy or patients in whom embolus is very large, resulting in acute cardiopulmonary compromise Insertion of vena caval filter or umbrella to trap emboli from lower extremities; it is used most often when anticoagulation fails to prevent recurrent emboli or is contraindicated; pulmonary emboli produce severe cardiopulmonary compromise; recurrent emboli occur in presence of septic pelvic thrombophlebitis and as adjunct to pulmonary embolectomy; intracaval umbrella has particular advantages over plication of large vein in that it is inserted with local anesthesia and produces gradual rather than acute obstruction of inferior vena cava, with progressive development of venous stasis in lower extremity Plication, ligation, or clipping of large vein that is source of recurrent emboli; plication of large vein requires major surgery and results in abrupt, pronounced venous stasis in lower extremity
■ Coronary embolus, MI	■ Absence of MI Cardiac output within normal limits	■ Monitor for severe, crushing precordial or substernal chest pain (unrelated to movement); ECG changes—S-T elevation, followed by T wave inversion and finally Q waves; arrhythmias; hypotension and tachycardia; diaphoresis; cold, clammy skin; restlessness; anxiety; shortness of breath; faintness; indigestion; and elevated cardiac enzyme levels If problem occurs, see Standard 12, *Acute myocardial infarction*
■ Cerebral embolus, cerebrovascular infarct	■ Absence of cerebral embolus, infarct Mental status remains clear; patient oriented to time, place, and people	■ Monitor for Sudden dizziness Altered mental status progressing to coma, aphasia, dysphasia, seizures, unilateral weakness, paralysis, ptosis of eyelids, nystagmus, visual loss, ptosis of mouth, incontinence with concurrent elevated BP and bradycardia Notify physician for any of these abnormalities If problem occurs, institute therapy as ordered
■ Renal artery embolism, renal infarct	■ Absence of renal artery embolus, renal infarct Indices of renal function within normal limits	■ Monitor for costovertebral angle back pain, lower back pain, persistent hematuria, pyuria and/or oliguria, edema, and lab values indicating impaired renal function, embolism/infarction Monitor intake and output, for electrolyte imbalance and for acid-base imbalance very closely Notify physician of abnormalities Administer supportive therapy as ordered If renal failure occurs, see Standard 52, *Acute renal failure*
■ Mesenteric artery thrombosis, embolus; infarction of part of intestine	■ Absence of mesenteric artery thrombosis, embolus, or infarction of intestine Bowel function within normal limits	■ Monitor For fever and lower abdominal discomfort Pain and bloody diarrhea For shock—pallor, diaphoresis, cold and clammy extremities, tachycardia, hypotension Lab results including elevated WBC count, ESR, and LDH Notify physician for any of these abnormalities If problem occurs Administer supportive therapy as ordered Prepare patient for arteriography and/or surgery if planned

POTENTIAL PROBLEMS	EXPECTED OUTCOMES	NURSING ACTIVITIES
■ Splenic artery thrombosis, embolus; splenic infarction	■ Absence of splenic artery thrombosis, embolus, and splenic infarction Splenic function, particularly regarding RBC destruction, within normal limits	■ Monitor for Signs and symptoms of splenic infarction, including pain in left upper quadrant of abdomen, which may radiate to left shoulder, and pleural friction rub Lab values indicating elevated WBC count or ESR; anemia Notify physician if any of these abnormalities occur Administer supportive therapy as ordered; prepare patient for arteriography and/or surgery if ordered
■ Fat embolism, including diffuse shower of fat microemboli to various end organs; is commonly associated with Trauma, particularly in presence of long bone fracture; signs and symptoms of diffuse shower of fat emboli occur 24 to 48 hours after traumatic injury Infections such as Osteomyelitis Septicemia Metabolic abnormalities such as Diabetes Acute pancreatitis Alcoholism Burns Anesthesia CPB Fat emboli and petechiae impair microcirculatory flow, resulting in tissue hypoxia, anoxia, and hemorrhagic infarcts	■ Absence of or resolution of fat emboli Respiratory, neurological, renal function within normal limits Absence of petechiae	■ Carefully assess patient's baseline Respiratory status, then repeat serially; note rate and ease of respirations Neurological status; LOC Renal status—urine volume, specific gravity; test for presence of fat in urine may be ordered Prevent by Immobilizing fractures Monitoring for and administering therapy to prevent fluid and blood loss, dehydration, hypovolemia, and hemoconcentration Monitor for Signs and symptoms of fat embolism, particularly in patients with long bone fractures; signs and symptoms are primarily result of diffuse shower of fat microemboli resulting in local circulatory insufficiency Signs and symptoms of fat emboli in the following organ systems Pulmonary Dyspnea, tachypnea, signs of hypoxia, duskiness, bubbling rales Chest radiograph often reveals diffuse haziness, interstitial edema (inflammatory response to fat microemboli) Arterial blood gas results may reveal hypoxemia Signs of sympathetic response to hypoxia, particularly tachycardia Cerebral: sudden development of urinary incontinence, abusiveness, restlessness, disorientation, irritability, delirium; occasionally neuromuscular dysfunction (e.g., twitching) and even convulsion and coma may occur NOTE: Craniocerebral trauma should be ruled out in trauma victim; compared to trauma, cerebral fat embolism syndrome has a long lucid interval (18 to 24 hours), and when it does develop, confusion is more severe, deterioration is more rapid, and localizing signs are usually absent Skin Cyanosis Petechiae (caused by endothelial damage of skin capillaries and/or thrombocytopenia); seen often on chest, upper arms, base of neck, in axilla, and in conjunctiva Renal Hematuria Oliguria Intestinal Diarrhea Abdominal discomfort Gastric: hematemesis Low-grade fever Lab results indicating Decreased Hgb, platelet levels Free fat in urine; impaired kidney function Fat globules in sputum Elevated serum lipase level

POTENTIAL PROBLEMS	EXPECTED OUTCOMES	NURSING ACTIVITIES
		Notify physician of any of these abnormalities
		If fat embolism occurs, administer therapy as ordered, which may include
		Humidified O_2
		Chest physiotherapy q2-4 hr
		Repositioning patient q1-2 hr
		Intubation with mechanical ventilation
		See Standard 6, *Mechanical ventilation*
		PEEP may be required during mechanical ventilation; see Standard 7, *Positive end-expiratory pressure*
		Diuretics (osmotic diuretics for cerebral emboli)
		Fluids to prevent hemoconcentration, shock, decreased capillary blood flow
		Anticoagulation (usually heparin sodium) in intermittent doses or as continuous infusion, as soon as fat embolic process is highly suspected, if ordered
		Heparin if ordered; monitor for signs of bleeding, particularly in trauma patient (observe and test skin, urine, sputum, emesis, feces for presence of blood)
		Corticosteroids, if ordered, with concurrent antacid or H_2 antagonist
		Low molecular weight dextran if ordered; monitor closely for signs of fluid overload, CHF, pulmonary edema, and impaired renal function (oliguria)
		Lytic enzymes and antibiotics if ordered
		Monitor
		Arterial blood gas results for resolving hypoxemia, hypercapnia or hypocapnia, and acidosis
		Chest radiograph results for resolution of pulmonary emboli and areas of atelectasis
■ Air embolus, which may be related to air entry through arterial line, left atrial line, hemodialysis tubing	■ Absence of air in any line entering patient Absence of or resolution of large embolus in heart or lungs or smaller air emboli in coronary, pulmonary, carotid, renal, mesenteric, or peripheral artery Absence of signs and symptoms of circulatory insufficiency and impaired function of end organs	■ Prevent by
		Inserting lines into large central veins with patient in Trendelenburg position (if patient can tolerate this position)
		Avoiding air entry while making connections in all tubings going to patient and in drawing blood samples
		Ensuring absence of air in fluid bag and tubing of all pressurized fluid infusions
		Monitor for
		Air in tubings going to patient
		Signs of ischemic tissue distal to arterial embolus
		An arterial embolus in cardiopulmonary system, manifested by hemodynamic instability
		Arterial embolus in brain; signs and symptoms may be similar to stroke
		If venous air embolus is suspected, monitor BP, P, and LOC
		If large venous air embolus is suspected
		Immediately place patient in left lateral position, with head of bed lowered; head of bed and patient should not be elevated for any reason for 24 to 48 hours or as ordered; this position helps to keep air in right atrium, allows adequate pulmonary artery blood flow, and prevents air from entering cerebral circulation
		Monitor pulmonary status closely; air may move into pulmonary artery, seriously impairing blood flow, oxygenation, and hemodynamic stability
		Monitor serial arterial blood gas levels frequently during acute period
		If aforementioned measures fail, assist in emergency thoracotomy or direct needle aspiration in right atrium if either of these procedures becomes necessary

POTENTIAL PROBLEMS	EXPECTED OUTCOMES	NURSING ACTIVITIES

■ Recurrent embolization	■ Absence of recurrent emboli
	Resolution of existent emboli
		■ Implement prescribed therapy to prevent further embolization
		Anticoagulants
		  Administer heparin IV, if ordered, either as continuous drip or by intermittent IV or subcutaneous injections; continuous IV infusion provides consistent anticoagulant effect with steady blood level; if subcutaneous heparin injections are given, do not massage injection site
		  Monitor site for hematoma formation
		  Doses are determined by APTT; monitor these levels
		  Administer warfarin, if ordered, for long-term anticoagulation; doses are determined by PT and clotting times (maintaining them at approximately 1½ to 2½ times control values)
		  Anticoagulants are usually continued until lung scan demonstrates further improvement and evidence of deep vein thrombosis subsides
		  For medications that patient is receiving that enhance or diminish activity of warfarin
		    Monitor chart for results of coagulation studies
		    Closely monitor patient for internal/external bleeding
		  If bleeding occurs
		    Protamine sulfate may be ordered to reverse effects of heparin
		    Vitamin K may be ordered to block action of warfarin
		  Administer antiplatelet medications if ordered, which may include aspirin, dipyridamole (Persantine), or dextran
		  Administer proteolytic enzymes if ordered
		Monitor for further thrombophlebitis; serially test legs for Homans sign, pain, swelling, tenderness, erythema of extremity
		Monitor for recurrent thrombosis of or embolization to pulmonary, cerebral, coronary, mesenteric, renal, or peripheral artery
		Prepare patient for serial radiographs, scans as ordered
		Surgical therapy may be accomplished for
		  Large pulmonary emboli
		    Prepare patient for emergency surgery for removal of large pulmonary embolus
		    This is usually reserved for patients with associated significant reduction in cardiac output and hypoxemia
		  Recurrent emboli
		    Partial venous interruption of vena cava, using umbrella to filter out large emboli; this is usually reserved for patients in whom
		      Anticoagulation fails to prevent recurrent emboli or anticoagulation is contraindicated
		      Pulmonary emboli are producing severe cardiopulmonary compromise
		      Recurrent emboli occur in presence of septic pelvic thrombophlebitis (as adjunct to pulmonary embolectomy)
		    Plication of femoral vein or vena cava, which helps to trap emboli in femoral venous system; may be done for patients with
		      Mesenteric thrombi, emboli, and associated infarction of intestine
		      Splenic emboli, infarction
		      Renal artery emboli, infarction
		      Pulmonary emboli

■ Hemodynamic instability, which may be related to
Hypotension, inadequate fluid replacement
Hemorrhage
Heart failure
Arrhythmias
	■ Hemodynamic stability; BP, P within normal limits; other indices of adequate cardiac output within normal limits
	Absence or resolution of arrhythmias
		■ Prevent by administering fluids and blood products as ordered to maintain hemodynamic stability and adequate cardiac output
		Prevent arrhythmias by providing for
		  Adequate oxygenation
		  Pain relief
		  Comfort
		  Psychological support

POTENTIAL PROBLEMS	EXPECTED OUTCOMES	NURSING ACTIVITIES
		Monitor (q1 hr and prn until stable) 　BP 　Pulses for rate, quality 　ECG—continuously if possible; if arrhythmias occur, note perfusion of and overall hemodynamic effect 　CVP and PAP/PCWP if available 　For jugular venous distention 　Urine output with specific gravity 　Color for signs of reduced peripheral circulation 　Mentation 　Hgb, Hct levels 　Coagulation studies 　Weight Notify physician of any clinical abnormalities If hypotension occurs 　Administer fluids as ordered, closely monitoring patient's hemodynamic response 　Administer inotropic agent, if ordered, to increase cardiac output of compromised heart If hemorrhage occurs, monitor serial Hgb and Hct levels and administer blood and blood products as ordered If heart failure occurs, see Standard 15, *Heart failure (low cardiac output)* If arrhythmias occur, see Standard 21, *Arrhythmias*
■ Insufficient knowledge to comply with discharge regimen*	■ Before discharge patient/family is able to Describe regimen for medications Identify several precautionary measures to avoid bruising, inadvertent bleeding Describe exercises, accurately perform them, and describe precautions in activities Describe precautionary measures for specific discharge medications Describe several signs, symptoms requiring medical follow-up	■ Assess patient/family's understanding of discharge regimen Instruct the patient/family in the following 　Leg exercises that are designed to decrease venous stasis and enhance circulation 　Medications, including their identification, route, dose, frequency, timing, and potential adverse effects 　If warfarin sodium is ordered, take it at same time every day 　Not to take over-the-counter medications without consulting physician first 　Foods that are high in vitamin K should be omitted altogether or eaten in a regular, consistent pattern (particularly yellow and green leafy vegetables); a list of these foods should be shared with patient/family 　To tell dentist or any other doctor that he/she is receiving anticoagulant medication 　To report diarrhea, vomiting, or any febrile illness, which may indicate coagulation testing and require temporary increment in warfarin sodium dosage; review potential signs and symptoms requiring medical attention 　To avoid bruises or falls and active "contact" activities 　To report bruises that enlarge, cuts that do not stop bleeding, red or brown urine, red or dark brown stool, nosebleed that does not stop with moderate pressure, flank or abdominal pain, headaches, unusual joint pain 　When skin is cut, to apply direct pressure and maintain for several minutes until clotting occurs 　Helpful guidelines to avoid accidents, including 　　Wearing gloves while gardening 　　Using electric shaver 　　Using soft bristle toothbrush (avoid using Water Pik) 　　Using nonslip mat in bathtub 　　Avoiding use of oil in bath water 　　Hazards of going barefoot 　　Avoiding use of power tools, particularly those with blades

*If responsibility of critical care nurse includes such follow-up care.

POTENTIAL PROBLEMS	EXPECTED OUTCOMES	NURSING ACTIVITIES

		To avoid the following
		    Remaining in one position for a long time
		    Constricting clothing such as girdles, garter belts
		    Massaging or rubbing legs
		    Extremes of hot or cold; extremities should be kept dry and warm
		    Smoking
		Patient should wear medical alert bracelet and carry card with patient's name, name of drug, and phone number of who to contact in emergency
		Describe follow-up plan of care, including when and where to go, who to see, and what specimens to bring; briefly explain purpose and format of follow-up visits
		Provide opportunity for and encourage patient/family's questions
		Assess potential compliance of patient/family with discharge regimen

Neurological

STANDARD 32

INCREASED INTRACRANIAL PRESSURE

Intracranial pressure (ICP) is the pressure exerted by the constituents of the brain, namely the brain tissue, cerebrospinal fluid (CSF), and intravascular blood, which are contained within the rigid skull. The relationship between the cranial cavity and its contents largely determines the ICP. The normal volume ratios of the cranial cavity are brain tissue, 85%; CSF, approximately 10%; and intravascular blood, 2% to 11%. The expansion of one volume is at the expense of the other constituents (by subtracting from their volume), and the resulting alterations in volume and pressure eventually affect cerebral functioning and integrity and increase ICP.

ICP normally ranges from 110 to 140 mm H_2O or 0 to 10 mm Hg. Pressures above 200 mg H_2O or 15 mm Hg usually signify increased ICP. Compensatory mechanisms occur when the volume of any one constituent increases in an effort to protect the brain against damage and interference with cerebral functioning. For instance, the growth of an intracranial mass may initiate a reduction in the volume of CSF and a lesser decrease in intracranial blood volume. As long as these fluids can be displaced, the ICP remains within normal limits. However, eventually a critical point is reached at which no further displacement is possible, and the ICP rises.

For adequate cerebral functioning a continual and effective blood supply, circulation, and perfusion are necessary. Cerebral blood flow is equal to the mean arterial pressure minus the intracranial pressure (Cerebral blood flow = MAP − ICP). Other factors such as vascular resistance and venous flow also affect the flow. The term *cerebral perfusion pressure (PP)* may also be used to determine the status of the cerebral circulation. Under normal conditions PP in cerebral vessels is approximately equal to the MAP. Any increase in ICP must be subtracted from the MAP in determining the effective PP; the resulting decrease in PP reduces cerebral blood flow. Cerebral blood flow ceases when ICP equals cerebral PP.

Two major problems associated with increased ICP are the nonuniform expansion of the brain and the interference with adequate blood supply. If the increased ICP significantly lowers the effective PP, resulting in decreased cerebral blood flow, two compensatory mechanisms are activated. In *autoregulation,* the cerebral vasculature compensates by altering vascular resistance through controlled vasodilatation to maintain cerebral blood flow by decreasing arterial resistance. If ineffective, the further decrease in PP and cerebral blood flow causes Cushing phenomenon to occur, possibly as a result of brainstem ischemia. In *vasomotor control,* the smooth muscle responds to altered arterial pressures of oxygen and particularly carbon dioxide. The CNS ischemic response produces a marked rise in systemic arterial pressure. Vasodilatation also occurs in an attempt to improve cerebral blood flow. The prognosis of increased ICP can become worse if there is a complete loss of autoregulation or the development of vasoparalysis and cerebral edema. If ICP continues to increase and cannot be controlled or treated, the progression of cerebral pathology may culminate in herniation and irreversible brain damage or death.

Many processes can lead to or cause increased ICP. Among these are head trauma; brain tumors; cerebral hemorrhages, infarcts, infections, and abscesses; CSF overproduction, flow obstruction, or impaired absorption; metabolic disturbances; and toxic factors such as poisons and lead ingestion. The extent and progression of increased ICP and cerebral damage incurred vary with each individual. Some of the factors contributing to this variability include cerebral areas involved, preinsult functioning of cerebral tissue and circulation, effectiveness of collateral circulation, time period of increasing ICP (slow increase versus sudden pressure rise), effectiveness of compensatory mechanisms, amount and distribution of increased pressure and compression, and selective vulnerability of certain areas in the brain. The classical triad of symptomatology associated with increased ICP is headache, vomiting (with or without nausea), and papilledema. However, symptomatology may be varied, ranging from a single symptom to a myriad of symptoms.

Clinical symptoms of increased ICP may not be evident until the ICP has increased well above normal levels. An ICP monitor may be employed to provide for early detection and treatment of elevations.

ASSESSMENT

1. Onset, progression, duration, frequency, and specific description of neurological symptoms, including
   a. Headache: location, severity, association with specific activity/movement, time-related occurrence, any associated concurrent neurological symptoms
   b. Vomiting (with or without nausea), any projectile emesis, precipitating factors or associated symptoms, time-related patterns
   c. Papilledema; visual disturbances including diplopia, nystagmus, blurred vision, ocular palsies or impairments, pupillary changes
   d. Ataxia (severity, locality)
   e. Changes in behavior; including inattentiveness, irritability, personality changes, hallucinations
   f. Changes in LOC including forgetfullness, memory impairment, disorientation, confusion, sleepiness, or lethargy
   g. Motor/sensory dysfunctions
   h. Alterations in communication abilities
   i. Seizures
2. Previous head trauma incident; specific description of event, treatment, clinical course
3. Previous infection, particularly meningitis/encephalitis
4. Previous ingestion of poisons, toxins, or drug overdose
5. Previous symptomatology/treatment for increased ICP; neurological treatment or neurosurgical procedure
6. Medications taken for neurological status, including anticonvulsants, steroids, pain medications; effects and side effects of therapies
7. Presence of excessive thirst or urination
8. Presence of any medical problems and medications/ treatments prescribed and followed
9. Patient's perceptions and reaction to diagnosis, therapeutic modalities and anticipated surgical intervention if planned
10. Presence of any alterations in body image; fears of permanent disability or deficit; altered roles in family, normal occupation, ADL
11. Baseline parameters status
    a. Neurological
    b. Respiratory
    c. Cardiovascular
    d. Metabolic
    e. Hydration
    f. Fluid/electrolyte
    g. Skin integument (rash, ecchymosis, open areas, edema)
    h. Urine output pattern
    i. Vital signs
    j. Weight
    k. Handedness (right or left)
12. Diagnostic test results, including
    a. Skull films
    b. Tomograms
    c. CT scan
    d. Cerebral angiography
    e. Pneumoencephalogram
    f. EEG
    g. Brain scan
    h. Lumbar puncture
    i. NMR scan
13. Results of
    a. Serum electrolyte levels
    b. CSF determinations
    c. Urinalysis, culture, specific gravity, osmolality, electrolytes
    d. Arterial blood gas levels
    e. Clotting profile
    f. Serum anticonvulsant levels
    g. Hgb and Hct, platelet count, WBC count and differentiation
    h. Toxin screens
    i. Chest radiograph
    j. ECG

GOALS

1. Optimal neurological functioning
2. Optimal independence in ADL
3. Adequate alveolar ventilation and perfusion
4. Adequate cardiac output
5. Serum electrolytes and fluid balance within normal limits
6. Hgb and Hct stable and within normal limits
7. Acid-base balance within normal limits
8. Reduction in patient/family's anxiety with provision of information, demonstrations, support
9. Before discharge, patient/family is able to
   a. Describe medication, activity, exercise, and dietary regimens
   b. Describe any treatments/therapeutic measures prescribed
   c. Demonstrate safety measures and techniques; proper use of any equipment/devices prescribed
   d. Describe signs and symptoms requiring medical attention
   e. State necessary information regarding follow-up care

POTENTIAL PROBLEMS	EXPECTED OUTCOMES	NURSING ACTIVITIES

■ Progressive increased ICP related to
  Further volume expansion
  Cerebral edema
  Loss of autoregulation
  Vasoparalysis
  Cerebral herniation
	■ Absence or control of complications
	Control or resolution of increased ICP (if possible)
	Maximal neurological functioning
		■ Establish neurological baseline and vital signs on admission; ongoing assessments of status and specific symptomatology/deficit q1 hr; monitor in particular extent and degree of
		  Altered LOC
		  Pupillary changes (size, equality, light reactivity)
		  Motor/sensory system dysfunctions
		  Cranial nerve dysfunctions
		  Ocular palsies/impaired extraocular movements
		  Classical triad of increased ICP—headache, vomiting, papilledema
		  Personality changes such as restlessness, irritability
		  Ataxia
		  Diplopia/nystagmus
		  Dysphagia
		  Alterations in communication abilities, speech quality
		  Visual alterations
		  Alterations in reflex status
		  For development of Cushing phenomenon—increasing systolic BP with widening pulse pressure, decreasing pulse, and change in respiratory pattern
		  Abnormal posturing
		  In infants (if fontanelles are open, this allows greater area for brain expansion)—increased head circumference, bulging fontanelles, split sutures, irritability, somnolence, high-pitched cry, decreased feeding, sunsetting, nystagmus, vomiting
		Monitor for precipitating factors that may further increase cerebral edema and ICP such as hypoxia, hypercapnia, fever, hypotension, hypertension, myocardial damage, shock, Valsalva maneuver; if controllable, institute measures to prevent such as
		  Assist patient with positioning and turning; instruct patient not to hold breath
		  Prevent constipation by establishing bowel regimen as individually warranted
		  Avoid sharp angling of neck, which can obstruct venous outflow
		Monitor for any signs/symptoms that could initiate factor development such as hypoventilation, infection, ECG abnormalities
		Maintain head of bed as ordered; frequently it is elevated to promote venous drainage and aid in decreasing ICP
		Administer medications/treatments as ordered; monitor effects and side effects; if patient is receiving steroids, monitor for side effects including GI bleeding, glycosuria
		Monitor and accurately record intake and output as ordered (frequently q1-2 hr); assess for any imbalance
		Monitor serum electrolytes, arterial blood gas values for any abnormalities
		Have emergency equipment and medications readily available, including
		  Ventricular tap set and appropriate drill sets
		  Osmotic diuretics
		Notify physician immediately of any
		  Change in baseline neurological status whether appearance of new deficit or increasing severity of prior symptomatology such as headache, restlessness, projectile vomiting
		  Vital sign abnormality
		  Presence/potential precipitating factor occurrence
		  Fluid/electrolyte balance abnormality
		  Arterial blood gas value abnormality
		Initiate and maintain hypothermia as ordered
		Prepare patient/family for any diagnostic tests/procedures necessary
		Monitor ICP values and waveforms if patient has intracranial monitoring line inserted
		  Maintain patency/sterility of system
		  Monitor effects of other treatments or therapies on ICP including coughing, turning, suctioning, chest physiotherapy

POTENTIAL PROBLEMS	EXPECTED OUTCOMES	NURSING ACTIVITIES
		Space therapies if possible to minimize increases in ICP
		Monitor neurological status correlated with ICP values and notify physician
		If ordered, assist physician with drainage of amount of CSF fluid to maintain ICP at specific level determined; record fluid amount drained each time; monitor effects on ICP value, correlation between neurological status and CSF drainage
		Hyperventilate patient as ordered by physician for specific ICP level increase
		Administer medications/treatments as ordered; monitor effects/side effects on status and ICP; osmotic diuretics are commonly ordered prn or as ongoing therapy
		Notify physician immediately of any increase in ICP/wave recording; frequently physician will specify maximal ICP levels
		Monitor ventricular drainage system or other external drain if patient has one inserted
		Prevent compression, kinking, pulling, or tension on tubing by proper positioning; if necessary, restrain patient's hands
		Maintain patency/sterility of system
		Maintain at specific level ordered by physician
		Measure and record pressure, amount, and quality of drainage as ordered
		Check dressing q1 hr; monitor for leakage around needle or catheter site, swelling/edema
		If patient is on ICP monitoring, record pressures and drain amount of fluid specified by physician to maintain pressure values
		Monitor neurological status correlated with fluid pressure/quantity
		Administer antibiotics as ordered
		Send CSF specimens to lab as ordered and monitor results
		Monitor serum electrolytes as Na$^+$ values may decrease from loss of CSF by drainage
		Notify physician of results and replace fluids as ordered (frequently CSF fluid is ordered replaced milliliter for milliliter)
		Notify physician immediately of any change in neurological status; fluid pressure, amount/quality varying from norm specified or expected; nonpatency of system or abnormal lab values
		Monitor for signs of epidural hematoma (potential complication of drain); see Standard 33, *Head trauma*, Problem, Epidural hematoma
		If ordered, clamp tubing as specified by physician, maintaining precise time schedule and recording time, pressure, fluid drainage, amount/quality; notify physician immediately of any change in neurological status or signs of increased ICP; unclamp drain as per physician's standing or stat order
		After removal of ventricular drain by physician, monitor neurological status and vital signs frequently; drain site for bleeding, oozing, drainage/edema; monitor for signs of increased ICP
		See appropriate standard for identified etiology or surgical intervention planned, e.g.
		Standard 33, *Head trauma* Standard 42, *Meningitis/encephalitis* Standard 36, *Supratentorial craniotomy* Standard 37, *Infratentorial craniotomy* Standard 38, *Internalized shunting procedures*
■ Presence of neurological signs/symptoms	■ Maximal neurological functioning Absence of complications	■ Establish baseline neurological assessment on admission with specific documentation of status; continue ongoing assessments as ordered; implement care plan based on individual needs/deficit
		Notify physician immediately of any increase in initial deficit, progression, increased severity of symptoms, or symptomatology/deficit appearance

POTENTIAL PROBLEMS	EXPECTED OUTCOMES	NURSING ACTIVITIES
Decreased LOC		Close observation; siderails at all times when patient is alone Reorient patient frequently to time, place, and person Have family bring familiar pictures, objects for bedside Reaffirm to family relationship between patient's behavior, LOC, and neurological condition Assess family's level of anxiety related to patient's decreased LOC Encourage family's verbalization of fears and concerns Support and realistically reassure family If patient becomes restless/combative, restrain as ordered by physician if absolutely necessary to protect from injury to self or others Explain reasons for restraints to family Check restraints frequently for proper placement; monitor effectiveness, skin integrity, and circulation Reapply q4 hr and prn Remove restraints as soon as possible If patient is not moving spontaneously Turn and position properly q2 hr Apply measures to aid in prevention of complications of immobility, including sheepskin or flotation pads to promote skin integrity maintenance; monitor skin surfaces frequently for signs of impaired circulation; massage skin and pad skin areas prone to irritation
Nausea/vomiting; possible dehydration		Assess frequency/degree, association with other neurological symptoms Monitor for any abnormality Accurately record intake and output as ordered State of hydration Presence/quality of gag, cough, swallowing reflexes Serum electrolytes Hct values Administer medications as ordered; monitor effects; notify physician if control of nausea/vomiting is ineffective Notify physician if reflexes are decreased or absent Keep patient NPO Administer IV fluids/NG feedings as ordered Frequent oral hygiene
Paresis or paralysis of extremity		Assess location/degree of weakness ROM exercises as ordered by physician; passive to active dependent on patient's status q2 hr Institute measures to prevent complications such as contractures, subluxations, wrist-drop/foot-drop; may include footboard, splint, sling, handrolls Obtain order for physiotherapy referral as indicated Instruct and supervise patient/family in exercise program when status allows
Impaired sensation of extremity		Assess for nature, location/extent of impaired sensation Protect from injury and potential complications including abrasions, decubitus ulcers, burns Turn and position patient as necessary q2 hr Monitor skin integument q2 hr for any signs of impaired circulation When status allows, assist and supervise patient in necessary safety measures required by deficit such as Testing of water temperature by nurse/family Avoiding use of heating pads or other temperature devices
Ataxia		Assess location/degree of ataxia Assist and supervise patient in ADL and ambulation as necessary Apply safety measures such as siderails while patient is in bed, safety belt for wheelchair Maintain safe environment Remove as many obstacles or objects that might cause falls as possible Obtain appropriate safety equipment

POTENTIAL PROBLEMS	EXPECTED OUTCOMES	NURSING ACTIVITIES
		Obtain physician's order for physiotherapy referral as warranted
		Explain to patient/family reasons for assistance, special measures to promote safety
Headache		Assess location, degree, duration, and frequency of headache, association with any other neurological symptoms
		Maintain as quiet an environment as possible; prevent unnecessary disturbances
		Administer medication as ordered by physician (narcotics are usually not ordered)
		Monitor effectiveness
		Notify physician if headache persists
■ Fluid and electrolyte imbalance related to Increased ICP producing alterations in normal mechanism of production/release of antidiuretic hormone (ADH) Disruption/imbalances of normal hormonal control mechanism of salt and water balance	■ Fluid and electrolyte balance within normal or prescribed limits	■ Monitor and accurately record intake and output; urine specific gravity, osmolality as ordered (frequently q2 hr)
		Monitor for signs of dehydration or overhydration such as
		Poor skin turgor
		Dry mucous membranes
		Peripheral edema
		Excessive thirst
		Change in LOC
		Monitor for
		Abnormal vital signs, Hgb and Hct values
Osmotic diuretic medication administration		Abnormal serum electrolyte/osmolality values, urine electrolyte values
Plasma hyponatremia—causes of hypoosmolality include water intoxication, excess vasopressin (inappropriate ADH) either from overadministration of vasopressin or inappropriate secretion of ADH from cerebral injury or disease		Weight alterations
		Temperature elevations
		Insensible fluid losses including respiratory, diaphoresis, secretions
		Presence/degree of nausea and vomiting; effectiveness of medications ordered
		Changes in neurological status
		Monitor for signs of decreased or increased production/release of ADH (or vasopressin)
		Decreased ADH; monitor for
		Hypernatremia
		Hyperosmolality
		Dehydration
		Diabetes insipidus—polyuria, polydipsia
Plasma hypernatremia—causes of hyperosmolality include dehydration without corresponding loss of Na^+, impaired secretion of ADH from cerebral injury or disease		Cerebral dysfunction (usually occurs above 160 serum Na^+ level) including irritability, restlessness, hypertonicity, twitching, seizures, and nystagmus
		Increased ADH (inappropriate ADH); monitor for
		Hyponatremia
		Hypoosmolality
		Overhydration
		Water retention/intoxication
		Cerebral dysfunction (usually occurs below 130 serum Na^+ level) including lethargy, inattention, slight confusion, nausea/vomiting
		Administer IV fluids, NG feedings as ordered
		Administer medications as ordered; monitor effects and side effects; if patient is receiving steroids, monitor urine glucose and acetone levels as ordered
		Notify physician of any fluid imbalance or electrolyte abnormality, signs of cerebral dysfunction from ADH disorders
		If patient is receiving osmotic diuretics such as mannitol and urea, monitor
		Hourly urine output
		Serum electrolytes frequently for serious imbalances resulting from rapid diuresis of water and electrolytes
		For signs of congestive heart failure
		For dehydration or hypovolemia (may be masked)
		Notify physician of effects of therapy
		If po is allowed, maintain patient on fluid restriction or encouragement regimen as ordered by physician

POTENTIAL PROBLEMS	EXPECTED OUTCOMES	NURSING ACTIVITIES

■ Respiratory insufficiency related to
CNS dysfunction
Edema
Cranial nerve dysfunction
Pneumonia
Atelectasis
Pulmonary emboli
Cerebral dysfunction may decrease or abolish normal respiratory control mechanisms effected by chemoreceptors in aortic and carotid vessels and in medulla
If cerebral dysfunction occurs in brainstem, different respiratory abnormalities result that may not be adequate to maintain adequate ventilation and perfusion
Area and respiratory pattern
  Forebrain: posthyperventilation apnea
  Internal capsule and basal ganglia: Cheyne-Stokes respirations
  Midbrain: central neurogenic hyperventilation
  Pons: apneustic
  Medulla: ataxic, loss of automatic breathing
Respiratory acidosis can produce additional cerebral hypoxia and cerebral edema; both systemic hypoxia and hypercapnia can promote increased cerebral blood flow and cause further increase in ICP by increased volume of blood compartment
	■ Patent airway
	Adequate alveolar ventilation and perfusion
	Arterial blood gas levels within patient's normal limits
		■ Ongoing assessment of respiratory status q1 hr and prn; monitor for any abnormality/decline
		Respiratory rate, quality, and pattern
		Patency of upper airway and patient's ability to handle secretions
		Presence/strength of gag, cough, and swallowing reflexes
		Cranial nerve functioning, particularly presence/strength of nerves IX to XII
		Skin color, nail beds, peripheral pulses, and skin warmth
		Breath sounds bilaterally for quality of aeration; signs of obstruction (rales, rhonchi)
		For signs of pulmonary edema (neurogenic may occur related to increased ICP) including tachycardia, dyspnea, wheezing, peripheral edema, weight gains, decreased urinary output
		Arterial blood gas values
		Chest radiograph results
		Signs/symptoms of thrombophlebitis, pulmonary emboli
		Maintain patent airway by
		Turning and positioning to prevent obstruction or aspiration of secretions q2 hr and prn
		Deep breathing and coughing q1 hr and prn (if allowed)
		Suctioning prn
		Adequate oxygenation and humidification as ordered
		Chest physiotherapy/pulmonary toilet if warranted and not contraindicated by physician's order
		If reflexes (gag, cough, swallowing) are decreased or absent, keep patient NPO as ordered by physician; when reflexes are stronger and patient is started on po, stay with patient for initial feedings, monitor swallowing effectiveness, and assess for any signs of choking/nasal regurgitation
		Apply antithromboembolic stockings or Ace bandages as ordered, reapply every shift and prn, and monitor for constriction/looseness, condition of skin
		Instruct and supervise patient in performing leg exercises and ROM exercises as status and physician's order allow
		Increase activity level/progression when allowed
		Notify physician immediately of any change in respiratory/neurological status or signs of complication potential/occurrence
		If respiratory problem occurs, assist with emergency measures to maintain patent airway and adequate ventilation
		Administer medications/treatments as ordered; monitor effects and side effects
		Monitor neurological status closely as both hypoventilation/hyperventilation may increase ICP
		
		See STANDARD 6 *Mechanical ventilation*
		
		Explain procedures and reasons for equipment/respiratory assistance to patient/family; provide reassurance and support
		Establish alternate means of communication as needed
		If embolism occurs, see Standard 31, *Embolic phenomena*

■ Hemodynamic instability	■ BP, P, within patient's normal or prescribed limits	■ Monitor BP as ordered for any variance from minimal or maximal acceptable level specified by physician Administer medications as ordered to maintain BP level; monitor effects and side effects Notify physician immediately of BP variance or ineffectiveness of medications Monitor for Hypotension—signs of bleeding, falling Hgb levels Hypertension—signs of Cushing phenomenon Alterations in neurological status Monitor and record pulse rate and quality as ordered; notify physician immediately if patient suddenly develops symptoms of bradycardia

POTENTIAL PROBLEMS	EXPECTED OUTCOMES	NURSING ACTIVITIES
		ECG monitoring as warranted Monitor serum electrolyte values for any abnormalities, particularly in K^+ Administer medications as ordered; monitor effects and side effects
■ Fever related to Infection Disruption in normal temperature regulation by hypothalamus from increased ICP	■ Normal body temperature	■ Prevent precipitating factors such as urinary retention, pulmonary congestion-aspiration Maintain strict sterile technique for procedures such as catheterization, endotracheal/tracheostomy tube care/management Monitor Temperature as ordered and prn for any fever IV sites frequently for any signs of redness, tenderness, phlebitis WBC count (may be falsely elevated if patient is receiving steroids) For possible drug reactions, presence of skin rash For signs of meningitis For alterations in neurological status; fever may increase ICP Notify physician immediately of any temperature elevation/signs of infection Monitor possible infection sources, including urine and sputum cultures, chest radiograph results, CSF determinations Administer medications/treatments as ordered; monitor effects and side effects Maintain hypothermia blanket as ordered; institute measures to prevent complications of therapy; monitor effects and side effects Maintain hypothermia balnket as ordered; institute measures to prevent complications of therapy; monitor effects and side effects If infection occurs, monitor for resolution or progression If problem occurs, see Standard 42, *Meningitis/encephalitis*
■ Seizures	■ Absence or control of seizures	■ Prevention of precipitating factors in seizure occurrence including fever, hypoxia, H_2O intoxication, electrolyte disturbances Notify physician of potential/presence of any factors Seizure precautions (if indicated) Padded siderails up at all times when patient is alone Bed height at lowest level Padded tongue blade and airway at bedside Emergency medications and equipment readily available Close observation and supervision Administer anticonvulsant medications as ordered; monitor effects and side effects, serum anticonvulsant levels If seizure occurs, monitor and record seizure activity; notify physician *See* STANDARD 41 *Seizures*
■ GI bleeding related to CNS factors Stress Steroid administration	■ Absence or resolution of GI bleeding	■ Monitor vital signs q2-4 hr; Hgb and Hct; Hematest of stools three times a week; Hematest of aspirate, emesis, and urine for any abnormalities Obtain order for antacid administration as soon as patient able to take po Monitor for signs of GI bleeding, including abdominal tenderness/distention, hypotension, sudden tachycardia Notify physician immediately if any abnormality occurs If problem occurs, see Standard 49, *Acute upper gastrointestinal bleeding*
■ Patient/family's anxiety related to Limited understanding of clinical problem, diagnostic procedures, therapeutic measures Threat of continued neurological deficit	■ Patient/family's behavior demonstrates decreased anxiety with provision of information	■ Ongoing assessment of level of anxiety Encourage patient/family's verbalization of questions, fears, concerns Collaborate with physician in providing realistic information and reassurance appropriate to level of understanding Explain relationship between condition and clinical symptoms, status, course Explain reasons/necessity for frequent assessments

POTENTIAL PROBLEMS	EXPECTED OUTCOMES	NURSING ACTIVITIES
		Explain and prepare patient/family for treatments, diagnostic tests/procedures, therapeutic measures, anticipated operative intervention (if planned)
		Collaborate medical plan of care and nursing care plan if expected prognosis is known
		If complete recovery is expected, reassure patient/family
		If partial recovery is expected, support and encourage verbalization of fears, angers, questions; see problem, Continued presence of neurological deficit
■ Continued presence of neurological deficit Patient/family's fears, anxiety, anger related to deficit and possible alterations in life-style	■ Maximal neurological functioning* Maximal independence in ADL (within capabilities) Patient/family verbalizes concerns	■ Assess patient's specific neurological deficit Collaborate with physician regarding prognosis, possible degree of recovery Implement individualized plan of care based on patient's needs and deficits Assist as needed in ADL Monitor potential for independent functioning and obtain equipment to maximize function and promote safety Obtain orders for appropriate referrals such as physiotherapy; speech and occupational therapy; social services Encourage verbalization of patient/family's fears, anxieties, and other reactions—level and degree Answer questions realistically Encourage their participation in care planning, implementation, evaluation, and decision making Realistically reassure and support patient/family Reinforce any gains or independence patient achieves Plan, instruct, demonstrate, supervise, and evaluate patient/family's demonstration of needed information/skills for maximal independent functioning such as Measures to prevent complications Assistance necessary—type, amount, degree Proper use of therapeutic devices/equipment Monitor level of achievement toward maximizing potentials and independence; means to promote as "normal" a life-style as possible

*If responsibility of critical care nurse includes this stage of care.

POTENTIAL PROBLEMS	EXPECTED OUTCOMES	NURSING ACTIVITIES
■ Insufficient knowledge to comply with discharge regimen*	■ Patient/family demonstrates or verbalizes understanding of discharge regimen	■ Assess patient/family's level of understanding of neurological problem and therapy received Explain relationship between patient's neurological status and therapies prescribed If present, explain relationship of increased ICP occurrence to head injury, toxin exposure or drug overdose; explore with patient/family measures to prevent recurrence of condition, importance of controlling precipitating factors Instruction of patient/family regarding required information/skills so that before discharge patient/family is able to

	Patient/family accurately describes medication, activity, and dietary regimens	Describe medication regimen
		  Name and purpose
		  Route, dosage, frequency, times
		  Side effects
		  Special precautions necessary including drugs, foods, beverages contraindicated or regulated in quantity; factors potentiating/decreasing effects or side effects; physical restrictions; safety measures
		Describe dietary regimen
		Describe activity regimen, exercise program
		Describe and demonstrate any special therapeutic measures prescribed

	Patient/family describes means to achieve maximal independence in ADL, promote safety, and prevent complications	Describe and demonstrate proper use of equipment or therapeutic devices
		  Reasons for using
		  Time, method, and duration of use
		  Precautions/safeguards
		  Necessary maintenance (type, frequency)
		  Measures to promote optimal functioning, upkeep/duration

	Patient/family describes signs/symptoms requiring medical attention	Describe signs/symptoms of neurological status requiring medical care
	Patient/family describes follow-up care regimen	Describe plan for follow-up care, including purpose of appointment, when and where to go, who to see, what to expect

*If responsibility of critical care nurse includes such follow-up care.

HEAD TRAUMA

The causes of head trauma are multiple and include motor vehicle accidents, falls, and gunshot and stab wounds. Head injuries may be penetrating or nonpenetrating wounds. Cerebral trauma may result in a wide range of pathology, diversity, and complexity from a mild injury with spontaneous, complete recovery to massive brain injury with irreversible damage culminating in cerebral death. Factors influencing the variable pathological consequences include patient's age and prior status; force, duration, location, and nature of the injury; adequacy of emergency on-the-scene treatment; and functioning of other bodily systems. Common cerebral damage produced by head trauma includes contusions, concussion, skull fractures, epidural hematomas, intracerebral hematomas/hemorrhages, subdural hematomas, cranial nerve injury, and metabolic injury of neurons and brain cells (see Table 33-1 for specifics of the more common pathologies). Brain injury may occur at the time of initial trauma insult or develop days to weeks later.

Priorities of treatment and management of head trauma include maintenance of adequate airway; adequate pulmonary ventilation and perfusion; treatment of shock; prevention/control of metabolic disturbances, which cause cerebral damage that exceeds the direct traumatic effects on neuron functioning; and control of increased ICP and cerebral edema. Cerebral edema is a common complication of head injury, possibly because of an alteration in the blood-brain barrier and paralysis of autoregulation. Any patient with head trauma should initially be handled as having a potential cervical cord injury until this is ruled out.

A complete assessment is necessary to establish if there are any other injuries or complicating factors. If multiple trauma is the case, priority focuses on the injury that is most immediately life threatening (see Standard 63, *Multiple trauma*). Complications of head injury that commonly occur and that must be controlled (especially since they can mimic head injury signs/symptoms) include respiratory acidosis, cerebral fat embolism, dehydration/water intoxication, and pneumonia. Injuries in other body areas may have indirect effects on CNS functioning and may increase the progression and extent of cerebral damage. Direct cardiac damage or excessive blood loss and shock may affect the vascular system and produce cerebral hypoxia and injury. Respiratory acidosis from chest injury, pulmonary hemorrhage, and aspiration or other ventilatory problems may produce cerebral hypoxia and damage. The head injury itself frequently causes a depression of respiratory drive and promotes development of respiratory acidosis.

Head trauma requires critical observations, assessments, recognition, and prompt interventions to prevent development/progression of cerebral damage, complications, and irreversibility of pathology. No head injury can be treated "lightly," for even a seemingly insignificant head trauma incident may progress or may mask significant and severe cerebral damage or potential for damage. The treatment of head injury (see Table 5) may be medical management, immediate emergency surgical intervention, or elective surgical procedures. Surgical intervention is usually necessary for severe depressed skull fractures; hematomas; hemorrhages; persistent or recurrent rhinorrhea, otorrhea, or meningitis. Many head trauma patients, with proper nursing and medical management/interventions, can recover fully or achieve the highest possible degree of recovery within the limitations of their residual deficit.

ASSESSMENT

1. Specific description of head trauma occurrence/sequelae, including
   a. Time
   b. Nature of, such as fall, blow, car accident; if blow, instrument involved; if fall, object or distance struck
   c. Area/side of head involved, force, and duration
   d. Patient status at time of trauma and afterward, including any loss of consciousness (when, length, recovery period); headache (location, severity, concurrent neurological symptoms); nausea/vomiting (severity, amount); confusion; agitation/irritability; seizures (onset, progression, type, locality, length, postictal status)
   e. Patient awareness/amnesia of incident, events before/after; last event patient remembered
   f. Cuts, abrasions, swelling, ecchymosis, skull deformity, or scalp damage (location, severity)
   g. Amount of bleeding or other drainage from injury

TABLE 33-1. Common cerebral pathology

TYPE	CLINICAL MANIFESTATION	CLINICAL COURSE/MANAGEMENT
Concussion Occurs most commonly with blunt, non-penetrating minor head injury (patients who do not regain consciousness usually have severe damage; those who regain consciousness after trauma but then become unconscious usually require immediate surgery for evacuation of clot/hemorrhage, relief of massive cerebral swelling)	Transient loss of consciousness, which is immediate and of varying duration (from seconds to hours) Depression/suppression of reflexes Transient cessation of respiration Brief period of bradycardia and hypotension	Usually resolves spontaneously and rapidly Vital signs quickly return to normal Reflexes start returning Slow regaining of consciousness through successive levels/stages Patient may remain amnesic of injury but usually regains full recovery awareness of present situation Commonly duration of amnesia is indicative of concussion severity
Skull fracture Pathological considerations involve 　Site and potential severity of brain damage 　Pathways for influx of bacteria/air, efflux of CSF Depression—location and extent	May have drowsiness, headache, confusion, numbness and weakness of legs with Babinski sign present, temporary blindness Basal skull fractures commonly manifest cranial nerve dysfunctions particularly olfactory, optic, oculomotor, trigeminal, trochlear, facial, and auditory If underlying meninges are torn or basal fracture passes through posterior wall of nasal sinus, bacteria or air may enter cranial cavity with resulting meningitis, abscess, or air within ventricles Fractures of base of skull with dural tear 　Rhinorrhea (anterior fossa) 　Otorrhea (posterior fossa)	Depressed skull fractures become significant when underlying dura is lacerated by bone fragments or brain is compressed Surgical reelevation is usually done if fracture depression is greater than one half of skull thickness Persistence or recurrence of rhinorrhea, otorrhea, or meningitis usually requires surgical repair
Contusion Occurs most often with closed blunt injury Bruising of brain, disruption of brain tissue 　Coup lesion—directly below site of impact 　Contrecoup lesion—opposite side of brain from impact	Variable, depending on location, degree, effects on brain integrity/functioning; amount of cerebral edema; increased ICP	Mild contusions commonly resolve spontaneously Severe contusions commonly require surgical intervention to correct pathology and to decrease edema/ICP
Intracerebral hematoma/hemorrhage Commonly occurs with penetrating or open head wounds	Variable, depending on size, location, progression, amount of cerebral edema and increased ICP Focal signs of damage common (see Table 6, Standard 36, *Supratentorial craniotomy)* If subarachnoid hemorrhage is present, see Standard 34, *Subarachnoid hemorrhage*	If amenable to surgical evacuation supratentorial craniotomy or infratentorial craniotomy is done See Standard 36, *Supratentorial craniotomy;* Standard 37, *Infratentorial craniotomy*
Subdural hematoma May be acute or chronic	See Standard 35, *Subdural hematoma*	See Standard 35, *Subdural hematoma*

Continued.

TABLE 33-1. Common cerebral pathology—cont'd

TYPE	CLINICAL MANIFESTATION	CLINICAL COURSE/MANAGEMENT
Epidural hematoma Clot is usually produced by temporal or parietal fracture crossing groove containing middle meningeal artery and lacerating or rupturing artery Bleeding is usually arterial, rapid, and forceful Enlarging clot pushes medially, causing shift of brain tissue toward tentorial opening, or notch; progresses to displacement of uncal portion of temporal lobe through notch, called *uncal* or *tentorial herniation*	*Syndrome of uncal herniation* Early third nerve stage: oculomotor (third) nerve compressed at point where it exits from midbrain by uncus pushing through notch, producing dilatating ipsilateral pupil that reacts sluggishly to light Late third nerve stage: midbrain dysfunction from rapid encroachment of brainstem by herniating hippocampal gyrus; may exhibit stupor or coma, decreased or absent oculovestibular responses, contralateral hemiparesis and Babinski sign (from cerebral peduncle compression on herniation side) progressing to ipsilateral as opposite cerebral peduncle is compressed Midbrain–upper pons stage: opposite pupil dilatates and fixes; sustained hyperventilation, bilateral decerebrate rigidity	Immediate surgical evacuation of epidural hematoma in early stages of uncal herniation is necessary to prevent progression of syndrome

h. CSF leak from nose (rhinorrhea) or ear (otorrhea)—location, duration, frequency, amount, association with any other symptoms or certain activities (such as bending over, coughing, sneezing)

i. Neurological status at time of injury and following trauma

j. Treatment, emergency procedures administered

k. Other injuries or signs/symptoms of trauma areas (see Standard 63, *Multiple trauma*)

2. Onset, duration, progression, frequency, and specific description of neurological symptoms, particularly
   a. Alterations in LOC, including forgetfulness, drowsiness, irritability, agitation
   b. Changes in behavior or personality including fatigability, insomnia, nervous instability
   c. Headache
   d. Nausea/vomiting
   e. Alterations in motor/sensory abilities
   f. Pupillary alterations, impaired extraocular movements
   g. Visual disturbances including field cuts, photophobia, diplopia, nystagmus, decreased vision
   h. Cranial nerve dysfunctions
   i. Dizziness/ataxia
   j. CSF leak from nose or ear
   k. Nuchal rigidity, neck movement limitation

l. Decrease in communication abilities
m. Incontinence
n. Neurological status from trauma occurrence to admission; any fluctuations in status

3. Previous seizures—exact description including onset, progression, type, locality, length, aura, incontinence
   a. Postictal status; any injury incurred
   b. Presence of any precipitating factors such as fever, emotional upset
   c. Frequency of seizures
   d. If multiple seizures, whether seizure activity is varied or similar
   e. If patient is receiving anticonvulsants, whether prescribed regimen has been adhered to

4. Previous neurological treatment or neurosurgical procedure

5. Medications taken for neurological problem such as anticonvulsants, steroids, pain medications; effects of medications on clinical course/status

6. Presence of alcohol or drug abuse

7. Presence of any medical problems and medications/treatments prescribed and followed

8. Patient's perceptions and reaction to trauma occurrence, diagnosis, therapeutic modalities, anticipated surgical intervention (if planned)

9. Presence of any alterations in body image; fears of

permanent disability or deficit; altered role in family, normal occupation/performing ADL
10. Baseline parameters status
    a. Neurological
    b. Respiratory/pulmonary
    c. Cardiovascular
    d. Metabolic
    e. Renal
    f. Hydration
    g. Hemodynamic
    h. Fluid and electrolyte
    i. Other injury
    j. Vital signs
    k. Weight
    l. Urine output pattern
    m. Handedness (right or left)
11. Diagnostic test results, including
    a. CT scan
    b. Cerebral angiography
    c. Skull radiographs
    d. Cervical spine radiographs
    e. Chest radiographs
    f. Abdominal radiographs
    g. EEG
    h. Lumbar puncture
    i. Pneumoencephalogram
    j. Brain scan
    k. NMR scan
12. Results of
    a. Serum electrolyte levels
    b. Hgb and Hct, platelet count, WBC count with differential

c. Arterial blood gas levels
d. Clotting profile
e. CSF determinations
f. Serum drug/alcohol levels
g. Anticonvulsant drug levels
h. Blood typing and cross matching
i. Urinalysis, gravity, culture, osmolality, electrolytes
j. ECG

GOALS

1. Maximal neurological functioning
2. Maximal independence in ADL
3. Adequate alveolar ventilation and perfusion
4. Adequate cardiac output
5. Serum electrolyte levels and fluid balance within normal limits
6. Hgb and Hct stable and within normal limits
7. Acid-base balance within normal limits
8. Infection free
9. Absence or resolution of CSF leak
10. Reduction in patient/family's anxiety with provision of information, demonstrations, support
11. Before discharge patient/family is able to
    a. Describe medication, activity, exercise, and dietary regimens
    b. Demonstrate safety measures and techniques; proper use of any equipment/therapeutic devices prescribed
    c. Describe signs and symptoms requiring medical attention
    d. State necessary information regarding follow-up care

POTENTIAL PROBLEMS	EXPECTED OUTCOMES	NURSING ACTIVITIES
■ Increased ICP/decline in neurological status related to Hematoma Hemorrhage Skull fracture Cerebral edema Vasospasm Concussion/contusion	■ Absence of complications Maximal neurological functioning Control or resolution of increased ICP (if possible)	■ Establish neurological baseline and vital signs on admission; ongoing assessments of status and specific symptomatology/deficit q1 hr; in particular, monitor extent and degree of LOC (arousal and content components) alterations, especially subtle changes Change in personality, behavior, mental abilities Pupillary changes (size, equality, light reactivity); impaired extraocular movements, ocular palsies Appearance of or increase in restlessness, agitation, irritability, headache, nausea/vomiting, papilledema Motor/sensory system dysfunctions Cranial nerve dysfunctions Decline in communication abilities Decline in visual abilities including diplopia, nystagmus Alterations in vital signs, especially development of Cushing phenomenon Alterations in reflex status Abnormal posturing; decerebrate/decorticate to stimuli or spontaneously Monitor q1-2 hr For any CSF leakage—location, amount, quality For any bloody head drainage—location, amount

POTENTIAL PROBLEMS	EXPECTED OUTCOMES	NURSING ACTIVITIES
		For any swelling, edema, bulging of cranium—location, degree
		For any ecchymosis, open areas, tenderness, bone depression/protrusion
		For any signs/symptoms of subdural hematoma, intracranial hemorrhage, embolism, or cerebral infarction; for specifics see Standard 35, *Subdural hematoma;* Standard 36, *Supratentorial craniotomy;* Standard 31, *Embolic phenomena*
		Avoid precipitating factors of increased ICP such as hypoxia, hypercapnia, fever, Valsalva maneuvers
		Assist patient with positioning
		Instruct patient not to hold breath, blow nose vigorously, or reach for bedside articles (if there is CSF leak or skull fracture of sinus, instruct patient not to blow nose)
		Monitor for any signs/symptoms that could initiate development of factors such as hypoventilation/constipation
		Notify physician of factor presence/potential
		Administer IV fluids, medications/treatments as ordered; monitor effects and side effects
		Maintain head gatch and activity (usually bed rest) as ordered
		Accurately record intake and output as ordered (frequently q2 hr); monitor for any imbalance; notify physician if imbalance occurs
		Monitor serum electrolytes, CBC, and arterial blood gas levels for any abnormalities; notify physician if any abnormality occurs
		Notify physician immediately of any change in neurological status, vital signs, signs/symptoms of cerebral complications
		Prepare patient for any diagnostic tests/procedures ordered
		If surgery is necessary, see appropriate standard, i.e., Standard 35, *Subdural hematoma;* Standard 36, *Supratentorial craniototmy;* Standard 37, *Infratentorial craniotomy*
		Assist with emergency measures/treatments as necessary
		If patient has ICP line inserted, monitor values and waveforms
		Maintain patency/sterility of system
		Monitor effects of other therapies on ICP including coughing, turning, chest physiotherapy, suctioning
		Space therapies if possible to minimize increases in ICP
		Monitor neurological status correlated with ICP values and notify physician
		If ordered, assist physician with drainage of CSF amount to maintain ICP at specific level determined; record fluid amount drained each time; monitor effects on ICP value, correlation between neurological status and CSF drainage
		Hyperventilate patient as ordered by physician for specific ICP level increase
		Administer medications/treatments as ordered; monitor effects and side effects on status and ICP; frequently osmotic diuretics are ordered prn or as ongoing therapy
		Notify physician immediately of any increase in ICP/wave recording; frequently physician will specify maximal ICP limit
		See STANDARD 32 *Increased intracranial pressure*
■ Epidural hematoma	■ Absence or resolution of uncal herniation (by prompt clot evacuation) Maximal neurological functioning	■ See Problem, Increased ICP/decline in neurological status, for specific activities
		In addition, monitor in particular for
		History of brief episode of loss of consciousness followed by lucid interval progressing to unconsciousness (from hematoma enlargement and impending/actual uncal herniation)
		Subtle change in LOC including slightly more restless, agitated, or irritable behavior; thought content slightly impaired; patient slightly more difficult to arouse
		Increase in headaches, nausea/vomiting
		Change in vital signs especially development of hypertension, bradycardia, altered respiratory rate and quality

POTENTIAL PROBLEMS	EXPECTED OUTCOMES	NURSING ACTIVITIES
		Dilatating ipsilateral pupil, which reacts sluggishly to light (from third cranial nerve dysfunction); cardinal early sign of uncal herniation
		Notify physician immediately of any change in neurological status/ vital signs; dilatating ipsilateral pupil warrants immediate surgical evacuation of clot
		Administer emergency medications and treatments as ordered (osmotic diuretics are frequently ordered)
		Prepare patient for surgery as ordered
		For postoperative specifics see Standard 36, *Supratentorial craniotomy* or Standard 37, *Infratentorial craniotomy*
■ Depressed LOC, restlessness/agitation	■ Safe patient environment Absence of injury complications	■ Close observation—siderails up at all times when patient is alone
		Maintain as quiet an environment as possible, reducing excessive external stimuli to minimum
		Establish baseline and continue ongoing assessments of LOC and reflex status monitoring
		For signs of restlessness/agitation, noting degree, frequency, extent
		Components of consciousness—arousal and content
		Presence/quality of reflexes including corneal, gag, cough, swallow; if reflexes are decreased or absent, institute preventive measures such as protecting cornea with eye drops; lid taping/ closure; suctioning equipment at bedside
		Monitor for other possible causes of restlessness such as bladder/ abdominal distention, headache, hypoxia
		Notify physician if any of aforementioned occurs
		Administer medications/treatments as ordered; monitor effects
		Reorient patient frequently to time, place, person, head trauma occurrence, and necessity of hospitalization
		Apply restraints as ordered by physician if this is only alternative to protect patient from injury
		Explain to patient/family reasons for restraints
		Reassure family of necessity for restraints and relationship between patient's behavior and head trauma
		Check restraints frequently for proper placement; monitor effectiveness, skin integrity, and circulation
		Reapply q4 hr and prn
		Frequently reevaluate need for continuing restraints
		Notify physician immediately if there is sudden appearance or increase in degree of restlessness, irritability, agitation, and/or headache or change in reflex/cranial nerve status
■ Shock	■ Absence or resolution of shock Adequate cardiac output Hemodynamic stability	■ Monitor for
		Hypotension, tachycardia, diaphoresis, oliguria, skin warmth, elevated temperature q1 hr and prn
		Abnormal respiratory rate and quality, arterial blood gas values
		Falling Hgb/Hct values
		Decreasing CVP q1 hr (if available)
		Any ECG abnormality/arrhythmia
		Any external signs of bleeding and note location, amount, force, duration; apply external pressure to control bleeding; assist physician with any procedures and note effects
		Notify physician of any abnormality
		Administer medications/treatments as ordered
		Monitor blood transfusions; note effects
		Monitor for resolution/progression of problem; if shock persists, cause is usually not head injury (unless massive open bleeding head wound is present); monitor for other possible trauma sources including chest, abdomen
		See STANDARD 63 *Multiple trauma*

POTENTIAL PROBLEMS	EXPECTED OUTCOMES	NURSING ACTIVITIES
■ Respiratory insufficiency related to CNS dysfunction Edema Cranial nerve dysfunction Pneumonia Atelectasis Pulmonary emboli	■ Patent airway Normal respiratory rate and pattern Adequate alveolar ventilation and perfusion Arterial blood gas levels within patient's normal limits	■ Ongoing assessment of respiratory status q1 hr and prn; monitor for any abnormality/decline Respiratory rate, quality, and pattern Patency of upper airway and patient's ability to handle secretions Presence/strength of gag, cough, and swallow reflexes Cranial nerve functioning, particularly presence/strength of ninth to twelfth nerves Skin color, nail beds, peripheral pulses, and skin warmth Breath sounds bilaterally for quality of aeration, signs of obstruction (rales, rhonchi) For signs of pulmonary edema (neurogenic may occur related to head injury) including tachycardia, dyspnea, wheezing, peripheral edema, weight gains, decreased urinary output Arterial blood gas values Chest radiograph results Signs/symptoms of thrombophlebitis, pulmonary emboli Maintain patent airway by Turning and positioning to prevent obstruction or aspiration of secretions q2 hr and prn Deep breathing and coughing q1 hr and prn (if allowed) Suctioning prn (check with physician before nasotracheal suctioning to determine potential for basal skull fracture) Adequate oxygenation and humidification as ordered Chest physiotherapy/pulmonary toilet if warranted and not contraindicated by physician's order If reflexes (gag, cough, swallow) are decreased or absent, keep patient NPO as per physician's order; when reflexes are stronger and patient is started on po, stay with patient for initial feedings; monitor swallowing effectiveness and assess for any signs of choking/nasal regurgitation Apply antithromboembolic stockings or ACE bandages as ordered; reapply every shift and prn; monitor for constriction/looseness, condition of skin Instruct and supervise patient in performing leg exercises and ROM exercises as status and physician's order allow Increase activity level/progression when allowed Notify physician immediately of any change in respiratory/neurological status or signs of complication potential/occurrence If respiratory problem occurs, assist with emergency measures to maintain patent airway and adequate ventilation Administer medications/treatments as ordered, monitoring effects and side effects Monitor neurological status closely as both hypoventilation and hyperventilation may increase ICP See Standard 6, *Mechanical ventilation* Explain procedures and reasons for equipment/respiratory assistance to patient/family; reassure and support Establish alternate means of communication as needed If embolism occurs, see Standard 31, *Embolic phenomena*
■ Fluid and electrolyte imbalance related to Cerebral trauma commonly producing positive balance of Na⁺ and H₂O—salt retention from overproduction of aldosterone; water retention from overproduction of ADH or vasopressin Osmotic diuretic medication administration	■ Fluid and electrolyte balance within normal or prescribed limits	■ Monitor and accurately record intake and output, urine specific gravity, osmolality as ordered (frequently q2 hr) Monitor for signs of dehydration/overhydration such as Poor skin turgor Dry mucous membranes Peripheral edema Excessive thirst Change in LOC Monitor for Abnormal vital signs, Hgb/Hct values Weight alterations Abnormal serum/urine electrolyte values, particularly Na⁺, K⁺ Abnormal serum/urine osmolalities

POTENTIAL PROBLEMS	EXPECTED OUTCOMES	NURSING ACTIVITIES
		Temperature elevations
		Insensible fluid losses including respiratory, diaphoresis, secretions
		Presence/degree of nausea and vomiting; effectiveness of medications ordered
		Changes in neurological status
		Monitor for signs of increased production/release of ADH (inappropriate ADH), including
		Hyponatremia
		Hypoosmolality
		Overhydration
		Water retention/intoxication
		Cerebral dysfunction
		Administer IV fluids, NG feedings, as ordered
		Administer medications as ordered; monitor effects and side effects; if patient is receiving steroids, monitor urine glucose and acetone levels as ordered
		Notify physician of any fluid imbalance or electrolyte abnormality; signs of cerebral dysfunction from ADH disorder
		If patient is receiving osmotic diuretics such as mannitol, urea, monitor
		Hourly urine output
		For signs of congestive heart failure
		For serious imbalances from rapid diuresis of H_2O and electrolytes
		For dehydration or hypovolemia (may be masked)
		Notify physician of effects of therapy
		If patient is allowed po, maintain fluid restriction or encouragement regimen as ordered by physician

■ Seizures related to
  Head injury
  Irritative effect of blood
  Cerebral edema
  Cerebral ischemia
	■ Absence or control of seizures	■ Prevention of precipitating factors in seizure occurrence including fever, hypoxia, H_2O intoxication, electrolyte disturbances; notify physician of potential/presence of any of these factors

		Seizure precautions (if indicated)
		Padded siderails up at all times when patient is alone
		Bed height at lowest level
		Padded tongue blade and airway at bedside
		Emergency medications and equipment readily available
		Close observation and supervision
		Administer anticonvulsant medication as ordered; monitor effects and side effects, serum anticonvulsant levels
		If seizure occurs, monitor and record seizure activity; notify physician; See Standard 41, *Seizures*

■ CSF leakage related to
  Skull fracture
  Tearing/laceration of
    meninges from bone
    fragments or stress
  Penetrating or open head
    wounds
	■ Absence or resolution of CSF leak	■ If there is basal skull fracture, avoid nasotracheal suctioning or any nasal treatments

		Monitor for any signs of CSF leak, particularly rhinorrhea (with anterior fossa fractures) and otorrhea (posterior fossa fractures)
		If CSF leak occurs, try to collect specimen and test for presence of glucose (result positive if CSF)
		Monitor site, amount, and quality of drainage
		Notify physician immediately
		Administer medications/treatments as ordered
		Monitor for persistence/resolution of CSF leak
		Monitor for signs/symptoms of meningitis; if problem occurs, see Standard 42, *Meningitis/encephalitis*
		If CSF leak/meningitis is persistent or recurrent, surgical intervention is usually performed; see Standard 36, *Supratentorial craniotomy* for postoperative specifics

■ Infection related to
  Skull fracture
  Penetrating or open head
    wounds
  Other sources of infection
	■ Absence or resolution of infection	■ Keep patient's hands from any open head wounds, CSF leak sites

		Prevent precipitating factors such as urinary retention, pulmonary congestion/aspiration
		Maintain strict sterile technique for procedures such as wound irrigations, dressing changes, catheterization, endotracheal/tracheostomy tube care/management

POTENTIAL PROBLEMS	EXPECTED OUTCOMES	NURSING ACTIVITIES

		Monitor
		    Temperature q2-4 hr for any elevation
		    IV sites frequently for any signs of redness, tenderness, phlebitis
		    Wounds for any signs of redness, bulging, tenderness, drainage quantity/quality
		    Neurological status and vital signs for any decline/abnormality
		    For any signs of meningitis
		    WBC count (may be falsely elevated if patient is receiving steroids)
		Notify physician of any signs of infection
		If signs of infection are present
		    Administer medications/treatments as ordered; monitor effects and side effects
		    Monitor wound culture results
		    Monitor for other possible infection sources if warranted, including urine and sputum cultures, chest radiograph results, CSF determinations
		    Institute measures if possible to promote resolution of infection source
		    Monitor for resolution/progression of infection
		If problem occurs, see Standard 42, *Meningitis/encephalitis*

■ Presence of neurological deficit	■ Absence of complications Maximal neurological functioning	■ On admission establish and implement nursing care plan based on individual needs and specific deficit present; ongoing assessments of effectiveness of interventions Institute measures to promote optimal muscular tone, functioning, and maintenance; skin integrity; and circulation Prevent complications such as contractures, foot-drop/wrist-drop, decubiti by measures such as sheepskin/air mattress, footboard, handrolls/splints, ROM exercises from active to passive as status allows, frequent turning, and proper positioning Keep skin clean, dry, and pressure free; monitor skin integrity, circulation, and potential pressure sites q2 hr and prn Obtain orders for appropriate referrals/equipment such as physiotherapy/occupational therapy

■ Patient/family's fear, anxiety, anger related to
Limited understanding of diagnostic tests/procedures
Head trauma occurrence
Presence of neurological deficit or potential development/worsening
	■ Patient/family's behavior indicates decreased anxiety with provision of information
	Patient/family verbalizes fears, angers, concerns
		■ Ongoing assessment of level of anxiety and other reactions
		Encourage patient/family's verbalization of questions, fears, anger
		Collaborate with physician in providing realistic information and reassurance appropriate to level of understanding
		    Explain relationship between pathology and clinical symptoms, status, course
		    Explain anticipated treatments, therapeutic measures, and clinical course/prognosis (if known)
		    Explain and prepare patient/family for diagnostic tests or procedures, operative intervention if planned
		    Explain reasons for frequent monitoring of neurological status and vital signs
		If patient/family expresses anger regarding head trauma (especially if it was induced by violence), encourage them to express feelings and support them in dealing with stages and reactions and accepting reality of present situation
		Obtain appropriate referrals such as religious personnel, social services

■ Posttraumatic nervous instability/psychiatric disorders
Patient/family's anxiety, anger related to presence
	■ Patient/family verbalizes concerns
	Patient/family's behavior indicates decreased anxiety with provision of information
		■ Ongoing assessment of patient behavior, signs/symptoms, patient/family's anxiety
		Explain relationship of behavior, signs/symptoms to head trauma
		Reassure patient/family that status will gradually improve with time
		Establish plan of care and instruct family in appropriate interventions based on individual patient needs such as
		    Maintain calm, quiet, supportive environment
		    Reduce environmental/emotional stresses, external stimuli as much as possible

POTENTIAL PROBLEMS	EXPECTED OUTCOMES	NURSING ACTIVITIES
This posttraumatic syndrome commonly occurs and usually lessens or disappears over a period ranging from months to years Persistent amnesia of trauma incident, headache, impaired memory capabilities, fatigability, and insomnia are common symptoms		Repeat explanations frequently and simply Support and reassure patient in progression of recovery according to individual rate of recovery; avoid "pushing" or "demand pressuring" Avoid taxing mental energies Reorient patient to reality and circumstances of present and past experiences; have family bring in familiar pictures, objects Assist and support patient in gradually returning to "normal" lifestyle, role, ADL Assist patient in judgments, perceptions, reorientation to space and time, etc., as needed Protect patient from self-injury as needed Encourage patient/family to maintain support, patience; encourage family acceptance of behavior by reinforcing pathological causes
■ GI bleeding related to CNS factors Stress Steroid administration	■ Absence or resolution of GI bleeding	■ Monitor vital signs q2-4 hr, Hgb and Hct, stools for Hematest three times a week, Hematest of aspirate, emesis and urine for any abnormalities Obtain order for antacid administration as soon as patient is able to take po Monitor for signs of GI bleeding including abdominal tenderness/distention, hypotension, sudden tachycardia Notify physician immediately if any abnormality occurs; if problem occurs, see Standard 49, *Acute upper gastrointestinal bleeding*
■ Dizziness when activity increase initiated	■ Control of dizziness Patient ambulates safely	■ When patient increases activity level, monitor vital signs and assess for dizziness Gradually increase head gatch level Have patient dangle legs at side of bed for short periods Assist/supervise patient in getting out of bed and ambulating as needed Provide rest periods between activities to gradually increase activity tolerance levels/strengths
■ Continued presence of neurological deficit Patient/family's fears, anxiety, anger related to deficit and possible alterations in life-style	■ Maximal neurological functioning* Maximal independence in ADL (within capabilities) Patient/family verbalizes concerns	■ Assess patient's specific neurological deficit; collaborate with physician regarding prognosis, expected degree of recovery Implement individualized plan of care based on patient's needs and deficits Assist as needed in ADL Monitor potential for independent functioning, and obtain equipment to maximize function and promote safety Obtain orders for appropriate referrals such as physiotherapy; speech and occupational therapy; and social services Encourage verbalization of patient/family's fears, anxieties, and other reactions—level and degree Answer questions realistically Encourage patient/family's participation in care planning, implementation, evaluation, and decision making Realistically reassure and support patient/family Reinforce any gains or independence that patient achieves Plan, instruct, demonstrate, supervise, and evaluate patient/family's demonstrations of needed information/skills for maximal independent functioning such as Measures to prevent complications Assistance necessary—type, amount, degree Proper use of therapeutic devices/equipment Monitor level of achievement toward maximizing potentials and independence; means to promote as "normal" a life-style as possible

*If responsibility of critical care nurse includes this stage of care.

POTENTIAL PROBLEMS	EXPECTED OUTCOMES	NURSING ACTIVITIES
▪ Insufficient knowledge to comply with discharge regimen*	▪ Patient/family demonstrates or verbalizes understanding of discharge regimen	▪ Assess patient/family's level of understanding of neurological problem and therapy received Explain relationship between patient's neurological status and therapies prescribed If factors/circumstances in head trauma can be controlled, explain to patient/family relationship of factors to head trauma and importance of controlling them to prevent recurrence of trauma; some individual factors may include alcohol intake, drug ingestion, safety precautions/measures, safety devices/equipment; obtain appropriate referrals and counseling services as needed Instruction of patient/family regarding required information and skills so that before discharge patient/family is able to

	Patient/family accurately describes medication, activity, and dietary regimens	Describe medication regimen
		  Name and purpose
		  Route, dosage, frequency, times
		  Side effects
		  Special precautions necessary, including drugs, foods, beverages contraindicated or regulated in quantity; factors potentiating/decreasing effects or side effects; physical restrictions; safety measures
		Describe dietary regimen
		Describe activity regimen, exercise program
		Describe and demonstrate any special therapeutic measures prescribed

	Patient/family describes means to achieve maximal independence in ADL, promote safety, and prevent complications	Describe and demonstrate proper use of equipment or therapeutic devices
		  Reasons for using
		  Time, method, and duration of use
		  Precautions/safeguards
		  Necessary maintenance (type, frequency)
		  Measures to promote optimal functioning, upkeep/duration

	Patient/family describes signs/symptoms requiring medical attention	Describe signs/symptoms of neurological status requiring medical care
	Patient/family describes follow-up care regimen	Describe plan for follow-up care including purpose of appointment, when and where to go, who to see, what to expect

*If responsibility of critical care nurse includes such follow-up care.

SUBARACHNOID HEMORRHAGE

The subarachnoid space lies between the pia mater and the arachnoid membranes. The brain and spinal cord are suspended in CSF, which fills the subarachnoid space surrounding them. A subarachnoid hemorrhage (SAH) occurs when blood escapes from a cerebral artery to the subarachnoid space. Causes of SAH include head trauma, rupture of an intracranial aneurysm, bleeding from arteriovenous malformations, and hemorrhage into brain tumors.

Diagnosis of a subarachnoid hemorrhage is suspected from the patient's history and presenting signs and symptoms. Confirmation is usually obtained by performing a lumbar puncture. Significant findings confirming a SAH include an elevation of CSF pressure (often greater than 300 mm H_2O); presence of blood on an atraumatic tap; a high CSF erythrocyte count on the first and last specimens; and/or xanthochromic appearance of the spinal fluid. The protein content of the CSF may be elevated above normal levels because of the presence of cells.

Signs and symptoms of SAH may range from a minimal to a severe neurological deficit. Some of the factors affecting the symptomatology variability include type of pathology, size and extent of the bleeding, areas involved in the bleeding, presence and degree of vasospasm, and/or hydrocephalus. Signs/symptoms that frequently occur with SAH include the following:

1. Headache—usually sudden, severe, and associated with activity
2. Alteration in consciousness—patient may have brief loss of consciousness and then become alert or drowsy
3. Mental dysfunctions such as confusion, apathy, restlessness, irritability
4. Meningeal irritation from blood in the spinal fluid, possibly with irritation of nerve roots, resulting in irritability, photophobia, nuchal rigidity (neck stiffness and resistance to passive motion), and fever
5. Nausea/vomiting
6. Focal neurological signs such as motor weakness, sensory disturbances, speech disorders, seizures, visual disturbances, and diplopia

On admission the immediate goal of therapy is to prevent further hemorrhage and promote recovery of neurological functioning. The therapeutic intervention decided on for the future depends on the cause of the SAH. Surgical intervention may be performed for some patients, whereas for others medical treatment is preferable. The following assessment and standard apply to any patient with an SAH, regardless of the cause or possible future surgical intervention.

ASSESSMENT

1. Onset, duration, progression, and specific description of neurological symptoms, including
   a. Headache
   b. Nuchal rigidity
   c. Alterations in LOC
   d. Changes in behavior or personality
   e. Changes in motor/sensory functioning
   f. Communication deficits
   g. Nausea/vomiting
   h. Visual disturbances
   i. Pupillary changes; ptosis of eyelid
   j. Seizures
2. Previous head trauma or injury—exact description of incident, clinical course, treatment, sequelae
3. Previous neurological treatment or neurosurgical procedure; medications taken, effects on clinical course/status
4. Presence of any medical problems and medications/treatments employed
5. Patient's perceptions of and reaction to diagnosis and treatment modalities
6. Presence of any alterations in body image; fear of permanent disability or deficit; altered role in family, normal occupation, performance of ADL
7. Baseline parameters status
   a. Neurological
   b. Respiratory
   c. Cardiac
   d. Circulatory and vascular
   e. Metabolic
   f. Hydration/nutritional
   g. Vital signs
   h. Weight
   i. Handedness (right or left)

8. Diagnostic test results, including
   a. CT scan
   b. Lumbar puncture
   c. Cerebral angiography
   d. Brain scan
   e. EEG
   f. NMR scan
9. Results of
   a. Serum electrolyte levels
   b. Hgb and Hct, platelet count
   c. Clotting profile
   d. Anticonvulsant drug levels
   e. CSF determinations
   f. Urinalysis, culture, gravity, osmolality
   g. ECG
   h. Chest radiograph
   i. Arterial blood gas levels

GOALS

1. Maximal neurological functioning
2. Optimal independence in ADL within physical limitations (when allowed)
3. Adequate alveolar ventilation
4. Serum electrolytes and fluid balance within normal limits
5. Hgb and Hct stable within normal limits
6. Acid-base balance within normal limits
7. Infection free
8. Reduction in patient/family's anxiety with provision of information, demonstrations, support
9. Before discharge patient/family is able to
   a. Describe medication, activity, exercise, and dietary regimens
   b. Demonstrate safety measures and techniques; proper use of any equipment, therapeutic devices
   c. Describe any special precautions/measures to decrease rebleeding potential (especially if SAH is the result of head trauma)
   d. Describe signs and symptoms requiring medical attention
   e. State necessary information regarding follow-up care

POTENTIAL PROBLEMS	EXPECTED OUTCOMES	NURSING ACTIVITIES
■ Rebleeding Greatest potential for rebleeding is usually 1 to 2 weeks after initial bleeding	■ Absence or resolution of rebleeding Absence of complications Minimal external stimulation	■ Establish neurological baseline and vital signs on admission Follow physician's policy/orders regarding minimization of external stimuli; may include Single, quiet, dark room Absolute bed rest Feeding, turning, and bathing patient Limitation of visitors to immediate family; certain number, time period Minimization of patient's talking Head of bed elevated at angle specified (usually 15 to 20 degrees) Siderails in position when patient is alone No smoking in patient's room or by patient Restriction or no use allowed of telephone, television, radio Restriction of coffee/tea, very hot/cold foods No rectal temperatures or treatments Prevent constipation by establishing bowel regimen when patient is admitted Assess patient's normal elimination pattern, food likes, aids in elimination Obtain necessary orders from physician such as stool softeners, laxatives Accurately record bowel movements, amount, consistency Monitor neurological status and vital signs as ordered and prn, especially for changes in LOC Motor and sensory functioning Behavior or personality Pupil equality, size, reaction; extraocular movements; ptosis Visual abilities including acuity, diplopia, nystagmus, photophobia Presence/extent of headache, nausea or vomiting, nuchal rigidity Communication abilities Cranial nerve functioning Monitor for factors that could increase anxiety/agitation such as bladder and abdominal distention; notify physician if not resolved

POTENTIAL PROBLEMS	EXPECTED OUTCOMES	NURSING ACTIVITIES

		Administer medications as ordered; monitor effect and side effects
		  Sedation is usually ordered for patient
		  Notify physician of effectiveness; monitor serum drug levels
		Caution family to avoid discussing condition, potential complications, or prognosis with patient
		Notify physician immediately of any change in neurological status or vital signs

■ Increased ICP related to
  Hematoma formation
  Hydrocephalus
  Cerebral edema from
    vasospasm
  Ischemic infarction/re-
    bleeding
	■ Absence or resolution of
	  increased ICP
		■ Avoid precipitating factors in increased ICP such as hypoxia, hypercapnia, fever, Valsalva maneuver
		  Assist patient in positioning and turning
		  Instruct patient not to hold breath, blow nose vigorously, or reach for bedside articles
		  Monitor for any signs/symptoms that could initiate development of factors such as hypoventilation, constipation
		  Notify physician of potential/presence of any factors
		Maintain head gatch and bed rest as ordered
		Monitor neurological status and vital signs as ordered and prn (see Problem, Rebleeding: monitor neurological status and vital signs [nursing activities] for specifics)
		Administer medications, treatments, and IV fluids as ordered; monitor effects and side effects
		Accurately record intake and output; monitor for any imbalance
		Monitor serum electrolyte levels, CBC, arterial blood gas values for any abnormalities
		Notify physician of any change in neurological status or vital signs or of abnormal fluid balance/lab values
		If problem occurs, see Standard 32, *Increased intracranial pressure*

■ Presence of neurological
  deficit
	■ Absence of complications
	  Maximal neurological
	    functioning
		■ On admission establish and implement nursing care plan based on individual needs and specific deficit present
		Implement interventions based on needs/deficit such as
		  Diplopia: provide and institute alternating eye patch
		  Headache: provide quiet environment; medicate as per physician's order; monitor effects and notify physician if measures are ineffectual
		  Restricted activity/movement: turn and position properly q2 hr; use sheepskin or air mattress; monitor skin and bony prominences frequently for any abnormalities
		  Weakness or paralysis: maintain proper limb alignment to prevent foot-drop, subluxation/contractures; measures may include footboard, splints, sling, handrolls, ROM exercises if allowed
		  Communication deficits: establish alternate means of communication if possible
		Ongoing assessments and evaluations of neurological status and effectiveness of interventions
		Notify physician of any signs/symptoms of complications

■ Hypertension	■ BP within normal or pre- scribed limits	■ Maintain minimal amount of external stimuli/emotional stress Monitor and record BP as ordered (usually q1-2 hr) Administer medications as ordered; monitor effects, side effects, and relevant serum level values Notify physician immediately of any increase in BP above specified maximal level

■ Seizures	■ Absence or control of sei-
	  zures
		■ Prevention of precipitating factors in seizure occurrence, including fever, hypoxia, H_2O intoxication, electrolyte disturbances
		  Notify physician of potential/presence of any factors
		Seizure precautions (if indicated)
		  Padded siderails up at all times when patient is alone
		  Bed height at lowest level
		  Padded tongue blade and airway at bedside
		  Emergency medications and equipment readily available
		  Close observation and supervision

POTENTIAL PROBLEMS	EXPECTED OUTCOMES	NURSING ACTIVITIES
		Administer anticonvulsant medications as ordered; monitor effects and side effects, serum anticonvulsant levels
		If seizure occurs, monitor and record seizure activity; notify physician; see Standard 41, *Seizures*
■ Fluid and electrolyte imbalance	■ Fluid and electrolyte balance within normal limits	■ Monitor and accurately record intake and output, urine specific gravity as ordered
		Monitor for signs of dehydration or overhydration such as
		Poor skin turgor
		Dry mucous membranes
		Peripheral edema
		Excessive thirst
		Change in LOC
		Monitor for
		Abnormal vital signs, Hgb/Hct values
		Abnormal serum electrolyte values
		Weight alterations
		Temperature elevations
		Insensible fluid losses including respiratory, diaphoresis, secretions
		Presence/degree of nausea and vomiting; effectiveness of medications ordered
		Administer IV fluids, NG feedings as ordered
		Administer medications as ordered; monitor effects and side effects; if patient is receiving steroids, monitor urine glucose and acetone levels four times a day
		Notify physician of any fluid imbalance or electrolyte abnormality

■ Respiratory insufficiency related to
  CNS dysfunction
  Pneumonia
  Atelectasis
  Pulmonary emboli
	■ Patent airway
	  Adequate alveolar ventilation
	  Normal respiratory rate and quality
	  Arterial blood gas levels within patient's normal limits
		■ Ongoing assessment of respiratory status q2 hr and prn

		Assess and monitor for any abnormality/decline
		Respiratory rate, quality, and pattern
		Patency of upper airway and patient's ability to handle secretions
		Skin color, nail beds, peripheral pulses, and skin warmth
		Presence/strength of gag, cough, and swallow reflexes
		Breath sounds bilaterally for quality of aeration; signs of obstruction (rales, rhonchi)
		Arterial blood gas values
		Chest radiograph results
		Signs/symptoms of thrombophlebitis, pulmonary emboli, pulmonary edema
		Maintain patent airway by
		Turning and positioning to prevent obstruction or aspiration of secretions q2 hr
		Deep breathing, gentle suctioning, and coughing prn if not contraindicated by physician's orders
		Adequate oxygenation and humidification as ordered
		Apply antithromboembolic stockings or Ace bandages as ordered; reapply every shift and prn; monitor for constriction/looseness, condition of skin
		Instruct and supervise patient in performing leg exercises (if allowed by physician)
		Increase activity level/progression when allowed
		Notify physician immediately of any change in respiratory/neurological status
		If problem occurs, assist with emergency measures to maintain patent airway and adequate ventilation; see Standard 6, *Mechanical ventilation*
		If emboli occur, see Standard 31, *Embolic phenomena*
■ Infection	■ Absence or resolution of infection	■ Prevent precipitating factors such as urinary retention, pulmonary congestion/aspiration
		Maintain strict sterile technique for procedures such as catheterization; endotracheal/tracheostomy tube care, management, suctioning

POTENTIAL PROBLEMS	EXPECTED OUTCOMES	NURSING ACTIVITIES

		Monitor
		    Temperature (usually ordered orally) q4 hr and prn for any elevation
		    IV sites frequently for any signs of redness, tenderness/phlebitis
		    For potential infection sources including pulmonary, urinary, exposure to infection sources
		    WBC count (may be falsely elevated if patient is receiving steroids)
		If temperature elevation or sign of infection occurs, notify physician and culture possible infection sources
		    Monitor sputum/urine cultures, chest radiograph results, CSF cultures
		    Continue accurate recording of intake and output; monitor for dehydration/overhydration
		    Institute measures to promote resolution of infection source if possible
		    Administer medications and treatments as ordered
		If CSF infection occurs, see Standard 42, *Meningitis/encephalitis*

■ GI bleeding related to CNS factors Stress Steroid administration	■ Absence or resolution of GI bleeding	■ Monitor vital signs q2-4 hr, Hgb and Hct, stools for Hematest three times a week; Hematest of aspirate, emesis, and urine for any abnormalities Obtain order for antacid administration as soon as patient able to take po Monitor for signs of GI bleeding including abdominal tenderness/distention, hypotension, sudden tachycardia Notify physician immediately if any abnormalities occur If problem occurs, see Standard 49, *Upper gastrointestinal bleeding*

■ Patient/family's anxiety related to
Fear of disability/death
Uncertain prognosis
Potential/presence of deficit
	■ Minimal emotional stress
	Family verbalizes fears/concerns away from patient
		■ Ongoing assessment of patient/family's level of anxiety
		Reduce external stimuli and stress factors to patient
		    Explain to family reasons for avoiding stress
		    Instruct family not to question patient or discuss stressful issues
		Collaborate with physician in providing realistic information and reassurance to family
		    Encourage verbalization of fears and concerns
		    Answer questions appropriate to level of understanding
		If patient is to undergo surgery, see Standard 36, *Supratentorial craniotomy*, but check with physician regarding what specific information and preparation of patient is allowed (physician may not want any done or only minimal to avoid preoperative stress)
		If patient is being treated conservatively, is progressing toward plans of discharge, and is stable
		    Encourage verbalization of fears/concerns
		    Answer questions appropriate to level of understanding
		    Provide time and support
		    Ongoing assessment of level of anxiety; potential for independent functioning in ADL; and reactions to hospitalization, diagnosis/treatments

■ Continued presence of neurological deficit
Patient/family's fears, anxiety, anger related to deficit and possible alterations in life-style
	■ Maximal neurological functioning*
	Maximal independence in ADL (within capabilities)
	Patient/family verbalizes concerns
		■ Assess patient's specific neurological deficit
		Implement individualized plan of care based on patient's needs and deficits
		    Assist as needed in ADL
		    Monitor potential for independent functioning and obtain equipment to maximize function and promote safety
		    Obtain orders for appropriate referrals such as physiotherapy, speech and occupational therapy; social service
		Encourage verbalization of patient/family's fears, anxieties, and other reactions—level and degree
		    Answer questions realistically
		    Encourage their participation in care planning, implementation, evaluation, and decision making
		    Realistically reassure and support patient/family

*If responsibility of critical care nurse includes this stage of care.

POTENTIAL PROBLEMS	EXPECTED OUTCOMES	NURSING ACTIVITIES
		Reinforce any gains or independence patient achieves
		Plan, instruct, demonstrate, supervise, and evaluate patient/family's verbalization/performance of needed information/skills for maximal independent functioning such as
		Measures to prevent complications
		Assistance necessary—type, amount, degree
		Proper use of therapeutic devices/equipment
		Monitor level of achievement toward maximizing potentials and independence; means to promote as "normal" a life-style as possible
■ Insufficient knowledge to comply with discharge regimen*	■ Patient/family demonstrates or verbalizes understanding of discharge regimen	■ Assess patient/family's level of understanding of neurological problem and therapy received
		Explain relationship between patient's neurological status and therapies prescribed
		If appropriate, explain relationship between head injury occurrence and SAH
		Encourage patient/family to discuss means, measures, alterations, precautions to decrease potential for head injury recurrence
		Explain safety precautions to prevent head injury recurrence
		Instruct patient/family regarding required information and skills so that before discharge patient/family is able to
	Patient/family describes medication, activity, and dietary regimens	Describe medication regimen
		Name and purpose
		Route, dosage, frequency, times
		Side effects
		Special precautions necessary including drugs, foods, beverages contraindicated or quantity regulated; factors potentiating/decreasing effects or side effects; physical restrictions; safety measures
		Describe dietary regimen
		Describe activity regimen, exercise program
		Describe and demonstrate any special therapeutic measures prescribed
	Patient/family describes and demonstrates means to achieve maximal independence in ADL, promote maximal safety, and prevent complications	Describe and demonstrate proper use of equipment or therapeutic devices
		Reasons for using
		Time, method, and duration of use
		Precautions/safeguards
		Necessary maintenance (type, frequency)
		Measures to promote optimal functioning, upkeep/duration
	Patient/family describes signs/symptoms requiring medical attention	Describes signs/symptoms of neurological status requiring medical care
	Patient/family describes follow-up care regimen	Describes plan for follow-up care including purpose of appointment, when and where to go, and who to see, what to expect

*If responsibility of critical care nurse includes this stage of care.

SUBDURAL HEMATOMA

A subdural hematoma is a collection of blood, which may be mixed with blood pigments and proteins, that accumulates in the subdural space (the area in which the dura and arachnoid membranes meet). Subdural hemorrhage is usually a consequence of head trauma. The hemorrhages are mainly venous in origin, so bleeding and accumulation are slower than in epidural hemorrhages. The common sources of subdural bleeding are cortical hemorrhagic contusions involving tearing of the arachnoid and lacerations or tears of the dura. Approximately one third of hemorrhages result from rupture of bridging veins. Subdural hemorrhage is most common over the lateral and upper aspects of the hemispheres and in the temporal regions. The hematomas may be unilateral or bilateral.

Subdural hematomas are more common in the elderly (especially if cortical atrophy is present, allowing a larger area in the subdural space for accumulation), alcoholics, and patients receiving anticoagulant therapy. Cause is unknown in approximately one tenth of hematoma occurrence.

The two main types or classifications of subdural hematoma are acute and chronic.

An *acute* subdural hematoma is usually associated with a severe head injury. Frequently the hematoma is accompanied by cerebral contusion and laceration. The most common symptoms are headaches, drowsiness, confusion, slowness in thinking, and sometimes agitation. The symptoms worsen progressively, and in later stages hemiparesis or focal signs may occur. Acute subdural hematomas evolve rapidly, because they mainly involve tearing of bridging veins, and symptoms result from direct compression of the brain by the fresh, expanding clot. The bleeding may cease when the ICP rises, compressing the veins, so the progression of symptoms is usually not as rapid as with an epidural hematoma. Rarely, a subdural hematoma may occur in the posterior fossa, causing symptoms of headache, vomiting, dysphagia, cranial nerve palsies, and anisocoria (pupil inequality).

In patients with *chronic* subdural hematoma the traumatic etiology is often more obscure—the injury may have been so slight that the person is unaware of or has forgotten the incident. The bleeding usually spreads thinly and widely over the hemisphere for a period extending from weeks to months. The blood clot organizes and then becomes encased by fibrous membranes. As red cells hemolyze and blood proteins disintegrate, the osmotic pressure rises, resulting in fluid entrance into the hematoma and producing an enlargement of the hematoma and increased compression of brain tissue. This stage of membrane formation around the hematoma usually occurs within 4 to 8 weeks after the initial insult. The common symptoms that occur weeks after the injury include headache, diffuse mental changes, personality changes, confusion, and occasionally seizures and hemiparesis. The symptoms commonly fluctuate from day to day, possibly because of alterations in the delicate balance between compensation and decompensation of neural and vascular structures around the tentorial notch.

The diagnosis of subdural hematoma is commonly suspected based on the patient's history, clinical status and symptoms, and past or recent head injury. Treatment of a subdural hematoma is surgical—burr holes are placed over the appropriate brain lobe and the clot is evacuated. Surgical evacuation can prevent further progression of neurological deterioration from cerebral compression and displacement.

ASSESSMENT

1. Previous head injury or trauma—exact description of incident, clinical course, treatment, sequelae
2. Presence of external physical signs of head injury, including ecchymosis, swelling, lacerations—location, severity, duration
3. Onset, progression, frequency, duration, fluctuations, and specific description of neurological symptoms, including
   a. Headache
   b. Mental changes
   c. Personality changes
   d. Alterations in LOC
   e. Alterations in communication abilities
   f. Motor weakness
   g. Sensory disturbances
   h. Nausea/vomiting
   i. Ataxia
   j. Pupillary changes
   k. Visual deficits/alterations

l. Seizures

4. Previous neurological treatment or neurosurgical procedure; medications taken, effects on clinical course/status
5. Presence of any potentially related medical problems especially blood dyscrasias, emboli, alcoholism, hypertension; medications taken, particularly anticoagulants; therapies employed
6. Patient's perceptions and reaction to diagnosis, treatment modalities, surgical intervention
7. Presence of any alterations in body image; fears of permanent disability or deficit; altered role in family, normal occupation, performing ADL
8. Baseline parameters status
   a. Neurological
   b. Respiratory
   c. Circulatory and vascular
   d. Cardiac
   e. Metabolic
   f. Hydration/nutritional
   g. Vital signs
   h. Weight
   i. Handedness (right or left)
9. Diagnostic test results, including
   a. CT scan
   b. Cerebral arteriography
   c. Skull radiographs
   d. Tomography
   e. EEG
   f. Brain scan
   g. Lumbar puncture
   h. NMR scan

0. Results of
   a. Serum electrolyte levels
   b. Hgb and Hct, platelet count
   c. Clotting profile
   d. Arterial blood gas levels
   e. Anticonvulsant drug levels
   f. Type and cross-matching
   g. Urinalysis, osmolality, gravity, culture
   h. ECG
   i. Chest radiograph
   j. If indicated; alcohol levels, liver/renal function tests, lung scan/thrombophlebitis studies

GOALS

1. Maximal neurological functioning
2. Optimal independence in ADL
3. Serum electrolytes and fluid balance within normal limits
4. Hgb and Hct stable within normal limits
5. Acid-base balance within normal limits
6. Burr hole sites well-healed and infection free
7. Reduction in patient/family's anxiety with provision of information, demonstrations, support
8. Before discharge patient/family is able to
   a. Describe medication, activity, exercise, and dietary regimens
   b. Demonstrate safety measures and techniques; proper use of any equipment, therapeutic devices
   c. Describe any special precautions/measures to aid in prevention of hematoma recurrence
   d. Describe signs and symptoms requiring medical attention
   e. State necessary information regarding follow-up care

POTENTIAL PROBLEMS	EXPECTED OUTCOMES	NURSING ACTIVITIES
Preoperative		
■ Increased ICP/decline in neurological functioning related to suspected/confirmed subdural hematoma	■ Absence/resolution of increased ICP Maximal neurological functioning	■ Establish neurological baseline and vital signs on admission Prevent precipitating factors of increased ICP such as hypoxia, hypercapnia, fever, Valsalva maneuvers Monitor for any signs/symptoms that could initiate development of factors such as hypoventilation, constipation Assist patient with positioning; instruct patient not to hold breath Notify physician of potential/presence of any factors Monitor neurological status and vital signs as ordered and report any change to physician immediately, especially Subtle alteration in LOC, personality, mental abilities; may have drowsiness, inattentiveness, forgetfulness, confusion, withdrawal, etc. Appearance of or increase in restlessness, agitation, irritability Appearance of or increase in headache, nausea/vomiting (severity, frequency, duration) Decline in motor, sensory, or communication abilities/functioning Pupillary changes, decreased visual abilities Alterations in vital signs Appearance of or increased ataxia Fluctuations in status; monitor specific symptomatology onset, progression, duration, appearance of or increased headache

POTENTIAL PROBLEMS	EXPECTED OUTCOMES	NURSING ACTIVITIES
		Maintain activity level and head gatch as ordered
		Monitor for any imbalance/abnormality; notify physician if any imbalance/abnormality occurs
		Intake and output
		Serum electrolytes
		Hgb and Hct
		Arterial blood gas levels
		Temperature
		Administer medications/treatments as ordered; monitor effects and side effects
		Establish and record neurological baseline immediately before surgery (if possible) to provide for comparison postoperatively
■ Restlessness and agitation	■ Safe patient environment Absence of injury complications	■ Close observation; siderails up at all times when patient is alone
		Monitor for other possible causes of restlessness/agitation such as abdominal/bladder distention, headache, hypoxia
		Notify physician if any of the aforementioned occurs
		Administer analgesics, comfort measures, treatments as ordered
		Monitor for signs/degree of restlessness and agitation; notify physician immediately regarding sudden appearance or increase in degree
		Reorient patient to reality—time, place, and person; reasons for hospitalization, treatments
		Reduce external stimuli to minimum, maintaining room as quiet and dark as feasible
		Apply restraints as per physician's order if this is only alternative to protect patient from self-injury; before applying restraints, try explanations and reasons for necessary care, orders, procedures to patient
		If restraints are necessary
		Explain to patient/family reasons for restraints
		Reassure family of necessity for restraints and of relationship between patient's behavior and pathology
		Check restraints frequently for proper placement; monitor effectiveness, skin integrity, and circulation
		Reapply q4 hr and prn
		Frequently reevaluate need for continuing restraints
■ Seizures	■ Absence or control of seizures	■ Prevention of precipitating factors in seizure occurrence including fever, hypoxia, H_2O intoxication, electrolyte disturbances
		Notify physician of potential/presence of any factors
		Seizure precautions (if indicated)
		Padded siderails up at all times when patient is alone
		Bed height at lowest level
		Padded tongue blade and airway at bedside
		Suctioning and O_2 equipment readily available
		Emergency medications available
		Close supervision and observation
		Administer anticonvulsant medications as ordered; monitor effects, side effects, and serum drug levels
		If seizure occurs, monitor and record seizure activity; notify physician; see Standard 41, *Seizures*
■ Presence of neurological deficit	■ Absence of complications Maximal neurological functioning	■ On admission establish and implement nursing care plan based on individual needs and specific deficit present
		Ongoing assessments and evaluations of effectiveness of interventions

POTENTIAL PROBLEMS	EXPECTED OUTCOMES	NURSING ACTIVITIES
■ Patient/family's anxiety related to 　Limited understanding of diagnostic tests, procedures, anticipated surgery, postoperative course 　Potential/presence of neurological deficit; fears of disability or worsened deficit	■ Patient/family's behavior indicates decreased anxiety with provision of information	■ Ongoing assessment of level of anxiety, knowledge base, and understanding 　Encourage patient/family's verbalization of questions and fears; collaborate with physician in providing realistic information and reassurance appropriate to level of understanding 　Explain relationship between symptoms and neurological problems—reasons for therapies 　Explain and prepare patient for procedures, tests, preoperative routines 　If hair is to be shaved, assess anxieties regarding hair loss and possible altered body image; save hair if patient desires; provide information on means to deal with hair loss, such as wigs 　Explain postoperative care anticipated, including routines, setting, monitoring equipment, IVs, drains, length of stay, visiting policy 　Explain reasons for frequent neurological assessments and vital sign monitoring 　Instruct patient in deep breathing and leg exercises; evaluate patient's performance 　Provide time needed for support and instruction of patient/family 　Notify unit in which patient will be after surgery of any special problems or items patient needs such as 　　Eyeglasses: for vision, to evaluate visual fields/acuity 　　Dentures: for patient comfort, to evaluate facial symmetry 　　If language barrier is present: effort should be made to have interpreter available postoperatively

Postoperative

POTENTIAL PROBLEMS	EXPECTED OUTCOMES	NURSING ACTIVITIES
■ General immediate postoperative complications	■ Absence or resolution of complications	■ Monitor for recovery from anesthesia; notify physician if patient is not recovered in expected time period 　Monitor for recovery from any special measures induced during surgery; such as hypotension/hypothermia 　Monitor for signs/symptoms of potential complications including hypovolemia, shock, hypostatic pneumonia, pulmonary emboli, thrombophlebitis, abdominal ileus, nausea/vomiting, oliguria/urinary retention 　Notify physician immediately of any signs/symptoms of complication 　　Administer medications and treatments as ordered 　　Monitor effects and side effects and for resolution or progression of complication 　See appropriate standard for identified complication such as Standard 31, *Embolic phenomena;* Standard 17, *Shock*
■ Increased ICP/neurological deficit; appearance of deficit related to 　Edema 　Hemorrhage 　Hematoma 　Air formation	■ Absence or resolution of increased ICP 　Maximal neurological functioning 　Absence or resolution of complications	■ Establish neurological baseline postoperatively and compare to preoperative baseline; notify physician immediately if there is any decrease in status 　Neurological assessments and vital signs as ordered (usually q15 min until stable, q30 min until stable, then q1-2 hr) 　Monitor 　　Closely LOC, pupils (size, equality, light reactivity, and ocular movements); motor/sensory systems; communication abilities and speech quality; BP, P, respiratory rate, pattern and quality; for any abnormality/decline 　　For any increase in headache, nausea/vomiting above usual postoperative expectation 　　Notify physician immediately of any change in neurological status or vital signs 　See Problem, Increased ICP (preoperative) for all other activities and more detailed neurological assessments as status allows 　Maintain patency of subdural drain if present 　See Problem, Nonpatent subdural drain

POTENTIAL PROBLEMS	EXPECTED OUTCOMES	NURSING ACTIVITIES

■ Nonpatent subdural drain Potential reaccumulation of subdural hematoma	■ Patent subdural drain Absence/resolution of hematoma accumulation	■ Frequent neurological assessments and vital signs as ordered; notify physician of any change in status
		Maintain head position as ordered by physician; patient is frequently kept flat for 2 to 3 days postoperatively to aid in prevention of reaccumulation
		Prevent pulling, tension, or compression of tubing by
		  Properly securing and positioning tubing
		  Assisting patient with positioning
		  Restraining patient as per physician's order if absolutely necessary (first try explanations of reasons, dangers of pulling)
		Monitor frequently
		  Patency of drainage tubing, ensuring that it is kink/compression free
		  Bottle or collection apparatus for position maintenance as ordered
		  Amount and quality of drainage; record accurately
		  Drain site for intactness; any oozing or bleeding/bulging around site; fluid leakage/swelling
		  If dressing is in place, check for any leakage of blood or other fluid
		  Any correlation between amount of drainage and neurological status; if physician orders tubing clamped, maintain specific interval schedule ordered and closely monitor correlations
		Notify physician immediately if drain is not patent or oozing/leakage occurs at site
		  Have new equipment needed for drainage change
		  Assist physician with procedure
		When subdural drain is removed by physician
		  Record total output and quality
		  Send specimens as ordered and monitor results
		  Monitor drain site for any oozing, fluid leakage/bulging
		  Monitor for any signs of reaccumulation

■ Leakage or infection at burr hole sites	■ Burr hole sites sealed, well-healed, and infection free	■ Restraints applied as per physician's order if necessary to prevent patient touching burr hole sites
		Monitor
		  Burr hole sites for any leakage, drainage (amount, quality); edema; redness; or exudate
		  Temperature q4 hr and prn for any elevation
		  WBC count (may be falsely elevated if patient is receiving steroids)
		Administer antibiotics as ordered; monitor effects and side effects
		Notify physician if any abnormality occurs
		  Monitor culture results of exudate
		  Assist physician with treatments/suturing of site

■ Fluid and electrolyte imbalance	■ Fluid and electrolyte balance within normal limits	■ Monitor and accurately record intake and output, urine specific gravity as ordered
		Monitor for signs of dehydration or overhydration such as
		  Poor skin turgor
		  Dry mucous membranes
		  Peripheral edema
		  Excessive thirst
		  Change in LOC
		Monitor for
		  Abnormal vital signs, Hgb/Hct values
		  Abnormal serum electrolyte values
		  Weight alterations
		  Temperature elevations
		  Insensible fluid losses including respiratory, diaphoresis, secretions
		  Presence/degree of nausea or vomiting; monitor effectiveness of medications ordered
		Administer IV fluids as ordered

POTENTIAL PROBLEMS	EXPECTED OUTCOMES	NURSING ACTIVITIES
		Administer medications as ordered; monitor effects and side effects; if patient is receiving steroids, monitor urine glucose and acetone levels four times a day Notify physician of any fluid imbalance or electrolyte abnormality
■ Seizures	■ Absence or control of seizures	■ See problem, Seizures (preoperative)

■ Thrombophlebitis/pulmonary emboli
 May be related to withdrawal of anticoagulation therapy patient was previously receiving
	■ Absence or resolution of thrombophlebitis/pulmonary emboli	■ Apply antithromboembolic stockings or Ace bandages as ordered; reapply every shift and prn; monitor for constriction/looseness, condition of skin
		 Instruct and supervise patient in leg exercises, ROM exercises
		 Increase activity level/progression when allowed
		 Explain to patient/family the reasons why anticoagulants are being withheld
		 Monitor q4 hr and prn
		   Respiratory rate, quality, and pattern for any dyspnea, tachypnea
		   Breath sounds bilaterally for quality of aeration, signs of obstruction
		   Extremities for increase in warmth/girth, tenderness, Homans sign
		   Vital signs for tachycardia, hypotension
		   For patient complaints of chest pain, leg cramps, increasing anxiety/apprehension
		   If indicated, serial measurements of both calves and thighs daily in same spot
		 Notify physician immediately if any abnormalities occur
		 Prepare patient/family for any diagnostic procedures ordered
		 If problem occurs, see Standard 31, *Embolic phenomena*

■ GI bleeding related to CNS factors Stress Steroid administration	■ Absence or resolution of GI bleeding	■ Monitor vital signs q2-4 hr, Hgb and Hct; stools for Hematest three times a week; Hematest of aspirate, emesis, and urine for any abnormalities Obtain order for antacid administration as soon as patient is able to take po Monitor for signs of GI bleeding, including abdominal tenderness/distention, hypotension, sudden tachycardia Notify physician immediately if any abnormalities occur If problem occurs, see Standard 49, *Upper gastrointestinal bleeding*

■ Continued presence of neurological deficit
 Patient/family's fears, anxiety, anger related to deficit and possible alterations in life-style
	■ Maximal neurological functioning*
	 Maximal independence in ADL (within capabilities)
	 Patient/family verbalizes concerns
		■ Assess patient's specific neurological deficit
		 Implement individualized plan of care based on patient's needs and deficits
		   Assist as needed in ADL
		   Monitor potential for independent functioning and obtain equipment to maximize function and promote safety
		   Obtain orders for appropriate referrals such as physiotherapy, speech and occupational therapy, social services
		 Encourage patient/family's verbalization of fears, anxieties, and other reactions—level and degree
		   Answer questions realistically
		   Encourage their participation in care planning, implementation, evaluation, and decision making
		   Realistically reassure and support patient/family
		 Reinforce any gains or independence patient achieves
		 Plan, instruct, demonstrate, supervise, and evaluate patient/family's verbalization/performance of needed information/skills for maximal independent functioning such as
		   Measures to prevent complications
		   Assistance necessary—type, amount, degree
		   Proper use of therapeutic devices/equipment
		 Monitor level of achievement toward maximizing potentials and independence; means to promote as "normal" a life-style as possible

*If responsibility of critical care nurse includes this stage of care.

POTENTIAL PROBLEMS	EXPECTED OUTCOMES	NURSING ACTIVITIES
■ Insufficient knowledge to comply with discharge regimen*	■ Patient/family demonstrates or verbalizes understanding of discharge regimen	■ Assess patient/family's level of understanding of neurological problem and therapy received Explain relationship between patient's neurological status and therapies prescribed If appropriate, explain relationship between head injury occurrence and subdural hematoma; other contributing factors Encourage patient/family to discuss means, measures, alterations, precautions to decrease potential for head injury recurrence; if patient is alcoholic, secure appropriate resources for assistance in dealing with problem Explain safety precautions to prevent/minimize falls Instruct patient/family regarding required information/skills so that before discharge patient/family is able to
	Patient/family accurately describes medication, activity, and dietary regimen	Describe medication regimen Name and purpose Route, dosage, frequency, times Side effects Special precautions necessary including drugs, foods, and beverages contraindicated or quantity regulated; factors potentiating/decreasing effects/side effects; physical restrictions; safety measures
	Patient/family describes means to achieve maximal independence in ADL, promote safety, and prevent complications	Describe activity regimen, exercise program Describe dietary regimen Describe and demonstrate any special therapeutic measures prescribed; safety precautions Describe and demonstrate proper use of equipment or therapeutic devices Reasons for using Time, method, and duration of use Precautions/safeguards Necessary maintenance (type, frequency) Measures to promote optimal functioning, upkeep, duration
	Patient/family describes signs/symptoms requiring medical attention	Describe signs/symptoms of neurological status requiring medical care
	Patient/family describes follow-up care regimen	Describe plan for follow-up care including purpose of appointment, when and where to go, who to see, what to expect

*If responsibility of the critical care nurse includes such follow-up care.

SUPRATENTORIAL CRANIOTOMY

Supratentorial craniotomy is a surgical procedure in which the cranium is incised above the tentorium (the fold of the dura mater that separates the cerebral cortex from the cerebellum and brainstem). This type of operative approach is commonly performed in adults, since approximately two thirds of cerebral conditions requiring surgical intervention are located above the tentorium. The pathological conditions for which a supratentorial craniotomy may be performed are numerous. They commonly include complete or partial removal of a brain tumor or arteriovenous malformation, clipping or wrapping of an intracerebral aneurysm, excision of abscess, evacuation of clot, elevation of depressed skull fractures, tissue biopsy, and temporal lobectomy for seizure control. Whatever the pathological entity involved, a supratentorial craniotomy may be performed to correct or attempt to control the potential presence or progression of cerebral damage, disturbance, or impaired functioning.

The diverse pathological conditions warranting operative therapy manifest widely variable neurological symptoms ranging from no symptoms or subtle signs to a sudden cerebral herniation syndrome. Many factors influence the presence, extent, type, and progression of neurological symptoms exhibited. These factors include location and area of pathological conditions, onset of pathological conditions (slow growing versus abrupt onset); effectiveness of compensatory mechanisms; effects on ICP, cerebral blood flow, and cerebral edema; effects on CSF dynamics; extent of displacement and compression of cerebral tissue; invasion of other areas; and extent and degree of cerebral damage. Some common neurological signs manifested by the myriad of pathological conditions include headache, vomiting, altered LOC, mental changes, visual defects, seizures, and papilledema.

There are some common focal neurological signs occurring with pathology in specific lobes of the brain (see Table 36-1). The signs are not absolute indicators of pathology location, but their presence would increase the probability of certain areas as suspected pathological sites. In some instances, a strong correlation does exist between the area involved in pathology and the clinical signs manifested. However, symptoms alone from a certain focal area of the cerebral cortex cannot be absolutely equated with the func-

tions distributed to that area. The brain is a complex structure whose normal functioning depends on many associative areas, integrative areas, feedback systems, and interrelationships. Dysfunction in one cerebral area may produce a wide range of signs from the physiological and pathological effects on other areas and overall cerebral functioning. In general, supratentorial motor and sensory functioning are manifested and effected on the opposite side of the body from the hemisphere. The right cerebral hemisphere controls motor and sensory functioning of the left side of the body; the left hemisphere controls functioning of the right side of the body. The term *contralateral* refers to the opposite body side from the hemisphere involved in the pathological condition; for instance, a right frontal tumor may result in left arm/leg weakness or paralysis (contralateral motor signs, that is, opposite to side of hemisphere pathological condition). The term *ipsilateral* refers to the same body side as the hemisphere involved, for instance, right hemisphere pathology producing signs that are manifested on the right side of the body (ipsilateral signs). The dominant hemisphere for the majority of the population is thought to be the left; speech center functions also are usually located on this side. Frequently invasive treatments or tests are performed in the nondominant hemisphere (usually right), if feasible, to minimize damage or interference with functioning.

ASSESSMENT

1. Onset, duration, progression, and specific description of neurological symptoms, especially any alterations in
   a. LOC
   b. Behavior or personality
   c. Motor system
   d. Sensory system
   e. Pupils and extraocular movements
   f. Visual abilities
   g. Communication skills
2. Presence or history of headache including location, severity, frequency, duration, precipitating factors or time-related occurrence, association with other neurological symptoms; nausea/vomiting including frequency, severity, time-related factors
3. Previous seizures—exact description including onset,

TABLE 36-1. Common focal signs of lobe pathology

Frontal lobe damage

1. Mental changes such as personality changes, impaired memory, lack of initiative, mood changes
2. Motor weakness or spastic paralysis on contralateral side
3. Presence of sucking and grasping reflexes
4. Expressive (Broca) aphasia if dominant hemisphere is involved (left hemisphere for most people)
5. Seizures—jacksonian or generalized motor
6. Agraphia
7. Apraxia

Temporal lobe damage

1. Visual field defect of upper contralateral quadrant
2. Auditory illusions and hallucinations
3. Personality changes—psychotic behavior
4. Seizures—psychomotor or generalized
   a. Dreamy state—unicinate epilepsy
   b. May have auditory hallucinations alone or with visual, gustatory hallucinations
   c. Masticatory movements
   d. Disturbances in time perception
5. In dominant hemisphere involvement (usually left)
   a. Receptive (Wernicke) aphasia
   b. Difficulty in tests of verbal material presented through auditory sense
6. In nondominant hemisphere involvement
   a. Difficulty judging spatial relationships
   b. Difficulty in tests of nonverbal material presented through visual sense

Parietal lobe damage

1. Sensory disturbances
   a. Loss of two-point discrimination
   b. Loss of ability to judge size and shape of objects (astereognosis)
   c. Hypoesthesia/paresthesia—contralateral side
   d. Impairment or loss of position sense
2. Motor weakness—contralateral side
3. Homonymous hemianopia or visual inattention
4. Seizures—sensory type
5. Inattentiveness
6. Impaired memory
7. If dominant lobe involvement
   a. Language disorders, especially alexia
   b. Gerstmann syndrome
      (1) Difficulty writing (agraphia)
      (2) Difficulty doing math (acalculia)
      (3) Finger agnosia
      (4) Right/left confusion
   c. Apraxia—ideomotor
8. If nondominant hemisphere involvement
   a. Memory loss
   b. Neglect of one half of body (anosognosia)
   c. Dressing apraxia

Occipital lobe damage

1. Homonymous hemianopia—contralateral
2. Visual illusions and hallucinations
3. Cortical blindness
4. Visual agnosia—cannot name or identify use of object seen
5. Defects in visual perceptions with loss of topographic memory
6. Loss of color perception

progression, type, locality, length, aura, incontinence
   a. Postictal status; any injury incurred
   b. Presence of any precipitating factors such as fever, emotional upset
   c. Frequency of seizures
   d. If multiple seizures, any variation in seizure activity or similar episodes
   e. If patient is receiving anticonvulsants, whether prescribed regimen has been adhered to
4. Medications taken for neurological problem such as anticonvulsants, steroids, pain medications; effects and side effects of drug therapies
5. Previous neurological treatment or neurosurgical procedure
6. Presence of any medical problems and medications/treatments prescribed and followed
7. Patient's perceptions and reaction to diagnosis, therapeutic modalities, anticipated surgical intervention
8. Presence of any alterations in body image; fears of permanent disability or deficit; altered roles in family,

normal occupation, performing ADL; fears of tumor regrowth or recurrence of pathological condition
9. Baseline parameters status
   a. Neurological
   b. Respiratory
   c. Cardiovascular
   d. Hydration
   e. Vital signs
   f. Weight
   g. Handedness (right or left)
   h. Urine output pattern
10. Diagnostic test results, including
   a. CT scan
   b. Cerebral angiography
   c. Skull radiographs
   d. Brain scan
   e. EEG
   f. Pneumoencephalogram
   g. Lumbar puncture
   h. NMR scan

11. Results of
    a. Serum electrolyte levels
    b. Hgb and Hct, platelet count, WBC count and differentiation
    c. Type and cross-matching
    d. Urinalysis, culture, specific gravity, osmolality, electrolytes
    e. Arterial blood gas levels
    f. Clotting profile
    g. Anticonvulsant drug levels
    h. CSF determinations
    i. Chest radiograph
    j. ECG

GOALS

1. Optimal neurological functioning
2. Optimal independence in ADL
3. Adequate alveolar ventilation

4. Serum electrolytes and fluid balance within normal limits
5. Hgb and Hct stable within normal limits
6. Acid-base balance within normal limits
7. Incision well-healed
8. Infection free
9. Reduction in patient/family's anxiety with provision of information, demonstrations, support
10. Before discharge patient/family is able to
    a. Describe medication, activity, exercise, and dietary regimens
    b. Demonstrate safety measures and techniques; proper use of any equipment/therapeutic devices prescribed
    c. Describe signs and symptoms requiring medical attention
    d. State necessary information regarding follow-up care

POTENTIAL PROBLEMS	EXPECTED OUTCOMES	NURSING ACTIVITIES
Preoperative		
■ Patient/family's anxiety related to Limited understanding of diagnostic tests, procedures, anticipated surgery, postoperative course Potential/presence of neurological deficit; fears of disability or worsened deficit	■ Patient/family's behavior indicates decreased anxiety with provision of information	■ Ongoing assessment of level of anxiety, knowledge base, and understanding Encourage patient/family's verbalization of questions and fears; collaborate with physician in providing realistic information and reassurance appropriate to level of understanding (if surgery is to be performed for aneurysm, physician may allow provision of only limited information; see Standard 34, *Subarachnoid hemorrhage*, if this occurs) Explain relationship between symptoms and neurological problem; reasons for therapies Explain and prepare patient for procedures, tests, preoperative routines If hair is to be shaved, assess anxieties regarding hair loss and possible altered body image; save hair if patient desires; provide information on means to deal with hair loss, such as wigs Explain anticipated postoperative care including routines, setting, monitoring equipment, IVs, drains, length of stay, visiting policy Explain reasons for frequent neurological assessments and vital sign monitoring Instruct in deep breathing and leg exercises; evaluate patient's performance Provide time needed for support and instruction of patient/family Notify unit in which patient will be after surgery of any special problems or items patient needs, such as Eyeglasses: for vision; to evaluate visual fields/acuity Dentures: for patient comfort; to evaluate facial symmetry If language barrier is present: effort should be made to have interpreter available postoperatively
■ Increased ICP with possible development or worsening of neurological deficit	■ Absence of complications Maximal neurological functioning	■ Establish neurological baseline and vital signs on admission; ongoing assessments as ordered of status and specific symptomatology, monitoring especially for extent and degree of Headache Nausea/vomiting Altered LOC Mental changes such as disorientation, impaired memory

POTENTIAL PROBLEMS	EXPECTED OUTCOMES	NURSING ACTIVITIES
		Pupillary changes
		Visual defects
		Papilledema
		Motor/sensory system dysfunctions
		Communication ability deficits
		Personality changes such as restlessness, irritability, apathy
		Avoid precipitating factors in increased ICP such as hypoxia, hypercapnia, fever, Valsalva maneuvers
		Assist patient with positioning and turning; instruct patient not to hold breath
		Prevent constipation by establishing bowel regimen as individually warranted; ensure that patient has bowel movement preoperatively
		Monitor for any signs/symptoms that could initiate factor development such as hypoventilation
		Notify physician of potential/presence of any factors
		Maintain head gatch and activity as ordered
		Administer medications and treatments as ordered; monitor effects and side effects
		Accurately record intake and output; monitor for any imbalance
		Monitor serum electrolyte levels for any abnormalities
		Notify physician immediately of any change in neurological status, vital signs, or abnormal fluid/electrolyte balance
		If problem occurs, see Standard 32, *Increased intracranial pressure*
■ Presence of neurological deficit	■ Absence of complications	■ On admission establish and implement nursing care plan based on individual needs and specific deficit present
		Ongoing assessments and evaluations of effectiveness of interventions
		Establish neurological baseline immediately preoperatively to provide for comparison postoperatively
■ Seizures	■ Absence or control of seizures	■ Prevention of precipitating factors in seizure occurrence including fever, hypoxia, H_2O intoxication, electrolyte disturbances
		Notify physician of potential/presence of any factors
		Seizure precautions (if indicated)
		Padded siderails up at all times when patient is alone
		Bed height at lowest level
		Padded tongue blade and airway at bedside
		Emergency medications and equipment readily available
		Close observation and supervision
		Administer anticonvulsant medications as ordered; monitor effects and side effects, serum anticonvulsant levels
		If seizure occurs, monitor and record seizure activity; notify physician
		See STANDARD 41, *Seizures*
Postoperative		
■ General postoperative complications immediately after surgery	■ Absence or resolution of complications	■ Monitor for
		Recovery from anesthesia; notify physician if patient has not recovered in expected time period
		Potential hypovolemia, shock, hypostatic pneumonia, pulmonary emboli, thrombophlebitis, abdominal ileus, nausea/vomiting, oliguria/urinary retention
		Recovery from any special measures induced during surgery such as hypotension/hypothermia
		Notify physician immediately of any signs/symptoms of complication
		Administer medications and treatments as ordered
		Monitor effects and side effects
		Continue monitoring for resolution or progression of complication
		See appropriate standard for identified complication such as Standard 31, *Embolic phenomena*; Standard 17, *Shock*

POTENTIAL PROBLEMS	EXPECTED OUTCOMES	NURSING ACTIVITIES

■ Increased ICP/increased neurological deficit/appearance related to
Edema
Hemorrhage
Hematoma formation
	■ Absence or control of increased ICP
	Maximal neurological functioning
		■ Establish neurological baseline postoperatively and compare to pre-operative baseline
		See Problem, Increased ICP (preoperative) for all specific activities
		In addition, monitor
		  Neurological assessments and vital signs as ordered and prn (usually q15 min until stable, q30 min until stable, q1 hr until stable, and then q2 hr)
		  Particularly LOC; pupil size, equality, and reactivity; extraocular movements; motor and sensory systems; communication abilities and speech quality; respiratory rate, pattern, and quality; BP and P for any abnormalities
		  For any increase in headache, nausea/vomiting above usual postoperative expectation
		  For signs of epidural hematoma (see Standard 33, *Head trauma,* Problem, Epidural hematoma)
		  For more detailed and specific assessments as patient's status allows
		  Head dressing with neurological assessments for any bleeding or oozing, elevation in surgical site or edema in other sites, unusual constriction or looseness
		Maintain head gatch as ordered (usually elevated to promote venous drainage)
		If Hemovac (or other drainage collection apparatus) is used
		  Prevent any tension or pulling on drainage tubing by proper positioning of patient and securing of drainage tubing; if necessary, restrain patient's hands to prevent pulling or tension of tubing (first try explanations of reasons necessary/purposes of drain)
		  Maintain Hemovac as per physician's order such as suction or gravity drainage (if frontal sinus is incised intraoperatively, suction is usually avoided postoperatively)
		  Monitor
		    And accurately record amount and quality of drainage; notify physician immediately if amount is more than expected or quality differs from normal
		    Functioning of system
		    Drain site for any oozing or bleeding around area
		    For patency of drain and intactness
		    Notify physician of any signs of drainage malfunctioning
		  When drain is removed by physician, monitor
		    And accurately record output
		    Drain site for oozing, bleeding, or edema
		    Results of any specimens obtained
		Notify physician immediately of any decline in neurological status from preoperative status, or change in status or vital signs postoperatively; of any increase in symptoms or worsening deficit
		  Administer medications/treatments as ordered; monitor effects and side effects
		  Prepare patient/family for any diagnostic tests/procedures ordered

■ Respiratory insufficiency related to CNS dysfunction Pneumonia Atelectasis Pulmonary emboli	■ Patent airway Adequate alveolar ventilation and perfusion Normal respiratory rate and quality Arterial blood gas levels within patient's normal limits	■ Ongoing assessments of respiratory status q2 hr and prn; monitor for any abnormality/decline Respiratory rate, quality, and pattern Patency of upper airway and patient's ability to handle secretions Skin color, nail beds, peripheral pulses, and skin warmth Presence/strength of gag, cough, and swallow reflexes Breath sounds bilaterally for quality of aeration; signs of obstruction (rales, rhonchi) Arterial blood gas values Chest radiograph results Signs/symptoms of thrombophlebitis, pulmonary emboli, pulmonary edema

POTENTIAL PROBLEMS	EXPECTED OUTCOMES	NURSING ACTIVITIES

		Maintain patent airway by
		  Turning and positioning to prevent obstruction or aspiration of secretions q2 hr and prn; (if bone flap has been removed, patient may not be permitted to lie on one side of head)
		  Deep breathing and coughing q1 hr and prn (if allowed)
		  Suctioning prn (if frontal sinus was incised intraoperatively, nasal suctioning is usually contraindicated)
		  Adequate oxygenation and humidification as ordered
		  Chest physiotherapy/pulmonary toilet if warranted and not contraindicated by physician's order
		Apply antithromboembolic stockings or Ace bandages as ordered; reapply every shift and prn; monitor for constriction/looseness, condition of skin
		Instruct and supervise patient in performing leg exercises, ROM exercises
		Increase activity level/progression when allowed
		Notify physician immediately of any change in respiratory/neurological status or signs of complication potential/occurrence
		If problem occurs, assist with emergency measures to maintain patent airway and adequate ventilation
		  Administer medications/treatments as ordered; monitor effects and side effects
		See Standard 6, *Mechanical ventilation;* if emboli occur, see Standard 31, *Embolic phenomena*

■ Fluid and electrolyte imbalance	■ Fluid and electrolyte balance within normal limits	■ Monitor and accurately record intake and output, urine specific gravity as ordered
		Monitor for signs of dehydration or overhydration, such as
		  Poor skin turgor
		  Dry mucous membranes
		  Peripheral edema
		  Excessive thirst
		  Change in LOC
		Monitor for
		  Abnormal vital signs, Hgb/Hct values
		  Abnormal serum electrolyte values (retention of Na^+ from increased aldosterone effect with increased release of ADH frequently occurs postoperatively, resulting in decreased serum Na^+ values)
		  Weight alterations
		  Temperature elevations
		  Insensible fluid losses including respiratory, diaphoresis, secretions
		  Presence/degree of nausea/vomiting; effectiveness of medications ordered
		  Presence/quality of bowel sounds for any abnormality
		Administer IV fluids, NG feedings as ordered
		Administer medication as ordered; monitor effects and side effects; if patient is receiving steroids, monitor urine glucose and acetone levels four times a day
		Notify physician of any fluid imbalance or electrolyte abnormality

■ Headache/incisional pain	■ Absence or control of pain	■ Administer pain medications as ordered; monitor effects and side effects Notify physician if medication is not effective Monitor dressing for increased tightness/constriction Maintain environment at quietest level possible

■ Seizures	■ Absence or control of seizures	■ See Problem, Seizures (preoperative), for all activities
		In addition
		  Phenytoin (Dilantin) is frequently ordered postoperatively; if given IV, monitor ECG for any abnormalities, BP for any hypotension
		  Prevent, if possible, exposure to potential fever sources, since elevated temperature can precipitate seizure activity

POTENTIAL PROBLEMS	EXPECTED OUTCOMES	NURSING ACTIVITIES
		Monitor and report to physician signs of other factors predisposing patient to postoperative seizures such as hypoxia, hypoglycemia, H_2O intoxication, hyperventilation Administer medications/treatments as ordered; monitor effects and side effects; monitor appropriate lab test results
■ Hypotension or hypertension	■ BP within patient's normal or prescribed limits	■ Monitor 　BP as ordered for any abnormality 　For signs of hypovolemia/hypervolemia 　For signs of shock 　Neurological status for any decline q1-2 hr Maintain BP at level ordered by physician by administration of prn medications ordered 　Monitor effects and side effects 　Notify physician if medication regimen is not resulting in desired BP level Notify physician immediately of any abnormality
■ Infection	■ Infection free 　Incision well-healed	■ Keep patient's hands from operative site/drain Maintain sterility of head dressing/drainage apparatus Administer antibiotics as ordered; monitor effects and side effects (frequently ordered postoperatively prophylactically) Monitor 　Temperature as ordered and prn for any elevation 　Dressing/incision site q2 hr for any signs of redness, tenderness, bulging, separation, or drainage (amount and quality) 　If drainage apparatus is present, monitor amount and quality for any abnormality 　Neurological status and vital signs for any decline/abnormality 　IV sites frequently for any signs for redness, tenderness, phlebitis 　WBC count (may be falsely elevated if patient is receiving steroids) 　For any signs/symptoms of meningitis Notify physician immediately of any signs/symptoms of infection Administer medications/treatments as ordered Monitor wound culture results Monitor for other possible infection sources if warranted, including urine, sputum, chest radiograph results, CSF determinations Monitor for resolution/progression of infection If problem occurs, see Standard 42, *Meningitis/encephalitis*
■ GI bleeding related to CNS factors Stress Steroid administration	■ Absence or resolution of GI bleeding	■ Monitor vital signs q2-4 hr, Hgb and Hct, stools for Hematest three times a week; Hematest of aspirate, urine, and emesis for any abnormalities Obtain order for antacid administration as soon as patient is able to take po Monitor for signs of GI bleeding, including abdominal tenderness/distention, hypotension, sudden tachycardia Notify physician immediately if any abnormality occurs If problem occurs, see Standard 49, *Acute upper gastrointestinal bleeding*
■ Continued presence of neurological deficit Patient/family's fears, anxiety, anger related to deficit and possible alterations in life-style	■ Maximal neurological functioning* Maximal independence in ADL (within capabilities) Patient/family verbalizes concerns	■ Assess patient's specific neurological deficit; collaborate with physician regarding prognosis, possible degree of recovery Implement individualized plan of care based on patient's needs and deficits Assist as needed in ADL Monitor potential for independent functioning and obtain equipment to maximize function and promote safety Obtain orders for appropriate referrals such as physiotherapy, speech or occupational therapy; social services

*If responsibility of critical care nurse includes this stage of care.

POTENTIAL PROBLEMS	EXPECTED OUTCOMES	NURSING ACTIVITIES
		Encourage verbalization of patient/family's fears, anxieties, and other reactions—level and degree
		Answer questions realistically
		Encourage their participation in care planning, implementation, evaluation, and decision making
		Realistically reassure and support patient/family
		Reinforce any gains or independence patient achieves
		Plan, instruct, demonstrate, supervise, and evaluate patient/family's verbalization/performance of needed information/skills for maximal independent functioning such as
		Measures to prevent complications
		Assistance necessary—type, amount, degree
		Proper use of therapeutic devices/equipment
		Monitor level of achievement toward maximizing potentials and independence; means to promote as ''normal'' a life-style as possible
■ Insufficient knowledge to comply with discharge regimen*	■ Patient/family demonstrates or verbalizes understanding of discharge regimen	■ Assess patient/family's level of understanding of neurological problem and therapy received
		Explain relationship between patient's neurological status and therapies prescribed
		If cerebral pathological condition was caused by head injury or trauma, explore with patient/family measures to decrease injury recurrence potential and importance of controlling factors precipitating head injury
		Instruct patient/family regarding required information and skills so that before discharge patient/family is able to
	Patient/family accurately describes medication, activity, and dietary regimens	Describe medication regimen
		Name and purpose
		Route, dosage, frequency, times
		Side effects
		Special precautions necessary including drugs, foods, beverages contraindicated or quantity regulated; factors potentiating/decreasing effects or side effects; physical restrictions; safety measures
		Describe dietary regimen
		Describe activity regimen, exercise program
		Describe and demonstrate any special therapeutic measures prescribed
	Patient/family describes means to achieve maximal independence in ADL, promote safety, and prevent complications	Describe and demonstrate proper use of equipment or therapeutic devices
		Reasons for using
		Time, method, and duration of use
		Precautions/safeguards
		Necessary maintenance (type, frequency)
		Measures to promote optimal functioning, upkeep/duration
	Patient/family describes signs/symptoms requiring medical attention	Describe signs/symptoms of neurological status requiring medical care
	Patient/family describes follow-up care regimen	Describe plan for follow-up care including purpose of appointment, when and where to go, who to see, what to expect

*If responsibility of critical care nurse includes such follow-up care.

INFRATENTORIAL CRANIOTOMY

Infratentorial craniotomy is a surgical procedure in which the cranium is incised below the tentorium (the fold of the dura mater that separates the cerebral cortex from the cerebellum and brain stem). The areas below the tentorium that may be involved in pathological conditions are numerous. Tumors, hemorrhages, and clots may reside in the midbrain, pons, medulla, fourth ventricle, cerebellum, and cerebellar pontine angle (particularly acoustic neurinomas and meningiomas). Infratentorial craniotomies are usually longer and more complex than supratentorial craniotomies because of a less accessible operative site, the difficult positioning required, the need to avoid many vital structures in the infratentorial area such as respiratory and reticular activating system, the common presence of increased ICP, the common compression of additional areas by displacements from original pathological site, and so on. In general, recovery from infratentorial craniotomy takes longer than recovery from supratentorial craniotomy.

The symptoms manifested when a pathological condition exists in the brainstem, cerebellum, or fourth ventricle vary with each individual. Some of the factors contributing to this variability include size, location, rate of growth, quality, and extent of tumor or clot; effectiveness of compensatory mechanisms; location, amount and degree of compression of other cerebral structures; and effects on ICP and CSF dynamics. There are common symptoms associated with certain areas of the brainstem, cerebellum, and fourth ventricle (Table 37-1). The presence of these symptoms does not pinpoint the original site of the pathological condition in all cases, since the dysfunction could be caused by compression or displacement from another area.

A pathological condition in the brainstem commonly produces cranial nerve dysfunctions by an interference with the nuclei or processes for effecting cranial nerve function. Cranial nerve nuclei located within the brainstem include hypoglossal (XII), spinal accessory (XI), glossopharyngeal (IX), and vagus (X) in the medulla; trigeminal (V), abducens (VI), facial (VII), and acoustic (VIII) in the pons; and oculomotor (III) and trochlear (IV) in the midbrain.

Unilateral lesions of the cerebellum produce signs on the same side of the body as the lesion (ipsilateral) because of the double pathway–crossing mechanism of cerebellar output. The signs of cerebellar dysfunction are caused by a loss of the usual cerebellar influences, resulting in centers released from normal modulating controls. Incoordination, impaired balance, and disorders of equilibrium and gait are common signs of cerebellar dysfunction. Clinical signs may also include hypotonia, decomposition of movement, asthenia (muscles tire easily), adiadochokinesia (impaired ability to perform alternating repetitive movements rapidly), tremor (usually intention), dysmetria (inability to stop at desired point), ataxia, scanning speech or dysarthria, and nystagmus.

Pathological disorders in the fourth ventricle, either from a primary source or as a result of compression from another area, commonly produce hydrocephalus. This CSF accumulation, from overproduction or interference with normal reabsorption and circulation, may increase the ICP. Further increases in ICP may result in additional damage by displacement and compression. Herniation syndromes, both upward through the tentorial notch and downward through the foramen magnum, may occur with infratentorial lesions. Frequently a burr hole is placed, either preoperatively or intraoperatively, in the lateral ventricle for relief of increased ICP by insertion of a ventriculostomy drain for ventricular fluid drainage. This external ventricular drainage system may be left in place for a time postoperatively to relieve the pressure and also provide a parameter for assessing the amount of pressure and fluid within the ventricular system. If long-term hydrocephalus is a problem, an internalized shunting mechanism will usually be inserted.

Other considerations in infratentorial pathophysiology relate to the functioning of important vital structures and systems. The medulla has centers for vomiting, respiration, vasomotor control, and swallow reflex. The vagal system is composed of reflexes normally used for protection and compensation, including the carotid sinus reflex, carotid body reflex, and cough, gag, and swallow reflexes. Damage or compression of these vital centers may obliterate normal protective mechanisms and further increase the potential for cerebral damage or death. The brainstem contains a reticular formation composed of multiple neurons and fibers, which are involved with consciousness and wakefulness. Interference with this reticular activating system can result in altered LOC and various stages of coma.

TABLE 37-1. Common symptoms of brainstem lesions

Medulla

Hypoglossal nerve (XII) damage, producing lower motor neuron paralysis on ipsilateral side; initially fasciculations of tongue may occur followed by atrophy; on protrusion, tongue deviates to paralyzed side

Corticospinal tract of pyramid (motor) and medial lemniscus (discriminative general senses) damage, producing upper motor neuron paralysis and loss of position and muscle and joint sense, impaired tactile discrimination, and loss of vibratory sense on contralateral side of body (lesion interrupts tracts above level of decussation)

Spinothalamic tract damage, producing loss of senses of pain and temperature on opposite side of body

Spinal trigeminal tract and nucleus damage, producing loss of senses of pain and temperature on same side of face and in nasal and oral cavities

Vagal, glossopharyngeal, and spinal portions of accessory nerves damage, producing dysphagia, hoarseness, and loss of gag reflex on same side

Midbrain

Weber syndrome: damage to oculomotor nerve (III) on same side, producing ptosis; diplopia; external strabismus; dilated pupil; inability to gaze up, down, and in; corticospinal tract damage producing upper motor neuron paralysis of contralateral side

Corticobulbar and corticoreticular fiber damage, producing lower facial expression weakness on opposite side

Benedikt syndrome: damage to oculomotor nerve (III), producing lower motor neuron paralysis of extraocular muscles and dilated pupil on ipsilateral side; red nucleus and fibers of superior cerebellar peduncle damage, producing signs of cerebellar damage on contralateral side; spinothalamic tract and medial lemniscus damage, resulting in loss of senses of pain and temperature and discriminative senses on opposite side of body

Pons

Abducens nerve (VI) damage, producing inability to abduct eye to same side as lesion and horizontal diplopia (which worsens when patient attempts to gaze toward side of lesion)

Corticospinal fibers and medial lemniscus damage, producing contralateral upper motor neuron paralysis and loss of discriminative senses (position, muscle and joint, vibration)

Medial longitudinal fasciculus damage, producing disturbance of conjugate horizontal eye movements (abduction and adduction)

Trigeminal nerve (V) damage, producing loss of sensation on ipsilateral side of face, forehead, nasal and oral cavities; absence of corneal sensation and reflex; lower motor neuron paralysis of muscles of mastication with chin deviating to lesion side when mouth is opened

Lateral lemniscus damage, producing decrease in hearing that is more pronounced on opposite side

Pontocerebellar fibers interrupted, producing cerebellar signs on same side

Cerebellopontine angle

Acoustic nerve (VIII) damage, producing tinnitus followed by progressive deafness on same side as lesion; abnormal labyrinthine responses including tilting and rotating of head with chin pointing to lesion side

Cerebellar peduncle damage, producing coarse intention tremor, ataxic gait, dysmetria on lesion side

Spinal trigeminal tract damage, producing loss of senses of pain and temperature on ipsilateral side of face, oral cavity, and nasal cavity

Spinothalamic tract damage, producing loss of pain and temperature on contralateral side of body

Facial nerve (VII) injury, producing lower motor neuron paralysis of muscles of facial expression (Bell palsy) and loss of taste on anterior two thirds of tongue ipsilaterally

ASSESSMENT

1. Onset, progression, frequency, duration, and specific description of neurological symptoms, including
   a. Cranial nerve dysfunctions
   b. Cerebellar signs; disturbances of balance and coordination
   c. Headache—location, severity, association with specific activity/movement, time-related pattern or occurrence, any associated concurrent neurological symptoms
   d. Nausea/vomiting
   e. Papilledema
   f. Pupillary alterations; impaired extraocular movements
   g. Visual disturbances including diplopia, blurred vision, nystagmus, field defects
   h. Hearing defects including diminished or loss of hearing, tinnitus, vertigo
   i. Motor/sensory dysfunctions
2. Medications taken for neurological problem such as steroids, antiemetics, pain medications; effects and side effects of therapies
3. Previous head trauma or injury; specific description of incident, treatment, clinical course
4. Previous neurological treatment or neurosurgical procedure
5. Presence of any medical problems and medications/treatments prescribed and followed
6. Patient's perceptions and reaction to diagnosis, therapeutic modalities, anticipated surgical intervention
7. Presence of any alterations in body image; fears of permanent disability or deficit; altered roles in family, normal occupation, performing ADL; fears of tumor regrowth or recurrence of pathological condition
8. Baseline parameters status
   a. Neurological

b. Respiratory
c. Cardiovascular
d. Hydration
e. Urine output pattern
f. Vital signs
g. Weight
h. Handedness (right or left)
9. Diagnostic test results including
   a. CT scan
   b. Cerebral angiography
   c. Pneumoencephalogram
   d. Skull radiographs
   e. Brain scan
   f. Lumbar puncture
   g. Ventriculogram
   g. Hearing acuity testing
   i. NMR scan
10. Results of
    a. Serum electrolyte levels
    b. Hgb and Hct, platelet count, WBC count with differentiation
    c. Type and cross-matching
    d. Urinalysis, culture, specific gravity, osmolality, electrolytes
    e. Arterial blood gas levels
    f. Clotting profile

g. CSF determinations
h. Chest radiograph
i. ECG

GOALS

1. Optimal neurological functioning
2. Optimal independence in ADL
3. Adequate alveolar ventilation and perfusion
4. Adequate cardiac output
5. Serum electrolytes and fluid balance within normal limits
6. Acid-base balance within normal limits
7. Hgb and Hct stable within normal limits
8. Incision well-healed
9. Infection free
10. Reduction in patient/family's anxiety with provision of information, demonstrations, support
11. Before discharge patient/family is able to
    a. Describe medication, activity, exercise, and dietary regimens
    b. Demonstrate safety measures and techniques; proper use of any equipment/therapeutic devices prescribed
    c. Describe signs and symptoms requiring medical attention
    d. State necessary information regarding follow-up care

POTENTIAL PROBLEMS	EXPECTED OUTCOMES	NURSING ACTIVITIES
Preoperative		
■ Patient/family's anxiety related to Limited understanding of diagnostic tests, procedures, anticipated surgery, postoperative course Potential/presence of neurological deficit; fears of disability or worsened deficit	■ Patient/family's behavior indicates decreased anxiety with provision of information	■ Ongoing assessment of level of anxiety, knowledge base, and understanding Encourage patient/family's verbalization of questions and fears; collaborate with physician in providing realistic information and reassurance appropriate to level of understanding Explain relationship between symptoms and neurological problem; reasons for therapies Explain and prepare for procedures, tests, preoperative routines If hair is to be shaved, assess anxieties regarding hair loss and possible altered body image; save hair if patient desires; provide information on means to deal with hair loss, such as wigs Explain anticipated postoperative care including routines, settings, monitoring equipment, IVs, drains, length of stay, visiting policy Explain reasons for frequent neurological assessments and vital sign monitoring Instruct in deep breathing and leg exercises; evaluate patient's performance Provide time needed for support and instruction of patient/family Notify unit where patient will be after surgery of any special problems or items patient needs, such as Eyeglasses: for vision; to evaluate visual fields/acuity Dentures: for patient comfort; to evaluate facial symmetry If language barrier is present: effort should be made to have interpreter available postoperatively

POTENTIAL PROBLEMS	EXPECTED OUTCOMES	NURSING ACTIVITIES
■ Increased ICP with possible development or worsening of neurological deficit	■ Absence of complications Maximal neurological functioning	■ Establish neurological baseline and vital signs on admission; ongoing assessments as ordered of status and specific symptomatology, especially monitoring for extent and degree Headache Nausea/vomiting Visual problems such as diplopia, blurred vision, nystagmus, field defects Hearing defects such as diminished or loss, tinnitus, vertigo Cranial nerve dysfunctions Cerebellar disturbance signs such as ataxia, tremor, falling to one side, hypotonia, disorders or equilibrium, incoordination, dizziness, vertigo, dysarthria, muscle weakness/fatigability Presence/quality of gag, cough, and swallowing reflexes Papilledema Altered LOC Motor/sensory system dysfunctions Pupil size, equality, light reactivity; extraocular movements Balance and coordination Communication ability deficits Avoid precipitating factors in increased ICP such as hypoxia, hypercapnia, fever, Valsalva maneuvers Assist patient with positioning and turning; instruct patient not to hold breath Prevent constipation by establishing bowel regimen as individually warranted; ensure that patient has bowel movement preoperatively Monitor for any signs/symptoms that could initiate factor development such as hypoventialtion Notify physician of potential/presence of factors Maintain head gatch and activity as ordered Administer medications and treatments as ordered; monitor effects and side effects Accurately record intake and output; monitor for any imbalance Monitor serum electrolytes for any abnormalities Notify physician immediately of any change in neurological status, vital signs, or abnormal fluid/electrolyte balance If problem occurs, see Standard 32, *Increased intracranial pressure*
■ Presence of neurological deficit	■ Absence of complications	■ On admission establish and implement nursing care plan based on individual needs and specific deficit present Ongoing assessments and evaluations of effectiveness of interventions Establish neurological baseline immediately preoperatively to provide for comparison postoperatively
■ Ataxia—impaired balance and coordination	■ Ambulates safely with assistance	■ Assess degree, location, and extent of ataxia Assist and supervise patient in ADL and ambulation Apply safety measures such as siderails while patient is in bed, safety belt in wheelchair Maintain safe environment Remove as many obstacles or objects with the potential for causing falls as possible Obtain appropriate safety equipment Explain to patient/family reasons for assistance, special measures to promote safety
Postoperative ■ General immediate postoperative complications	■ Absence or resolution of complication	■ Monitor for Recovery from anesthesia; notify physician if patient has not recovered in expected time Potential hypovolemia, shock, hypostatic pneumonia, pulmonary emboli, thrombophlebitis, abdominal ileus, nausea/vomiting, oliguria/urinary retention

POTENTIAL PROBLEMS	EXPECTED OUTCOMES	NURSING ACTIVITIES
		Recovery from any special measures induced during surgery, such as hypotension/hypothermia Notify physician immediately of any signs/symptoms of complication Administer medications and treatments as ordered Monitor effects and side effects Continue monitoring for resolution or progression of complication See appropriate standard for identified complication such as Standard 31, *Embolic phenomena;* Standard 17, *Shock*

■ Increased ICP related to
Edema
Hematoma
CSF obstruction
Possible upward or downward cerebral herniation from increased ICP
	■ Absence or control of increased ICP
	Maximal neurological functioning
		■ Establish neurological baseline postoperatively and compare to preoperative baseline
		See Problem, Increased ICP (preoperative), for all specific activities
		In addition, monitor
		  Neurological assessments and vital signs as ordered and prn (usually q15 min until stable, q30 min until stable, and then q1 hr)
		  Particularly LOC; pupil size, equality, and reactivity; extraocular movements; motor and sensory systems; communication abilities and speech quality; respiratory rate, pattern, and quality; BP and P for any abnormalities
		  For any increase in headache, nausea/vomiting above usual postoperative expectation
		  For any sudden appearance or increase in diplopia, nystagmus, ataxia, cerebellar dysfunctions, cranial nerve dysfunctions
		  For more detailed and specific assessments as patient's status allows
		  Operative site q1-2 hr for any signs of bleeding, bulging, or tenseness
		Maintain head gatch as ordered (usually elevated 30 to 45 degrees)
		Accurately record intake and output q1-2 hr; monitor for signs of dehydration/overhydration; see Problem, Fluid and electrolyte imbalance
		Avoid hyperflexion or extension of neck
		  Support head when turning or lifting patient
		  Frequently neck collar may be ordered; maintain in proper position
		  If pillow is allowed, position with type to avoid aforementioned (such as horseshoe)
		Notify physician immediately of any decline in neurological status from preoperative baseline or change in status or vital signs postoperatively; of any increase in symptoms or worsening deficit
		  Administer medications/treatments as ordered; monitor effects and side effects
		  Prepare patient/family for any diagnostic tests/procedures ordered
		If ventricular drainage system is continued postoperatively
		  Prevent any compression, kinking, pulling, or tension on tubing by proper positioning of patient; if necessary restrain patient's hands to prevent pulling or tension of tubing (first try explanations of necessary reasons/purposes for drain)
		  Monitor drainage system q1 hr for patency; fluid should be fluctuating in tubing or draining into collection apparatus
		  Maintain sterility of system
		  Maintain at specific level ordered by physician
		  Measure and record as ordered pressure, amount, and quality of drainage; notify physician if variable from norm specified; (physician will usually specify acceptable ranges of pressure and amount)
		  Notify physician immediately of any cloudiness of CSF
		  Check dressing q1 hr; monitor for any leakage around drain site, swelling, or edema
		  Monitor neurological status correlated with fluid pressure/quantity
		  If patient is on ICP monitoring, record pressures and drain fluid amount specified by physician's order to maintain pressure values; monitor effects of certain treatments on ICP such as coughing, turning, and suctioning; space activities if possible to minimize increases in ICP

POTENTIAL PROBLEMS	EXPECTED OUTCOMES	NURSING ACTIVITIES
		Administer antibiotics as ordered; monitor effects and side effects
		Send CSF specimens as ordered and monitor results
		Monitor serum electrolyte levels as Na$^+$ values may decrease from loss of CSF by drainage; notify physician of results and replace fluid as ordered (frequently CSF fluid is ordered replaced milliliter for milliliter)
		Monitor for signs of epidural hematoma (see Standard 33, *Head trauma*, Problem, Epidural hematoma) and meningitis (see Standard 42, *Meningitis/encephalitis*)—both potential problem complications of ventricular drainage
		If ordered, clamp tubing as specified by physician, such as may be ordered when coughing and turning patient
		Notify physician immediately of any change in neurological status; fluid pressure, amount or quality abnormality; nonpatency of system; or abnormal lab values
		If clamping schedule is ordered, clamp tubing as specified, maintaining precise time schedule and recording of time, pressure, fluid drainage amount/quality; notify physician of any change in neurological status or signs of increased ICP; unclamp drain as per physician's standing or stat order
		After removal of ventricular drain by physician, monitor neurological status and vital signs frequently; burr hole sites for oozing, bleeding, drainage/edema; for signs of increased ICP; have emergency ventriculostomy set, medications readily available; report to physician immediately any abnormality/decline; if internal shunting procedure is necessary, see Standard 38, *Internalized shunting procedures*
■ Respiratory insufficiency related to CNS dysfunction Edema Cranial nerve dysfunction Pneumonia Atelectasis Pulmonary emboli	■ Patent airway Adequate alveolar ventilation and perfusion Normal respiratory rate and quality Arterial blood gas levels within patient's normal limits	■ Ongoing assessment of respiratory status q1 hr and prn; monitor for any abnormality/decline Respiratory rate, quality, and pattern Patency of upper airway and patient's ability to handle secretions Presence/strength of gag, cough, and swallow reflexes Cranial nerve functioning, particularly presence/strength of nerves IX to XII Skin color, nail beds, peripheral pulses, and skin warmth Breath sounds bilaterally for quality of aeration; signs of obstruction (rales, rhonchi) Arterial blood gas values Chest radiograph results Signs/symptoms of thrombophlebitis, pulmonary emboli, pulmonary edema Maintain patent airway by Turning and positioning to prevent obstruction or aspiration of secretions q2 hr and prn Deep breathing and coughing q1 hr and prn (if allowed) Suctioning prn Adequate oxygenation and humidification as ordered Chest physiotherapy/pulmonary toilet if warranted and not contraindicated by physician's order Apply antithromboembolic stockings or Ace bandages as ordered; reapply every shift and prn; monitor for constriction/looseness, condition of skin Instruct and supervise patient in performing leg exercises, ROM exercises Increase activity level/progression when allowed Notify physician immediately of any change in respiratory/neurological status or signs of complication potential/occurrence If patient electively remains intubated postoperatively, see Standard 6, *Mechanical ventilation* (this is commonly done if surgery was performed near or in medulla, edema was found intraoperatively or is anticipated postoperatively, or severe cranial nerve dysfunctions are expected)

POTENTIAL PROBLEMS	EXPECTED OUTCOMES	NURSING ACTIVITIES
		Explain procedures and reasons for equipment/respiratory assistance to patient/family; reassure and support
		Establish alternative means of communication
		When patient is extubated, closely monitor respiratory/neurological status and vital signs
		If respiratory problem occurs, assist with emergency measures to maintain patent airway and adequate ventilation
		Administer medications/treatments as ordered; monitor effects and side effects
		See STANDARD 6 *Mechanical ventilation*
		If emboli occur, see Standard 31, *Embolic phenomena*
■ Cranial nerve dysfunction	■ Absence of complications	■ Ongoing assessments of cranial nerve functioning—presence, strength, and quality—q1-2 hr
		Specifically monitor any symptoms of dysfunction
		Notify physician of any increase in cranial nerve dysfunction
		Monitor for improvement or decline
		Plan and implement individualized care based on patient's status; ongoing assessments and evaluations of effectiveness of interventions
Oculomotor (III)		Monitor pupil size, equality, and reactivity; extraocular movements
Trochlear (IV)		Monitor for ptosis/nystagmus—degree/extent
Abducens (VI)		If diplopia occurs, apply alternating eye patch
Nystagmus, ptosis, decreased extraocular movements, diplopia		
Trigeminal (V)		Monitor facial sensation
Loss of facial sensation		If decreased, protect from injury by removal of sharp objects on pillow, pads for cushioning
Trigeminal (V) and facial (VII)		Monitor for presence/strength of corneal reflex bilaterally
Loss of corneal reflex		If decreased or absent
		Obtain order for protective eyedrops and lubricants
		Tape eyelid on affected side shut to prevent corneal abrasion, which may occur because of inability to close eyelid
Facial (VII)		Monitor for facial weakness/asymmetry
Decreased facial muscle strength/facial expression		If present, determine patient's chewing ability
		Assess patient's food likes and preferences
Facial weakness/paralysis		Assist patient in diet selection within chewing capabilities
Patient/family's anxiety related to body image from distortion of mouth		Have patient chew on unaffected side
		Stay with patient during mealtimes, assessing and evaluating chewing abilities and diet appropriateness
		Monitor for facial droop, which may cause drooling of saliva from affected side
		Excellent oral hygiene
		Frequent removal of secretions
		Instruct and supervise in facial exercises
		If patient has dentures, assess if refitting is necessary and obtain order for appropriate referral
		Assess level of patient's anxiety and altered body image related to facial nerve weakness, droop/drooling from mouth
		If speech is impaired from facial weakness/paralysis, establish alternate means of communication
		Encourage patient's verbalization of fears, concerns, feelings, since decreased facial strength may inhibit normal facial expression conveyance
Acoustic (VIII)		Assess hearing loss
Decreased hearing		Obtain hearing aid if patient possesses one and insert it
		Speak to patient from unaffected side; assess volume level necessary
		Face patient when speaking
		If hearing loss is bilateral, establish alternate means of communication such as magic slate, pad, word board

POTENTIAL PROBLEMS	EXPECTED OUTCOMES	NURSING ACTIVITIES
Disturbance of balance and equilibrium		Assess degree of ataxia and location (may be more pronounced falling to one side) Determine measures necessary for safety and implement such as Assist patient in getting out of bed Assist in ambulation Maintain safe environment by removing obstacles Assess for nystagmus Obtain equipment to help patient toward independence, instructing and supervising in use Obtain order for physiotherapy consultation Reassure and support patient, praising frequently for progress achieved
Dizziness		Have patient move slowly and cautiously when changing position Dangle for 5 to 10 minutes before standing Assist in ambulation and activities as needed

Glossopharyngeal (IX)
Vagus (X)
  Decreased or absent gag, swallowing, and cough reflexes
  Dysphagia/aspiration
  Nasal, dysarthric speech
		Assess presence and quality of gag, cough, and swallow reflexes; ability to handle secretions
		If reflexes are absent/diminished, maintain interventions to prevent complications
		Suction prn
		Position to prevent obstruction or aspiration of secretions
		Keep patient NPO
		Administer IV fluids/NG feedings as ordered; monitor NG tube for patency and proper placement; NG feedings for absorption/retention
		Frequent oral hygiene
		Explain necessity for NG or IV feedings, reasons NPO
		If gag reflex is adequate, start po fluids slowly as per physician's order
		Stay with patient at mealtimes, monitoring swallowing ability and effectiveness
		Assess foods patient tolerates best and assist with diet selection
		Continually assess for any choking/nasal regurgitation
		Assess for nasal speech and hoarseness; obtain order for speech consultation if indicated; if dysarthria is a problem, establish alternate means of communication
		Reassure and support patient/family; encourage verbalization and answer questions

Hypoglossal (XII) Decreased tongue strength		Assess for tongue position and muscle strength; monitor for any deviation or tongue tremor (location and degree) Provide for frequent oral hygiene Instruct and supervise patient in exercise programs for strengthening
Spinal accessory (XI) Impaired/absent shoulder shrug and head turning to side		Assess ability to shrug shoulder, turn head, and bend forward Assist with ADL as needed Place objects within field of head turning capability and vision Instruct and supervise in exercise program

■ Cardiac arrhythmia related to
  Vagal stimulation
  Brainstem edema
	■ Normal sinus rhythm
	Absence or control of arrhythmia
	Adequate cardiac output
		■ Monitor
		ECG recording for any abnormality
		Vital signs including apical and radial pulses q1 hr
		Serum electrolyte levels for any abnormality
		Adequacy of cardiac output and perfusion
		Avoid vagal stimulation such as Valsalva maneuver, neck vein compression
		Notify physician of any arrhythmia or abnormality
		Administer medications/treatments as ordered
		Monitor for resolution or progression of ECG abnormality
		Notify physician if therapy is not effective

See STANDARD 21   *Arrhythmias*

POTENTIAL PROBLEMS	EXPECTED OUTCOMES	NURSING ACTIVITIES

▪ Fluid and electrolyte imbalance related to
Ventricular fluid loss
CNS pathology
Medications administered
	▪ Fluid and electrolyte balance within normal limits	▪ Monitor and accurately record intake and output, urine specific gravity q1-2 hr; if there is ventricular drainage, record and report amount
		Monitor for signs of dehydration or overhydration such as
		    Poor skin turgor
		    Dry mucous membranes
		    Peripheral edema
		    Excessive thirst
		    Change in LOC
		Monitor for
		    Abnormal vital signs, Hgb/Hct values
		    Abnormal serum electrolytes
		    Weight alterations
		    Temperature elevations
		    Insensible fluid losses including respiratory, diaphoresis, secretions
		    Presence/degree of nausea and vomiting; effectiveness of medications ordered
		    Presence/quality of bowel sounds for any abnormality
		Monitor for signs of fluid imbalance, which may occur because of decreased or increased production/release of ADH (vasopressin); either condition can occur postoperatively
		    Decreased ADH: monitor for
		        Hypernatremia
		        Hyperosmolality
		        Dehydration
		        Diabetes insipidus: polyuria, polydipsia
		        Alterations in LOC such as irritability, increased muscle tone, hyperactive reflexes, muscle twitching, convulsions, decerebrate rigidity
		    Increased ADH (inappropriate ADH): monitor for
		        Hyponatremia
		        Hypoosmolality
		        Overhydration
		        H_2O retention/intoxication
		        Nausea/vomiting
		        Apathy, muscle twitching, irritability, disorientation
		Administer IV fluids, NG feedings as ordered
		Administer medications as ordered; monitor effects and side effects; if patient is receiving steroids, monitor urine glucose and acetone levels four times a day
		Notify physician of any fluid imbalance or electrolyte abnormality, any signs of ADH disorder
		    Administer medications/treatments as ordered
		    Maintain intake at specific level ordered
		    Monitor hourly intake and output
		    Explain to patient reasons for fluid restriction or encouragement; plan oral intake based on regimen ordered, assessing fluid preferences

▪ Infection	▪ Infection free
	Incision well-healed
		▪ Keep patient's hands from operative site/drain
		Maintain sterility of head dressing/drainage apparatus
		Monitor
		    Temperature as ordered and prn for any elevation
		    Dressing, incision site, drainage site q2 hr for any signs of redness, tenderness, bulging, separation, or drainage (amount and quality)
		    If ventricular drain is present, monitor CSF amount and quality for any abnormality
		    Neurological status and vital signs for any decline/abnormality
		    IV sites frequently for any signs of redness, tenderness, phlebitis
		    WBC count (may be falsely elevated if patient is receiving steroids)
		    For any signs/symptoms of meningitis

POTENTIAL PROBLEMS	EXPECTED OUTCOMES	NURSING ACTIVITIES
		Administer antibiotics as ordered; monitor effects and side effects (frequently ordered prophylactically postoperatively) Notify physician immediately of any signs/symptoms of infection Administer medications/treatments as ordered Monitor wound culture results, CSF determinations Monitor for other possible infection sources if warranted, including urine, sputum, chest radiograph results Monitor for resolution/progression of infection If problem occurs, see Standard 42, *Meningitis/encephalitis*
■ GI bleeding related to CNS factors Stress Steroid administration	■ Absence or resolution of GI bleeding	■ Monitor vital signs q2-4 hr, Hgb and Hct, stools for Hematest three times a week; Hematest of aspirate, urine, and emesis for any abnormalities Obtain order for antacid administration as soon as patient is able to take po Monitor for signs of GI bleeding, including abdominal tenderness/distention, hypotension, sudden tachycardia Notify physician immediately if any abnormality occurs; if problem occurs, see Standard 49, *Acute upper gastrointestinal bleeding*
■ Cerebellar dysfunction Ataxia, loss of balance and coordination	■ Patient ambulates safely with assistance Patient performs ADL safely with maximal possible independence	■ Monitor cerebellar functioning Establish and implement plan of care based on individual needs and specific deficit Focus plan of care on maintaining safety while promoting maximal possible independence Involve patient/family in planning care and decision making Encourage verbalization by patient/family; answer questions realistically; reassure and support gains/realistic goals Instruct and evaluate patient/family in necessary information and skills required to deal with problem/deficit, such as Safety precautions Exercise program Special equipment Assistance needed (type, amount, degree)
■ Continued presence of neurological deficit Patient/family's fears, anxiety/anger related to deficit and possible alterations in life-style	■ Maximal neurological functioning* Maximal independence in ADL (within capabilities) Patient/family verbalizes concerns	■ Assess patient's specific neurological deficit Collaborate with physician regarding prognosis, possible degree of recovery Implement individualized plan of care based on patient's needs and deficits Assist as needed in ADL Monitor potential for independent functioning and obtain equipment to maximize function and promote safety Obtain orders for appropriate referrals such as physiotherapy, speech or occupational therapy; social services Encourage verbalization of patient/family's fears, anxieties, and other reactions—level and degree Answer questions realistically Encourage their participation in care planning, implementation, evaluation, and decision making Realistically reassure and support patient/family Reinforce any gains or independence patient achieves Plan, instruct, demonstrate, supervise, and evaluate patient/family's verbalization/performance of needed information/skills for maximal independent functioning such as Measures to prevent complications Assistance necessary—type, amount, degree Proper use of therapeutic devices/equipment Monitor level of achievement toward maximizing potentials and independence; means to promote as "normal" a life-style as possible

*If responsibility of critical care nurse includes this stage of care.

POTENTIAL PROBLEMS	EXPECTED OUTCOMES	NURSING ACTIVITIES
■ Insufficient knowledge to comply with discharge regimen	■ Patient/family demonstrates or verbalizes understanding of discharge regimen*	■ Assess patient/family's level of understanding of neurological problem and therapy received Explain relationship between patient's neurological status and therapies prescribed If cerebral pathology was caused by head injury or trauma, explore with patient/family measures to decrease potential injury recurrence, importance of controlling factors precipitating head injury Instruct patient/family regarding required information/skills so that before discharge patient/family is able to
	Patient/family accurately describes medication, activity, and dietary regimens	Describe medication regimen 　Name and purpose 　Route, dosage, frequency, times 　Side effects 　Special precautions necessary including drugs, foods, beverages contraindicated or quantity regulated; factors potentiating/decreasing effects or side effects; physical restrictions; safety measures Describe dietary regimen Describe activity regimen, exercise program Describe and demonstrate any special therapeutic measures prescribed
	Patient/family describes and demonstrates means to achieve maximal independence in ADL, promote safety, and prevent complications	Describe and demonstrate proper use of equipment or therapeutic devices 　Reasons for using 　Time, method, and duration of use 　Precautions/safeguards 　Necessary maintenance (type, frequency) 　Measures to promote optimal functioning, upkeep/duration Describe and demonstrate safety precautions in performing ADL
	Patient/family describes signs/symptoms requiring medical attention	Describe signs/symptoms of neurological status requiring medical care
	Patient/family describes follow-up care regimen	Describe plan for follow-up care including purpose of appointment, when and where to go, who to see, what to expect, what specimens to bring

*If responsibility of critical care nurse includes such follow-up care.

INTERNALIZED SHUNTING PROCEDURES

Internalized shunt insertions are usually performed when the patient's clinical status demonstrates an enlargement of part or all of the ventricular system of the brain. *Hydrocephalus,* or "water on the brain," is a term commonly used to denote this ventricular enlargement produced by an overproduction of CSF or obstruction of CSF flow. Increased ICP frequently results from the CSF accumulation and retention. Internalized shunt insertion does not correct the original condition that is producing the overproduction or obstruction, but rather removes and diverts the excessive CSF away from the brain in an effort to decrease the dilatated and enlarged ventricular size and diminish the increased ICP. The shunting devices commonly inserted consist of a catheter placed in a lateral ventricle, a reservoir for fluid accumulation, a one-way valve to maintain flow out of the ventricle, and a catheter to transfer the CSF to the internal jugular vein, heart, or peritoneum. Shunt insertion is frequently done in the right lateral ventricle, since the right hemisphere is the nondominant side for the majority of the population. The purpose of the shunt insertion and functioning is to remove the excess CSF from the ventricles and transfer the fluid to other circulatory pathways, thereby reducing or eliminating the degree of hydrocephalus within the brain.

HYDROCEPHALUS

Two types of hydrocephalus are commonly identified. *Communicating* hydrocephalus results from increased production of CSF with normal absorptive rate or impairment of CSF absorption back into the circulating blood. It may also occur as the result of a block in the CSF pathways distal to the foramina of Magendie and Luschka. In this situation fluid reaches the subarachnoid space but does not circulate over the surface of the brain and is therefore not reabsorbed in sufficient quantities to prevent ventricular dilatation. *Noncommunicating* hydrocephalus is caused by blockage in the CSF pathway between formation in the ventricular system and proximal to the foramina of Magendie and Luschka.

Three common processes that cause hydrocephalus either singly or in combination are as follows:

1. Overproduction of CSF from choroid plexus papillomas and other tumors; also associated with the condition known as *pseudotumor cerebri.*
2. Obstruction of normal CSF flow (most common cause of hydrocephalus). The blockage or obstruction of the CSF results in accumulation of the fluid and ventricular dilatation. Common sites of obstruction include the foramina of Monro (frequently from third ventricular tumors); aqueduct of Sylvius (frequently from congenital or inflammatory obliterations, brainstem lesions); fourth ventricle foramina (frequently from displacement of medulla by lesions, congenital malformations, or meningeal fibrosis); and subarachnoid pathways (frequently from congenital malformations, inflammation, hemorrhage, or adhesions in subarachnoid space).
3. Impaired or failed absorption at arachnoid villi and granulations. Absorption problem as a primary cause of hydrocephalus is rare but can occur when the blood breakdown products from a SAH flow to the arachnoid villi where they then impair absorption of CSF.

Many etiologies can produce the process that causes hydrocephalus, including tumors, infections, hemorrhages, congenital malformations, and adhesions. Hydrocephalus may also occur as a postoperative complication, especially following posterior fossa operations and shunting procedures for previously diagnosed hydrocephalus (whether initial shunt insertion, revision, or removal of a shunt system or component). The extent and degree of hydrocephalus or ventricular dilatation depends on many factors. These factors affecting the clinical variability include primary/secondary causes of hydrocephalus; duration, progression, and location of pathological condition; and compensatory mechanisms and effectiveness. Hydrocephalus is a clinical syndrome for which causes are numerous, variable, and frequently unknown.

Normal pressure hydrocephalus is a clinical syndrome usually characterized by dementia, gait apraxia, and urinary incontinence. Enlargement of the cerebral ventricles is present, but ICP is not increased. Diagnostic procedures demonstrate accumulation of CSF in the lateral ventricles, indicating impairment/failure of normal CSF circulation. Shunt insertion may be performed to relieve the CSF accumulation.

ASSESSMENT

1. Onset, progression, duration, frequency, and specific description of neurological symptoms, including
   a. Headache
   b. Nausea/vomiting
   c. Changes in behavior/personality
   d. Changes in mental abilities
   e. Pupillary/visual alterations, including diplopia, ocular palsies, nystagmus, blurred vision, papilledema
   f. Alterations in LOC
   g. Changes in motor/sensory functioning
   h. Difficulty ambulating; ataxia; falls
   i. Incontinence
   j. Alterations in communication abilities
   k. Seizures
2. Previous history of head trauma/injury, congenital anomalies, delayed growth and development milestones, CNS infections
3. Previous neurological treatment or neurosurgical procedure; medications taken and effects on clinical course and status
4. If prior shunt insertion was performed
   a. Number, type, placement, and duration of previous shunt systems
   b. Effects on clinical status
   c. Complications, both immediate and long-term; if shunt malfunction occurred, cause and treatment/ surgical intervention
   d. Any special therapeutic measures prescribed to promote shunt functioning such as pumping of shunt system valve or reservoir, shunt taps by physician
   e. Follow-up care regimen of shunt insertion and clinical course
5. Presence of any medical problems and medications/ treatments prescribed and followed
6. Patient's perceptions and reaction to diagnosis, treatment modalities, surgical interventions
7. Presence of any alterations in body image; fears of shunt insertion, functioning/malfunctioning; fears of permanent disability or deficit; altered role in family, normal occupation/performing ADL
8. Baseline parameters status
   a. Neurological
   b. Respiratory
   c. Cardiovascular
   d. Hydration/nutritional
   e. Metabolic
   f. Skin integument
   g. Infection
   h. Vital signs
   i. Weight
   j. Urine output pattern
   k. Handedness (right or left)
9. Diagnostic test results, including
   a. CT scan
   b. Skull radiographs
   c. Lumbar puncture
   d. Cisternal puncture, isotope cisternography
   e. Subdural taps
   f. Brain scan, isotopic scanning
   g. Pneumoencephalogram
   h. Ventriculogram
   i. Shunt injections and scanning
   j. Cerebral angiography
   k. NMR scan
10. Results of
   a. Serum electrolyte levels
   b. Hgb and Hct, platelet count, WBC count with differentiation
   c. Type and cross-matching
   d. CSF determinations
   e. Urinalysis, culture, specific gravity, osmolality, electrolytes
   f. Arterial blood gas levels
   g. Clotting profile
   h. Anticonvulsant drug levels
   i. Chest radiograph
   j. ECG

GOALS

1. Optimal neurological functioning
2. Optimal independence in ADL
3. Serum electrolyte levels and fluid balance within normal limits
4. Hgb and Hct stable within normal limits
5. Incisions well-healed without any external protrusion of shunt system
6. Shunt system patent and functioning
7. Infection free
8. Reduction in patient/family's anxiety with provision of information, demonstrations, support
9. Before discharge patient/family is able to
   a. Describe medication, activity, exercise, and dietary regimens
   b. Demonstrate safety measures and techniques; proper use of any equipment/therapeutic devices prescribed
   c. Demonstrate and describe any special therapeutic measures; shunt care, maintenance, or treatments prescribed
   d. Describe signs and symptoms requiring medical attention
   e. State necessary information regarding follow-up care

POTENTIAL PROBLEMS	EXPECTED OUTCOMES	NURSING ACTIVITIES
Preoperative ■ Patient/family's anxiety related to Limited understanding of diagnostic tests, procedures, anticipated surgery, postoperative course Potential/presence of neurological deficit; fears of disability or worsened deficit	■ Patient/family's behavior indicates decreased anxiety with provision of information	■ Ongoing assessment of level of anxiety, knowledge base, and understanding Encourage patient/family's verbalization of questions and fears; collaborate with physician in providing realistic information and reassurance appropriate to level of understanding Explain relationship between symptoms and neurological problem; reasons for therapies Explain and prepare for procedures, tests, preoperative routines If hair is to be shaved, assess anxieties regarding hair loss and possible altered body image; save hair if patient desires; provide information on means to deal with hair loss, such as wigs Explain anticipated postoperative care including routines, setting, monitoring equipment, IVs, drains, length of stay, visiting policy Explain reasons for frequent neurological assessments and vital sign monitoring Instruct in deep breathing and leg exercises; evaluate patient's performance Provide time needed for support and instruction of patient/family Notify unit in which patient will be after surgery of any special problems or items patient needs, such as Eyeglasses: for vision; to evaluate visual fields/acuity Dentures: for patient comfort; to evaluate facial symmetry If language barrier is present: effort should be made to have interpreter available postoperatively
■ Increased ICP with possible development or worsening of neurological deficit/symptomatology	■ Absence of complications Maximal neurological functioning	■ Establish neurological baseline and vital signs on admission; ongoing assessments, as ordered, of status and specific symptomatology; especially monitor extent and degree of Headache Nausea/vomiting Papilledema Mental changes such as disorientation, impaired memory Personality changes such as irritability, restlessness, apathy Pupillary changes and ocular palsies, particularly abducens nerve (VI) dysfunction Blurred vision; diplopia; nystagmus Incontinence Alterations in LOC Difficulty ambulating, ataxia Alterations in motor/sensory functioning Alterations in communication abilities, speech quality In infants: increased head circumference, bulging fontanelles, split sutures, irritability, somnolence, high-pitched cry, decreased feeding, sunsetting, nystagmus, vomiting Avoid precipitating factors in increased ICP such as hypoxia, hypercapnia, fever, Valsalva maneuvers, sharp angling of neck (may block venous outflow) Assist patient with positioning and turning; instruct patient not to hold breath Prevent constipation by establishing bowel regimen as individually warranted; ensure that patient has bowel movement preoperatively Monitor for any signs/symptoms that could initiate factor development, such as hypoventilation Notify physician of potential/presence of precipitating factors Maintain head gatch and activity as ordered Administer medications and treatments as ordered; monitor effects and side effects Accurately record intake and output; monitor for any imbalance Monitor serum electrolyte levels for any abnormalities

POTENTIAL PROBLEMS	EXPECTED OUTCOMES	NURSING ACTIVITIES
		Notify physician immediately of any change in neurological status, vital signs, or abnormal fluid/electrolyte balance If problem occurs, see Standard 32, *Increased intracranial pressure*
■ Presence of neurological deficit	■ Absence of complications	■ On admission establish and implement nursing care plan based on individual needs and specific deficit present Ongoing assessments and evaluations of effectiveness of interventions Establish neurological baseline immediately preoperatively to provide for comparison postoperatively
■ Seizures	■ Absence or control of seizures	■ Prevention of precipitating factors in seizure occurrence including fever, hypoxia, H_2O intoxication, electrolyte disturbances Notify physician of potential/presence of any factors Seizure precautions (if indicated) 　Padded siderails up at all times when patient is alone 　Bed height at lowest level 　Padded tongue blade and airway at bedside 　Emergency medications and equipment readily available 　Close observation and supervision Administer anticonvulsant medications as ordered; monitor effects and side effects, serum anticonvulsant levels If seizure occurs, monitor and record seizure activity; notify physician *See* STANDARD 41 *Seizures*
■ Skin breakdown	■ Skin integument intact	■ Ongoing assessments of skin integument and intactness q2 hr and prn Prevent skin breakdown by instituting measures such as 　Turn and position q2 hr 　Change head position frequently; use pillows to prevent pressure areas 　Monitor all skin areas frequently; massage, rub, apply protective lubricants and lotions as needed 　Keep skin clean and dry 　Obtain devices to prevent skin breakdown such as sheepskin, air mattress, padding Notify physician immediately of any signs/symptoms of skin abrasion, decreased skin circulation 　Administer medications and treatments as ordered; monitor effects and side effects 　Notify physician of results, resolution/progression
■ Nausea/vomiting	■ Control of nausea/vomiting Absence of complications	■ Initial assessment of presence, extent, duration of nausea/vomiting; ongoing assessments as ordered and prn Prevent aspiration by 　Suctioning equipment readily available 　Monitor closely presence/quality of gag, cough, and swallow reflexes; keep patient NPO if decreased or absent 　If nausea/vomiting occurs, turn patient on side and position properly; suction prn Notify physician immediately of presence, new appearance, or increased severity of nausea/vomiting 　Keep patient NPO as ordered 　Administer medications/treatments as ordered; monitor effects and side effects 　Administer IV fluids as ordered 　Accurately record intake and output 　Monitor neurological status closely; assess for any associated neurological symptoms or vital sign changes preceding, concurrent with, or following nausea/vomiting

POTENTIAL PROBLEMS	EXPECTED OUTCOMES	NURSING ACTIVITIES

Postoperative

POTENTIAL PROBLEMS	EXPECTED OUTCOMES	NURSING ACTIVITIES
■ General immediate postoperative complications	■ Absence or resolution of complication	■ Monitor for Recovery from anesthesia; notify physician if patient has not recovered in expected time Potential hypovolemia, shock, hypostatic pneumonia, pulmonary emboli, thrombophlebitis, abdominal ileus, nausea/vomiting, oliguria/urinary retention Recovery from any special measures induced during surgery such as hypotension/hypothermia Notify physician immediately of any signs/symptoms of complication Administer medications and treatments as ordered Monitor effects and side effects Continue monitoring for resolution or progression of complication See appropriate standard for identified complication such as Standard 31, *Embolic phenomena;* Standard 17, *Shock*
■ Increased ICP/increased neurological deficit/appearance related to Shunt obstruction/malfunction Hematoma/air formation Edema	■ Absence or control of increased ICP Maximal neurological functioning	■ Establish neurological baseline postoperatively and compare to preoperative baseline See Problem, Increased ICP (preoperative), for all specific activities In addition, monitor Neurological assessments and vital signs as ordered (usually q15 min until stable, q30 min until stable, q1 hr until stable, and then q2 hr) Particularly LOC; pupil size, equality, and reactivity; extraocular movements, motor and sensory systems; communication abilities and speech quality; respiratory rate, pattern, and quality; BP, P; cranial nerve functioning; cerebellar functioning for any abnormality/decline For any increase in headache, nausea/vomiting above usual postoperative expectations Maintain head level position as ordered (frequently flat or small degree of elevation) Notify physician immediately of any decline from preoperative baseline or change in neurological status or vital signs postoperatively If shunt pumping is ordered by physician, pump as specifically ordered including location, frequency, and duration; maintain schedule regimen and recording of pumping, effects and side effects Prepare patient/family for any diagnostic procedures/tests ordered Monitor for shunt functioning (see Problem, Shunt obstruction/malfunction)
■ Shunt obstruction/malfunction One of the greatest problems associated with procedure, clinical prognosis, and outcomes; patients frequently require repeated surgical interventions either immediately or over a period of years to correct shunt malfunction Common causes of shunt malfunction include Malposition of catheters Detachment of shunt system components	■ Absence or resolution of shunt obstruction/malfunction Shunt patent and functioning	■ Ongoing assessments as ordered of neurological status, vital signs and monitoring for signs/symptoms of increased ICP Monitor sites of shunt system placement q2 hr and prn For any signs of redness, tenderness, fluid collection, bulging, edema, skin opening/protrusion of shunt system components For any signs of CSF "tracking" or accumulation/cranial depression Dressings for any signs of bleeding or other drainage Maintain head position as ordered by physician; patient is frequently kept flat for 1 to 2 days to prevent too rapid decompression or potential accumulation of subdural hematoma/air formation Position patient as ordered to prevent compression of shunt tubing; frequently patient may only be allowed to lie on one side of head Explain to patient/family reasons for bed and head positions ordered Increase head gatch as specifically ordered by physician Monitor neurological status, vital signs, shunt site/functioning with head elevations Monitor for any headache, nausea/vomiting, dizziness; notify physician if any of these occur

POTENTIAL PROBLEMS	EXPECTED OUTCOMES	NURSING ACTIVITIES
Infection of shunt system (see Problem, Infection of shunt system/insertion site) Plugging or obstruction of shunt system		Activity progression as ordered; monitor closely for any ataxia Notify physician immediately of any change in neurological status, vital signs or any signs/symptoms of shunt malfunctioning Administer medications/treatments as ordered; monitor effects and side effects Explain and prepare patient/family for any diagnostic tests or procedures ordered Assist physician with any procedures or tests necessary such as shunt taps, CSF specimen collections If problem occurs, see Standard 35, *Subdural hematoma*

■ Fluid and electrolyte imbalance	■ Fluid and electrolyte balance within normal limits	■ Monitor and accurately record intake and output, urine specific gravity as ordered
		Monitor for signs of dehydration or overhydration such as
		  Poor skin turgor
		  Dry mucous membranes
		  Peripheral edema
		  Excessive thirst/urine output
		  Change in LOC
		Monitor for
		  Abnormal vital signs, Hgb/Hct values
		  Abnormal serum electrolyte values
		  Weight alterations
		  Temperature elevations
		  Insensible fluid losses including respiratory, diaphoresis, secretions
		  Presence/degree of nausea and vomiting; effectiveness of medications ordered
		Assess presence and quality of bowel sounds especially if peritoneal shunt system has been placed
		  Keep NPO as per physician's order
		  Begin fluids slowly when allowed
		  Monitor for signs/symptoms of paralytic ileus, abdominal tenderness/distention, peritonitis
		  Monitor abdominal site and dressing if peritoneal shunt is in place
		  Notify physician immediately of any signs/symptoms of abdominal obstruction or infection
		Administer IV fluids, NG feedings as ordered
		Administer medications as ordered; monitor effects and side effects; if patient is receiving steroids, monitor urine glucose and acetone levels four times a day
		Notify physician of any fluid imbalance or electrolyte abnormality

■ Infection of shunt system/ insertion sites	■ Infection free
	Incision sites well-healed
		■ Keep patient's hands from operative sites
		Administer antibiotics as ordered; monitor effects and side effects (frequently ordered prophylactically postoperatively)
		Monitor shunt insertion and system placement site frequently for
		  Intactness of suture line and containment of shunt system
		  Any signs of edema, bulging, redness, tenderness
		  Any drainage; note amount, quality
		  Any signs of CSF "tracking" or accumulation
		  Any signs of abdominal distention, ileus, pain, peritonitis if peritoneal shunt is in place
		Monitor
		  Temperature q4 hr and prn for any elevation (commonly low grade or spikes)
		  Neurological status and vital signs for any decline/abnormality
		  WBC count (may be falsely elevated if patient is receiving steroids)
		  For any general systemic complaints
		  For any signs/symptoms of meningitis

POTENTIAL PROBLEMS	EXPECTED OUTCOMES	NURSING ACTIVITIES
		Notify physician immediately of any signs/symptoms of suspected shunt infection Administer medications and treatments as ordered; monitor effects and side effects Explain and prepare patient/family for any diagnostic tests or procedures ordered Assist physician with procedures such as shunt tap, lumbar puncture Monitor results of CSF determinations and cultures If problem occurs, see Standard 42, *Meningitis/encephalitis*
■ Seizures	■ Absence or control of seizures	■ See Problem, Seizures (preoperative), for all activities
■ GI bleeding related to CNS factors Stress Steroid administration	■ Absence or resolution of GI bleeding	■ Monitor vital signs q2-4 hr; Hgb and Hct; stools for Hematest three times a week; Hematest of aspirate, emesis, and urine for any abnormalities Obtain order for antacid administration as soon as patient is able to take po Monitor for signs of GI bleeding including abdominal tenderness/distention, hypotension, sudden tachycardia Notify physician immediately if any abnormalities occur; if problem occurs, see Standard 49, *Acute upper gastrointestinal bleeding*
■ Continued presence of neurological deficit Patient/family's fears, anxiety, anger related to deficit and possible alterations in life-style	■ Maximal neurological functioning* Maximal independence in ADL (within capabilities) Patient/family verbalizes concerns	■ Assess patient's specific neurological deficit; collaborate with physician regarding prognosis, possible degree of recovery Implement individualized plan of care based on patient's needs and deficits Assist as needed in ADL Monitor potential for independent functioning and obtain equipment to maximize function and promote safety Obtain orders for appropriate referrals such as physiotherapy, speech or occupational therapy; social services Encourage patient/family's verbalization of fears, anxieties, and other reactions—level and degree Answer questions realistically Encourage their participation in care planning, implementation, evaluation, and decision making Realistically reassure and support patient/family Reinforce any gains or independence patient achieves Plan, instruct, demonstrate, supervise, and evaluate patient/family's verbalization/performance of needed information/skills for maximal independent functioning such as Measures to prevent complications Assistance necessary—type, amount, degree Proper use of therapeutic devices/equipment Monitor level of achievement toward maximizing potentials and independence; means to promote as "normal" a life-style as possible
■ Insufficient knowledge to comply with discharge regimen†	■ Patient/family demonstrates or verbalizes understanding of discharge regimen	■ Assess patient/family's level of understanding of neurological problem and therapy received Explain relationship between patient's neurological status and therapies prescribed Describe reasons for shunt insertion, purpose of shunt, expected effects, type of shunt inserted, and mechanism of action; common problems occurring, short- or long-term; diagrams or pictures may enhance explanations Instruct patient/family regarding required information and skills so that before discharge patient/family is able to

*If responsibility of critical care nurse includes this stage of care.
†If responsibility of critical care nurse includes such follow-up care.

POTENTIAL PROBLEMS	EXPECTED OUTCOMES	NURSING ACTIVITIES

	Patient/family accurately describes medication, activity, and dietary regimens	Describe medication regimen
		  Name and purpose
		  Route, dosage, frequency, times
		  Side effects
		  Special precautions necessary including drugs, foods, beverages contraindicated or quantity regulated; factors potentiating/decreasing effects or side effects; physical restrictions; safety measures
		Describe dietary regimen
		Describe activity regimen, exercise program
		Describe and demonstrate any special therapeutic measures prescribed such as shunt pumping (when, where, how)

	Patient/family describes means to achieve maximal independence in ADL, promote safety, and prevent complications	Describe and demonstrate proper use of equipment or therapeutic devices
		  Reasons for using
		  Time, method, and duration of use
		  Precautions/safeguards
		  Necessary maintenance (type, frequency)
		  Measures to promote optimal functioning, upkeep/duration

	Patient/family describes signs/symptoms requiring medical attention	Describe signs/symptoms of neurological status requiring medical care; signs/symptoms of shunt malformation, obstruction/infection
	Patient/family describes follow-up care regimen	Describe plan for follow-up care including purpose of appointment, when and where to go, who to see, what to expect, what charting or recorded data to bring

CAROTID ENDARTERECTOMY

Carotid endarterectomy is an operative procedure in which a plaque is removed from an artery and a graft is performed, using either synthetic substances or a graft from the patient's own body. The purposes of the operation are to restore normal circulation to the brain and to prevent the development of a stroke and irreversible neurological damage. Plaques may occur in numerous arteries within the cerebral circulatory system. Commonly they form in the internal and external carotid arteries, vertebral arteries, and the innominate, common carotid, and subclavian arteries. Plaques narrow the lumen of the vessel and restrict blood flow. If uncorrected, the obstruction of blood flow eventually results in thrombosis and occlusion.

Controversy exists regarding the benefits of carotid endarterectomy procedures, but most authorities recommend operative intervention if the plaque can be surgically removed and if the patient has experienced transient ischemic attacks (TIAs). Several studies have documented that, if untreated, one third of patients who have experienced a TIA will develop a severe neurological deficit within 5 years. Carotid endarterectomy may be the procedure of choice if the plaque is accessible for removal and if the occlusion can be surgically corrected.

TIA refers to the onset and disappearance of a neurological deficit within 24 hours because of a temporary disruption of blood supply to the brain. Usually recovery is complete within a few minutes to hours. The signs and symptoms and extent of recovery after this disturbance of the blood supply to a local area of the brain depend on how quickly and effectively the individual's collateral blood supply can provide adequate circulation and perfusion to the area. There are some typical signs and symptoms that occur with TIA, depending on the artery that is involved (see Table 39-1).

ASSESSMENT

1. History of any previous TIA
   a. Exact description of symptomatology including onset, duration, progression, and resolution (time and extent of recovery)
   b. Frequency of occurrence
   c. Whether episodes of TIA are of similar symptomatology or of variable symptoms or degree
   d. Precipitating factors in attacks such as activity, sharp angling of neck, rapid position change
2. Presence of any residual neurological deficit—specific description
3. Presence of medical factors prominent in stroke-prone profile such as cardiac abnormalities, hypertension, diabetes, hyperlipidemia; medications/treatments prescribed and followed
4. Presence of other factors identified in stroke-prone profile such as family history, smoking, gout, platelet aggregation, oral contraceptive use, obesity
5. Medications taken for neurological problem such as anticoagulants, vasodilators
6. Previous neurological treatment or neurosurgical procedure
7. Patient's perceptions and reaction to diagnosis, treatment modalities, surgical intervention
8. Presence of any alterations in body image; fears of permanent disability or deficit; altered roles in family, normal occupation, performance of ADL
9. Baseline parameters status
   a. Neurological
   b. Vital signs including BP recording on both arms in lying and standing positions
   c. Cardiac; circulatory and vascular
   d. Respiratory/pulmonary
   e. Handedness (right or left)
   f. Weight
   g. Hydration
10. Diagnostic test results, including
    a. Cerebral angiography
    b. Thermogram
    c. EEG
    d. CT scan
    e. Digital venous infusion (DVI)
    f. NMR scan
11. Results of
    a. Serum electrolyte levels
    b. Hgb and Hct, platelet count
    c. Clotting profile
    d. Arterial blood gas levels
    e. ECG

f. Chest radiograph

g. Urinalysis, specific gravity, culture

h. Type and cross-matching

GOALS

1. Optimal neurological functioning
2. Optimal independence in ADL
3. Adequate alveolar ventilation
4. Adequate cardiac output
5. Artery involved remains patent after operative procedure
6. Serum electrolyte levels within normal limits
7. Hgb and Hct stable within normal limits
8. Fluid balance within normal limits
9. Incision well-healed
10. Infection free

11. Reduction in patient/family's anxiety with provision of information, demonstrations, support
12. Before discharge patient/family is able to
    a. Describe medication, activity, exercise, and dietary regimens
    b. Demonstrate safety measures and techniques; proper use of any equipment, therapeutic devices if prescribed
    c. Identify, if present, risk factors of patient and importance of controlling or eliminating to decrease potential for recurrent plaque formation
    d. Describe signs and symptoms requiring medical attention
    e. State necessary information regarding follow-up care

TABLE 39-1. Transient ischemic attacks

Carotid arterial system

The classical history consists of a swift onset of contralateral weakness or numbness of arms or legs, dysphasia (difficulty in speaking or understanding) if dominant hemisphere is involved (for about 80% of population left hemisphere is dominant), and impaired vision of eye on side of diminished carotid blood flow

1. Internal carotid: typically patient experiences fleeting blindness of one eye, known as *amaurosis fugax*
2. On physical examination there may be evidence of arterial disease such as decreased pulsation in carotid artery or bruit over carotid artery

Middle cerebral artery

1. Contralateral paralysis or weakness of side, limb, face—worse in upper extremities
2. Impairment of sensation—numbness or hypesthesia
3. Blindness in one half of visual field (hemianopsia)
4. Dysphasia
5. Inability to recognize persons and things (agnosia)

Anterior cerebral artery

1. Contralateral paralysis or weakness of lower extremities
2. Mental change—impaired judgment and insight
3. Clumsiness in walking
4. Grasping and sucking reflexes on opposite side
5. Incontinence

Posterior cerebral artery

1. Inability to recognize or comprehend written words (alexia)
2. Mental change with memory impairment
3. Blindness in one half of visual field
4. Inability to recognize people and things
5. Weakness or paralysis of cranial nerve III (oculomotor)

Vertebrobasilar artery system

1. Impaired sense of touch on the face
2. Vertigo—dizziness, sensation of revolving movement
3. Vomiting
4. Difficulty swallowing (dysphagia)
5. Loss of muscle coordination on same side as paralysis or weakness
6. Weakness or paralysis of all limbs
7. Stammering and inability to articulate (dysarthria)
8. Double vision (diplopia) and visual field defects or blindness
9. Temporary loss of consciousness (syncope)
10. "Drop attacks"—falling caused by sudden loss of postural tone without loss of consciousness
11. Contralateral loss of pain and temperature sensations

POTENTIAL PROBLEMS	EXPECTED OUTCOMES	NURSING ACTIVITIES
Preoperative		
■ Development of neurological deficit; possibility of stroke	■ Maintenance of neurological functioning Absence of complications	■ Establish neurological baseline and vital signs on admission; ongoing assessments as ordered and prn Assess and immediately notify physician if patient experiences any TIAs 　Instruct patient to inform nurse immediately if TIA occurs; reassure and reemphasize importance and necessity of patient reporting any symptoms of TIA 　Monitor episode for exact description of symptoms, onset, progression, location, duration, resolution time period, frequency 　Monitor vital signs as ordered and prn 　Monitor for any precipitating factors enhancing TIA occurrence, and institute measures to control factors if possible Maintain BP in prescribed range ordered by physician by administration of standing and prn medications ordered for BP control Administer medications/treatments as ordered 　Explain reasons for therapy to patient/family 　Monitor effects and side effects 　Monitor clotting profile results Notify physician immediately of any neurological deficit development 　Prepare patient/family for any tests or procedures ordered Assess and document neurological status and vital signs immediately preoperatively to provide baseline for comparison postoperatively
■ Presence of neurological deficit on admission	■ Maximal neurological functioning Absence of complications	■ On admission establish and implement nursing care plan based on individual needs and specific deficit present Ongoing assessments and evaluations of effectiveness of interventions Monitor neurological status frequently; notify physician of any change in status Monitor and document preoperatively specific deficit patient has to provide for comparison postoperatively
■ Patient/family's anxiety related to 　Limited understanding of diagnostic tests and procedures 　Anticipated surgery 　Lack of knowledge regarding expected postoperative course 　Fears of disability or worsened deficit	■ Patient/family's behavior indicates decreased anxiety with provision of information	■ Ongoing assessment of level of anxiety, knowledge base, and understanding Encourage patient/family's verbalization of questions and fears; collaborate with physician in providing realistic information and reassurance appropriate to level of understanding 　Explain relationship between neurological problem and symptoms; reasons for therapies 　Explain and prepare for tests, procedures, preoperative routines 　If patient is receiving anticoagulation therapy, medication will usually be stopped 24 to 48 hours before surgery; explain reasons for medication cancellation 　Explain anticipated postoperative care including setting, routines, monitoring equipment, ECG recording, IVs, neck dressing, length of stay, visiting policy 　Explain reasons for frequent neurological assessments and vital sign monitoring 　Instruct in deep breathing, leg exercises; evaluate patient's performance 　Provide time needed for support and instruction of patient/family Notify unit in which patient will be after surgery of any special problems or items patient needs such as 　Eyeglasses: for patient vision; to evaluate visual abilities 　Dentures: for patient comfort; to evaluate facial symmetry 　Communication problems: if language barrier is present, effort should be made to have interpreter available postoperatively; if communication deficit is present, assess what aids or measures have assisted patient in improving abilities to communicate

POTENTIAL PROBLEMS	EXPECTED OUTCOMES	NURSING ACTIVITIES
Postoperative		
■ General immediate postoperative complications	■ Absence or resolution of complications	■ Monitor for Recovery from anesthesia; notify physician if patient has not recovered in expected time period Signs/symptoms of hypovolemia, shock, hypostatic pneumonia, pulmonary emboli, thrombophlebitis, abdominal ileus, nausea/vomiting, oliguria/urinary retention Recovery from any special measures induced during surgery such as hypotension/hypothermia Notify physician immediately of any signs/symptoms of complication Administer medications and treatments as ordered Monitor effects and side effects Continue monitoring for resolution or progression of complication See appropriate standard for identified complication such as Standard 31, *Embolic phenomena;* Standard 17, *Shock*
■ Neurological deficit related to decreased cerebral blood flow	■ Maintenance or improvement of neurological status from preoperative baseline	■ Establish neurological baseline postoperatively and compare to preoperative baseline status; ongoing neurological assessment and vital sign monitoring q15 min until stable, q30 min until stable, and then q1 hr Monitor for any abnormalities in LOC; motor and sensory functioning; pupil size, equality, and light reactivity; extraocular movements; cranial nerve functioning; and communication system Notify physician immediately of any worsening of preoperative neurological deficit/status, new deficit appearance, or significant change in vital signs Administer medications and treatments as ordered; monitor effects and side effects Maintain BP in specific range ordered by physician Prepare patient/family for any tests or procedures ordered Continue monitoring neurological status closely for improvement/resolution of deficit or worsening Explain to patient necessity for frequent assessments and reasons for specific tests being done Monitor for more detailed and specific neurological assessments as patient's status allows
■ Lack of patency of artery operated on related to Hematoma Occlusion Bleeding Embolus	■ Artery patent and functioning normally External pulses easily palpable and strong	■ Monitor with ongoing neurological assessments and vital signs; see Problem, Neurological deficit, for specific activities Appropriate external pulses for presence, strength, quality, and bilateral symmetry If operation was performed on internal carotid arteries, palpate temporal pulses bilaterally; if vertebral artery was operated on, palpate radial pulses bilaterally For any correlations between external pulse status and neurological status; BP levels and neurological status Operative site for any bleeding, swelling, or hematoma development; record amount, quality, and degree Notify physician immediately if external pulse is absent or diminished or hyperpulse develops; of any abnormality in operative site and/or any decrease in neurological status or correlations with signs/symptoms of abnormalities Administer medications and treatments as ordered; monitor effects and side effects Maintain BP within specific range ordered by physician Prepare patient/family for any tests ordered Continue monitoring for resolution or progression of abnormality

POTENTIAL PROBLEMS	EXPECTED OUTCOMES	NURSING ACTIVITIES

■ Hypotension related to Carotid sinus manipulation
Distensibility of carotid artery after removal of plaque
	■ BP within patient's normal or prescribed limits	■ Maintain head of bed at degree ordered
		Monitor and record BP as ordered and prn
		Maintain BP at specific level ordered by physician
		  Administer and titrate prn medications ordered by physician to maintain BP level; monitor effects and side effects; notify physician if not effective for control
		  If prn medication not ordered for maintaining BP, notify physician immediately if BP above or below specified level
		  Monitor for any correlation between BP levels and neurological status; notify physician if occurs

■ Bleeding, hematoma, or swelling at operative site	■ BP, P within normal limits
	Surgical site free of bleeding, swelling, or hematoma
	Hgb and Hct stable
		■ Monitor
		  Ongoing neurological assessments for any decline in neurological status
		  BP and P as ordered for any abnormalities or deviations from specified acceptable range
		  Surgical site for any bleeding, swelling, or hematoma (amount, quality, degree)
		  For any decrease in Hgb/Hct levels
		  For any signs of hypovolemia, bleeding, shock
		  Clotting profile if indicated
		Notify physician immediately of any abnormalities at operative site, signs/symptoms of bleeding
		  Administer medications/treatments as ordered; monitor effects and side effects
		  Assist physician with procedures such as resuturing

■ Respiratory insufficiency related to
Vagal nerve (X) edema or manipulation
Shift of trachea
Pneumonia
Atelectasis
Pulmonary emboli
	■ Patent airway
	Normal respiratory rate and quality
	Adequate alveolar ventilation
	Arterial blood gas levels within patient's normal limits
		■ Ongoing assessment of respiratory status q1 hr and prn
		Assess and monitor for any abnormality
		  Respiratory rate, quality, and pattern
		  Patency of upper airway and patient's ability to handle secretions
		  Position of trachea
		  Operative site for any bleeding, swelling, or hematoma development
		  Breath sounds bilaterally for quality of aeration; signs of obstruction (rales, rhonchi)
		  Presence/strength of gag, cough, and swallowing reflexes
		  Skin color, nail beds, peripheral pulses, and skin warmth
		  Arterial blood gas values
		  Chest radiograph results
		  Signs/symptoms of thrombophlebitis, pulmonary emboli, pulmonary edema
		Maintain patent airway by
		  Turning and positioning to prevent obstruction or aspiration of secretions q2 hr and prn
		  Deep breathing and coughing q1 hr and prn
		  Suctioning prn
		  Adequate oxygenation and humidification as ordered
		  Chest physiotherapy/pulmonary toilet if warranted and not contraindicated by physician's order
		Apply antithromboembolic stockings or Ace bandages as ordered; reapply every shift and prn; monitor for constriction/looseness, condition of skin
		Instruct and supervise patient in leg exercises, ROM exercises
		Increase activity level/progression when allowed
		Notify physician immediately of any change in respiratory/neurological status or signs/symptoms of complication occurrence or potential
		If problem occurs, assist with emergency measures to maintain patent airway and adequate ventilation
		See Standard 6, *Mechanical ventilation*
		If emboli occur, see Standard 31, *Embolic phenomena*

POTENTIAL PROBLEMS	EXPECTED OUTCOMES	NURSING ACTIVITIES
■ Difficulty swallowing related to edema, bleeding, or manipulation around glossopharyngeal (IX) and vagus (X) nerves	■ Gag reflex present and strong bilaterally Patient swallows without difficulty	■ Monitor patient's gag reflex and swallowing ability q1-2 hr and prn Ongoing assessments of presence/quality Notify physician immediately if any decrease in gag reflex or difficulty in swallowing develops Explain necessity for frequent assessments and interventions to patient Encourage verbalization of fears and answer questions Reassure patient that reflexes will return; explain relationship between surgery and diminished reflex ability Keep patient NPO until gag and swallow reflexes return to normal Suction secretions prn Start po fluids as per physician's order when reflexes are strong; stay with patient when initially beginning po fluids Reassess presence/quality of reflexes
■ Hoarseness from edema of recurrent laryngeal nerve/intubation	■ Absence or resolution of hoarseness Voice tone and strength normal	■ Monitor patient's voice for signs of hoarseness Notify physician if hoarseness develops or progresses Administer medications and treatments as ordered; monitor effects and side effects Obtain order for throat lozenges Reassure patient that hoarseness will resolve Explain relationship between surgery and hoarseness Encourage patient to rest voice until hoarseness resolves Continue monitoring voice until tone and strength are normal
■ Fluid and electrolyte imbalance Oliguria or retention	■ Fluid and electrolyte balance within normal limits Voiding is satisfactory	■ Administer IV fluids, medications as ordered; monitor effects and side effects Monitor Accurate recording of intake and output, urine specific gravity as ordered For any signs of urine retention or oliguria Presence/degree of nausea or vomiting; effectiveness of medications ordered Quality of bowel sounds; start po fluids as per physician's order when warranted Abnormal vital signs, Hgb/Hct values Abnormal serum electrolyte values Temperature elevations Signs of dehydration or overhydration Neurological status for any decline in LOC Notify physician of any fluid imbalance or electrolyte abnormality Administer medications/treatments as ordered; monitor effects and side effects
■ Arrhythmia related to Preexisting cardiac abnormalities Carotid sinus manipulation intraoperatively Vagal nerve (X) edema or manipulation intraoperatively	■ Absence or control of arrhythmia	■ Monitor Bedside ECG recording for any abnormalities Pulse rate and quality for bradycardia/tachycardia, irregularity; if indicated compare apical pulse rate to radial pulse and assess for perfusion irregularities For patient complaints of chest pain/discomfort, angina, arm pain, and radiation Notify physician immediately of any abnormality Administer medications and treatments as ordered; monitor effects and side effects If problem is not resolved, see appropriate standard, e.g., Standard 21, *Arrhythmias;* Standard 11, *Angina pectoris;* Standard 12, *Acute myocardial infarction*
■ Dizziness when head gatch is elevated Potential orthostatic hypotension	■ Patient can sit, stand, and ambulate without dizziness	■ Gradually elevate head of bed when physician's order permits Check BP frequently Monitor for any signs of dizziness or headache Slowly raise head of bed if BP is stable and patient is without dizziness until head is fully elevated

POTENTIAL PROBLEMS	EXPECTED OUTCOMES	NURSING ACTIVITIES
		Have patient dangle at side of bed for 5 to 10 minutes before assisting patient out of bed
		Initially assist patient and supervise until patient can ambulate safely and independently
		If problem occurs with hypotension or dizziness, notify physician
		Maintain head gatch at level that supports normal BP and prevents dizziness
		Slowly and gradually increase gatch level and activity progression within tolerance limits
■ Infection	■ Infection free Incision well-healed	■ Keep patient's hands away from operative site
		Monitor
		Temperature as ordered and prn for any elevation
		Incision site for any signs of redness, tenderness, swelling, separation, or drainage (amount and quality)
		Graft site, if present, for any abnormalities
		Notify physician of any signs of infection
		Administer medications/treatments as ordered; monitor effects and side effects
		Monitor wound culture results
		Monitor for other possible infection sources if warranted including sputum, urine, chest radiograph results
		Monitor WBC counts for elevations; if elevated, monitor serially for resolution or progression
■ Continued presence of neurological deficit Patient/family's fears, anxiety, anger related to deficit and possible alterations in life-style	■ Maximal neurological functioning* Maximal independence in ADL (within capabilities) Patient/family verbalizes concerns	■ Assess patient's specific neurological deficit
		Implement individualized plan of care based on patient's need and deficits
		Assist as needed in ADL
		Monitor potential for independent functioning and obtain equipment to maximize function and promote safety
		Obtain orders for appropriate referrals such as physiotherapy, speech or occupational therapy, social services
		Encourage verbalization of patient/family's fears, anxieties, and other reactions—level and degree
		Answer questions realistically
		Encourage their participation in care planning, implementation, evaluation, and decision making
		Realistically reassure and support patient/family
		Reinforce any gains or independence patient achieves
		Plan, instruct, demonstrate, supervise, and evaluate patient/family's verbalization/performance of needed information/skills for maximal independent functioning such as
		Measures to prevent complications
		Assistance necessary—type, amount, degree
		Proper use of therapeutic devices/equipment
		Monitor level of achievement toward maximizing potentials and independence; means to promote as "normal" a life-style as possible
■ Insufficient knowledge to comply with discharge regimen†	■ Patient/family demonstrates or verbalizes understanding of discharge regimen	■ Assess patient/family's level of understanding of neurological problem and therapy received
		Explain relationship between patient's neurological status and therapies prescribed
		If present, explain relationship of patient's risk factors to plaque formation and importance of controlling/eliminating factors to decrease potential for recurrent plaque formation

*If responsibility of critical care nurse includes this stage of care.
†If responsibility of critical care nurse includes such follow-up care.

POTENTIAL PROBLEMS	EXPECTED OUTCOMES	NURSING ACTIVITIES

	Patient/family accurately describes medication, activity, and dietary regimens	Instruction of patient/family regarding required information/skills so that before discharge patient/family is able to
		Describe medication regimen
		  Name and purpose
		  Route, dosage, frequency, times
		  Side effects
		  Special precautions necessary including drugs, foods, beverages contraindicated or quantity regulated; factors potentiating/decreasing effects or side effects; physical restrictions; safety measures
		Describe activity regimen, exercise program
		Describe dietary regimen
		Describe and demonstrate any special therapeutic measures prescribed

	Patient/family describes and demonstrates means to achieve maximal independence in ADL, promote safety, and prevent complications	Describe and demonstrate proper use of equipment or therapeutic devices
		  Reasons for using
		  Time, method, and duration of use
		  Precautions/safeguards
		  Necessary maintenance (type, frequency)
		  Measures to promote optimal functioning, upkeep/duration

	Patient/family describes signs/symptoms requiring medical attention	Describe signs/symptoms of neurological status requiring medical care
	Patient/family describes follow-up care	Describe plan for follow-up care including purpose of appointment, when and where to go, who to see, what to expect

TRANSSPHENOIDAL HYPOPHYSECTOMY (PITUITARY TUMORS)

The pituitary gland (hypophysis) is a small gland located in the sella turcica at the base of the brain. A circular fold of dura mater, the *diagphragm sella*, forms the roof of this fossa and contains an opening through which the pituitary stalk (infundibulum) passes. The pituitary stalk is the connecting pathway between the pituitary gland and the hypothalamus. The pituitary gland contains two lobes: the anterior lobe, known as the *adenohypophysis;* and the posterior lobe, or *neurohypophysis*.

The pituitary gland is the principal regulator of most of the glands of internal secretion by its own secretion of many important hormones. Pituitary secretion is controlled mainly by signals transmitted from the hypothalamus. Secretion from the anterior lobe is regulated by neurosecretory substances secreted by the hypothalamus. Posterior lobe secretion is controlled by nerve fibers originating in the hypothalamus and terminating in the posterior lobe.

The hormones secreted by the anterior pituitary (adenohypophysis) stimulate target organs and glands. Some of the major hormones include human growth hormone (HGH); adenocorticotropic hormone (ACTH); thyrotropin (TSH); gonadotropic hormones—follicle-stimulating hormone (FSH); luteinizing hormone (LH); luteotropic hormone (LTH); melanocyte-stimulating hormone (MSH); and prolactin.

The posterior lobe (neurohypophysis) is a storage area for the neurosecretory system of the hypothalamus that includes the supraoptic and paraventricular nuclei. The axons of these nuclei travel from the hypothalamus through the supraoptic hypophyseal tract of the stalk to storage areas in the posterior lobe. The two main hormones secreted and transported by these nuclei are ADH, also known as vasopressin, and oxytocin. The main function of ADH is the control of water reabsorption by the kidneys, which is effected by altering the permeability of the renal tubules. The release of ADH from the posterior lobe is controlled by a feedback regulatory mechanism that senses and responds to the plasma osmotic pressure. Normally this mechanism functions to maintain a normal range of osmolality and osmotic pressure. Hypothalamic osmoreceptors monitor the serum osmolality and respond to changes in the normal range by either stimulating or suppressing the release of ADH from the posterior lobe storage cells in an attempt to restore the osmolality to a normal level, as in the following:

Dehydration: hyperosmolality results in stimulation of ADH release to promote kidney reabsorption of water.

Overhydration: hypoosmolality results in suppression of ADH release to promote kidney excretion of water through urinary diuresis.

PITUITARY TUMORS

Because the pituitary gland secretes many important hormones, patients with lesions of the gland frequently have endocrine dysfunctions or symptoms of dysfunctions. The anatomical relationship of the pituitary gland to the optic chiasm is important in the consideration of pituitary tumors and their effects. The optic chiasm lies just above the anterior portion of the diaphragm sella. At the optic chiasm the fibers from each nasal retina (which carry temporal vision) cross over to join the fibers from the temporal retina (which carry nasal vision) of the other eye. The two sets of fibers then form the optic tract. Compression of the optic chiasm by a pituitary tumor produces various types of visual defects. The type of visual defect depends on the position of the chiasm in relation to the pituitary gland and the direction of growth of the tumor. If the tumor grows beyond the sella, the optic nerve may be compressed, producing optic atrophy and eventual loss of vision in the affected eye.

Pituitary tumors are located mainly in the anterior lobe (adenohypophysis). Their expansion and growth may erode surrounding bone; cause atrophy or distortion of the optic nerves, chiasm, or tracts; or produce pressure on the hypothalamus or impinge on the third ventricle. The pituitary tumors arising in the anterior lobe are usually benign and slow growing. The majority are adenomas, which frequently are partly cystic. They may cause hypofunctioning of the gland or secretion of abnormally high amounts of pituitary hormones.

Common signs and symptoms

1. Visual loss or failure: visual field defects—more than one half of patients with pituitary adenomas receive med-

ical attention because of the occurrence of this symptom
  a. Frequently the visual loss involves a partial or complete bitemporal hemianopsia that has developed gradually; the superior quadrants of the visual fields are usually affected first
  b. In cases of long-standing visual disorder, some degree of optic atrophy is present
2. Headache
3. Endocrine syndromes
  a. Hypopituitary signs—may include impotency, amenorrhea, loss of body hair; hypothyroidism and adrenal insufficiency may also be present
  b. Hormone-secreting pituitary tumors
    (1) Prolactin-secreting pituitary tumors—patient may have galactorrhea, amenorrhea
    (2) HGH-secreting pituitary tumors—patient may have gigantism and acromegaly
    (3) ACTH-secreting pituitary tumors—patient may have Cushing syndrome
4. Ocular palsies may occur if the cavernous sinus is compressed
5. Rarely, patient may have seizures, rhinorrhea, diabetes insipidus, hypothermia/somnolence

The treatments for pituitary tumors are numerous and include radiotherapy, medical management by drug regimens, and surgical removal. The two available surgical approaches are craniotomy or transsphenoidal hypophysectomy. The transsphenoidal hypophysectomy is a more recently perfected approach and is frequently the preferable choice. The following standard focuses on postoperative care following this approach.

ASSESSMENT

1. Onset, duration, progression, and specific description of neurological symptoms, particularly
  a. Visual loss or defect
  b. Alterations in pupil size, equality, and reaction; extraocular movements
  c. Headache
  d. Nausea/vomiting
  e. Diplopia, nystagmus
  f. Ataxia
  g. Seizures
2. Presence of any endocrine problems or signs/symptoms of dysfunction such as
  a. Impotence
  b. Amenorrhea
  c. Loss of body hair
  d. Galactorrhea
  e. Gigantism, acromegaly
  f. Cushing syndrome
  g. Diabetes insipidus (polyuria, polydipsia)
  h. Hypothyroidism
  i. Adrenal insufficiency
  j. Excessive weight gain
  k. Intolerance to cold
3. Medications taken for neurological/endocrine problem such as steroids, hormonal replacement, anticonvulsants, and pain medications
4. Previous neurological treatment or neurosurgical procedure
5. Presence of any alterations in body image; fears of permanent disability or deficit; altered role in family, normal occupation/performance of ADL; fears of tumor regrowth
6. Patient's perceptions and reaction to diagnosis, treatment modalities, surgical intervention
7. Presence of any other medical problems and medications/treatments prescribed and followed
8. Baseline parameters status
  a. Neurological
  b. Endocrine
  c. Metabolic
  d. Vital signs
  3. Weight
  f. Visual ability
  g. Hydration, urine output and pattern
9. Diagnostic test results, including
  a. Skull radiographs
  b. Tomograms of sella
  c. CT scan
  d. Pneumonencephalogram
  e. Lumbar puncture
  f. EEG
  g. Cerebral angiography
  h. Visual field studies
  i. Endocrine studies such as HGH, prolactin, plasma ACTH, TSH, hydrocortisone and ketosteroids, urine for gonadotropic hormone
  j. NMR scan
10. Results of
  a. Serum electrolyte levels
  b. Type and cross-matching
  c. Hgb and Hct, platelet count
  d. Urinalysis, specific gravity, osmolality, electrolytes
  e. Thyroid, pituitary/adrenal function tests if indicated
  f. Clotting profile if indicated

GOALS

1. Optimal neurological functioning
2. Optimal independence in ADL
3. Serum electrolyte levels within normal limits
4. Hgb and Hct stable within normal limits
5. Fluid balance within normal limits—diabetes insipidus controlled
6. Acid-base balance within normal limits
7. Incision healed without CSF leak
8. Infection free

9. Endocrine function controlled within normal limits
10. Reduction in patient/family's anxiety with provision of information, demonstrations, support
11. Before discharge patient/family is able to
    a. Describe medication, activity, and dietary regimens
    b. Describe any special therapeutic measures such as recording and balancing fluid intake/output; urine testing of glucose and acetone, specific gravity; weight recording
    c. Demonstrate safety measures and techniques; proper use of any equipment, therapeutic devices
    d. Describe, if present, relationship between neurological problem and endocrine dysfunction
    e. Describe signs/symptoms requiring medical attention
    f. State necessary information regarding follow-up care

POTENTIAL PROBLEMS	EXPECTED OUTCOMES	NURSING ACTIVITIES
Preoperative		
■ Decreased vision Visual loss/visual field defect	■ Maximal independence in ADL Safety of patient	■ Monitor visual ability; assess acuity, field cut, color loss Specifically monitor and document baseline visual loss/field defects Monitor for any increase in visual loss and notify physician if this occurs Promote independent functioning in ADL by Placing within patient's field of vision objects such as food, telephone, hygiene items Tell patient location of objects Have patient turn head to compensate for visual defects Obtain eyeglasses if patient has pair and uses them to improve visual ability Promote patient safety Assist with activities as needed to maintain safety Place call light within field of vision; inform patient of location Assist with ambulation as needed Siderails up if necessary to prevent falls
■ Patient/family's anxiety related to Limited understanding of diagnostic tests and procedures Anticipated surgery Lack of knowledge regarding expected postoperative course Fears of disability or worsened deficit	■ Patient/family's behavior indicates decreased anxiety with provision of information	■ Ongoing assessment of level of anxiety, knowledge base, and understanding Encourage patient/family's verbalization of questions and fears; collaborate with physician in providing realistic information and reassurance appropriate to level of understanding Explain relationship between neurological problem and symptoms, endocrine disorders; reasons for therapies Explain and prepare for tests, procedures, preoperative routines Explain anticipated postoperative care including setting, routines, monitoring equipment, IVs, Foley catheter, nasal packing, visiting policy, length of stay Explain reasons for frequent neurological assessments and vital sign monitoring Instruct in mouth breathing, leg exercises; evaluate patient's performance Provide time needed for support and instruction of patient/family Notify unit in which patient will be after surgery of any special problems or items patient needs such as Eyeglasses: for patient vision; to evaluate visual fields/acuity Visual field defect: notify unit of specific deficit as this could prevent having patient restricted to viewing wall postoperatively if bed selection can be flexible and chosen appropriately If language barrier is present: effort should be made to have interpreter available postoperatively
Postoperative		
■ General immediate postoperative complications	■ Absence or resolution of complication	■ Monitor for Recovery from anesthesia; notify physician if patient has not recovered in expected time period Signs/symptoms of hypovolemia, shock, hypostatic pneumonia, pulmonary emboli, thrombophlebitis, abdominal ileus, nausea/vomiting, oliguria/urinary retention

POTENTIAL PROBLEMS	EXPECTED OUTCOMES	NURSING ACTIVITIES
		Recovery from any special measurements induced during surgery such as hypotention/hypothermia Notify physician immediately of any signs/symptoms of complication Administer medications and treatments as ordered Monitor effects and side effects Continue monitoring for resolution or progression of complication See appropriate standard for identified complication such as Standard 31, *Embolic phenomena;* Standard 17, *Shock*
■ Increased ICP/potential neurological deficit related to Hemorrhage Hematoma Edema	■ Absence or resolution of increased ICP Maximal neurological functioning	■ Establish neurological baseline postoperatively and compare to preoperative baseline; notify physician immediately if there is any decrease in status Neurological assessments and vital signs as ordered and prn (usually q15 min four times, q30 min four times, then q1 hr); monitor particularly Pupil size, equality, and light reactivity—both direct and consensual; extraocular movements; visual acuity and fields LOC; motor and sensory functioning; communication abilities For any increase in headache, nausea/vomiting above usual postoperative expectation Notify physician immediately of any change in neurological status or vital signs Administer medications and treatments as ordered; monitor effects and side effects Prepare patient/family for any tests or procedures ordered If increased ICP occurs see Standard 32, *Increased intracranial pressure*
■ Excessive bloody nasal drainage	■ Normal amount of nasal drainage Absence or resolution of excessive amount	■ Prevent by No nasal treatments or suctioning Ice bag to nose as per physician's order Keep patient's hands from nose/packing; restrain if absolutely necessary as per physician's order Instruct patient to not use toothbrush for 10 days Provide oral hygiene q2 hr and prn Monitor Amount of bloody drainage on packing/oozing from nose; notify physician if above usual expectation For falling Hgb/Hct levels For hypotension, tachycardia Notify physician of any abnormality
■ CSF leak	■ Absence or resolution of CSF leak	■ Instruct patient to not blow nose or sneeze (if preventable); explain reasons why it is necessary to avoid these Assist physician with lumbar puncture, which may be done to decrease potential for CSF leak Explain procedure to patient Send CSF specimens as per physician's order; monitor results Monitor Amount and type of nasal drainage; if quality is suspicious (clear), obtain specimen and test for glucose (result usually positive for sugar if specimen is CSF); monitor for CSF "circle" on bed linen For complaints of severe, continuous headache Temperature as ordered for any elevation For signs of meningitis Notify physician immediately of any signs/symptoms of CSF leak (headache, fever, clear nasal drainage/positive dextrose result) Administer medications as ordered; monitor effects and side effects Monitor CSF culture results Monitor WBC count (may be falsely elevated if patient is receiving steroids) If meningitis occurs, see Standard 42, *Meningitis/encephalitis*

POTENTIAL PROBLEMS	EXPECTED OUTCOMES	NURSING ACTIVITIES
■ Fluid and electrolyte imbalance Diabetes insipidus*	■ Fluid and electrolyte balance within normal or prescribed limits Diabetes insipidus controlled	■ Monitor Hourly intake and output accurately and record on graph sheet Specific gravity q1 hr or with each voiding Notify physician immediately of any increased output or decreased specific gravity deviating from levels specified by physician's order that establishes fluid balance maintenance Daily weights or as ordered for any alterations, particularly weight loss For signs of polydipsia Serum electrolytes for any abnormalities particularly hypernatremia, hyperglycemia Urine glucose and acetone determinations as ordered Presence/degree of nausea and vomiting; effectiveness of medications ordered Hgb and Hct values for any abnormalities Administer IV fluids as ordered If problem occurs, notify physician immediately Administer medications as ordered; monitor effects and side effects; frequently vasopressin may be ordered; insulin coverage for glucose and acetone determinations Maintain intake at specific level ordered Monitor results of urine osmolality/electrolytes, serum osmolality values If patient is taking po fluids, determine fluid preferences and offer these frequently if po is encouraged by physician Explain to patient relationship between surgery and diabetes insipidus
■ GI bleeding related to CNS factors Stress Steroid administration	■ Absence or resolution of GI bleeding	■ Monitor vital signs q2-4 hr, Hgb and Hct; stools for Hematest three times a week; Hematest of aspirate, emesis, and urine for any abnormalities Obtain order for antacid administration as soon as patient is able to take po Monitor for signs of GI bleeding including abdominal tenderness/distention; hypotension, sudden tachycardia Notify physician immediately if any abnormality occurs If problem occurs, see Standard 49, *Acute upper gastrointestinal bleeding*
■ Continued presence of decreased vision Visual loss/visual field defect	■ Maximal independence in ADL Safety of patient	■ See Problem, Decreased vision (preoperative), for nursing activities Collaborate with physician regarding prognosis for recovery or improvement in vision (physician may have expectations for prognosis based on operative findings) Provide realistic information and reassurance to patient/family Encourage verbalization of anxieties and fears if visual loss is permanent Assess level of anxiety related to potential altered body image/role Support patient/family in verbalizing concerns, anger Instruct patient/family in measures to promote maximal independence and safety Obtain orders for appropriate referrals such as social services, vocational training

*Diabetes insipidus is characterized by polyuria and polydipsia. Specific gravity frequently falls to 1.000 to 1.005. Urine output rises well above the fluid intake. Restriction of intake, which in the normal functioning body mechanism would stimulate release of ADH from the pituitary gland (in response to hyperosmolality) and end diuresis, does not occur in patients with diabetes insipidus. This disruption of normal stimulation of ADH secretion mechanism is related to surgical manipulation or edema near the hypothalamus or supraoptic hypophyseal tract.

POTENTIAL PROBLEMS	EXPECTED OUTCOMES	NURSING ACTIVITIES
■ Insufficient knowledge to comply with discharge regimen*	■ Patient/family demonstrates or verbalizes understanding of discharge regimen	■ Assess patient/family's level of understanding of neurological problem and therapy received Explain relationship between patient's neurological status and therapies prescribed If endocrine symptoms or dysfunctions are present, explain relationship to neurological status and reasons, importance, and necessity of complying with hormonal replacement medication regimen Instruction of patient/family regarding required information and skills so that before discharge patient/family is able to

	Patient/family describes medication, activity, and dietary regimens	Describe medication regimen
		  Name and purpose
		  Route, dosage, frequency times
		  Side effects
		  Special precautions necessary, including drugs, foods, beverages contraindicated or quantity regulated; factors potentiating/decreasing effects or side effects; physical restrictions; safety measures
		Describe dietary regimen
		Describe activity regimen, exercise program

	Patient/family describes special therapeutic measures	Describe and demonstrate any special therapeutic measures prescribed such as
		  Accurate monitoring, recording, and graphing of intake and output
		  Monitoring and recording urine specific gravity, glucose, and acetone determinations
		  Maintenance of intake and output at prescribed level by adjustment of fluid intake, use of medications ordered prn
		  Weight monitoring and recording
		  Describe and demonstrate any visual therapeutic devices, techniques/measures prescribed

	Patient/family describes signs/symptoms requiring medical attention	Describe signs/symptoms of neurological status requiring medical care; signs of endocrine/metabolic status requiring care if present
	Patient/family describes follow-up care regimen	Describe plan for follow-up care including purpose of appointment, when and where to go, who to see, what to expect, what recorded information, charts, and specimens to bring

*If the responsibility of the critical care nurse includes such follow-up care.

SEIZURES

A seizure can be basically described as a sudden, excessive, disorderly discharge of cerebral neurons that produces an intermittent derangement of the nervous system. For a variety of reasons certain neve cells may fire or discharge an excessive amount of sudden impulses, resulting in electrical disturbances in the brain and instigating seizure occurrence. This abnormal discharge activity commonly results in disturbances of sensation, loss of consciousness or psychic function, motor disturbances, convulsive movements, or varied combinations of symptoms.

A seizure indicates that the nervous system has been affected by disease disturbance. Most authorities propose that an isolated seizure is a symptom of an underlying pathological condition, and they suggest that the term *epilepsy* be restricted to describing recurrent or repeated seizure occurrence. Subdivisions of epilepsy include *primary* (recurrent seizures of unknown cause) and *secondary* (recurrent seizures of known cause).

Seizures may be caused by a variety of pathological conditions including brain tumors, trauma, clots; meningitis and encephalitis; electrolyte disorders; alcohol and drug overdose/withdrawal; metabolic disorders; uremia; overhydration; toxic substances; and cerebral anoxia. Seizures are also a major potential complication of various neurosurgical procedures. In the majority of seizure disorders the cause of the recurrent seizure activity is unknown; this type is termed *idiopathic epilepsy.*

Seizures have been classified in various ways according to site, EEG correlates, symptomatology, therapy responses, and so on. Some common types of seizures that nurses frequently encounter include generalized seizures such as grand mal and petit mal; minor motor seizures such as akinetic and myoclonic; and focal seizures such as psychomotor, jacksonian, focal somatic sensory, and focal visual. *Status epilepticus* denotes a series of seizures occurring without complete recovery between attacks or a continuing seizure attack usually lasting longer than 30 minutes. See Table 41-1 for common seizure types and clinical signs/presentation.

The treatment of seizures is aimed at determining and removing the cause if possible; effective anticonvulsant drug control (either short-term or long-term, depending on necessity); prevention of precipitating factors; and promotion and regulation of physical and mental hygiene. A complete workup will be done on most patients to determine if there is an underlying pathological cause that can be corrected or controlled. In some cases the cause of the seizure symptomatology may be surgically removed, such as with a brain tumor or clot. Other pathological conditions causing seizures may be controlled by medical management and treatment, such as metabolic or electrolyte disturbances and renal dysfunctions.

ASSESSMENT

1. Specific description of any previous seizure, including
   a. Time of first occurrence
   b. Frequency of seizures; any increase in seizure activity
   c. Onset, duration, progression, type, locality, length of seizure
   d. Any aura, incontinence, eye/head deviation, tongue biting, mouth frothing, chewing-sucking movements, eye rolling, pupillary status
   e. Respiratory status and skin color
   f. Postictal status; any injury incurred
   g. Patient amnesic or aware of seizure, events before and after
   h. If patient has been receiving anticonvulsant drugs, whether schedule has been adhered to
   i. Presence of any precipitating factors such as fever, emotional/physical stress
   j. Whether seizures were associated with any other symptoms such as headaches, nausea/vomiting
   k. If multiple seizures, any variation in activity or similarity of episodes
2. Onset, duration, and progression of any other neurological symptoms; if present, whether there is any association between symptom appearance and seizure occurrence
3. Previous head trauma or injury; specific description and details
4. Previous toxin ingestion or exposure such as metals, carbon monoxide

5. Previous infectious process such as meningitis, encephalitis
6. Previous drug/alcohol abuse or withdrawal
7. Presence of congenital anomaly, delayed growth and development milestones, birth injury
8. Previous metabolic, electrolyte, or renal disturbances; any anoxic episodes
9. Medications taken for neurological problem such as anticonvulsants, steroids
10. Previous neurological treatment or neurosurgical procedure
11. Presence of any medical problems; medications/treatments prescribed and followed
12. Presence and degree of any physical/emotional stress
13. Nutritional habits and dietary regimen
14. Patient's perceptions and reactions to diagnosis, treatment modalities; level of anxiety related to hospitalization
15. Level of patient/family's knowledge of seizure disorder, treatments, medication regimens, precipitating factors, and so on if seizures are not new occurrence
16. Presence of any alterations in body image; fears of permanent disability or deficit; altered role in family, normal occupation/performance of ADL; restrictions caused by disorder; ''stigma'' reactions
17. Baseline parameters status
    a. Neurological
    b. Seizure history
    c. Respiratory
    d. Metabolic

TABLE 41-1. Types of seizures: common clinical signs and presentation

GENERALIZED
Grand mal (tonic clonic)
Frequently preceded by aura, loss of consciousness
 Tonic phase: jaw snapped shut; frequently tongue biting; respiratory muscles caught in tonic spasm—cyanosis of skin and mucous membranes; pupils dilatated and unreactive; frequently incontinence; usual length is 10 to 15 seconds
 Clonic phase: generalized trembling progressing to violent muscle contractions of entire body; eye rolling; tachycardia; excessive salivation; facial grimacing; profuse diaphoresis; respirations jerky; usual length from 1 to 2 minutes
 Postictal: loss of consciousness persists from minutes to hours; pupils begin to react; muscles relax and breathing becomes quiet and regular; patient awakens, usually startled and confused, and then falls asleep
 Patient may remember aura but not seizure occurrence; may have headache, muscle stiffness, and fatigue following seizure

Petit mal (absence attacks)
Consists of sudden, brief episode of interruption of consciousness in which patient seems to be daydreaming, staring and is motionless and stops in middle of conversation
 May have brief period of eyelid fluttering, clonus of facial muscles/fingers
 Automatisms—lip smacking and chewing—are common
 Postural tone may be decreased or increased but usually patient does not fall
 Patient may or may not be aware of attacks

MINOR MOTOR
Akinetic
Momentary lapse of consciousness; loss of postural tone

Myoclonic
Sudden onset of brief muscle contractions/jerks

FOCAL (from lesion in certain area of cerebral cortex)
Psychomotor (commonly from temporal lobe involvement)
Aura: frequently hallucination or perceptual illusion
Behaves in confused manner and is amnesic of this
Hallucinations: usually visual and auditory; infrequently olfactory
Illusions/distortion of perceptions
Psycognitive states: increased reality/familiarity (déjà vu) or unfamiliarity/strangeness
Automatisms: lip smacking, sucking/chewing movements or repetition of inappropriate acts
May proceed to tonic spasms

Jacksonian (commonly from lesion of frontal lobe)
Tonic contraction of fingers/face/foot on one side, which may spread to involve entire same side and progress to clonic movements
Eye and head turning/deviation usually to side opposite irritative focus (looking at convulsing side)
May have sensory signs
May progress to grand mal

Somatic sensory (commonly from lesion of parietal lobe)
Numbness and tingling initially of lips, fingers, and toes; then spreads

Visual (frequently from lesion of occipital lobe)
Visual sensations of darkness/spots
Visual hallucinations

e. Renal
f. Fluid/electrolyte
g. Cardiovascular
h. Nutritional
i. Emotional
j. Vital signs
k. Weight
l. Handedness (right or left)
m. Growth and developmental level
n. Associated congenital anomalies

18. Diagnostic test results, including
   a. EEG
   b. CT scan
   c. Cerebral angiography
   d. Brain scan
   e. Skull radiographs
   f. Lumbar puncture
   g. Psychological testing
   h. NMR scan

19. Results of
   a. Serum electrolyte levels
   b. Serum Ca^{++} and phosphorus levels, BUN levels
   c. Anticonvulsant drug levels
   d. Amino acid screen
   e. Alcohol/drug levels
   f. Toxin screens
   g. Urine specific gravity, osmolality, analysis, culture, electrolytes
   h. Serum osmolality
   i. Hgb and Hct, platelet count, WBC count and differential

j. Clotting profile
k. Arterial blood gas levels
l. Chest radiograph
m. ECG

GOALS

1. Optimal neurological functioning
2. Optimal seizure control and safety maintenance
3. Optimal independence in ADL within safety restrictions/limitations
4. Adequate alveolar ventilation
5. Serum electrolyte levels within normal limits
6. Acid-base balance within normal limits
7. Fluid balance within normal range
8. Hgb, Hct, and platelet levels stable within normal limits
9. Anticonvulsant drug levels within therapeutic range
10. Reduction in patient/family's anxiety with provision of information, demonstrations, support
11. Before discharge patient/family is able to
    a. Describe medication, activity, and dietary regimens
    b. Describe safety measures, necessary restrictions, safety techniques
    c. Describe methods to maintain seizure threshold
    d. Describe appropriate interventions if seizure occurs at home
    e. Describe signs and symptoms requiring medical attention
    f. State necessary information regarding follow-up care

POTENTIAL PROBLEMS	EXPECTED OUTCOMES	NURSING ACTIVITIES
■ Recurrence of seizure	■ Seizure control Absence of complications	■ Assess seizure history of patient on admission (see Assessment, item 1, for specifics); establish baseline neurological status and vital signs If patient commonly has aura before seizure, instruct patient to call nurse immediately if aura occurs; stress importance of patient notifying nurse, and ensure that call light is within patient's reach Close observation and supervision Seizure precautions (especially if potential grand mal); may include Padded tongue blade and airway at bedside Bed height at lowest level Padded siderails up at all times when patient is alone Call light within easy reach Suction and O_2 equipment readily available Emergency medications and respiratory assistance equipment readily available Plastic eating utensils and dishes; no straws No smoking by patient when unsupervised Instruct patient to call nurse immediately if "focal" seizure occurs; stress importance of notifying and reasons why Administer anticonvulsants as ordered Monitor effects and side effects Monitor serum anticonvulsant levels; other tests ordered for evaluation of therapeutic dosage levels

POTENTIAL PROBLEMS	EXPECTED OUTCOMES	NURSING ACTIVITIES
		Prevention of precipitating factors including
		Hypoxia: monitor respiratory rate, quality and pattern; adequacy of alveolar ventilation and perfusion; for any signs of hypoventilation or other abnormalities
		Hyperventilation: encourage patient to breathe slowly and deeply; reassure and support
		Hypoglycemia: assess patient's food preferences and assist in selection of well-balanced meals; monitor for signs/symptoms of hypoglycemia including decreased serum glucose levels, restlessness, weakness, faintness
		Overhydration: monitor and accurately record intake and output; monitor for any signs/symptoms of fluid imbalance
		Electrolyte disorders: monitor serum electrolytes including Ca^{++}; phosphorus, BUN levels for any abnormalities
		Hyperthermia: protect patient from possible sources of infection; monitor temperature for any elevation q4 hr and prn; maintain sterile technique as warranted; institute and maintain hypothermia blanket as ordered
		Metabolic disorder: monitor amino acid screen for any abnormalities; monitor for signs/symptoms of disturbances
		Extreme fatigue: provide rest periods between activity; encourage good night's sleep
		Emotional stress: try to minimize stressful situations; consistently reassure and support
		Notify physician immediately if any precipitating factors occur or potential is present
		Administer medications and treatments as ordered
		Monitor effects and side effects
		Monitor for resolution or progression of factor
		If seizure occurs, stay with patient and call for help (see Problems, Patient self-injury during seizure, and Respiratory distress during seizure, for specific problems occurring with seizures)
		Monitor
		Seizure activity for onset, progression, type, focus, and duration
		Pupil size, equality, and reactivity
		For eye/head deviation; gaze preference
		For chewing/sucking movements, eye rolling, mouth frothing
		For presence of aura or incontinence
		Notify physician of seizure and specific description
		Administer medications as ordered; monitor effects and side effects
		Accurately record specific description of seizure and medications administered; effects on seizure activity
		Monitor postictal status q15 min or as ordered, including
		LOC
		Vital signs
		Neurological status
		Patient's awareness or amnesia of seizure occurrence; events before and after
		Presence of headache, muscle soreness, or stiffness
■ Patient self-injury during seizure	■ Absence or control of injury Absence of complications	■ Stay with patient
		If jaws are not clenched, insert tongue blade to prevent possible tongue biting
		If patient is wearing dentures, remove if possible, if jaws are not clenched
		Protect patient's head by placing pillow, other soft object, or hands under head
		Loosen any tight or restrictive clothing
		Do not attempt to restrain patient, as this may result in limb fractures
		Move dangerous objects, sharp furniture away from patient

POTENTIAL PROBLEMS	EXPECTED OUTCOMES	NURSING ACTIVITIES
		When seizure ceases, remain with patient; inform patient about what has happened; reassure and support Monitor for any signs of injury such as cuts, bruises; notify physician if any occurred and administer therapy as ordered
■ Respiratory distress during seizure	■ Patent airway Normal respiratory rate and pattern Adequate alveolar ventilation	■ Maintain patent airway Turn and position patient on side to prevent aspiration Position head to maintain airway Insert airway if needed Suction secretions as needed Administer O₂ prn Monitor respiratory status Period of apnea Color of skin and mucous membranes Respiratory rate, pattern, and quality Vital signs If respiratory distress continues, call for emergency equipment and notify physician Assist with emergency measures to maintain patent airway and adequate alveolar ventilation Administer medications and treatments as ordered; monitor effects and side effects If unresolved, see Problem, Status epilepticus: respiratory insufficiency, for specific activities
■ Patient/family's anxiety related to potential or actual seizure occurrence	■ Patient/family verbalizes fears	■ Ongoing assessment of level of anxiety Encourage verbalization of fears, anxieties, and questions Collaborate with physician in providing realistic information and reassurance appropriate to level of understanding Explain, if present, relationship between seizures and underlying pathology Explain routines, precautions, and medication regimens; reaffirm that medication control of seizures requires time to determine adequate regimen Explain reasons for frequent monitoring of neurological status and vital signs Explain and prepare for treatments, tests, therapeutic measures Provide continuing time, support, and explanations Reassure that patient does not have to become upset about "losing control"
■ Status epilepticus Status epilepticus is a medical emergency and must be controlled to prevent potential cerebral anoxia, damage, and ischemia EEG during status epilepticus usually demonstrates extreme discharging by neurons of reticular activating system and cerebral cortex	■ Absence of complications Resolution or control of status epilepticus	■ Monitor initially same activities as in Problems, Recurrence of seizure; Patient self-injury during seizure; and Respiratory distress during seizure Notify physician immediately of recurrent seizures without full recovery or of prolonged single seizure Have emergency equipment and medications readily available Intubation equipment and mechanical ventilator will usually be needed because of further respiratory depression from medications administered Medications commonly administered IV include diazepam (Valium), phenytoin (Dilantin), phenobarbital, and paraldehyde Monitor vital signs, respiratory and neurological status, seizure activity q5 min or as ordered Monitor ECG recording for any abnormalities Assist physician with administration of emergency medications; monitor for effectiveness of seizure control and side effects including Phenytoin (Dilantin): monitor for hypotension, cardiovascular collapse, arrhythmias Diazepam (Valium): monitor for respiratory depression, hypotension, cardiac arrest Phenobarbital: monitor for respiratory depression, cumulative effect, prolonged coma, delayed action

POTENTIAL PROBLEMS	EXPECTED OUTCOMES	NURSING ACTIVITIES
		Continue monitoring neurological status and vital signs q1 hr or as ordered; monitor for any signs of seizure activity and notify physician immediately if recurs Monitor 　Anticonvulsant drug levels for therapeutic range maintenance 　Serum electrolytes including Ca^{++}, glucose, phosphorus for any abnormalities Control precipitating factors in seizure occurrence whenever possible including hypoxia, hyperventilation, hyperthermia
■ Status epilepticus: respiratory insufficiency related to 　Medication administration 　CNS pathology	■ Patent airway 　Normal respiratory rate and quality 　Adequate alveolar ventilation and perfusion 　Arterial blood gas values within patient's normal limits	■ Ongoing assessments of respiratory status q1-2 hr and prn; monitor for any abnormality/decline 　Respiratory rate, quality, and pattern 　Patency of upper airway and patient's ability to handle secretions 　Skin color, nail beds, peripheral pulses, and skin warmth 　Breath sounds bilaterally for quality of aeration, signs of obstruction (rales, rhonchi) 　Presence/strength of gag, cough, and swallow reflexes 　Arterial blood gas values 　Chest radiograph results 　For signs/symptoms of thrombophlebitis, pulmonary emboli, pulmonary edema Monitor neurological status frequently, particularly LOC, seizure activity, focal deficits Maintain patent airway by 　Turning and positioning to prevent obstruction or aspiration of secretions q2 hr and prn 　Artificial airway if needed 　Suctioning prn 　Chest physiotherapy/pulmonary toilet q2 hr if not contraindicated 　Adequate oxygenation and humidification as ordered Apply antithromboembolic stockings or Ace bandages as ordered; reapply every shift and prn; monitor for constriction/looseness, condition of skin Notify physician immediately of any decline in respiratory status, neurological status, or seizure control 　Assist with emergency measures to maintain patent airway and adequate ventilation 　See Standard 6, *Mechanical ventilation* 　Administer medications and treatments as ordered; monitor effects and side effects When seizure control is achieved and respiratory effects of medications are eliminated, monitor 　For improvement in LOC 　Respiratory status, adequacy of ventilation and perfusion
■ Status epilepticus: fluid and electrolyte imbalance	■ Fluid and electrolyte balance within normal limits	■ Monitor and accurately record intake and output, urine specific gravity, and osmolality as ordered Monitor for signs of dehydration or overhydration such as 　Poor skin turgor 　Dry mucous membranes 　Peripheral edema 　Change in LOC Monitor for 　Abnormal vital signs, Hgb/Hct values 　Abnormal serum electrolyte values, particularly glucose, Ca^{++}, and phosphorus levels (disorders may potentiate or prolong status occurrence) 　Insensible fluid losses including respiratory, diaphoresis, secretions 　Weight alterations 　Acute renal failure if status is result of anoxia; see Standard 52, *Acute renal failure*

POTENTIAL PROBLEMS	EXPECTED OUTCOMES	NURSING ACTIVITIES
		Monitor temperature q2 hr and prn for any elevation, because fever can potentiate seizures If elevation occurs, notify physician immediately Monitor and culture possible sources Institute and maintain hypothermia blanket as ordered Administer IV fluids and medications as ordered; if patient is receiving steroids, monitor urine glucose and acetone levels four times a day Notify physician immediately of any fluid imbalance or electrolyte abnormality Administer medications and treatments as ordered Monitor for resolution or progression of abnormality and notify physician of results
■ Status epilepticus: family's fears and anxiety related to patient in status epilepticus	■ Family verbalizes fears	■ Encourage verbalization of fears and concerns Collaborate with physician in providing realistic information and reassurance to family Explain Pathology and relationship to present status Reasons for medications and treatments; importance of controlling seizures Reasons patient's LOC/respiratory functioning is depressed Reasons for certain therapies and mechanical assistance at this time Anticipated course and prognosis Ongoing support of family; provide time, explanations, and reassurance
■ Continued potential or presence of seizure activity Patient/family's anxiety and fears related to Lack of knowledge Threat of seizure Altered life-style and restrictions	■ Patient/family verbalizes concerns* Patient/family demonstrates or verbalizes required knowledge and skills	■ Ongoing assessments of patient/family's level of anxiety Encourage verbalization of fears, concerns, anger related to potential continuation of seizure disorder Collaborate with physician in providing realistic information and reassurance based on expected prognosis Encourage patient/family's verbalization and questions regarding restrictions imposed by threat of potential seizure and effects on life-style; restrictions of prior activities or job responsibilities may include revocation of driver's license, constant supervision for certain activities, restriction on using electrical equipment at home/job Assess patient/family's reactions to restrictions and alterations; effects on usual life-style and responsibilities, role, and ADL Explore ways patient/family can cope with condition; capabilities to maximize potential for independent functioning within confines of necessary safety precautions Stress importance of and support and encourage patient/family in accepting seizure disorder reality and adopting positive attitude toward coping; monitor reactions, acceptance level, degree of control expected Reaffirm that although there is no cure for seizure disorder, a nearly ''normal'' life can continue by adherence to control measures and regimens Reinforce that potential for maximal control of seizure disorder and independence is promoted by acquisition of knowledge and skills; implementation and adherence to prescribed regimens, precaution; and confidence in dealing and coping with disorder Assess and monitor level of understanding of seizure disorder and needed information and skills Promote collaboration of patient/family and health team in achieving maximal control, independence, positive attitude, and as ''normal'' a life-style as possible Provide facts and realistic information to correct fallacies and misconceptions including dealing with ''stigma'' misperceptions

*If responsibility of critical care nurse includes this stage of care.

POTENTIAL PROBLEMS	EXPECTED OUTCOMES	NURSING ACTIVITIES
		Obtain orders for appropriate referrals such as social services, vocational training, National Epilepsy Foundation
		Stress variability of achieving seizure control with each individual
		Reassure and support patient/family
		Instruct, demonstrate, and evaluate patient/family's knowledge acquisition and performance in needed information/skills such as
		What seizure is; reason for occurrence if related to pathology
		Knowledge of seizure disorder
		Patient's own specific seizure manifestations; if aura is present, what to do if occurs
		Identification of precipitating factors and importance of controlling; includes excessive fatigue, poor nutrition, electrolyte imbalance, fever, emotional stress/strain
		Verbalization of means to control precipitating factors; appropriate actions to take if precipitating factors occur
		Provision of realistic facts and information, correction of fallacies and myths
		Necessary interventions if seizure occurs including airway maintenance, safety measures, monitoring and recording of specific activity
		Restrictions necessitated by seizure disorder including dietary, activity, alcohol intake, seizure precautions
		Importance of good oral hygiene
		Explain and reinforce to patient/family
		Necessary reasons for restrictions
		Threats/dangers of noncompliance
		Necessity of wearing medical alert identification
		Explore with patient/family alternate means/measures to maintain as ''normal'' a life-style as possible
		Promote maintenance of usual routines, activities, and relationships within limits of restrictions
		Means to deal with other family members, friends, social occasions
		Avoidance of overdependence and overprotection within family and outside family
■ Insufficient knowledge to comply with discharge regimen*	■ Patient/family demonstrates or verbalizes understanding of discharge regimen	■ Assess patient/family's level of understanding of neurological problem and therapy received
		Explain relationship between patient's neurological status and therapies prescribed
		Importance of and identification of means to maintain seizure threshold
		Specific disorder; restrictions necessary
		Reasons and importance of compliance to control seizure; prevention of precipitating factors
		Instruction of patient/family regarding required information and skills so that before discharge patient/family is able to
	Patient/family accurately describes medication, activity, and dietary regimens	Describe medication regimen
		Name and purpose
		Route, dosage, frequency, times
		Side effects
		Special precautions necessary including drugs, foods, alcohol contraindicated or quantity regulated; factors potentiating/decreasing effects or side effects; physical restrictions; safety measures
		Measures to promote effectiveness and minimize side effects
		Blood tests required; reasons and importance
		Scheduling of regimen to enhance compliance
		Times when medication addition/adjustment may be needed
		If patient is to adjust own regimen: when, how often, effectiveness

*If the responsibility of the critical care nurse includes such follow-up care.

POTENTIAL PROBLEMS	EXPECTED OUTCOMES	NURSING ACTIVITIES
		Describe dietary regimen
		Describe activity regimen, exercise program
		Describe and demonstrate any special therapeutic measures prescribed
	Patient/family describes means to achieve maximal independence in ADL, promote safety, and prevent complications	Describe restrictions, precautions, control of precipitating factors
		Describe proper interventions, observations/recording if seizure occurs
	Patient/family describes signs/symptoms requiring medical attention	Describe signs/symptoms of seizure disorder/control requiring medical attention
	Patient/family describes follow-up care regimen	Describe plan for follow-up care including purpose of appointment, when and where to go, who to see, what to expect, specimens to bring, charting or recording to bring

MENINGITIS/ENCEPHALITIS

Meningitis and encephalitis are common infectious processes of the CNS that may occur as primary diseases or secondary complications of neurosurgery, certain diagnostic procedures, trauma, ear/sinus infections, systemic infections, and so on. A large variety of bacteria and viruses can be responsible for the primary infections of the CNS.

MENINGITIS

Bacterial meningitis (leptomeningitis) is mainly an infection of the pia mater and arachnoidea and the fluid in the space they enclose. The subarachnoid space is continuous around the brain, spinal cord, and optic nerves. An infective organism that enters the subarachnoid space can extend and spread throughout the entire space and reach the ventricles of the brain. The effect of bacteria in the subarachnoid space is to cause an inflammatory response in the pia mater, arachnoidea, CSF, and ventricles. Blood vessels become engorged and may rupture or thrombose. The subarachnoid exudate is increased by the irritative effects of the bacteria, which promote vascular congestion and increased capillary permeability. The exudate accumulation may spread into cranial and spinal nerves or obstruct the normal flow route of the CSF, resulting in the development of hydrocephalus. Secondary encephalitis and neuronal degeneration may occur if the brain surface adjacent to the meninges becomes involved.

Bacteria enter the CNS through two major routes: hematogenous spread (emboli of bacteria or infected thrombi) or spread from cranial structures (ears, sinuses, cranial trauma). A small proportion of infections are iatrogenic, having been introduced by lumbar puncture needles. Factors that promote the bloodstream invasion by the bacteria to reach the meninges are not fully known but may include a preceding viral infection of the upper respiratory tract or lung. The disruption of the normal blood-brain barrier may contribute to the entry of bacteria into the subarachnoid space. Skull fractures and dural tears from head trauma may promote meningitis development. Occasionally, a brain abscess may infect the meninges if it ruptures into the subarachnoid space or ventricles.

The early clinical manifestations of bacterial meningitis are signs of meningeal irritation. These include fever, severe headache, nuchal rigidity, generalized convulsions, and altered LOC. Two signs that are frequently present are the Kernig (inability to completely extend the legs) and Brudzinski signs (forward flexion of head causing hip and knee flexion response). Focal signs of cerebral damage and cranial nerve abnormalities may occur with meningitis because of the various bacteria involved and the diversity of stages. A diagnosis of bacterial meningitis is suspected from the clinical signs and confirmed by examination of the CSF. Features of the CSF usually include pleocytosis, elevated spinal fluid pressure, elevated protein levels, and decreased glucose content. Cultures and gram stains of the CSF usually identify the infective organism, and treatment of meningitis consists of antibiotic administration. Some cases may be caused by a mixture/combination of organisms, and administration of multiple antibiotic drugs may be required. The resolution of the inflammatory process and degree of recovery depend largely on the stage at which the infection is controlled, with potential complete recovery greatest in the early stages. If the meningitis continues, the chances for further progression of inflammation and resulting cerebral damage increase.

Aseptic meningitis is a term used to describe a clinical symptomatology entity that can be produced by a variety of infective agents, the majority of which are viral. Common symptoms are fever, headache, and other signs of meningeal irritation. Photophobia and pain with ocular movements commonly occur, whereas the Kernig and Brudzinski signs are usually absent. The common viruses involved are enteroviruses, paramyxovirus, and herpes simplex virus (type 2). Many times the specific virus cannot be isolated. Data that may assist in the differential diagnosis of viral meningitis include immunizations, past infectious diseases, family outbreaks, animal bites, recent travel, epidemic outbreaks, and seasonal/geographical distributions. Viral meningitis is usually benign and lasts 1 to 2 weeks with complete recovery afterward.

ENCEPHALITIS

Encephalitis is a syndrome characterized by an acute febrile state; signs of meningeal involvement; and signs/symptoms of dysfunction of the cerebrum, brainstem, or cerebellum. It is usually caused by a viral infection. The onset of neurological signs is commonly preceded by a prodromal illness of a few days' duration with fever, headache, malaise, aches, sore throat, nausea, and vomiting resulting from organism invasion. Within the CNS viral infections cause inflammation that can involve the cortex, white matter, meninges, and so on. The resultant pathological condition may include destruction of neurons, demyelination, diffuse edema, hemorrhage, and necrosis.

The main types of encephalitis are caused by arboviruses, acute herpes simplex (type 1), animal bites, infectious mononucleosis, and aftermaths of prophylactic inoculations. A variety of pathological effects can result from the viral infection because of the variations in susceptibility of nervous tissue areas and the diversity of viral organisms. Invasion of the CNS usually occurs by the hematogenous (blood) and peripheral nerve (retrograde axoplasmic spread) pathways. The neurological dysfunctions may include weakness, aphasia, ataxia, involuntary movements, myoclonic jerks, ocular palsies, nystagmus, facial weakness, and coma.

Patients with herpes simplex, in addition to signs of acute encephalitis, usually manifest signs that include bizarre behavior, olfactory/gustatory hallucinations, temporal lobe seizures, and anosmia. The frontal and temporal lobes are commonly affected.

Herpes zoster (shingles) produces an acute inflammatory reaction in spinal or cranial sensory ganglia, the posterior grey matter of the spinal cord, and adjacent meninges. Clinical signs include rash, pain, palsies, itching, and burning or tingling sensations.

The prognosis of viral encephalitis is widely variable and frequently unpredictable during its early clinical course. The death and morbidity rates vary greatly, and residual neurological deficits occur in about one fifth of patients after the infection. In some cases the virus may not be isolated, whereas in others an antiviral agent may not be available or effective for an identified virus.

ASSESSMENT

1. Onset, progression, frequency, duration, and specific description of neurological symptoms, including
   a. Headache
   b. Nuchal rigidity
   c. Fever
   d. Alterations in LOC
   e. Changes in behavior or personality
   f. Alterations in motor/sensory abilities
   g. Alteration in communication abilities
   h. Ocular palsies, photophobia, nystagmus, ptosis
   i. Cranial nerve palsies
   j. Alterations in visual abilities, hearing acuity
   k. Kernig/Brudzinski signs
   l. Seizures

   m. Medullary symptoms: vomiting, tachyardia, respiratory difficulties, arrhythmias
2. Recent preceding viral illness or infectious disease; past history of disease, rash
3. Recent inoculations, immunizations, exposure to infection/viral disease
4. Recent travel, insect bites, contact with animals, bites
5. Family outbreaks, geographical outbreaks, work/social contacts; exposure to or presence of infection/disease
6. Previous head trauma or injury: incident; clinical course, treatment, sequelae; any skull fracture, dural tear, CSF leak
7. Previous/present ear, sinus infections or recurrent infections
8. Previous ingestion of poisons, drug overdose, toxin exposure
9. Previous neurological treatment or neurosurgical procedure; medications taken, effects on clinical course/status
10. Presence of any medical problems and the therapy employed; risk factors that have been identified as contributing to the development of meningitis/encephalitis include debilitation, alcoholism, diabetes mellitus, long-term radiation therapy, immunosuppressive therapy, immunoglobulin deficiency, reticuloendothelial system malignancies, and renal failure
11. Patient's perceptions and reaction to diagnosis, disease progression, treatment modalities
12. Presence of any alterations in body image; fears of permanent disability or deficit; altered role in family, normal occupation, performance of ADL
13. Baseline parameters status
    a. Neurological
    b. Respiratory/pulmonary
    c. Cardiovascular
    d. Metabolic
    e. Renal
    f. Hydration/nutritional
    g. Fluid/electrolyte
    h. Infection
    i. Vital signs
    j. Temperature
    k. Weight
    l. Handedness (right or left)
14. Diagnostic test results, including
    a. Lumbar puncture
    b. Skull radiographs
    c. EEG
    d. CT scan
    e. Cerebral angiography
    f. Brain scan
    g. Brain biopsy
    h. NMR scan

15. Results of
    a. CSF determinations
    b. Serum electrolyte levels
    c. Hgb, Hct, platelet count, WBC count/differential
    d. Sedimentation rate
    e. Urinalysis, culture, osmolality, gravity
    f. Amino acid screen
    g. Antibody detection
    h. Clotting profile
    i. Arterial blood gas levels
    j. Anticonvulsant drug levels
    k. Toxin screens
    l. C and S including blood, sputum, urine, nasal secretions, wound/sinus drainage, CSF
    m. ECG
    n. Chest radiograph

GOALS

1. Maximal neurological functioning
2. Optimal independence in ADL

3. Resolution of acute infectious process; infection free systemically, in CSF, and in specific body systems
4. Afebrile, normal blood values
5. Adequate alveolar ventilation and perfusion
6. Serum electrolyte levels and fluid balance within normal limits
7. Hgb and Hct stable within normal limits
8. Acid-base balance within normal limits
9. Seizures controlled
10. Reduction in patient/family's anxiety with provision of information, demonstrations, support
11. Before discharge patient/family is able to
    a. Describe medication, activity, exercise, and dietary regimens
    b. Demonstrate safety measures and techniques; proper use of any equipment, therapeutic devices prescribed
    c. Describe signs and symptoms requiring medical attention
    d. State necessary information regarding follow-up care

POTENTIAL PROBLEMS	EXPECTED OUTCOMES	NURSING ACTIVITIES
■ Increased ICP Decline in neurological status related to acute infection—swelling, inflammatory process/hydrocephalus	■ Absence or resolution of signs of increased ICP Maximal neurological functioning	■ Avoid precipitating factors in increased ICP such as hypoxia, hypercapnia, fever, Valsalva maneuver Assist patient with positioning and turning Instruct patient not to hold breath, blow nose vigorously, or reach for bedside articles Monitor for any signs and symptoms that could initiate development of factors such as hypoventilation, constipation Notify physician of potential/presence of any factors Establish baseline and ongoing assessments of neurological status and vital signs q1 hr; monitor especially LOC Headache locality/severity Motor, sensory, and communication systems functioning/deficits Cranial nerve functioning Visual abilities and functioning; field cuts, photophobia, nystagmus, ptosis Auditory system functioning Nausea/vomiting Kernig/Brudzinski signs Ataxia, myoclonic jerks Reflex status Pupil size, equality; direct and consensual light responses; extraocular movements Behavior and personality alterations (in infants, decreased feeding, high-pitched cry) Posturing spontaneously or stimuli response, decerebrate/decorticate Administer medications, treatments, and IV fluids as ordered; monitor effects and side effects Maintain head gatch/bed rest as ordered Accurately record intake and output; monitor for any imbalance Monitor serum electrolytes, CBC, arterial blood gas values for any abnormalities Notify physician of any change in neurological status, vital signs, or abnormal fluid balance/lab values Initiate and maintain hypothermia as ordered

POTENTIAL PROBLEMS	EXPECTED OUTCOMES	NURSING ACTIVITIES
		If patient has ICP line inserted, monitor values and waveforms Maintain patency/sterility of system Monitor effects of other treatments or therapies on ICP including coughing, turning, chest physiotherapy, suctioning Space therapies if possible to minimize increases in ICP Monitor neurological status correlated with ICP values and notify physician If ordered, assist physician with drainage of CSF fluid amount to maintain ICP at specific level determined; record fluid amount drained/time; monitor effects on ICP value, correlation between neurological status and CSF drainage Hyperventilate patient as ordered by physician for specific ICP level increase Administer medications/treatments as ordered; monitor effects and side effects on status and ICP; frequently osmotic diuretics are ordered prn or as ongoing therapy Monitor ventricular drainage system or other external drain if patient has one inserted Prevent compression, kinking, pulling, or tension on tubing by proper positioning; if necessary, restrain patient's hands to prevent pulling or tension of tubing (first try explanations of reasons/purposes for drain) Maintain patency/sterility of system Maintain at specific level ordered by physician Measure and record as ordered pressure, amount and quality of drainage Check dressing q1 hr; monitor for leakage around needle or catheter site, swelling/edema If patient is on ICP monitoring, record pressures and drain fluid amount specified by physician's order to maintain pressure values Monitor neurological status correlated with fluid pressure/quantity Administer antibiotics as ordered Send CSF specimens as ordered and monitor results Monitor serum electrolytes as Na$^+$ values may decrease from loss of CSF by drainage; notify physician of results and replace fluids as ordered (frequently CSF fluid is ordered replaced milliliter for milliliter) Monitor for signs of epidural hematoma (potential complication of drain); see Standard 33, *Head trauma*, Problem, Epidural hematoma Notify physician immediately of any change in neurological status; fluid pressure, amount/quality varying from norm specified or expected; nonpatency of system or abnormal lab values If ordered, clamp tubing as specified by physician, maintaining precise time schedule and recording time, pressure, fluid drainage amount/quality; notify physician of any change in neurological status or signs of increased ICP; unclamp drain as per physician's standing or stat order After removal of ventricular drain by physician, monitor neurological status and vital signs frequently; drain site for bleeding, oozing, drainage/edema; for signs of increased ICP; have emergency ventriculostomy set/medications available *See* STANDARD 32 *Increased intracranial pressure* If internalized shunting procedure is necessary, see Standard 38, *Internalized shunting procedures*
▪ Infection progression	▪ Resolution of infection Maximal neurological functioning	▪ Ongoing assessments of neurological status and vital signs q1 hr and prn (see Problem, Increased ICP: avoid precipitating factors in increased ICP, and establish baseline and ongoing assessments of neurological status and vital signs [nursing activities])

POTENTIAL PROBLEMS	EXPECTED OUTCOMES	NURSING ACTIVITIES

		Maintain strict isolation procedures/precautions as warranted by specific pathogen
		    Post procedure on door of patient's room
		    Restrict visitors
		    Instruct/supervise visitors in correct procedures
		Maintain strict sterile procedure where required
		Monitor
		    Temperature q1-2 hr and prn
		    Skin integument frequently for presence/extent of rash, petechiae, open skin areas
		    Culture results and drug sensitivities of CSF, urine, sputum, blood specimens
		    For signs of toxemia/septicemia, including decreased LOC, hypotension
		    WBC counts for elevations (may be falsely elevated if patient is receiving steroids)
		    Drug levels
		    IV sites frequently for any signs of redness, tenderness/phlebitis
		Administer
		    Antipyretic medications as ordered
		    Cooling blankets as ordered; institute measures to prevent complications of hypothermia
		    Tepid sponges as ordered
		    Antibiotic medications at precise time ordered
		    Frequent skin and oral hygiene
		Assist physician with treatments/diagnostic procedures
		    Anticipate frequent lumbar punctures; explain necessity to patient/family
		    Monitor pressure levels of CSF with each lumbar puncture; correlation with neurological status
		    Monitor CSF specimen results including cultures, protein, glucose, cell counts for resolution/progression of infectious process
		Notify physician immediately of any change in neurological status, abnormal lab values, signs of complications, or appearance of new culture pathogen/drug resistance

■ Depressed/altered LOC, restlessness, agitation/irritability	■ Safe patient environment
	Absence of injury complications
		■ Close observation; siderails up at all times when patient is alone
		Maintain as quiet an environment as possible, reducing excessive external stimuli to minimum
		    Provide rest periods between activities
		    Dark room
		Establish baseline and continue ongoing assessments of LOC and reflex status; monitor
		    For signs of restlessness/agitation; note degree, frequency, extent
		    Components of consciousness—arousal and content
		    Presence/quality of reflexes including corneal, gag, cough, swallow; if reflexes are absent or decreased, institute preventive measures such as protecting cornea with eyedrops, lid taping/closure; suctioning equipment at bedside
		Monitor for other possible causes of restlessness such as bladder/abdominal distention, headache, hypoxia
		    Notify physician if any of these occurs
		    Administer analgesics, comfort measures, treatments as ordered
		Reorient patient frequently to time, place, person; reasons for hospitalization; pathology and relationship to symptoms
		    Have family bring familiar objects, pictures to aid in orientation
		    Continually reassure patient
		    Support family; reaffirm frequently relationship between LOC and pathology
		Apply restraints as per physician's order if this is only alternative to protect patient from injury
		    Explain to patient/family reasons for restraints

POTENTIAL PROBLEMS	EXPECTED OUTCOMES	NURSING ACTIVITIES
		Reassure family of restraint necessity; relationship between patient's behavior and pathology
		Check restraints frequently for proper placement; monitor effectiveness, skin integrity, and circulation
		Reapply q4 hr and prn
		Frequently reevaluate need for continuing restraints
		Notify physician immediately of sudden appearance or increase in prior restlessness, irritability, agitation, headache, or change in reflex status/neurological functioning
■ Presence of neurological symptoms/deficit	■ Absence of complications Maximal comfort	■ On admission establish and implement care plan based on individual needs and specific symptoms/deficit present
		Institute measures to promote maximal comfort and prevent complications; common symptoms/deficits include
		Headache: maintain quiet, dark environment; ice bag, analgesics as ordered
		Nuchal rigidity: reposition frequently, supporting with pillows for comfort; massage and apply lotion
		Vomiting: keep NPO; turn slowly and carefully; prn medication as ordered
		Motor deficit: ROM, turn and reposition properly to promote optimal muscular tone, functioning, maintenance, and circulation; sheepskin, air mattress, handrools, splints, etc.
		Sensory deficit: hypoalgesia/hyperalgesia—monitor skin integument frequently; administer frequent skin care to keep skin clean and dry; change linen frequently; if rash is present, keep skin free of friction, apply lubricants to decrease itching, medications prn; if aches/pains, neuritis are present, administer medications as ordered
		Communication deficits: evaluate and implement effective alternate means of communication such as magic slate, word board, pictures if feasible
		Visual deficits: if field cut, approach patient and place objects within visual field; if diplopia is present, use alternating eye patch; if photophobia is present, keep room dark and provide glasses for patient
		Auditory deficits: approach patient from greater hearing side; establish alternate means of communication
		Cranial nerve dysfunctions/decreased reflexes: measures to prevent complications such as corneal abrasions, aspiration
		Reflex status alteration: hyporeflexia/hyperreflexia—protect from injury
		Altered LOC: prevention and control of hazards of immobility; promotion of safety maintenance
		Ongoing assessments and evaluations of patient status/effectiveness of interventions; readjust plan based on status alterations
		Collaborate with physician regarding anticipated prognosis for extent of recovery from deficit (if known); provide realistic information and reassurance
		Assist as needed with ADL
		Provide frequent rest periods between activities
		Provide explanations to patient/family for specific interventions; even if full recovery from deficit is expected, complication prevention must be instituted from admission to promote optimal recovery and functioning
■ Seizures	■ Absence or control of seizures	■ Prevention of precipitating factors in seizure occurrence including fever, hypoxia, H_2O intoxication, electrolyte disturbances
		Notify physician of potential/presence of any factors
		Seizure precautions for any patient with suspected meningitis/encephalitis
		Padded siderails up at all times when patient is alone

POTENTIAL PROBLEMS	EXPECTED OUTCOMES	NURSING ACTIVITIES
		Bed height at lowest level Padded tongue blade and airway at bedside Suction and O_2 equipment readily available Emergency medications/equipment readily available Close supervision and observation Administer anticonvulsant medications as ordered; monitor effects, side effects, serum anticonvulsant levels If seizure occurs, monitor and record seizure activity; notify physician; see Standard 41, *Seizures*

■ Fluid and electrolyte imbalance	■ Fluid and electrolyte balance within normal limits	■ Monitor and accurately record intake and output, urine specific gravity as ordered
		Monitor for signs of dehydration or overhydration such as
		  Poor skin turgor
		  Dry mucous membranes
		  Peripheral edema
		  Excessive thirst
		  Change in LOC
		Monitor for
		  Abnormal vital signs, Hgb/Hct values
		  Abnormal serum electrolyte values
		  Weight alterations
		  Temperature elevations
		  Insensible fluid losses including respiratory, diaphoresis, secretions
		  Presence/degree of nausea or vomiting, emesis quality; monitor effectiveness of medications ordered
		  Presence/quality of gag, cough, and swallow reflexes; if depressed, keep patient NPO and notify physician
		Administer IV fluids, NG feedings as ordered
		Administer medications as ordered; monitor effects and side effects if patient is receiving steroids, monitor urine glucose and acetone levels four times a day
		If po is allowed and tolerated, assist patient with diet selection within chewing capabilities, food likes, and nutritionally well-balanced meals
		Notify physician of any fluid imbalance or electrolyte abnormality

■ Respiratory insufficiency related to
  CNS dysfunction
  Pneumonia
  Atelectasis
  Pulmonary emboli
	■ Patent airway
	Adequate alveolar ventilation and perfusion
	Normal respiratory rate and quality
	Arterial blood gas levels within patient's normal limits
		■ Ongoing assessment of respiratory status q2 hr and prn; monitor for any abnormality/decline
		  Respiratory rate, quality, and pattern
		  Patency of upper airway and patient's ability to handle secretions
		  Skin color, nail beds, peripheral pulses, and skin warmth
		  Presence/strength of gag, cough, and swallow reflexes
		  Breath sounds bilaterally for quality of aeration; signs of obstruction (rales, rhonchi)
		  Arterial blood gas values
		  Chest radiograph results
		  Signs/symptoms of thrombophlebitis, pulmonary emboli, pulmonary edema
		Maintain patent airway by
		  Turning and positioning to prevent obstruction or aspiration of secretions q2 hr and prn
		  Deep breathing and coughing q1 hr and prn
		  Suctioning prn
		  Adequate oxygenation and humidification as ordered
		  Chest physiotherapy/pulmonary toilet if warranted and not contraindicated by physician's order
		Apply antithromboembolic stockings or Ace bandages as ordered; reapply every shift and prn; monitor for constriction/looseness, condition of skin
		Instruct and supervise patient in performing leg exercises, ROM exercises

POTENTIAL PROBLEMS	EXPECTED OUTCOMES	NURSING ACTIVITIES
		Increase activity level/progression when allowed
		Notify physician immediately of any change in respiratory/neuro-logical status or signs of complication potential/occurrence
		If problem occurs, assist with emergency measures to maintain patent airway and adequate ventilation
		Administer medications and treatments as ordered; monitor effects and side effects
		Explain procedures and reasons for equipment/respiratory assistance to patient/family; reassure and support
		Establish alternate means of communication as needed
		See STANDARD 6 *Mechanical ventilation*
		If emboli occur, see Standard 31, *Embolic phenomena*
■ Bradycardia	■ Absence or resolution of bradycardia	■ Monitor and record pulse rate and quality with neurological assessments; assess for any correlation between pulse rate/quality and neurological status
		Monitor serum electrolyte values; especially note hypokalemia/hyperkalemia
		Notify physician immediately if patient develops pulse rate less than 60
		Administer medications and treatments as ordered; monitor effects and side effects
■ Bowel/bladder dysfunction	■ Urinary output adequate No bladder distention Normal bowel elimination	■ Assess patient's prior elimination patterns: usual voiding pattern, bowel pattern, problems, dietary/medication measures for elimination
		Monitor
		Accurate recording of intake and output
		For any signs/symptoms of urinary retention, overflow voiding, or residual; notify physician if any of these occurs and administer medications/treatments as ordered; monitor effects and side effects
		Bowel movements (amount, consistency, frequency)
		Bowel sounds, presence/quality; signs/symptoms of paralytic ileus
		Establish and implement individualized bowel regimen based on patient's needs, pattern, previous measures, preferences/effectiveness
		Involve patient in planning
		Obtain orders for administration of stool softeners, cathartics, enemas as needed
		Assess effectiveness of regimen; readjust as needed
		When patient is allowed po, assist in food selection to promote bowel elimination

■ GI bleeding related to
  CNS factors
  Stress
  Steroid administration
	■ Absence or resolution of GI bleeding	■ Monitor vital signs q2-4 hr, Hgb and Hct; stools for Hematest three times a week; Hematest of aspirate, emesis, and urine for any abnormalities

		Monitor for signs of GI bleeding including abdominal distention, tenderness; hypotension, sudden tachycardia
		Obtain order for antacid administration as soon as patient is able to take po
		Notify physician of any abnormalities; if problem occurs, see Standard 49, *Upper gastrointestinal bleeding*
■ Patient/family's anxiety, fears, anger related to Limited understanding of disease, diagnostic tests/procedures	■ Patient/family's behavior indicates decreased anxiety with provision of information Patient/family verbalizes fears, angers, concerns	■ Ongoing assessments of level of anxiety
		Encourage patient/family's verbalization of questions, fears, concerns
		Collaborate with physician in providing realistic information and reassurance appropriate to level of understanding
		Explain relationship between pathology and clinical symptoms, status, course

POTENTIAL PROBLEMS	EXPECTED OUTCOMES	NURSING ACTIVITIES
Presence of neurological deficit or potential continuation, development, worsening Possible alterations in life-style		Explain anticipated treatments, therapeutic measures, and clinical course prognosis (if known) If prognosis is unknown, explain reasons why course is obscure Provide continuing time, support, and explanations to patient/family; maintain calm, accepting attitude of their reactions to lengthy disease course, undetermined prognosis Support family's acceptance of patient's behavior alterations by reinforcing pathological causes Explain and prepare patient/family for all diagnostic tests/procedures Involve patient/family in decision making, care planning, participation, and evaluation As status improves, promote patient progression from dependent to independent functioning Slowly and progressively increase activity as status and tolerance levels allow Stress any positive gains or improvements in status Encourage participation in diversional interests/activities Encourage verbalization of family/patient's perceptions of possible alterations in life-style; means to promote as ''normal'' a life-style as possible Obtain appropriate referrals such as religious personnel, counseling services Evaluate for reduction in level of anxiety
■ Continued presence of neurological deficit Patient/family's fears, anxiety, anger related to deficit and possible alterations in life-style	■ Maximal neurological functioning* Maximal independence in ADL (within capabilities) Patient/family verbalizes concerns	■ Assess patient's specific neurological deficit Collaborate with physician regarding prognosis, possible degree of recovery Implement individualized plan of care based on patient's needs and deficits Assist as needed in ADL Monitor potential for independent functioning and obtain equipment to maximize function and promote safety Obtain orders for appropriate referrals such as physiotherapy, speech or occupational therapy; social services Encourage verbalization of patient/family's fears, anxieties, and other reactions—level and degree Answer questions realistically Encourage their participation in care planning, implementation, evaluation, and decision making Realistically reassure and support Reinforce any gains or independence patient achieves Plan, instruct, demonstrate, supervise, and evaluate patient/family's verbalization/performance of needed information/skills for maximal independent functioning such as Measures to prevent complication Assistance necessary—type, amount, degree Proper use of therapeutic devices/equipment Monitor level of achievement toward maximizing potentials and independence; means to promote as ''normal'' a life-style as possible
■ Insufficient knowledge to comply with discharge regimen†	■ Patient/family demonstrates or verbalizes understanding of discharge regimen	■ Assess patient/family's level of understanding of neurological problem and therapy received Explain relationship between patient's neurological status and therapies prescribed If pathological condition is related to factors such as head trauma, toxin exposure/drug overdose, explain relationship and importance of patient/family controlling identified individual factors to prevent disease recurrence

*If responsibility of critical care nurse includes this stage of care.
†If responsibility of the critical care nurse includes such follow-up care.

POTENTIAL PROBLEMS	EXPECTED OUTCOMES	NURSING ACTIVITIES
		Instruction of patient/family regarding required information/skills so that before discharge patient/family regarding required information/skills so that before discharge patient/family is able to

	Patient/family accurately describes medication, activity, and dietary regimens	Describe medication regimen
		  Name and purpose
		  Route, dosage, frequency, times
		  Side effects
		  Special precautions necessary including drugs, foods, beverages contraindicated; factors potentiating/decreasing effects/side effects; physical restrictions; safety measures
		Describe activity regimen, exercise program
		Describe dietary regimen
		Describe and demonstrate any special therapeutic measures prescribed

	Patient/family describes means to achieve maximal independence in ADL, promote safety, and prevent complications	Describe and demonstrate proper use of equipment or therapeutic devices
		  Reasons for using
		  Time, method, and duration of use
		  Precautions/safeguards
		  Necessary maintenance (type, frequency)
		  Measures to promote optimal functioning, upkeep/duration

	Patient/family describes signs/symptoms requiring medical attention	Describe signs/symptoms of neurological status requiring medical care
	Patient/family describes follow-up care regimen	Describe plan for follow-up care including purpose of appointment, when and where to go, who to see, what to expect

MYASTHENIA GRAVIS (INCLUDING THYMECTOMY)

Myasthenia gravis is a neuromuscular weakness that primarily involves the skeletal muscles. Its onset may be precipitous or insidious, and it usually progresses slowly after the initial onset of symptoms. Clinical features of myasthenia gravis include exhaustion of muscle strength and paresis in response to repetitive or constant activity/stimulation.

Myasthenia gravis is a disease that is unpredictable in course and prognosis and is frequently characterized by periods of remissions and exacerbations. The voluntary muscles commonly involved in the weakness are as follows:

1. Extraocular—ocular palsies, drooping eyelid, and intermittent diplopia (most commonly affected)
2. Facial expression—altered mobility/expression
3. Mastication—difficulty chewing
4. Swallowing—dysphagia
5. Speech—dysarthria
6. Jaw
7. Neck

If muscular involvement of the limbs and trunk is present, the proximal muscles are affected more than the distal. Myasthenia gravis may range from mild ocular involvement to severe muscular involvement including the diaphragm, intercostal muscles, and abdominal and external sphincters. The common clinical manifestations of myasthenia gravis are usually a fluctuating ocular, facial, and bulbar palsy. Muscular weakness of the bulbar cranial nerves may produce dysphagia, dysarthria, dyspnea, facial drooping, and jaw weakness. Two life-threatening symptoms of myasthenia gravis are dyspnea and dysphagia, which frequently occur in crisis situations and increase the potential threat of aspiration and acute respiratory failure.

The cause of myasthenia gravis is unknown, but the defect is generally presumed to occur at the neuromuscular junction. Multiple theories of etiology have been advanced, but to date no single one has been firmly established. Proposed theories of etiology include the following:

1. Decreased formation/release of acetylcholine
2. Increased formation/release of acetylcholinesterase
3. Muscle fiber defect of motor end plate
4. Marked reduction of acetylcholine receptors in the muscle end plates

5. Autoimmune response—most popular theory to date because of
   a. Frequent association of thymic hyperplasia and thymoma in myasthenia gravis patients
   b. A high percentage of myasthenia gravis patients have thyrotoxicosis and other autoimmune disorders (e.g., rheumatoid arthritis, lupus erythematosis, and polymyositis)
   c. Frequent presence of antiacetylcholine antibody (against acetylcholine receptor) in postsynaptic membrane—immunological reaction to destroy the receptor

The diagnosis of myasthenia gravis is suspected based on the clinical history of signs/symptoms. Myasthenia gravis is highly suspected in patients with a clinical history of muscle weakness developing after repetitive or consistent activity and partial strength restoration after rest. Some muscle weakness may be present at all times but is usually made worse by activity. Confirmation of myasthenia gravis is attempted by use of a variety of diagnostic tests including electromyogram, edrophonium chloride (Tensilon) test, neostigmine test, curare test, and immunological studies.

The medical management of myasthenia gravis includes medication therapy control using anticholinesterases and corticosteroids. Surgical intervention, or thymectomy, is performed in some cases of myasthenia gravis. Recently, plasma-electrophoresis has been used as a therapeutic modality for patients with myasthenia gravis.

Thymectomy consists of removal of the thymus gland, either by a sternal-split or transcervical approach. Thymectomy is usually performed if a thymoma is present, which occurs in approximately one fifth of myasthenia gravis patients. Hyperplasia of the thymic gland is found in a large number of remaining patients. Thymectomy is also frequently performed in cases of bulbar myasthenia gravis that are poorly responsive to medical therapy/management. Postoperatively, remission or an improvement in clinical status may not occur immediately. Following thymectomy the patient may still require medical management with medication regimens, but the amount of medications may be decreased and/or effectiveness of medication control may be enhanced. The surgery is considered successful if less ongoing medication is required and less supplementary medication is needed during periods of stress such as infection and menses. Surgical results are best in patients who have had myasthenia gravis for a shorter time (1 to 2 years).

ASSESSMENT

1. Onset, duration, progression, and description of neuromuscular symptoms, especially
   a. Ocular—impaired extraocular movements/palsies, drooping eyelid/ptosis, diplopia, weakened eyelid closure
   b. Facial weakness/alterations in facial expression
   c. Difficulty chewing; choking/nasal regurgitations
   d. Difficulty swallowing (dysphagia)
   e. Alterations in speech abilities, voice tone, quality; nasal and dysarthric speech
   f. Jaw weakness
   g. Neck weakness
   h. Muscle weakness of trunk or limbs, motor functioning
   i. External sphincter weakness—bowel/bladder
   j. Dyspnea
2. Time-related presence, extent, severity of neurological symptoms
   a. Association with activity—type, extent, length
   b. Association with time of day, fatigue
   c. Fluctuations in symptomatology
3. Presence of any precipitating factors in symptomatology occurrence such as infection, emotional upset, stress
4. Previous clinical course of disease (if prior diagnosis)
   a. Disease management/control
   b. Adequacy of treatment/control
   c. Any "crisis" occurrences—when, type, duration, treatment, any precipitating factors; postcrisis status
   d. Any previous intubation/tracheostomy—when, type, duration, status after procedure
5. Medications taken for neurological problem including anticholinesterases, corticosteroids
   a. Dosage, frequency, schedule
   b. Length of time medication taken
   c. Effects and side effects
   d. Alterations in regimen—if on demand schedule, what factors necessitate medication adjustment; effectiveness of demand scheduling
6. Previous neurological treatment or neurosurgical procedure
7. Presence and degree of any physical/emotional stress
8. Nutritional habits and dietary regimen
9. Activity regimen and sleep habits
10. Presence of any alterations in body image; fears of permanent disability or deficit; altered role in family, normal occupation/performance of ADL; restrictions caused by myasthenia gravis
11. Level of anxiety related to hospitalization; if patient was previously hospitalized, reactions, coping mechanisms, etc.
12. Level of patient/family's knowledge of myasthenia gravis—medications, precipitating factors, treatments, potential complications, etc.
13. Presence of any medical problems; medications/treatments prescribed and followed
14. Baseline parameters status
    a. Neurological
    b. Myasthenia gravis disease history, course
    c. Respiratory
    d. Cardiac; circulatory and vascular
    e. Metabolic
    f. Nutritional
    g. Hydration
    h. Emotional
    i. Weight
    j. Vital capacity
    k. Inspiratory force/forced expiratory volume
15. Diagnostic test results, including
    a. Electromyography
    b. Edrophonium chloride (Tensilon), neostigmine/curare tests
    c. Tomography
    d. Thyroid function tests
    e. Pulmonary function tests
    f. Immunological studies
16. Results of
    a. Serum electrolyte levels
    b. Hgb and Hct, platelet count
    c. Serum Ca^{++} level
    d. Arterial blood gas levels
    e. Urine output, specific gravity, osmolality, urinalysis
    f. Chest radiograph
    g. ECG
    h. Clotting profile
    i. Cultures if indicated—sputum, urine
    j. Parathyroid hormone levels if indicated

GOALS

1. Optimal neurological functioning
2. Optimal independence in ADL within safety restrictions, tolerance levels/limitations
3. Adequate alveolar ventilation and perfusion
4. Adequate cardiac output
5. Acid-base balance within normal limits
6. Fluid balance within normal range
7. Serum electrolyte levels within normal limits
8. Hgb, Hct, and platelet levels stable and within normal limits
9. Medication regimen control at optimal management level of disease
10. Infection free

11. If thymectomy is performed, well-healed incision, without signs of infection
12. Reduction in patient/family's anxiety with provision of information, explanations, demonstrations, support
13. Before discharge patient/family is able to describe
    a. Medication regimen
    b. Activity regimen
    c. Dietary regimen
    d. Safety measures, necessary restrictions/precautions, safety techniques
    e. Methods to promote optimal disease control/management
    f. Appropriate interventions if complication, crisis occurs at home
    g. Demonstrate any special therapeutic measures prescribed
    h. Signs and symptoms requiring medical attention
    i. Necessary information regarding follow-up care

POTENTIAL PROBLEMS	EXPECTED OUTCOMES	NURSING ACTIVITIES
Medical management		

■ Muscle weakness Increased muscle weakness with fatigue	■ Optimal muscle strength	■ Establish baseline and continue ongoing assessments as ordered and prn of
		Neurological status: monitor
		  Muscle strength of all groups with repetitive activity; establish specific testing modalities and record on flow sheet q2-4 hr and prn
		  Ability to raise/lower eyelids completely; location/degree of ptosis if present
		  Facial (cranial nerve VII) muscular strength bilaterally
		  Extraocular movements; presence, degree, and location of ocular palsies, nystagmus, diplopia
		  Presence/quality of chewing and swallowing abilities; foods manageable, ability to handle secretions; signs and symptoms of dysphagia
		  Presence/quality of gag and cough reflexes
		  Speech quality and ability; degree of dysarthria if present
		  Cranial nerve functioning
		Respiratory status: monitor for any abnormality/decline
		  Vital signs including respiratory rate, quality/pattern
		  Bilateral breath sounds for signs of obstruction/decreased aeration (rales, rhonchi, etc.)
		  Strength of diaphragmatic and intercostal muscles
		  Presence/quality of cough, gag, and swallow reflexes
		  Presence, amount/quality of secretions and saliva and ability to handle secretions
		  For any signs/symptoms of dysphagia, dyspnea (at rest or exertional), dysarthria
		  Vital capacity measurement q2-4 hr and prn using same spirometer, proper position, and recording technique; inflate cuff if tracheostomy tube is in place; if jaw weakness caused by facial muscle involvement is present, prevent air leak while using mouthpiece; position in sitting position for measurement if feasible
		Maintain flow sheet recording of vital capacities
		  Serial arterial blood gas levels
		  Chest radiograph results
		Close observation—place patient close to nurse's station
		Avoid precipitating factors in myasthenic crisis such as emotional upset, physical stress, infection, constipation
		Develop care plan based on individual patient needs/status—involve patient/family in planning
		  Assess adjustments in ADL regimen that patient has made and adapt to hospital setting
		  Ongoing evaluations of effectiveness of interventions
		  If muscle weakness/paralysis is present, prevent complications by measures including turning, positioning, ROM exercises, coughing, deep breathing

POTENTIAL PROBLEMS	EXPECTED OUTCOMES	NURSING ACTIVITIES
		Always anticipate and be prepared for sudden worsening in neurological/respiratory status especially aspiration/respiratory failure
		Suctioning equipment, O_2, airway at bedside
		Emergency ventilation, intubation, mechanical ventilator, medications readily available
		Administer anticholinesterases, corticosteroids, and other medications as ordered at precise time specified
		Prevent or minimize GI side effects by giving with small amount of food or after meals (if mealtime is flexible); medications such as atropine may also be ordered to minimize side effects
		Monitor and record on flow sheet muscle strength status related to medication
		Effects and side effects
		Duration
		Peak action effect (usually optimal 1 to 2 hours after medication)
		Minimal action effect (usually 3 to 4 hours after medication)
		Assess patient's evaluation of strength and motor ability related to medication regimen
		Monitor vital capacity measurements and relate to medication time effects
		If patient experiences worsening of symptoms, notify physician immediately as this may be sign of overdosage or ineffective medication regimen
		Plan activities around peak effect levels of medications, arranging for meal consumption 45 minutes to 1 hour after medication; plan treatments and major activities early in the day
		Prevent overexertion or greater than usual fatigue
		Provide uninterrupted rest periods between activities
		Space activities to correlate with peak effects of medication
		Provide calm, quiet, supportive environment
		Minimize physical stress by maintaining activity within tolerance limitation levels
		Minimize emotional stress; See Problem, Patient/family's anxiety
		Notify physician immediately of any decline in neurological or respiratory status; any decrease in vital capacity below minimal acceptable level individually specified

■ Bulbar cranial nerve (V, VII, IX, X, XII) dysfunction/weakness
Facial (VII)
Trigeminal (V)
  Decreased facial muscle strength/facial expression
  Difficulty chewing
  Inability to close eyelid
  Decreased/absent corneal reflex
Glossopharyngeal (IX)
Vagus (X)
Hypoglossal (XII)
  Decreased or absent swallow, gag, and cough reflexes
  Dysphagia/aspiration
  Dyspnea/respiratory failure
  Dysarthria
	■ Absence or resolution of dysfunction
	Absence of complications
		■ Assess chewing ability; assist patient in diet selection within chewing capabilities; instruct patient to chew on unaffected side; stay with patient during mealtime

		Assess facial droop; provide excellent oral hygiene, frequent removal of secretions
		If ability to completely close eyelids is decreased/absent, obtain order for protective drops, maintain eyelid closure, and monitor for any signs of corneal irritation/abrasion
		Encourage verbalization of patient's fears, concerns, and feelings, since decreased facial strength may inhibit normal facial expression conveyance
		Assess level of patient's anxiety/altered body image related to facial nerve weakness, droop/drooling from mouth
		Monitor presence/strength of swallow, gag, and cough reflexes; ability to handle secretions and po
		Schedule meals when strength is maximum; stay with patient at mealtimes; monitor swallowing effectiveness
		Assess for any choking/nasal regurgitation
		Avoid fluids that enhance saliva production such as milk
		Assess foods that patient tolerates best and assist with diet selection
		If any impairment in swallow, gag, or cough reflexes is present, keep patient NPO and notify physician; suction secretions prn; prevent aspiration by positioning, maintaining patent airway; and closely monitor respiratory status/functioning; see Problem, Respiratory insufficiency

POTENTIAL PROBLEMS	EXPECTED OUTCOMES	NURSING ACTIVITIES
		If dysarthria is a problem, establish alternate means of communication; evaluate effectiveness and readjust prn; see Problem, Altered communication ability
■ Respiratory insufficiency/ arrest related to weakness or paralysis of respiratory muscles caused by Pneumonia Atelectasis Aspiration Dyspnea/dysphagia	■ Patent airway Adequate alveolar ventilation Normal respiratory rate and quality Clear breath sounds Arterial blood gas levels within patient's normal limits	■ Ongoing assessment of neurological and respiratory status q2 hr and prn; see Problem, Muscle weakness Assess and monitor for any abnormality/decline Patency of upper airway and patient's ability to handle secretions Skin color, nail beds, peripheral pulses, and skin warmth For signs/symptoms of thrombophlebitis, pulmonary emboli, pulmonary edema, dyspnea/dysphagia Maintain patent airway by turning and positioning to prevent obstruction or aspiration of secretions q2 hr and prn; deep breathing, coughing, and suctioning prn; chest physiotherapy; adequate oxygenation and humidification as ordered Apply antithromboembolic stockings or Ace bandages as ordered; reapply every shift and prn; monitor for constriction/looseness, condition of skin Instruct and supervise patient in leg exercises, ROM exercises Prevent precipitating factors in respiratory failure; patient is especially vulnerable if either of the following is present Severe dysphagia—ongoing monitoring of swallow reflex, keep patient NPO if necessary to prevent potential aspiration Respiratory tract infection—protect from potential infection sources; vigorous suctioning, chest physiotherapy to maintain patent airway; position for proper ventilation/lung expansion Notify physician immediately of any change in respiratory/neurological status or development of potential complication If respiratory problem occurs, assist with emergency measures and procedures to maintain patent airway and ventilation; see Standard 6, *Mechanical ventilation* When neurological/respiratory status improves, begin to slowly wean patient for short periods of time Wean periods at peak medication time effectiveness Stay with patient; give frequent reassurance and support Reaffirm that ventilator assistance will not be withdrawn until patient can breathe independently Assess patient/family's reactions to respiratory problem occurrence/ experience Progressively increase activity; monitor effects on neurological/respiratory status and notify physician of results; limit activity to tolerance level
■ Crisis—worsening of muscle weakness with potential respiratory failure/aspiration Myasthenic—sudden worsening in status; drug regimen ineffective for unknown reasons Cholinergic—worsening in status from overdose of myasthenic drugs	■ Resolution of crisis Absence of complications	■ Prevent precipitating factors in crisis such as infection, emotional crisis, constipation Careful observations and frequent assessments of neurological/respiratory status Administer medications and treatments as ordered at precise time; monitor Effects by flow sheet record; correlate medication time specifics on graded muscle strength; cranial nerve functioning; swallow, gag, and cough reflexes Presence/degree of dysphagia, dyspnea, dysarthria Respiratory status Vital capacities Side effects Monitor for signs/symptoms of crisis Common manifestations of both myasthenic and cholinergic (present in either type) Increased skeletal muscular weakness Anxiety, restlessness Dyspnea, dysphagia, dysarthria

POTENTIAL PROBLEMS	EXPECTED OUTCOMES	NURSING ACTIVITIES

		Differentiating signs of crisis type
		  Myasthenic: ocular palsies, ptosis, diplopia development/worsening
		  Cholinergic: fasciculations/fine twitching; abdominal cramps and diarrhea, nausea/vomiting; increased secretions including salivation, sweating, lacrimation, bronchial secretions; blurred vision; most ominous sign is increased weakness 1 hour after medication instead of expected improvement
		Notify physician immediately of any signs/symptoms of crisis
		  Assist with emergency measures and procedures to maintain patent airway and ventilation
		  Assist physician with tests (usually edrophonium chloride [Tensilon] test done to differentiate crisis type) and have emergency medications available (i.e., atropine, prostigmine) in anticipation of worsened crisis; if patient is in myasthenic crisis, status usually improves with edrophonium chloride (Tensilon) injection (positive test result), whereas if patient is in cholinergic crisis, status worsens
		Assessments/interventions common to either crisis
		  Maintain patent airway and adequate ventilation, mechanical ventilator as ordered; see Problem, Respiratory insufficiency/arrest
		  Monitor respiratory status and vital capacity q1 hr
		  Monitor neurological status q1 hr including muscle strength grading; cranial nerve functioning; swallow, cough, and gag reflexes; presence/extent of dysphagia, dyspnea, dysarthria
		  Accurate recording of intake and output
		  Administer IV fluids/NG feedings as ordered
		  Bed rest; prevent complications of immobility by turning and positioning, ROM exercises, skin care, etc.
		  Establish alternate means of communication if ability is altered
		    Explain all tests, procedures, measures to patient/family and necessary reasons
		    Explain reasons why medications are being withheld, anticipated restarting time, and course
		  Provide rest periods between activity to prevent fatigue or overexertion
		  When medication regimen is restarted, continue to closely monitor effects/side effects, neurological/respiratory status
		  When activity progression is allowed, slowly increase to tolerance levels
		  As status improves, promote patient assuming independence in appropriate activities
		    Slowly wean from dependent position/role
		    Encourage self-participation in care, decisions, medication evaluation; assist as needed in ADL
		  Continually provide explanations, support, reassurance, understanding to patient/family throughout crisis period/duration
		    Try to assign individual nurse to consistently care for patient
		    Encourage verbalization/other means of communication of patient/family's fears, angers, concerns, depression; help them to cope with crisis threat and promote positive attitude that status will improve
		  Maintain calm, consistent, and supportive attitude/environment
		Specific interventions in myasthenic crisis
		  Maintain endotracheal/tracheostomy tube in proper position, patency, and with proper care techniques; mechanical ventilator as ordered
		  Chest physiotherapy and pulmonary toilet; vigorous regimen to maintain patent airway and adequate ventilation
		  Strict sterile technique maintained when necessary including suctioning, catheterization
		  See Problem, Respiratory insufficiency/arrest, and Standard 6, *Mechanical ventilation* for more specifics

POTENTIAL PROBLEMS	EXPECTED OUTCOMES	NURSING ACTIVITIES
		Specific interventions in cholinergic crisis 　Monitor for GI signs/symptoms—presence, degree/frequency 　Administer medications ordered; monitor effects/side effects and notify physician of results 　Frequent and scrupulous skin care to prevent complications of increased secretions from sweating, diarrhea, lacrimation, etc.; keep skin clean, dry, and intact; monitor all surfaces frequently for integument maintenance
■ Fluid and electrolyte imbalance	■ Fluid and electrolyte balance within normal limits	■ Monitor 　Vital signs, Hgb and Hct for any abnormality 　Serum electrolytes for any abnormality 　Weight determinations as ordered 　Accurate recording of intake and output; urine specific gravity as ordered 　Insensible fluid losses including respiratory, diaphoresis, secretions 　For presence, degree of nausea/vomiting; administer medications and notify physician if ineffectual 　For presence/degree of dysphagia, difficulty chewing, nasal regurgitation; keep NPO if severe dysphagia is present 　For signs of dehydration/overhydration such as poor skin turgor, peripheral edema, dry mucous membranes, excessive thirst, change in LOC Administer IV fluids, NG feedings as ordered Notify physician of any fluid/electrolyte abnormality; if ordered 　Monitor and record hourly intake and output 　Maintain intake at specific amount ordered 　Send specimens and monitor results
■ Altered communication ability related to 　Cranial nerve dysfunction 　Motor paralysis 　Endotracheal/tracheostomy tube insertion	■ Alternate means of communication established	■ Monitor communication abilities If ability is altered, establish alternate means of communication based on individual patient needs/status such as writing tablet, word or letter board, eye-blinking system Convey alternate means to other staff and family, assisting prn in effective use Anticipate patient's needs Establish means for patient to get nurse's attention quickly and easily Encourage staff/family to speak to patient even if he/she is unable to respond Evaluate effectiveness of alternate means of communication with patient/family 　Involve patient/family in planning care; reevaluate/readjust alternate means as necessary 　Try to find means that are least physically, mentally, and emotionally taxing to patient 　Accept frustrations patient frequently experiences from altered ability and resulting depression; try to minimize frustrations by anticipating needs, giving constant supervision, having same nurse provide care
■ Bowel/bladder dysfunction	■ Adequate urine output Absence of bladder distention Normal bowel elimination	■ Monitor Accurate recording of intake and output Patient's prior elimination pattern—usual voiding, bowel problems, dietary/medication measures For any signs/symptoms of urinary retention, overflow voiding, or residual; notify physician if problem occurs and administer medications, treatments as ordered; monitor effects and side effects; intermittent catheterization may be ordered Bowel movements (amount, consistency, frequency) Bowel sounds, presence/quality; signs/symptoms of paralytic ileus Establish and implement individualized bowel regimen based on patient's needs, pattern, prior measures Involve patient in planning bowel regimen program, time for elimination/treatments based on patient's preference and effectiveness

POTENTIAL PROBLEMS	EXPECTED OUTCOMES	NURSING ACTIVITIES
		Obtain physician's orders for stool softener, cathartics, enemas as needed
		When patient is allowed po, assist in food selection to promote bowel elimination
		Assess effectiveness of bowel regimen; reevaluate and readjust prn
■ GI bleeding related to CNS factors Stress Steroid administration	■ Absence or resolution of GI bleeding	■ Monitor vital signs, Hgb and Hct; stools for Hematest three times a week; Hematest of aspirate, emesis, and urine for any abnormality
		Monitor for signs of GI bleeding including abdominal tenderness, pain, distention; hypotension, sudden tachycardia
		Obtain order for antacid administration as soon as patient able to take po
		Notify physician of any abnormalities; if any abnormalities occur, see Standard 49, *Acute upper gastrointestinal bleeding*
■ Complications of cortico-steroid therapy	■ Absence or resolution of complications	■ Monitor for any complications of corticosteroid therapy, especially GI irritation
		Development or exacerbation of diabetes mellitus
		Increased susceptibility to infection
		Psychoses, behavioral changes
		Hypokalemia
		Hypertension
		Osteoporosis
		Acne
		Moon face
		Ongoing assessments and implementation of measures to prevent complications; instruction of patient/family in monitoring and preventing such as
		Control of GI irritation; see Problem, GI bleeding
		Prevent exposure to sources of infection
		Prevent potential osteoporosis by ROM exercises, encouraging activity within fatigue limitations when allowed; notify physician of any complaints of bone, radicular pain and monitor bone radiograph results
		Careful and frequent skin cleansing to decrease acne occurrence/potential
		Report immediately any mental, emotional/behavioral changes
		Monitor urine determinations of glucose and acetone, serum glucose levels, signs/symptoms of diabetes
		Monitor serum electrolytes for hypokalemia; BP q2 hr and prn for hypertension
		Notify physician of any abnormality
		Monitor neurological/respiratory status frequently; be aware of danger of exacerbation of weakness that may occur usually between 4 to 10 days of treatment initiation but must be monitored for from day 1
		Report immediately any signs/symptoms of exacerbation
		If exacerbation occurs, see Problem, Crisis (Medical management)
■ Infection	■ Absence or resolution of infection	■ Prevent precipitating factors such as urinary retention, pulmonary congestion/aspiration
		Maintain strict sterile technique for procedures such as catheterization; endotracheal/tracheostomy tube care management, suctioning; ventilator maintenance
		Monitor
		Temperature q4 hr and prn for any elevation
		IV sites frequently for any signs of redness, tenderness/phlebitis
		For potential infection sources including pulmonary, urinary, exposure to infection sources
		WBC count (may be falsely elevated if patient is receiving steroids)

POTENTIAL PROBLEMS	EXPECTED OUTCOMES	NURSING ACTIVITIES
		If temperature elevation or other sign of infection occurs, notify physician and culture possible infection sources Monitor sputum/urinary cultures, chest radiograph results Continue accurate recording of intake and output; monitor for dehydration/overhydration Institute measures to promote resolution of infection source if possible Administer medications/treatments as ordered; monitor effects
■ Patient/family's anxiety related to lack of understanding of diagnostic tests, treatments, disease process, therapeutic interventions	■ Patient/family's behavior indicates decreased anxiety with provision of information	■ Ongoing assessment of level of anxiety and knowledge base/understanding of patient/family Collaborate with physician in providing realistic information to patient/family Provide information relevant to level of understanding Explain all diagnostic tests, procedures, therapeutic interventions, regimens, and necessary reasons Explain relationship between symptoms and disease process Explain reasons for frequent neurological assessments, vital signs and vital capacity monitoring Encourage patient/family's verbalization of questions, fears, concerns Provide time and support Answer questions realistically Assess patient/family's comprehension and acceptance of information Explain and continually reinforce that optimal medication control and determination take time to achieve and require frequent reevaluations, readjustments, and periods of medication withdrawal to best control disease and potential crisis occurrence Explain relationship between medication regimen and status; peak and minimal effect times Explain relationship between fatigue/time of day and status If crisis occurs, explain reasons for procedures, treatments, tests Continually support, provide explanations, answer questions Reinforce that cause of crisis is often unknown, but that patient/family will be taught preventive measures to try to decrease potential for crisis and appropriate information/interventions for identification and management of crisis if it occurs See Problem, Patient/family's fear, anger, depression
■ Patient/family's fear, anger, depression related to disease Alteration in body image/life-style Dependency; threat of disease crisis Fear of home care management	■ Patient/family verbalizes fear, anger, depression* Patient/family verbalizes required care	■ Ongoing assessments of level of anxiety, knowledge base of disease/problems, and other reactions Collaborate with physician regarding disease prognosis/control in promoting patient/family's acceptance of disease and regarding necessity of patient/family's knowledge acquisition and implementation to promote optimal control and potential independent functioning Encourage verbalization of patient/family's fears and reactions Provide time and support; accept reactions and stage of emotions Reassure patient/family that reactions and behavior are "normal" in confrontation with disease Reassure patient/family that depression, frustration, anger, fear are natural reactions and occur frequently Assess patient/family's strengths/weaknesses in disease confrontation, potential for coping with acceptance, management of disease threat, and attitude Support patient/family with calm, reassuring, and accepting manner Assess patient/family's normal life-style, occupation, interests, living situation

*If responsibility of critical care nurse includes this stage of care.

POTENTIAL PROBLEMS	EXPECTED OUTCOMES	NURSING ACTIVITIES
		Implement plan of care and intervention based on individualized patient status, patient/family's needs and potentials
		Encourage patient/family's participation in care and decisions regarding short- and long-term goals
		Monitor patient/family's potential for achieving maximal independence in ADL
		Obtain orders for appropriate referrals such as physiotherapy and occupational therapy, social services
		Obtain appropriate equipment to promote maximal independence in ADL and safety maintenance
		Encourage patient's maximal independence in ADL within capabilities/limitations; readjust interventions as status progresses from dependent to independent functioning
		Reinforce any gains patient achieves
		Promote patient/family's acceptance of disease and realities
		Reaffirm that best control potential occurs with patient/family's knowledge of disease, problems, and appropriate management
		Reaffirm that reactions are normal experiences but that patient/family's acceptance of disease and positive attitude toward control/management may enhance maximal independence and as "normal" a life-style as feasible
■ Insufficient knowledge to comply with discharge regimen*	■ Patient/family verbalizes and demonstrates necessary information and skills to comply with discharge regimen	■ Assess patient/family's level of understanding of neurological problem and therapies received
		Explain relationship between patient's neurological status and therapies prescribed
		Assess alterations in usual life-style necessitated by individual patient's status, severity/control of disease
		Try to promote as normal a life style as possible by collaboration with patient/family and other health team members in planning regimens such as medications, acitvity
		Involve patient/family to maximal degree possible in planning, decision making, establishing regimen schedules
		Continually reassure and support patient/family that they will be provided with needed knowledge, skills, information to optimally cope with/manage disease and problems
		Collaborate with physician in providing realistic information and reassurance regarding control potential, prognosis, disease process
		Promote positive aspects of medication adjustments, demand schedule regimens
		Continually assess patient/family's potential for assuming responsibility in control/management of disease; promote strengths and abilities to cope and assume control
		Reaffirm that patient/family can best control disease by maximal knowledge acquisition/implementation
		Encourage patient/family's participation in assessing home situation, necessary alterations; decisions regarding home care and management
		Instruct and evaluate patient/family's acquisition/demonstration of necessary information and skills to comply with discharge regimen and promote maximal disease control
		Institute teaching program for patient/family, including
		Precipitating factors in crisis—stress, fatigue, infection, constipation
		Avoid infections and exposure, strenuous exercise
		Patient/family's identification of own factors and measures to prevent occurrence

*If responsibility of critical care nurse includes such follow-up care.

POTENTIAL PROBLEMS	EXPECTED OUTCOMES	NURSING ACTIVITIES
	Patient/family describes activity and dietary regimen	Importance of regular, well-balanced diet
		Planning of daily activities to provide rest periods; prevention of fatigue/overexertion
	Patient/family describes means to achieve maximal independence in ADL, promote safety, and prevent complications	Promotion of maximal independence within capabilities and frustration levels
		Proper use of equipment
		Assistance necessary (type, amount, degree)
		Safety measures
		Prevention of complications
		Importance of 8 hours of sleep or appropriate amount
		Emergency measures that should be implemented for prevention
		Medical alert identification
		Working telephone in home
		Establish ambulance service, police service, fastest local routes to hospital
		Telephone numbers of accessible means to hospital
		If appropriate, home availability/proper use of airway, suctioning equipment, resuscitative equipment and technique
		Signs/symptoms of myasthenic or cholinergic crisis—what to do
		Avoidance of all over-the-counter medications including cold preparations, aspirin; strong cathartics, enemas
	Patient/family describes medication regimen	Medication regimen
		Name and purpose
		Route, dosage, frequency, times
		Side effects and when to notify physician
		Special precautions necessary including drugs, foods, beverages contraindicated or quantity regulated; factors potentiating/decreasing effects/side effects
		If feasible, demand scheduling for medication use to promote optimal management; collaborate with physician in providing necessary information
		Instruct in peak effect times of medications; encourage patient/family planning of ADL at optimal effect times
		Appropriate resources including Myasthenia Gravis Foundation
		Importance of ongoing medical care and regular checkups; that any physician or health facility should be fully informed of disease history, medications
		Proper use of any equipment or therapeutic devices
		If respirator assistance is prescribed for home use, teach use, care/maintenance, potential problems/interventions, preventive measures
		Special therapeutic measures prescribed/maintained
		If tracheostomy tube is in place on discharge, teach proper care techniques/maintenance, prevention of complications, signs/symptoms of problems and measures to overcome, when and who to notify for medical intervention
		If vital capacity recordings are indicated, teach method, times, proper equipment use/maintenance, values necessitating notification of physician
		If indicated, teach muscle strength testing, grading, and recording
	Patient/family describes signs/symptoms requiring medical attention	Signs and symptoms of neurological status/medication control requiring medical attention
	Patient/family describes follow-up care regimen	Plan for follow-up care including purpose of appointment, when and where to go, who to see, what to expect, any data recording to bring

POTENTIAL PROBLEMS	EXPECTED OUTCOMES	NURSING ACTIVITIES

THYMECTOMY
Preoperative period

■ Respiratory distress, insufficiency, which may be related to
Pulmonary infection
Withholding anticholinesterase drugs in hours immediately preceding surgery
Thoracic and/or oropharyngeal muscle weakness
Excess tracheobronchial secretions

■ Respiratory function sufficient for adequate oxygenation and ventilation in order to achieve PaO_2 and $PaCO_2$ levels within patient's normal limits
Absence of pulmonary infection
Effective mobilization of secretions
Patent airway

■ Administer systematic, thorough pulmonary toilet, including chest physiotherapy, timed to coincide with peak activity of anticholinesterase medication
Administer anticholinesterases as ordered; time activities (e.g., eating, ambulation) to occur at peak activity of medication
Administer antibiotics and ultrasonic nebulization treatments as ordered
Administer steroid medication preoperatively if ordered
Administer long-acting anticholinesterase medication (time-span capsule) on night before surgery or a few hours preoperatively, as ordered
Administer atropine for control of secretion production
If respiratory insufficiency and production of secretions are marked, nurse or physician should accompany patient to operating room with manual breathing bag and portable suction system

■ Patient/family's anxiety, fears, regarding
Hospitalization
Disease process
Diagnostic procedures
Therapeutic regimen
Surgery
Dependence, altered life-style imposed by myasthenia gravis

■ Reduction in patient/family's anxiety with provision of information, explanations, and encouragement

■ Assess level of patient/family's anxiety regarding impending diagnostic procedures, surgery
Assess level of understanding of anticipated diagnostic procedures and surgery
Describe purpose of planned diagnostic procedures and what patient will experience
Prepare and support patient before and during procedures
Describe purpose of surgery and, in collaboration with physician, expected outcomes
Prepare patient for surgery and provide support and encouragement for patient/family as needed
Describe perioperative experiences, including
Preoperative
Chest physiotherapy
Coughing and deep breathing
Incentive spirometry
Shave
Light dinner, then NPO after midnight
Medication for sleep if needed
Morning bath/shower
Preoperative medications
Hospital gown
Care of valuables
Ride to operating room
Scrub suits, masks, and hats worn by operating room staff
Anesthesia
Postoperative
Waking up in recovery room/intensive care unit
Describe general environment (size of unit, room, etc.)
Nurse always nearby
Dull, continuous noises
Breathing tube may be temporarily in place to ease work of breathing
Incision with bandage
IV, arterial lines
Chest tubes, if anticipated
ECG monitoring, if anticipated
Medicine for discomfort, pain
Policy on family visits
As patient progresses
Tubes out
Deep breathing, coughing, and chest physiotherapy
Eating again
Getting stronger, ambulation
Assess reduction in level of patient/family's anxiety

POTENTIAL PROBLEMS	EXPECTED OUTCOMES	NURSING ACTIVITIES
	Patient/family demonstrates understanding of disease process, therapeutic regimen, and physical limitations imposed by disease	Ongoing assessment of patient/family's level of anxiety, specific fears, and concerns Encourage verbalization of fears and concerns; provide information, support as needed
	Patient achieves independence in normal ADL Patient accepts degree of dependence dictated by disease	Assess patient/family's normal life-style, level of activity Obtain orders for appropriate referrals such as social service, occupational therapy, physiotherapy, Myasthenia Gravis Foundation Encourage and provide for maximal independence in ADL within capabilities, limitations Promote patient/family's realistic acceptance of disease, recognizing therapy available and inherent physical limitations See Medical management

Postoperative period
■ Respiratory insufficiency related to
  Muscular weakness associated with disease process
  Phrenic nerve injury
	■ Respiratory function adequate for sufficient oxygenation and ventilation; Pao_2 and $Paco_2$ levels within patient's normal limits
	Diaphragmatic movements active and within normal limits
	Effective expectoration of secretions, patent airway
	Pulmonary function tests compatible with spontaneous breathing
	Patent chest tube drainage system
		■ Ongoing assessment of
		  Quality of respirations; note presence of respiratory distress
		  Respiratory muscle strength; observe diaphragmatic movement, excursion
		  Secretions
		    Volume
		    Nature of
		    Ability of patient to expectorate
		  Breath sounds
		  Results of pulmonary function tests, including inspiratory force, vital capacity
		  Arterial blood gas levels; deterioration indicates respiratory insufficiency and may herald respiratory failure
		  Results of chest radiograph for
		    Infiltrates, atelectasis
		    Gross diaphragmatic abnormalities
		Maintain patency of chest tube drainage system
		Monitor amount and nature of chest tube drainage
		Note presence of hemorrhage or air leak; notify physician if either occurs

Pulmonary interstitial edema	Absence of pulmonary interstitial edema Weight returns to preoperative baseline level within a few days postoperatively	Keep careful intake and output records Administer fluids and diuretics as ordered, avoiding fluid overload, weight gain, and pulmonary interstitial edema Monitor weight daily for gain or loss Maintain patient on assisted mechanical ventilation; see Standard 6, *Mechanical ventilation* Provide stiff (tonsillar) suction catheter for patient to aspirate oral secretions as frequently as necessary; patient with myasthenia gravis is usually able to lift hand enough to use these stiff catheters Administer antibiotics as ordered (aminoglycoside medications should not be given) Administer steroids if ordered (as continuation of preoperative therapy)
	Patient successfully weaned from ventilator	Carefully, systematically wean patient from ventilator (usually begins 36 to 48 hours postoperatively) Stay with patient continuously during weaning process; provide for support and encouragement Use intermittent mandatory ventilation system for gradual weaning, if ventilator is so equipped; positive end-expiratory pressure (2 to 4 cm H_2O pressure) is usually employed in system May use T-tube/T-piece system, if ordered, whereby patient is removed from ventilator and allowed to breathe humidified O_2 through wide-bore tubing, using own respiratory muscular effort exclusively Precipitous changes in blood gas values may occur when this method is used

POTENTIAL PROBLEMS	EXPECTED OUTCOMES	NURSING ACTIVITIES
		Pao₂ values greater than 60 and pH values greater than 7.3 are usually acceptable; Paco₂ levels may become elevated because of respiratory muscle weakness and hypoventilation; mild elevation is usually acceptable
		The T-tube/T-piece system is usually applied for 20 to 40 minutes according to patient's clinical status and arterial blood gas levels
	Vital capacity and inspiratory force measurements steadily increase during weaning process	Monitor serial strength, vital capacity, and inspiratory force measurements during weaning process; if measurements indicate poor patient toleration of weaning effort, notify physician
		Administer anticholinesterase medication if ordered during period of weaning
		Monitor effect of medication q15-30 min
		Anticholinesterase medication is often avoided during weaning process because of associated increased secretion production
		Since patient cannot swallow a pill, first dose of anticholinesterase medication is given IV or IM; first dose is usually about one-half of preoperative dose, with increments according to patient's response
Copious secretions Respiratory, oropharyngeal muscle weakness	Effective mobilization and expectoration of secretions	Monitor amount and nature of secretions associated with autonomic (muscarinic) effects of anticholinesterase medication
		Monitor patient's ability to handle (expectorate) secretions, and if marked difficulty is present, notify physician
		Administer atropine if ordered and closely monitor for decrease in secretion production
		During and after weaning procedure, administer vigorous chest physiotherapy and aspirate secretions as necessary
		Closely monitor patient's respiratory status q15-30 min or as patient's condition dictates
		Monitor patient's respiratory status continuously during first 12 to 24 hours after extubation
		After extubation, monitor patient's ability to phonate, since inability to phonate properly usually indicates ineffective cough
		If patient cannot be weaned within 5 to 7 days postoperatively, prepare patient for and assist with tracheotomy according to surgical plan of care, if ordered
■ Hypocalcemia, which can result from inadvertent removal of parathyroid glands lodged within thymus gland	■ Serum Ca⁺⁺ levels within normal limits	■ Monitor
		For signs and symptoms of hypocalcemia including neuromuscular irritability, twitching, Chvostek sign, Trousseau sign
		Serum Ca⁺⁺ levels
		Notify physician of abnormalities
		Administer Ca⁺⁺ supplements as ordered
■ Tracheal injury, which may be related to Mechanical stress Infection	■ Proper amount of air maintained in cuff; air leak around tracheal cuff is apparent on sigh breath	■ Prevent by
		Maintaining minimal amount of air in cuff—permitting leak with sigh (and minimal leak with each inspiration) if low-pressure cuff used; if high-pressure cuff used, regularly deflate (e.g., 5 minutes every hour)
	An air leak may be permitted with normal tidal volumes	Recording volume of air in cuff; alert physician if requirements increase, especially if requirements exceed 8 to 10 ml
	Tracheal tube secured in place	Avoiding movement of tracheal tube
		Note centimeter marking at teeth or nares and record
		Tape tube securely in place
		Note placement of tube on radiograph
		If any change occurs, recheck centimeter marking on tube in relation to mouth and nares
		Using aseptic technique in care of tracheal tube and in suctioning procedures (see Problem, Infection)

POTENTIAL PROBLEMS	EXPECTED OUTCOMES	NURSING ACTIVITIES
■ Infection	■ Absence of or resolution of infection Prompt recognition and intervention if infection occurs	■ Prevent by Averting factors such as urinary retention, pulmonary congestion/aspiration Maintaining strict sterile technique for procedures such as catheterization, endotracheal/tracheostomy tube care, suctioning, ventilator maintenance Monitor Temperature q4 hr and prn IV sites frequently for any signs of redness, tenderness, phlebitis For potential infection sources including pulmonary and urinary and exposure to possible sources of infection WBC count (may be falsely elevated if patient is receiving steroids) If signs of infection occur, notify physician For other measures, see Medical management
■ Crisis—excessive muscle weakness associated with too much or too little medication, including the following two types Myasthenic—sudden muscular weakness; drug regimen ineffective for unknown reasons Cholinergic—worsening status from overdose of myasthenic drugs	■ Immediate recognition of impending crisis occurrence and intervention Patent airway Adequate ventilation, with Paco₂ levels within patient's normal limits	■ Careful observations and frequent assessments of neurological/respiratory status Keep emergency equipment and medications readily available—intubation, suctioning equipment; O₂; hand ventilator; airway; mechanical ventilator; cardiopulmonary drugs; etc.—always anticipate potential crisis occurrence Prevent by Administering medications and treatments as ordered at precise time and regimen Monitoring Effects—maintain flow sheet correlating medication time effectiveness on graded muscle strength, cranial nerve functioning, reflexes of swallow, gag, cough Closely for presence/degree of dysphagia, dyspnea, dysarthria Respiratory status—rate, quality, pattern Vital capacity measurements Averting precipitating factors for crisis such as infection, emotional crisis, constipation Monitor for signs and symptoms of crisis Common manifestations of both myasthenic and cholinergic crisis (present in either crisis): skeletal muscular weakness, increased anxiety, restlessness, dyspnea, dysphagia, dysarthria Differentiating signs according to crisis type Myasthenic: ocular palsies, ptosis, development/worsening of diplopia Cholinergic: fasciculations/fine twitching; abdominal cramps and diarrhea, nausea/vomiting; increased secretions—salivation, sweating, lacrimation, bronchial; blurred vision; most ominous sign is increased weakness instead of expected improvement 1 hour after medication is administered Notify physician immediately of any signs and symptoms of crisis Administer emergency measures as ordered; see Medical management
■ Inordinate weakness and fatigue	■ Optimal muscle strength Early recognition of increased muscle weakness Minimization of fatigue	■ Establish neurological baseline on admission Monitor ongoing neurological status Muscle strength of all groups with repetitive activity Ability to raise/lower eyelids completely; if ptosis is present, note location and degree Facial muscular strength (cranial nerve VII) bilaterally Extraocular movements—presence/degree, location of ocular palsies, nystagmus, diplopia Presence/degree of gag and cough reflexes Presence/quality of chewing ability Speech quality and ability

POTENTIAL PROBLEMS	EXPECTED OUTCOMES	NURSING ACTIVITIES
		Monitor respiratory parameters (establish baseline on admission)
		Vital signs—respiratory rate, quality, and pattern
		Breath sounds for decreased or absent sounds and presence of rales and/or rhonchi
		Vital capacity measurements
		Muscle strength of diaphragmatic and intercostal muscles
		Presence/quality of cough, gag, and swallow reflexes
		Presence, amount/quality of secretions/saliva and patient's ability to handle effectively
		Arterial blood gas levels
		Chest radiograph results
		Patient's history established
		See Medical management for pertinent historical information that should be collected
		Ongoing assessment of neurological and respiratory status
		Provide for close observation; place patient close to nurse's station
		Monitor
		Muscle strengths and vital capacities q2-4 hr and prn
		Maintain flow sheet of muscle strength; establish specific testing modalities for repetitive muscle strength/fatigue assessments
		Maintain flow sheet of vital capacities; use same spirometer and proper position and measurement technique
		Presence/quality of bulbar functioning; facial, hypoglossal, vagal, and glossopharyngeal muscle strength and status
		Presence/quality of gag, swallow, and cough reflexes
		Presence/quality of extraocular movements and strength of eyelid opening and closure
		For presence/degree of ptosis, diplopia, corneal reflex
		For any signs/symptoms of dysphagia, dyspnea (exertional or at rest), dysarthria—presence, quality, and degree
		Notify physician immediately of any decline in neurological/respiratory status
		Notify physician immediately of any decrease in vital capacity below minimal acceptable level specified for individual patient
		Administer therapy as ordered to improve neurological/respiratory status
		See Problem, Muscle weakness (Medical management)
	Patient demonstrates steady increase in neuromuscular function and strength in postoperative period	Ambulate patient as soon as tolerated; if peripheral weakness is marked, ambulation may have to be delayed until anticholinesterase medication is resumed
		Apply bra for women with large breasts for support and to avoid stretch/stress on incision

Subacute postoperative period

POTENTIAL PROBLEMS	EXPECTED OUTCOMES	NURSING ACTIVITIES

■ Respiratory insufficiency/arrest related to Weakness/paralysis of respiratory muscles caused by Pneumonia Atelectasis Dysphagia/aspiration Decreased or absent swallow, gag, and cough reflexes Dysarthria Dyspnea/respiratory failure	■ Adequate alveolar ventilation
	Patent airway
	Respiratory rate and quality within patient's normal limits
	Arterial blood gas levels within normal limits
	Swallow, gag, and cough reflexes at least as good as baseline preoperative level
	Absence of dysarthria or dysphagia
	Absence of pulmonary infection/pneumonia
		■ Prevention
		Maintain patent airway
		Turn and reposition patient q1-2 hr; position to prevent airway obstruction and aspiration of secretions
		Assist patient with coughing and deep breathing
		Administer chest physiotherapy q2-4 hr as needed
		Administer humidified O_2 as ordered to achieve adequate oxygenation and liquefaction of secretions
		Prevent precipitating factors in respiratory failure, especially
		   Severe dysphagia: ongoing monitoring of swallow reflex and status; keep patient NPO if risk of aspiration is high
		   Respiratory tract infection: protect from potential infection sources; vigorous suctioning and chest physiotherapy to maintain patent airway

POTENTIAL PROBLEMS	EXPECTED OUTCOMES	NURSING ACTIVITIES

		Prevent aspiration by
		  Assessing foods that patient tolerates best and assisting with diet selection
		  Avoiding fluids that enhance saliva production such as milk
		  Scheduling meals when strength is maximum
		  Staying with patient at mealtimes; monitoring effectiveness of swallowing
		Prevent pulmonary embolism by
		  Instructing and supervising patient in leg exercises, ROM exercises
		  Applying antithromboembolic stockings or Ace bandages as per physician's order; rewrap or reapply every shift and prn; avoid constriction or looseness
		Monitor neurological and respiratory status q2 hr and prn, including
		  Muscle strength; cranial nerve functioning; swallow, cough, gag reflexes
		  For any choking/nasal regurgitation
		  Vital signs—respiratory rate, quality, and pattern
		  Vital capacities
		  Muscle strength of respiratory muscles (diaphragm and intercostal muscles)
		  Breath sounds for decrease in or absence of sounds and for signs of obstruction (rales, rhonchi, etc.)
		  Patency of upper airway and patient's ability to handle secretions
		  Skin color, nail beds, peripheral pulses, and skin warmth
		  For signs and symptoms of thrombophlebitis, pulmonary emboli, pulmonary edema, dyspnea/dysphagia
		  Arterial blood gas levels and chest radiograph results
		If any impairment in swallow, gag, or cough reflexes is present, keep patient NPO and notify physician; suction secretions prn; prevent aspiration by positioning, maintaining patent airway
		Have emergency equipment and medications readily available if respiratory problem occurs
		Notify physician immediately of any change in respiratory/neurological status
		  Administer medications and treatments as ordered
		  Monitor effects and side effects of therapy; notify physician of results
		If respiratory problem occurs, see Medical management

■ Altered communication ability, which may be related to cranial nerve dysfunction, motor paralysis, endotracheal or tracheostomy tube insertion	■ Means for patient to communicate needs are established and in use	■ Monitor communication abilities
		If ability to communicate is altered, establish alternate means of communication based on individual patient needs/status
		Develop alternative communication modes that are least physically, mentally, and emotionally taxing to patient
		Establish means for patient to get nurse's attention
		Evaluate effectiveness of alternative communication modes with patient/family
		  Involve patient/family in planning care
		  Involve patient/family in reevaluation/readjustment of modes of communication as necessary
		Anticipate patient's needs
		Encourage staff/family to speak to patient, even if patient cannot respond

■ Bowel or bladder dysfunction	■ Urinary output within normal limits
	Absence of bladder distention
	Pattern of bowel elimination within patient's normal limits
		■ Assess patient's prior elimination patterns
		Usual voiding pattern
		Bowel pattern, problems, dietary/medication measures for elimination
		Monitor
		Intake and output measurements
		Bowel movements—amount, consistency, frequency
		  Assess bowel sounds for presence/quality
		  Monitor for signs and symptoms of paralytic ileus; notify physician immediately if any signs/symptoms occur

POTENTIAL PROBLEMS	EXPECTED OUTCOMES	NURSING ACTIVITIES
		For any signs and symptoms of urinary retention, overflow voiding, or residual; notify physician if any of these occur Administer medications as ordered Implement treatments as ordered, such as intermittent catheterization Monitor effects and side effects of interventions and notify physician of results Continue monitoring urinary output Establish and implement individualized bowel/bladder regimen based on patient needs, pattern, previous measures, etc. See Medical management
■ GI bleeding related to CNS factors Stress Steroid administration	■ Absence or control of GI bleeding	■ Prevent by Minimizing factors in environment that contribute to patient's stress level Helping patient deal with anxiety (see Problem, Patient/family's anxiety) Administering antacid as soon as patient is able to take po, if ordered Monitor Vital signs, Hgb, Hct Stools for Hematest three times a week Hematest of aspirate, emesis, urine For signs of GI bleeding such as abdominal tenderness, pain, distention If patient is receiving steroids, monitor urine glucose and acetone four times a day and prn or as ordered; notify physician of results Report immediately to physician any signs and symptoms of GI bleeding If problem occurs, see Medical management; see Standard 49, *Acute upper gastrointestinal bleeding*
■ Complications of corticosteroid therapy	■ Prompt recognition of any complications and notification of physician	■ Monitor for any complications of corticosteroid therapy, including Signs of GI irritation Development or exacerbation of diabetes mellitus Increased susceptibility to infection Psychosis; behavioral changes Hypokalemia Hypertension Osteoporosis Acne For other precautionary measures for the use of steroid therapy in the myasthenic patient, see Medical management
■ Insufficient knowledge to comply with discharge regimen*	■ Sufficient information to comply with discharge regimen Before discharge patient/family accurately Describes medication, activity, and dietary regimens Describes precautionary measures for postoperative period Is able to demonstrate proper care for suture line Verbalizes procedure for follow-up visits	■ Assess patient/family's knowledge regarding disease process, discharge regimen, and follow-up plan of care Consult with physician regarding discharge regimen; ascertain what has been discussed with patient Describe patient's disease process and rationale for discharge regimen Instruct patient/family in medications Name and identification of drug Purpose Indications for use of prn drug Dosage/number of pills and schedule Precautionary measures Potential adverse effects and how to minimize Avoidance of over-the-counter medications that can change activity of prescribed medications and to consult physician before using any of these products Describe postdischarge activity progression, precautions Encourage patient to exercise in regular, moderate amounts, with frequent rest periods

*If the responsibility of the critical care nurse includes follow-up care.

POTENTIAL PROBLEMS	EXPECTED OUTCOMES	NURSING ACTIVITIES
		More strenuous activities should be planned for approximately ½ to 2 hours after anticholinesterase medication is given
		Light activities such as walking, climbing stairs, or cooking are all acceptable in early postoperative period
		If sternotomy approach was used, encourage patient to avoid activities requiring strenuous chest muscle activity for several months; examples of activities that should be avoided in the first few weeks at home include
		Driving a car
		Vacuuming
		Lifting a window
		More vigorous activities should be avoided for several months, including tennis, swimming, golf, and vigorous manual skills such as carpentry work
		Explain that ''remission'' (or need for less anticholinesterase medication to accomplish daily activities) may not occur for several months postoperatively; occurrence and significance of remission cannot be predicted
		Demonstrate and describe care of suture line; provide opportunity for return demonstration
		Review plan for follow-up care, including purpose of follow-up visits; when and where to go; who to see; what specimens to bring
		Assess potential compliance with discharge regimen

GUILLAIN-BARRÉ SYNDROME

Guillain-Barré syndrome is an inflammatory disease process that involves dymyelination and degeneration of the myelin sheath and cylinder of peripheral nerves and the anterior (ventral) and posterior (dorsal) roots at spinal segmental levels. Patients with Guillain-Barré syndrome usually present clinically with a rapidly ascending motor and sensory deficit along with cranial nerve involvement. The progression of the disease process is usually complete within 10 to 12 days after symptoms begin. Strangely enough, the progression can stop at any one level without any further deterioration or progression.

Treatment of Guillain-Barré syndrome is supportive. Recovery occurs spontaneously, and the patient regains prior motor and sensory function, often in a stepwise fashion. The speed of recovery varies with each individual, but recovery commonly occurs over weeks or months. Complete recovery of normal function occurs in the majority of cases, with only a small percentage of patients retaining mild residual defects.

The cause of Guillain-Barré syndrome is not known. Two theories of causation are the infective and the immunological. A virus has not been isolated in Guillain-Barré syndrome but is considered a strong possibility as the cause of the polyneuritis. The immunological theory involves the autoallergic response of body cells to antibodies formed against infectious agents. The clinical history in 50% of Guillain-Barré patients involves the occurrence of a mild respiratory or GI infection 1 to 3 weeks before the appearance of neurological symptoms. This high incidence of preceding infection heightens suspicion that a viral agent may be responsible.

SIGNS AND SYMPTOMS

1. Paresthesias: numbness, tingling, and other abnormal sensations, commonly beginning in the feet. Pain, temperature, proprioception, vibration, and touch are also diminished in the affected areas because of inflammation and degeneration of the posterior (dorsal) roots of the spinal cord.
2. Paresis/paralysis: the motor involvement is usually a complete lower motor neuron paralysis with flaccidity, decreased or absent deep tendon reflexes, and hypotonia

or atonia of muscles. The motor involvement usually corresponds to the areas involved in the sensory deficits and progresses in the same pattern. Weakness usually appears first bilaterally and then progresses to paralysis of involved areas. The motor deficits are caused by inflammation and degeneration of the motor neuron axons that exit from the spinal cord in the anterior (ventral) roots. Commonly, the motor paralysis progresses from legs to trunk, arm, and cranial muscles, attaining peak severity within 10 to 14 days. The motor paralysis of intercostal and phrenic nerves, if it occurs, results in respiratory failure, which is the greatest threat and primary cause of mortality in patients with Guillain-Barré syndrome.
3. Cranial nerve dysfunction: the cranial nerves commonly involved in pathology are
   a. Facial (VII)—lower motor neuron weakness or paralysis of facial muscle control unilaterally or bilaterally
   b. Glossopharyngeal (IX), vagus (X), and hypoglossal (XII)—lower motor neuron bulbar palsy causes nasal, dysarthric speech; dysphagia; impaired gag and cough reflexes; and sympathetic dysfunction with postural hypotension, episodes of hypertension, flushing, sweating, and tachycardia
   c. Oculomotor (III) and abducens (VI)—produce diplopia, nonconjugate eye movements, ptosis
   d. Spinal accessory (XI)—produces impaired shoulder shrug and head turning to side

The diagnosis of Guillain-Barré syndrome is based on the clinical history, clinical presentation of signs/symptoms, progression, and clinical course. A lumbar puncture is performed to aid in diagnosis. The CSF is under normal pressure and contains a normal leukocyte count with an elevated protein count (this increased protein content and normal leukocyte count is called albuminocytological dissociation). The elevated protein count usually appears several days after the onset of symptoms; the protein level continues to rise, reaching a peak in 4 to 6 weeks. This increased CSF protein content is thought to result from the release of plasma proteins from the inflammation, degeneration, and damage of the nerve roots.

ASSESSMENT

1. Onset, duration, progression, and description of neurological symptoms, especially
   a. Motor system: weakness or paralysis, tone, muscles involved
   b. Sensory system: numbness, tingling; pain, temperature, proprioception, vibratory sensations status
   c. Cranial nerve dysfunctions
   d. Reflex system and status
   e. Respiratory symptoms of muscular weakness such as dyspnea, tachypnea
2. Any previous respiratory or GI infection: when, symptoms of, and duration
3. Previous neurological treatment or neurosurgical procedure
4. Presence of any medical problems and therapy employed
5. Any previous vaccination or immunization received: when, specific type, effects, and side effects
6. Patient's perceptions of and reaction to diagnosis, disease progression, treatment modalities
7. Presence of any alterations in body image; fears of permanent disability or deficit; altered role in family, normal occupation/performance of ADL
8. Baseline parameters status
   a. Neurological
   b. Respiratory
   c. Cardiac
   d. Circulatory and vascular
   e. Fluid and electrolyte levels
   f. Hydration/nutritional
   g. Metabolic
   h. Vital capacity
   i. Vital signs
   j. Weight
9. Diagnostic test results, including
   a. Lumbar puncture
   b. Electromyography
10. Results of
    a. CSF determinations
    b. Serum electrolyte levels
    c. Hgb, Hct, platelet count, WBC count/differential
    d. Arterial blood gas levels
    e. Clotting profile
    f. Urinalysis, culture, specific gravity, osmolality
    g. Chest radiograph
    h. ECG

GOALS

1. Optimal neurological functioning
2. Optimal recovery extent and rate; absence of complications
3. Optimal independence in ADL
4. Adequate alveolar ventilation and perfusion
5. Acid-base balance within normal limits
6. Adequate cardiac output
7. Serum electrolyte levels and fluid balance within normal limits
8. Hgb and Hct stable within normal limits
9. Infection free
10. Normal bladder and bowel function
11. Behavior demonstrates reduction of patient/family's anxiety with provision of information, demonstrations, support
12. Before discharge patient/family is able to
    a. Describe medication, activity, exercise, and dietary regimens
    b. Demonstrate safety measures and techniques; proper use of any equipment, therapeutic devices
    c. Describe signs and symptoms requiring medical attention
    d. State necessary information regarding follow-up care

POTENTIAL PROBLEMS	EXPECTED OUTCOMES	NURSING ACTIVITIES
■ Increasing severity and level of motor/sensory deficits Progression is usually rapidly ascending motor and sensory deficit, but cases have occurred in which progression is descending	■ Maximal neurological functioning Absence or resolution of neurological deficit (after disease course) Absence of complications	■ Establish neurological baseline on admission and continue ongoing assessments of neurological status q1 hr and prn; monitor And specifically record deficit present, degree, level, extremities involved especially motor and sensory functioning; cranial nerve functioning and reflex status (presence and quality) LOC; pupil size, equality, light reactivity; extraocular movements Presence and quality of swallow, cough, and gag reflexes Vital signs for any abnormalities Notify physician immediately of any decline in neurological status—either worsening severity or progression of level Institute measures and administer supportive treatments and interventions as physician's order and patient's status necessitate

POTENTIAL PROBLEMS	EXPECTED OUTCOMES	NURSING ACTIVITIES

■ Respiratory insufficiency related to weakness/paralysis of intercostal and diaphragmatic muscles	■ Patent airway
	Adequate alveolar ventilation and perfusion
	Normal respiratory rate, pattern, and quality
	Vital capacity within normal limits
	Arterial blood gas values within patient's normal limits
		■ Establish baseline respiratory status and continue ongoing assessments q1 hr and prn
		Monitor for any abnormality/decline
		  Respiratory rate, quality, and pattern
		  Vital signs
		  Neurological status, particularly muscle strength/functioning of respiratory muscles (intercostal, diaphragmatic)
		  Vital capacity
		  Patency of upper airway and patient's ability to handle secretions
		  Presence/quality of gag, cough, and swallow reflexes
		  Breath sounds bilaterally for quality of aeration; signs of obstruction
		  Skin color, nail beds, peripheral pulses, and skin warmth
		  Arterial blood gas values
		  Chest radiograph results
		  Signs/symptoms of thrombophlebitis, pulmonary emboli, pulmonary edema
		Maintain patent airway by
		  Turning and positioning to prevent obstruction or aspiration of secretions q2 hr and prn
		  Deep breathing and coughing q1 hr and prn
		  Suctioning prn
		  Chest physiotherapy and pulmonary toilet q2 hr and prn
		  IPPB as ordered
		  Adequate oxygenation and humidification as ordered
		Apply antithromboembolic stockings or Ace bandages as ordered; reapply every shift and prn; monitor for constriction/looseness, condition of skin
		Assist patient or perform passive ROM exercises
		Notify physician immediately of any decline in respiratory status, neurological status, vital capacity, vital signs
		If problem occurs
		  Assist with emergency measures to maintain patent airway and adequate ventilation
		  Administer medications/treatments as ordered; monitor effects and side effects
		  Patient will be intubated or tracheostomy will be performed if respiratory muscles are involved in paralysis development/progression; ensure proper positioning of endotracheal tube q2 hr
		  Maintain mechanical ventilator as ordered
		  See Standard 6, *Mechanical ventilation*
		  Provide explanations and support to patient/family; explain relationship between neurological status and respiratory insufficiency; necessity for respiratory assistance/interventions; see Problem, Patient/family's anxiety
		Establish alternate means of communication; see Problem, Altered communication ability

■ Flaccid paralysis, paresthesias related to motor and sensory deficits	■ Absence of complications
	Full ROM of all extremities
	Skin intact
	Absence of contractures
		■ Establish and implement care plan based on individual needs and status; ongoing assessments of motor and sensory deficits/functioning
		Institute measures to prevent complications such as contractures, decubiti, foot-drop/wrist-drop
		  Turn and position properly q2 hr and prn; maintain alignment and decrease gravity pull
		  Sheepskin or air mattress to decrease pressure factors
		  ROM to all extremities from passive to active exercises as status warrants; maintain exercise regimen within pain limits without stretching or resistance
		  Meticulous skin care and inspection of all skin surfaces q2 hr; massage skin and bony prominences

POTENTIAL PROBLEMS	EXPECTED OUTCOMES	NURSING ACTIVITIES
		Obtain devices to prevent deformities, such as handrolls, footboard, hand/foot splints
		Obtain order for appropriate referrals, such as physiotherapy
		Monitor sensory deficits and administer medications and treatments, as ordered, such as analgesics, bed cradle, warm moist packs; turn gently and position comfortably
		Increase activity level/progression as status improves; see Problem, Long rehabilitative phase, for further specifics
■ Cranial nerve dysfunction Oculomotor (III) Abducens (VI) Diplopia, impaired extraocular movements/nonconjugate eye movements	■ Absence of complications	■ Ongoing assessments of cranial nerve functioning Assess pupil size, equality, reactivity; extraocular movements; presence/degree of ptosis Apply alternating eye patch if diplopia is present Place objects within field of vision according to extraocular movements functioning
Facial (VII)—lower motor neuron Facial weakness/paralysis, impaired mouth/lip movement control, decreased or absent corneal reflex		Assess facial muscle functioning and strength, chewing ability, presence and quality of corneal reflex, speech ability If corneal reflex is decreased or absent, obtain order for administration of protective eyedrops and maintain lid closure on affected side by tape, butterfly patch, etc. Ongoing assessments for corneal irritation, abrasions Frequent eye care If patient is allowed po, help select foods that patient can chew Frequent oral hygiene and removal of saliva from drooling If speech is impaired from facial weakness/paralysis, establish alternate means of communication; see Problem, Altered communication ability

Glossopharyngeal (IX)
Vagus (X)
Hypoglossal (XII)
Lower motor neuron bulbar palsy causing nasal, dysarthric speech; dysphagia; absent/diminished swallow, gag, and cough reflexes
		Assess presence and quality of swallow, cough, and gag reflexes; speech quality; tongue strength/position
		If reflexes are absent/diminished, maintain interventions to prevent complications
		  Suction prn; position to prevent obstruction or aspiration of secretions
		  Keep patient NPO
		  Administer IV fluids/NG feedings as ordered; monitor NG tube for proper placement and patency; if endotracheal/tracheostomy tube is in place, inflate cuff for 30 minutes before and after feedings
		When po is allowed, elevate head of bed, and start slowly monitoring quality and effectiveness of swallowing ability
		Progress diet slowly

Spinal accessory (XI) Impaired/absent shoulder shrug and head turning to side abilities		Assess ability to shrug shoulders, turn head to each side If ability to turn head to side is impaired, place objects within field of vision according to head-turning ability/degree

■ Unstable vasomotor function	■ Absence of complication
	Resolution of vasomotor instability
		■ Maintain absolute bed rest as ordered; change position slowly
		Apply antithromboembolic stockings/Ace bandages as ordered
		Monitor ECG recording continually for any abnormality
		Monitor vital signs q2 hr and prn
		Monitor for hypotension, hypertension, sweating, flushing; notify physician immediately if any of these occurs
		  Administer medications and treatments as ordered; monitor effects and side effects; notify physician of results
		When neurological status allows
		  Tilt table if needed
		  Slowly increase head gatch and activity

POTENTIAL PROBLEMS	EXPECTED OUTCOMES	NURSING ACTIVITIES

■ Patient/family's anxiety related to
Neurological disease
Neurological deficit and progression
Fears of permanent disability or deficit
	■ Patient/family's behavior demonstrates decreased anxiety with provision of information	■ Ongoing assessment of level of patient/family's anxiety, fears, concerns
		  Collaborate with physician in providing realistic information appropriate to level of understanding
		    Explain usual signs/symptoms, progression, and clinical course of syndrome
		    Explain that cause is unknown; that shock, fear, frustrations, anger are normal reactions to this insidious, rapid disease onset; accept reactions and help patient/family to deal realistically with reactions
		    Explain usual prognosis expected; that spontaneous recovery occurs over time with recovery onset and speed of recovery varying with each individual
		  Encourage verbalization of questions, fears, anxieties, and other concerns/reactions
		    Answer questions realistically
		    Provide time and support
		    Reinforce that treatment is supportive, that recovery will occur spontaneously and progress, and that no interventions or "pushing" will promote initiation of recovery
		    Continually reassure and reinforce that recovery from disease will occur
		  Explain reasons for frequent respiratory/neurological assessments, vital signs and vital capacity monitoring
		  Explain reasons why all treatments, measures, interventions are necessary
		  Explain tests to patient/family; prepare and support patient during tests such as lumbar punctures, muscle testing
		  If possible, provide one nurse to care for patient exclusively; have same nurses provide care
		  Involve patient in planning of care and goals; encourage patient to make decisions regarding care when possible
		  Involve family in care planning, decision making, maintaining communication

■ Altered communication ability related to
Cranial nerve dysfunction
Motor paralysis
Endotracheal or tracheostomy tube insertion
	■ Alternate means of communication established	■ Monitor communication abilities
		  If ability is altered, set up alternate means of communication based on individual patient needs/status such as writing tablet, word or letter board, eye-blinking system
		  Convey alternate means of communication used to other staff, family; assist in effective use of means
		  Anticipate patient's needs
		  Establish means for patient to get nurse's attention
		  Continue verbal stimulation of patient even if patient is unable to respond; encourage family to talk to patient to maintain stimulation, interests, and contact with reality
		  Evaluate effectiveness of alternative communication means with patient/family
		    Involve patient/family in planning care
		    Involve patient/family in reevaluation/readjustment of alternative communication means as necessary
		    Try to find alternative communication means that are least physically, mentally, and emotionally taxing to patient
		    Accept frustrations patient frequently experiences from altered communication ability and resulting depression; try to minimize frustrations by anticipating needs, constant supervision, having same nurses provide care, etc.

POTENTIAL PROBLEMS	EXPECTED OUTCOMES	NURSING ACTIVITIES

■ Fluid and electrolyte imbalance	■ Fluid and electrolyte balance within normal limits	■ Monitor and accurately record intake and output, urine specific gravity as ordered
		Monitor for signs of dehydration or overhydration such as
		  Poor skin turgor
		  Dry mucous membranes
		  Peripheral edema
		  Excessive thirst
		  Change in LOC
		Monitor for
		  Abnormal vital signs, Hgb/Hct values
		  NOTE: Retention of Na⁺ from effects of increased aldosterone with increased release of ADH may occur as well as K⁺ depletion from immobility
		  Weight alterations
		  Temperature elevations
		  Insensible fluid losses including respiratory, diaphoresis, secretions
		  Presence/degree of nausea and vomiting; effectiveness of medications ordered
		  Presence/quality of gag and swallow reflexes
		Administer IV fluids, NG feedings as ordered
		Administer medications as ordered; monitor effects and side effects; if patient is receiving steroids, monitor urine glucose and acetone levels four times a day
		Notify physician of any fluid imbalance or electrolyte abnormality

■ Bowel/bladder dysfunction	■ Urinary output adequate
	No bladder distention
	Normal bowel elimination
		■ Assess patient's prior elimination patterns—usual voiding pattern, bowel pattern, problems, dietary/medication measures for elimination
		Monitor
		  Accurate recording of intake and output
		  For any signs/symptoms of urinary retention, overflow voiding, or residual; notify physician if any of these occurs and administer medications/treatments as ordered; monitor effects
		  Bowel movements (amount, consistency, frequency)
		  Bowel sounds, presence/quality; signs/symptoms of paralytic ileus
		Establish and implement individualized bowel regimen based on patient needs, pattern, previous measures, preferences/effectiveness
		Involve patient in planning
		Obtain orders for administration of stool softeners, cathartics, enemas as needed
		Assess effectiveness of regimen; readjust as needed
		When patient is allowed po, assist in food selection to promote bowel elimination

■ Infection	■ Absence or resolution of infection	■ Prevent precipitating factors such as urinary retention, pulmonary congestion/aspiration
		Maintain strict sterile technique for procedures such as catheterization; endotracheal/tracheostomy tube care, management, suctioning; ventilator maintenance
		Monitor
		  Temperature q4 hr and prn for any elevation
		  IV sites frequently for any signs of redness, tenderness, phlebitis
		  For potential infection sources including pulmonary, urinary, exposure to infection sources
		  WBC count (may be falsely elevated if patient is receiving steroids)
		If temperature elevation or sign of infection occurs, notify physician and culture possible infection sources
		Monitor sputum/urinary cultures, chest radiograph results
		Administer medications/treatments as ordered; monitor effects and side effects
		Continue accurate recording of intake and output; monitor for dehydration/overhydration
		Monitor for resolution/progression
		Institute measures to promote resolution of infection source if possible

POTENTIAL PROBLEMS	EXPECTED OUTCOMES	NURSING ACTIVITIES
▪ GI bleeding related to Stress Steroid administration Anticoagulation regimen complication	▪ Absence or resolution of GI bleeding	▪ Monitor vital signs q2-4 hr, Hgb and Hct; stools for Hematest three times a week; Hematest of aspirate, emesis, and urine for any abnormalities If patient is receiving anticoagulants, monitor for effects and side effects; notify physician of results Monitor clotting profile results and appropriate coagulation values as ordered Obtain order for antacid administration as soon as patient is able to pake po Monitor for signs of GI bleeding including abdominal tenderness/distention, hypotension, sudden tachycardia Notify physician immediately if any abnormality occurs; if problem occurs, see Standard 49, *Acute upper gastrointestinal bleeding*
▪ Long rehabilitative phase Patient/family's anxiety, anger, frustrations, depression related to Lengthy rehabilitative phase Slow resolution of neurological deficits	▪ Maximal neurological functioning* Maximal level of independence Patient/family verbalizes fears, frustrations, and other concerns Patient/family copes with lengthy rehabilitative process Patient/family demonstrates required care	▪ Ongoing assessment of neurological status—implementation of individualized plan of care and interventions based on patient's needs and status; plan care in collaboration with physician and department of physiotherapy based on disease phase Acute phase: rehabilitative aspects include complete bed rest, prevention of complications, passive ROM exercises within pain limits, exercise regimen without stretching or resistance Condition stabilization phase but without return of function: exercise regimen progresses to gentle stretching and active exercise with avoidance of overstretching weakened muscles Recovery phase: exercise regimen progresses to active-resistant as muscle strength and reflexes return; activity regimen is initiated Provide explanations, time, support, reassurance to patient/family of interventions and necessary reasons; ongoing assessment of patient/family's level of anxiety, anger, and other reactions; see Problem, Patient/family's anxiety, for nursing activities In addition Explain relationship between phases and interventions Explain that vigorous exercise during acute phase will not promote function/recovery but may promote damage of muscles; overstretching exercises during phase of stability before recovery phase can cause permanent damage Reevaluate and readjust care plan as patient's status/needs necessitate and phase progression occurs Implement individualized plan of care to promote maximal neurological functioning, independence in ADL, and patient/family involvement in planning, giving care, and decision making Assist patient as needed in performing ADL; promote personal hygiene Monitor potential and encourage self-care as patient's rehabilitative phase status allows; encourage return to independence Provide rest periods between activities Increase activity to tolerance level Obtain appropriate referrals such as physiotherapy/occupational therapy, social services Obtain appropriate equipment/devices to maximize potential for independent functioning and safety Try to assist patient/family in coping with illness; channel reactions to positive potentials/interventions to promote maximal independence Encourage patient/family to maintain prior interests as feasible such as reading, hobbies, social visits Reinforce and reassure any progression in rehabilitative/recovery phase Reinforce any gains in muscle strength/functioning, independence achieved

*If responsibility of the critical care nurse includes this stage of care.

POTENTIAL PROBLEMS	EXPECTED OUTCOMES	NURSING ACTIVITIES
		Plan, instruct, demonstrate, and evaluate patient/family's verbalization/performance of needed information/skills for maximal independent functioning such as
		Proper use of therapeutic devices/equipment
		Measures to prevent complications
		Assistance necessary: type, amount, and degree
		Assess patient/family's progress toward maximizing potential and independence in ADL
		Monitor level achieved
		If residual deficit is anticipated; coping means, reactions, knowledge, skills demonstrated by patient/family
		If full recovery is anticipated: level achieved by patient/family toward attainment
		Encourage verbalization of perceptions of possible alterations in life-style whether temporary/permanent
		Assess means to promote as "normal" a life-style as possible and encourage striving for attainment
■ Insufficient knowledge to comply with discharge regimen*	■ Patient/family demonstrates or verbalizes understanding of discharge regimen	■ Assess patient/family's level of understanding of neurological problem and therapy received
		Explain relationship between patient's neurological status and therapies prescribed
		Instruction of patient/family regarding required information and skills so that before discharge patient/family is able to
	Patient/family accurately describes medication, activity, and dietary regimens	Describe medication regimen
		Name and purpose
		Route, dosage, frequency, times
		Side effects
		Special precautions necessary including drugs, foods, beverages contraindicated or quantity regulated; factors potentiating/decreasing effects or side effects; physical restrictions; safety measures
		Describe dietary regimen
		Describe activity regimen, exercise program
		Describe and demonstrate any special therapeutic measures prescribed
	Patient/family describes means to achieve maximal independence in ADL, promote safety, and prevent complications	Describe and demonstrate proper use of equipment or therapeutic devices prescribed
		Reasons for using
		Time, method, and duration of use
		Precautions/safeguards
		Necessary maintenance (type, frequency)
		Measures to promote optimal functioning, upkeep/duration
	Patient/family describes signs/symptoms requiring medical attention	Describe signs/symptoms of neurological status requiring medical care
	Patient/family describes follow-up care regimen	Describe plan for follow-up care including purpose of appointment, when and where to go, who to see, what to expect

*If the responsibility of the critical care nurse includes such follow-up care.

Gastrointestinal

PERITONITIS

Peritonitis is an inflammation of the peritoneum associated with an irritative or infective offending agent.

Primary peritonitis is an infection de novo, resulting from a blood-borne or lymph-borne spread of an infectious organism that "seeds" the peritoneum. It occurs most commonly in patients with cirrhosis and ascites. It also occurs in patients with a compromised resistance and immunity to infective organisms. Immunological compromise occurs in patients receiving immunosuppressive therapy or chemotherapy. Chronic diseases that reduce host immunity include cancer, kidney disease (e.g., uremia, nephrotic syndrome), liver disease (e.g., postnecrotic cirrhosis), cystic fibrosis, and lupus erythematosus.

Secondary peritonitis results from direct extension of irritative or infective substances from a ruptured organ or infection outside the peritoneum. Etiological factors may include rupture of a viscus (e.g., from trauma, ulcer disease, ulcerative colitis); gangrenous bowel; extension of an extraperitoneal infection (e.g., pyonephrosis); or pancreatitis.

Postoperative peritonitis occurs occasionally after surgery on the biliary tract, stomach, pancreas, and intestine, particularly if difficulties were encountered during surgery.

Nutritional depletion, fluid and electrolyte imbalance, and the aforementioned risk factors for primary and secondary peritonitis increase the likelihood of postoperative peritonitis.

The pathogenesis of peritonitis may involve the entry of bacteria and other offending agents* into the peritoneum where they are normally phagocytosed by macrophages, polymorphonuclear leukocytes, and opsonins and cleared from the blood by the reticuloendothelial system and other systemic defense systems. However, the bacteria and their

*Viral, tuberculous, or fungal organisms occasionally infect the peritoneum.

endotoxins may proliferate in the peritoneal cavity, particularly in hosts with impaired immunity and in the presence of the exudation of a large amount of fibrin-containing serous fluid. In the acute phase the systemic defense mechanisms may be exhausted, resulting in septic, endotoxin shock and a high probability of death.

Chemical peritonitis results from the abnormal entry of bile, gastric acid, urine, pancreatic juice, and other body substances into the peritoneum.

Pain is the predominant symptom of peritonitis and is accompanied by rebound tenderness and abdominal muscle rigidity. Abdominal pain, nausea, and vomiting often occur together, with systemic symptoms of fever and chills. Bowel sounds are decreased or absent, representing an evolving paralytic ileus.

In making the diagnosis of peritonitis, a leukocyte count may be helpful, although these levels are of equivocal value in patients with acquired immunological deficiency. In cases of suspected or actual trauma an initial lavage with a peritoneal catheter can be useful in diagnosis. One liter of Ringer lactate is infused into the peritoneum, allowed to remain for 5 minutes, and then withdrawn. If the WBC count is greater than $500/mm^3$ or the RBC count is greater than $50,000/mm^2$, intraperitoneal disease is considered present. When the lavage is done, the results are correlated with other lab values (e.g., peritoneal, blood, urine amylase levels) and with the patient's clinical picture to permit the development of an appropriate therapeutic regimen.

An abdominal radiograph may reveal free air in the abdomen in the case of a perforated viscus and/or a diffuse ileus. A chest radiograph is done to rule out pneumonia and to detect atelectasis or a sympathetic pleural effusion.

Medical therapy and nursing care are supportive in nature and include restoration of plasma volume, fluid and electrolyte replacement, pain medication (only after a diagnosis and therapeutic regimen have been formulated), systemic and local (via peritoneal lavage) antibiotics, control of the fever, GI decompression (with an NG tube), respiratory support, and provision of adequate nutrition, often with hyperalimentation.

Surgery may be indicated to remove foreign material (e.g., after trauma), to drain an abscess or to repair a ruptured abdominal viscus, which can involve the creation of a colostomy. Drains are placed to drain discrete abscesses.

The principal complications of peritonitis are respiratory insufficiency, hypovolemia, and renal dysfunction. The principal late complication is the formation of intraperitoneal abscess. The anatomical spaces that tend to collect intraperitoneal fluid, and thereby tend to be sites of abscess formation, are the right and left subphrenic spaces, the right hepatic space, and the pelvis, although abscesses may develop anywhere in the peritoneal cavity. Abscesses stimulate the formation of adhesions, which may lead to intestinal obstruction.

Pelvic abscesses are easier to treat and tend to be associated with lower morbidity. For this reason, patients with peritonitis are placed in semi- to high Fowler position to encourage fluid to drain into the pelvic area. This positioning also improves respiratory excursion and ventilation.

Evidence of an evolving abscess includes a general deterioration in the patient's postoperative progress, a pale and weak appearance, anorexia, abdominal distention, and vomiting. Body temperature, WBC count, and fever increase.

If an abscess develops, treatment includes administration of fluids and antibiotics. Surgical drainage is generally required.

ASSESSMENT

1. History of
   a. Abdominal trauma
   b. Abdominal surgery
   c. Abdominal complaints
2. History, presence, and nature of
   a. Chronic disease(s)
   b. Current or chronic infections
3. Dietary habits
4. Medications taken, particularly corticosteroids, antibiotics, analgesics
5. Physical signs/symptoms
   a. Location, severity of discomfort/pain
   b. Radiation, rebound tenderness, and/or rigidity
   c. Nausea and vomiting
   d. Bowel function abnormalities
   e. Decreased or absent bowel sounds

f. Inability to pass flatus or feces
g. Fever
h. Hypotension, tachycardia, tachypnea; signs and symptoms of dehydration
i. Thirst and oliguria
6. Results of lab and diagnostic tests, including
   a. Serum protein, albumin levels
   b. WBC count
   c. Amylase levels
   d. Sedimentation rate
   e. Chest and abdominal radiographic studies, which may reveal a perforated viscus as the cause of the peritonitis, dilatation of the large and small bowel with edema of the small bowel wall, or some other abnormality associated with peritonitis
   f. Paracentesis
7. Level of patient/family's anxiety concerning disease process, hospitalization, diagnostic procedures, and therapy employed

GOALS

1. Patient/family's behavior indicates reduction in anxiety with provision of information, explanations and encouragement
2. Infection free, afebrile
   a. Absence of or minimal formation of adhesions
   b. Wound intact; no evisceration
   c. Absence of new infection at drain sites
   d. Absence of abscess formation or septic shock
3. Normal bowel function; no ileus
4. Fluid and electrolyte balance within normal limits; weight responds in the desired direction
5. Respiratory function sufficient to maintain
   a. Serum PaO_2 and $PaCO_2$ within normal limits
   b. Absence of atelectasis, pulmonary infection, pneumonia
   c. Absence of pleural effusion, "shock lung" (adult respiratory distress syndrome)
6. Nutritional intake sufficient to maintain body weight, positive nitrogen balance, and adequate wound healing
7. Before discharge patient/family is able to
   a. Describe specific wound, suture line care as ordered with return demonstration as appropriate
   b. Describe dietary regimen
   c. Describe activity regimen
   d. Describe medication regimen
   e. Identify signs and symptoms requiring medical attention
   f. State necessary information regarding follow-up care

POTENTIAL PROBLEMS	EXPECTED OUTCOMES	NURSING ACTIVITIES
▪ Patient/family's anxiety related to Hospitalization Disease process Signs and symptoms Diagnostic procedures Therapeutic regimen Altered family roles Dependency	▪ Reduction in level of anxiety with provision of information, explanations, and encouragement	▪ Ongoing assessment of level of patient/family's anxiety Assess level of knowledge and understanding of disease process, diagnostic procedures, and therapy employed Explain relationship of disease process to signs/symptoms patient is experiencing Explain in simple terms disease process and rationale for various therapeutic interventions Describe diagnostic procedures and what patient will experience; prepare patient for each Provide opportunity for and encourage questions, verbalization of fears and anxieties Provide comfort measures Encourage participation in care as tolerated Assess reduction in level of patient/family's anxiety with provision of information, explanations, and encouragement
▪ Infection, which may be associated with Peritonitis Abscess formation localized in subphrenic spaces, pelvis, retroperitoneum Wound evisceration Sepsis Septic shock Failure of resolution or localization of peritonitis	▪ Afebrile Infection free Bowel function within normal limits (bowel sounds, flatus)	▪ Prevent by Using aseptic technique when indicated Providing oral hygiene q2 hr Administering prophylactic antibiotics after certain procedures and surgeries if ordered Monitor for Fever, hypotension, tachycardia in patients at high risk for development of infection, particularly those who are debilitated and/or malnourished Presence, nature, and progression of abdominal discomfort, pain; carefully document and report Quality of all drainage (e.g., serous, serosanguineous, pustular, bloody) Nausea and vomiting Decreased or absent bowel sounds, bowel function Altered LOC Abnormal results of laboratory and diagnostic tests, including WBC count with differential, sedimentation rate Serum amylase Serial blood, sputum, throat, urine, and if abdominal suture line/wound is present, wound cultures Chest and abdominal radiograph results Notify physician of abnormalities in aforementioned If problem occurs Serially repeat all cultures Administer antibiotics as ordered Monitor progression of fever and other signs/symptoms Administer wound care using aseptic technique Monitor Serial measurements of abdominal girth For progression, alleviation of abdominal discomfort, pain (local or diffuse) Progression/alleviation of tenderness and rigidity of abdomen Intake and output q1 hr Daily weights Hemodynamic measurements q1 hr until stable (e.g., BP, P, CVP, and PAP if available; urine output, peripheral circulation) Notify physician of abnormalities in aforementioned measurements Administer fluid replacement as ordered Administer peritoneal dialysis with antibiotics if ordered To prevent continuing unresolved peritonitis, monitor for presence of ulcer, excess peritoneal exudate; necrotic, infected bowel; appendicitis; localized abscess(es) Prepare patient for additional diagnostic tests as ordered Surgery may be performed to plicate an ulcer, to remove excess peritoneal exudate, for bowel resection, for appendectomy, or to drain localized abscess(es) Prepare patient for surgery according to plan of care

POTENTIAL PROBLEMS	EXPECTED OUTCOMES	NURSING ACTIVITIES

■ Paralytic ileus	■ Bowel sounds within normal limits	■ Prevent by administering therapy to treat peritonitis as ordered
		Monitor for
		  Presence of peritonitis
		  Bowel sounds, bowel function, flatus
		  Abdominal girth q4-8 hr for distention
		  Volume of NG aspirates
		  Weight gain or loss
		If ileus occurs
		  Monitor bowel function, abdominal girth, and weight
		  Maintain and ensure patency of NG tube as indicated (e.g., status after ulcer plication, intestinal anastomosis)
		  Assist with insertion of intestinal tube for decompression, as indicated
		  Administer agents such as suppositories, enemas, neostigmine (Prostigmin) to stimulate bowel function if ordered

■ Respiratory insufficiency related to
Discomfort
Abdominal distention
Atelectasis
Pleural effusion
Acute respiratory distress syndrome or pulmonary interstitial edema—may be associated with septicemia; large protein losses into peritoneum, which thus decrease serum oncotic pressure; or result from vigorous fluid resuscitation
	■ Adequate oxygenation and ventilation with arterial blood gas levels within normal limits
	Chest radiograph reveals full lung expansion, without atelectasis, interstitial edema
	No dyspnea
		■ Prevent by
		  Placing patient in Fowler position (NOTE: This position encourages inflammatory exudate to collect in pelvis rather than subphrenic space; it is felt that pelvic abscesses, should they occur, are easier to treat than subphrenic abscesses)
		  Administering pain medication sufficient to permit adequate breathing and coughing
		  Administering chest physiotherapy q2-4 hr while patient is on bed rest; thereafter administering as needed
		  Turning at least q2 hr
		Monitor respiratory status
		  Quality of respirations q1 hr; note tachypnea, dyspnea
		  Serial arterial blood gas determinations for hypoxemia, hypercapnia, acidosis q6-12 hr
		  Breath sounds q1-2 hr for decreased or absent sounds and presence of rales and/or rhonchi
		  Serial chest radiograph results for atelectasis, pleural effusion, and other abnormalities
		  Serial sputum C and S results
		Monitor daily weights for gain or loss
		Notify physician of any abnormalities
		If respiratory insufficiency occurs
		  Assess nature, extent of problem
		  Administer humidified O_2 as ordered
		  Provide for vigorous chest physiotherapy to affected areas of lung
		  Assist with aspiration of pleural effusion, if procedure is necessary
		  Assist with intubation if needed (see Standard 6, *Mechanical ventilation*)
		  Administer antibiotics and/or steroids as ordered
		  Administer diuretics if ordered; closely monitor patient's response

■ Fluid and/or electrolyte imbalance related to
Fluid losses into peritoneum
GI fluid losses related to decompression and, if present, wound losses
May be associated with development of renal failure
	■ Weight within normal limits
	Normovolemia with hemodynamic parameters within normal limits
		■ Prevent by
		  Administering fluid replacement according to serial weights, hemodynamic parameters, as ordered
		  Administering electrolyte replacement according to calculated losses and measured serum levels, as ordered
		Monitor
		  Daily weights for loss or gain
		  Indices of intravascular volume, including serial measurements of BP, P, CVP, PAP, urine output, peripheral circulation, and mentation; correlate with changes in abdominal girth
		  Serum electrolyte levels q6-12 hr
		  For signs/symptoms of electrolyte imbalance including weakness, lethargy, irritability
		Notify physician of abnormalities
		If fluid and electrolyte imbalance occurs, administer plasma, fluids, diuretics, and/or electrolytes as ordered; closely monitor patient's response

POTENTIAL PROBLEMS	EXPECTED OUTCOMES	NURSING ACTIVITIES
■ Malnutrition, metabolic abnormalities related to Increased catabolism with loss of muscle mass Glucose intolerance	■ Weight within normal limits for patient Positive nitrogen balance Body muscle mass remains stable or increases in size	■ Assess nutritional status Diet history State of muscle mass, skin turgor, mucous membranes, hair Prevent metabolic abnormalities, malnutrition by Monitoring blood and urine glucose levels and notifying physician of abnormalities Administering glucose supplements and insulin as ordered and closely monitoring patient's response If oral intake of nutrients is limited or absent for an extended period of time, administer IV hyperalimentation early in course of therapy as ordered Monitor Blood protein levels (e.g., albumin) Daily weights for gain or loss Serial blood, urine glucose; urine acetone levels for signs/symptoms of hyperglycemia and hypoglycemia If malnutrition or metabolic abnormalities occur, provide nutrients orally by NG tube or IV TPN as ordered
■ Renal failure related to decreased perfusion of kidneys	■ Renal function within normal limits	■ Prevent by Administering adequate fluid intake Administering therapy to provide for adequate cardiac output and renal blood flow Monitor For hypovolemia by assessing hemodynamic parameters q1-2 hr Note hypotension, tachycardia, low CVP and pulmonary pressure, and signs of peripheral hypoperfusion Serial weights for gain or loss Fluid intake and output q1 hr; note oliguria BUN and serum creatinine levels daily Urine electrolyte levels Notify physician of significant abnormalities If renal failure occurs, see Standard 52, *Acute renal failure*
■ Insufficient information for compliance with discharge regimen*	■ Before discharge patient/family accurately describes Activity progression Dietary management Medication regimen Plan for follow-up care	■ Assess patient/family's level of understanding of peritonitis and therapy employed Explain relationship between peritonitis and therapy prescribed Describe follow-up plan for Activity levels Diet Medications Purpose Identification Route Dosage Frequency, timing Describe untoward signs/symptoms requiring medical attention (individualize description according to patient's problem and need to know), including Fever, flushed feeling Abdominal pain, discomfort Tight abdominal muscles Abdominal distention Decreased bowel function and fewer bowel movements Nausea, vomiting Loss of appetite Describe follow-up plan of care, including purpose of follow-up appointments, where and when to go, what specimens to bring, and what activities will be included in follow-up visit Encourage patient/family to ask questions Assess potential compliance of patient/family with discharge regimen

*If responsibility of critical care nurse includes this type of follow-up care.

LIVER FAILURE/DECOMPRESSIVE PORTOVENOUS SHUNTING PROCEDURES

LIVER FAILURE

Liver failure is the derangement of one or all of the functioning units of the liver. The extent of derangement depends on how much each unit has been affected, including (1) parenchymal cells, (2) reticuloendothelial cells, and (3) biliary ducts.

The liver aids in initial digestion and emulsification by secreting bile. It controls carbohydrate, protein, and fat metabolism (both anabolism and catabolism) to supply energy to meet the body's needs, build up muscle tissue, and supply proteins and enzymes to perform many important bodily functions. The liver acts as a warehouse by storing glycogen, iron, minerals and metals, and some vitamins (A, B_6, B_{12}, D, E, K, folic acid). The liver metabolizes nitrogenous waste products into ammonia, urea, and bilirubin. Hormones are conjugated in the liver and secreted in bile. The liver protects the body by removing bacteria and by detoxifying endotoxins and drugs.

The liver has a remarkable regenerative power that allows it to recover from such major insults as hepatitis and to regenerate tissue after a major resection. Approximately 70% of the hepatic parenchymal tissue must be damaged before the liver function tests become consistently abnormal. The associated liver dysfunction involves a disturbance in all the normal hepatic functions described before.

Liver failure may result from indirect or direct hepatotoxins or as part of a disease process. Indirect hepatotoxins interfere with a specific metabolic pathway, with a variable latent period followed by hepatitis. Excessive alcohol intake produces an indirect toxic effect by accelerating triglyceride synthesis, which produces an increase in smooth endoplasmic reticulum and intracellular fat deposits, resulting in alcoholic hepatitis with hepatocellular necrosis. Some drugs act as indirect hepatotoxins and, in persons with a hypersensitivity response, produce a similar picture.

Diseases that can produce hepatic dysfunction and failure include hepatitis, Wilson disease, Budd-Chiari syndrome, metastatic cancer, schistosomiasis, venoocclusive disease, extrahepatic vein thrombosis, postanesthesia hepatic failure, glycogen storage diseases, homozygous-familial hypercho-

lia, tularemia, and cryptogenic hepatic failure.

Advanced liver failure is manifested by ascites, hypersplenism, gastric and esophageal varices, hypoproteinemia, and abnormal coagulation studies. Severe portal hypertension may result in variceal bleeding and increase circulatory levels of nitrogenous products.

Prognosis varies according to the severity of liver dysfunction and other body variables. Mortality is high in patients with encephalopathy, ascites, renal failure, and certain lab abnormalities, (i.e., prolonged prothrombin time [PT], hyperbilirubinemia, high BUN levels, and leukocytosis).

DECOMPRESSIVE PORTOVENOUS SHUNTING PROCEDURES

The objective of surgery is to reduce the risk of esophageal and gastric bleeding by lowering the portal esophageal and gastric venous pressures. Venous blood that would normally traverse the portal vein is diverted into another vein that eventually empties directly into the vena cava. The systemic load of nitrogenous waste products is thereby increased, usually producing some degree of encephalopathy.

Shunts that provide the greatest reduction in the risk of bleeding also divert a greater proportion of blood away from the esophagogastric veins and from the liver and are associated with the greatest incidence of encephalopathy (e.g., portacaval shunts). Other decompressive shunts provide less diversion of blood away from varices and less reduction in the risk of bleeding, but are also associated with a less severe encephalopathy (e.g., mesocaval, splenorenal, coronary/left gastric–caval, splenocaval).

Potential candidates for surgery are rated on the presence of certain prognostic parameters. Parameters that reflect a good surgical risk include albumin levels greater than 3 g/100 ml, bilirubin level less than 2 mg/100 ml, normal or only slightly prolonged PT, transaminase levels less than 80 units, alkaline phosphatase level normal or only slightly elevated, absence of ascites and advanced encephalopathy, and good nutritional status.

A new surgical procedure called the *Sugiura procedure*

may be an alternative to the shunting operations. This surgical procedure was developed in Japan with the major goal of preventing bleeding from esophageal and gastric varices. The esophagus is first denuded of its varices. (This procedure requires a thoracic approach; therefore the patient will have chest tubes postoperatively.) Later, a second operation is performed to remove the gastric varices. (This procedure uses an abdominal approach.) The success rate for preventing rebleeding from varices is presently being studied in the United States.

ASSESSMENT

1. History of
   a. Any disease affecting the liver
   b. Amount of alcohol intake on a daily/weekly basis
   c. Exposure to toxins such as carbon tetrachloride
   d. Any injections in the past 6 months, including blood tests, dental treatments, tattoos
   e. Signs and symptoms that suggest cholelithiasis or choledocholithiasis
   f. Dark urine and light stools; jaundice and pruritus; icteric sclera
   g. Anemia; splenectomy, cholecystectomy; congenital or familial hyperbilirubinemia; tremors or neurological abnormalities
   h. Medications taken recently—note those known to affect liver function
   i. Adverse reactions to any drugs taken
2. Presence and extent of
   a. Jaundice—hues
      (1) Muddy yellow may indicate hemolysis of RBC
      (2) Orange may indicate parenchymal disease
      (3) Deep greenish may indicate prolonged biliary obstruction
   b. Icteric sclera
   c. Cachexia, wasting of extremities
   d. Dilatated veins in flank, anteroabdominal region; hemorrhoids
   e. Enlarged, nodular, firm liver; or atrophied, small liver
   f. Tender hepatic margins
   g. Enlarged gallbladder (Courvoisier sign)
   h. Splenomegaly
   i. Asterixis, any neurological abnormalities
   j. Mental, personality changes
   k. Stigmata of cirrhosis
   l. Parotid gland enlargement
   m. Dupuytren contracture
   n. Gynecomastia
   o. Diminished axillary or pubic hair
   p. Skin ecchymosis
   q. Palmar erythema, spider angiomas; scratch marks, pruritus
   r. Clubbing of nails
   s. Xanthomas
3. Lab values
   a. Serum proteins, including total protein, albumin levels; albumin-globulin ratio
   b. Immunoglobulins; gamma globulin
   c. Coagulation studies, including clotting factors and platelets
   d. Hct, Hgb
   e. WBC count
   f. Bilirubin (total, indirect, direct)
   g. Ammonia
   h. Lipids; esterified cholesterol
   i. Flocculation and turbidity tests
   j. Serum enzymes: SGOT, SGPT, LDH
4. If indicated
   a. Bromosulfophthalein (BSP) excretion study
   b. Ceruloplasmin and copper levels
   c. Schistosomal levels
   d. Antigen for hepatitis B
   e. Urine levels of
      (1) Conjugated bilirubin—glucuronide (note levels above 0.4 mg/100 ml)
      (2) Urobilinogen
      (3) Electrolytes
5. Results of diagnostic tests
   a. Abdominal radiography
   b. Liver-spleen scan (scintiscan)
   c. Angiography, venography
   d. Splenoportography
   e. Barium studies of the GI tract
   f. Emergency celiac angiography and endoscopy for emergency bleeding
   g. Endoscopy
   h. Laparoscopy
   i. Liver biopsy
   j. Cholecystography and cholangiography
   k. Portal and hepatic vein manometry
6. Anxiety about and understanding of disease process, diagnostic procedures, purpose of hospitalization, therapy planned; if appropriate, surgery and the expected outcome and what the patient will experience in the perioperative period
7. Patient's perception of and reaction to the diagnosis and therapy

GOALS

1. Reduction in patient/family's anxiety with provision of information, explanations, and encouragement
2. Liver dysfunction does not further deteriorate; absence or resolution of coagulation abnormalities
3. Absence or resolution of GI bleeding
4. Hemodynamic stability
5. Absence or no exacerbation of encephalopathy
6. Absence or resolution of ascites

7. Electrolyte levels within normal limits
8. Renal function within normal limits; absence of hepatorenal syndrome
9. Respiratory function sufficient to maintain adequate oxygenation, ventilation
10. Absence of emboli
11. Adequate nutritional intake, positive nitrogen balance

12. Patent decompressive shunt
13. Before discharge patient/family is able to describe discharge regimen, including
    a. Medication, dietary, and activity regimens
    b. Identify untoward signs and symptoms requiring medical attention
    c. Describe plan for follow-up care

POTENTIAL PROBLEMS	EXPECTED OUTCOMES	NURSING ACTIVITIES
Medical management		
■ Patient/family's anxiety related to Hospitalization Disease process Therapy prescribed Diagnostic procedures	■ Reduction in patient/family's anxiety with provision of information, explanations, and encouragement	■ Ongoing assessment of anxiety Assess patient/family's knowledge of disease process, therapy prescribed, and diagnostic procedures Explain disease process and its relationship to therapy employed Describe rationale for planned diagnostic tests; prepare patient for and, if appropriate, assist with diagnostic tests Provide opportunity for and encourage patient/family's questions, verbalization of fears and anxieties Assess reduction in level of patient/family's anxiety
■ Ascites related to Increased portal hydrostatic pressure Decreased plasma colloid osmotic pressure associated with decreased albumin synthesis Hypovolemia, which may stimulate increased aldosterone production and retention of Na^+ and H_2O by kidney Increased lymph formation in cirrhosis and in hepatic venous obstruction Loss of newly formed albumin into free peritoneal space	■ Absence of or resolution of ascites; abdominal girth remains stable or decreases in size Weight remains stable Serum protein, albumin levels within normal limits	■ Administer plasma, colloids as ordered to maintain oncotic pressure, serum protein and albumin levels within normal limits Promote/support liver function (see Problem, Unresolved progressive liver failure: nursing activities, for prevention of liver failure) Salt and/or H_2O restriction if ordered Monitor for Anasarca; presence and extent of edema in various body areas Daily weight changes Serial abdominal girths; note progression of ascites Abnormal serum protein and albumin levels Abnormal serum electrolytes, particularly Na^+ levels Notify physician if aforementioned abnormalities occur Employ the following measures as ordered Salt restriction, which may be limited to 500 mg Na^+/day (occasionally is limited to 250 mg Na^+/day); because salt restriction limits protein intake to some degree, administer protein supplements in the form of powdered milk low in Na^+ if ordered H_2O restriction is employed for some patients with impaired free H_2O clearance to help prevent dilutional hyponatremia; may be limited to 1500 ml/day in adults as ordered Administer diuretics as ordered; diuretics should be given cautiously so that depletion of extracellular fluid volume does not occur; since capacity to absorb ascitic fluid is limited to about 800 ml/day, depletion of extracellular fluid volume should not proceed at a rate greater than this Monitor for electrolyte loss and imbalance associated with diuretic administration q12-24 hr Bed rest may be ordered for patients with ascites; after diuresis has begun, gradual increase in activity is usually permitted Assist with paracentesis, which may be done if abdominal distention is severe; not more than 1000 to 1500 ml of fluid should be withdrawn at a time or hypotension, shock, and encephalopathy may ensue Monitor vital signs q1-2 hr Monitor for potential complications of paracentesis—hemorrhage, protein depletion, shock Protein supplementation Administer salt-poor albumin—25 g/day IV for 3 to 4 days, if ordered, to augment intravascular osmotic pull and to enhance movement of ascitic fluid into intravascular space, thus promoting diuresis

POTENTIAL PROBLEMS	EXPECTED OUTCOMES	NURSING ACTIVITIES
		Corticosteroids In addition to diuretics, administer corticosteroids, if ordered, to augment free H_2O clearance in patients in whom extracellular fluid volume is markedly expanded and hyponatremia is severe; corticosteroids are usually administered for 7 to 10 days in moderate to large doses, then discontinued

■ Encephalopathy precipitated by
  Medications that require liver metabolism
  GI bleeding with increased protein load
  Hypotension, shock
  Diuretic therapy with associated hypokalemic alkalosis, which increases ammonia production
  Abnormal cerebral metabolism of glucose associated with high ammonia levels
	■ Absence and/or resolution of encephalopathy
	  BUN levels remain stable or decrease
	  LOC, mentation, behavior, gait, speech, and neuromuscular function remain same or improve
		■ *Avoid* the following abnormalities and therapies that can increase ammonia production
		  Administration of ammonium chloride
		  Diuresis of more than 1 to 2 kg/day
		  Dehydration, shock
		  Sedatives, narcotics, tranquilizers
		  Anesthesia, decompressive shunting procedures
		  Infection
		  Acid-base, electrolyte imbalance (avoid hypokalemic alkalosis); if acidification is needed, lactulose may be ordered to acidify bowel
		Prevent by
		  Administering lactulose, if ordered, to induce movement of ammonia from blood to colon; lactulose also has laxative action that promotes excretion of ammonium ion
		  Administering poorly absorbed antibiotics, if ordered (orally, by enema), to reduce nitrogen-forming intestinal bacteria
		  Administering antacids and/or anti-H_2 medication, if ordered, to reduce risk of GI bleeding
		  NOTE: If GI bleeding is present, institute therapy to control it; see Standard 49, *Acute upper gastrointestinal bleeding*
		  Administering fluid volume repletion as ordered, usually including salt-poor albumin
		Monitor
		  Blood ammonia and BUN levels; assist in titrating patient's protein intake to level that does not raise circulating ammonia and BUN to unacceptable levels
		  Patient's LOC, mentation, speech, behavior, gait, and neuromuscular function
		  Results of EEG, which may reflect diffuse slowing
		If encephalopathy occurs
		  Maintain safe environment
		  Reorient patient frequently to time, place, and person
		  Explain procedures simply and clearly
		  Avoid medications that depend heavily on liver metabolism: ammonia-containing drugs, amino compounds
		    If sedation is needed, phenobarbital and chloral hydrate are preferred; occasionally diazepam is given in very small quantities
		  Administer a cathartic such as sorbitol in H_2O or magnesium citrate, as ordered, to reduce intestinal flora
		  Reduce dietary intake of protein while providing adequate calories as ordered
		    Low-protein tube feedings are available such as Lipomul-Oral*
		    When protein intake is resumed, start with 20 to 40 g protein/day or as ordered and increase by 10 to 20 g q2-4 days as tolerated in adults
		  Administer lactulose (adults: 35 to 70 g/day), if ordered, to produce acidic colonic pH, which favors movement of ammonia into stool
		    Arginine or glutamic monochloride is sometimes ordered in effort to inactivate excess ammonia

*The Upjohn Co., Kalamazoo, Mich.

POTENTIAL PROBLEMS	EXPECTED OUTCOMES	NURSING ACTIVITIES
■ Unresolved, progressive liver failure related to Viral hepatitis—may follow fulminant course Drug sensitivity Phosphorous poisoning Reye syndrome	■ Liver dysfunction does not further deteriorate Absence of clotting abnormalities, encephalopathy	■ Monitor For signs/symptoms of liver failure, including progressive jaundice, encephalopathy Serial liver function tests, including serum bilirubin and transaminase levels (usually 2 times a week in acute phase), prothrombin levels For abnormal coagulation studies For signs/symptoms of bleeding, including petechiae and ecchymoses Assist with liver biopsy (done if diagnosis is unclear or patient has prolonged or relapsing hepatitis) If bleeding occurs, notify physician; administer therapy as ordered, which may include fresh whole blood, fresh frozen plasma, or products containing only clotting factors and platelets; monitor for transfusion reaction Administer corticosteroids if ordered; may be given to patients with chronic, active hepatitis and hepatic necrosis, and/or in presence of anorexia, encephalopathy, and clotting abnormalities Effect of steroids on healing and on progression of necrotic process has not been conclusively determined Institute bed rest until acute liver failure episode subsides (if it does) or until fever abates, abnormal liver function tests begin to show return to normal, and clinical improvement occurs, as ordered Monitor results of liver function tests Administer or assist with unusual supportive measures as ordered, including exchange blood transfusions, plasma exchanges, hemodialysis or peritoneal dialysis, saline washout, extracorporeal pig liver perfusion, or cross-circulation with human volunteers or primates
■ Malnutrition related to fulminant liver failure and associated with Insufficient intake of protein Impaired absorption of fat-soluble vitamins Macrocytic anemia, vitamin B_{12} deficiency related to Hepatitis Chronic, active hepatic necrosis Acute alcoholic hepatitis Anorexia, encephalopathy Clotting abnormalities	■ Sufficient intake of protein for liver regeneration, but not so much that blood nitrogenous waste product levels significantly increase Liver function within normal limits With medications tailored to specific liver dysfunction, liver function tests return toward normal and clotting abnormalities and/or encephalopathy, if present, subside	■ Patient's dietary intake of protein should be titrated to toleration for nitrogen load; if tolerated, intake may be as much as 100 to 125 g protein/day and 3000 calories/day, with approximately one half of total calories supplied as carbohydrates; if encephalopathy develops, notify physician; protein load should be reduced accordingly If patient is in fulminant liver failure, protein intake may be as little as 20 to 40 g/day, with increments of 10 g every 2 to 3 days if liver failure is resolving; remainder of diet is moderate in fat, high in carbohydrates; salt restriction is usually needed to limit fluid retention If anorexia impairs food intake, tube feedings may be administered as ordered If adequate intake of nutrients is impossible using these methods, IV hyperalimentation may be employed; see Standard 57, *Total parenteral nutrition* Administer vitamins, particularly A, D, and K as ordered; B vitamins are often ordered, particularly if macrocytic anemia is present
■ Hepatorenal syndrome Acute renal failure in advanced liver disease may be related to Circulating pressor substance that cannot be detoxified by impaired liver Production of vasoactive substances by dysfunctional liver Decreased effective plasma volume associated with ascites	■ Absence and/or resolution of hepatorenal syndrome Renal function within normal limits BUN and creatinine levels are within normal limits Absence of hypotension and oliguria Serum Na^+ levels within normal limits Urinary creatinine and creatinine clearance within normal limits Absence of proteinuria	■ Observe measures to prevent decreased renal blood flow, including Slow removal of ascitic fluid during abdominal paracentesis with careful fluid, albumin repletion as needed Avoidance of vigorous diuretic therapy Preparing patient for Levine shunt, which may be placed to connect peritoneal space, where much of ascitic fluid lies, with vena cava, thus permitting recirculation of ascitic fluid Administer therapy as ordered to improve liver function Monitor for signs of portal hypertension: ascites, encephalopathy, jaundice, and oliguria; notify physician if any of these occurs; conditions such as urinary obstruction or prerenal failure should be ruled out as causes of oliguria, and treatment should be altered accordingly

POTENTIAL PROBLEMS	EXPECTED OUTCOMES	NURSING ACTIVITIES

AV shunts (which may be surgically created)		Monitor
		  Intake and output, especially urine output
		  Serum electrolyte levels for hyponatremia
		  Serum creatinine concentrations (0.7 to 1.5 mg/100 ml is normal)
		  Urine creatinine excretion (25 mg/kg/24 hours is normal)
		  Creatinine clearance (ml/minute), which is urine concentration × urine volume ÷ plasma concentration (normal creatinine clearance is 90 to 140 ml/minute)
		  For proteinuria
		Administer dopamine in low doses, if ordered, to augment renal blood flow and to produce natriuresis and diuresis
		Administer antibiotics, if ordered, to reduce circulating ammonia levels
		  In presence of renal dysfunction, antibiotic doses should be appropriately reduced

■ Bleeding resulting from
  Esophageal and gastric varices, esophageal laceration, peptic ulcer, gastritis, and, occasionally, carcinoma of esophagus
  Hepatic disease
    Deficient production of clotting factors; coagulopathy
	■ Absence or resolution of bleeding (e.g., GI)
	  Hct, Hgb remain stable or, with supplementation of blood products, return to normal limits
		■ Prevent by administering therapy to support/promote liver function and to limit portal hypertension (see Problem, Unresolved progressive liver failure)
		Monitor for
		  Hematemesis
		  Hematest-positive stools and vomitus/NG aspirate
		  Dropping Hct
		  Hypotension, tachycardia
		Notify physician of any abnormality
		If bleeding occurs
		  Administer fluids and blood products to maintain hemodynamic parameters and Hct within normal limits
		  Control bleeding as ordered with iced saline NG lavages and, if necessary, esophagogastric pressure balloons—maintain air pressure in balloons at predetermined level; see Standard 49, *Acute upper gastrointestinal bleeding*
		Prepare patient for and assist with endoscopy and other diagnostic tests or therapeutic procedures as ordered
		Prepare patient for surgery if planned

■ Emboli
  Pulmonary
  Mesenteric
  Renal
  Cerebrovascular
  Coronary
	■ Absence of emboli
	  Absence of signs, symptoms of ischemia or infarction of pulmonary, intestinal, renal, cerebral, or myocardial tissue
		■ Administer fluids and blood products as ordered to prevent low, sluggish blood flow and associated ischemia
		Administer low-dose heparinization, if ordered, in high-risk surgical patients
		Provide for early mobilization and ambulation as ordered
		Monitor for
		  Signs of thrombophlebitis, including Homans sign (calf pain or dorsiflexion)
		  Signs of peripheral arterial emboli
		  Signs and symptoms of various types of emboli (e.g., coronary, pulmonary, mesenteric, renal, and cerebrovascular)
		If embolus occurs, administer therapy as ordered
		For other preventive, monitoring activities and the therapeutic interventions, see Standard 31, *Embolic phenomena*

■ Insufficient information to comply with discharge regimen*	■ Sufficient information to comply with discharge regimen	■ Assess patient/family's knowledge and understanding of discharge regimen
		Instruct patient/family as needed in
		  Medications, including identification, dosage, frequency, timing, and precautionary measures
		  Dietary regimen
		  Activity progression
		  Specific therapeutic measures, such as dressings, if appropriate; provide opportunity for practice and return demonstration

*If this type of follow-up care is the responsibility of the critical care unit nurse.

POTENTIAL PROBLEMS	EXPECTED OUTCOMES	NURSING ACTIVITIES
	Before discharge patient/ family is able to Verbalize knowledge of discharge regimen, including medications, dietary regimen, and activity progression and is able to perform specific therapeutic interventions Identify untoward signs/ symptoms requiring medical attention Describe plan for follow-up care, including purpose of visits, when and where to go, who to see, what specimens to bring	Describe signs and symptoms that require attention Describe plan for follow-up care, including purpose of visits, when and where to go, who to see, and what specimens to bring Provide opportunity for and encourage patient/family to ask questions Assess patient's potential compliance with discharge regimen

SURGICAL MANAGEMENT: DECOMPRESSIVE PORTOVENOUS SHUNTING PROCEDURES
Preoperative

■ Patient/family's anxiety related to Diagnostic, preparatory tests before surgery Surgery, its expected outcomes, and potential problems	■ Reduction in patient/family's anxiety with provision of information, explanations, and encouragement Patient/family verbalizes anxiety and asks questions Absence of nonverbal responses suggestive of anxiety	■ Ongoing assessment of patient/family's level of anxiety Assess patient/family's knowledge and understanding of certain diagnostic tests, rationale for these tests, and what patient will experience Explain, in simple terms, disease process, need for surgery, expected outcomes (and associated benefits), and potential problems Explain purpose of diagnostic tests and what patient will experience Encourage patient/family to verbalize fears and to ask questions Assess reduction in level of anxiety with provision of information, explanations, and encouragement

Postoperative

■ Hemodynamic instability related to Hemorrhage Fluid depletion from Loss of ascitic fluid when abdomen is surgically opened and/or during paracentesis Loss of lymphatic fluid during surgery Prolonged NG suctioning	■ Hemodynamic stability; BP, P, CVP, PAP, urine output, peripheral circulation, and mentation within normal limits	■ Monitor for (q½-1 hr) Hypotension Tachycardia Low CVP and PAP Reduced peripheral circulation Restlessness Signs and symptoms of hemorrhage including Bloody aspirate from NG tube or other drains Increasing tenseness of abdomen and size of abdominal girth Hct, Hgb, platelet, and albumin levels q6-12 hr until stable Daily weights Excessive amounts of NG drainage Notify physician of any abnormality If hemodynamic instability occurs Administer fluids, fresh whole blood, fresh frozen plasma, platelets, clotting factors, and/or vitamin K as ordered Closely monitor patient's response
■ Shunt closure related to Small caliber of shunt Low blood flow through shunt (hypotension)	■ Patent decompressive shunt Severe portal hypertension does not recur	■ Administer fluids, blood products as ordered Monitor for hypotension, increasing abdominal girth, recurring ascites, increasing weight, progressive encephalopathy, signs of increased pressure in esophageal varices, esophageal bleeding Monitor indices of liver function for the following Decreasing protein, albumin, and fibrinogen levels Abnormal coagulation studies Elevated bilirubin, ammonia levels Elevated liver enzyme levels (alkaline phosphatase, transaminases) Notify physician of significant abnormalities in any of aforementioned measurements

POTENTIAL PROBLEMS	EXPECTED OUTCOMES	NURSING ACTIVITIES
■ Abnormal electrolyte levels Hyponatremia Hypokalemia—often associated with diuretic therapy	■ Electrolyte levels within normal limits Absence of signs/symptoms of electrolyte imbalance	■ Monitor for Signs and symptoms of electrolyte imbalance Serum and urine electrolyte levels q12-24 hr Notify physician of any abnormality Administer electrolyte replacement as ordered
■ Progressive liver dysfunction related to Decreased circulation to liver, which can produce central lobular necrosis with marked deterioration in liver function within 36 hours after surgery Slow progressive deterioration in liver function that may result from deficient hepatic blood supply associated with bypass operation	■ Liver function tests reveal no postoperative deterioration Absence of encephalopathy, ascites, and bleeding (coagulation disorders)	■ If possible, decompressive shunt is chosen that does not significantly impair hepatic blood flow, such as renal-splenic shunt Progressive liver dysfunction is prevented with careful postoperative maintenance of blood flow to liver by administering fluids and blood products as ordered Monitor for parameters indicating liver dysfunction (encephalopathy, jaundice, bleeding, ascites) Notify physician of any abnormality If liver failure occurs, see Medical management
■ Coagulation abnormalities related to Liver dysfunction with reduction of prothrombin, clotting factors Administration of stored blood in perioperative period, particularly in presence of low circulating levels of clotting factors, prothrombin	■ Hgb, Hct levels remain stable without exogenous blood administration Coagulation studies within normal limits Absence of bleeding from mucous membranes or petechiae, ecchymoses	■ Prevent bleeding by using small-gauge needles for injections; maintain indwelling catheters for regular collection of blood specimens Provide for safe environment Padded siderails can be employed to prevent trauma, hematoma formation Administer vitamin K as ordered to assist in synthesis of prothrombin Assess extent of coagulation abnormality: presence of ecchymoses, petechiae, any spontaneous bleeding from mucous membranes or puncture sites Monitor (q6-12 hr until stable) PT, APTT Hct, Hgb, and platelet levels Hematest results on all drainages or specimens including NG aspirates, urine, and stool Notify physician of any abnormality If coagulation abnormalities occur, administer replacement in form of fresh blood, fresh frozen plasma, and/or platelets as ordered
■ Encephalopathy related to Venous blood, carrying nitrogenous waste products, is shunted away from liver Protein (nitrogen) load from surgical blood loss and blood remaining in GI tract from preoperative bleeding Anesthetics	■ Minimal or no encephalopathy after decompressive liver shunt Patient oriented to place and person	■ See Medical management
■ Respiratory insufficiency related to Cerebral depression from anesthesia Encephalopathy Splinting from incisional pain Diaphragmatic elevation from ascites	■ Absence of respiratory insufficiency Full diaphragmatic excursion and lung expansion sufficient to maintain Pao_2 and $Paco_2$ levels within normal limits	■ Prevent by Encouraging patient to cough and deep breathe q1 hr Repositioning patient q1-2 hr Administering chest physiotherapy q3-4 hr or as needed Administering incentive spirometry and/or IPPB as ordered Administering supplemental humidified O_2 as ordered Administering analgesics as ordered for pain relief and to permit effective pulmonary physiotherapy Administering analgesics that require little liver metabolism, with decreased dosages to prevent mental or respiratory depression

POTENTIAL PROBLEMS	EXPECTED OUTCOMES	NURSING ACTIVITIES

		Monitor patient's ongoing respiratory status, particularly noting presence of
		  Dyspnea, tachypnea, shallow breathing
		  Difficulty in effective deep breathing, coughing, and/or turning
		  Signs/symptoms of hypoxia
		  Arterial blood gas results indicating hypoxemia, hypercapnia
		Notify physician of any abnormality
		If respiratory insufficiency occurs, see Standard 2, *Acute respiratory failure*

■ Malnutrition	■ Positive nitrogen balance Weight stability or weight gain in form of muscle mass, not ascites	■ See Medical management Maintain NG aspiration, as ordered, for first few postoperative days until bowel sounds return Administer antacids to neutralize gastric hyperacidity associated with hypersecretion if ordered Administer nutrients as ordered after surgery (to prevent sustained negative nitrogen balance)

■ Insufficient information to comply with discharge regimen*	■ Sufficient information to comply with discharge regimen
	Before discharge patient/family is able to
	Verbalize knowledge of discharge regimen, including schedule for medications, dietary regimen, activity levels; and perform specific therapeutic interventions
	Identify untoward signs/symptoms require demonstration
	Describe signs and symptoms that requiring medical attention
	Describe plan for follow-up care, including purpose for visits, when and where to go, who to see, and what specimens to bring
		■ Assess patient/family's knowledge and understanding of discharge regimen
		Instruct patient/family as needed in
		  Medications, including identification, dosage, frequency, timing, and precautionary measures
		  Dietary regimen
		  Activity progression
		  Specific therapeutic measures (e.g., dressings); provide opportunity to practice and for return demonstration
		Describe signs and symptoms that require medical attention
		Describe plan for follow-up care, including purpose of visits, when and where to go, who to see, and what specimens to bring
		Provide opportunity for and encourage patient/family's questions
		Assess patient's potential compliance with discharge regimen

*If critical care nurse is responsible for this type of follow-up care.

PANCREATITIS

Pancreatitis is an inflammation of the pancreas that may occur with a mild or fulminant course. There are varying degrees of severity, which range from acute edema to hemorrhagic (necrotic) inflammation.

Acute edematous pancreatitis includes interstitial pancreatic edema with escape of enzymes into nearby tissues and peritoneal entry. Peritoneal fluid accumulates and is accompanied by tenderness across the upper abdomen, abdominal and back pain, and nausea and vomiting. Lipase causes fatty necrosis of the omentum; blood lipase and amylase levels are elevated.

Acute interstitial pancreatitis may become hemorrhagic where enzymatic digestion of the pancreas is more widespread. Blood escapes into the pancreatic tissue and into the retroperitoneum, resulting in more severe abdominal and back pain, often with clinical signs and symptoms of peritonitis. The peripancreatic tissue becomes necrotic.

The pancreas is a gland and an accessory organ of digestion. The normal exocrine function of the pancreas is to produce digestive enzymes for protein, carbohydrate, and fat metabolism. The normal endocrine function of the pancreas is responsible for production of insulin and glucagon, which regulate glucose metabolism. Both the endocrine and exocrine functions may be altered in the patient with pancreatitis, resulting in digestive and metabolic abnormalities.

There are many different causes of pancreatitis. Biliary tract disease is the most common disorder associated with the development of pancreatitis. It is postulated that gallstones may block the ampulla of Vater, causing a reflux of bile into the pancreas. The bile activates the pancreatic enzymes, and autodigestion of the pancreatic tissues takes place. The histological damage caused by biliary tract disease is usually not permanent.

Pancreatitis can also be induced by alcohol abuse. The exact etiological mechanism is not known, but two major theories exist. One theory postulates that alcohol increases gastric and pancreatic secretions, induces duodenal wall inflammation, and stimulates edema and spasm of the ampulla of Vater, thereby producing partial obstruction. Alcohol intake also causes a decreased gastric pH, which stimulates constant secretion of pancreatic juices in the face of a partially obstructed ampulla, resulting in acute edematous pancreatitis and eventually in hemorrhagic pancreatitis and/or in fibrosis. The second theory postulates that alcohol ingestion produces a metabolic effect on the pancreatic tissue. With prolonged use of alcohol, histological changes in the duct system occur that impede drainage of the enzymes. Tissue changes also may cause irregularity in the production of insulin and glucagon. The histological changes associated with prolonged alcohol ingestion are usually permanent and not reversible, even if alcohol ingestion is curtailed.

Other abnormalities that are associated with and can precipitate pancreatitis include the following:

1. Vasculitis of the different vessels in systemic lupus erythematosus
2. Steroid and/or thiazide therapy
3. Infectious organisms from the blood stream, i.e., mumps, scarlet fever
4. Staphylococcal food poisoning
5. Hyperlipemia, hyperparathyroidism
6. Dietary indiscretion with higher fat intake
7. Trauma (blunt or penetrating injury in upper abdominal trauma)
8. Iatrogenic causes (surgical)
9. Complications of pregnancy
10. Genetic disorders, i.e., defects in renal tubular reabsorption of lysine and cystine
11. Heredity

ASSESSMENT

1. History that includes
   a. Alcohol intake—type and amount
   b. Biliary tract disease (''gallstone'')
   c. Duodenal ulcer
   d. Recent abdominal surgery
   e. Recent trauma to abdomen
   f. Hereditary pancreatitis
   g. Hyperlipemia
   h. Any other diseases present
   i. Medications, particularly steroids, diuretics
   j. Onset of infectious disease, e.g., mumps
2. Presence, nature, and severity of
   a. Nausea and vomiting
   b. Abdominal distention, adynamic ileus, constipation

413

c. Peritonitis

d. Fever

e. Severe intense abdominal pain; determine the location of pain to assist in localizing the lesion in the head, body, or the tail of the pancreas; lesions in the tail are associated with left upper quadrant pain, those in the body are associated with epigastric pain, and those in head are associated with epigastric or right upper quadrant pain

f. Weakness

g. Distress, restlessness, anxiety

h. Dyspnea (diaphragmatic instability)

i. Hypotension, tachycardia, diaphoresis, even shock, with an associated oliguria

j. Mottled skin, cold extremities

k. Weight gain or loss

l. Nutritional status, including dietary history, appearance of mucous membranes, general strength, degree of muscle atrophy

3. Presence of the following signs (most often seen in hemorrhagic pancreatitis and related to extravasation of sloughing tissue)

   a. Grey Turner sign: bluish green, brown discoloration in the flank (blood in retroperitoneal routes)

   b. Cullen sign: bluish discoloration around umbilicus (blood dissecting beneath anterior abdominal muscles)

   c. Tetany: tonic spasm of any muscle with occasional generalized convulsions (calcium binds with free lipids)

4. Results of lab and diagnostic tests

   a. Blood amylase, lipase levels

   b. CBC: Hgb, Hct, WBC levels (neutrophils elevated in 90% of patients with pancreatitis)

   c. Electrolyte levels; hyperglycemia or hypoglycemia, abnormal protein, albumin, globulin, bilirubin, and calcium levels

   d. Urine amylase levels—note diagnostic elevation of more than 500 μm/hour in patients with acute interstitial pancreatitis; no elevation in amylase output may be present in patients with hemorrhagic pancreatitis

e. Urine glucose and fat levels

f. Fecal fat and trypsin levels, particularly if steatorrhea is present

g. Chest radiograph for elevation of the left side of diaphragm and left pleural effusion

h. Abdominal radiograph for presence of distended, gas-filled loops of intestine, signs of paralytic ileus

i. Arteriography

j. Biliary tract studies, IV cholangiography

k. Sonogram studies

l. ECG for presence of transient S-T segment depression, T wave changes

5. Level of patient/family's anxiety related to the disease process, accompanying signs and symptoms, diagnostic and lab tests, therapeutic regimen, and prognosis

GOALS

1. Reduction in patient/family's anxiety with provision of information and explanations

2. Hemodynamic stability

3. Pancreatic stress minimized; function adequate for digestion of nutrients, maintenance of blood glucose within normal limits

4. Adequate intake of nutrients, vitamins to meet calculated daily requirements, weight stabilization or weight gain

5. Respiratory sufficiency, with Pao_2 and $Paco_2$ within normal limits

6. Absence of pleural effusions, pulmonary interstitial edema, or pulmonary microemboli

7. Infection free—absence of peritonitis

8. Electrolyte levels and acid-base balance within normal limits

9. Absence or resolution of potential problems, including pseudocyst, cyst, or abscess formation

10. Before discharge patient/family correctly verbalizes postdischarge regimen, including

    a. Medications

    b. Dietary management

    c. Activity progression

    d. Plan for follow-up visits

POTENTIAL PROBLEMS	EXPECTED OUTCOMES	NURSING ACTIVITIES
■ Patient/family's anxiety related to insufficient knowledge of disease process, planned therapeutic intervention, and/or diagnostic procedures	■ Reduction in patient/family's anxiety with provision of information regarding disease process, therapy, and/or diagnostic procedures	■ Assess patient/family's level of anxiety Assess patient/family's understanding of disease process and therapy employed Explain in simple terms disease process and its relationship to therapy employed Assess patient/family's understanding of diagnostic procedures and results Explain purpose of planned diagnostic procedures and what patient will experience Evaluate reduction in anxiety

POTENTIAL PROBLEMS	EXPECTED OUTCOMES	NURSING ACTIVITIES
■ Hemodynamic instability, which may be associated with 　Fluid loss into peritoneum, retroperitoneal space 　Serum, plasma, albumin, blood loss into peritoneum, peritoneal space 　Fever 　Dehydration from nausea and vomiting 　Coagulation defects, with blood loss associated with DIC	■ Hemodynamic stability 　BP, P, CVP, PAP, peripheral circulation, urine output within normal limits 　Stable Hct and Hgb 　Absence of bleeding 　Afebrile	■ Monitor for 　Extent of hemodynamic instability: BP, P, CVP, and PAP if available (q2-4 hr); daily weight; urine output; peripheral circulation; and mentation 　Signs of internal bleeding (hemorrhagic pancreatitis) 　　Low Hgb, Hct levels q6-12 hr 　　Cullen sign 　　Grey Turner sign 　　Measure for increasing abdominal girth q4-8 hr, depending on rate of progression 　Notify physician of any abnormality 　If problem occurs 　　Administer fluid, blood, or blood products as ordered 　　Administer vitamin K as ordered 　　Administer antipyretic agents as ordered 　　See Standard 65, *Disseminated intravascular coagulation*
■ Pancreatic dysfunction with altered production of digestive enzymes, insulin, and glucagon	■ Minimal pancreatic stress; function adequate for digestion of nutrients and maintenance of blood glucose within normal limits	■ Monitor for (q6-12 hr) 　Serial serum amylase, lipase levels 　Urine amylase levels 　Serial blood glucose levels 　Signs of hyperglycemia: polydipsia, polyuria, polyphagia, weakness 　Urine for elevated glucose, acetone levels 　Digestive disturbances 　Steatorrhea 　Nature, severity of clinical signs/symptoms of pancreatitis, i.e., nausea, and vomiting, pain, fever 　Notify physician of any abnormality 　Administer therapy to include 　　NPO in acute phase 　　NG tube to continuous low suction; note character and amount of drainage q2-4 hr; maintain patency 　　Frequent mouth care; apply lubricant around NG tube and nares 　　Evaluate for presence of earaches and parotitis if use of NG tube is prolonged 　　Nonabsorbable antacids q1-2 hr 　　Cimetidine or another H$_2$ antagonist as ordered 　　Anticholinergics as ordered 　　Antipyretics if needed, as ordered; alcohol sponges, cooling blanket as needed 　　Calm and quiet environment 　Reduce metabolic requirements to minimum 　　Keep patient resting; bed rest in acute phase 　　Administer sedation if needed, as ordered 　　O$_2$ therapy if hypoxia develops (reduces respiratory effort) 　Provide adequate nutritional intake with minimal stimulation of pancreas; may be done with IV hyperalimentation 　Administer supplemental insulin and/or enzyme preparations if needed, as ordered 　Administer other medications/agents as ordered 　　Steroids 　　5-Fluorouracil: decreases metabolism of pancreatic cells and production of enzymes 　　Propylthiouracil: decreases metabolism of pancreatic cells and production of enzymes 　　Bile salts to prevent loss of fat in stool and to facilitate digestion and absorption of vitamins A, D, E, and K

POTENTIAL PROBLEMS	EXPECTED OUTCOMES	NURSING ACTIVITIES
■ Malnutrition related to Alcoholism Low vitamin and nutrient intake Abnormal, inefficient metabolism	■ Absence or resolution of malnutrition Weight gain or maintenance Positive nitrogen balance	■ Assess nutritional status and general appearance for presence of Dry, flaky, and cracked skin Tongue—dry and discolored Sunken eyeballs Loss of appetite Lethargy Poor skin turgor; flaccidity Decreased muscle control; tremors and twitching Provide adequate nutritional intake as ordered IV hyperalimentation may be employed in acute phase, followed by bland, low-fat, high-calorie diet, or if fed via enteral tube, elemental diet, e.g., Vivonex, Vital, is preferred as tube feeding Avoidance of coffee, tea, alcohol, and spicy, hot, or rich foods Supplementary pancreatic enzyme preparations (pancreatin [Viokase], pancrelipase [Cotazym]) and/or insulin may be ordered Vitamin supplements, including vitamin K, may be ordered Ongoing assessment of nutritional status and therapy, including Weight loss or gain Muscle atrophy, weakness Changes in skin turgor Altered mental status—restlessness, irritability, confusion
■ Respiratory failure related to Pain, producing splinting and hypoventilation Atelectasis Respiratory distress syndrome (pulmonary interstitial edema) related to inflammatory process and vigorous fluid administration Pleural effusion with exudation of serous fluid from pancreatic area Microemboli	■ Respiratory sufficiency with adequate oxygenation and ventilation (PaO_2 and $PaCO_2$ within normal limits) Absence and/or resolution of pleural effusion, pulmonary interstitial edema, or pulmonary microemboli	■ Administer analgesics (usually meperidine and dihydromorphinone [Dilaudid]) as ordered for pain to prevent splinting and hypoventilation; morphine is usually contraindicated, as it may cause spasm of sphincter of Oddi Administer vigorous chest physiotherapy q2-4 hr Reposition q1-2 hr Monitor chest radiograph results for presence of atelectasis, pleural effusion, pulmonary interstitial edema, and microemboli every day Provide cool, oxygenated vapor therapy as ordered for adequate oxygenation and humidification of secretions If microemboli are suspected, monitor results of coagulation studies Monitor For pain and associated splinting Respirations for rate and quality q1-2 hr; note tachypnea, dyspnea, wheezing Breath sounds q1-2 hr; note decreased or absent breath sounds or presence of adventitious breath sounds Secretions for amount, consistency, and color Chest radiograph results for atelectasis, interstitial edema Arterial blood gas results for hypoxemia, hypercapnia, or acidosis If problem occurs, see Standard 2, *Acute respiratory failure,* and, if appropriate, Standard 6, *Mechanical ventilation;* Standard 7, *Positive end-expiratory pressure*
■ Peritonitis related to leakage of pancreatic enzymes into peritoneum causing inflammation and infection	■ Absence and/or resolution of peritonitis Afebrile	■ Monitor for signs and symptoms of peritonitis, including abdominal pain, rigidity; fever, elevated WBC count daily If problem occurs, see Standard 45, *Peritonitis*
■ Electrolyte imbalance related to Hypocalcemia—fatty acids combine with Ca^{++} Hyperkalemia/hypokalemia from diuretics, vomiting and NG suctioning	■ Electrolyte levels within normal limits Absence of signs, symptoms of electrolyte imbalance	■ Monitor serial serum electrolyte levels Monitor for signs/symptoms of electrolyte imbalance: weakness; altered mental status (e.g., lethargy, irritability); arrhythmias; tetany, particularly from second or third day in episode of acute pancreatitis Notify physician of any abnormality If problem occurs, administer electrolyte replacement as ordered

POTENTIAL PROBLEMS	EXPECTED OUTCOMES	NURSING ACTIVITIES

■ Ketoacidosis, which may be related to low insulin levels and diabetes, with incomplete fat metabolism and ketosis	■ Absence and/or resolution of ketoacidosis	■ Monitor (q 6-12 hr)
		    Blood and urine pH levels
		    Abnormal electrolyte levels
		    For glucose and acetone in urine
		Notify physician of any abnormality
		If ketoacidosis occurs, see standard 56, *Diabetic ketoacidosis*

■ Pseudocyst—capsule of cellular debris and irritating substances that may lead to
Cysts in pancreas (collection of fluid usually rich in pancreatic enzymes and necrotic tissue, which is enclosed by fibrous wall)
Abscess
Bleeding
	■ Absence of pseudocyst, cyst, abscess formation	■ Administer antibiotics as ordered to prevent or combat secondary infection and secondary abscess formation
		Monitor for
		    Pattern (location and intensity), progression of pain and abdominal discomfort
		    Fever q1-2 hr
		    Leukocytosis q6-12 hr
		    Signs/symptoms of large cyst pressing against stomach or colon
		Notify physician of any abnormality
		If pseudocyst, cyst, or abscess occurs, surgery may be employed for drainage
		    Prepare patient for procedure

■ Insufficient information to comply with discharge regimen*	■ Sufficient information to comply with discharge regimen
	Patient/family correctly verbalizes postdischarge medication, dietary, and activity progression regimen
	Patient/family describes signs and symptoms that require medical follow-up
	Patient/family correctly describes plan for follow-up visits
		■ Assess patient/family's level of understanding regarding discharge regimen
		Explain in simple terms what pancreatitis is and purpose of therapy employed
		If appropriate, teach about hazards of continued alcohol intake; Alcoholics Anonymous may be recommended
		If diabetes is present, teach patient how to control this disease (see Standard 56, *Diabetic ketoacidosis*)
		Describe signs and symptoms of recurrent attack of pancreatitis and indicate how and where patient should get help
		Discuss dietary modifications, including avoidance of spicy, hot foods; heavy meals (eat smaller, more frequent meals); alcohol, tea, and coffee
		Discuss the medication regimen, including
		    Identification, dosage, frequency, timing
		    Pancreatic supplement
		    Antibiotics, if being continued
		    Analgesic, if needed and ordered
		    Insulin, if needed
		Describe progression in level of activity in postdischarge period
		Discuss plan for follow-up care, including purpose of visits, when and where to go, who to see, and what specimens to bring
		Provide opportunity for and encourage questions and verbalization of anxiety regarding discharge regimen
		Assess potential compliance with discharge regimen

*If critical care nurse is responsible for this type of follow-up care.

PANCREATIC SURGERY

Pancreatic surgery involves partial or total removal of the pancreas and resection/repair of contiguous organs. It may be performed for several pathophysiological problems, including tumors (e.g., carcinomas), hemorrhagic pancreatitis unresponsive to medical therapy, recurrent relapsing pancreatitis, and complications of acute pancreatitis unresponsive to medical therapy, recurrent relapsing pancreatitis, and complications of acute pancreatitis such as abscess, pseudocyst, and pancreatic ascites.

A *Whipple operation* is a surgical procedure in which a tumor of the head of the pancreas, the adjacent stomach, and the distal portion of the common bile duct are removed. The remaining portion of the common bile duct is sutured to the end of the jejunal segment, and the remaining pancreas and gastric remnant are anastomosed to the side of the jejunal loop. This procedure is performed for tumors invading contiguous organs including adenocarcinomas, beta or alpha cell tumors, and cystoadenocarcinomas. If a Whipple operation is not possible, obstruction and jaundice may be relieved by a cholecystojejunostomy or choledochojejunostomy to divert bile from the gallbladder into the jejunum.

Radiotherapy and chemotherapy may be employed to shrink the tumor and achieve pain relief. Low cure rates associated with partial pancreatectomy have resulted in increasing employment of total pancreatectomy to achieve removal of all cancer cells. This surgery results in less frequent anastomotic disruption but often produces a brittle type of diabetes.

Surgical intervention for hemorrhagic pancreatitis not responding to medical therapy may include debridement of necrotic pancreatic tissues, a choledochotomy, insertion of a T tube for any common bile duct obstruction, and placement of large drains near the pancreas. Surgery may be considered for chronic relapsing pancreatitis to establish a free flow of bile into the duodenum and to eliminate obstruction of the pancreatic duct. This is accomplished by sphincterotomy, or dilatation of the sphincter of Oddi, or reimplantation of the distal end of the duct into a limb of the jejunum.

A vagotomy may be performed to reduce the volume of gastric acid, which can ulcerate a fresh anastomosis.

Trauma may result in formation of a persistent pancreatic fistula or delayed formation of a pseudocyst. Fistulas can be surgically treated by implantation of the duct or tract into the duodenum or jejunum; a pseudocyst can be simply drained externally or internally with a cystogastrostomy or cystojejunostomy.

Whenever pancreatic surgery is performed, a gastrostomy attached to suction/gravity drainage may be employed to decrease gastric contents in the duodenum and reduce stimulation of pancreatic secretion. A jejunostomy may be placed for feedings to prevent duodenal stimulation of pancreatic function and/or to bypass duodenal obstruction.

ASSESSMENT

1. Presence, nature, and extent of
   a. Abscess: episodic temperature elevations; elevated WBC count, ESR; chest and abdominal radiographs may indicate subdiaphragmatic collection
   b. Pseudocyst: left upper quadrant mass; chest and abdominal radiographs may indicate subdiaphragmatic mass
   c. Pancreatic ascites: abdominal ascites and distention
2. Result of lab and diagnostic data
   a. Elevated alkaline phosphatase, bilirubin levels if common duct obstruction or hepatic metastasis is present; neoplastic obstruction produces higher bilirubin levels than are seen with benign biliary obstruction
   b. Diagnostic secretin stimulation of pancreatic secretions may induce release of malignant cells, collected in the duodenum
   c. Upper GI series may reveal invasion (filling defect) by tumor
   d. Angiography of the pancreas often reveals distortion of pancreatic vessels by the tumor and increased vascularization within the tumor
   e. Transhepatic cholangiogram or retrograde cannulation of biliary system may reveal common bile duct obstruction
3. Patient/family's knowledge regarding operative therapy—what they have been told, their expectations, fears regarding surgery and the outcomes, previous experiences with surgery, if any

4. Information and detail surgeon has provided about the need for surgery, the actual surgery to be done, and the expected outcome
5. Patient/family's level of anxiety related to surgery and prognosis

GOALS

1. Reduction in patient/family's anxiety with provision of information and explanations
2. Pancreatic secretory function kept at a minimum, yet adequate for digestion of nutrients and maintenance of blood glucose levels within normal limits
3. Hemodynamic stability
   a. Absence of intraoperative, postoperative hemorrhage
   b. Anastomosis intact
4. Respiratory function sufficient to maintain adequate oxygenation and ventilation
5. Adequate intake of nutrients; weight gain or weight stabilization
6. Infection free—absence of wound infection, peritonitis, or sepsis
7. Prevention of or resolution of potential problems, including pseudocyst, cyst, or abscess formation
8. Before discharge patient/family is able to verbalize
   a. Medication regimen, dietary management, and activity progression
   b. Signs and symptoms necessitating medical attention
   c. Plan for follow-up visits

POTENTIAL PROBLEMS	EXPECTED OUTCOMES	NURSING ACTIVITIES
Preoperative		
■ Patient/family's anxiety related to insufficient information regarding Disease process Medical therapy employed Anticipated diagnostic procedures Surgical intervention	■ Reduction in patient/family's anxiety with provision of information, explanations	■ Assess patient/family's level of anxiety Assess patient/family's understanding of disease process and ongoing medical therapy Explain disease process and its relationship to medical therapy employed in simple terms Assess patient/family's understanding of diagnostic procedures and results Explain purpose of diagnostic procedures and what patient will experience Describe preoperative experiences and therapeutic regimen, including Preoperative Orient patient to chest physiotherapy (call therapist if available) Coughing and deep breathing Incentive spirometry Postural drainage Shave Light dinner, then NPO after midnight Morning bath/shower Preoperative medications Hospital gown Care of valuables Ride to operating room Scrub suits, masks, and hats worn by operating room staff Anesthesia Postoperative Waking up in recovery room/critical care unit Describe general environment (size of unit, room, etc.) Dull, continuous noises If anticipated, breathing tube that may be temporarily in place Incision with bandage IV, arterial lines ECG monitoring Medicine for discomfort, pain Policy on family visits As patient progresses Tubes out Ambulation Coughing and deep breathing, chest physiotherapy Describe responsibility of patient in achieving speedy recovery by taking active role in coughing and deep breathing to keep lungs clear, etc. Encourage patient/family's questions

POTENTIAL PROBLEMS	EXPECTED OUTCOMES	NURSING ACTIVITIES
		Encourage verbalization of anxiety, fears related to hospitalization, diagnostic procedures, therapeutic regimen, surgery, and anticipated surgical outcomes Evaluate reduction in patient/family's level of anxiety

■ Malnutrition	■ Weight gain, at least back to preoperative baseline level
	Positive nitrogen balance
	Absence or resolution of any signs of malnutrition
		■ Assess nutritional status including
		  Dietary history
		  History of weight loss
		  Appearance of mucous membranes
		  Skin turgor; dry, flaky skin; spongy gums that bleed easily
		  Swollen joints, muscle atrophy
		Notify physician of presence of these abnormalities
		Administer nutrients and IV hyperalimentation as ordered
		
		See STANDARD 57 *Total parenteral nutrition*

■ Dehydration	■ Absence and/or resolution of dehydration
	Patient's appearance, including eyes, skin, and mucous membranes, indicates good level of hydration
		■ Assess state of hydration, including
		  History of nausea and vomiting
		  History of acute weight loss (over hours to 2 to 3 days)
		  Appearance of mucous membranes
		  Poor skin turgor
		  Dull sunken eyes
		Monitor
		  Intake and output q1 hr
		  BP, P, CVP, PAP, urine output, and peripheral circulation q½-1 hr until stable
		  Daily weights
		  LOC q2-3 hr
		Notify physician of any abnormalities
		If dehydration occurs, administer fluids as ordered

Postoperative
■ Hemorrhage related to leakage of pancreatic enzymes, digestive acids during and after surgery, causing breakdown of vascular (capillary) membranes
	■ Absence of hemorrhage
	Hct and Hgb within normal limits
	Adequate cardiac output
	Hemodynamic stability with BP, P within normal limits
		■ Monitor
		  Vital signs q1-2 hr and prn until stable
		  Note hypotension, tachycardia
		  CVP and PAP q1-2 hr; note low values
		  Intake and output q1 hr; note oliguria
		  Hct and Hgb levels q6 hr and more frequently if signs of bleeding occur
		Notify physician of abnormalities
		If hemorrhage occurs
		  Administer blood and blood products as ordered; carefully monitor patient's response
		  Monitor for continued bleeding

■ Pancreatic insufficiency secondary to
Initial excessive production/release of enzymes, insulin, glucagon
Deficient production of enzymes, insulin, glucagon
	■ Blood glucose, urine glucose and acetone levels within normal limits	■ Monitor
		  Serum amylase levels daily
		  Serial blood glucose levels q6-12 hr and prn
		  Urine glucose and acetone levels q1 hr
		Notify physician of abnormalities in aforementioned
		If problem occurs
		  Administer glucose and/or insulin as ordered; carefully monitor patient's response
		
		See STANDARD 47 *Pancreatitis*

POTENTIAL PROBLEMS	EXPECTED OUTCOMES	NURSING ACTIVITIES
■ Peritonitis Occurs in approximately 30% of pancreatectomy patients May result from Preoperative peritonitis Leakage of irritating pancreatic enzymes and exudate into peritoneum during surgery	■ Absence of or resolution of peritonitis Abdomen undistended, supple/soft, and pain free Afebrile Absence of pancreatic enzymes leakage Intact anastomosis	■ Prevention Administer prophylactic antibiotics if ordered Surgery may be planned before preoperative peritonitis ensues Monitor For signs and symptoms of peritonitis q1 hr, particularly fever, general abdominal discomfort, nausea and vomiting Notify physician of any abnormalities If signs and symptoms of peritonitis occur Assist in careful insertion of drains into operative area, which may reveal exudate indicative of anastomotic rupture, formation of fistulas Assist in dye studies to document further anastomotic defect If problem occurs, administer appropriate antibiotics if ordered and assist with local drainage if instituted *See* STANDARD 45 *Peritonitis*
■ Peritonitis associated with ileus and/or abscess formation	■ Bowel function within normal limits Absence of or resolution of abscess formation	■ Prevention Encourage and assist in early ambulation Provide for patent NG tube and maintain on low suction Monitor for Presence and nature of bowel sounds q6-12 hr Serial measurements of abdominal girth daily and more often if signs of peritonitis occur Presence/absence of flatus and stool q12 hr Pain pattern q2 hr indicative of peritonitis, ileus, and/or abscess Complete blood count q6 hr for leukocytosis and increased sedimentation rate (during acute phase) Chest and abdominal radiograph daily for detection of subdiaphragmatic and peritoneal abscesses Notify physician of any abnormality If peritonitis occurs, see Standard 45, *Peritonitis*
■ Metabolic/digestive abnormality	■ Absence of and/or resolution of metabolic/digestive abnormality	■ Prevention Provide for preoperative nutritional supplementation, which may include IV hyperalimentation as ordered Administer pancreatic enzyme supplements, if ordered, just before meals Administer insulin as ordered Monitor for digestive disturbances q12-24 hr Indigestion Steatorrhea (persistent fatty diarrhea) Weight loss Notify physician of presence of any of these, and implement changes in therapy as ordered If problem occurs, see Standard 47, *Pancreatitis*
■ Fluid and electrolyte imbalance	■ Fluid and electrolyte levels within normal limits	■ Prevention Provide proper hydration and electrolyte replacement if needed, as ordered Monitor For signs and symptoms of electrolyte imbalance q1-2 hr Serial serum electrolyte levels q6 hr Accurate intake and output q1-2 hr; daily weights Notify physician of any abnormality If problem occurs, administer therapy as ordered *See* STANDARD 50 *Gastrointestinal surgery* STANDARD 47 *Pancreatitis*

POTENTIAL PROBLEMS	EXPECTED OUTCOMES	NURSING ACTIVITIES

■ Liver dysfunction related to
  Obstruction of splenic vein by tumor, causing splenomegaly and segmental portal hypertension with bleeding esophageal varices
  Obstruction of hepatic veins may cause Budd-Chiari syndrome (thrombosis of hepatic veins)
	■ Liver function tests within normal limits
	  Coagulation studies, transaminase levels within normal limits
	  Absence of hepatomegaly, icteric sclera
		■ Prevention by early detection of precipitating cause and implementation of therapy as indicated
		  Monitor
		   Liver function tests, including total protein, serum albumin levels; fibrinogen, prothrombin levels, coagulation studies; transaminase levels q6-12 hr during acute phase
		   For hepatomegaly, jaundice, icteric sclera q6-12 hr
		  Notify physician of any abnormality
		  If problem occurs, see Standard 46, *Liver failure/decompressive portovenous shunting procedures*

■ Wound and skin irritation, breakdown, which may result from
  Contact with irritating pancreatic drainage
  Malnutrition with poor healing
	■ Wound intact, without erythema, pain, and drainage
	  Skin intact, without signs of irritation (redness, swelling)
	  Adequate intake of nutrients, sufficient to maintain weight, considering age and pathophysiological abnormalities
		■ Prevention and management
		  Monitor for reddened excoriated skin
		  Administer alimentation for adequate nutritional requirement as ordered
		  Keep skin around wound dry
		  Protect skin by applying
		   A protective agent on skin that repels drainage
		   Peristomal (Stomahesive) pad to form an occlusive protective covering
		   Ostomy bag if drainage is leaking around as well as through sump drain

■ Pancreatic and duodenal fistulas including biliary fistulas related to
  Partial anastomotic disruption
  Distal obstruction
  Total disruption of anastomosis caused by inadequate blood supply to jejunal limb
  Pancreatic fistula
	■ Pancreatic and duodenal membrane intact
	  Absence of or resolution of fistula formation
		■ Maintain continuous patent suction system
		  Monitor for
		   Continued large volume drainage (400 to 600 ml) for more than 5 to 8 days
		   Skin breakdown (from activation of bile and pancreatic enzymes present)
		   Presence of obstruction as evidenced by plain abdominal radiography and upper GI series with contrast media results
		   Signs of subhepatic abscess and/or obstructive jaundice indicating anastomotic disruption
		  Notify physician of any of these abnormalities
		  If problem occurs
		   Administer alimentation as ordered, often including IV hyperalimentation; see Standard 57, *Total parenteral nutrition*
		   Administer skin care around fistula, including application of protein powder or agents to protect skin
		   Prepare patient for reconstructive surgery if planned

■ Intraabdominal abscess related to inadequate drainage and collection of fluid in subphrenic or subhepatic space	■ Absence of or resolution of intraabdominal abscess	■ Maintain continuous patent suction system
		  Monitor for
		   Spiking fevers; check vital signs, and temperature q1-2 hr
		   Ileus; note quality of bowel sounds q2 hr
		   Abdominal pain and tenderness q6-12 hr
		   Presence of pleural effusion, elevated diaphragm and collection of fluid in abdomen, and distended bowel as evidenced in daily chest and abdominal radiograph results; note sonogram results if procedure done
		   Elevation in bilirubin and alkaline phosphatase daily
		  Notify physician of any abnormality
		  If intraabdominal abscess occurs
		   Administer antibiotics and fluids as ordered
		   Administer sufficient nutrients, often via hyperalimentation, as ordered; see Standard 57, *Total parenteral nutrition*
		   Prepare patient for surgery if planned

POTENTIAL PROBLEMS	EXPECTED OUTCOMES	NURSING ACTIVITIES
■ Malnutrition related to prolonged absence of adequate nutritional intake Abnormal metabolism of nutrients caused by pancreatic dysfunction	■ Weight stable or gain Appearance and character of skin indicates good hydration, sufficient nutrient intake Moist, pink mucous membranes Muscle mass remains stable or increases in size and is firm	■ Determine presence of recent weight loss or gain Assess patient's dietary, beverage intake history Note adequacy of nutritional intake and intake of foods, beverages that may be related to present pathophysiology requiring surgery (e.g., amount of alcohol intake and amount of sugar-glucose in diet) Assess present nutritional status, including weight and appearance and character of skin, mucous membranes, muscle mass Monitor daily weights; intake of nutrients as ordered Provide for intake of required/needed nutrients If malnutrition occurs, administer nutrients as ordered, which may include hyperalimentation in presence of (or anticipation of) extended periods of NPO See Standard 47, *Pancreatitis*, or Standard 57, *Total parenteral nutrition*, as appropriate
■ Insufficient information to comply with discharge regimen*	■ Sufficient information for compliance with discharge regimen Patient/family correctly verbalizes postdischarge regimen regarding medications, diet, fluid intake, and progression in activity levels Patient/family describes signs and symptoms that require medical follow-up Patient/family correctly describes plan for follow-up visits	■ Assess level of patient/family's understanding of discharge regimen Explain patient's pathophysiological problem and rationale for postdischarge regimen in simple terms If appropriate, explain hazards of continued alcohol intake; Alcoholics Anonymous may be recommended Discuss importance of dietary modifications, including avoidance of spicy, hot foods, heavy meals, alcohol, tea, and coffee If diabetes is present, teach patient how to control this disease (see Standard 56, *Diabetic ketoacidosis*) Instruct patient/family about prescribed medications, including identification, dosage, frequency, timing Pancreatic supplement Antibiotic, if being continued Analgesic, if needed Insulin, if needed Discuss signs and symptoms of recurrence and indicate how/where patient should seek medical attention Explain plan for follow-up care, including purpose of visits, when and where to go, who to see, and what specimens to bring Assess patient/family's potential compliance with discharge regimen

*If responsibility of critical care nurse includes discharge teaching.

ACUTE UPPER GASTROINTESTINAL BLEEDING

Patients bleeding from the upper GI tract are always at risk of death from exsanguination and shock.

The clinical manifestation of upper GI bleeding varies with the underlying disease and extent of bleeding. Overt clinical manifestations are usually present, including hematemesis, melena, and hematochezia (which is the passage of bright red blood from the rectum).

Hematemesis of bright red or dark red blood indicates that the origin of bleeding is above the ligament of Treitz, usually in the stomach and esophagus. Hematemesis indicates a rapidly bleeding lesion, and surgery is required in a high percentage of patients. Coffee ground vomitus is blood that has been in the stomach long enough for the gastric acid to convert hemoglobin to methemoglobin. This does not indicate origin or time of bleeding.

Melena (the passage of tarry black stools) indicates bleeding from the upper GI tract. The appearance of melena is not, however, an accurate gauge of the time in which bleeding has occurred. It is thought that melena is the product of oxidation of heme by intestinal and bacterial enzymes.

Hematochezia may occur as a result of rapid intestinal transit of blood from the GI tract. The presence of blood in the stomach often produces increased gastric motility with gastric retention, vomiting, and hematochezia.

Orthostatic changes in BP and P and a low-value Hct are reliable indices of hemodynamic compromise in acute bleeding but may indicate an underestimated fluid loss. Renewed or major loss of circulating blood volume is evidenced by tachycardia; restlessness; pallor; diaphoresis; cool, clammy skin; and thirst.

The more common causes of upper GI hemorrhage include the following:

Esophagus—esophageal varices; Mallory-Weiss syndrome

Stomach—gastritis secondary to alcohol and drug intake; gastric ulcers; gastric varices

Duodenum—duodenal ulcer

Esophageal or gastric varices are frequently related to the portal hypertension associated with liver cirrhosis. Although bleeding tends to be massive and abrupt, minor bleeding may occur for days before detection.

The Mallory-Weiss syndrome is a longitudinal laceration of the mucosa near the esophagogastric junction associated with nonbloody vomiting followed by hematemesis after episodes of forceful retching.

Gastritis can include either generalized or localized erosions or ulcerations of the gastric mucosa associated with hyperacidity related to alcohol intake, drug ingestion, or stressful situations.

Ulcers are the most common cause of upper GI bleeding. The majority of these ulcers are found in the duodenum. About 25% of patients with ulcers will have at least one episode of GI bleeding.

Therapy is directed toward maintaining intravascular volume, stopping the hemorrhage, and defining the source of bleeding within a reasonable period of time.

ASSESSMENT

1. Baseline data regarding clinical history of
   a. Ulcer disease or epigastric pain relieved by food, milk, or antacid
   b. Previous bleeding episodes, vomiting, diarrhea, cramps, weight loss, fever, bleeding from other sites, i.e., skin, mucous membrane, etc.
   c. Family history of intestinal disease or hemorrhagic diathesis
   d. Recent ingestion of drugs known to irritate gastric mucosa
   e. Alcoholism; recent alcoholic binge
   f. Jaundice
   g. Forceful retching before hematemesis
   h. Frequent stressful and anxiety-provoking situations
   i. Smoking; number of packs per day
   j. Dietary habits
   k. Seasonal occurrence
   l. Associated diseases including hyperparathyroidism, polycythemia vera, chronic liver disease, chronic respiratory disease, uremia, and any malignancy, i.e., presence of rectal shelf, etc.
2. Presence, extent, and/or nature of
   a. Nonintestinal source of bleeding, i.e., rule out hemoptysis, epistaxis, and any pharyngeal lesions
   b. Associated conditions including signs of liver disease: jaundice, telangiectasia, spider angiomas, hepatomegaly, ascites, edema, and unusual skin pigmentation

c. Abdominal masses, nodes, and hepatosplenomegaly
d. Dilatated veins in flank, anteroabdominal region; hemorrhoids
e. Any obvious neurological or personality abnormalities
f. Frequency and character of vomitus and bowel sounds
g. Cachexia, especially of extremities
3. Baseline lab and diagnostic data for
   a. Abnormal serial blood counts, particularly leukocytosis; low Hct and Hgb; and red cell morphological abnormalities
   b. Abnormal serum electrolytes
   c. Serial BUN measurements for elevation
   d. Abnormalities in clotting studies
   e. Extent of positive Hematest of gastric aspirate, vomitus, and stool
   f. Results of endoscopic procedures
   g. Angiography and upper GI studies if done
   h. Abdominal radiograph for any visible free air
4. Patient/family's perception of and reaction to disease process, symptoms, diagnostic procedures, and therapy planned
5. Patient/family's understanding of disease process, purpose of hospitalization, therapy planned, expected prognosis, and, if appropriate, the surgery, expected outcome, and what the patient will experience in the perioperative period; if patient is an alcoholic, assess psychosocial effect on patient/family

GOALS

1. Reduction of patient/family's anxiety with provision of information and explanations
2. Absence and/or resolution of GI bleeding
3. Absence and/or resolution of any complications including pulmonary edema, renal failure, and coagulopathy
4. Hemodynamic stability
5. CBC, acid-base balance, and electrolyte levels within normal limits
6. Absence of any further deterioration of associated diseases related to upper GI bleeding
7. Nutritional intake sufficient to maintain body weight and positive nitrogen balance
8. Before discharge patient/family is able to
   a. Describe medication regimen
   b. Describe dietary regimen
   c. Describe activity regimen
   d. List signs and symptoms requiring medical attention
   e. State necessary information regarding follow-up care

POTENTIAL PROBLEMS	EXPECTED OUTCOMES	NURSING ACTIVITIES

■ Anxiety related to Hemorrhage	■ Patient demonstrates decreased level of anxiety with provision of emotional support and information	■ Assess level of anxiety
		Demonstrate interest and concern
		  Reassure and stay with patient
		  Explain all procedures before administering them
		  Perform procedures in unhurried manner
		  Maintain calm and pleasant manner when providing care
		Encourage verbalization of any anxiety or fears related to hemorrhage
		Prepare patient for and assist with diagnostic procedures
		Provide environment conducive to mental, physical, and emotional rest
		  Keep patient dry, warm, and comfortable
		  Allow for rest periods between treatments
		  Limit visitors according to patient's needs; inform visitors to avoid stressful conversations

Insufficient knowledge of Disease process Diagnostic procedures Therapy employed	Patient/family's behavior demonstrates decreased level of anxiety with provision of information and explanations Patient/family verbalizes understanding of disease process and its relationship to therapy employed Patient/family participates actively in planning and implementing care	Ongoing assessment of anxiety Describe nature of disease process and rationales for various therapeutic interventions Explain anticipated procedures involved in diagnostic process/plan of care and what patient will experience Assure that proper preparation is made before any diagnostic procedures Encourage patient/family's questions, verbalization of fears and anxieties Involve patient/family in planning for care

POTENTIAL PROBLEMS	EXPECTED OUTCOMES	NURSING ACTIVITIES

■ Hemorrhage	■ Control or resolution of hemorrhage
	Absence of blood volume deficit
	Normal circulating blood volume
		■ Monitor for
		  Any transfusion reactions
		  Hypoperfusion or hemodynamic instability including
		    Orthostatic vital signs and temperature q30 min until stable or as often as indicated by condition
		    Measurement of CVP, cardiac output, pulmonary pressures if available until stable q1 hr
		    Presence of tachycardia, diaphoresis, cold, clammy extremities, daily weights below what is expected
		    Oliguria, hourly intake and output until stable
		    Frequency, amount, nature of hematemesis and melena
		  Signs and symptoms of respiratory distress
		  Giddiness, restlessness, syncope, and any alterations in LOC
		  Arrhythmias, especially atrial arrhythmias
		  Serial blood count; Hct, and Hgb
		  Serial electrolytes; elevated BUN, ESR, etc.
		  Presence or absence and nature of bowel sounds
		  Clinical manifestations of perforation, including
		    Severe persistent abdominal pain, increasing in intensity
		    Pain radiating to shoulder
		    Boardlike rigidity, extremely tender abdomen
		    Abdominal radiographs showing presence of free air under diaphragm
		Notify physician of any abnormalities
		Administer continuous chilled saline lavage until clear with continuous suction via NG tube; norepinephrine (Levophed) may be added to iced saline lavage to effect localized vasoconstriction at bleeding site in stomach
		Administer parenteral fluids, blood expanders, and blood, as ordered
		Administer medications, i.e., vitamins K and B_{12}, sedatives, antacids, and H_2 inhibitors, as ordered
		Maintain patent airway, position to sides, aseptic suctioning if necessary; administer O_2 if ordered; frequent oral hygiene
		Reassure and stay with patient
		Endoscopy and angiography may be done to determine cause of hemorrhage and to tailor therapy
		  Explain procedure
		  Assist with procedure
		If surgery is indicated, see Standard 50, *Gastrointestinal surgery*

■ GI distress related to
 	
  Gastritis secondary to alcohol and drug abuse
  Ulcers—gastric and duodenal
	■ Absence or remission of
	
	  Gastritis
	
	  Ulcers
		■ Refer to Problem, Hemorrhage, for parameters permitting detection of hemorrhage and activities for control
		Intraarterial or IV infusion of vasopressin (Pitressin) may be ordered specifically for patients with gastritis
		Monitor for vasopressin side effects, including
		  Facial pallor, discomfort, abdominal colic, hypertension, abnormal ECG, chest pain, abdominal tenderness and distention, oliguria, and hyponatremia, H_2O intoxication
		  Catheter insertion site for infection, thrombosis, and embolism
		Administer cimetidine and H_2 inhibitor if ordered
		Administer antacid (that does not contain aluminum hydroxide and/or calcium carbonate) q1 hr as directed
		Administer anticholinergic drugs and sedatives if ordered specifically for patients with ulcers
		If surgery is indicated, see Standard 50, *Gastrointestinal surgery*
		Institute dietary regimen appropriate for gastric problem
		Provide environment conducive to physical and mental rest
		  Allow for rest periods between treatments
		  Limit visitors; inform them of need to avoid stressful conversations
		Monitor effectiveness of therapy/intervention
		Evaluate for health teaching regarding control of excessive drug and/or alcohol intake

POTENTIAL PROBLEMS	EXPECTED OUTCOMES	NURSING ACTIVITIES

Mallory-Weiss syndrome	Complete occlusion of tear either by embolization or surgical repair	Refer to Problem, Hemorrhage, for parameters permitting detection of hemorrhage and activities for control
		If embolization therapy is required
		  Explain procedure to patient
		  Prepare and shave area as ordered
		  Postembolization monitoring activity same as in Problem, Hemorrhage, with decreasing frequency as condition stabilizes
		If surgery is required, see Standard 50, *Gastrointestinal surgery*

Varices—esophageal and/or gastric	Absence or resolution of bleeding from varices	Refer to Problem, Hemorrhage, for control of hemorrhage
		Monitoring activity same as in Problem, Hemorrhage, with decreasing frequency as condition stabilizes
		Administer arterial or IV infusion of vasopressin if ordered
		Monitor for side effects of vasopressin therapy (see Problem, GI distress: Nursing activity—monitor for vasopressin side effects)
		Sengstaken-Blakemore (SB) tube may be used for active bleeding from esophageal and/or gastric varices
		Assist with insertion of SB tube
		  Check gastric and esophageal balloons for weak spots and leaks under H_2O after air inflation
		  Check patency of each lumen
		  Explain procedure to patient
		  Monitor patient's vital signs during insertion procedure
		  Stay with and reassure patient while tube is being inserted
		Once SB tube is in place, ensure proper inflation and stabilization
		SB tube has three ports; two ports are labeled "balloon," and each is inflated with air to compress bleeding varices in esophagus and/or fundus of stomach; third port; labeled "gastric aspirate," is drainage tube used to decompress or irrigate stomach.
		Esophageal balloon
		  Inflated to 20 to 40 mm Hg with air; check inflation pressure with sphygmomanometer; then clamp to prevent air escape
		Gastric balloon
		  Inflated with 200 to 500 cc of air; after inflation, clamp to prevent air leakage
		Gastric aspirate port
		  Drainage port that is used to decompress or irrigate stomach; this port should be attached to low intermittent suction; patency must be ensured
		NOTE: It is necessary for additional NG tube to be passed through nares into back of mouth to drain oropharyngeal secretions, since patient cannot swallow or cough; this tube should be connected to low suction and labeled "Do not irrigate—in back of mouth" to prevent accidental lavaging of tube and possible aspiration
		Secure SB tube in place; use slight traction
		Keep pair of scissors taped at bedside for emergency deflation of SB tube in case of acute respiratory distress secondary to occlusion of airway by balloon
		Assist with radiograph to verify proper placement of SB tube
		Monitor for respiratory distress
		Maintain traction on SB tube, as ordered
		Irrigate SB tube (gastric aspirate port) q1 hr and prn for patency with iced sterile saline; note color, amount, and nature of aspirate; continuous gastric lavage may be ordered; keep gastric port patent
		Check for prescribed pressure readings q½-1 hr and that lumens of SB tube are secured properly
		Deflate and inflate esophageal balloon if ordered
		Monitor for
		  Gross bleeding q1 hr
		  Abnormal vital signs q15-30 min
		  Lethargy, drowsiness, confusion, and unconsciousness
		  Chest pain, any respiratory distress
		  Serial Hct, Hgb, and electrolyte levels

POTENTIAL PROBLEMS	EXPECTED OUTCOMES	NURSING ACTIVITIES
		Keep head of bed elevated to 30 degrees unless patient is in shock
		Mouth and nares care q1 hr and prn
		Position to sides q1-2 hr and provide skin care
		Instruct patient not to gag, cough, or strain
		Reassure patient/family
		Encourage deep breathing exercise q1 hr
		Assist in removal of SB tube, usually 24 hours after bleeding has been controlled
		Assist in removal of SB tube
		Esophageal and gastric ports are usually deflated for a few hours before removal of tube to ensure that patient will not rebleed
		Notify physician of any abnormality
		If surgery is indicated, see Standard 50, *Gastrointestinal surgery*

■ Pulmonary edema caused by fluid overload	■ Absence or resolution of pulmonary edema
	Normal respiration pattern
	No obvious sign of chest congestion
		■ Prevent by cautious administration of colloid and crystalloid solution with careful monitoring of hemodynamic response
		Monitor for
		  Sudden coughing, restlessness, and anxiety
		  Marked dyspnea and orthopnea, tachycardia
		  Cyanosis, audible wheezing, and rales throughout lung fields
		  White or pink-tinged frothy sputum
		  Abnormal arterial blood gas levels
		  Any tachyarrhythmias
		  Hypotension and/or hypertension
		  Accurate intake and output, daily weights
		  Abnormal CVP, cardiac output, and pulmonary pressures if available
		  Notify physician of any abnormalities
		If problem occurs, see Standard 2, *Acute respiratory failure*

■ Coagulopathy and/or continued bleeding as result of massive transfusion reaction	■ Absence of and/or control of coagulopathy
	No continued bleeding
	Bleeding stops and does not recur
		■ Prevent by administration of platelets and fresh frozen plasma (about 1 unit per 3 to 4 units of banked blood) to replace factors necessary for coagulation
		Monitor for
		  Serial blood counts for leukocytosis, low Hgb and Hct; abnormal prothrombin and thrombin time, fibrinogen levels, bleeding tests, and immunoassays
		  Continuous gross bleeding: hematemesis and hematochezia
		  Any spontaneous skin discoloration including petechiae, bruises
		  Prolonged bleeding or oozing of injection sites, hematoma
		  Presence of hematuria
		  Notify physician of any abnormality
		If problem occurs, see Standard 65, *Disseminated intravascular coagulation*

■ Encephalopathy precipitated by GI bleeding with increased protein load	■ Absence or resolution of encephalopathy	■ Avoid the following abnormalities and therapies that can increase ammonia production
		  Administration of ammonium chloride
		  Diuresis of more than 1 to 2 kg/day
		  Dehydration, shock
		  Sedatives, narcotics, tranquilizers
		  Anesthesia, decompressive shunting procedures
		  Infection
		  Acid-base, electrolyte imbalance (avoid hypokalemic alkalosis); if acidification is needed, lactulose may be ordered to acidify bowel
		Prevent by
		  Administering lactulose, if ordered, to induce movement of ammonia from blood to colon; lactulose also has laxative action that promotes excretion of ammonium ion
		  Administering poorly absorbed antibiotics, if ordered (orally, by enema), to reduce nitrogen-forming intestinal bacteria
		  Administering antacids and/or anti-H_2 medication, if ordered, to reduce risk of GI bleeding

POTENTIAL PROBLEMS	EXPECTED OUTCOMES	NURSING ACTIVITIES
		NOTE: If GI bleeding is present, institute therapy to control it; maintain patient NPO; see Standard 46, *Liver failure/decompressive portovenous shunting procedures*
		Administering fluid volume repletion as ordered, usually inculding salt-poor albumin
		Monitor
		Blood ammonia and BUN levels; assist in titrating patient's protein intake to level that does not raise circulating ammonia and BUN to unacceptable levels
		Patient's LOC, mentation, speech, behavior, gait, and neuromuscular function
		Results of EEG, which may reflect diffuse slowing
		If encephalopathy occurs
		Maintain safe environment
		Reorient patient frequently to time, place, and person
		Explain procedures simply and clearly
		Avoid medications that depend heavily on liver metabolism: ammonia-containing drugs, amino compounds
		If sedation is needed, phenobarbital and chloral hydrate are preferred; occasionally diazepam is given in very small quantities
		Administer cathartic such as sorbitol in H_2O or magnesium citrate, as ordered, to reduce intestinal flora
		Reduce dietary intake of protein while providing adequate calories as ordered
		Low-protein tube feedings are available such as Lipomul-Oral
		When protein intake is resumed, start with 20 to 40 g protein/ day or as ordered and increase by 10 to 20 g q2 to 4 days as tolerated in adults
		Administer lactulose (adults: 35 to 70 g/day), if ordered, to produce acidic colonic pH, which favors movement of ammonia into stool
		Arginine or glutamic monochloride is sometimes ordered in effort to inactivate excess ammonia
■ Renal failure related to decreased renal perfusion	■ Absence and/or resolution of renal failure	■ Prevent by
		Careful administration of colloid and crystalloid solution
		Monitoring for adequate urine output
		Monitor for
		Hypotension, BP q1 hr until stable
		Oliguria and/or polyuria; accurate hourly intake and output
		Abnormal CVP, cardiac output, and PAP if available
		Serial blood and urinary electrolyte levels
		Serial increase in BUN and creatinine levels
		Any alterations in LOC
		Presence of albumin in urine, high specific gravity, and urine-to-plasma creatinine concentration (ratio is usually greater than 20)
		Notify physician of any abnormality
		If problem occurs, see Standard 52, *Acute renal failure*
■ Insufficient information to comply with discharge regimen*	■ Sufficient information to comply with discharge regimen	■ Assess patient/family's level of understanding and ability to comprehend; determine any physical limitations regarding follow-up plan of care or discharge regimen
	Patient/family verbalizes dietary, medication, and activity regimens	Describe discharge regimen, including
		Dietary regimen—antacids may be ordered to prevent mucosal irritation between meals
		Explain therapeutic diet and need for good eating habits, including
		Nutritionally adequate diet
		Meals to be eaten in quiet, relaxed environment
		Frequent small feedings; do not miss a meal

*If critical care nurse is responsible for this type of follow-up care.

POTENTIAL PROBLEMS	EXPECTED OUTCOMES	NURSING ACTIVITIES
		Foods to be chewed well
		Avoidance of irritating and hard-to-digest foods including fried foods, coffee, highly seasoned foods, and alcohol
		Need for bland diet and foods high in fat to neutralize acid
		Assist patient/family in planning diet
		Adjust diet to cultural and socioeconomic needs
		Vitamins may be ordered
		Medication regimen
		Names of drugs and purpose
		Specific dosage schedule in hours, considering patient's eating habits
		Expected adverse side effects, how to deal with them, and when to report to physician
		Avoidance of medications that will irritate esophageal and gastric mucosa, including aspirin, etc.; if necessary take them with meals, milk, or crackers
		Avoidance of over-the-counter medications
		Activity regimen
		Planned and regular exercise and rest activities; avoidance of fatigue
		Avoidance of certain activities such as eating a heavy meal
		Avoidance of straining at stool and constipation, heavy lifting, severe coughing, and vomiting
		Avoidance of smoking to prevent increase of gastric acid
		Encourage family involvement with activity progression
	Patient/family describes signs and symptoms that will require medical intervention	Identify signs and symptoms of
		Early bleeding
		Dizziness and blurred vision
		Coffee ground vomitus
	Patient/family verbalizes information on Alcoholics Anonymous association	Sudden or gradual weakness
		Dark stool, heme positive on testing
		Common colds and/or respiratory distress requiring medical attention
	Patient/family accurately describes plans for follow-up care	Provide information and referral services for available community resources to patient/family (e.g., Alcoholics Anonymous)
		Describe follow-up visits including reason for, when and where to go, who to see, and what specimens to bring
		Provide opportunity for and encourage patient/family's questions and verbalization of anxiety regarding discharge regimen
		Assess patient/family's potential compliance with discharge regimen

GASTROINTESTINAL SURGERY

GI surgery is performed when medical management is inadequate to control the adverse signs and symptoms of certain GI abnormalities. Surgery may also resolve or at least halt the progress of GI problems.

Operative therapy may be used to treat gastric or duodenal ulcers* in patients with intractable ulcers (recurrent despite therapy) and in the presence of perforation, hemorrhage, or gastric outlet obstruction. A duodenal ulcer may be treated with pyloroplasty and vagotomy, antrectomy with vagotomy, or gastroenterostomy with vagotomy. A gastric ulcer is treated by plication or by a partial or total gastrectomy with either a gastroduodenostomy (Billroth I) or gastrojejunostomy (Billroth II).

Tumors are removed if they are malignant or if they are benign but causing bleeding, obstruction, and/or intussusception. Gastric neoplasms are removed by partial or total gastrectomy. Small adenomas and mucosal excrescences may be removed by surgical excision using cold forceps and diathermy if they are not amenable to endoscopic removal.

Surgery is commonly required to resolve obstructive conditions of the GI tract, including simple mechanical obstruction and strangulation obstruction. Lesions that can produce bowel necrosis may also require surgery, such as a hernia, volvulus, intussusception, obturation, and complete obstruction caused by chronic adhesions. Surgery may also be necessary for a partial obstruction that does not respond adequately to medical decompressive efforts.

A superior mesenteric artery embolus can cause a "vascular obstruction" and necrosis of the bowel in that region. Early surgical intervention may permit adequate resolution with a mesenteric embolectomy, although a resection of the severely ischemic or necrotic bowel is usually required.

Regional enteritis, including regional ileitis, regional enterocolitis, and Crohn disease are inflammatory diseases that commonly occur in the terminal ileum, although they may occur anywhere along the GI tract. Surgery is indicated when medical management fails to control symptoms or

*For medical management of ulcers, see Standard 49, *Acute upper gastrointestinal bleeding.*

when complications such as obstruction, bleeding, colonic perforation, or fistula formation occur. If surgery becomes necessary in a period of acute exacerbation, a temporary ileostomy may be created.

Diverticulosis and diverticulitis are treated with surgery if any of the following occur: perforation, obstruction, fistula formation to surrounding tissue, massive hemorrhage, and chronic/recurrent symptoms. In general, surgery is avoided during an acute attack. Rather, antibiotics are administered and the inflammatory process is given time to subside. (If surgery appears to be necessary, it is postponed for 3 to 6 months whenever possible.) *If* acute symptoms persist for 1 week or more or there is evidence of acute perforation or abscess formation, surgery is usually indicated and may include the establishment of a transverse colostomy and drainage of any collections or abscesses present.

Essential components of the postoperative regimen include GI decompression of the bowel (until function resumes) and careful fluid and electrolyte replacement. Much of the nursing care is focused on prevention of and monitoring for potential postoperative problems, with appropriate revision of the plan of care should any occur.

ASSESSMENT

1. History, presence, and nature of
   a. Factors that predispose to intestinal obstruction
      (1) Previous abdominal surgery
      (2) Presence of marked adhesions
      (3) Abdominal injuries or wounds
      (4) Peritonitis
      (5) Volvulus, intussusception, diverticulitis, adenoma, or carcinoma of colon or rectum
      (6) Hernias
      (7) Other
   b. Factors that predispose to paralytic ileus
      (1) Recent abdominal surgery
      (2) Blunt trauma to abdomen
      (3) Electrolyte or metabolic abnormalities
   c. Factors that predispose to vascular obstruction
      (1) Aneurysm of aorta
      (2) Severe atherosclerosis of aorta

(3) Low cardiac output, atrial fibrillation, congestive heart failure

(4) Dehydration

d. Inflammatory diseases that can produce an obstruction and/or require primary resection

(1) Ulcerative colitis

(2) Regional enteritis

(3) Diverticulitis and diverticulosis

(4) Ulcer disease

(5) Appendicitis

e. Abnormalities that require primary resection or surgical revision

(1) Upper GI hemorrhage

(2) Peptic ulcer disease

(3) Appendicitis

(4) Diverticula

(5) Familial intestinal polyposis

(6) Small bowel fistulas

2. Signs and symptoms, including

a. Abdominal pain—manner of onset, location, radiation and intensity; note pain that is

(1) Continuous—may indicate strangulation, peritonitis

(2) Crampy

b. Abdominal tenderness, rebound tenderness

c. Abdominal rigidity (muscles over area of inflammation become spastic)

d. Abdominal distention

e. Bowel sounds—hyperactive, borborygmus, diminished, or absent

f. Anorexia, nausea and/or vomiting

g. GI bleeding

(1) Hematemesis

(2) Bloody mucus in rectum (may indicate intus-
suseption—more common in children)

(3) Bloody diarrhea (mesenteric infarction)

(4) Melena

h. Signs of recent abdominal trauma—wounds, contusions, lacerations

i. Signs of rupture of hollow viscus (bladder, peritoneum)

j. Signs of rupture of solid viscus ([spleen, liver, kid-
ney] see Standard 63, *Multiple trauma)*

k. Fever

l. Tachycardia

m. Jaundice

n. Constipation, obstipation

o. Diarrhea (nonbloody)

3. Lab and diagnostic data, including

a. WBC count with differential—note presence of leukocytosis

b. Electrolyte imbalance

c. Stool test positive for occult blood

d. Chest radiograph (upright, posterior, anterior) and
abdominal radiograph (upright and supine)—note results indicating free air or intestinal obstruction

e. Peritoneal lavage after abdominal trauma; note presence of blood and results of gram stain, culture, and
amylase determination

f. Urinalysis for WBC and RBC counts

g. Liver function tests (particularly in the presence of
GI bleeding)

(1) Coagulation study results

(2) Transaminase levels

(3) Alkaline phosphatase levels

(4) Serum total protein, albumin levels

(5) Albumin-globulin ratio

(6) Blood ammonia levels

h. Esophagogastroscopy

i. Gastroduodenoscopy

j. Fiberoptic endoscopy (if patient is not bleeding mas-
sively)

k. Abdominal scans

l. Arteriograms (e.g., done in trauma, vascular obstruction)

m. Dye studies (e.g., done in ulcer disease, occasionally
in obstruction)

4. Patient/family's understanding and level of anxiety regarding disease process, purpose of hospitalization, and
therapy planned, including potential surgery and expected outcome

5. Patient/family's knowledge regarding operative therapy

a. What they have been told

b. Their expectations

c. Previous experiences with surgery

GOALS

1. Reduction in patient/family's anxiety with provision of
information, explanations, and encouragement

2. GI function within normal limits

a. Anastomosis intact

b. Normal peristalsis—absence of ileus

c. Absence of intestinal obstruction, marginal ulceration, dumping syndrome, or ''nine-day'' syndrome

3. Hemodynamic stability

a. BP, P within patient's normal limits

b. Absence of intraoperative or postoperative hemorrhage

4. Respiratory function sufficient to maintain Pao_2 and
$Paco_2$ within patient's normal limits

5. Infection free; patient afebrile; no wound infection, peritonitis, or sepsis

6. Patient/family verbalizes understanding of disease condition, signs and symptoms, and specific therapy prescribed

7. Before discharge patient/family is able to describe accurately
   a. Medication regimen
   b. Dietary alterations
   c. Activity progression
   d. Signs and symptoms requiring medical attention
   e. Plan for follow-up visits

POTENTIAL PROBLEMS	EXPECTED OUTCOMES	NURSING ACTIVITIES
Preoperative		
■ Patient/family's anxiety related to Disease process Medical therapy Need/purpose for surgery Expected surgical outcomes Diagnostic procedures	■ Patient/family demonstrates decreased anxiety with provision of emotional support, encouragement, and explanations Patient/family verbalizes understanding of disease process and its relationship to therapy employed Patient/family participates actively in planning and implementing care	■ Ongoing assessment of patient/family's level of anxiety Assess patient/family's level of understanding of disease process and therapeutic regimen Explain disease process, medical management, need/purpose for surgery, and expected outcomes in simple terms Describe purpose of diagnostic procedures and what patient will experience in simple terms Encourage verbalization of questions, anxieties, and fears Provide emotional support, appropriate encouragement Encourage patient/family's participation, including decision making, in care Evaluate for reduction in level of patient/family's anxiety
■ Obstruction Small bowel obstruction related to Adhesions (account for 30% to 40% of small bowel obstruction) Volvulus Intussusception Internal hernia Large bowel obstruction related to Neoplasm Volvulus of sigmoid colon Incarcerated hernia (groin)	■ Absence and/or resolution of small bowel obstruction Absence and/or resolution of large bowel obstruction	■ Prevention Evaluate progression of signs and symptoms of patient with "acute abdomen" Correlate signs and symptoms to assist in diagnostic process and for appropriate therapeutic intervention Monitor for Signs and symptoms indicating bowel obstruction q1 hr and prn, including Persistent and/or crampy abdominal pain Continuous pain, which suggests strangulation or peritonitis Tenderness, which may be diffuse or localized Bowel sounds, hyperactive borborygmus (may decrease after prolonged course), tympany Abdominal distention Nausea and vomiting Absence of and inability to pass gas or stool Fever (more common if strangulation or peritonitis is present) Dehydration; note hypotension, tachycardia, low CVP, oliguria, high urine specific gravities, and ketonuria Abnormal results of lab and diagnostic data, including Metabolic acidosis; check arterial blood gas results q1-2 hr Hemoconcentration—increased Hct, Hgb WBC count for leukocytosis (suggests strangulation/peritonitis) q4-8 hr or as ordered Electrolyte imbalance (Na^+, K^+, Cl^-, CO_2, and BUN abnormalities); check electrolyte levels q4-8 hr or as ordered Abdominal radiographs daily or as ordered (upright or lateral decubitus) for presence of free air in abdomen, dilated bowel, fluid levels in bowel Notify physician of any abnormality Administer medical therapy for patient stabilization while need for surgery is evaluated, as ordered Keep NPO Administer fluids for volume repletion NG tube to low suction Monitoring activities as given previously Prepare patient for surgery if needed, as ordered

POTENTIAL PROBLEMS	EXPECTED OUTCOMES	NURSING ACTIVITIES
▪ Strangulation of bowel related to 　Paralytic ileus—often associated with 　　Surgery 　　Acute peritonitis 　　Local trauma 　Acute peritonitis—often associated with 　　Acute pancreatitis 　　Perforation and/or necrosis of GI tract	▪ Bowel function within normal limits 　Absence of strangulation, paralytic ileus, or acute peritonitis	▪ Monitor (q1-2 hr) for signs and symptoms of strangulation 　Constant, severe abdominal pain 　Signs of peritonitis 　Fever 　Tachycardia 　Increasing leukocytosis 　Blood in rectum 　Associated abdominal, pelvic, rectal mass 　Notify physician of aforementioned signs and symptoms; administer therapy as ordered and monitor patient's response 　Monitor (q1-2 hr) for signs and symptoms of paralytic ileus 　Silent abdomen, absent bowel sounds 　Absence of cramping 　Radiographic evidence of gas throughout small and large intestines 　Notify physician if aforementioned occur and administer therapy as ordered; monitor patient's response 　Monitor (q1-2 hr) for signs and symptoms of acute peritonitis 　Malaise 　Abdominal discomfort, pain 　Rebound tenderness, with muscular rigidity over primary area of inflammation 　Leukocytosis 　Fever 　Nausea, vomiting 　Fluid and electrolyte imbalance 　Notify physician of aforementioned abnormalities and administer therapy as ordered; monitor patient's response 　If problem occurs, see Standard 45, *Peritonitis* 　Prepare patient for surgery if necessary, as ordered
▪ Vascular obstruction related to 　Mesenteric arterial thrombosis associated with aortic aneurysms, severe aortic atherosclerosis 　Mesenteric vasoconstriction, hypoxia, and vasospasm of mesenteric artery associated with low cardiac output 　Mesenteric venous thrombosis, which may be associated with appendicitis, strangulation hernia, abdominal hernia, and other abnormalities	▪ Vascular sufficiency 　Bowel sounds within normal limits	▪ Monitor for 　Signs and symptoms of arterial mesenteric occlusion q1 hr 　Occult blood in stools 　Hypotension, tachycardia, fever 　Signs and symptoms of mesenteric venous occlusion q1 hr 　Patient complaints of pain that is out of proportion to physical findings (early in course) 　Tender abdomen 　Diminished or absent peristalsis; reduced/absent bowel sounds 　Gradually developing distention 　Vital signs, including temperature; note hypotension, fever 　Lab reports for leukocytosis; check CBC results for WBC count q12-24 hr 　Note results of abdominal tap, if done, indicating presence of blood in peritoneum (may indicate infarcted bowel) 　Notify physician of any of these abnormalities 　If vascular obstruction occurs, administer therapy as ordered, which may include 　Fluid, electrolyte, and blood replacement 　Antibiotics 　Preparation of patient for surgery to resect infarcted bowel or to perform an embolectomy or thrombectomy of artery, vein involved
▪ Diverticulitis	▪ Absence or resolution of diverticulitis and associated problems	▪ Monitor for 　Progression of characteristic signs and symptoms of *chronic* diverticulitis q1 hr 　Altered bowel habits, e.g., constipation, diarrhea, flatulence 　Recurrent left lower quadrant pain and tenderness 　Rectal bleeding (occasional) 　Signs and symptoms of *acute* sigmoid diverticulitis q1 hr 　Rapid onset of marked lower left quadrant pain 　Lower abdominal tenderness, peritoneal irritation

POTENTIAL PROBLEMS	EXPECTED OUTCOMES	NURSING ACTIVITIES

		Fever—check vital signs including temperature
		Leukocytosis; note CBC results
		Mass in area of acute pain
		Notify physician of any abnormality
		Prepare patient for barium enema, sigmoidoscopy as ordered
		Administer low-residue diet if ordered
		Administer anticholinergic drugs to promote bowel function if needed, as ordered
		For patients with *acute* diverticulitis
		  Administer antibiotics as ordered
		  Prepare patient for surgery if procedure is necessary (if medical measures do not sufficiently arrest inflammatory process or if abscess is documented)

▪ Ulcerative colitis	▪ Absence or resolution of signs and symptoms of ulcerative colitis	▪ Monitor for
		Severe diarrhea that may be bloody; determine frequency and amount
		Fever; check vital signs, including temperature q1 hr and prn
		Weight loss
		Accurate intake and output q1 hr
		BP, P; CVP, PAP readings q1 hr, if available
		Electrolyte imbalance; note serum electrolyte levels as well as signs and symptoms of electrolyte abnormality
		Specific signs and symptoms of acute fulminating ulcerative colitis, including
		  Abdominal pain and distention
		  Leukocytosis; monitor CBC
		  Toxemia
		  Peritonitis
		  Bloody diarrhea
		  Toxic dilatation of colon
		Notify physician of any abnormality
		Prepare for and assist with sigmoidoscopy, barium enema as ordered
		For patients with *fulminating ulcerative* colitis
		  Administer fluids, antibiotics, blood transfusions as ordered
		  Administer analgesics and sedatives if needed, as ordered
		  For persisting acute symptoms, administer steroids as ordered
		For patients with *chronic debilitating* colitis
		  Administer bland diet as ordered
		  Administer anticholinergic, antidiarrheal agents, corticosteroids, and sedatives if needed, as ordered

▪ Diaphragmatic hernia, which may be one of two types Esophageal hiatal hernia	▪ Resolution of diaphragmatic hernia	▪ Monitor for progression of signs and symptoms of esophageal hiatal hernia, including Esophagitis Substernal or epigastric distress and heartburn, made worse by patient being in reclining position after eating Nausea, vomiting, dysphagia (occur occasionally) Bleeding; check vital signs q1 hr and prn Hematest-positive stools and vomitus Notify physician of any abnormality Prepare patient for barium study, esophagoscopy as ordered Administer bland diet, antacids, anticholinergic drugs if ordered Place head of bed in semiupright position, particularly after patient eats Prepare patient for surgery if ordered
Traumatic diaphragmatic hernia		Monitor for signs and symptoms of traumatic diaphragmatic hernia, particularly respiratory distress, nausea and vomiting, evidence of intestinal obstruction Notify physician of any abnormality Prepare patient for radiograph, barium study, and/or esophagoscopy as ordered Prepare patient for surgery if procedure is necessary

POTENTIAL PROBLEMS	EXPECTED OUTCOMES	NURSING ACTIVITIES
Postoperative		
■ Hemodynamic instability Hemorrhage related to Bleeding arteriole DIC Hypotension related to Insufficient fluid ad- ministration Inadequate myocardial function	■ Hemodynamic stability	■ Intraoperatively, administer blood products and fluids to replace blood losses as ordered; observe for transfusion reaction Monitor BP, P q1-2 hr; note hypotension, tachycardia CVP, PAP, cardiac output, if available Urine output with specific gravity q1 hr Peripheral circulation, mentation; note signs of reduced perfusion, restlessness; cool, blanched extremities, oliguria Hct and Hgb, coagulation studies; note low Hct, Hgb, abnormal coagulation studies Drainage (e.g., NG, wound) for presence and amount of blood; weigh dressing if wound drainage is copious and include in fluid output totals Abdomen for tenseness q1 hr and girth q4-8 hr and prn Notify physician of any abnormality Maintain accurate fluid intake with accurate intake and output records including specific gravity; daily weights If hemodynamic instability occurs, administer fluids and blood products as ordered; closely monitor patient's hemodynamic response and urine output
■ Respiratory insuffi- ciency—atelectasis re- lated to Anesthesia and pro- longed immobility during surgery Pain, splinting, and de- creased diaphragmatic movement NG tube producing sore throat and difficulty with effective cough	■ Patient breathes without distress; respiratory rate within normal limits Adequate oxygenation, ventilation, with Pao_2 and $Paco_2$ within normal limits Clear lungs determined by auscultation, radiograph	■ Monitor for Restlessness, agitation, confusion, somnolence Fever, tachypnea, tachycardia, and hypertension; check vital signs including temperature q1 hr Decreased chest wall movement on affected side Amount, color, consistency of secretions Presence of rales, rhonchi, and other adventitious breath sounds Elevated diaphragm on one or both sides Presence of atelectasis, local or diffuse infiltrates, pleural effusion; check chest radiograph results daily Infection: note presence of purulent, copious secretions; monitor results of sputum C and S Acidosis; note arterial blood gas results q12 hr and prn Decreasing LOC Notify physician of any abnormality Chest physiotherapy q2-4 hr and prn in early postoperative period; nasotracheal suction if patient is unable to cough up secretions Administer pain medication, as needed, for effective coughing and breathing exercises Assist patient with use of spirometer Ambulate as soon as possible according to plan of care If aforementioned measures fail, prepare for and assist with intubation; see Standard 6, *Mechanical ventilation*
■ Pulmonary emboli, throm- bophlebitis related to Venous stasis associated with immobility Hypercoagulability asso- ciated with stress of surgery	■ Absence of pulmonary em- boli, thrombophlebitis	■ Prevention Apply antithromboembolic stockings or external pneumatic boots Assist patient with ROM exercises, isometric exercises, ambulation Administer low-dose anticoagulation therapy, if ordered, for high-risk surgical patients Monitor for Signs and symptoms of thrombophlebitis of lower extremities q4-8 hr Calf tenderness Homans sign (pain when patient's foot is dorsiflexed) Swelling, redness along vein Signs and symptoms of pulmonary embolism Chest pain Tachypnea, dyspnea Hemoptysis

POTENTIAL PROBLEMS	EXPECTED OUTCOMES	NURSING ACTIVITIES
		Elevated BP, tachycardia; determine vital signs, including temperature, q1 hr and prn Notify physician if these signs and symptoms occur If pulmonary emboli, thrombophlebitis occur, see Standard 31, *Embolic phenomena*

■ Fluid and electrolyte imbalance related to
Large GI, wound, ostomy losses
Hypovolemia caused by inadequate fluid replacement in preoperative and intraoperative periods
Hypervolemia caused by vigorous fluid replacement
Inordinate electrolyte losses and/or inadequate electrolyte replacement
	■ Fluid intake and output in balance
	Weight approximates preoperative baseline level
	Serum electrolyte levels within normal limits
		■ Monitor
		  Fluid intake and output records q1-2 hr (including GI, wound, ostomy losses)
		  Daily weights for significant gain or loss
		  For signs and symptoms of electrolyte imbalance q4-8 hr: lassitude, irritability, weakness, nausea, vomiting, neuromuscular abnormalities, twitching
		  Serum electrolyte levels q24 hr or prn
		Notify physician of any abnormalities
		If fluid and electrolyte imbalance occurs
		  Administer fluid and electrolyte replacement as ordered; closely monitor patient's response
		  Administer special therapy according to causal factors, e.g., low-residue diet; antidiarrheal/H_2 antagonist medication in patients with ileostomy

■ Infection: wound	■ Infection free, afebrile
	Wound clean and dry, intact (healing well)
		■ Prevention
		  Aseptic wound care and dressing change
		  Provide for adequate intake of nutrients to facilitate wound healing
		Monitor for
		  Appearance of incision line and surrounding tissues; note redness, warmth, and swelling; any complaints of localized tenderness, pain
		  Wound drainage—amount, color, and odor
		  Results of wound C and S if infection is suspected
		  Leukocytosis; check CBC results every day
		  Fever; note vital signs including temperature q2 hr and prn
		Notify physician of any abnormalities
		If wound infection occurs
		  Administer antibiotics as ordered
		  Administer wound care as ordered
		
		See STANDARD 61 *Infection control in the critical care unit*

■ Infection: peritonitis related to
Duodenal stump leakage
Leakage of bile, bowel during surgery
Necrotic bowel resulting from deficient blood supply
Intussusception of bowel, often related to polyp or growth that causes herniation of one part of bowel into another, followed by decreased blood supply to that segment of bowel and necrosis
	■ Absence and/or resolution of peritonitis
	Intact anastomosis
	GI, bowel function within normal limits including
	Normal bowel sounds
	Bowel movements that begin soon after patient resumes dietary intake
		■ Prevention
		  Careful aseptic wound care
		  Adequate intake of nutrients to facilitate healing as ordered
		Monitor for signs and symptoms of peritonitis q1-2 hr, including
		  Continuing large NG drainage
		  Fecal or bilious contents in wound drainage
		  Distended, rigid, tender abdomen with rebound tenderness
		  Increasing size of abdominal girth
		  Presence and characteristics of pain; note constant, increasingly intense discomfort
		  Fever, tachycardia; check vital signs including temperature q1-2 hr until stable
		  Elevated WBC count and ESR
		  Acidosis
		  Nausea and vomiting
		Notify physician of any abnormality
		If peritonitis occurs
		  Monitor accurate intake and output q1-2 hr
		  Monitor daily weights
		  Administer fluids as ordered
		  Send cultures of wound drainage, blood as ordered
		  Administer antibiotics as ordered
		  Assist in peritoneal dialysis if ordered
		  See Standard 45, *Peritonitis;* Standard 53, *Peritoneal dialysis*

POTENTIAL PROBLEMS	EXPECTED OUTCOMES	NURSING ACTIVITIES
■ Infection: localized abdominal abscess, subphrenic abscess	■ Infection free; afebrile Absence of signs of localized abdominal infection	■ Monitor for Elevation of diaphragm, obliteration of costophrenic angle in chest radiograph results Discomfort and pain q2 hr; note localization of pain Fever q2 hr often occurring in late afternoon or evening Leukocytosis, elevated ESR Scans and ultrasonography results, if tests done Notify physician of any abnormality If localized abdominal or subphrenic abscess occurs Administer antibiotics Prepare for surgery if necessary, as ordered
■ Infection: sepsis	■ Infection free; afebrile	■ Monitor (q1-2 hr) for signs and symptoms of sepsis Shock Diaphoresis, hyperthermia, hypothermia Altered LOC and malaise Fever Notify physician of any abnormality If sepsis is suspected, obtain cultures as ordered If sepsis occurs, administer antibiotics as ordered, and monitor for resolution
■ Paralyic ileus related to operative stress and manipulation	■ Normal GI function Bowel sounds present 1 to 2 days after surgery	■ Monitor for signs and symptoms of paralytic ileus q2 hr Large gastric output per NG tube Absent or diminished bowel sounds Absent or diminished passage of flatus Increasing abdominal girth; measure q4-8 hr and prn Notify physician of any of these abnormalities If paralytic ileus occurs Administer suppository, enema, or neostigmine (Prostigmin) if ordered (to stimulate peristalsis) Administer oral/IV nutrients as ordered
■ Marginal ulceration related to Damage of tissue along anastomosis from acidic gastric secretions or alkaline pancreatic secretions Incomplete vagotomy	■ Intact surgical anastomosis	■ Monitor for signs and symptoms of ulceration with bleeding Gastric discomfort, pain Hematest-positive stool and NG aspirates Hypotension; take vital signs including temperature q1-2 hr Low Hct and Hgb Notify physician of any abnormality If marginal ulceration occurs, administer antacid or H_2 antagonist as ordered; prepare patient for surgery if procedure is necessary
■ Obstruction, retention in GI tract, which may include Dilatation of gastric remnant after partial gastrectomy Gastric retention following Billroth I or II operation associated with Constricting anastomosis Edema and subsequent scarring and stricture of proximal loop Ileus, atony	■ Absence or resolution of obstruction Intact anastomosis without signs and symptoms of gastric dilatation, retention	■ Prevent by Ensuring continuous function of NG tube; irrigate as necessary Avoiding removal of NG tube Monitor q1-2 hr for Nausea, vomiting Hiccups Continued large NG aspirate Distended upper abdomen Signs and symptoms of shock and pulmonary embolus if dilatation is severe Monitor abdominal radiograph results (flatplate and upright) Notify physician of presence of any of these abnormalities If obstruction/retention occurs Administer fluid and electrolyte replacement as ordered Check for patency of NG tube q½-1 hr to ensure continuous gastric decompression Replace GI losses as ordered

POTENTIAL PROBLEMS	EXPECTED OUTCOMES	NURSING ACTIVITIES

Dumping syndrome consists of nausea caused by intake of high-carbohydrate food, which pulls large amount of fluids into intestinal tract, resulting in dehydration, nausea, diaphoresis, diarrhea, and cramping	GI function within normal limits
	No nausea and/or vomiting
	Nutrient intake consists of low-medium carbohydrate concentration and is isotonic
		Prevent dumping syndrome by
		  Administering nutrients with low-medium carbohydrate content and isotonic osmolality
		  Administering frequent small meals
		Monitor for
		  Any complaints of nausea, diaphoresis, diarrhea, cramping
		  Tachycardia, weakness, dizziness
		  Accurate intake and output q1-2 hr
		  Serial serum electrolyte levels
		Notify physician of any abnormality
		If dumping syndrome occurs
		  Administer fluid, electrolyte replacement as ordered
		  Reevaluate content of patient's nutritional intake and alter as indicated and ordered

Adhesion formation promoted by extensive surgical manipulation, infection, and peritonitis	Absence and/or resolution of symptoms related to adhesion formation	Monitor for evidence of adhesion formation
		  Adequacy of bowel function
		  Presence, nature of bowel sounds
		  Presence of flatus
		  Suppleness/rigidity of abdomen
		  Patient's complaints of specific area of tenderness, signs/symptoms of peritonitis
		  Changes in abdominal girth
		  Weight loss/gain
		  Amount, character of NG aspirates
		  Abdominal radiograph results (flatplate and upright)

Intussusception of bowel related to
Polyp or tumor
	Absence and/or resolution of intussusception	Monitor for signs and symptoms of complete intestinal obstruction
		  Nausea and vomiting
		  Pain, tenderness
		  Distended abdomen
		  Increased, then decreased bowel sounds
		  Air and fluid levels (by radiograph) proximal to point of obstruction

Duodenal stump ''blow-out'' or anastomotic breakdown (occurs about tenth postoperative day)		Notify physician of any abnormality
		If adhesion formation, intestinal obstruction, intussusception, or anastomotic breakdown of bowel occurs
		  Monitor progress of signs and symptoms
		  Maintain decompression of GI tract with NG tube or long intestinal tube (Miller-Abbott, Cantor)
		  Serial measurements of abdominal girth q4-8 hr and prn
		  Maintain scrupulous fluid intake, output records q1 hr
		  Monitor serum electrolyte levels
		  Administer fluid, electrolyte replacement as ordered
		  Monitor for signs of systemic infection: note temperature, vital signs, mentation, lab values—WBC count, sedimentation rate
		  Provide optimal chest physiotherapy
		  Maintain patient in semi-Fowler position
		  Reposition at least q2 hr
		  Ensure effective deep breathing and coughing; administer pain medication as ordered, if needed
		  Monitor arterial blood gas values
		  Prepare patient for surgery for lysis of adhesions and/or resection of portion of gangrenous bowel if necessary

■ Jaundice related to
Edema of duodenal stump in Billroth I and II surgeries, causing occlusion of common bile duct
Surgical occlusion of common bile duct
	■ Absence or resolution of jaundice	■ Monitor for
		  Jaundice, icteric schlera
		  Presence of upper abdominal pain (every shift)
		  Bilious drainage (q2 hr)
		  Results of liver function tests; note elevated bilirubin levels
		Notify physician of any abnormality
		If jaundice occurs, administer therapy as ordered

POTENTIAL PROBLEMS	EXPECTED OUTCOMES	NURSING ACTIVITIES
Hemolysis of RBC in stored blood administered in perioperative period (occurs in patient requiring many units of blood)		

■ Wound dehiscence, evisceration related to obesity, malnutrition, debilitation
Dehiscence involves disruption of several layers of wound (e.g., peritoneum, outer fascia)
Evisceration is the escape of abdominal viscera through wound and is associated with inadequate support from all fascial layers
	■ Suture line intact, healing well, and without signs of dehiscence, evisceration	■ Perioperative use of abdominal binders may be useful for some obese patients
		Monitor for sudden discharge of serosanguineous fluid, which may indicate dehiscence
		Patient may complain of "popping" sensation during coughing
		If dehiscence is suspected
		  Notify physician
		  Cover wound with sterile dressing or towels
		  Place patient on immediate, strict bed rest
		  Instruct patient to avoid further straining
		  Prepare patient for surgery as ordered
		Monitor for appearance of abdominal contents in wound subsequent to dehiscence, indicating that evisceration is occurring
		Notify physician
		If dehiscence/evisceration occurs, cover with sterile towels
		Prepare patient for surgery if necessary, as ordered

■ Malnutrition, negative nitrogen balance	■ Weight maintenance or weight gain (unless patient is obese)
	Positive nitrogen balance
		■ Monitor for
		  Return of bowel sounds after surgery q4-8 hr
		  Daily weight (without adequate nutrition, 0.5 pound [0.23 kg] of muscle mass can be lost per day)
		  Nitrogen balance results if done
		  Evidence of malnutrition
		    Weight loss
		    Muscle wasting
		    Weakness, lethargy, malaise
		    Poor skin turgor
		Notify physician of any of aforementioned and administer therapy as ordered; monitor patient's response
		Administer alimentation as ordered
		  Through oral intake, gastrostomy, or jejunostomy tube
		  For parenteral alimentation, see Standard 57, *Total parenteral nutrition*

■ Prolapse
Rectal—related to inadequate abdominal support
Of ileostomy or colostomy—related to weak abdominal ring or to inadequate internal fixation of ileum
	■ Absence or resolution of intestinal prolapse	■ Prevent by instructing patients not to strain excessively at stool; if difficulty with defecation is present, stool softeners and small enemas may be useful
		Monitor for rectal prolapse
		  Mass felt by patient, particularly when walking or during defecation
		  Soiling of clothing from discharge, bleeding, fecal incontinence
		  Visible appearance of rectum through anal ring
		Notify physician of these abnormalities
		Prepare patient for diagnostic modalities to document problem
		Monitor for prolapse of ileostomy
		  Appearance of additional intestinal mucosa/lining through ileostomy opening, which often appears superficially infected, edematous and ulcerated
		Notify physician if aforementioned signs occur
		Prepare patient for surgery if ordered

POTENTIAL PROBLEMS	EXPECTED OUTCOMES	NURSING ACTIVITIES

■ In hiatal hernia or esophagogastrectomy *reflux* from incompetent cardiac sphincter, which may result in aspiration of gastric contents into the lungs	■ Minimal to no reflux of gastric contents into esophagus
	Absence of aspiration of gastric contents into lungs
		■ Prevention
		    Place patient in semi-Fowler position unless contraindicated
		    When oral intake resumes, administer small, frequent meals that are low in bulk and easily digested
		Monitor for
		    Patient's complaints of gastric acidity, discomfort, and heartburn associated with reflux of acidic gastric contents into upper esophagus/throat
		    Aspiration of gastric contents into lungs
		Notify physician of these abnormalities
		If reflux of gastric contents occurs
		    Reevaluate patient's position and dietary intake and revise appropriately
		If aspiration of gastric contents into lung occurs
		    Notify physician immediately
		    Immediately suction patient's airway
		    Administer humidified O_2, as ordered
		See Problem, Respiratory insufficiency (postoperative)

■ Undue gastric fullness occurring with surgery that includes vagotomy, in which stomach becomes atonic and empties more slowly, permitting food fermentation	■ Absence of undue gastric fullness after meals	■ Prevent by providing for small, frequent meals
		Monitor for
		    Patient's complaints of fullness, discomfort after eating
		    Gastric distention
		    Inordinate flatus, diarrhea
		If problem occurs reevaluate patient's dietary intake and alter accordingly, as ordered

■ Skin irritation
    Occurs most frequently in patients with diversion of fecal material to skin (e.g., ileostomies)
	■ Skin intact and dry	■ Prevent by protecting skin with properly fitted ileostomy/colostomy appliance and meticulous skin care
		Monitor for reddened, irritated skin around ileostomy site
		If problem occurs
		    Alter skin care to provide additional protection and permit healing to occur
		    If skin irritation is severe, notify physician and administer therapy as ordered

■ Insufficient information for compliance with discharge regimen*	■ Sufficient information for compliance with discharge regimen
	Before discharge patient/family
	    Verbalizes knowledge of discharge program, including medication regimen, dietary management, activity progression
	    Is able to perform specific therapeutic interventions
		■ Assess patient/family's knowledge and understanding of discharge regimen
		Instruct patient/family as needed in
		    Therapeutic interventions such as dressings; provide opportunity for practice
		    Medication regimen, including
		        Purpose
		        Identification
		        Dosage
		        Frequency and timing
		        Potential adverse effects
		        Precautions
		    Dietary management
		        For all patients after GI surgery, slow progression in diet with small frequent meals is recommended
		        Avoid foods high in roughage, residue in early postoperative period
		        Dietary alterations are made according to specific GI surgery done and individual tolerance

*If responsibility of critical care nurse includes this type of follow-up care.

POTENTIAL PROBLEMS	EXPECTED OUTCOMES	NURSING ACTIVITIES

		For gastrectomy and hiatal hernia repair patients
		  Resumption of oral intake should occur gradually with small frequent meals consisting of food that is easily digested, mild, and low in bulk and residue (ulcer-type diet works well)
		  Advise patient not to eat for several hours before bedtime
		For hiatal hernia patients with dysphagia from residual postoperative esophageal edema, encourage patient to eat slowly and chew food well; encourage patient to avoid certain meats that are hard to swallow, eggs, fresh bread, spicy or hot foods, salads, and carbonated beverages until dysphagia subsides
		If patient has signs/symptoms of dumping syndrome
		  Low-carbohydrate, high-protein (meat, eggs, cheese), moderately high-fat diet is recommended
		  Foods to avoid include those high in sugar (e.g., sweets), alcohol, sweet carbonated beverages
		  Fluids are taken between meals, at least 1 hour before and 1 hour after meals
		Activity progression
		  Avoid lifting heavy objects (over 15 pounds) in first few postoperative months
		  Activities that require vigorous abdominal muscular effort should be avoided (e.g., opening stuck windows, tennis)
		  Straining at stool should be avoided

	Identifies untoward signs and symptoms requiring medical attention Describes plan for follow-up care	Describe untoward signs and symptoms that require medical attention, according to specific type of GI surgery performed Discuss plan for follow-up care, including purpose of the visits, when and where to go, who to see, and what specimens to bring Provide opportunity for and encourage patient/family's questions Assess patient's potential compliance with discharge regimen

JEJUNAL-ILEAL AND GASTRIC BYPASS SURGERIES

Morbid obesity is a major health problem in the United States. The incidence of medical problems related to obesity is high and includes cardiac and cardiovascular disease, diabetes, osteoarthritis, and pickwickian syndrome (somnolence, hypoventilation, and hypoxia). The hazards of the continued presence of these medical problems if surgery is not performed should be weighed against the disadvantages of surgery. The two most common surgeries used are the jejunal-ileal bypass and the gastric bypass procedures.

A jejunal-ileal bypass operation involves resection of 14 inches of jejunum and 4 inches of ileum (or 12 and 6 inches, respectively) to reduce the intestinal absorption of nutrients consumed, resulting in weight loss.

Gastric restriction procedures as a surgical solution to morbid obesity have gained increasing popularity over the jejunal-ileal bypass procedure. All the gastric restrictive surgeries involve the creation of a small proximal gastric pouch, which limits the amount of food that can be ingested at any one time. The gastric pouch can hold approximately 45 to 100 ml of food. Outflow from the pouch can be accomplished by two methods: (1) gastrojejunostomy, as in the gastric bypass or (2) a channel in the distal stomach, as in the gastroplasty or gastric partition surgery.

Relative indications for surgery include the presence of morbid obesity for most of the patient's lifetime (at least 5 years). Morbid obesity is defined as 100 pounds over ideal weight. Surgery is considered when medical measures for modifying the obesity have failed, including psychosocial counseling, behavior modification programs, weight reduction groups, and various dietary and medication regimens. The surgical candidate should be free of endocrine imbalances such as hypothyroidism and Cushing disease as well as alcohol abuse. Relative contraindications for gastric bypass surgery include a history of hiatal hernia with gastric reflux, duodenal ulcers, or GI disease.

Psychosocial evaluation of a morbidly obese patient often reveals a negative body image, a feeling of helplessness in dealing with an obsessive eating habit, depression, and a dependent type of personality. These individuals often describe feelings of isolation. Surgical success is enhanced by a psychosocial evaluation that reveals sufficient stability and motivation to comply with the discharge regimen. The patient should be able to tolerate the psychosocial changes associated with significant weight loss and the potential problems associated with the specific surgical procedure.

Complications associated with jejunal-ileal bypass surgery include the psychosocial adjustment to weight loss, diarrhea, easy fatigability, progressive hepatic dysfunction caused by fatty necrosis, renal stone formation, hyperuricemia, and arthritic symptoms (probably related to circulating cryoproteins formed by colonic bacteria). There is also a small operative mortality.

The incidence of complications with gastric bypass is relatively lower than that of jejunal-ileal bypass. The major complication is emesis while the patient is trying to adjust to the small stomach pouch. The incidence of ulceration, dumping syndrome, and reflux esophagitis has been reported as low. Gastric perforation and anastomotic leaks have decreased since the introduction of the newer stapling devices. Gastric bypass patients do not have the diarrhea that is seen in jejunal-ileal bypass patients. Electrolyte deficiencies and liver dysfunction are rare complications of gastric bypass surgery. One-year weight loss is comparable with the two surgeries.

Postoperative care is focused on achieving adequate oxygenation and ventilation and on managing the problems associated with the specific procedure. To assist the patient adjust successfully to the many changes that take place postoperatively, the patient and family are encouraged to verbalize their fears and anxieties. Encouragement and support from the staff and a plan of care that provides for patient and family participation in its planning and delivery can enhance the surgical outcome.

ASSESSMENT

1. History, presence, nature, and severity of medical problems commonly associated with sustained obesity, including
   a. Cardiac and cardiovascular abnormalities
      (1) Heart failure
      (2) Angina
      (3) Hypertension
      (4) Symptoms of pulmonary edema
      (5) Shortness of breath, dyspnea on exertion

b. Pulmonary abnormalities
   (1) Pulmonary disease
   (2) Respiratory distress
   (3) History of smoking
c. GI abnormalities (Specific for gastric bypass)
   (1) Hiatal hernia
   (2) Duodenal ulcer
   (3) GI disease

2. Nature of weight gain
  a. Actual weight
  b. Amount of recent weight loss or gain
  c. Length of time and pattern of weight gain
  d. Pertinent circumstances related to weight gain
  e. Weight loss programs employed
  f. Typical food and alcohol intake
  g. Medications taken; note those that may impair liver function

3. Previous and current medical therapy; past surgical procedures

4. Psychosocial factors that are pertinent to patient's sustained obesity and that are also important factors in the postoperative period
  a. Feelings about weight gain
  b. Factors that precipitate eating
  c. Previous counseling in weight reduction, including formal weight reduction programs
  d. Pertinent psychosocial factors in family background, support systems
  e. Employment history
  f. Educational and comprehension level

5. Results of lab tests that affect surgical outcome, including
  a. Liver function tests—alkaline phosphatase, transaminase, and bilirubin levels
  b. Protein and albumin levels
  c. Coagulation studies
  d. Indices of kidney function, particularly BUN, creatinine
  e. Pulmonary function tests
  f. Arterial blood gas values
  g. Chest radiograph results

6. Patient/family's anxiety regarding hospitalization and altered family roles

7. Patient/family's knowledge regarding operative therapy
  a. What they have been told
  b. Their expectations and fears regarding surgery and the outcomes
  c. Previous experiences with surgery, if any

8. Information and detail surgeon has provided about the need for surgery, the actual surgery to be done, and the expected outcomes

9. Patient/family's level of anxiety related to the surgery and prognosis

GOALS

1. Reduction of patient/family's anxiety with provision of information, explanations, and encouragement
2. Hemodynamic stability
3. Respiratory function sufficient to maintain arterial blood gas levels within patient's normal limits
4. Fluid balance adequate to maintain hemodynamic stability and adequate urine output; electrolyte levels within normal limits
5. Blood glucose levels within normal limits
6. Infection free
  a. Wound heals without infection, dehiscence, or evisceration
  b. Absence of pulmonary infection
7. Absence of thrombophlebitis, pulmonary emboli, cerebral emboli, or other types of emboli
8. Specific for jejunal-ileal bypass
  a. Liver function tests within normal limits, including serum protein, bilirubin, and enzyme levels and coagulation studies
  b. Bowel function within normal limits; diarrhea controlled
  c. Urinary function within normal limits; absence of urinary calculi
  d. Absence of arthralgia
  e. Hair thickness at approximately baseline levels
9. Reduction in GI complications in gastric bypass patient
10. Patient/family accurately verbalizes discharge regimen, including dietary management, medication regimen, activity progression, and plan for follow-up visits

POTENTIAL PROBLEMS	EXPECTED OUTCOMES	NURSING ACTIVITIES

In both surgeries

- Patient/family's anxiety related to
  Obesity and associated complications
  Hospitalization
  Diagnostic procedures
  Therapeutic regimen
  Anticipated surgery and expected outcomes

- Reduction in patient/family's anxiety with provision of information, explanations, and encouragement

- Ongoing assessment of level of patient/family's anxiety
  Assess patient/family's knowledge and understanding of surgery, expected outcomes, potential problems, postoperative medical regimen
  Assess patient/family's response to hospitalization
  Arrange for psychiatric consult and follow-up as ordered
  Encourage participation in care as tolerated
  Perform treatments in unhurried manner
  Provide comfort measures
  Explain anticipated diagnostic procedures and what patient will experience
  Assist in preparing patient for diagnostic procedures
  Explain rationale for intestinal bypass procedure
  Teach patient about medical regimen to enhance success of surgery
    No alcohol intake
    Dietary modifications
    Demonstrate respiratory exercises; teach and encourage patient until he/she is able to exercise properly
  Describe perioperative experience, including
    Preoperative
      Orient patient to chest physiotherapy (call therapist for assistance if available)
        Coughing and deep breathing
        Incentive spirometry
        Postural drainage
      Shave and prep
      Light dinner, then NPO after midnight
      Medication for sleep if needed
      Morning bath/shower
      Preoperative medications
      Hospital gown
      Care of valuables
      Ride to operating room
      Scrub suits, masks, and hats worn by operating room staff
      Anesthesia
    Postoperative
      Waking up in recovery room/critical care unit
      Describe general environment (size of unit, room, equipment)
      Nurse always nearby
      Dull, continuous noises
      Breathing tube temporarily in place to ease patient's work of breathing and load on heart
      NPO until "breathing tube" removed
      Incision with bandage
      IV, arterial lines
      ECG monitoring
      Medicine for discomfort, pain
      Policy on family visits
    As patient progresses
      Tubes out
      Eating again
      Getting stronger, ambulation
      Chest physiotherapy
      Diarrhea expected with therapy to control (with jejunal-ileal bypass)
  Describe responsibility of patient in achieving speedy recovery by taking active role in coughing and deep breathing to keep lungs clear
  Encourage patient/family's questions
  Encourage verbalization of anxiety, fears related to hospitalization, diagnostic procedures, therapeutic regimen, surgery, and anticipated surgical outcomes

POTENTIAL PROBLEMS	EXPECTED OUTCOMES	NURSING ACTIVITIES
■ Hemodynamic instability, which may be related to Low cardiac output Heart failure Increased metabolic requirements of obesity with increased O₂ needs Angina, myocardial ischemia, and possibly MI Arrhythmias	■ Hemodynamic stability Absence of Low cardiac output/ heart failure Angina Myocardial ischemia and MI Arrhythmias ECG within normal limits	■ Prevent hemodynamic instability by Carefully monitoring hemodynamic parameters, fluid intake and output measurements, and weight Administering fluids and diuretics to keep these parameters within normal limits Administering humidified supplemental O₂ as ordered to prevent tachycardia associated with hypoxemia Administering measures to prevent emboli formation, which contributes to hemodynamic instability (see Problem, Embolus formation) Early, gradual ambulation as ordered Monitor BP, P q½-1 hr until stable; CVP and PAP if available q½-1 hr until stable Urine output with specific gravity q1 hr; note oliguria with high specific gravities Indices of peripheral circulation and mentation; note signs of reduced peripheral circulation and altered mentation Daily weights for gain or loss For chest pain ECG and/or apical and radial pulse for arrhythmias, signs of myocardial ischemia, MI Notify physician of abnormalities in aforementioned If problem occurs Administer fluids, blood, and blood products as ordered; carefully monitor patient's response in terms of hemodynamic parameters and fluid intake and output measurements Administer inotropic/vasopressor medications if necessary, as ordered If arrhythmias, heart failure, angina, or myocardial infarction occur, see Standard 21, *Arrhythmias;* Standard 15, *Heart failure (low cardiac output);* Standard 11, *Angina pectoris;* Standard 12, *Acute myocardial infarction,* as appropriate
■ Respiratory insufficiency related to Atelectasis Pneumonia Pulmonary interstitial edema Emboli	■ Full lung expansion Arterial blood gas levels within patient's normal limits No abnormal or adventitious breath sounds Clear chest radiograph	■ Prevention Place patient in semi-Fowler position Careful fluid intake and output records Notify physician of imbalance, and adjust fluid intake and/or administer diuretic agent as ordered Turn, reposition q1-2 hr Administer chest physiotherapy q2 hr Administer humidified O₂ supplementation as ordered Monitor Respirations for sudden dyspnea or tachypnea and for restlessness and tachycardia; composite of these symptoms may indicate pulmonary embolus Serial arterial blood gas levels for hypoxemia, hypercapnia Breath sounds q1-2 hr for decreased or absent sounds or presence of rales, rhonchi, and wheezes Chest radiograph results for atelectasis, pneumonia Quality and amount of secretions Serial sputum cultures as ordered, particularly when character of the sputum suggests infection Temperature for elevation (q2 hr) Notify physician of abnormalities in aforementioned If respiratory insufficiency occurs Administer antibiotics as ordered Continue preventive and monitoring activities as described before If acute respiratory insufficiency is suspected, monitor arterial blood gas results for hypoxemia, hypercapnia, and acidemia Monitor and document patient's pattern of respiratory insufficiency; note progression of respiratory parameters

POTENTIAL PROBLEMS	EXPECTED OUTCOMES	NURSING ACTIVITIES
■ Fluid imbalance	■ Fluid administration adequate to maintain BP, P, CVP, PAP, urine output, peripheral circulation, and mentation within normal limits Steady loss of weight after first few postoperative days	■ Prevention 　Careful administration of fluids, as ordered, according to patient's intake and output record; BP, P; CVP, PAP (if available); and daily weight changes 　Monitor 　　Fluid intake and output q1 hr; correlate with hemodynamic parameters and weight changes 　　Daily weights 　　Hemodynamic parameters: BP, P; CVP, PAP (if available) q1 hr and prn until stable 　Notify physician of abnormalities in any of these parameters 　If fluid imbalance occurs 　　Restrict fluid intake or administer additional fluids as ordered; closely monitor patient's response 　　Administer diuretics as ordered; closely monitor urine output and hemodynamic indices
■ Abnormal glucose metabolism, diabetes	■ Blood glucose levels within normal limits	■ Monitor daily 　Urine glucose and acetone levels 　For signs and symptoms of hyperglycemia and hypoglycemia 　Serial blood glucose levels 　Notify physician of any abnormality 　If hyperglycemia occurs, administer insulin and institute dietary alterations as ordered 　If hypoglycemia occurs, administer glucose as ordered; institute dietary changes as appropriate
■ Wound infection related to 　Delayed, poor healing of suture line because of inadequate blood flow through thick layers of abdominal fat 　Wound dehiscence 　Hypoalbuminemia associated with liver failure	■ Infection free 　Wound heals without infection, dehiscence	■ Prevent by 　Applying abdominal binder for support as needed and as ordered 　Employing careful aseptic technique with dressing changes, wound care as indicated 　Carefully cleaning and assisting patient to clean skin folds 　Monitor 　　Nature of wound drainage; note presence of any purulent drainage, notify physician, and obtain wound culture, as ordered 　　For fever q2 hr; signs of local wound infection daily; note presence of erythema, local discomfort, inflammation, and/or abnormal drainage 　　WBC levels daily for leukocytosis; note 　　For increase in abdominal pain 　　For restlessness 　　For change in vital signs 　Notify physician of any abnormality 　If wound infection occurs 　　Continue monitoring as outlined 　　Assist with or administer local irrigation as ordered; change dressing frequently, as needed 　　Administer antibiotics as ordered
■ Embolus formation, which may be related to 　Thrombophlebitis 　Obesity 　Immobility	■ Absence or resolution of emboli	■ Prevent by 　Early mobilization, ambulation 　Applying antithromboembolic stockings/intermittent pressure stockings 　Administering prophylactic anticoagulation if ordered 　Monitor for signs and symptoms of 　　Thrombophlebitis 　　　Positive Homans sign with dorsiflexion 　　　Pain in calf muscles 　　　Redness, warmth along vein 　　　Swelling distal to suspected site of embolus 　　Plumonary emboli 　　　Sharp chest pain 　　　Dyspnea, tachypnea 　　　Restlessness

POTENTIAL PROBLEMS	EXPECTED OUTCOMES	NURSING ACTIVITIES
		Signs and symptoms of hypoxemia, including tachycardia, restlessness
		If suspected, arterial blood gas sample should be drawn immediately to determine presence of hypoxemia and significant drop in Pao_2
		Cerebral emboli
		Altered LOC, restlessness, aphasia, dysphasia
		Unilateral weakness, ptosis
		Other types of emboli including renal, mesenteric, splenic; see Standard 31, *Embolic phenomena*
In jejunal-ileal bypass		

■ Electrolyte imbalance related to
NG suction in the early postoperative period
Diarrhea
	■ Blood electrolyte levels within normal limits	■ Prevent by administering electrolytes as ordered to replace electrolytes lost in NG drainage, diarrhea
		Monitor
		  Serum electrolyte levels q24 hr and prn
		  For signs and symptoms of electrolyte imbalance: neuromuscular irritability, weakness, lassitude
		Notify physician of these abnormalities
		If electrolyte imbalance occurs
		  Administer electrolyte supplements as ordered
		  Administer therapy for cause of electrolyte loss as ordered, e.g., antidiarrheal agents

■ Liver dysfunction related to
Malabsorption as a result of creation of shunt and consequent reduced intestinal surface area for absorption
Fatty degeneration
Toxic substances may be produced by shunted remnant of intestine
	■ Liver function tests within normal limits
	Coagulation studies and serum protein levels within normal limits
		■ Prevent by
		  Administration of special diet as ordered, usually low-fat and low-oxalate; protein levels are titrated to toleration of patient's liver for protein load, monitored by ammonia and BUN levels
		  Administering amino acid preparation if ordered
		Monitor daily
		  Liver function tests, including alkaline phosphatase, transaminase levels
		  Bilirubin, ammonia, and BUN levels
		  Serum protein levels
		  Coagulation studies
		Notify physician of abnormalities in aforementioned
		If problem occurs, see Standard 46, *Liver failure/decompressive portovenous shunting procedures*

■ Diarrhea; occurs in nearly every jejunal-ileal bypass patient	■ Absence or resolution of diarrhea	■ Monitor
		  Stool for consistency, frequency, color
		    Note frequent loose stools
		  For presence of occult blood and chart results
		If diarrhea occurs
		  Notify physician regarding nature of diarrhea
		  Administer antidiarrheal agent as ordered
		  Administer IV fluids and electrolytes as ordered
		  Note presence of associated rectal excoriation; cleanse and apply lubricant
		  Support patient/family psychologically; assure them that diarrhea is common, can be treated, and will decrease as intestine adjusts to its new length
		  Keep careful intake and output records, including diarrheal losses
		  Monitor serial electrolyte determinations, because electrolyte losses can be significant with diarrhea

■ Metabolic imbalance and associated problems
Urinary calculi, oxalate renal stones
	■ Urine function within normal limits
	Urinary tract remains patent
		■ Assess metabolic status
		  Diet history, weight
		  Physical appearance including skin turgor, mucous membranes, hair
		Prevent by
		  Administering and teaching patient/family about low-oxalate diet
		  Administering cholestyramine therapy and increased Ca^{++} intake if ordered

POTENTIAL PROBLEMS	EXPECTED OUTCOMES	NURSING ACTIVITIES

		Administering fluids as ordered to provide adequate fluid intake and urine output
		Monitor for signs and symptoms of urinary calculi
		   Flank pain
		   Nausea and vomiting (in some cases)
		   Fever, if secondary infection is present
		   Dysuria, if stone is present in neck or outlet area of bladder
		Notify physician of abnormalities in aforementioned
		If problem occurs
		   Determine any deviations from prescribed diet, and notify physician and dietitian
		   Instruct patient in revised diet
		   Administer supportive therapy for urinary calculi as ordered

Arthralgia related to
   Increased circulating levels of cryoproteins
   Altered activity of colonic bacteria
	Musculoskeletal function within normal limits
	Absence of athralgia
		Prevent by administering antianaerobic antibiotic, if ordered, which is prophylaxis against intestinal syndrome that often precedes arthralgia
		Monitor for
		   Signs and symptoms of arthralgia: achiness, pain in one or more joints, bones; evidence of arthralgia may be preceded by watery diarrhea, fever, lower abdominal discomfort, pain, diffusely tender abdomen, and distended lower abdomen
		Notify physician if any of these occur
		If problem occurs
		   Apply soaks if needed, as ordered
		   Administer analgesic and/or antiinflammatory agent as ordered
		   Administer antianaerobic antibiotic, if ordered, for relief of intestinal syndrome and arthritic symptoms

Hair loss related to
   Altered carbohydrate metabolism
   Decreased blood proteins
	Hair thickness at baseline, preoperative level	Prevention
		   Minimize metabolic abnormality by providing sufficient intake of nutrients for building of body proteins, including hair
		Monitor for hair thickness, hair loss
		Monitor levels of serum proteins and nitrogenous waste products
		Notify physician of abnormalities in aforementioned
		If problem occurs
		   Assure patient/family that with resumption of more normal metabolism, hair usually grows back to its original thickness
		   Provide for high-protein, moderate-carbohydrate diet, as ordered, if liver can handle protein load
		   If nitrogenous metabolite levels increase (e.g., creatinine, BUN), protein intake may need to be decreased

In gastric bypass		

▪ Alterations in GI function related to surgery
   Nausea and vomiting
   Bile reflux
   Marginal ulceration
   Peritonitis
	▪ Minimal GI complications	▪ Monitor for
		   Nausea and vomiting
		   Bilious emesis
		   Signs and symptoms of peritonitis
		      Pain
		      Rebound tenderness
		      Nausea and vomiting
		      Fever
		      Chills
		      Decreased or absent bowel sounds
		      See Standard 45, *Peritonitis*
		   Signs and symptoms of dumping syndrome, e.g., diarrhea, cramping, diaphoresis
		   Signs and symptoms of ulceration, e.g., bleeding
		   Hematest all emesis or NG aspirate
		Notify physician of aforementioned abnormalities
		Administer therapy as ordered, which may include
		   Titrating antacids or administering H$_2$ antagonist as ordered
		   Instructing patient to eat small amounts to prevent emesis
		   Giving antibiotics for peritonitis

POTENTIAL PROBLEMS	EXPECTED OUTCOMES	NURSING ACTIVITIES
In both surgeries		
■ Psychological dependence, depression	■ Patient progresses from dependent role to more independent one	■ Ongoing assessment of patient's psychological status and stress level Arrange for psychiatric consult and follow-up as ordered Determine nature of current stresses and patient's ability to cope with them; assist patient in mobilization of resources to deal with these problems; enlist support of family/significant others Carefully encourage and provide opportunity for patient progression from dependent role to more independent one by the time of discharge from critical care area Encourage patient's decision making and participation in his/her care Include family in care; encourage their support of patient Provide emotional support and encouragement; acknowledge patient's progress Encourage verbalization of anxieties, fears, and feelings of depression

■ Insufficient knowledge to comply with discharge regimen*	■ Before discharge patient/family is able to
	Accurately verbalize discharge regimen regarding dietary management, medication regimen, and activity progression
	Describe signs and symptoms requiring medical attention
	Accurately describe plan for follow-up care
		■ Assess patient/family's understanding of discharge regimen
		Arrange for dietary consult
		Instruct patient/family in
		  Diet
		    For jejunal-ileal bypass patient
		      Foods to avoid
		      Vitamin B supplements, other vitamins
		      Fluids avoid alcohol—describe hazard regarding increased risk of liver dysfunction
		    For gastric bypass patient
		      Calorie restriction
		  Weight
		    Explain that weight loss does not occur for several days postoperatively; that steady weight loss will occur during first year; for jejunal-ileal bypass patient after first year weight may plateau because bowel progressively dilatates and thereby adjusts to its new length
		  Medication
		    Identification of dosage, timing/frequency; potential adverse effects, precautionary measures
		    For jejunal-ileal bypass patient
		      Medications may include antidiarrheal agent, vitamins
		      Oral contraceptives are usually not recommended because absorption is unreliable
		Encourage patient/family's communication of feelings regarding weight loss
		Review signs and symptoms requiring medical attention
		Review plan for follow-up visits, including when and where to go, who to see, and what specimens to bring
		Briefly review purpose and importance of follow-up visits
		Provide opportunity for and encourage patient/family's questions

*If responsibility of critical care nurse includes this type of follow-up care.

Renal

ACUTE RENAL FAILURE

Acute renal failure is a sudden onset of kidney dysfunction caused by impaired renal blood flow or glomerular/tubular damage. The function of the kidney in excreting nitrogenous waste products is impaired, resulting in azotemia with high BUN, uric acid, and creatinine levels.

Acute renal failure is characterized by the onset of a variable period of oliguria or anuria, acidosis, and electrolyte abnormalities. In some cases of acute renal failure, it is possible to have normal or large amounts of urine in the early period, although this is rare. The period of oliguria is followed by polyuria and, finally, recovery of renal function. Acute renal damage is usually reversible, although renal function may not return to a normal baseline.

The etiological factors of renal failure can be categorized into prerenal, renal, and postrenal events. The *prerenal* event includes physiological abnormalities that cause diminished renal perfusion such as decreased cardiac output, dehydration, and bilateral renal vascular obstruction. These conditions may result in oliguria or anuria, and azotemia.

The *renal* event is caused by two major types of conditions: (1) ischemic insult, which is secondary to severe prolonged volume depletion as in hypotension, severe dehydration, and "third spacing" as in third-degree burns and sepsis and following major vascular surgery; and (2) direct, chemical damage by toxins taken by ingestion, injection, or inhalants such as chemotherapeutic agents, exogenous toxins, drugs, organic solvents, or heavy metals.

The *postrenal* event is caused by lower urinary tract obstruction, such as renal calculi and prostatic hypertrophy.

Both the prerenal and the postrenal causes, if uncorrected, may lead to acute renal failure. However, if therapy is immediate, renal perfusion and urine output usually will be restored, thus ensuring continued kidney function.

The diagnosis of acute renal failure is based on clinical findings, lack of increased urine output in response to a fluid or a diuretic challenge, and characteristic abnormalities in the urinalysis. The tubular dysfunction accompanying acute renal failure results in inefficient concentrating ability. Other common findings are urinary sodium greater than 20 mEq/liter and specific gravity less than 1.015. The prerenal type of acute renal failure will be evidenced by urine sodium less than 20 mEq/liter and specific gravity greater than 1.020.

The patient in acute renal failure appears critically ill, very lethargic, and sometimes confused. Anorexia, nausea, vomiting, and diarrhea are often present. Physical findings in acute renal failure are variable and relate to the cause. Skin and mucous membranes may provide evidence of volume depletion (prerenal) or volume excess (e.g., edema). Urine output may be scanty, normal, or high. Specific gravity of urine suggests the state of hydration of the patient as well as the quality of tubular function and therefore may vary widely.

The three clinical phases of acute renal failure include the oliguric, diuretic, and convalescent phases. The oliguric phase, in which the urine output is less than 400 to 600 ml/24 hours, is accompanied by an increase of serum concentration of elements usually excreted by the kidney (urea, creatinine, uric acids, and the intracellular cations potassium and magnesium).

The oliguric phase is usually followed by a phase of high urine output called the diuretic phase of renal failure. In "high output failure" nitrogenous waste products are retained even though 2 to 3 liters of urine are excreted daily. In some patients the oliguric phase is transient, and the high output phase is the primary clinical sign of renal dysfunction. The third phase, or period of convalescence, is marked by improvement of renal function, a process that occasionally takes 6 to 12 months.

Acute renal failure is often a catastrophic complication of illness and/or surgery and is associated with a high mortality. Prevention of acute renal failure is a paramount responsibility of health care professionals, especially in critical care units. This responsibility includes identification of patient who are at high risk for developing acute renal failure, recognition of the clinical settings in which acute renal failure is likely to develop, and systematic assessment for early detection of the onset of acute renal failure.

Patients at high risk for development of acute renal failure include elderly patients, patients with preexisting renal insufficiency or exposure to nephrotoxic agents, diabetic patients who have undergone diagnostic radiology procedures such as IV pyelogram or cholangiogram, and patients with obstructive jaundice.

Clinical settings that further predispose the patient to development of acute renal failure include cardiovascular surgery, hemmorrhage, extensive burns, prolonged hypotension, (particularly when vasopressor agents are used), and sepsis.

Preventive measures recommended for patients at high risk include efforts to maintain optimal renal perfusion: maintaining adequate BP; maintaining adequate intravascular volume; maintaining urine flow at 50 ml/hr; monitoring the use of nephrotoxic agents, especially aminoglycoside drugs; and using caution in scheduling procedures that use iodine-based dye.

Early detection of acute renal failure is of particular importance, because reversibility of the conditions that give rise to renal failure may prevent lasting renal damage. Careful assessment of urine output (each 8 hours) and patient weight (daily) are particularly useful. Daily examination of urine quality and serum creatinine are recommended. Other assessment parameters are outlined in this standard.

ASSESSMENT

1. History, presence, and nature of
   a. Chronic renal disease
   b. Previous radiation therapy
   c. Infection involving kidneys
   d. Diseases/conditions that are associated with low kidney perfusion, causing renal ischemia
   e. Ingestion/injection/inhalation of various nephrotoxins; any drugs patient has recently taken
   f. Recent hypersensitivity response
   g. Disease of glomeruli and small blood vessels, including diabetes, collagen vascular disease
   h. Major blood vessel disease
   i. Lower urinary tract obstruction; presence of wide fluctuations in urine output; enlarged prostate; distended bladder
   j. Massive hemorrhage, trauma
   k. Cardiac disease
   l. Pulmonary insufficiency
   m. Hypertension

n. Hepatomegaly, jaundice, ascites
o. Exposure to radio-iodide contrast media
2. Signs/symptoms (if any) of chronic renal failure complications
   a. General appearance
      (1) Anemia, pallor
      (2) Peripheral edema of eyelids, feet, legs, hands, lumbar-sacral area
      (3) Pruritus
      (4) Poor skin turgor
      (5) Dry mucous membranes
   b. Cardiovascular
      (1) Pericarditis
      (2) Hypertension
      (3) Retinopathy
   c. Respiratory
      (1) Deep sighing, Kussmaul respirations
      (2) Urine smell on breath
      (3) Chest radiograph signs of hilar pneumonitis
   d. Urinary—urine produced may reflect proteinuria, hematuria, pyuria, casts
   e. GI—hiccups, anorexia, nausea and vomiting, coated tongue, patient's complaints of ammonia taste
   f. CNS—headache, lassitude, confusion, disorientation, drowsiness, insomnia, muscle twitching, weakness
3. Parameters to include
   a. BP, P, noting orthostatic changes
   b. Pallor
   c. LOC
   d. Pattern of urine output, urine volumes, specific gravity, state of hydration
   e. Weight
4. Results of lab and diagnostic tests
   a. Urinalysis; urinary sediment, osmolality, creatinine, electrolytes
   b. Serum creatinine, uric acid, bilirubin, BUN, electrolyte, Mg^{++}, Ca^{++} and phosphorous levels
   c. Coagulation studies
   d. Hct, Hgb, platelets, WBC with differential
   e. Liver function studies particularly serum albumin and protein levels, liver enzymes
   f. Blood type with cross-matching
   g. Abdominal flat plate radiogram
   h. Tomography
   i. Renal scan
   j. IV pyelogram
   k. Cystoscopy
   l. Arteriogram
   m. Renal biopsy
   n. Echogram (for kidney size)
5. Patient's perception of and reaction to the diagnosis and therapy

GOALS

1. Normovolemia, removal of excess body fluids
2. Hct, Hgb, and coagulation studies within normal limits
3. Blood levels of nitrogenous waste substances within normal limits
4. Serum electrolyte levels and acid-base balance within normal limits
5. Infection free
6. Nutrition adequate to prevent protein catabolism, achieve positive nitrogen balance
7. Normal cardiovascular, GI, neuromuscular, and integumentary function
8. Patient's behavior demonstrates decreased anxiety with provision of information, encouragement
9. Patient oriented to time, place, and person; clear sensorium
10. Before discharge,* patient/family is able to
    a. Explain relationship between renal dysfunction and therapy prescribed
    b. Successfully identify all medications, dosage/number of pills, schedule, and potential adverse effects and precautions
    c. Briefly describe signs/symptoms of chronic renal dysfunction
    d. Describe and follow prescribed diet
    e. Describe follow-up regimen
    f. Ask pertinent questions

*Applies when chronic management and/or prevention is required.

POTENTIAL PROBLEMS	EXPECTED OUTCOMES	NURSING ACTIVITIES
■ Patient/family's anxiety related to limited understanding of renal dysfunction, its effects on body, and diagnostic procedures	■ Patient/family's behavior demonstrates decreased anxiety with provision of information, encouragement Patient asks questions and demonstrates understanding of disease	■ Ongoing assessment of level of anxiety Describe nature of patient's renal disease and its relationship to signs/symptoms patient is experiencing in simple terms Explain relationship of renal failure to plan of care Explain briefly diagnostic procedures involved in plan of care Encourage patient/family's questions, verbalization of fears

■ Hypervolemia	■ Normovolemia
	Restoration of normal volume status
		■ Careful administration of fluid replacement
		Maintain diet with sodium restriction when appropriate
		Strict intake and output q1-2 hr; daily weights
		Monitor for presence of
		  Moist rales
		  Dyspnea, tachycardia
		  Pulmonary congestion
		  Edema, distended neck veins
		  Increased CVP, cardiac output, PAP, and PCWP
		  Hypertension
		  Abnormal skin turgor
		Notify physician of any abnormality
		If hypervolemia occurs
		  Administer diuretics as ordered
		  Monitor pressures (BP, CVP, PAP, PCWP, and cardiac output, if available) q½-1 hr
		  Head gatch at 45-degree angle
		  Dialysis may be ordered; see Standard 53, *Peritoneal dialysis;* Standard 54, *Hemodialysis*

■ Metabolic acidosis	■ Serum pH and bicarbonate within normal limits	■ Monitor for presence of Acidemia, anion gap Hyperkalemia Serum bicarbonate < 20 mEq/liter Deep, sighing respirations (Kussmaul) If acidemia occurs Administer or assist with dialysis, if ordered and according to hospital's protocol; see Standard 53, *Peritoneal dialysis;* Standard 54, *Hemodialysis*

POTENTIAL PROBLEMS	EXPECTED OUTCOMES	NURSING ACTIVITIES
■ Electrolyte imbalance Hyperkalemia Hypernatremia Hyponatremia Other ions, including Low serum Ca^{++} levels Elevated serum Mg^{++} levels Elevated serum phosphate levels	■ Electrolyte levels within normal limits	■ Monitor for presence of Acidosis—check arterial blood gas levels q4-8 hr Abnormal skin turgor, flaccid paralysis, and anxiety Arrhythmias Ventricular tachycardia Conduction defect Presence of peaked T wave Abnormal serum electrolyte levels Hypertension Congestive heart failure Tetany Notify physician of any abnormality If electrolyte imbalance occurs, administer therapy as ordered Antacid-phosphate binders Vitamin D Sodium polystyrene sulfonate (Kayexalate) to bind K^+ Infusion of sodium bicarbonate, calcium solutions, glucose and insulin; instillation of cation-exchange resins Restriction of potassium intake Restriction of sodium intake (when hypernatremic or fluid overloaded) Replacement of sodium (when hyponatremic) Continuous cardiac monitoring may be ordered Monitor electrolyte levels q4 hr Assess effect of therapy Assist in dialysis if ordered; see Standard 53, *Peritoneal dialysis;* Standard 54, *Hemodialysis*
■ Infection	■ Infection free	■ Prevention Administer good hygiene Observe appropriate aseptic technique Employ protective isolation technique if patient's WBC count is very low, if ordered Administer Foley catheter care every shift and prn Change IV dressings q24 hr and prn; ensure site change after 2 days (*maximum* 3 days) Remove urinary catheter if anuric/oliguric Pulmonary physiotherapy q2-4 hr Monitor for presence of General malaise Hypothermia/hyperthermia; check T, P, R q2-4 hr Abnormal WBC counts Signs of local infection Positive C and S results of blood or urine Notify physician of any abnormality If infection occurs Appropriate cultures redone as ordered Administer antibiotic therapy as ordered *See* STANDARD 61 *Infection control in the critical care unit*
■ Cardiovascular disorders: hypertension related to Fluid retention Renin angiotensin system disturbance	■ Resolution of hypertension BP within normal limits	■ Monitor for Diastolic pressure greater than 100 mm Hg Possible seizures Headache and restlessness Notify physician of any abnormality

POTENTIAL PROBLEMS	EXPECTED OUTCOMES	NURSING ACTIVITIES
		If hypertension occurs 　Monitor vital signs q½ hr and prn 　Maintain low-sodium diet as ordered 　Strict intake and output q1 hr; daily weights 　Administer antihypertensive medications as ordered 　Administer antihypertensive medications as ordered 　Administer diuretics and sedatives as ordered 　Assist in dialysis if ordered; see Standard 53, *Peritoneal dialysis;* 　　Standard 54, *Hemodialysis*
■ Cardiovascular disorders: pericarditis associated with toxic effects of systemic uremia	■ Adequate cardiac output 　Normal pericardium	■ Monitor for presence of 　Chest pain, discomfort on deep inspiration and change of position 　Paradoxical pulse 　Pericardial friction rub 　Arrhythmias Notify physician of any abnormality If pericarditis occurs 　Monitor arterial pressure and cardiac activity continuously 　Position for comfort 　Administer medication for chest pain 　Assist in dialysis or pericardiocentesis as ordered, if needed; see 　　Standard 18, *Pericarditis;* Standard 53, *Peritoneal dialysis;* 　　Standard 54, *Hemodialysis*
■ Pulmonary disorder related to pulmonary edema	■ Intravascular volume within normal limits 　Breath sounds normal 　Arterial blood gas levels within patient's normal limits	■ Monitor 　Intake and output 　Daily weight 　Breath sounds q8 hr 　For evidence of adequate oxygenation; note signs/symptoms of 　　hypoxia, e.g., tachycardia, restlessness 　Arterial blood gas levels for hypoxemia 　For peripheral edema Notify physician of any abnormality If problem occurs 　Assist with dialysis, if necessary, as ordered 　Observe for adequate oxygenation
■ Uremia: encephalopathy 　Disorientation 　Confusion	■ Patient is oriented to time, place, and persons 　Clear sensorium	■ Prevention 　Orientation of patient to time, place, date, and persons 　Placement of clock and calendar in room 　Planning and participation in own care if able 　Passive and active ROM exercises Monitor for 　Inability to concentrate 　Periods of agitation, excitation, and depression 　Changes in LOC Notify physician of any abnormality If encephalopathy occurs administer therapy as ordered 　Reemphasize aforementioned preventive measures 　Position for comfort 　Protect patient against injury, i.e., restraints if needed, as ordered 　Administer physiotherapy if needed, as ordered
■ Uremia: GI manifestations 　Nausea 　Ulcers 　Bleeding	■ Normal GI function 　Absence of nausea, vomiting, ulcers, bleeding	■ Test vomitus or NG aspirate and stool for Hematest Monitor for Hct and Hgb daily Observe for anorexia, nausea, vomiting Notify physician of any abnormality If GI manifestation of uremia occurs 　Alter diet therapy if ordered 　Administer antiemetic drugs if needed, as ordered 　Provide frequent mouth care 　Administer iron supplement (with meals) as ordered 　Administer blood transfusion if ordered and observe for transfusion 　　reaction

POTENTIAL PROBLEMS	EXPECTED OUTCOMES	NURSING ACTIVITIES
■ Uremia: hematopoietic system disturbances Normochromic, normocytic anemia Coagulation abnormalities	■ Hct, Hgb, and coagulation studies within normal limits Reticulocyte count increased toward normal or within normal limits	■ Monitor: Hgb and Hct daily; Hct may fall to 11% to 12% if untreated Platelet count daily For subcutaneous hemorrhage For pale skin, mucosa, and nail beds Weakness and fatigability Notify physician of any abnormality If hematopoietic system disturbances occur Blood transfusion may be ordered; observe for transfusion reaction
■ Uremia: integumentary system disturbances Pruritus Petechiae	■ Skin reflects good turgor and hydration Absence of pruritus	■ Provide frequent mouth care and good skin care; apply lotion Reposition frequently Administer calamine lotion for pruritus Administer antihistaminic if needed, as ordered
■ Malnutrition	■ Nutrition adequate to prevent protein catabolism Positive nitrogen balance Weight maintained or weight gain if appropriate	■ Assess baseline nutritional status Set required therapeutic diet and fluids with physician and dietitian Monitor for signs and symptoms of malnutrition; increased BUN daily Monitor strict intake and output every shift, daily weights Provide frequent oral care Ensure intake of therapeutic diet and fluid required Provide for small frequent feedings if necessary Mobilize, ambulate as soon as possible to decrease tissue catabolism Provide good hygiene Administer anabolic steroids if ordered Administer hyperalimentation if ordered; see Standard 57, *Total parenteral nutrition*
■ Insufficient knowledge to comply with discharge regimen*	■ Sufficient knowledge to comply with discharge regimen Patient/family accurately describes dietary, medication, and activity regimens	■ Assess patient/family's level of understanding, ability to comprehend follow-up plan of care or discharge regimen Discuss Prescribed therapeutic diet and fluids Medications including purposes, side effects, route, dose, schedules/times, and precautions Activity progression: avoid overfatigue; allow for rest and relaxation
	Patient/family identifies signs and symptoms of acute and chronic renal dysfunction requiring immediate medical attention	Describe signs and symptoms of acute and chronic renal dysfunction
	Patient/family accurately describes plans for follow-up care	Describe follow-up plan of care, clinic visits, when and where to go, who to see, and what specimens to bring Provide opportunity for and encourage questions and verbalization of anxiety regarding discharge regimen Arrange follow-up care with community health organization if necessary

*If this type of follow-up care is the responsibility of the critical care unit nurse.

PERITONEAL DIALYSIS

Dialysis is a method of removing metabolic waste products, electrolytes, and excess body fluid during renal failure. Certain toxic substances may be similarly removed when the kidney is inadequate to perform the task. Dialysis is based on the principle that a substance present in different concentrations on two sides of a semipermeable membrane moves from the side of greater concentration to that of lesser concentration (diffusion).

Peritoneal dialysis uses the patient's peritoneum as the semipermeable membrane, permitting transfer of nitrogenous waste products and other substances from the blood through the peritoneum into the dialysate, a solution composed of dextrose and electrolytes in concentrations that facilitate this transfer. The glucose in the dialysate creates an osmotic gradient such that the solvent (water) moves from an area of greater water concentration to one of lesser water concentration.

A peritoneal catheter may be inserted at the bedside, or a permanent indwelling catheter (Tenckoff catheter) may be inserted in the operating room. If a temporary (acute) catheter is to be placed, the equipment needed for the procedure includes the peritoneal dialysis catheter, cutdown tray, sterile towels, surgical gloves, dialysis fluid (dialysate) of a specified osmolarity, either a 1.5% or 4.25% glucose solution, and administration tubing. Both solutions are hypertonic to normal plasma and will provide an osmotic gradient for the passage of fluid through the peritoneal membrane into the dialysate, with the 4.25% solution providing the greater osmotic gradient. Generally, 1.5% is used initially; if a greater or faster body fluid loss is required, 1.5% and 4.25% solutions may be used alternately, or 4.25% may be used continuously (in adults).

Potassium may be added to the dialysate, even in the presence of hyperkalemia, to allow a more gradual rate of potassium ion diffusion and loss.

Heparin may be added to the dialysis fluid to prevent coagulation at the catheter tip and to ensure free flow of the solution.

Under some conditions, peritoneal dialysis may be preferred to hemodialysis because it uses a simpler technique and produces a more gradual physiological change. Peritoneal dialysis, however, is less useful when rapid removal of toxic substances, metabolites, body fluid, and/or electrolytes is necessary. The technique is also less useful when the peritoneal membrane surface is not intact and cannot retain the dialysate, such as occurs in the early postoperative period after abdominal surgery. Peritoneal dialysis is associated with an increased risk of infection, particularly pulmonary and peritoneal; significant protein (albumin) loss; and patient discomfort.

Careful observation of the patient during and immediately after peritoneal dialysis is an important aspect of this procedure. Various changes in the regimen may be based on these observations according to metabolic, fluid, and electrolyte changes that occur. Problems that arise may also require alterations in the therapeutic regimen, including difficulties with the peritoneal dialysis system, respiratory embarrassment, hemodynamic instability, and infection.

ASSESSMENT

1. History of ingestion/injection of drugs or other toxic substances
2. History, presence, and nature of the following
   a. Cardiac decompensation and other abnormalities that decrease renal blood flow
   b. Coronary heart disease; "cardiac" medications taken, such as digitalis, antianginal agents, beta-blocking agents
   c. Hypertension—antihypertensive medications taken
   d. Lower urinary tract obstruction
   e. Kidney disease
   f. Previous peritoneal dialysis
   g. Previous surgery, particularly abdominal surgery
   h. Related medical problems
   i. Malnutrition
   j. Uremia and related problems
      (1) Anemia
      (2) Metabolic bone disease
      (3) Gout
      (4) Coronary artery disease
      (5) Cardiovascular complications
      (6) Infections
      (7) Neuromuscular complications
      (8) GI complications—ulcers, bleeding

(9) Metabolic acidosis

(10) Electrolyte abnormalities, e.g., hyperkalemia

k. Other health problems

3. Signs and symptoms of kidney/bladder dysfunction—costovertebral pain (flank pain, lower back discomfort); hematuria; dysuria

4. Lab and diagnostic tests, including indices of renal function

   a. Urine specific gravity
   b. Urine osmolality
   c. Urine sediment
   d. Urine electrolytes
   e. Urine creatinine
   f. Serum electrolytes
   g. Serum creatinine, uric acid, BUN
   h. Blood levels of certain toxic substances based on patient's history
   i. WBC count
   j. Liver function studies including transaminase levels and coagulation studies; serum protein levels
   k. Chest radiograph results
   l. Abdominal flat plate radiograph results
   m. Kidney, ureter, and bladder radiograph results
   n. Cystoscopy
   o. Arteriogram
   p. Ultrasonography

5. Hemodynamic/respiratory status

   a. BP, P, peripheral circulation, temperature, respirations for rate and quality
   b. Urine volume

6. Weight

7. Level of patient/family's anxiety regarding patient's renal dysfunction, the need for peritoneal dialysis, the procedure itself, and other related concerns

GOALS

1. Reduction of patient/family's anxiety with provision of information, explanations, and encouragement
2. Minimal discomfort associated with peritoneal dialysis
3. Infection free; absence of peritonitis
4. Respiratory function adequate to maintain blood gas levels within patient's normal limits, without pulmonary infection
5. Cardiovascular stability—BP and P within patient's normal limits; no ectopic beats
6. Normovolemia—desired alteration in body fluid volume achieved
7. Efficient dialysis, adequate to achieve levels of nitrogenous waste products (BUN, creatinine, uric acid) within normal limits, serum electrolyte values within normal limits and adequate to remove toxic substances (drugs, etc.); normoglycemia; and adequate blood protein/albumin levels are maintained
8. Acid-base parameters in balance
9. Nutrition adequate to prevent protein catabolism and to maintain positive nitrogen balance
10. Before discharge patient/family is able to
    a. Properly care for catheter insertion site
    b. Identify each medication and describe the administration regimen, precautionary measures
    c. Keep accurate fluid intake and output records
    d. Accurately record daily weight
    e. Consume proper diet and describe dietary guidelines
    f. Maintain progressive activity level in the hospital and describe expected daily schedule after discharge
    g. Describe plan for follow-up visits

POTENTIAL PROBLEMS	EXPECTED OUTCOMES	NURSING ACTIVITIES
■ Patient/family's anxiety related to insufficient information regarding Hospitalization Disease process Diagnostic procedures Therapy employed	■ Patient/family's behavior demonstrates decreased anxiety with provision of explanations and encouragement	■ Assess level of patient/family's anxiety and understanding of procedure Evaluate psychosocial dynamics of family If complex problems are present, mobilize other resources, which may include social worker, clergy, and psychiatrist for consults and follow-up Explain in simple terms patient's disease process and need for dialysis Explain procedure to patient/family Encourage and provide opportunity for patient/family to ask questions and verbalize fears and anxieties Encourage and comfort patient/family during procedure; reassure them that certain responses during dialysis are normal (e.g., feeling of fullness) Assess reduction in level of patient/family's anxiety with provision of information, explanations, and encouragement

POTENTIAL PROBLEMS	EXPECTED OUTCOMES	NURSING ACTIVITIES
■ Improper choice and/or preparation of dialysate	■ Dialysis solution properly prepared with dialysate able to dialyze patient efficiently to achieve Normovolemia and desired weight changes Acid-base parameters and electrolyte levels within normal limits	■ Ongoing assessment of 　BP, P 　CVP if available 　Weight 　Acid-base balance 　Temperature 　Parameters of kidney function 　　Urine output 　　Specific gravity 　　Urine sediment 　　Osmolality—serum, urine 　　Electrolytes—serum, urine 　　Creatinine—serum, urine 　　Serum uric acid, BUN 　Serum levels of certain toxic substances based on patient's history 　Hgb, Hct 　Serum albumin 　Liver function studies, including transaminase levels, coagulation studies, and serum protein levels Prevent by 　Properly preparing patient for dialysis 　　Ensure empty bladder by having patient void or by placing bladder catheter 　　Place patient in supine position with slight head elevation 　　Assist physician during catheter insertion 　Properly preparing dialysate and equipment 　　Add medications ordered to dialysate bottle and label it with additives, number of exchange, date, and time 　　Warm dialysate to 37° C (98.6° F) 　　Connect administration set to dialysate bottle and prime tubing with dialysate 　　Connect primed administration tubing to peritoneal catheter 　Ascertaining and implementing prescribed regimen for dialysis; guidelines should include 　　Type of dialysate to be used 　　Times for inflow/equilibration/outflow (usually 10 minutes/20 to 30 minutes/20 to 30 minutes) 　　Total number of exchanges (usually 48 to 72), medications to be added (usually potassium, heparin) 　　Frequency of weights; specimens to be sent, i.e., blood electrolyte levels and culture of dialysate
■ Traumatic insertion of catheter Bleeding	■ Atraumatic insertion Blood-tinged returns subside after first few runs	■ Monitor for frank bloody drainage that continues past first few runs (blood-tinged drainage normally subsides after first few runs) Notify physician immediately of significant bleeding If bleeding occurs 　Pressure dressing, sandbags, ice packs may be applied 　Area in which bleeding arteriole is suspected may be infiltrated with solution containing epinephrine 　Monitor BP, P closely
Bowel perforation	Absence or resolution of bowel perforation	Monitor for 　Fecal contents in dialysate returns 　Urge for defecation, eventually producing stool mixed with large amounts of fluid 　Hypotension, tachycardia If evidence of bowel perforation occurs 　Notify physician immediately; stop dialysis 　Antibiotic is usually added to dialysate with antibiotic lavage continuing for several days 　Monitor BP, P, q15-30 min 　A surgical repair of tear may be done immediately, then lavage started; prepare patient for procedure, as ordered 　Notify physician if pronounced hypotension, tachycardia occur

POTENTIAL PROBLEMS	EXPECTED OUTCOMES	NURSING ACTIVITIES

Bladder perforation	Absence/resolution of bladder perforation	Monitor for
		  Intense urge to urinate with large urine outputs
		  Production of large amounts of urine through bladder catheter; if this occurs, test for high glucose concentration
		If evidence of bladder perforation occurs
		  Notify physician of signs/symptoms
		  Stop dialysis as ordered
		  Assist with removal of catheter as needed

■ Leakage of dialysate from insertion site of peritoneal catheter, resulting in Excoriation of skin
 	
Inaccurate intake and output records
	■ Absence of or minimal leakage of dialysate around catheter insertion site
	Absence of excoriation of skin around catheter insertion site
	Accurate dialysate inflow/outflow records
		■ Monitor for frequent need to change dressing and for dialysate leakage around insertion site
		If dialysate leakage occurs
		  Weigh dressing and include in record of fluid loss
		  Assist physician to tighten and/or place suture in skin around catheter insertion site
		  Change dressing at catheter insertion site as frequently as needed
		  Protect skin at insertion site by applying spray that forms barrier to irritating dialysate outflow

■ Ileus, usually related to irritation/inflammation from dialysis procedure	■ Normal bowel function	■ Monitor for any of the following that persist after day of catheter insertion
		  Absence of bowel sounds
		  No bowel movements
		  Malaise, loss of appetite
		  Abdominal distention
		  Large NG aspirates if NG tube in place
		Notify physician if aforementioned abnormalities occur
		If ileus occurs
		  Apply warm packs to help stimulate peristalsis
		  Administer medications to increase bowel activity as ordered
		  Provide for adequate nutritional intake as ordered either by oral or IV/central venous route

■ Pain, irritation, discomfort occurring during and/or immediately after catheter placement related to	■ Absence of/or minimal discomfort during dialysis treatment	■ Assess presence, nature, and severity of discomfort, pain
		Monitor for
		  Pain occurring at point of catheter insertion into abdomen
		  Localized pain in region of catheter tip
		  Complaints of pain in lower abdomen, perineal region or discomfort localized in bladder, vagina, or at root of penis; referred pain to shoulder

Catheter in place too long; catheter irritation of bladder, vagina, root of penis, diaphragm	Absence and/or resolution of irritation	Notify physician of these abnormalities
		If irritation, discomfort, pain occur
		  Administer analgesics if needed, as ordered
		  If pain occurs at time of insertion, catheter will be repositioned by physician
		    Short length of catheter is usually pulled out to alleviate discomfort
		    With repositioning, discomfort should subside shortly
		  Note alleviation of mild discomfort

Cold dialysate	Absence of or minimal discomfort during dialysis treatment	Prevent by warming dialysate to 37° C (98.6° F) If inadequate warming is suspected Monitor for presence and nature of pain that begins when inflow is intiated and continues through much of equilibration phase
Acidic dialysate		Monitor for pain that starts during inflow and continues during equilibration phase If this type of pain occurs, add bicarbonate to dialysate or into administration tubing before the run; procaine may also be added to tubing as ordered
Distention of peritoneum, abdomen with dialysate		Monitor for pain that starts during inflow and continues during equilibration phase

POTENTIAL PROBLEMS	EXPECTED OUTCOMES	NURSING ACTIVITIES

		If distention of peritoneum, abdomen with dialysate occurs
		  Assure patient that discomfort usually lessens after first few runs
		  Place patient in semi-Fowler position
		  Administer analgesics if needed, as ordered
		  For significant continuing discomfort, notify physician; smaller infusion volumes may be ordered

Air infusion through administration tubing		Prevent by allowing no air entry during connections and by using administration set with drip chamber and rubber diaphragm (that closes over tubing when chamber is empty) Monitor for symptoms that include pain in shoulder blade area If air infusion occurs, air can sometimes be removed from peritoneum through catheter with patient in knee-chest or Trendelenburg position
Intraperitoneal infection		Monitor for severe continuing pain, which may indicate infection in peritoneum (peritonitis); see Problem, Peritonitis

■ Peritonitis
  Bacterial
  Nonbacterial
  NOTE: Sterile peritonitis is an inflammatory process and may occur in response to composition of dialysate
	■ Absence of peritonitis
	  Afebrile
		■ Prevent infection by
		  Changing administration tubing according to hospital protocol
		  Changing dressing frequently, because small amounts of dialysate inevitably leak around insertion site
		  Cleansing insertion site and surrounding skin with antiseptic solution; protective skin barrier spray or cream may be applied to protect skin
		  Between dialysis treatments, assisting physician in removal of dialysis catheter and aseptic replacement with peritoneal button to keep tract open *or* disconnecting administration tubing from peritoneal catheter and placing cap on hub of catheter; then placing sterile dressing over catheter
		  After catheter or peritoneal ''button'' is removed, ensuring that wound is completely closed with Steri-strips or butterfly bandages and sterile dressing
		Monitor
		  Temperature q2 hr and prn for elevation
		  For persistent cloudy dialysate returns
		  For persistent unexplained localized or diffuse tenderness, particularly if in association with elevated WBC count in dialysate returns
		  Results of serial cultures of dialysate returns
		  For unexplained fever and malaise
		  For elevated WBC count in dialysate returns (300 cells/mm^3 or more)
		  Elevated serum WBC levels for elevation
		  Catheter tract or insertion site for infection
		  For late catheter obstruction that cannot be corrected by irrigation
		If peritonitis occurs, implement the following, if ordered
		  Send stat sample of dialysate returns for C and S determination
		  Monitor results of stat blood cultures, if done
		  Add antibiotics to the dialysate
		  Administer systemic antibiotics (often given if septicemia is documented)
		  Administer local antibiotic with short half-life in dialysate

■ Pulmonary insufficiency
  Pulmonary infection, pneumonia
  Dialysate elevates diaphragm, which decreases diaphragmatic excursion and tidal volumes, producing respiratory embarrassment
	■ Breathing without respiratory distress
	  Adequate exchange of blood gases, with Pao_2 and $Paco_2$ within normal limits
	  Absence of atelectasis, respiratory infection
		■ Prevention
		  Place patient in semi-Fowler position
		  Provide respiratory support to maintain adequate oxygenation and ventilation, which may include humidified O_2 through mask or artificial ventilation, if necessary
		  Turn side to side q1-2 hr
		  Administer chest physiotherapy as indicated
		  Assist extubated patient with deep breathing and coughing, breathing exercises, incentive spirometry

POTENTIAL PROBLEMS	EXPECTED OUTCOMES	NURSING ACTIVITIES

Uremic patient is particularly susceptible as result of
Depressed cough reflex and respiratory effort caused by CNS depression
Increased viscosity of pulmonary secretions caused by dehydration and mouth breathing
Pulmonary congestion and "shock lung"
		Monitor
		  Quality of respirations q½ hr until stable; note tachypnea, dyspnea, shortness of breath, shallow breathing
		  Breath sounds q1 hr and prn
		    Note decreased, absent, or adventitious breath sounds
		  Amount, color, and consistency of secretions
		  Arterial blood gas results; note hypoxemia, hypercapnia
		  Chest radiograph results
		  Serial body weights
		  Temperature q1-2 hr for fever
		Notify physician of clinical abnormalities
		If pulmonary insufficiency occurs
		  Augment activities to keep lungs clear (see prevention activities)
		  Administer humidified O_2 support as ordered
		  Assist with intubation if procedure is necessary (see Standard 6, *Mechanical ventilation*)
		If pneumonia occurs
		  Administer antibiotic therapy as ordered
		  Monitor sputum C and S results
		  Monitor temperature q1 hr until stable
		  Administer antipyretics if needed, as ordered
		Provide for quiet, restful environment
		Reassure patient that nurse is always nearby

■ Hemodynamic instability related to hypotension, resulting from
Rapid removal of intravascular fluid
Vena caval compression (children are more susceptible to this)
	■ Hemodynamic stability with BP, P within normal limits	■ Prevent by
		  Withholding or decreasing dosage of cardiac drugs and antihypertensive medications in presence of renal failure; adjust dosages at time of dialysis, as ordered
		  Avoiding rapid fluid shifts and loss by administering 1.5% dialysate, at least for first few runs
		Monitor
		  Weight every 6 to 10 runs; weigh patient when peritoneum is empty
		  BP and P q15 min during first complete run of dialysis; thereafter monitor BP and P q1-2 hr
		  Monitor ECG continuously if monitor is available
		  CVP and PAP if available
		  Urine output with specific gravity q1 hr
		Notify physician of significant abnormalities in these parameters
		If *mild* hypotension occurs
		  Open drainage tubing and begin outflow phase to reduce pressure exerted by fluid on vena cava
		  Turn patient to side in effort to reduce direct vena caval pressure and enhance outflow phase
		If *marked* hypotension occurs, perform aforementioned activities and Notify physician
		  Alter dialysate regimen, as ordered, which may include changing from exclusive use of 4.25% dialysate to regimen of alternating 4.25% and 1.5% (in adults)
		  Reduce volume of each run (infusion), as ordered

■ Hemodynamic instability related to hypertension associated with
Discomfort, pain
Hypervolemia secondary to fluid retention
	■ Hemodynamic stability with BP, P within normal limits	■ Monitor BP q½-1 hr during dialysis; note hypertension
		If significant hypertension occurs, notify physician
		  Evaluate level of discomfort; alleviate any cause of pain (see Problem, Traumatic insertion of catheter)
		  Evaluate for fluid overload, particularly if 1.5% concentration has been used, weight gain has occurred, and overall dialysis fluid balance is positive
		Notify physician of these abnormalities and administer therapy as ordered

POTENTIAL PROBLEMS	EXPECTED OUTCOMES	NURSING ACTIVITIES

■ Arrhythmias
  Premature beats associated with cold dialysate, respiratory distress (diaphragmatic elevation caused by dialysate)
  Bradyarrhythmias related to overdistention with dialysate (may be reflex response)
	■ Absence or resolution of arrhythmias, bradyarrhythmia
	  Adequate cardiac output
	  Hemodynamic stability
		■ Prevent by
		    Minimizing discomfort associated with peritoneal dialysis by
		      Positioning for ease in breathing, comfort
		      Implementing measures to prevent respiratory distress
		      Warming dialysate
		    Administering humidified O_2 supplements to provide for adequate oxygenation if needed, as ordered
		    Administering therapy to achieve acid-base parameters and electrolyte levels within normal limits
		  Monitor
		    ECG continuously via bedside monitor if possible
		    For arrhythmias
		      Ectopic beats
		      Premature beats
		    P q1 hr and prn for bradycardia
		    Arterial blood gas results for hypoxemia, acidosis
		    Serum electrolyte levels for imbalance
		  Notify physician of any significant incidence of ectopic beats (more than 4 to 6/minute) or significant drop in pulse rate
		  If arrhythmias and/or bradycardia occur
		    Administer antiarrhythmic agent as ordered; closely monitor patient's response
		    Decrease size of dialysate infusion volume if ordered
		    Administer therapy to correct predisposing factors such as hypoxia, acid-base imbalance, or electrolyte abnormalities as ordered

■ Hypervolemia, fluid overload related to
  Hyponatremia (dilutional) occurring just before dialysis treatment
  Sole use of 1.5% dialysate, particularly in adults
	■ Normovolemia
	  Desired alteration in body fluid volume and weight is achieved
		■ Prevent by
		    Keeping accurate record of intake and output, providing for even or negative balance, as patient's plan of care requires
		    Administering salt-poor albumin as ordered
		  Monitor
		    Serial body weights (q8 hr) during dialysis therapy
		    For positive fluid balance (patient retaining fluid)
		    For elevated BP, P, CVP, and PAP
		    For elevated urine output
		    For confusion or disorientation
		    Serum electrolyte results; note low Na^+ levels
		  Notify physician of abnormalities
		  If hypervolemia occurs
		    Alter dialysate regimen as ordered; proportion of runs using dialysate of 4.25% glucose concentration may be increased
		    If electrolyte imbalance is present, administer therapy to correct as ordered

■ Inefficient dialysis related to difficulties in drainage of dialysate (outflow phase)	■ Efficient dialysis sufficient to achieve
	  Normovolemia—desired alteration in body fluid volume (desired weight change achieved)
	  Acid-base balance within normal limits
	  Blood levels of nitrogenous waste products within normal limits, including BUN, creatinine, uric acid
		■ Monitor for signs of difficulty in drainage or protracted outflow phase
		  Monitor for occlusion of catheter by fibrin or blood clots; heparin may be added to dialysate
		  If difficulty in drainage occurs, enhance drainage of dialysate
		    By turning patient from side to side
		    By pressing hands against patient's retroperitoneal spaces (use this method particularly if turning is not well tolerated)
		    By sitting patient up in bed (if patient's physiological status permits)

POTENTIAL PROBLEMS	EXPECTED OUTCOMES	NURSING ACTIVITIES

■ Inefficient dialysis related to difficulties in inflow caused by
Obstructed catheter
  Clots
  Fibrin
  Fat deposits
Malpositioned catheter
  Catheter may be nestled in area of dense adhesions from previous surgery or peritonitis
	■ Peritoneal dialysis system patent and optimal inflow/outflow phases of dialysis achieved	■ Prevent catheter obstruction by adding heparin to dialysate, if ordered, in effort to prevent occlusion of catheter with fatty, fibrin aggregates
		Monitor for slow or absent progress in infusion of dialysate
		If catheter is obstructed, assist physician with irrigation of catheter; add heparin to dialysate, if ordered
		If catheter malposition is apparent, notify physician
		Assist with repositioning catheter if needed

Kinks in catheter, tubing	Patent catheter	Prevent kinks in administration tubing, catheter; anchor catheter such that good inflows/outflows are achieved
		Monitor for difficulty in both inflow and outflow phases
		If kinks in catheter and/or tubing occur
		  Note external position of catheter; change angle at which it enters skin, if necessary, to achieve better catheter alignment, obviate kinking
		  If aforementioned maneuvers do not work, notify physician and assist with catheter replacement, if necessary

Catheter occluded by loop of bowel		Monitor for difficulty in both inflow and outflow phases If catheter is presumed to be occluded by loop of bowel, administer mild cathartic and/or enemas, if ordered, to stimulate bowel movement; this effect may resolve catheter occlusion
Dialysate bottle not high enough		Drip chamber of dialysate administration tubing should be 4 feet above patient
Air in administration tubing		Prevent air entry into administration tubing during connections If outflow tubing becomes partly or completely filled with air, release air through outflow tubing and reprime with dialysate from inflow tubing

Peritonitis (see Problem, Peritonitis)	Peritoneum free of infection	Prevent peritonitis (see Problem, Peritonitis)
		Monitor for evidence of peritonitis
		  Abdominal discomfort, pain
		  Rebound tenderness, regidity of abdominal muscles
		  Decreased or absent bowel sounds
		  Fever, malaise
		  Cloudy dialysate returns
		  Elevated WBC count in dialysate returns (300 cells/mm³ or more)
		If peritonitis develops
		  Add antibiotics to dialysate if ordered
		  Administer systemic antibiotics if ordered

Adhesions may develop subsequent to repeated intraperitoneal instillation of dialysate	Peritoneum free of adhesions	Observe for difficulties in both inflow/outflow phases; adhesions should be suspected if patient has had previous abdominal surgery, peritonitis, peritoneal dialysis or if catheter has been in place for several days or longer
		If problem occurs
		  Notify physician
		  Assist with catheter replacement, if necessary
		  Prepare patient for hemodialysis if ordered

■ Hyperglycemia related to infusion of 4.25% glucose dialysate solution, which can lead to cellular dehydration, confusion, and eventually coma	■ Blood glucose level within normal limits	■ Monitor
		  Blood glucose levels using blood glucose monitoring strips (at bedside)
		  Serial blood glucose determinations q6 hr when dialysis is initiated
		  Urine glucose levels for glycosuria
		  For clinical signs of hyperglycemia
		Notify physician of abnormalities
		If hyperglycemia occurs
		  Alternate dialysate concentrations—4.25% and 1.5% if ordered
		  Add insulin to dialysate bottle or give subcutaneously as ordered
		  Monitor serial K⁺ levels closely (hypokalemia should be avoided, particularly if patient is receiving digoxin)

POTENTIAL PROBLEMS	EXPECTED OUTCOMES	NURSING ACTIVITIES
■ Protein loss	■ Serum protein/albumin levels within normal limits	■ Monitor Serum albumin/protein levels as ordered Dialysate returns for protein levels If significant protein loss occurs Administer salt-poor albumin to replace albumin lost through peritoneum, as ordered Administer nutritional replacement of protein/albumin as ordered; if po diet is possible, 80 g protein diet is often instituted in adults
■ Malnutrition, protein catabolism, which may be related to Anorexia Nausea and vomiting Altered mentation, malaise with decreased food intake Decreased absorption of Ca^{++} and iron Stomatitis	■ Adequate nutritional intake Positive nitrogen balance Weight maintenance or weight gain	■ Prevent by Controlling nausea and vomiting with medication, as ordered, if necessary Providing for adequate calories, essential amino acids Administering low-sodium, moderate- to high-protein (or as patient tolerates), high-carbohydrate diet, as ordered, with potassium and sodium restriction depending on BP and serum Na^+ levels (if patient can take po diet) Administering small, frequent meals Administering vitamins (particularly vitamin D), calcium, and iron supplements as ordered Administering phosphate binders, folic acid, and nandrolone decanoate (Deca-Durabolin) if ordered Monitor for signs/symptoms of malnutrition, e.g. Weight loss Loss of muscle mass Poor skin turgor Weakness, lethargy Notify physician of aforementioned abnormalities and administer therapy as ordered Reevaluate and alter aforementioned preventive activities, as ordered Administer sufficient calories/nutrients via peripheral or central venous catheter if ordered; see Standard 57, *Total parenteral nutrition* If malnutrition occurs, reevaluate and alter aforementioned preventive activities, as ordered; if needed, administer sufficient calories via peripheral or central venous catheter, as ordered
■ Insufficient knowledge to comply with discharge regimen*	■ Sufficient knowledge to comply with discharge regimen Before discharge patient/family is able to Do proper dressing of catheter insertion site if appropriate Identify each medication and describe regimen for administration and precautionary measures Keep accurate fluid intake and output records Describe dietary regimen	■ Discuss extended plan of care with physician and ascertain what has already been discussed with patient Collaborate with physician in patient/family explanations, teaching Assess patient's understanding of need for dialysis and his/her responsibilities in care *For patients undergoing long-term dialysis†* Discuss psychological, social, financial, and physical implications of long-term dialysis with patient; refer patient to special training program for patients undergoing dialysis at home for further discussion of these aspects Instruct patient in the following (patient may be able to assume many of these self-care activities while in hospital) Protection of peritoneal catheter and prosthesis, insertion site, and catheter tract Aseptic technique and prevention of infection Control of (and recording of) fluid intake and output Daily weights—to be done at same time of day using same scale Prescribed diet—adequate in calories and essential amino acids Medication regimen and precautions Reasonable activity level

*If critical care unit nurse is responsible for this type of follow-up care.
†If critical care unit nurse is responsible for preparing the patient for long-term dialysis.

POTENTIAL PROBLEMS	EXPECTED OUTCOMES	NURSING ACTIVITIES
	Describe activity progression	Describe preventive measures to avoid exacerbation of renal dysfunction
	Describe follow-up plan of care	If peritoneal dialysis is to be continued at home, refer patient to special teaching program designed to prepare patient/family to do dialysis safely and effectively at home
		Provide opportunity for patient/family to ask questions
		Describe plan for follow-up visits, including when and where to go, who to see, and what specimens to bring
	Patient successfully, accurately records daily weight on log form	On follow-up visits patient will be evaluated for signs/symptoms of protein and calorie malnutrition (weakness, apathy, weight loss, decreased serum albumin levels, and edema)
	Weight is maintained without significant incidence of edema	Fluid balance, including signs/symptoms of under or over hydration and weight, will also be assessed
		Assess patient/family's potential compliance with discharge regimen

HEMODIALYSIS

Dialysis is a method of removing metabolic waste products, electrolytes, and excess body fluid during renal failure or of removing toxic substances. Dialysis is based on the principle that a substance present in different concentrations on two sides of a semipermeable membrane moves from the side of greater concentration to that of lesser concentration.

During hemodialysis the patient's blood is drawn out from the body through tubing into the dialysis machine where it comes into contact with a semipermeable cellophane membrane. The dialysate is made of essential electrolytes in ideal concentrations, including sodium, potassium, calcium, and magnesium and the anions chloride and acetate. Through the process of diffusion, electrolytes move from the area of greater concentration to that of lesser concentration. Diffusion is responsible for removal of creatinine, urea, uric acid, potassium, magnesium, and phosphate. Similarly, calcium and acetate may be added to the blood by the same diffusion process. In addition, gradients in osmolality and hydrostatic pressure are created so that excess body fluid can be removed (by a process called ultrafiltration).

Various methods of vascular access are available. The external arteriovenous (AV) shunt was the first device available and is still used. It consists of Teflon cannulas inserted into the radial artery and an adjacent vein. There have been many problems and restrictions regarding the preservation of these shunts and their life span has been short (6 to 12 months).

Internal AV fistulas avoid many of the problems with external Teflon shunts and may last for several years. An artery, either radial or femoral, is connected by a side-to-side anastomosis to an adjacent vein. Internal fistulas can also be created from autogenous saphenous vein grafts, bovine grafts, and Dacron prostheses. After insertion of a graft or prosthesis, the vein into which it is inserted gradually dilatates and is able to accommodate blood flow into the dialyzer.

If hemodialysis is necessary and neither a mature internal fistula nor an external shunt is available, catheters may be inserted into a large artery and/or vein for the treatment.

Heparin is added to the blood to prevent coagulation. Special techniques for very low–dose heparinization can be used for patients with contraindications to systemic anticoagulation.

Careful observation of the patient during and immediately after hemodialysis is an important aspect of this procedure. Various changes in the regimen may be based on these observations according to metabolic, fluid, and electrolyte changes that occur. Problems that may require alterations in dialysis plans include malfunction of the shunt or fistula, hemodynamic instability, bleeding from any source, and angina.

ASSESSMENT

1. Etiology and/or history of
   a. Renal dysfunction
   b. Lower urinary tract obstruction
   c. Ingestion/injection of drugs or other toxic substances
2. History, presence, nature, and severity of
   a. Malnutrition
   b. Uremia and associated anemia, metabolic bone disease, gout, cardiovascular complications (pericarditis), neuromuscular complications, GI complications (particularly ulcers)
   c. Infections, hepatitis
   d. Signs/symptoms of kidney/bladder dysfunction—costovertebral pain, hematuria, dysuria, pyuria
   e. Signs and symptoms of chronic renal dysfunction
      (1) Costovertebral pain (flank pain, lower back discomfort)
      (2) Anemia, pallor
      (3) Eyelid swelling
      (4) Pruritus
      (5) Poor skin turgor
      (6) Dry mucous membranes
      (7) Gout
      (8) Malnutrition
   f. Cardiac and cardiovascular abnormalities
      (1) Coronary artery disease; use of medications such as nitroglycerin, digitalis preparations, propranolol (Inderal)
      (2) Hypertension—antihypertensive medications taken
      (3) Pericarditis

(4) Heart failure
g. Respiratory abnormalities
   (1) Deep sighing, Kussmaul respirations
   (2) Pulmonary edema
   (3) Chest radiograph for hilar pneumonitis
h. Renal abnormalities—if urine is produced, it may reflect proteinuria, hematuria, pyuria, casts
i. GI abnormalities—hiccups, anorexia, nausea and vomiting, coated tongue, complaints of taste of ammonia, ulcers, bleeding
j. CNS abnormalities
   (1) Headaches, lassitude
   (2) Confusion, disorientation
   (3) Drowsiness, insomnia
   (4) Muscle twitching, weakness
k. Retinopathy
3. Results of lab and diagnostic tests, including
a. Parameters of kidney function
   (1) Urine volume, specific gravity, and electrolytes
   (2) Serum electrolytes, creatinine, uric acid, BUN, calcium, and phosphorus
b. Liver function tests, particularly coagulation studies, serum protein, albumin levels
c. Hgb, Hct, and platelets levels; WBC count

GOALS

1. Patient/family's behavior demonstrates reduction in anxiety with provision of information, explanations, encouragement, and psychosocial/spiritual support
2. Hemodynamic stability, absence of arrhythmias or angina, absence of disequilibrium syndrome
3. Dialysis effectively achieves physiological levels of
a. Metabolic waste products
   (1) BUN
   (2) Creatinine
   (3) Uric acid

b. Toxic substances (drugs, etc.)
c. Electrolytes
d. Total fluid volume and intravascular volume within acceptable limits; excess body fluids removed; weight gain of approximately 0.5 kg/day in adults between treatments
4. Hct, Hgb, platelet levels within normal limits
5. Coagulation studies prolonged during hemodialysis
6. Fistula or shunt patent—fistula walls intact; tissue around shunt or fistula viable and intact
7. Infection free; without hepatitis
8. Nutrition adequate to prevent protein catabolism, to maintain/build body muscle mass, and to preserve protein/fat stores with reasonable blood levels of nitrogenous waste products and minimal uremic symptoms
9. Before discharge the patient is able to
a. Comply with dietary/fluid restrictions
b. Keep daily log of weight, fluid intake, and record of dietary intake if asked
c. For adults, keep daily weight gain between dialysis treatments at about 0.5 kg/day
d. Identify foods high in sodium and potassium that will be avoided altogether
e. Accurately take the proper dose of medications at the correct time and record it accurately on a chart (if hospital policy permits self-administration)
f. Properly care for shunt or fistula, using aseptic technique and providing for proper shunt alignment and prevention of injury to shunt or fistula
g. Properly ascertain shunt/fistula patency
h. Accurately describe precautionary measures that help to ensure longevity of shunt/fistula
i. Accurately describe sign/symptoms of complications of chronic renal failure and ways these complications can be prevented
j. Accurately describe plan for follow-up visits

POTENTIAL PROBLEMS	EXPECTED OUTCOMES	NURSING ACTIVITIES
■ Patient/family's anxiety related to limited understanding of disease and its relationship to need for dialysis and related therapy	■ Patient/family's behavior demonstrates decreased anxiety with provision of information, explanations, and encouragement	■ Ongoing assessment of level of anxiety Assess patient/family's understanding of disease process and its relationship to need for dialysis; explain in simple terms as needed Explain procedure for hemodialysis Reassure patient during procedure that certain responses are normal Encourage questions from patient/family
■ Dialysis procedure inadequate for patient's needs related to Improperly prepared hemodialysis system Inappropriate dialysis regimen Excessive ultrafiltration rate (excessively rapid removal of body fluid)	■ Effective dialysis sufficient to achieve Blood levels of metabolic waste products within normal limits Removal of desired amount of excess body fluid; desired weight loss during dialysis achieved; normovolemia	■ Prevention Before dialysis is started, perform observations or tests to ensure Intact electrical system Accuracy of dialysate concentrate Dialysate compatibility with blood Patency of blood tubing and membrane Secure connections Absence of air in tubing Sterile blood circuit (ensure that aseptic technique is used to make all connections)

POTENTIAL PROBLEMS	EXPECTED OUTCOMES	NURSING ACTIVITIES
		Before hemodialysis is started, ascertain the following guidelines for treatment, as ordered
		Type of equipment
		Frequency and length of dialysis
		Composition of dialysate
		Weight adjustment
		Fluid administration and/or replacement
		Transfusions to be administered if ordered
		Acceptable flow rates
		Degree of ultrafiltration
		Anticoagulation regimen; other medications to be administered
		Dietary management
		Lab requests, specimens to send
		Other special therapies during dialysis
		Ascertain guidelines for the following emergency situations
		Hypotension
		Hypertensive crisis
		Blood loss (dialyzer)
		Excessive bleeding and hematoma formation around fistula punctures or catheter sites
		Convulsion
		Monitor
		Serial weights for desired amount of weight loss with hemodialysis treatment
		Lab tests indicating levels of metabolic waste products: BUN, creatinine, uric acid
		Serum electrolyte levels
		Arterial blood gas results for acid-base balance
		Notify physician of any abnormality
		If problem occurs
		Examine dialysis system for leaks, air
		Change composition of dialysate as ordered
		Alter hemodialysis regimen if ordered (e.g., adjust flow rates; alter degree of ultrafiltration by decreasing positive pressure in blood chamber or by decreasing negative pressure in dialyzing bath, as ordered)

■ Inadequate dialysis with poor blood flow related to
  Vessel that goes into spasm easily
  Immature vessel or immature vessels around shunt
  Mature but small vessels
  Needle, cannula improperly positioned
  Flow rates set too high (in presence of satisfactorily functioning vessel, cannula)
  Incorrect needle gauge
	■ Desired degree of dialysis achieved
	  Blood levels of metabolic waste products within normal limits (BUN, creatinine, uric acid, ammonia)
	  Blood levels of electrolytes within normal limits
	  Removal of excess body fluid; desired weight loss achieved
	  Normovolemia
	  Acid-base balance within normal limits
		■ Prevention
		  Allow freshly placed arterial venous fistula to heal and "mature" before using it for dialysis (2 to 4 weeks)
		  For first few dialysis treatments, smaller needle sizes (fistulas) and slower blood flows may be employed; maintain flows sufficient to keep arterial side of tubing filled
		  In large adults fistula can usually accommodate large 14-gauge needle; fistula in smaller adults and children may not accept needle this large
		  Initiate dialysis by slowly increasing blood flows
		Monitor for indices of poor blood flow
		  Note low flowmeter readings
		  Collapsed tubing on arterial and/or venous side of dialysis tubing, indicating vessel spasm, improper positioning of one or both needles on sides of cannula, and/or too-high pump speed
		  Abnormalities at vessel cannulation sites, particularly during first few minutes of operation
		  For significant patient discomfort associated with poor blood flows, which may indicate placement of needle tip against vessel wall
		Notify physician of any of these abnormalities
		If vessel spasm occurs, patient may be instructed to immerse limb in warm/hot water before fistula venipuncture
		  Warm compresses may be continued during dialysis
		  Correct needle position or pump speed as needed

POTENTIAL PROBLEMS	EXPECTED OUTCOMES	NURSING ACTIVITIES
▪ Hypotension related to Diversion of approximately 300 ml of patient's blood into dialysis machine Hypovolemia related to ultrafiltration	▪ Hemodynamic stability Normovolemia	▪ Prevent by Priming dialysis machine with saline solution, albumin, or blood as ordered Avoiding weight loss of more than 3 to 4 kg during dialysis Monitor Weight before, during, and after hemodialysis for excessive weight loss BP, P, urine output, and peripheral circulation q15-30 min before, during, and after dialysis until stable; note hypotension, tachycardia, and evidence of peripheral vasoconstriction (e.g., cool, blanched extremities) CVP and PAP, if available, continuously during dialysis via monitor (or measure q15-30 min) Notify physician of abnormalities in the aforementioned If hypovolemia occurs Place patient in a more horizontal position, elevate legs Administer saline, albumin, blood, or blood products as ordered Administer vasopressor medication if ordered Adjust blood flows and ultrafiltration pressures according to protocol or as ordered
▪ Hypotension caused by antihypertensive medication When relative hypovolemia occurs during dialysis, antihypertensive medication may not permit sympathetic vasoconstriction to maintain BP within normal limits	▪ Hemodynamic stability BP within normal limits	▪ Physician may order omission of antihypertensive medication several hours before dialysis is begun Closely monitor BP, P, and peripheral circulation in patients receiving antihypertensive medication Notify physician if marked hypotension occurs during dialysis procedure Administer therapy as ordered, including fluids and adjustment of dosage of antihypertensive medication If dramatic hypotension occurs, administer vasopressor medication if ordered
▪ Hypotension caused by kinked tubing, vessel spasm, blood leaks in dialyzer	▪ Efficient dialysis Patent, unobstructed, intact dialysis system	▪ Prevent by Ensuring that all connections are tight before dialysis begins and that tubing is intact and unkinked Using mature, healed AV fistula Monitor For kinked tubing, vessel spasm For blood leaks in machine Blood leak detector, if machine is so equipped, and dialysate for evidence of blood leak Serial Hct results If tubing is kinked, straighten it and position so that kinking is not likely to recur If leak occurs, immediately clamp off cannula tubing and shut machine off; replace dialysate bath, replace extracorporeal tubing, ensure absence of leaks, and resume dialysis If vessel spasm occurs, reduce flow rate; if fistula/shunt is newly placed, reduced flow rates may be necessary for first few dialysis treatments
▪ Hemorrhage related to technical problems in fistula cannulation	▪ Hemodynamic stability Hemodialysis needles remain properly placed in fistula Hgb, Hct, and coagulation studies within normal limits or mildly prolonged during dialysis	▪ Prevent by Preventing needle dislodgement by securely taping needle in place; observe needle placement frequently Positioning patient's extremity to prevent abrupt movements and needle dislodgement Monitor Needle position and security throughout dialysis procedure BP, P, peripheral circulation, and other available hemodynamic parameters; notify physician of significant abnormalities For bleeding from needle puncture sites (fistula) Serial Hct levels

POTENTIAL PROBLEMS	EXPECTED OUTCOMES	NURSING ACTIVITIES
		If needle becomes dislodged, immediately clamp both arterial and venous lines; monitor BP, P closely; notify physician; apply pressure for 10 to 15 minutes or until bleeding stops; both needles may be removed; apply pressure dressing and leave in place for 3 to 4 hours; another needle(s) may be inserted and dialysis resumed
		If hematoma occurs, apply cool compress or ice bag until effects of heparin have worn off; then apply warm compress to relieve soreness and aid in resolution of hematoma
		Administer blood if needed, as ordered
		If needle is improperly positioned
		Slow blood flow (pump speed) temporarily and check needle/cannulas
		Pull needle back slightly and retape
		Needle/cannula may need to be lifted up by placing gauze square under hub of needle or cannula; decrease blood pump speed while doing this
■ Hemorrhage related to accidental disconnection of shunt between treatments	■ Shunt remains in situ without dislodgement Shunt cannulas remain connected and intact between treatments	■ Prevent by carefully dressing external shunts to protect them from accidental dislodgement Monitor for shunt disconnection If disconnection occurs, clamp both sides of cannula; notify physician immediately; follow protocol for aseptic reconnection If one cannula comes out of its insertion site, apply pressure to bleeding side and clamp cannula that is still in place; notify physician immediately
■ Hemorrhage related to Systemic heparinization with inadvertent hemorrhage related to altered coagulation times Repeated punctures of fistula through thin, dry skin Puncture of external shunt Tissue breakdown around cannula/fistula insertion sites Aneurysm formation around insertion site Cannula tip erosion through subcutaneous tissues or erosion of fistula vessel walls after repeated punctures	■ BP, P remain within normal limits Hgb, Hct remain within patient's normal limits, and no clinical signs of bleeding are evident Clotting times, PT, and APTT are moderately prolonged during dialysis No bleeding from puncture sites occurs External shunt intact Vessels around cannula tip are viable and intact without aneurysm formation Tissue around cannula tips is viable and intact	■ Prevent extraordinary pressure stress on extremity used for dialysis by preventing cuff BP measurements on extremity, both during dialysis and between treatments Apply pressure dressing after needle is removed; remove dressing after 3 to 4 hours; if bleeding/oozing continues, reapply pressure dressing for another 2 to 4 hours Apply shunt dressing to minimize stress on cannula insertion sites Instruct patient to avoid tight clothing on affected extremity Rotate fistula vessel puncture sites Permit no punctures of external shunt Monitor Serial clotting times, PT, and APTT during dialysis For signs/symptoms of external/internal bleeding during and after dialysis procedure Tissue around cannula insertion site and over point at which internal fistula joins patient's artery and vein for redness, swelling, discomfort, and dilatation Notify physician of any of these abnormalities If bleeding occurs Administer therapy as ordered, which may include removal of needles, discontinuation of dialysis, and application of pressure to insertion sites Administer blood if needed, as ordered If bleeding occurs in presence of systemic heparinization, notify physician; protamine sulfate, the antidote for heparin, is administered as ordered
■ Hypertension related to Body fluid overload Disequilibrium syndrome or disorientation caused by Cerebral edema Rapid dialysis or removal of serum solutes or fluid	■ Hemodynamic stability BP within patient's normal limits Weight gain not more than 0.5 kg/day in adults between dialysis treatments Absence of signs and symptoms of disequilibrium syndrome	■ Prevent by instituting the following as ordered Restrict fluid and sodium intake to avoid inordinate weight gain and fluid overload Individualize dialysate composition, blood flow rate, and dialysate bath flow rate Correct fluid and electrolyte imbalance slowly and cautiously Administer renin-releasing inhibitors such as propranolol

POTENTIAL PROBLEMS	EXPECTED OUTCOMES	NURSING ACTIVITIES

		Monitor
		  BP, P q15-30 min during treatment
		  CVP, if available
		  Weight (q8-24 hr, as appropriate)
		  For signs of disequilibrium syndrome (hypertension, headache, confusion, nausea and vomiting; in severe cases convulsions have occurred)
		If body fluid overload occurs
		  Alter dialysis treatment to remove excess fluid
		  Review with patient the necessary fluid and sodium restrictions
		If disequilibrium syndrome occurs, administer therapy as ordered, which may include
		  Reducing rate of solute/fluid movement during dialysis
		  Altering dialysate to be more compatible with patient's serum solute or fluid load

■ Angina pectoris, which may be related to
  Hypotension
  Excessive ultrafiltration rate
  Anxiety
	■ Absence of anginal pain	■ Prevent by slowly increasing blood flow rate (through dialysis machine)
		Monitor
		  BP, P q15-30 min during dialysis
		  For patient's complaints of chest pain
		If problem occurs, notify physician
		Alter regimen as ordered, including
		  Decreasing blood flow rate
		  Administering antianginal medication
		  Administering additional crystalloid or colloid fluids if needed, as ordered
		Reassure patient
		Sedative that requires little renal excretion may be ordered
		
		See STANDARD 11 *Angina pectoris*

■ Arrhythmias related to
  Rapid K^+ shifts
  Hypokalemia or other electrolyte imbalance
  Hypotension
	■ Absence of arrhythmias during dialysis
	Serum electrolyte levels within normal limits
		■ Prevent by
		  Maintaining K^+ concentration of dialysate bath at level that will minimize rapid K^+ shifts
		  Administering therapy to maintain physiological serum levels of other electrolytes: Na^+, Ca^{++}, magnesium, Cl^-, bicarbonate
		  Correcting cause of hypotension (increase in rate of fluid administration and/or decrease in ultrafiltration rate may increase BP)
		Monitor bedside ECG and apical and radial pulse for presence and incidence of serious, unperfused arrhythmias
		Notify physician of abnormalities
		If problem occurs
		  Administer antiarrhythmic medication as ordered
		  See Standard 21, *Arrhythmias*

■ Air embolus related to air entering tubing
  Large amounts of air in right ventricle interfere with pulmonary blood flow and oxygenation
  Can occur if IV bottle runs dry and blood pump continues to run, pulling air into tubing
	■ Intact hemodialysis system without air in system	■ Prevent by
		  Avoiding kinks in system; pay careful attention to alignment of tubing
		  Carefully taping all connections
		  Avoiding negative pressure between patient and pump; pay careful attention to blood flows
		  Hanging fresh IV bottle/bag before previous one is completely empty
		Monitor for
		  Air in dialysate tubing
		  Hemodynamic instability
		  Signs and symptoms of pulmonary air embolus
		    Chest pain
		    Cyanosis
		    Cough
		    "Mill wheel murmur" over precordium (sounds like whipping bubbles in motion)

POTENTIAL PROBLEMS	EXPECTED OUTCOMES	NURSING ACTIVITIES
		If significant amount of air is delivered to patient, put patient in Trendelenburg position and turn on left side; notify physician and turn off machine immediately
■ Electrolyte imbalance	■ Blood electrolyte levels within normal limits	■ Prevent by using dialysate bath tailored to patient's serum electrolyte values Monitor 　Serum electrolyte levels 　For signs/symptoms of electrolyte imbalance 　　Neuromuscular changes 　　Altered LOC (e.g., irritability, lethargy 　　Nausea Monitor particularly for evidence of hyperkalemia 　Spastic to flaccid muscle tone 　Irritability, restlessness 　Paresthesias 　Nausea, diarrhea 　ECG changes 　　Wide to absent P wave 　　Depressed S-T segment 　　Tall, peaked T wave 　　Prolonged Q-T interval 　High serum K^+ levels Monitor particularly for evidence of hypernatremia 　Dry, flushed skin 　Tachycardia, elevated BP 　Thirst 　Vomiting 　Weak, crampy and/or spastic muscle tone 　Irritability, excitability 　Lethargy, stupor 　High serum Na^+ levels Notify physician of abnormalities If problem occurs 　Alter dialysate bath as ordered 　Reduce ultrafiltration pressure as ordered
■ Infection 　Local 　　Shunt 　　Fistula 　Systemic	■ Absence or early resolution of local or systemic infection Afebrile	■ Prevent by 　Using aseptic technique in preparing dialysis machine, in making all connections 　Using scrupulous care to ensure uncontaminated dialysis machine tubing 　Using aseptic technique for daily shunt dressing 　Aseptically inserting needles into fistula Monitor for signs of local infection 　Swelling, redness, or warmth in skin temperature around shunt or fistula site 　Drainage of exudate around insertion sites of shunt cannulas 　Decreased circulation to extremity 　Fever Monitor for systemic sepsis 　Fever 　Shaking chills 　Hypotension, signs of peripheral vasoconstriction Notify physician of these clinical abnormalities If *local or systemic* infection occurs 　Monitor temperature q1-2 hr until stable 　Administer antipyretics if needed, as ordered If *systemic sepsis* occurs 　Administer antibiotics IV as ordered If local infection occurs 　Administer systemic and/or local antibiotic as ordered 　Monitor results of C and S of exudate around shunt/fistula insertion sites

POTENTIAL PROBLEMS	EXPECTED OUTCOMES	NURSING ACTIVITIES
		Apply warm soaks to affected extremity if ordered Prepare patient for and assist with drainage of infected local collection or shunt/fistula removal if either procedure is necessary

■ Shunt or fistula closure related to clotting	■ Patent shunt/fistula	■ Prevent shunt/fistula closure by
		  Administering fluids and pharmacological therapy to achieve adequate cardiac output and blood flow through shunt or fistula
		  Permitting no cuff BP readings or venipunctures in extremity with shunt or fistula
		  Instructing patient to avoid sleeping on affected extremity
		  For shunts in leg, avoiding weight bearing for 3 weeks or until edema subsides and healing is in progress
		  Elevating legs to relieve edema
		Monitor for patency frequently after shunt or fistula placement
		  Listen for bruit
		  Palpate for thrill by lightly depressing fistula or palpating above venous exit site of external shunt; note presence of weak or absent pulsation
		For shunts, frequently monitor color of blood in shunt, observing for
		  Uniform medium red color, indicating shunt patency
		  Dark purplish red color, which may indicate sluggish blood flow and beginning of clot
		  Dark reddish black color adjacent to clear yellow fluid, indicating full clot formation with separation of red cells from serum
		Feel shunt for warmth, indicating blood flow at body temperature
		Notify physician for abnormalities in aforementioned and administer therapy as ordered
		Prepare patient for surgery if necessary, as ordered; surgery may include clot removal or shunt/fistula removal

■ Secondary failure of fistula or shunt related to
  Repeated cannulation, inflammation, and/or clotting with sclerosis of the vessels
  Absence of normal dilatation of vessels around shunt or fistula
  Aneurysmal dilatation of vessels around fistula/shunt
  Infection at puncture sites (fistula) or shunt cannula insertion sites
	■ Patent fistula/shunt
	  Absence of aneurysmal dilatation of vessels around shunt insertion site or of fistula and surrounding vessels
		■ Prevent by
		  Maintaining flows within limits that will provide for efficient dialysis without complications
		  Using aseptic technique during cannulation and applying sterile pressure dressing after completion of hemodialysis treatment
		Monitor for
		  Signs of local infection of shunt or fistula site
		  Unusual warmth, erythema, inflammation, drainage from site
		  Dilatation of fistula or of vessels around shunt insertion site (some dilatation is expected; excessive dilatation represents weakening of vessel wall)
		  Patency of fistula/shunt
		  Note signs of fistula/shunt occlusion by clot
		Notify physician of abnormalities
		If local infection occurs
		  Administer local and/or systemic antibiotics as ordered
		  Administer antipyretic agent if needed, as ordered
		  Apply warm soaks
		If fistula/shunt clots prepare patient for and assist with clot removal (shunt)
		If clot removal is unsuccessful or if excessive aneurysmal vessel dilatation or infection occurs, prepare patient for surgery for fistula/shunt removal and for insertion of new fistula/shunt if necessary, as ordered

■ Secondary failure of shunt related to
  Kinking, bending, indentations, or roughening of shunt tip, thereby enhancing clot formation
	■ Patent shunt	■ Prevention
		  Silicone rubber cannulas and Teflon parts help to prevent clot formation
		  Discard bent, indented, roughened tip of connector and replace it
		  Handle shunt carefully; avoid malrotation, bending of shunt back or up
		  Apply dressings to achieve minimal tension on cannula sites

POTENTIAL PROBLEMS	EXPECTED OUTCOMES	NURSING ACTIVITIES

Irritation at shunt insertion site		Monitor
		  Results of radiograph revealing injury to Teflon tips inside vessel
		  For clotted shunt; see Problem, Shunt or fistula closure
		  For irritation at shunt insertion site
		If problem occurs, reevaluate and alter preventive activities; prepare patient for surgery, if necessary

■ Psychosocial difficulties related to
Depression
Dependency on machine for survival
Presence of "terminal" illness
Alteration of body image
Alteration of role in family
 	
In some cases
Breakdown of marital, family relationship(s)
Job loss
	■ Patient's behavior demonstrates decreased anxiety with psychosocial support and counseling, occupational counseling, and other support or counseling as indicated	■ Ongoing assessment of patient's level of anxiety
		Assess psychosocial adjustment in relation to
		  Renal failure
		  Dependence on hemodialysis machine
		  Altered family roles
		  Constant feelings of lethargy, fatigue
		Assess presence of
		  Loss of job
		  Impotence
		  Marital problems
		  Financial strain
		  Depression
		Allow patient to make decisions regarding scheduling and process of care as much as possible
		Provide for the following as needed
		  Psychosocial support from staff, physicians, social worker, clergy
		  Arrange for financial or marital counseling if needed; if signs of sexual problems are apparent, assess their nature and provide for counseling as necessary; support family and mobilize their psychosocial resources

■ Anemia with hemolysis of RBCs related to
Dialysate that is too warm or too cold
Inadequate heparinization
Dialysate of wrong concentration, composition
Increased RBC fragility; turbulent blood flows in dialysis machine
Decreased erythropoietin production by diseased kidneys
Splenomegaly with shortened RBC survival
Uremia
Transfusion reaction
	■ Hct, Hgb, platelet levels within normal limits
	Absence of bleeding during hemodialysis
		■ Prevent by
		  Warming dialysate bath to body temperature before dialysis treatment
		  Providing for adequate heparinization by monitoring serial clotting times, APTT during dialysis
		  Carefully regulating blood flows during dialysis treatment
		  Replacing frayed, bent parts of shunt
		  Transfusing patient with blood as necessary
		  Avoiding situations that increase RBC hemolysis, consumption of platelets
		  Minimizing uremia with dietary control of protein intake and regulating frequency of dialysis procedures
		Monitor the following before, during, and after dialysis
		  Serial Hct, Hgb, and platelet levels
		  Clotting times, APTT
		Monitor blood flows during dialysis and reduce flow if excessive
		Monitor dietary intake of protein and for evidence of uremia (e.g., confusion, disorientation; nausea, GI bleeding, anemia, pruritis, petechiae)
		Monitor slips and tags of all blood and blood products administered for compatibility with patient's blood; for transfusion reactions
		Notify physician of abnormalities
		If problem occurs
		  Reevaluate and revise preventive activities, as ordered
		  Administer blood products, as ordered
		  Monitor patient's response to therapy

■ Hepatitis acquired by
Transfusion with blood-borne hepatitis virus
Other sources
	■ Infection free, without hepatitis	■ Monitor serial liver function test results
		Periodically test patient for hepatitis B antigen, as ordered
		Periodically test staff for asymptomatic carriers of hepatitis virus
		If hepatitis occurs
		  Isolate patient
		  Administer supportive care as ordered
		  Monitor patient's liver function tests

POTENTIAL PROBLEMS	EXPECTED OUTCOMES	NURSING ACTIVITIES

▪ Congestive heart failure related to repeated hypervolemia between dialysis treatments	▪ Cardiac output remains within normal limits Weight gain of approximately 0.5 kg/day between treatments	▪ Prevent by
		  Restricting patient's fluid intake to amount prescribed during dialysis
		  Reviewing with patient the proper amount and type of fluids to be taken between treatments
		Monitor for signs/symptoms of heart failure, particularly low cardiac output and venous congestion
		  Evidence of decreasing cardiac function
		    Hypotension, pulsus alternans
		    Tachycardia
		    Decreased peripheral perfusion
		      Diaphoresis, cool skin
		      Restlessness, confusion
		      Cheyne-Stokes respirations
		      Oliguria
		  Evidence of pulmonary venous congestion
		    Dyspnea, tachypnea
		    Rales
		    Radiographic evidence of pulmonary congestion
		  Evidence of systemic venous congestion
		    Distended neck veins
		    Peripheral or sacral edema
		    Hepatic congestion (e.g., right upper quadrant tenderness, hepatomegaly)
		    Visceral congestion
		      Anorexia, nausea
		      Constipation
		      Bloating
		  ECG for changes indicative of ventricular hypertrophy
		Notify physician for abnormalities in aforementioned
		If problem occurs, see Standard 15, *Heart failure (low cardiac output)*

▪ Malnutrition related to
  Protein catabolism (negative nitrogen balance)
  Loss of protein, fat stores
  Loss of body muscle mass, weight
	▪ Nutrition adequate to prevent protein catabolism, maintain/build body muscle mass, and preserve protein, fat stores with reasonable BUN and creatinine levels and minimal uremic symptoms	▪ Prevent in hospital by
		  Administering diet and dietary supplements sufficient to meet patient's needs
		  Administering parenteral hyperalimentation if needed, as ordered
		
		See STANDARD 57 *Total parenteral nutrition*
		
		Assist in evaluation of patient's degree of renal dysfunction and uremic symptoms, which, together with age and physical activity, will determine prescription for protein intake
		  Take diet history
		  Assess home situation regarding food preparation
		  Ascertain dietary, fluid restrictions
		  Arrange with dietitian for dietary consult
		  Apply dietary restrictions to patient's dietary habits
		Monitor for evidence of malnutrition, e.g.
		  Weight loss
		  Muscle wasting
		  Weakness
		  Poor skin turgor
		Notify physician of any of aforementioned abnormalities and reevaluate patient's nutritional intake; alter patient's nutritional intake, as ordered
		Instruct patient/family in dietary regimen based on the following guidelines
		  Proteins
		    Usual prescription for adult is 0.5 to 1 g protein/kg/day (40 to 60 g); at least two thirds of this should be of high quality, that is, consist primarily of foods high in essential amino acids (eggs, milk, meat, fish, fowl); foods with protein that are low in these essential amino acids are vegetables and cereals

POTENTIAL PROBLEMS	EXPECTED OUTCOMES	NURSING ACTIVITIES
		Usual proportion of dietary calories composed of protein is about 15%
		Adequate protein intake reflected by BUN to serum creatinine ratio of approximately 10 to 1
		Carbohydrates
		Sufficient calories in the form of carbohydrates should be ingested to maintain body weight
		Recommended ratio of nonprotein (carbohydrates and fat) to protein calories is usually 5 to 1
		Total recommended calorie intake is 40 to 50 calories/kg ideal body weight for average adult
		Carbohydrates should be ingested within 4 hours of protein intake for protein-sparing effect on body
		Carbohydrate intolerance may be present, requiring curtailment of concentrated glucose preparations
		Fats
		It is usually recommended that less than 35% of diet consist of fats, with emphasis on intake of polyunsaturated fats to avoid hyperlipoproteinemia, hypertension, and vascular disease, which occur with higher incidence in patients with renal disease
		Prescribed proportion/amount of fat intake is reviewed with patient/family, with emphasis on polyunsaturated fats
		List of foods high in saturated and unsaturated fats may be shared with patient

■ High total body Na⁺ levels associated with
  Fluid overload
  Edema
  Hypertension
  Cardiac complications
	■ Serum Na⁺ levels within normal limits with no signs/symptoms of fluid overload, edema, and hypertension	■ Instruct patient/family according to the following guidelines regarding sodium
		  Provide list of foods/fluids with moderate sodium content; discuss those to be consumed in limited amounts
		  Exact sodium content may be included in list provided
		
		    1 g NaCl = 40 mg Na
		    1 mEq Na = 23 mg Na
		
		  No salt should be added to foods during cooking or at table
		  Salt substitutes should also be limited to some extent, since they contain potassium, which is also restricted
		  Water softeners often add sodium to tap water; should be considered in daily intake
		  Many medications contain sodium and should be considered in daily intake
		  Tips for improving palatability of food in light of salt restriction are shared (by dietitian if possible) including use of spices, herbs, and other seasonings

■ Fluid overload occurring between hemodialysis treatments	■ Normovolemia
	  BP, P within normal limits
	  Weight gain between treatments about 0.5 kg/day
		■ Instruct patient/family according to the following guidelines regarding fluids*
		  Discuss prescribed fluid intake with patient/family
		  Intake of fluids may vary according to patient's residual kidney function, body weight, physical activity, type of food intake (some foods such as ice cream are 90% fluid), ambient temperature, and tolerance to excess fluid accumulation between dialysis treatments
		  Acceptable daily weight gain is 0.5 kg/24 hours (adults)
		  Excess fluid gain may produce hypertension and edema
		  Usual fluid intake for adults is 500 to 800 ml plus urine volume for previous 24 hours in addition to fluids in foods; liquids low in both sodium and potassium are emphasized (e.g., H_2O; cranberry, grape, and apple juices)
		  Fluids should be carefully spaced and refreshingly cool to quench thirst
		  Frequent oral hygiene

*If critical care unit nurse is responsible for such follow-up care.

POTENTIAL PROBLEMS	EXPECTED OUTCOMES	NURSING ACTIVITIES
		Patient/family should be allowed and encouraged to tally intake of fluids and urine output while still in hospital Discuss with family signs of fluid overload, e.g. Weight gain of greater than 0.5 kg/24 hr Edema
■ Hyperkalemia	■ Serum K⁺ levels within normal limits	■ Instruct patient/family according to the following guidelines regarding potassium* Potassium restriction depends on residual kidney function and 24-hour loss of potassium Review foods that should be avoided altogether Protein restriction automatically reduces potassium intake The dietary potassium restriction is usually 40 to 70 mEq/day for adults (or approximately 1 mEq/kg of ideal body weight/day) 30 mg K = 1 mEq K 1200 mg K = 40 mEq K Patient/family may be encouraged to tally sodium and potassium intake while still in hospital Suggested meal plan may be shared and reviewed with patient/family
■ Insufficient knowledge to comply with discharge regimen*	■ Before discharge Patient accurately takes medications, maintains careful intake and output restrictions, and records and consumes sodium-restricted diet Patient describes potential problems related to long-term dialysis, how they will be prevented, and signs/symptoms by which they are recognized	■ Discuss extended plan of care with physician and ascertain what has already been discussed with patient Discuss psychological, social, financial, and physical implications of long-term dialysis with patient Arrange for assistance from social worker, vocational rehabilitation therapists, and clergy to counsel patient as appropriate Instruct patient in Careful recording of intake and output and daily weights Fluid and sodium restrictions Dietary restrictions in protein, cholesterol, and saturated fats Activities, which, in combination with diet, are designed to build muscle mass, maintain/build strength, ameliorate headaches, and improve psychological well-being Give information regarding discharge medications Name and purpose Dosage Frequency and schedule Side effects If home dialysis is to be done Instruct patient in procedure with emphasis on aseptic technique, prevention of infection, and careful preservation of vascular access Instruct patient that if unexplained bleeding occurs from around shunt/fistula site, to apply pressure dressing and perhaps BP cuff or other tourniquet to arm; patient should notify physician immediately and arrange transportation to appointed health facility for assessment/treatment of problem
■ Patient has limited understanding of how to safely care for shunt/fistula† Patency	■ Shunt/fistula remain patent, in situ, and infection free	■ Patency: shunt and fistula Instruct patient/family in how to monitor for shunt/fistula patency Palpate for *thrill* (pulsation) or ''buzzing'' sensation If it is difficult to palpate thrill, stethoscope can be used to hear *bruit* Monitor for indices of circulation to extremity (warmth, color)

*If critical care unit nurse is responsible for such follow-up care.
†If critical care unit nurse is responsible for preparing patient for long-term dialysis.

POTENTIAL PROBLEMS	EXPECTED OUTCOMES	NURSING ACTIVITIES
		Shunt patency
		Monitor for warmth of shunt, for uniform red, (not dark) color; for pain, tingling sensation under dressing
		Fistula patency
		Thrill with light depression of overlying skin
		If blood flow in *shunt* has decreased but is not completely occluded, instruct patient according to physician's order; guidelines may include
		Injection of heparin into the shunt every few hours
		Opening shunt, squeezing out few drops of blood, followed by aseptic reconnection of arterial and venous ends of cannula
		For *total shunt/fistula occlusion*
		Notify physician; declotting procedure is performed and may be followed by intermittent injection with heparin
		For *partial shunt occlusion*
		If one side of cannula is occluded, other side may be kept open by continuous or intermittent infusion until partially clotted side of cannula can be revised/replaced
		Instruct patient/family in situations that patient should avoid
		Constricting clothing
		Sleeping on arm with shunt or fistula, or acutely flexing extremity for long periods; cast or brace is sometimes helpful in developing habit of not sleeping on affected extremity
		Exposing extremity to extremes of heat and cold
		Situations in which shunt or fistula could be traumatized
		Fast movements with affected extremity; to avoid lifting heavy objects and doing strenuous activities with affected extremity
Infection		Instruct patient/family in proper shunt dressing, using aseptic technique
		Describe and demonstrate proper alignment of shunt; dressing must be kept dry
		Describe untoward signs
		Irritation, with skin rash around shunt resulting from sensitivity to iodine or Betadine; if this occurs, notify physician; solutions will be changed
		Signs/symptoms of local infection—redness, swelling, warmth, purulent drainage
		If these signs occur, encourage patient to notify physician so that cultures can be taken and infection treated
Shunt dislodgement		Demonstrate application of dressing such that tubing is not easily disconnected; two clamps should be carried on dressing at all times to be used to clamp shunt tubings should disconnection occur
		Should tubing come out of vessel, instruct patient/family to clamp cannula side that is still in place and to apply direct pressure to bleeding site
		Tourniquet (necktie or something like it will do) may be tightly tied above site; if BP cuff is available, it should be inflated to pressure just above patient's own systolic BP
		Instruct patient with *external shunt* in related self-care activities
		Whether bathing shunted extremity is permitted and, if so, whether protective waterproof covering is to be used
		If dressing becomes damp, patient is usually told to change it
		Prescribe physical activities on individual basis
		Encourage patient to wear medical alert bracelet

POTENTIAL PROBLEMS	EXPECTED OUTCOMES	NURSING ACTIVITIES

■ Patient/family has insufficient knowledge of complications of long-term renal failure including anemia, malnutrition, polyneuropathy, hyperparathyroidism, bony abnormalities	■ Patient identifies and, when appropriate, performs activities necessary to prevent potential long-term complications of hemodialysis
	
	Patient accurately records daily weight on log form
	
	Weight maintained without significant incidence of edema
		■ Review potential problems of long-term renal failure and care that will minimize associated problems
		   Anemia, unusual weakness, loss of energy, apathy, headache
		   Malnutrition, weight loss, nausea and vomiting
		   Polyneuropathy
		   Hyperparathyroidism
		   Bony abnormalities
		   Signs of fluid and electrolyte imbalance and acidosis—muscular irritability, twitching, weakness, lethargy
		Provide opportunity for patient/family to ask questions
		Describe plan for follow-up visits with patient/family, including when and where to go, who to see, and what specimens to bring
		   Explain that follow-up visits will include evaluation for
		      Signs/symptoms of protein and calorie malnutrition (weakness, apathy, weight loss, decreased albumin levels, and edema)
		      Weight changes; patient's daily weight log is reviewed
		      Fluid balance; signs of underhydration or overhydration

RENAL TRANSPLANTATION

In renal transplantation a functioning kidney is removed from one individual and used to replace a nonfunctioning kidney in another individual.

Renal transplantation is performed for a variety of reasons. Hemodialysis may be inadequate for control of renal failure. Medication and dietary management in the hemodialysis patient may not adequately control the signs/symptoms of renal failure. Psychosocial factors such as the realization of life-threatening aspects of renal failure, its ''terminal'' nature, and the concurrent dependency on the hemodialysis machine have an adverse effect on self-image and interpersonal relationships. Physiological effects of renal failure and hemodialysis, including fatigue, possible impotence, and job loss, further strain self-image and intimate relationships.

Renal transplantation can offer these persons a more normal life-style, an improved sense of well-being, and a more liberalized medication and dietary regimen than is possible with hemodialysis. Renal transplantation provides for a greater feeling of independence than is usually possible during hemodialysis therapy. Psychosocial difficulties that occur with long-term hemodialysis may also be ameliorated or avoided altogether. Potency may return in males, and libido may increase in women. Moreover, renal transplantation may result in decreased long-term financial cost.

Appropriate candidates for kidney transplantation include patients who anticipate long-term dialysis, are within a predetermined age range, and have had no cancer within a predetermined length of time.

In the early postoperative period, these patients are usually cared for in a surgical critical care unit or in a special transplant-dialysis unit.

Postoperatively, the goal of therapy is to prevent irreversible rejection of the donor kidney with the use of immunosuppressive agents. These medications depress the patient's immunological reaction against the donor tissue. Unfortunately, this therapy decreases the patient's ability to engulf and destroy unwanted bacteria, fungi, and viruses. The bacteria can multiply at an accelerated rate, producing a fulminant infection. Measures to prevent infection are thus an essential component of the postoperative regimen.

The nurse must monitor for infection and rejection on an ongoing basis. Should signs of either occur, the physician should be notified and the therapeutic regimen appropriately revised.

ASSESSMENT

1. History that includes
   a. Etiology, natural history of renal dysfunction
   b. Results of biopsies done
   c. Start and length of therapy with peritoneal dialysis and/or hemodialysis, including complications
   d. Presence and date of insertion of shunt and/or fistula
   e. Previous operations, particularly
      (1) Nephrectomy—left and/or right
      (2) Parathyroidectomy
      (3) Pericardiectomy
   f. Presence of chronic systemic disease or any disorders compromising life expectancy (e.g., cancer)
2. Signs and symptoms of chronic renal failure; see Standard 52, *Acute renal failure*
3. Hemodynamic status
   a. BP
   b. P
   c. Peripheral circulation
4. Results of lab and diagnostic tests, including
   a. Paramaters of kidney function
      (1) Urine (if present) volume, specific gravity
      (2) Urine sediment
      (3) Osmolality
      (4) Electrolytes
      (5) Blood—electrolyte levels particularly potassium, calcium, phosphorus levels; creatinine, uric acid, BUN; drug levels, if appropriate
   b. Liver function tests
      (1) Transaminase levels (SGOT, SGPT); alkaline phosphatase
      (2) Serum protein, albumin levels
      (3) Bilirubin levels (total, direct, indirect)
   c. Hct, Hgb, platelets, coagulation profile
   d. Australia antigen (serum hepatitis antigen)
   e. Viral studies (especially herpesvirus, cytomegalovirus)
   f. Blood type

481

g. Tissue type

h. Histocompatibility studies

    (1) Mixed lymphocyte cytotoxicity inhibition

    (2) Panel cross-match

    (3) Final cross-match with donor leukocytes

i. Complement levels

j. WBC count with differential

k. Immunological determinations

    (1) Blast cell count

    (2) Antibody titers

    (3) E-rosette levels

l. Baseline radiographs of major bone areas—shoulder, hips, joints

m. Tests performed to assure absence of cancer and ulcers

n. Cultures

    (1) Blood

    (2) Throat

    (3) Sputum

    (4) Urine

    (5) Stool or rectal

5. Level of patient/family's anxiety regarding hospitalization, transplant surgery, expected outcomes, and related therapy employed (e.g., immunosuppression)

6. Patient/family's knowledge regarding operative therapy
   a. What have they been told
   b. Their expectations
   c. Previous experience with surgery

7. Information and detail surgeon has provided patient/family about need for surgery, actual surgery to be performed, and expected outcome

GOALS

1. Reduction of patient/family's anxiety with provision of information, explanations, and encouragement

2. Physiological serum levels of
   a. Metabolic waste products (BUN, ammonia, uric acid, creatinine)
   b. Electrolytes
   c. Certain substances (drugs, etc.)

3. Hct, Hgb, and coagulation studies within normal limits

4. Normovolemia; hemodynamic stability

5. Acid-base balance within normal limits

6. Infection free

7. Nutrition adequate to prevent protein catabolism; positive nitrogen balance

8. Absence or alleviation of signs and symptoms of chronic renal failure

9. Normal cardiovascular, GI, neuromuscular, and integumentary function

10. Before discharge patient/family is able to describe
    a. Dietary and fluid management
    b. Activity progression
    c. Medication regimen
    d. Special procedures required (e.g., wound care)
    e. Untoward signs and symptoms
    f. Plan for follow-up care

11. Absence of long-term complications of immunosuppression

POTENTIAL PROBLEMS	EXPECTED OUTCOMES	NURSING ACTIVITIES
Perioperative		

■ Patient/family's anxiety related to
Disease process
Hospitalization
Diagnostic procedures
Therapeutic regimen
Anticipated surgery and expected outcomes
	■ Patient/family's behavior indicates reduction in anxiety with provision of information, explanations, and encouragement	■ Ongoing assessment of level of patient/family's anxiety
		Assess patient/family's knowledge and understanding of disease process and rationale for surgery
		Assess patient/family's understanding of diagnostic procedures, therapeutic regimen, anticipated surgery, expected outcomes
		Explain aforementioned as needed; individualize instruction in terms of approach, timing, and sequence
		Arrange for psychiatric consult and follow-up if needed, as ordered
		Encourage patient to participate in decisions regarding his/her care
		Encourage participation in care as tolerated
		Perform treatments in unhurried manner
		Provide comfort measures
		Describe perioperative experiences, including
		  Preoperative
		    Chest physiotherapy
		    Coughing and deep breathing
		    Incentive spirometry
		    Shave
		    Light dinner, then NPO after midnight
		    Morning bath/shower
		    Preoperative medications
		    Skin tests for immune status if appropriate

POTENTIAL PROBLEMS	EXPECTED OUTCOMES	NURSING ACTIVITIES
		Hospital gown
		Care of valuables
		Ride to operating room
		Scrub suits, masks, and hats worn by operating room staff
		Anesthesia
		Postoperative
		Waking up in the recovery room/critical care unit
		Describe general environment (size of unit, room, etc.)
		Nurse always nearby
		Dull, continuous noises
		Incision with bandage
		IV, arterial lines (if anticipated)
		ECG monitoring
		Medicine for discomfort, pain
		Policy on family visits
		Measures to prevent postoperative infection
		Protective isolation is planned
		Measures to keep lungs clear of secretions
		Use of immunosuppressive medications
		As patient progresses
		Tubes out
		Eating again
		Getting stronger, ambulation
		Chest physiotherapy, coughing, deep breathing
		Discuss long-term therapy of kidney transplantation, including
		Immunosuppression and possibility of rejection
		Prevention of infection
		Describe responsibility of patient in achieving speedy recovery by taking active role in coughing, deep breathing, etc.
		Encourage patient/family's questions
		Encourage verbalization of anxiety and fears related to hospitalization, diagnostic procedures, therapeutic regimen, surgery, and surgical outcomes
■ Inadequate stabilization of preoperative medical problems	■ Preoperative medical problems under control	■ Monitor
		Results of lab studies
		Hepatitis B antigen
		Viral titers (e.g., herpesvirus, cytomegalovirus)
		Hct, Hgb, platelet levels
		Coagulation profile
		WBC count with differential
		Electrolyte levels
		Temperature
		BP; note hypertension
		Notify physician of any of these abnormalities
		Administer therapy as ordered to correct acid-base imbalance, electrolyte abnormalities, and low Hgb/Hct and platelet levels
Postoperative		
■ Hemodynamic instability	■ Hemodynamic stability Cardiac output, BP, P within normal limits	■ Administer fluids and medications as ordered by physician to maintain BP and fluid balance within normal limits
		Note baseline preoperative BP, P, and CVP (if available)
		Monitor hemodynamic parameters (q15 min until stable, then q30 min four times; if stable, decrease frequency to q1 hr for duration of first postoperative day), including
		BP
		Pulses—note quality, fullness
		CVP (if available)
		Urine output; NOTE: Urine output of transplanted kidney may be very low in early postoperative period
		LOC

POTENTIAL PROBLEMS	EXPECTED OUTCOMES	NURSING ACTIVITIES
		Monitor for arrhythmias Notify physician of abnormalities in aforementioned and administer therapy as ordered; monitor patient's response

■ Fluid overload related to dysfunction of transplanted kidney	■ Normovolemia
	BP, P, CVP, weight, and urine output within normal limits
		■ Prevent by administering fluids as ordered; closely monitor urine output and other parameters of fluid balance (weight, BP, P, CVP, skin turgor)
		Monitor
		  BP, P, CVP, and PAP, if available, q½-1 hr until stable
		  Urine output q1 hr until stable
		  Daily weights
		  Skin turgor
		Notify physician of significantly decreased urine output or of increase in BP, CVP, and change of skin turgor
		If fluid overload occurs
		  Administer diuretics as ordered; closely monitor patient's response
		  Institute fluid restrictions as ordered
		  Prepare patient for and, if appropriate, assist with hemodialysis if procedure is necessary

■ Hypertension related to
  Hypervolemia
  Hypernatremia
	■ BP within normal limits
	  Serum Na⁺ levels within normal limits
		■ Prevent by
		  Preparing patient for bilateral nephrectomies, if necessary, to reduce circulating levels of renin; this is done several weeks before transplantation
		  Administering fluids as ordered to keep patient's weight, intake and output records, and hemodynamic parameters within prescribed limits
		  Administering sodium as ordered to keep serum Na⁺ levels within normal limits
		  Providing low-sodium diet if indicated, as ordered
		    Instruct patient/family in prescribed low-sodium diet
		Monitor
		  BP, P, CVP, and PAP, if available, q½-1 hr until stable
		  Urine output and specific gravity q1 hr
		  Daily weight
		  Serum and urine Na⁺ levels
		Notify physician of abnormalities in aforementioned parameters
		If hypertension occurs
		  Administer diuretics, if ordered
		  Readjust amount and type of fluid administered, as ordered
		  Alter levels of sodium administration as ordered
		  Administer antihypertensive medications if ordered; closely monitor patient's response

■ Pulmonary insufficiency, which may consist of
  Inadequate oxygenation
  Hypercapnia
  Atelectasis
  Pneumonia (see Problem, Infection)
	■ Adequate exchange of blood gases
	  Adequate oxygenation (arterial PaO₂ within normal limits)
	  Adequate ventilation (arterial PaCO₂ within normal limits)
		■ Prevent by
		  Administering vigorous chest physiotherapy, including
		    Turning at least q2 hr; early ambulation
		    Deep breathing and coughing
		    Chest physiotherapy in early postoperative period and later as indicated
		    Administration of humidified oxygenated air in early postoperative period and later, as indicated
		    An incentive spirometer, as ordered; assist patient to use and follow with encouragement to cough up mobilized secretions
		Monitor
		  Quality of respirations, secretions
		  Breath sounds serially for diminished or absent breath sounds and/or presence of rales, rhonchi, and other adventitious breath sounds
		  Serial arterial blood gas measurements, if needed
		  Note acidosis, hypoxemia, and/or hypercapnia
		  For signs/symptoms of hypoxia and/or hypercapnia including restlessness, altered mentation, tachypnea, tachycardia, and dusky color

POTENTIAL PROBLEMS	EXPECTED OUTCOMES	NURSING ACTIVITIES

		Notify physician of any abnormality, and alter therapy as ordered, which may include
		  Augmentation of aforementioned preventive activities (e.g., chest physiotherapy, oxygen)
		  Administration of antibiotics for infection
		  Intubation and mechanical ventilation if necessary; see Standard 6, *Mechanical ventilation*

▪ Renal dysfunction related to
  Obstructed urinary drainage system
	▪ Patent urinary drainage system	▪ Prevent by
		  Maintaining patent urinary drainage system: bladder catheters are connected to bag and maintained as closed, intact drainage system
		  Note presence of clots or other particles
		  If present, milk or aseptically irrigate the tubing and catheter as needed
		  Monitor for obstructed urinary drainage system
		    Urine output; note volume, color, odor, presence of particles (hematuria, casts)
		    Lower abdomen for distention
		    Bladder for distention
		  If obstructed urinary drainage system occurs, notify physician and prepare to assist with correcting obstruction, which generally includes replacement of catheter

▪ Acute renal failure, which may be related to
  Perioperative ischemia
  Kinking of ureter
  Kinking of renal artery
  Rupture of anastomosis (urine enters peritoneum)
  Renal vein thrombosis
  Perioperative ischemia
	▪ Absence of acute renal failure
	
	  Absence and/or resolution of ischemic damage before and during surgery
		▪ Prevent by administering fluids and, if needed, inotropic/vasopressor drugs such as dopamine or dobutamine to maintain adequate renal blood flow and urine output
		  Monitor
		    Urine output q1 hr in the early postoperative period
		    Daily weights
		    Kidney function tests
		      Urine and serum creatinine
		      Electrolyte levels
		      Osmolality
		      BUN
		    Spot urine samples as ordered for analysis of
		      RBC casts
		      Epithelial cells
		      WBC
		    Urine C and S results
		    For abdominal distention, which may result from kinking of renal artery or anastomotic rupture
		    Results of renograms
		  Notify physician of any of aforementioned abnormalities
		  If acute renal failure occurs, administer therapy, as ordered; see Standard 52, *Acute renal failure*

▪ Rejection caused by incompatibility of recipient and donor tissue	▪ Blood types A, B, and O (ABO) compatibility
	  Absence of signs of cytotoxicity
	  Immunological studies indicate optimal immunosuppression
		▪ Prevent rejection by assisting in verifying patient/donor tissue compatibility
		  Monitor results of histocompatibility studies, which may include
		    ABO compatibility studies
		    Result of tissue typing and comparison of human leukocyte antigen (HLA) constellations
		      Parents share one chromosome with patient, and siblings share two, one, or no chromosomes; siblings sharing both chromosomes are preferred donors
		      Cadaver donors are similarly tissue typed; recipient who is most closely matched from pool of potential recipients is chosen to receive cadaver kidney
		    Histocompatibility studies

POTENTIAL PROBLEMS	EXPECTED OUTCOMES	NURSING ACTIVITIES
		Mixed lymphocyte cytotoxicity inhibition—donor lymphocytes are put in contact with recipient lymphocytes in tissue culture to test for preformed cytotoxic antibodies; if marked aggregation occurs (antigen-antibody response), donor is incompatible with recipient
		Panel cross-match
		Final cross-match with donor leukocytes
		Immunological studies
		Antibody titers, blast cell count, E-rosette levels
		Prevent by administering immunosuppressive agents, as ordered, to suppress rejection of donor kidney
		Monitor lab indices of adequate immunosuppression, including
		Blast cell counts
		E-rosette levels
		Panel cross-match
		Mixed lymphocyte cytotoxicity inhibition
		Antibody titers
		Monitor tolerance of immunosuppression and for adverse effects
		Hct, Hgb, platelet, and reticulocyte levels; WBC count with differential; bleeding time, stool specimens for blood; liver function tests
		Note occurrence of the following
		Depression, anxiety, psychosis, other behavioral changes
		Increased BP
		Edema
		Visual changes
		Monitor for signs and symptoms of *hyperacute rejection,* which usually occurs within minutes to hours of surgery because of preformed cytotoxic antibodies to donor tissue; preoperative testing for such antibodies should prevent this type of rejection
		Monitor for *accelerated rejection* within 5 days of surgery (etiology not clear); treatment (usually including maximal steroid doses) may be unsuccessful
		Monitor for signs and symptoms of *acute cell-mediated rejection,* which appears from 1 week to 3 months after transplantation: fever, malaise, tenderness over graft site, deterioration in indices of renal function, Na⁺ retention, and reduction in creatinine clearance
		Treatment with high steroid doses and antithymocyte globulin may be successful in reversing such rejection
		Monitor for signs and symptoms of *chronic humoral antibody-mediated rejection:* progressive deterioration in indices of renal function, proteinuria, and hypertension; treatment is often unsuccessful
		Monitor for signs/symptoms of rejection, including
		Results of periodic renal scans, which may show deterioration of renal blood flow
		Pain over graft site
		Arthralgias
		Deteriorating parameters of renal function
		Elevated blood levels of Na⁺, BUN, creatinine
		Decreased urine output
		Concurrent
		Malaise and temperature elevation
		Increased BP
		If any of these signs/symptoms occur, notify physician
		Assist with plasmapheresis, which may be done to minimize patient's rejection of donor kidney tissue
		If rejection occurs
		Administer increasing dosages of immunosuppressive agents; gradually taper dosage as renal function improves
		Prepare patient for radiotherapy, if ordered

POTENTIAL PROBLEMS	EXPECTED OUTCOMES	NURSING ACTIVITIES
		Prepare patient for hemodialysis, if necessary If therapy for rejection is unsuccessful, removal of kidney may be necessary; prepare patient for procedure Keep patient informed of progress Give patient/family simple explanations Provide opportunity for expression of fears, anxieties Provide for kind, supportive care
■ Electrolyte imbalance, which may include Hypernatremia in oliguric phase of renal failure with concurrent administration of sodium Hyponatremia related to diuretic phase of renal failure or dilutional hyponatremia Hyperkalemia in oliguric phase of renal failure Hypokalemia In diuretic phase of renal failure With vigorous diuretic therapy	■ Serum electrolyte values within normal limits	■ Monitor serial blood and urine samples for electrolyte levels Notify physician of significant abnormalities Administer electrolyte replacement, which is ordered with consideration for urinary losses and concurrent therapeutic measures Monitor for signs/symptoms of electrolyte imbalance Neuromuscular changes: weakness, irritability, twitching, and/or (rarely) seizures Abnormal neurological signs: headaches, confusion, disorientation, restlessness, lethargy Skin alterations Temperature: warm or cold, clammy or dry Turgor: taut, firm, or loose Mucous membranes: moist, dry, cracked, or coated Daily weight for loss or gain
■ Metabolic abnormalities: acidosis associated with renal dysfunction/failure	■ Acid/base balance within normal limits	■ Monitor serial arterial blood gas samples for adequate oxygenation and acid-base balance Provide for adequate oxygenation with supplemental humidified O_2 and vigorous chest physiotherapy Institute therapy to correct primary abnormalities, as ordered Allow patient's body to compensate for metabolic imbalances with respiratory compensation Administer bicarbonate and electrolyte replacement, as ordered to correct metabolic disturbances
■ Infection of Wound Vascular access site Blood	■ Infection free	■ Prevent by Implementing protective isolation during period of maximal immunosuppressive therapy as indicated, according to hospital protocol Limiting contact of patient with personnel and extended family members Keep infected patients, visitors, and personnel away from patient Providing for scrupulous hygiene of mouth, perineum, and skin Providing for early ambulation Providing for adequate nutrition to promote healing, prevent infection Employing aseptic wound care Keeping vascular access for hemodialysis clean; change shunt dressing q24-48 hr using aseptic technique Monitor temperature; reculture patient for any significant temperature elevation, as ordered Monitor wound, vascular access sites for evidence of infection: erythema, inflammation, drainage Monitor culture results Notify physician of any of aforementioned abnormalities and administer therapy as ordered, which may include Local care Systemic antibiotics

POTENTIAL PROBLEMS	EXPECTED OUTCOMES	NURSING ACTIVITIES

■ Infection of
  Kidney
  Urinary tract
	■ Kidney and urinary tract
	  infection free
		■ Prevent by discontinuing bladder catheter as soon as possible
		  Monitor for
		    Patient's complaints of
		      Frequency
		      Dysuria or burning on urination
		      Lower back pain
		      Malaise
		    Cloudy urine
		  Notify physician of the presence of any of these symptoms, and send stat specimens for urinalysis and C and S determinations
		  Monitor
		    Urine WBC and bacterial levels (specimens usually sent every 1 to 2 days while catheter is in place, then two to three times a week or as ordered)
		    Urine C and S results (specimens usually sent every 1 to 2 days while catheter is in place, then 2 to 3 times a week)
		  If kidney, urinary tract infection occurs
		    Administer bladder catheter irrigation if ordered
		    Administer antibiotic therapy, as ordered

■ Pulmonary infection	■ Absence or resolution of
	  pulmonary infection
		■ Prevent pulmonary infection by
		    Providing for vigorous chest physiotherapy (see Problem, Pulmonary insufficiency)
		    Administering humidified O_2 supplements, as ordered, based on arterial blood gas measurements
		    Administering additional humidity and/or medications to liquefy secretions, if ordered
		    Repositioning patient q1-2 hr
		      Bed rest, with 30-degree head elevation, is usually ordered for first 2 to 3 days
		  Monitor for
		    Fever
		    Increased tenacity, amount, and abnormal color of secretions
		    Breath sounds q1-2 hr for decreased or absent breath sounds and for adventitious sounds (e.g., rales, rhonchi)
		    Signs of respiratory distress: tachypnea, dyspnea, shallow breathing
		    Chest radiograph results revealing areas of infiltrates, atelectasis, consolidation, or collapse
		  Notify physician of any of these abnormalities
		  If pulmonary infection occurs
		    Send additional sputum specimens for C and S, as ordered
		    Administer antibiotics, as ordered
		    Administer vigorous chest physiotherapy emphasizing affected areas of lung

■ Wound infection	■ Infection-free wound	■ Prevention
		    Aseptically care for wounds, puncture sites, and indwelling catheters
		    Monitor wound, puncture sites for erythema, discomfort or pain, and signs of infected drainage (odor, color, amount)
		    Notify physician of any signs of wound infection
		    Reculture wound/drainage when status changes, as ordered

■ Oral infection
  Herpesvirus
  Candida
	■ Infection-free mouth	■ Prevent by
		    Providing for scrupulous mouth care
		    Administering prophylactic antifungal mouthwash, if ordered, in effort to prevent candidal infection
		  Monitor for white coating in mouth, oral lesions
		  Notify physician if either of these occurs
		  If oral infection occurs, administer antifungal mouthwash or lozenges according to plan of care

POTENTIAL PROBLEMS	EXPECTED OUTCOMES	NURSING ACTIVITIES

■ Hyperglycemia related to Endogenous production of cortisone in response to stress of surgery
Large doses of exogenous steroids in early postoperative period
	■ Blood glucose levels within normal limits	■ Monitor
		  Serial blood glucose levels
		  Urine glucose and acetone levels
		  For signs and symptoms of hyperglycemia, including confusion, disorientation, dry mucous membranes
		Notify physician of any of these abnormalities
		If hyperglycemia occurs, administer insulin if ordered

■ Malnutrition	■ Nutrition adequate to prevent protein catabolism
	Positive nitrogen balance
		■ Arrange for dietary consult
		Administer postoperative diet according to kidney function (see Standard 52, *Acute renal failure*), as ordered
		After early postoperative renal dysfunction has subsided, diet progression as ordered
		If patient continues on high doses of steroids and/or is hypertensive, institute sodium restriction as ordered
		Monitor for evidence of malnutrition
		  Reduced muscle mass
		  Weight loss
		  Weakness, decreased exercise tolerance
		  Poor skin turgor
		  Altered LOC, e.g., restlessness, irritability, confusion
		If evidence of malnutrition occurs, notify physician; alter patient's diet and medications (e.g., vitamin supplements), as ordered

■ Insufficient knowledge to comply with discharge regimen*	■ Before discharge patient/family accurately verbalizes discharge regimen regarding
	Prevention of infection
	Activity progression
	Dietary management
	Fluid intake and output measurements
	Weights, BP measurements
	Medications
	
	Untoward signs and symptoms requiring medical attention
		■ Assess patient/family's understanding of discharge regimen
		Instruct patient/family regarding
		  Prevention of infection
		    Avoid contact with persons with respiratory infections, etc.
		    Demonstrate proper wound care
		    Describe signs of symptoms of infection
		  Activity progression
		  Dietary management
		    Fluid intake and output measurements (may be recorded daily in chart form)
		    Daily weights, BP measurement
		    Medications: purpose, dosage, timing, precautionary measures, and potential adverse effects
		Describe signs and symptoms requiring medical attention, including
		  Fever
		  Tenderness of implantation site
		  Anorexia
		  Malaise
		  Acute depression anxiety
		  Yellow-bronze color of skin
		  Yellowish tint in white of eyes (sclera)
		  Drug reaction
		  Decreased urine output
		  Significant changes in BP
		  Significant changes in weight
		According to medications patient is receiving, instruct in potential adverse effects of
		  Immunosuppression, including signs of cancer, infection
		  Long-term steroid therapy
		    Diabetes
		    Aseptic necrosis of bones
		    GI hemorrhage
		    Pancreatitis
		    Others

*If responsibility of the critical care nurse includes follow-up care.

POTENTIAL PROBLEMS	EXPECTED OUTCOMES	NURSING ACTIVITIES
		Cyclophosphamide therapy: hemorrhagic cystitis
		Azathioprine therapy
		Hepatitis
		Pancreatitis
	Patient accurately describes follow-up plan of care	Describe plan for follow-up care
		Location, date, times of appointments
		Specimens to bring
		Activities during visits
		Provide patient/family opportunity to discuss
		Family relationships
		Sexual adjustments
		Emotional problems
		Employ assistance of auxiliary services, as needed
		Social services
		Vocational rehabilitation
		Others
		Assess potential compliance with discharge regimen

Metabolic

DIABETIC KETOACIDOSIS

Diabetic ketoacidosis is an acute metabolic disorder that results primarily from a sustained lack of insulin and produces a condition called *hyperglycemia.*

Insulin is required to transport blood glucose for cell metabolism. Without insulin the glucose remains outside the cell and, despite the rising blood glucose levels, the cells "starve." Dehydration and metabolic abnormalities ensue.

Both intracellular and extracellular dehydration occur in the presence of hyperglycemia. Intracellular dehydration is the result of high extracellular osmolarity that causes a shift of intracellular water into the extracellular space. Extracellular dehydration is caused by an osmotic diuresis, and as glucose passes into the urine it obligates the loss of hypotonic fluid and electrolytes, particularly potassium and sodium.

Metabolic abnormalities include ketoacidosis and abnormal potassium and sodium levels.

Increased use of fats and proteins in place of glucose produces accumulation of free fatty acids. Free fatty acids are metabolized in the liver to ketone bodies (acetone, acetoacetic acid, and beta-hydroxybutyric acid), which can then be oxidized for energy. Production of ketone bodies in excess of their use and elimination results in ketosis and ketoacidosis.

The osmotic diuresis caused by glycosuria results in loss of potassium and a decrease in intravascular volume. The decrease in intravascular volume activates the renin-angiotensin system, releasing aldosterone and causing further loss of potassium. However, with acidosis intracellular buffer proteins release potassium ions into the serum, and serum potassium may be low, apparently normal, or high. Total body potassium is almost always low.

Total body sodium is usually low as a result of increased urinary losses. The serum sodium measurements in the presence of hyperglycemia are usually low. However, if dehydration is severe as a result of vomiting and excessive urinary loss of hypotonic fluid, the serum sodium may be normal or even high. Therefore a high or normal serum sodium in the presence of hyperglycemia is a clue to severe dehydration.

Other causes of ketoacidosis include salicylate intoxication and excessive alcohol intake. Salicylate intoxication alters normal metabolism and leads to production of organic acids including ketone bodies. Patients with salicylate intoxication may have ketones in serum and urine. Alcohol in the absence of starvation has been shown to cause increased serum ketones unrelated to diabetes. Unlike patients with diabetes, these patients have adequate endogenous insulin, but its release and action have been temporarily inhibited by alcohol and the humoral response to hypoglycemia. These patients will respond to glucose infusion, hydration, and small amounts of supplemental insulin.

Factors that can precipitate diabetic ketoacidosis include the following.
1. An undiagnosed diabetes
2. A known diabetic who has
   a. Failed to take prescribed insulin according to specified needs
   b. Not followed prescribed dietary requirement
   c. Severe infection
   d. Prolonged nausea and vomiting
   e. Concomitant illness; physiological stresses, i.e., trauma, surgery; emotional and mental stresses; and pregnancy
   f. Untreated renal insufficiency
   g. Insulin antibodies
3. A diabetic who is taking agents that can increase blood sugar levels (e.g., corticosteroids, diuretics)

These factors increase glucose use, impair glucose metabolism, and/or are associated with insufficient insulin availability.

Therapy in diabetic ketoacidosis is directed toward administration of insulin and treatment of dehydration, metabolic and electrolyte abnormalities, and correction of any underlying conditions that may have precipitated the ketoacidosis.

ASSESSMENT

1. Baseline information regarding history of
   a. Polydipsia, polyuria, and polyphagia related to dramatic weight fluctuations
   b. Number of years as diagnosed diabetic
   c. Family members with diabetes
   d. Inability to follow prescribed diabetic regimen and degree of adherence, i.e.
      (1) Omission of insulin intake
      (2) Failure to adhere to prescribed dietary and fluid requirements
   e. Recent conditions necessitating increased insulin intake including overeating, trauma, etc.
   f. Any associated illnesses including renal disease, pancreatitis, hepatitis, and endocrine disorders related to pregnancy, infection, obesity, cardiac disease
   g. Alcoholism
   h. Recent drug ingestion including salicylates, etc.
2. Physical signs and symptoms of
   a. Anorexia, nausea, vomiting
   b. Weakness, general malaise
   c. Abdominal pain and tenderness, which may be severe and can mimic surgical emergencies
   d. Abdominal distention, absence of bowel sounds
   e. Hepatomegaly
   f. Headache and visual disturbances
   g. Lethargy, drowsiness leading to coma, confusion
   h. Skin appearance
      (1) Flushed—results from local vasodilatation caused by ketone bodies
      (2) Dry—results from dehydration; may note "tenting" when skin is pinched and soft or sunken eyeballs
   i. Dry, crusty mucous membranes
   j. Tachycardia
   k. Hypothermia—may accompany coma and hypotension: suggestive of gram-negative sepsis
   l. Hyperthermia—may suggest sepsis
   m Air hunger with deep heavy respirations called *Kussmaul respirations*
   n. Acetone breath or fruity odor on breath
   o. Thirst
   p. Polyuria or oliguria
   q. Decrease or absence of reflexes

3. Lab and diagnostic data results, including
   a. Urine sugar and acetone, specific gravity, and osmolality
   b. Blood for electrolytes, ketones, BUN, and lipid levels; elevation and/or depletion of sodium, potassium, chloride, and bicarbonate; osmolality
   c. Blood glucose determination
   d. CBC for leukocytosis and elevated Hct
   e. Arterial blood gas results for acidosis
   f. ECG for any S-T segment and T wave abnormalities
   g. Results of throat, blood, sputum, urine, and stool cultures
4. Patient/family's knowledge and understanding of disease process, purpose of hospitalization, and therapy planned
   a. Assess patient/family's level of anxiety related to disease process, diagnostic procedures, and therapy planned
   b. Determine diabetic control regimen patient has been on at home, if any, and the degree of patient/family compliance

GOALS

1. Patient/family's behavior indicates reduction in level of anxiety with provision of information and explanations
2. Respiratory function within normal limits
   a. Respiratory assessment and arterial blood gas levels within patient's normal limits
   b. Absence of pulmonary edema
3. Hemodynamic stability
   a. Absence of arrhythmias
   b. Adequate cardiac output
4. Fluids, electrolytes, and CBC levels within normal limits; weight gain or loss in desired direction
5. Absence of and/or resolution of any complications including paralytic ileus secondary to hypokalemia, hypoglycemia, CHF
6. Prevention and/or resolution of associated medical problems precipitating diabetic ketoacidosis including infection, renal insufficiency, physiological stress, etc.
7. Before discharge patient/family is able to
   a. Describe cause, pathophysiology, diagnosis, therapy, and prognosis of diabetes
   b. Adhere to prescribed therapeutic diet, maintaining blood glucose and weight at desired levels
   c. Discuss early signs and symptoms of hypoglycemia and ketoacidosis, and what to do about them, including when to report them to physician
   d. Discuss signs and symptoms of infections that will require medical attention
   e. Verbalize and demonstrate, if appropriate, good health practices to prevent infections
   f. Describe and demonstraate, if appropriate, activity, dietary, medication, and follow-up regimens

POTENTIAL PROBLEMS	EXPECTED OUTCOMES	NURSING ACTIVITIES
■ Patient/family's anxiety related to insufficient knowledge of Disease process Diagnostic procedures Therapy employed	■ Patient/family's behavior demonstrates decreased level of anxiety with provision of information and explanations Patient/family verbalizes understanding of disease process and its relationship to therapy employed Patient/family participates actively in planning and implementing care	■ Ongoing assessment of level of anxiety Describe nature of disease process and its relation to signs and symptoms patient is experiencing Explain relationship of disease process to rationale for various therapeutic interventions Explain anticipated procedures involved in diagnostic process/plan of care and what patient will experience Assist in preparing patient for diagnostic procedures Encourage patient/family's questions, verbalization of fears and anxieties Involve patient/family in planning for care Demonstrate concern and warmth in providing care to patient Evaluate for decrease in level of anxiety with provision of information, explanations
■ Metabolic and electrolyte abnormalities Metabolic abnormalities Ketoacidosis as result of increased ketone bodies, causing decrease in bicarbonate	■ Absence or resolution of metabolic and electrolyte abnormalities Absence or resolution of ketoacidosis	■ Monitor and notify physician of abnormalities Vital signs including temperature q1 hr until stable; note presence of fever and hypotension Intake and output with glucose and acetone determination, specific gravity q1 hr until stable; daily weight Fingerstick glucose q1 hr to permit ongoing adjustment of insulin administration Lab blood glucose determination q2 hr CVP readings, if available, q1 hr Serum electrolytes and anions/cations such as ketones, phosphate q1 hr For presence of signs and symptoms of hyperkalemia, hypokalemia, hyponatremia, and hypophosphatemia BUN and creatinine levels q6-12 hr Serial arterial blood gas results for acidosis q1 hr until stable Serial complete blood count for leukocytosis and elevated ESR Chest radiograph to rule out infection Serial ECG for any T wave and/or S-T segment abnormalities Presence or absence of Kussmaul respirations and acetone breath Alterations in LOC, seizure activity, reflex status Skin color for cyanosis Absence or presence of bowel sounds and gastric dilatation
Compensatory respiratory alkalosis (Kussmaul) Hyperglycemia	Arterial blood gas levels within normal limits Regular and even respirations Absence or resolution of hyperglycemia Blood sugar within normal limits	If patient is comatose, other lab and diagnostic tests may be ordered and results monitored, including C and S of blood, sputum, urine, throat, stool, and cerebrospinal fluid Ca^{++}, amylase, lactic acid, serum and urine osmolalities Lumbar puncture for spinal fluid pressure and electrolyte determinations Appropriate samples for drug detection Type and cross-match Place patient on continuous cardiac monitor
Electrolyte abnormalities, particularly imbalance in K^+, Na^+, and abnormal phosphate levels	Serum electrolyte levels within normal limits, particularly K^+, Na^+, and phosphate	Administer parenteral infusion and plasma expanders as ordered Administer insulin, as ordered NOTE: Generally, initial fluid given is normal saline (0.9%), in large amounts, as ordered, to rehydrate patient; once blood volume is restored, half-strength normal saline (0.45%) is administered; at same time, loading dose of insulin is administered, followed by infusion at 4 to 8 units/hr (approximately 0.1 unit/kg/hr) or by intermittent subcutaneous, IM, or IV injections (blood glucose should be reduced *gradually;* rapid lowering of blood glucose promotes cerebral edema); when blood glucose level decreases to approximately 250 to 300 mg/dl, dextrose will be added to IV in most cases and insulin infusion will be reduced to 1 unit/hr or discontinued altogether Administer electrolyte replacements, i.e., K^+, Na^+, Cl^-, and anion phosphate, if ordered

POTENTIAL PROBLEMS	EXPECTED OUTCOMES	NURSING ACTIVITIES

		Check that blood specimens are drawn at specified time
		Insert Foley catheter and connect to closed gravity drainage, as ordered
		Administer O₂ therapy if ordered
		Maintain diabetic flow sheet, including glucose and acetone determinations, specific gravity, electrolytes (anion gap), arterial blood gas results, intake and output, and CVP results
		Keep patient NPO until nausea and ileus have cleared; then administer diet according to tolerance, as ordered
		Assist in NG tube insertion and connect to low continuous suction, if ordered
		Seizure precautions may be necessary; see Standard 41, *Seizures*
		Maintain low Fowler position unless contraindicated
		Administer skin care with position change q2 hr; check bony prominences and other areas for any skin breakdown
		Encourage deep breathing exercises q1 hr
		Oral hygiene q2 hr and prn
		Provide environment conducive to physical, mental, and emotional rest
		    Keep patient warm, dry, and comfortable
		    Allow for rest periods between treatments
		    Limit visitors according to patient's needs

■ Dehydration related to hyperglycemia and increased serum levels of ketone bodies	■ Fluid balance, CVP readings, urine output within normal limits for patient's age and size Weight remains within 5% of patient's normal baseline weight	■ Refer to Problem, Metabolic and electrolyte abnormalities, for parameters permitting detection of hyperglycemia and increased ketone bodies, and activities for control In addition, monitor serum osmolalities and Hct levels (elevated in diabetic ketoacidosis)

■ Hypoglycemia related to therapy	■ Absence and/or resolution of hypoglycemia
	Resolution of ketoacidosis with proper therapy
		■ Prevent by careful monitoring of parameters in Problem, Metabolic and electrolyte abnormalities, and activities for control of hyperglycemia
		Monitor or observe for signs and symptoms of hypoglycemia q1 hr, including
		    Sudden lowering of blood sugar level (usually below 60 mg/100 ml of blood)
		    Signs and symptoms of
		        Tachycardia
		        Slight increase in systolic BP
		        Sweating
		        Numbness
		        Dilatated pupils
		        Pallor
		        General weakness
		        Faintness
		    Cerebral manifestations
		        Nervousness
		        Apprehension
		        Visual disturbances
		        Headache
		        Thick speech
		        Muscle twitching
		        Tonic and clonic spasm
		        Urinary incontinence
		        Unconsciousness
		        Convulsions
		        Babinski reflex is often present
		    Unexpected behavioral reaction
		        Restlessness, negativism, personality changes, catatonia, and maniacal behavior

POTENTIAL PROBLEMS	EXPECTED OUTCOMES	NURSING ACTIVITIES
		If problem occurs
		Administer glucose IV, as ordered, (dextrose 50% is generally used for hypogycemic shock)
		If patient is able to swallow, orange juice with sugar, milk, or other sources of glucose can be given orally
		Administer glucagon if ordered and start IV 5% dextrose in water (D5W)
		Reevaluate and restandardize therapy to control and/or prevent hypoglycemia
		Monitor lab and diagnostic studies for control
■ Coma or altered mental status related to Metabolic and electrolyte abnormalities Sepsis, meningitis Embolic phenomenon caused by MI	■ Patient is alert and oriented to time, place, and person Absence and/or resolution of etiological factors	■ Refer to Problems, Metabolic and electrolyte abnormalities, and Dehydration, for parameters permitting detection of metabolic and electrolyte abnormalities and activities for control
		See Standard 42, *Meningitis/encephalitis;* Standard 31, *Embolic phenomena*
		Monitor for
		Weakness, general malaise
		Confusion
		Lethargy, dullness
		Drowsiness leading to coma
		If problem occurs
		Identify etiological factors and treat accordingly (see aforementioned problems)
		Provide for adequate airway patency, including
		Placing patient in semi-Fowler position; turn patient side to side q2 hr; suction q1 hr and/or prn; connect NG tube to suction to prevent aspiration
		Administering O$_2$ with humidification, as ordered
		Pulmonary toilet q2 hr and prn
		Auscultating for any abnormal breath sounds q2 hr
		Vital signs, including temperature, q2 hr until stable
		Serial arterial blood gas results q1-2 hr or as indicated
		If mechanical ventilation is indicated, see Standard 6, *Mechanical ventilation*
		Neurological assessment q2 hr
		Monitor LOC q2 hr
		Provide eye, ear, nose, mouth, and skin care q2 hr or as necessary
		Maintain proper body alignment and perform passive ROM exercises to all extremities q2 hr and prn
		Maintain seizure precautions
		Provide for elimination, i.e., perineal care, external catheter; check for bowel movement
		Maintain quiet environment
		Provide nursing support as indicated by patient's changing condition, i.e., restlessness
		Notify physician for any changes or abnormalities
		Provide emotional support to patient/family
■ Presence of precipitating factors, including Cardiac ischemia, i.e., MI Pancreatitis	■ Absence or resolution of Myocardial ischemia Pancreatitis	■ Monitor
		ECG for abnormalities—S-T segment and T wave changes and arrhythmias; notify physician if present
		If cardiac ischemia occurs, see Standard 11, *Angina pectoris;* Standard 12, *Acute myocardial infarction,* or Standard 21, *Arrhythmias*
		For moderate to severe left upper quadrant pain; notify physician if present
		If pancreatitis occurs, see Standard 47, *Pancreatitis*
Significant trauma or CNS catastrophe	Trauma or CNS dysfunction	For altered LOC (restlessness, agitation); pupils for inequality and unreactivity; notify physician if present
		If trauma or CNS catastrophe occurs, see Standard 33, *Head trauma*

POTENTIAL PROBLEMS	EXPECTED OUTCOMES	NURSING ACTIVITIES
Sepsis, i.e. 　Meningitis 　Pneumonia 　Cellulitis 　Pyelonephritis	Sepsis	For hypotension, hypothermia, hyperthermia, tachycardia, altered LOC; if present, notify physician If sepsis occurs, see Standard 17, *Shock*
■ Insufficient information to comply with discharge regimen*	■ Sufficient information to comply with discharge regimen	■ Assess patient/family's level of understanding, ability to comprehend, and any physical limitations regarding follow-up plan of care or discharge regimen Develop patient teaching and discharge regimen at patient/family's level of understanding Involve patient/family in planning for discharge regimen Describe patient teaching and discharge regimen
	Patient/family verbalizes understanding of patient teaching and discharge regimen, including Knowledge of diabetes Signs and symptoms, causes and treatment of hypoglycemia and hyperglycemia Importance of reporting early signs and symptoms to physician	Discuss disease process and fears, and correct misconceptions of diabetes Provide booklets and pamphlets from American Diabetes Association, Inc.† and pharmaceutical companies Describe early signs and symptoms of hyperglycemia and hypoglycemia, including causes of and actions to take

	Hyperglycemia	**Hypoglycemia**
Onset	Gradual	Sudden
Behavior	Drowsy	Excited
Breath	Fruity odor	Normal
Breathing	Deep and labored	Normal to rapid, shallow
Hunger	Absent	Present
Skin	Dry and flushed	Pale and moist
Sugar in urine	Large amount	Absence or slight
Thirst	Present	Absent
Tongue	Dry	Moist
Vomiting	Present	Absent

		If signs of hypoglycemia occur, instruct patient to drink glass of orange juice or milk (lactose in milk immediately increases blood sugar levels; it also provides protein, which keeps blood glucose elevated longer than nonprotein preparations) or suck on hard candies If signs of hyperglycemia occur, instruct patient to notify physician immediately
	Dietary and exercise regimen	Discuss importance of Regularity of diet and exercise Plan prescribed diet and substitutes with dietitian and patient/family, allowing for cultural and religious preference and economic status Same amount of exercise daily Importance of weight control Demonstrate how to do fingerstick blood glucose monitoring
	Patient/family is able to Test urine for sugar and acetone Administer insulin and oral hypoglycemics	Demonstrate how to test urine for sugar and acetone (fingerstick method for blood glucose monitoring is generally preferred since it provides more accurate reflection of blood glucose levels) Need to be consistent with type of testing equipment (tablets, reagent strip [dipstick], or test tape) Discuss dosage, frequency of administration, time effect begins, maximum action, duration, and side effects, i.e., skin reaction and hypoglycemia Discuss factors requiring adjustment of insulin dosage, and notify physician before adjusting dose Demonstrate proper technique of insulin administration with return demonstration from patient/family

*If responsibility of critical care nurse includes such follow-up care.
†American Diabetes Association, Inc., 18 East 48th St., New York, N.Y. 10017.

POTENTIAL PROBLEMS	EXPECTED OUTCOMES	NURSING ACTIVITIES

		Discuss importance of
		  Never missing a dose
		  Preventing dosage error
		  Recording dosage or pills taken
		  Insulin storage
		  Consulting physician before taking any other medications

	Patient/family's behavior indicates understanding of
	Importance of recognition and maintenance of proper health care
	Signs and symptoms of infections that may require medical intervention
	Patient/family accurately describes plans for follow-up care
		Discuss importance of and demonstrate
		  Good hygiene
		  Careful foot care
		  Regular routine activities of daily living
		  Regular physical check-up
		  Use of medical alert identification tag/bracelet
		Identify signs and symptoms of infection, including
		  Fever
		  Colds
		  Flu
		  Nausea and vomiting
		  Any reddened, swollen, and painful areas; wounds or cuts that do not heal
		  Difficulty or burning sensation with urination
		Discuss why diabetics are prone to infection and ways to prevent it
		Describe follow-up visits including purpose of, when and where to go, who to see, and what specimens to bring
		Provide opportunity for and encourage questions and verbalization of anxiety regarding discharge regimen
		Assess potential compliance with discharge regimen

TOTAL PARENTERAL NUTRITION

Total parenteral nutrition (TPN) is the method of delivering carbohydrates, proteins, minerals, vitamins, trace minerals, and fat through the IV route. Parenteral infusions administered via a central venous catheter can meet the total nutritional needs of patients who cannot ingest the needed nutrients or who cannot or should not absorb them from the GI system.

Parenteral infusions can be administered via a peripheral venous catheter in selected patients when central venous access is compromised or undesirable.

PARENTERAL NUTRITION THROUGH CENTRAL VENOUS ROUTE

Pathological conditions that necessitate the use of TPN in adult patients include (1) GI abnormalities, such as the malabsorption component of ulcerative colitis, regional enteritis, granulomatous colitis, fistulas, and surgical short-gut syndromes, (2) states in which the alimentary tract cannot be used, as in patients with CNS dysfunction for whom oral feedings are not possible and NG feedings are associated with a high incidence of aspiration, (3) situations in which bowel rest with resulting decreased GI secretions is desired, such as pancreatitis and some biliary problems, and (4) conditions in which the demand for nutrients is dramatically increased, as in trauma, burns, infection, and other hypermetabolic states.

The pathological conditions specific to pediatric patients include (1) congenital anomalies, (2) chronic diarrhea, (3) surgical short-gut syndromes, (4) prematurity, and (5) hypermetabolic states.

A TPN solution commonly formulated for adult patients is made by mixing a 50% dextrose solution and a 5% amino acid solution. Electrolytes, vitamins, minerals, and trace elements are added as required by the patient. The final solution is 25% dextrose with 6 grams of nitrogen and contains approximately 1000 calories per liter. Special solutions can be formulated for patients with renal, cardiac, or other metabolic problems. These solutions generally restrict fluid volume and modify dextrose, nitrogen, and electrolyte content. Additional calories are provided by increasing the dextrose concentration to 30% to 40%. IV fat preparations provide concentrated calories in a small fluid volume (1.1 to 2.0 calories/ml) as well as providing a source of required essential fatty acids. Essential fatty acids are particularly important to the long-term TPN patient with depleted stores of these nutrients.

TPN solutions for pediatric patients are more individualized than those for adults. The solution is based on the age of the infant or child and his/her requirements for growth and development in addition to the requirements created by the specific disease process. Hypertonic dextrose solution is mixed with amino acid solution, and appropriate dosages of electrolytes, vitamins, minerals, and trace elements are added as required by the patient. Calculations are done daily based on the patient's weight. Depending on this, 12% glucose solutions are initiated, then increased to 18%, and then increased as high as 25%, as tolerated. Approximately 25 to 30 grams of dextrose and 2.5 grams of protein per kilogram per day are given. Fat is essential for normal growth and development as well as to prevent fatty acid deficiencies. A 10% fat emulsion is administered daily with the dextrose/amino acid solution. Dosages range from 0.5 to 3.0 g/kg/day. The exact volume also depends on the weight of the patient. All TPN solutions must be administered by an infusion control device to ensure accurate delivery of volume and prevent metabolic complications.

Adequate monitoring of the patient is mandatory. This includes (1) close lab monitoring of electrolyte, mineral, serum glucose, protein, triglyceride, and cholesterol levels and liver and kidney function, every week as required by the patient's clinical status, (2) daily intake, with calorie counts and output records, (3) six hourly urine tests for sugar and acetone, (4) daily weights, (5) vital signs every shift, and (6) meticulous catheter care with daily tubing changes and regularly scheduled dressing changes.

PARENTERAL NUTRITION VIA PERIPHERAL VENOUS ROUTE

Peripheral parenteral nutrition (PPN) is the technique in which the administration of carbohydrates, protein, fat, and electrolytes through a peripheral vein provides nutrients to persons who cannot ingest or absorb the needed nutrients from the GI system. Feeding a patient by the peripheral venous route is different from TPN, because the blood flow through a peripheral vein is lower and therefore the osmotic density of the infusate must be lower. The final glucose concentration of the solution should not exceed 10% to 12%. Less-concentrated solutions provide fewer calories per unit of volume. Consequently, the total caloric needs of many patients cannot be met within physiologically acceptable fluid volumes.

The initial indications for PPN are similar to those for TPN in that they reflect the need to use an IV feeding method rather than the GI tract. There are, however, several important factors to be considered in choosing patients who could benefit from PPN. For adults, general indications include patients who (1) are mildly nutritionally depleted, (2) are not hypermetabolic, (3) will not require IV nutritional support for greater than 7 to 10 days, (4) have adequate peripheral veins, (5) do not have pulmonary, liver, or blood conditions in which large volumes of lipid are contraindicated, and (6) do not have cardiac or renal involvement and can tolerate 2 to 3 liters of infusate per day.

The indications for pediatric patients are essentially the same as those for adult patients, although PPN is contraindicated for neonates with hyperbilirubinemia (>10 mg/dl).

A commonly formulated PPN regimen for adults consists of 1000 to 1500 ml of 10% to 12% dextrose, 3% to 5% amino acids and electrolytes and trace minerals and 1000 to 1500 ml of a 10% fat emulsion. This provides approximately 1400 to 2000 calories/day. The osmolality of the lipid solution is significantly lower than the dextrose/amino acid solution. Administering both simultaneously helps to protect the vein wall and decrease the amount of phlebitis.

PPN solutions for pediatric patients vary in total volume. The range is from 120 to 160 ml/kg/day, depending on the patient's clinical condition. PPN solutions must be individualized for each pediatric patient.

The method of administration of PPN solutions also varies for adult and pediatric patients. For adult patients, administration is usually by gravity drip with a Y connector close to the peripheral access site. Infusion control devices are also used when available. For pediatric patients, infusion control is necessary to control fluid volumes accurately because of the tiny-bore catheters or needles that are used and because the incidence of catheter-related complications is greater with infants and children. Two devices are required, one for the dextrose/amino acid solution and one for the fat emulsion.

Patient monitoring for PPN is essentially the same as that for TPN with the exception of the less-frequent blood glucose levels needed in PPN. Hyperglycemia is not usually a problem because of the lower glucose concentrations. The insertion and care of the peripheral catheter is different in that insertion and removal are obviously simpler procedures. The major potential problem is the risk of local tissue damage from infiltration of the fluid. The risk of sepsis is reduced because the needle or peripheral catheter is changed more often than the central catheter. Care in preparation and delivery of the infusates, however, remains a major consideration.

• • •

The presence of a team of nutrition experts, including a physician, nurse, pharmacist, and dietitian has been shown to minimize complications in parenteral nutrition therapy. The functions that this group can serve include patient selection, nutritional assessment, catheter insertion, fluid preparation, metabolic monitoring, dressing changes, and staff education. A coordinated effort on the part of this team can maximize the success of parenteral nutrition therapy.

ASSESSMENT
Physical

1. History and presence of medical or surgical problem that would require total parenteral alimentation
   a. GI abnormalities
      (1) Major GI surgery
      (2) Impaired absorption of nutrients: ulcerative colitis, regional enteritis, granulomatous colitis, Crohn disease, intractable diarrhea in infancy
   b. Increased demand for nutrients, as in burn and trauma patients
   c. CNS dysfunction
   d. Pediatric patients with congenital GI abnormalities, chronic diarrhea, surgical short-gut syndrome, or, in some cases, prematurity

Nutritional

1. Anthropometric measurements in selected patients to establish lean body mass
2. Baseline lab tests to evaluate current patient status and contribute to formula and therapy plan
   a. Blood glucose
   b. Serum proteins
   c. Kidney function tests
   d. Liver function tests; cholesterol levels
   e. Serum electrolytes
   f. Acid-base determination
   g. Serum osmolalities
   h. Urine osmolality
   i. Urine glucose
3. Allergy skin testing in selected patients
4. Patient/family's level of anxiety related to disease condition and therapy prescribed

GOALS

1. Reduction of level of anxiety with provision of information, comfort, support
2. Absence of catheter-related sepsis
3. Blood glucose levels within normal limits
4. BUN and creatinine within normal limits

5. Serum electrolyte levels within normal limits
6. Absence of vitamin, mineral, fatty acid deficiency
7. Positive nitrogen balance; weight maintenance or weight gain without fluid retention; preservation of body's muscle mass, protein, and fat stores
8. Acid-base balance and blood gas values within normal limits
9. BP, P within normal limits
10. Urine output and renal function tests within normal limits
11. Liver function tests within normal limits
12. Intact infusion system, without air; no catheter dislodgement
13. Absence of signs/symptoms of emboli formation
14. Absence of psychological disturbances from change of feeding modality

POTENTIAL PROBLEMS	EXPECTED OUTCOMES	NURSING ACTIVITIES
■ Patient/family's anxiety related to Insufficient knowledge and understanding of TPN IV mode of nutrient intake Disease process requiring IV alimentation	■ Reduction in patient/family's anxiety with provision of information, explanations, and encouragement	■ Assess patient/family's level of anxiety Explain rationale for IV alimentation Explain method of TPN delivery and monitoring Provide opportunity for and encourage patient/family's questions, verbalization of anxieties, fears Support and encourage patient/family Provide for comfort measures Provide for diversional activities (e.g., reading, television) *Pediatrics* Particular attention should be paid to providing infants with adequate psychosocial stimulation

■ Inadequate preparation of patient/family for insertion of catheter	■ Patient/family properly prepared for catheter insertion	■ *Central*
		    Explain what patient will experience
		    Assess need for sedation
		    Shave chest for subclavian vein catheter and neck area for internal jugular vein catheter, as necessary
		Pediatrics
		    Catheters are inserted in operating room
		    Prepare infant or child as needed
		    Shave scalp of infant receiving external jugular vein catheter
		Adults
		    Catheters are inserted at bedside for adult patients
		    Procure all necessary equipment
		    Position patient in Trendelenburg position
		    Prep area
		    Maintain sterile technique throughout procedure
		    Monitor for
		        Complaints of tingling, numbness of fingers, which may indicate brachial plexus injury
		        Brisk bleeding during insertion procedure may indicate puncture of subclavian artery; if occurs, apply direct pressure for at least 10 to 15 minutes
		        Presence of respiratory distress or change in vital signs, which may indicate potential pneumothorax, hydrothorax, or hemothorax
		    Infuse hypertonic infusate only after proper position of central venous catheter is verified by chest radiograph
		    Prepare patient for insertion of Broviac/Hickman catheter if ordered; these catheters are employed for long-term therapy and inserted in operating room for adult and pediatric patients
		Peripheral
		    Explain that insertion of peripheral catheter will be similar to regular IV infusion needle placement
		    Remind patient/family to notify staff of any pain or swelling at insertion site
		    Check needle of peripheral catheter site regularly for evidence of infiltration

POTENTIAL PROBLEMS	EXPECTED OUTCOMES	NURSING ACTIVITIES

■ Infusion of improperly prepared solution	■ Infusion of properly prepared solution, free of precipitate, with proper formulation for patient's caloric and physiological needs	■ Check each new solution for clarity, proper constituents, and date mixed
		Change solution and administration tubing q24 hr
		Keep amino acid/dextrose solutions refrigerated and out of light until needed
		Store bottles out of light to prevent light-sensitive vitamin degradation
		For lipid administration
		  Check tubing during infusion for evidence of precipitate
		  Inspect bottles for separation of emulsion and any change from milky white color
		  Do not shake bottle as doing so may cause fat particles to aggregate
		  Follow instructions on bottle concerning need for refrigeration
		  Do not use filter on lipid line
		  Connect lipid line to primary line by Y connector at junction closest to insertion site, as it is not stable for long periods if mixed with other infusates
		  Hang lipid bottle (if gravity flow is used) higher than bottles of amino acid/dextrose solution to prevent backflow into amino acid/dextrose line caused by low specific gravity of lipids

■ Sepsis related to
 	
  TPN solution
 	
  Central catheter
 	
  Peripheral catheter
	■ Absence/resolution of infection	■ Maintain aseptic system
		Restrict use of line to nutritional infusates
		If contaminated solution is suspected, send infusate container and tubing for bacterial and fungal culture
		Maintain central catheter with moderate dextrose solution
		Send cultures of urine, wounds, sputum, and peripheral and central blood samples for bacterial and fungal culture
		Assist with catheter removal; culture tip
		Apply occlusive dressing over catheter exit site
		Administer antibiotics, as ordered
		Administer solution of moderate dextrose concentration (e.g., D10W) through peripheral vein, as ordered
		Monitor patient's response to therapy
		Stop PPN infusion, as ordered
		Remove catheter or needle
		Start IV infusion of low dextrose concentration in opposite arm, as ordered
		Send peripheral blood and site cultures, as ordered
		Administer antibiotics as appropriate, as ordered
		Apply dry, sterile dressing to peripheral site
		Monitor patient's vital signs

■ Complications related to presence of catheter
Vessel thrombosis/emboli
Vessel injury
	■ Absence/resolution of thrombosis/emboli	■ Filters may or may not be used for adult or pediatric patients depending on hospital policy
		Central
		  Monitor patient for swelling of head and chest above nipple line, which is indicative of superior vena cava syndrome
		  Monitor patient for edema along catheter route
		  Monitor patient for widened mediastinum on chest radiograph, which may indicate thoracic duct injury
		Peripheral
		  Observe peripheral needle or catheter site for local phlebitis and peripheral thrombosis/emboli
		
		See STANDARD 31 *Embolic phenomena*

Catheter displacement and infiltration	Catheter in place
	Absence of infiltration
		Central
		  Ensure that skin sutures are intact
		  Secure tubing from central line to skin with tape to minimize possibility of accidental dislodgement
		  Observe track of catheter for evidence of swelling or bleeding
		  Assess need for restraints for infants, toddlers, and delirious patients
		  Obtain radiograph of catheter track if displacement is suspected; use radiopaque solution to visualize catheter if necessary

POTENTIAL PROBLEMS	EXPECTED OUTCOMES	NURSING ACTIVITIES

Air embolism (air embolism is life-threatening problem)	Absence of air embolism	*Peripheral*
		Observe site and limb for local infiltration of infusate
		Central or peripheral
		Air elimination filter may or may not be used
		Secure connections of tubing well, and remove all air from tubing
		Have patient perform Valsalva maneuver during tubing changes or use Luer-Lok extension tubing with roller clamp
		If air enters tubing
		  Using aseptic technique, remove air from tubing while maintaining patency of line by slow sterile flush with appropriate dextrose solution
		  If air is suspected in right ventricle
		    Turn patient to left side and place in Trendelenburg position to keep air out of pulmonary artery; monitor vital signs frequently
		  Assist physician with aspiration of air through central line while patient performs Valsalva maneuver
		    If procedure is necessary, monitor for cardiopulmonary instability

■ Metabolic imbalance	■ Glucose and electrolyte levels within normal limits Absence of signs/symptoms of fatty acid deficiency, trace element deficiency, or fluid imbalance	■ Monitor established biochemical schedule closely and review results Establish nursing monitoring system Advance infusion rate gradually, as tolerated and ordered Control rate of infusion by infusion pump Check rate of infusion at least q1 hr to avoid any variance greater than 10% of rate ordered Wean patient from TPN solution over several days Physically assess patient daily

Hyperglycemia: dehydration	Serum glucose levels within normal limits	*Adults*
		Monitor urine glucose q4-6 hr during glucose infusion
		Monitor blood glucose levels q12-24 hr until stable infusion rate; then biweekly
		Pediatrics
		Monitor urine glucose with every voiding or q4 hr
		Monitor blood glucose levels q1 day for 3 days, then once a week
		In addition, for all patients
		Record intake and output every shift and total q24 hr
		Notify physician of 4+ glucosuria and excessive urinary output
		Watch for shallow breathing, restlessness, lethargy, or coma
		If hyperglycemic hyperosmolar, nonketotic dehydration occurs (blood glucose levels may range from 500 to 1000 mg/dl or higher)
		  Stop hypertonic dextrose solution and administer nondextrose saline solution
		  Give subcutaneous or IV insulin, as ordered
		  Monitor for electrolyte imbalances and correct, as ordered
		  Stay with patient or observe frequently until blood glucose levels are within normal limits

Hypoglycemia	Serum glucose levels within normal limits	Monitor urine glucose and specific gravity during glucose infusion Monitor blood glucose levels every day when infusion rates are decreased If infusion must be discontinued suddenly, administer moderate glucose solution by peripheral vein, as ordered Check administration tubing (including pump tubing) for regular flow Respond promptly to infusion pump alarms that stop infusion Monitor for signs of hypoglycemia including pallor, listlessness, dizziness, staring, muscular weakness, tremors, sweating If any of these occur, notify physician and alter therapy as ordered

POTENTIAL PROBLEMS	EXPECTED OUTCOMES	NURSING ACTIVITIES
Electrolyte imbalance	Serum electrolyte levels within normal limits	Monitor for signs of electrolyte imbalance, including 　Tremors 　Muscular cramping 　Irritability 　Restlessness 　Abnormal serum electrolyte levels If these signs/symptoms occur, notify physician and alter therapy as ordered
Fatty acid deficiency	Absence of signs/symptoms of fatty acid deficiency	Monitor for signs of fatty acid deficiency 　Dry, scaly skin 　Weight loss 　Increase in heart rate 　Hair loss Administer lipid solution routinely to patients receiving parenteral nutritional support 　For adults receiving TPN—200 or 500 ml bottle 1 to 2 times/week 　Lipid calories should be approximately 4% of total calories 　For pediatric patients receiving TPN—approximately 0.5 g/kg is administered daily 　Lipid is used as caloric source in PPN 　　For adults—1000 to 1500 ml/day 　　For pediatric patients—2 to 3 g/day Monitor for immediate adverse reaction to lipid solution, including 　Flushing 　Dyspnea 　Chest and back pain 　Nausea 　Dizziness 　Headache Monitor vital signs q10 min for first 30 minutes of infusion Monitor for delayed lipid intolerance reaction 　Headache 　Irritability 　Low-grade fever 　Abdominal pain 　Nausea 　Anemia 　Coagulopathy 　Turbid serum Monitor baseline and serial triglyceride levels Notify physician of abnormalities, and alter therapy as ordered
Trace element deficiency	Absence of signs/symptoms of trace element deficiency	Prevent by adding trace elements to TPN solution routinely Monitor for trace element deficiency after long-term TPN therapy
Zinc deficiency		Monitor for zinc deficiency 　Poor wound healing 　Loss of hair 　Hypogeusia
Copper deficiency		Monitor for copper deficiency 　Anemia 　Neutropenia 　Hypogeusia Notify physician of these signs and symptoms and alter therapy, as ordered

POTENTIAL PROBLEMS	EXPECTED OUTCOMES	NURSING ACTIVITIES

Acid-base imbalance	Absence of signs/symptoms of acid-base imbalance
	Arterial blood gas levels within normal limits
		Monitor for acid-base imbalance
		  Tachypnea
		  Headache
		  Mentation alterations (fatigue, drowsiness, restlessness, apathy, inattentiveness)
		Monitor arterial blood gas results for pH, bicarbonate, base excess, and CO_2 levels
		Note increased blood lactate levels
		Notify physician of abnormalities and alter therapy as ordered

Fluid overload	Absence of fluid imbalance
	Normovolemia
	Weight stable or weight gain consisting of increased muscle mass
		Weigh patient daily
		Note presence of edema
		Observe for
		  Respiratory distress
		  Signs of CHF
		Notify physician if either of aforementioned occurs; see Standard 15, *Heart failure (low cardiac output)*
		Administer diuretics, as ordered: closely monitor patient's response

■ Hepatomegaly	■ Absence of hepatomegaly
	Liver function tests within normal limits
		■ Monitor results of liver function tests for abnormalities, including SGOT, SGPT, alkaline phosphatase, gamma glytamyl transpeptidase, LDH, and bilirubin levels
		  Coagulation studies PT, APTT
		  Protein albumin/globulin levels
		Monitor for right upper quadrant fullness, elevated diaphragm on right side
		Notify physician of abnormalities and alter therapy, as ordered

BROVIAC/HICKMAN CATHETER

The Broviac/Hickman catheter is a silicone rubber, radiopaque, right atrium catheter (see Fig. 3). For patients receiving either intermittent or continuous IV therapy, the catheter is a vehicle for providing long-term venous access without repeated venipuncture. The distal end of the catheter lies in a position similar to that of a subclavian IV catheter, and the proximal portion is located in a tunnel of subcutaneous tissue along the anterior chest wall (see Fig. 4).

Placement of the catheter is a surgical procedure. Local anesthesia is commonly used, although general anesthesia is preferred for small children. The catheter is inserted into the circulatory system via a subcutaneous tunnel (see Fig. 4). Creation of the tunnel is accomplished with a long clamp that is inserted under the skin through a small incision at the deltopectoral groove to an exit site at the fourth or fifth intercostal space. The catheter is then drawn back up the tunnel, and the tip is drawn through the incision. At this time, the distance from the incision site to the right atrium is measured, and the catheter is trimmed to correspond to the patient's anatomy. The catheter is threaded through a venous cutdown or percutaneous puncture into the circulatory system under fluoroscopy. The cephalic vein is usually chosen; however, the internal or external jugular vein may also be used.* The tip of the catheter is then threaded into the superior vena cava via the subclavian vein and finally into the right atrium of the heart. Sutures at the cutdown site and the exit site hold the catheter in place until a Dacron cuff, which is located 30 centimeters from the hub, becomes overgrown by subcutaneous tissue. In this manner the cuff, which lies in the subcutaneous tunnel, reduces the incidence of dislodgement and infection and increases the longevity of the catheter. Once this overgrowth occurs (in approximately 10 days) the sutures may be removed. The catheter may be used immediately after placement.

The catheter was developed in 1973 by J. W. Broviac. Originally, it was placed in patients requiring long-term home parenteral nutrition as a result of extensive, chronic bowel diseases such as Crohn disease, short bowel syndrome, and congenital short bowel. Since the catheter proved successful in these patients, it is now being used in the treatment of a large variety of diseases. Modifications such as the larger-bore catheter designed by R. O. Hickman in 1975 and the double-lumen catheter designed in 1979 have also contributed to this expansion. Current uses of the catheter include patients who require repeated blood drawing and IV administration of chemotherapeutic agents, antibiotics, TPN solutions, and/or blood products.

The oncology patient, who requires most of these treatment modalities, has benefited the most from the Broviac/Hickman catheter. For example, these catheters have often been used for patients with leukemia or aplastic anemia who are undergoing bone marrow transplantation. Other patients who require long-term antibiotic therapy, such as those with cystic fibrosis, endocarditis, fungal infections, and osteomyelitis also benefit from this catheter. Another, less common use is the treatment of intractable pain by the administration of intrathecal morphine through a Broviac/Hickman catheter placed in the spinal epidural space.* The indications for inserting these catheters will undoubtedly continue to increase in the future, because research has demonstrated low complication rates for catheters that have been in place for as long as 1 year.

Whatever the purpose for insertion of the Broviac/Hickman catheter, safe and proper care of the catheter by the nurse ensures its successful use and longevity. Because the patient will also be caring for the catheter, it is vital that the nurse instruct the patient or family member in the following procedures before discharge.

First, the nurse must understand the purpose of catheter placement and the treatment modalities the patient will be receiving. If the patient is to continue his/her treatments at home, complete discharge instructions are required.

Second, to maintain the catheter properly its patency must be ensured. Patency is maintained by instilling the catheter with a sodium heparin–saline solution. Five to six milliliters

*Wade, J.K., et al.: Two methods for improved venous access in acute leukemia patients, JAMA **246:**144, 1981.

*Polette, C., et al.: Cancer pain relieved by long-term epidural morphine with permanent indwelling systems for self-administration, J. Neurosurg. **55:**582, 1981.

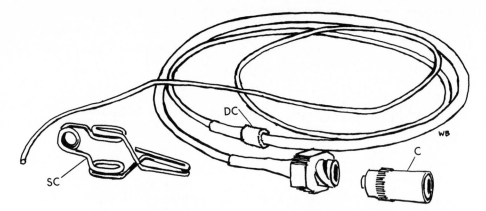

FIG. 3. Broviac/Hickman catheter. *DC,* Dacron cuff; *C,* injection cap; *SC,* stainless steel canula clamp.

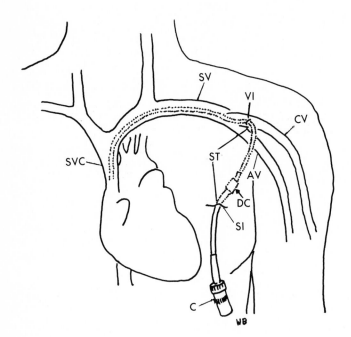

FIG. 4. Broviac/Hickman catheter in place. *SV,* Left subclavian vein; *CV,* left cephalic vein; *AV,* left axillary vein; *SI,* skin insertion site; *VI,* vein insertion site; *ST,* subcutaneous tunnel; *DC,* Dacron cuff; *SVC,* superior vena cava; *C,* injection cap.

of the solution is enough to clear the catheter completely; the exact dosage is ordered by the physician. Instillation must be done daily, whenever the catheter is capped, and after any IV therapy or blood drawing is completed. Because the heparin solution is instilled through the rubber of the male Luer-Lok cap, the use of a short, small-gauge needle, such as one 25 gauge × ⅝ inch, is preferred to prevent damage to the catheter itself.

Third, measures for prevention of infection are essential. Strict aseptic technique must be used when the catheter is opened to air for any reason. Whenever the patient is not receiving IV therapy, the catheter must be capped with a rubber-topped, male Luer-Lok cap to provide a sterile, closed system. This cap must fit securely to prevent any contamination, introduction of air emboli, or loss of blood. Because of the daily instillations of heparin solution the cap must be changed frequently, usually two to three times a

week, to prevent contamination of the catheter. In addition, a dry sterile dressing is always applied at the exit site to prevent infection. The exact dressing procedure will be determined by hospital policy. This usually includes cleaning of the site with hydrogen peroxide and/or povidone-iodine (Betadine) solution, application of a bacteriostatic ointment, and protection of the site with sterile dressing material. The dressing, like the cap, must be changed frequently. Whatever the exact regimen, the patient must be instructed to replace the dressing if it becomes loose or wet during a day's activity.

Finally, certain principles must be adhered to whenever caring for a Broviac/Hickman catheter. The catheter must always be clamped before the system is opened to prevent back flow of blood or introduction of air emboli. A smooth clamp, such as a stainless steel cannula clamp (never a sawtoothed clamp, such as a hemostat) is used. In addition, tape is placed on the catheter before the clamp is applied. The smooth clamp and the tape will prevent breaks in the integrity of the catheter. Other safety measures include coiling and taping any extra length of tubing on the dressing to prevent pulling on the catheter, which could cause displacement.

While the patient requires instruction concerning the use and maintenance of the Broviac/Hickman catheter, he/she also requires instructions about daily activities. The catheter itself actually has little impact on a patient's activity level. Patients usually may swim and shower once the sutures are removed and the exit site has healed. However, the presence of the underlying disease process may affect the patient's level of activity, and therefore instructions should be obtained from the physician.

Complications will be avoided by using proper technique in caring for a Broviac/Hickman catheter. It is significant to note that the rate of complications has been directly correlated to the patient's ability to correctly care for the catheter.* This indicates that complete patient/family education is a priority in the nursing plan of care if long-term maintenance of the Broviac/Hickman catheter is to be successful.

ASSESSMENT

1. Patient/family's knowledge of the disease process requiring Broviac/Hickman catheter
2. Patient's past history related to catheter placement
   a. Date of insertion
   b. Site of insertion
   c. Previous catheter placements
3. Patient/family's knowledge and understanding of the purpose and maintenance of the catheter
   a. Irrigation of the catheter
   b. Cap change
   c. Dressing change
   d. Correct use of clamp
   e. Use of aseptic technique

*Fleming, R., Witzke, D., and Beart, R.: Catheter-related complications in patients receiving home parenteral nutrition, Ann. Surg. **192:**598, 1980.

f. Home treatment regimen, if any; i.e., chemotherapy, home parenteral nutrition, etc.
4. Integrity and general function of the catheter
   a. Patency
   b. Placement
   c. Skin integrity
   d. Integrity of the catheter

GOALS

1. Absence or resolution of the following problems
   a. Infection
   b. Clot formation
   c. Air emboli
   d. Accidental blood loss
   e. Catheter displacement
   f. Break in catheter integrity
2. Patient demonstrates improved quality of life by
   a. A decrease in the length/frequency of hospitalizations
   b. Avoiding frequent, repeated venipuncture
   c. Attaining an element of control in the treatment of a chronic disease process
   d. Understanding that proper catheter maintenance promotes optimal health within the limits of a chronic disease process
3. Before discharge, the patient/family
   a. Describes and demonstrates specific catheter care procedures
      (1) Dressing change
      (2) Cap change
      (3) Drawing up of the heparin solution
      (4) Instillation of the heparin solution through the male Luer-lok injection cap
   b. Identifies problems that require emergency treatment and interim measures to take as medical attention is being sought
   c. Describes activity regimen
   d. States necessary information regarding follow-up care
   e. Describes and demonstrates specific treatment regimen that necessitated catheter insertion, i.e., chemotherapy, antibiotic therapy, etc.

POTENTIAL PROBLEMS	EXPECTED OUTCOMES	NURSING ACTIVITIES
■ Patient/family's anxiety related to insufficient knowledge and understanding of Broviac/Hickman catheter and/or underlying disease process	■ Reduction in patient/family's anxiety with provision of information, explanations, and encouragement	■ Assess patient/family's level of anxiety Explain rationale for insertion of Broviac/Hickman catheter Assess level of knowledge and understanding of disease process, diagnostic procedures, and therapy Allow for and encourage patient/family's questions and verbalization of anxieties and fears Explain in simple terms patient's disease and treatment regimen Encourage participation in care, as tolerated Assess patient/family's demonstration of routine of care of Broviac/Hickman catheter

POTENTIAL PROBLEMS	EXPECTED OUTCOMES	NURSING ACTIVITIES
		Dressing change technique Injection cap change Drawing up of heparin solution Instillation of heparin solution into catheter through injection cap Assess reduction in level of patient/family's anxiety with provision of information, explanations, and encouragement If insertion of Broviac/Hickman catheter is required, see Appendix B, *Surgical procedures: assessment*

▪ Infection related to
   Failure to maintain aseptic technique in caring for catheter
   Patient's debilitated or immunosuppressed state
	▪ Absence/resolution of infection	▪ Prevention
		  Maintain aseptic technique during
		    Injection cap change
		    Dressing change
		    Instillation of heparin solution
		    Drawing of blood from catheter
		    Administration of intermittent infusions
		  Cleanse insertion site with antiseptic solution and change dressing daily and prn
		  Change IV solution and tubing daily
		  Change cap twice a week and prn, if capped
		  Assess for signs and symptoms of infection
		Inspect insertion site and subcutaneous tunnel for the following
		  Pain on palpation
		  Drainage
		  Redness
		  Swelling
		  Local warmth
		  Elevated temperature
		Inspect Broviac/Hickman catheter for break in system
		  Pierced or cracked catheter
		  Loose cap connection
		  Catheter fatigue from repeated clamping at same site
		If infection is suspected
		  Draw one set of blood cultures from Broviac/Hickman catheter and one from peripheral site for comparison
		  Administer antibiotics, as ordered
		  Assist with removal of Broviac/Hickman catheter, if indicated
		    Give premedication
		    Place pressure over insertion site
		    Observe catheter for length to ensure that entire catheter is removed
		    Send catheter for C and S

▪ Break in integrity of Broviac/Hickman catheter	▪ Intact Broviac/Hickman catheter	▪ Prevention
		Educate patient, family, and staff to avoid situations in which integrity of catheter is potentially compromised
		  Avoid use of scissors or sharp instruments on or near catheter
		  Use ⅝ inch needles only
		    Introduce ⅝ inch needle through injection cap only
		  Protect catheter with tape before clamping
		  Rotate clamping sites
		  Use clamps without teeth, such as stainless steel cannula clamp (see Fig. 3)
		Monitor for break in integrity of Broviac/Hickman catheter
		  Fluid leaking from catheter
		  Blood backing up in catheter
		If problem occurs
		  Clamp below break with stainless steel cannula clamp over piece of tape
		  Notify physician
		  Insert 14-gauge, 2-inch Angiocath into catheter as temporary measure until catheter can be repaired, according to hospital protocol

POTENTIAL PROBLEMS	EXPECTED OUTCOMES	NURSING ACTIVITIES
		Obtain equipment for repair (commercially available kit is recommended*)
		Assist with repair procedure
■ Air embolism	■ Absence of air embolism	■ Remove all air from tubing
		Secure all connections with tape
		Inspect tubing and catheter for cracks
		For suspected air in right ventricle
		Turn patient on left side and place in Trendelenburg position to keep air out of pulmonary artery
		Monitor vital signs frequently
		Assist physician with aspiration of air through Broviac/Hickman catheter while patient performs Valsalva maneuver
		If this procedure is indicated, monitor for cardiopulmonary instability
		See STANDARD 31 *Embolic phenomena*
■ Hemorrhage related to accidental disconnection of system or displacement of catheter	■ Absence/resolution of hemorrhage	■ Prevention
		Secure and tape all connection sites in system
		Keep stainless steel cannula clamp at bedside at all times
		Avoid excess tubing, which can potentially catch
		Monitor for
		Displaced catheter
		Disconnection of catheter
		Bloody dressing
		Hypotension, tachycardia
		Restlessness
		Notify physician for abnormalities
		If hemorrhage occurs
		Monitor vital signs frequently
		Check Hgb, Hct
		Apply dressing and pressure over catheter insertion site
		Assist physician with catheter removal, if indicated
■ Obstructed aspiration of blood from Broviac/Hickman catheter related to catheter tip positioned against vessel wall	■ Free aspiration of blood from catheter	■ Ensure that clamp is removed
		Check for kinking of catheter
		Assess for difficulty in aspirating blood from catheter
		Instruct patient to take a deep breath, change body position, or raise one or both arms
		Notify physician if these measures are unsuccessful
		Assist with repositioning catheter, if indicated
■ Blocked catheter related to clotted blood or drug precipitate within catheter	■ Patent Broviac/Hickman catheter	■ Prevent catheter blockage by the following activities
		Maintain heparin lock after intermittent infusions
		Infuse IV solution at sufficient rate to maintain catheter patency
		Instill heparin solution at least q1 day into capped Broviac/Hickman catheter
		Clamp catheter while instilling last 0.5 ml of heparin solution; this maintains positive pressure and prevents back flow
		Flush catheter with normal saline between infusions that are incompatible
		Monitor for blocked catheter
		Inability to instill solution
		Inability to withdraw blood
		If problem occurs, the following activities will be performed according to hospital protocol
		Assist physician with serial instillations of heparin solution until clot can be aspirated from catheter
		Assist physician with instillation of streptokinase until clot can be aspirated from catheter

*The repair kit is available from Evermed, PO Box 296, Medina, WA 98039.

POTENTIAL PROBLEMS	EXPECTED OUTCOMES	NURSING ACTIVITIES

■ Vessel injury, vessel thrombosis/emboli related to presence of Broviac/Hickman catheter; more common in neonates	■ Absence/resolution of thrombosis/emboli	■ Monitor for superior vena cava syndrome, which is manifested by
		  Swelling of head and chest above nipple line
		  Edema along catheter route
		  Widened mediastinum on chest radiograph, which may indicate thoracic duct injury
		Notify physician of abnormalities
		Assist with removal of Broviac/Hickman catheter, if indicated

■ Pulmonary or cerebral embolus	■ Absence/resolution of emboli	■ Prevention
		  For capped Broviac/Hickman catheter
		    Instill heparin solution at least q1 day
		    Clamp catheter over piece of tape while instilling last ml of heparin solution to maintain positive pressure and prevent back flow
		    Maintain heparin lock after intermittent infusions or blood drawing
		  For catheters to constant IV infusion
		    Maintain IV flow rate at sufficient rate to ensure patency

Pulmonary embolus	Absence of pulmonary embolus, infarction
	Respiratory status remains stable and within normal limits
		Monitor for signs indicative of pulmonary embolus
		  Sudden restlessness, sense of impending doom
		  Respiratory distress—rapid, shallow breathing
		  Pain—pleuritic or substernal on inspiration
		  Decreased breath sounds
		  Altered arterial blood gas parameters indicating hypoxemia, hypercapnia or hypocapnia
		  Signs and symptoms of hypoxia—tachypnea, air hunger, anxiety, tachycardia, altered mental status, cyanosis
		  Cardiovascular instability
		    Dysrhythmias
		    Hypertension or hypotension
		    Reduced cardiac output
		    Engorged neck veins
		Notify physician of abnormalities and administer therapy, as ordered
		
		See STANDARD 31 *Embolic phenomena*

Cerebral embolus	Absence of cerebral embolus, infarction
	Mental status remains clear
	Patient oriented to time, place, person
		Monitor for signs indicative of cerebral embolus
		  Sudden dizziness
		  Altered mental status or LOC
		  Aphasia, dysphagia
		  Seizures
		  Weakness of extremities unilaterally
		  Paralysis
		  Ptosis of mouth, eyelids
		Notify physician of abnormalities and administer therapy, as ordered
		
		See STANDARD 31 *Embolic phenomena*

General

EMOTIONAL AND SPIRITUAL CARE
OF THE CRITICALLY ILL

It is unfortunate that the emotional and spiritual care of patients has low priority in most acute-care hospitals. In the critically ill patient, the physiological parameters are emphasized as the ultimate indicators of the overall condition of the patient and the success or failure of treatment regimens. The critical care nurse should therefore be particularly sensitive to the spiritual and emotional needs of the patient and should understand the interrelationship of these factors with the disease process. The critical care nurse deals with crisis, which commonly requires rapid interventions and leads to specific, short-term outcomes. There is a tendency to ignore the more chronic, complex emotional and spiritual background of the patient in whom the crisis emerged.

The symptoms of anger, denial, anorexia, loss, hopelessness, anxiety, need for high doses of pain medication, and refusal of medication in a seriously ill patient are often dealt with perfunctorily. The underlying causes of these symptoms requires an awareness of the patient's spiritual and emotional condition. Only with this awareness can the nurse formulate a comprehensive plan of treatment and care. The purposes of this standard are to call attention to the spiritual and psychological aspects of care for these patients and to provide a rationale for the application of this principle of care.

According to a 1975 Gallup poll, 94% of Americans believe in God. This "God-Man" relationship is personal, and it is different from the "I-You" relationship one has between oneself and others.* Spiritual care presumes and concerns itself with the patient's relationship to a higher being, i.e., God. Spiritual health can be defined as a dy-

*Christianity Today **XX:**(23)35, August 1976.

namic relationship with God in which hope, sense of meaning and purpose, love, and comfort are provided. A hospitalization, especially one of a critical nature, may cause one to become fearful of losing the things of high priority in life. It is natural to turn to God in times of crisis. The outcome in terms of peacefulness or sense of well-being may depend on the patient's relationship with God before the illness. In any case, if feelings of fear, uncertainty, guilt, isolation, and lack of meaning result, a spiritual crisis is present. The therapeutic challenge is to help reestablish the dynamic relationship with God that existed before the illness or, if there was no such relationship, to aid the patient in a spiritual search if the opportunity exists.

All people need and seek relationships outside themselves. When all is right with the world—ourselves, and the people in it—our emotional and psychological needs are met. We experience emotional and psychological crises when the people or things around us, which also provide hope, meaning, love, and comfort in our lives, are lost, changed, disturbed, or stressed. A serious illness and hospitalization can precipitate such an upheaval.

The relationship bond then is the basic distinction used here between spiritual and psychological needs. These relationships are both personal and private matters. The individual is solely responsible for his/her relationship to self, spouse, child, or God. But occasionally any intimate relationship may need the help of others for it to continue in a healthy, meaningful way.

Nursing is an intimate profession. A nurse will without hesitation inquire about bowel movements, menstrual periods, and sexual habits. Nurses are in the unique position of being more frequently present at the bedside than any other health care professional. Physicians, psychiatric liaison personnel, social service personnel, chaplains, visitors, and family are not available at the press of a call light, as nurses are. In a critical care setting, the nurse may spend virtually all 8, 10, or 12 hours of his/her tour of duty *in* the patient's room. The nurse is therefore in the best position to assess the spiritual and emotional condition of the patient and to monitor the impact made by an illness.

Often, despite severe illness and suffering, a patient will exhibit an amazing calm because he/she has found meaning and purpose in his/her circumstances. This patient will continue to have a strong hope system. On the other hand, patients whose physical condition is not critical often exhibit extreme emotional turmoil. This suggests that a dichotomy exists in *assessing* the true state of health or sickness in an individual, which represents a particular challenge in the critical care setting.

As humans we strive to understand the reason a particular life experience occurs—reason gives meaning to the experience. According to Friedrich Nietzsche, "He who has a *why* to live can bear with almost any *how*.* Nurses can assist an individual or family cope with the experience of illness and suffering and help them find meaning in these experiences.

Hope, on the other hand, is that glimmer of something better.† Hope makes life under stress tolerable and gives us a means of dealing with uncertainties. Critical illness produces such physical, emotional, and in some cases spiritual stress that without hope, despair can overwhelm a patient to the point of making recovery impossible. Hope is a vital ingredient in healing and wellness. Support of normostasis and optimal physical comfort in a patient in an atmosphere of decreased sensory stimulus allows for a patient's hope system to function best. Hope may not always be related to long-range goals or aspirations, or involve the hope to survive the critical illness. Hope may simply be manifested as a desire to see a loved one, write a letter, or be able to speak again after an illness that has prevented fulfillment of any of these needs.

The nurse also supports a patient's hope system when he/she makes it possible for the patient to carry out religious rituals, whether they involve praying, reading Scripture, or following dietary customs. Specifically, this is why addressing spiritual needs is not a frill but an integral component of total patient care. In these delicate areas the nurse as the primary caregiver can act as a channel for the patient and at times offer the patient's own background of faith as a reminder and tool to be used in dealing with illness or, ultimately, with dying. When the nurse feels he/she cannot directly meet the patient's spiritual needs, referral to another nurse or health team member is appropriate.

*In Frankl, V.E.: Man's search for meaning, New York, 1971, Washington Square Press, p. xiii.
†Fish, S., and Shelly, J.A.: Spiritual care: the nurse's role, Downer's Grove, Ill., 1978, Inter Varsity Press, p. 44.

Comprehensive spiritual care fosters hope, healing, and health. Yet having hope in God does not necessarily mean an abrupt end to a crisis. Hope in God is not dependent on God's ability to deliver a person from difficulty, but on God's control of the circumstances and His ability to support a person in the midst of them. Supporting a patient who does not have a belief in God through the crisis of illness is different, because the patient places ultimate hope for deliverance from a crisis in himself or other people. Because of this, the patient may place more demands on the nurse and medical staff. But by his/her very presence the nurse can contribute to the well-being of patients simply by caring, by using touch, by listening with empathy and compassion, by using self therapeutically, and by helping the patient maintain the relationships that foster meaning, purpose, and hope in his/her life.

The caring, astute nurse responding to verbal and nonverbal clues is aware that illness carries a host of expected emotional reactions. Fear is generally the overriding, glaring emotion. Even when patients are not dying, they may fear they are because they are hospitalized in a critical care unit. Aside from internal stresses, such as loneliness and powerlessness, the patient is bombarded with all the external stresses of hospital care, i.e., lack of privacy, loss of decision making, sensory overload, and sleep deprivation. The patient has little experience for coping in this setting. The patient is usually not the one to initiate direct discussions on emotional, psychological, or spiritual levels. The burden is on the nurse to explain virtually everything, to reassure, and to allay fears. By taking the initiative the nurse relieves the patient's anxiety, guilt, and fear for having problems coping with hospitalization.

Aside from the acute upheaval of illness, any number of problem situations can occur, including altered job or family roles, financial difficulties, altered body image, decreased mobility, abrupt goal changes, and strains in relationships with spouse, relatives, self, and God. In this case the nurse will initiate conversations with patients and their families based on observations concerning these specific situations. This will hopefully help the patient find solutions to concrete problems.

The nurse entering into care in these areas must still be guided by the patient's needs. These are made known by physical assessment, somatic complaints, remarks made during conversation, general attitude, and behavior. The nurse should also look at the patient's surroundings, made personal by books, belongings, articles, pictures, and cards. The specific problem may not be immediately known, even by the patient, but certain behavior will signal the need for spiritual and psychological help. The general principles of care involving the nursing process of observing, interpreting, planning, implementing, and evaluating (reobserving and reinterpreting) are also followed when addressing a patient's spiritual and psychological needs. Again, referral to other health team members is always appropriate when the nurse feels unable to meet the needs he/she has assessed.

It is imperative for the nurse who is stressed by working in a critical care setting to assess his/her own needs. Nurses also have the responsibility of maintaining their own optimal physical, psychological, and spiritual health. Proper rest, exercise, diet, hobbies, outside relationships, and relaxation and searching, building, or maintaining a dynamic relationship with God will ensure good patient care from a well–taken care of, well-rounded, whole person.

ASSESSMENT

1. History—medical, surgical, psychosocial
2. Patient profile, including religious affiliation; social status, i.e., married, single; key relationships and support systems; immediate social factors, i.e., job, family situation, life-style, habits; coping mechanisms previously used during stress; emotional stability
3. Patient's perception and reaction to diagnosis, progression of disease, and assessment and treatment modalities
4. Environment—family pictures, get-well cards, religious articles and literature, Bible
5. Physical symptoms not attributable to physical origin or contributed to by hospitalization
   a. Sleep deprivation
   b. Sensory overload
   c. Array of emotional responses, i.e., anger, denial, depression, stoicism, inappropriate joking
   d. Pain medication ineffective despite large doses; eating pattern alterations; bowel and bladder function alterations; tense upper back; increased pulse; tight throat; cool, perspiring hands; shallow respirations
6. Patient's general attitude and verbal comments expressing feelings of abandonment, loneliness, powerlessness, hopelessness, and fear of dying
7. Patient's general attitude and presence/absence of verbal comments concerning key persons in patient's life, including God

GOALS

1. Patient's realistic assessment of diagnosis, and progression of disease to facilitate self-help and care
2. Reestablishment or maintenance of support and coping systems, as indicated, e.g., patient's key relationships and relationship with God
3. Absence or decrease in physical manifestations of stress
4. Patient's behavior demonstrates reduction of anxiety
5. Promotion of patient satisfaction, health, and healing
   a. Patient finds meaning and purpose in face of illness
   b. Patient's hope system is intact
   c. Patient is prepared for discharge and able to cope with diagnosis with return to level of functioning beyond precrisis level
   d. Patient/family moves to acceptance stage of dying

POTENTIAL PROBLEMS	EXPECTED OUTCOMES	NURSING ACTIVITIES

■ Fear related to unknowns about illness
Role change
Change in life-style
Return to precrisis level of function
Dying
	■ Anxiety level decreased as evidenced by patient's behavior and decrease in symptoms of stress
	Maintenance of key relationships; establish or maintain relationship with God, as desired
	Verbalization of sense of optimism regarding expected outcomes of treatment, if appropriate
	Positive outlook and acceptance of possible change in role and activity level
	Verbalization of sense of ability to adjust to any necessary changes and understanding of why changes necessary
	Verbalization of fears and concerns
	Verbalization of confidence in purpose of equipment
	Verbalization of confidence in caregivers
		■ Ongoing assessment of level of anxiety
		Explain diagnosis, surroundings, equipment, and all procedures in calm, unhurried manner
		Reinforce any aspects indicative of positive progress
		Explore possible alternatives to current job role
		Administer sedation, as ordered
		Control environment to decrease sensory overload
		  Dim lights
		  Draw shades
		  Promote privacy
		  Lower level of auditory stimuli, i.e., monitors on low volume, staff talking outside patient's room
		Stay with patient when he/she appears upset
		Encourage use of relaxation techniques, e.g.
		  Meditation
		  Imagery technique
		  Slow, deep breathing
		Organize care to minimize sleep deprivation
		Encourage patient/family's participation in care, when appropriate
		Communicate concern and care through verbal and nonverbal means
		  Touch
		  Empathy
		  Compassion
		  Therapeutic use of self
		  Listening
		  Setting limits
		  Allowing for decision making when possible

POTENTIAL PROBLEMS	EXPECTED OUTCOMES	NURSING ACTIVITIES

	Maintenance of hope system and progression through stages of dying to acceptance in terminally ill patient	Encourage patient/family's coping mechanisms and hope system and comment on each to positively reinforce use as indicated
		Telephone calls to home
		Pictures of family in room
		Help and encourage patient to carry out religious practices
		  Clergy referral
		  Dietary regimen
		  Privacy to pray
		  Praying with patient
		  Scripture reading to patient
		Explore patient's relationship to God; use open-ended questions, e.g., "How is God helping you in this situation?"
		Organize care to allow for patient to verbalize specific fears concerning future and/or fear of dying
		NOTE: Specific fears concerning return to sexual function may especially plague patient after MI, CVA, or traumatic injury, i.e., burns or spinal cord involvement
		Reassure and teach patient and family most nonstressful intimate positions
		Emphasize holding, caressing, and touching rather than performance and climax
		Implement referrals to psychiatric liason, dietitian, and social services, as needed
		Provide reading material concerning needed changes in activity, habits, diet
		Initiate discussion of intimate topics, e.g., sex, God, death
		Using simple questions, allow patient to vent emotions, fears, and concerns
		  "Are you wondering about resumption of sexual activity?"
		  "This is all very frightening, how are you coping?"
		  "How does God fit into all this?"

■ Anger related to feelings of helplessness, loss of control, loneliness, and isolation
  May be associated with anorexia and insomnia
	■ Behavior indicative of decreased anger related to verbally venting angry, depressed feelings
	Verbalization of dislike for dependence and loss of control
	Verbalization of understanding of necessity for temporary isolation
	Cooperation in plan and care
	Restored sense of meaning and relatedness
	Maintenance of key relationships, hope system, and relationship with God, if desired
	Decrease in pain and physical symptoms of stress
	Adequate sleep and nutrition
		■ Allow patient to vent anger
		Assist patient in verbal venting of anger
		Protect patient, self, and other staff from bodily harm
		Be aware verbal abuse is "nothing personal"
		Do not withdraw from patient
		Assign same caretaker as frequently as possible
		Involve patient and family in care to constructively channel anger
		Support family, who also may be targets of anger
		Allow for extended visiting to decrease loneliness and isolation
		Encourage modification of environment with pictures, radio, books, personal belongings
		Monitor for and document
		  Refusal to cooperate with treatments
		  Verbal abuse to staff or family
		  Withdrawal
		  Frequent requests for pain medication and sedation
		Accept and acknowledge anger; comments such as, "If I were just told I have cancer, or an MI, or renal failure, or need surgery, etc., I would feel angry too."
		Assist angry patient to reestablish relationship with God, as situation dictates
		Be aware of clues and statements such as
		  "Why me?"
		  "How could this happen to me?"
		  "How could God do this to me?"
		  "God doesn't care about me."
		  "I've lost all hope and faith now."
		Use repetition of patient's words, as question to allow verbalization of concerns
		  "Your family doesn't care about you?"
		  "God doesn't care about you?"

POTENTIAL PROBLEMS	EXPECTED OUTCOMES	NURSING ACTIVITIES
		Resist banter about religion and ideologies
		Focus on patient's needs, not caregiver's beliefs
		Support patient silently by
		Listening without moralizing
		Using self therapeutically by giving backrubs, hand holding, massage
		Praying for and with patient, if patient desires
		Asking "Would you like me to pray with you?" "Can I read any Scripture meaningful to you?"
		Instruct in use of relaxation techniques
		Meditation
		Imagery
		Deep breathing
		Be aware of helpful literature that may benefit patient and family until out of acute angry phase e.g., *When Bad Things Happen to Good People* by Harold Kushner*
		Administer sedation, as ordered, to decrease anxiety, sensory overload, and sleep deprivation
		Do not focus on anorexia as problem; if present, it may be only means patient has of controlling environment
		Explore possible underlying causes, i.e., anger, depression, spiritual need, guilt, need for love and forgiveness
		Offer small feedings and favorite foods in calm, attractive atmosphere
		Remain as patient's advocate
		Promote understanding between staff and patient to decrease staff rejection, which further isolates angry patient

■ Denial related to
  Illness and possible need for life changes
    Changed body image and loss of self-esteem
    Dealing with dying
	■ Patient realistically appraises situation and view of self and future to promote health and healing
	Patient/family aware of diagnosis; asks pertinent questions related to disease
	Patient can answer questions related to illness
	Patient demonstrates renewed sense of self-esteem and acceptance of altered body image, i.e., active in care of
	  Colostomy
	  Peritoneal dialysis
	  Amputated limb
	  Mastectomy site
	  Prosthetic device
	  Artificial eye
	Terminally ill patient moves toward acceptance stage of dying
		■ Allow for certain amount of denial, which may be very helpful in patient's coping mechanism
		Implement referrals to psychiatric liason personnel, social services, ostomy nurse, or mastectomy groups, as needed
		Ongoing assessment of level of denial
		Reinforce teaching about diagnosis and self-care with eventual view toward discharge
		Support patient and family during denial phase of dying without fostering false hope
		Answer comments such as "I can't wait to take that vacation next year," (when patient has been told he/she has only few months to live) in supportive manner, appreciating desire for trip, and hoping patient will have desire fulfilled
		Minister to spiritual needs as they become apparent

■ Sensory overload related to
  Hospital environment
  Anxiety
  Sleep deprivation
  Agitation
  Pain
	■ Decrease in level of anxiety evidenced by patient's behavior, facial expression, body posture, and general attitude	■ Control environmental level of noise
		Afford as much privacy as possible
		Administer sedation and analgesics, as ordered
		See Problem, Fear

*Kushner, H.: When bad things happen to good people, New York, 1983, Avon Books. Other books that may be useful include Linn, M., and Linn, D.: Healing life's hurts: healing memories through five stages of forgiveness, New York, 1978, Paulist Press; and Tournier, P.: The healing of persons, New York, 1965, Harper & Row, Publishers Inc. (Translated by E. Hudson.)

POTENTIAL PROBLEMS	EXPECTED OUTCOMES	NURSING ACTIVITIES
	Adequate sleep Decrease in agitation Verbalization of sense of well-being and relief of pain	
■ Death	■ Patient moves through stages of dying to acceptance Physical comfort afforded Dignity afforded Peaceful death experience for patient and bereaved family	■ Be aware that stages of dying are not limited to patient but include family and staff Be aware that stages may merge and wax and wane over period of patient's dying 　Denial 　Anger 　Bargaining 　Depression 　Acceptance Organize care to stay with patient Allow venting of feelings associated with stages of dying, e.g. 　Patient says, "No, not me." 　　Allow patient denial; needs time to cope with awareness of impending death 　　When patient ready, supportive listener is needed 　Patient asks, "Why me?" 　　See Problem, Anger 　Patient says, "Yes, me . . . but. . . . " 　　Be aware that bargaining usually occurs between patient and God 　　Act as channel to encourage patient's reliance on and hope in God 　　Seek out clergy, family, significant others, or other staff members who are comfortable with ministering to patient's spiritual needs 　　Be aware that appropriate prayers for healing, peace, comfort, freedom from pain, and death are acceptable 　　Share with patient Scripture concerning God's faithfulness, as appropriate 　Patient says, "Yes, me." 　　Be aware that preparatory grief in depression may be more difficult for staff and family than for patient to accept 　　Resist remarks like, "Cheer up," or "It's not so bad." 　　Do not withdraw from patient 　　Rely on 　　　Therapeutic use of self 　　　Listening in silence 　Presence in silence Allow for extended family visits Decrease environmental noise Promote privacy Answer questions as accurately as possible when patient is not aware of imminent death Administer sedatives and analgesics, as ordered Discuss with physician concerning telling patient serious nature of illness Allow patient to bring up issue of death and dying Allow your nursing, caring art to help you say what feels right Admit your own feelings of helplessness, if present Assist patient maintain hope and find meaning in situation Seek to comfort with appropriate use of humor, not as "cop out" but as one normal way in which people relate Allow family participation

POTENTIAL PROBLEMS	EXPECTED OUTCOMES	NURSING ACTIVITIES
		After death
		Prepare patient by removing as much equipment and as many attachments as possible
		Stay with family in deceased patient's room
		Allow time and grieving behavior
		Support and protect family if screaming, weeping, or fainting occur
		Encourage family and inform them it is all right to touch deceased patient
		Ask if family would like to pray or carry out other significant religious rituals
		Pray with family, if desired
		Maintain personal resources as staff member, as appropriate
		Physical
		Weight
		Grooming
		Sleep
		Exercise
		Diet
		Routine medical, dental care
		Psychosocial
		Supportive relationships
		Socialization
		Hobbies
		Cultural enrichment
		Community involvement
		Professional growth
		Intellectual stimulation
		Relaxation
		Spiritual
		Church/synagogue affilation
		Personal prayer and Bible study
		Prayer partner
		Small-group fellowship

ICU SYNDROME

Throughout day-to-day life within the intensive care unit (ICU), critical care nurses have repeatedly noted alterations of mental status in previously lucid individuals who were subsequently subjected to the ICU environment. These alterations are of considerable concern, because they may inhibit recovery by placing additional stress on the patient's physical and psychological equilibrium. Referred to as the *ICU syndrome,* mental-status alteration in the critically ill patient has been documented in the literature since the early 1960s.

Patients presenting with ICU syndrome or ICU psychosis are less likely to survive in the hospital, more likely to spend more time in the ICU with associated increased cost, and more likely to have major complications (such as CHF, arrhythmias, incisional infection in surgery patients, and IV, arterial line, and PA line infections). Theoretically, if the nurse can intervene to decrease this delirium, a decrease in associated problems should result.

Delirium has been defined as an acute, *temporary,* organic alteration and dysfunction of the brain caused by a relative insufficiency of cerebral metabolism. If the cause for metabolic insufficiency can be removed, there is an excellent potential for recovery. The insult may be circulatory, infectious, metabolic, hormonal, primary, neurologic, traumatic, or toxic. Delirium may include hallucinations and delusions, which are found not only in patients with damaged brains but also in patients with damaged relation to reality. This delirium is characterized by progressive disorientation, first to time, then to place, and finally to person. Patients may experience various degrees of cognitive impairment. The delusions are often paranoid in nature. Nursing care for the delirious patient is directed toward normalizing the environmental stimuli and protecting the patient from self-harm.

Hallucinations are sensory perceptions in which there are no external stimuli. Hallucinations are commonly auditory in nature, but may also include the visual, tactile, and olfactory senses. Hallucinations are often motivated by the need to reduce anxiety and may help the patient to adjust to a reality which appears frightening. It is important that the nurse be alert for periods of hallucination. The nurse should try to bring the patient back to reality through interpersonal involvement and activities. Hallucinations should be responded to and connected with anxiety, because this explanation may prevent the escalating sequence of increased anxiety, increased hallucinations, and thus increased anxiety as a result of hallucinations.

The ICU environment has been likened to a tension-charged war bunker. "Sights of blood, vomitus and excreta, exposed genitalia, mutilated wasting bodies and unconscious and helpless people assault the sensibilities."* The patient is also exposed to an immediate, monotonous environment, sequestered in an enclosure, and surrounded by white sheets, walls, drapes, and ceilings. There are commonly no windows, and the environment is always "daylight." The individual's concrete ideas change, concentration becomes difficult, and, finally, hallucinations occur, accompanied by increased irritability and restlessness.

An important factor associated with this delirium is sleep deprivation, which has been shown to undermine the ability to maintain concentration. Sleep is divided into two types—rapid eye movement (REM) and non-REM.

REM sleep occurs in 70- to 90-minute cycles that increase in length as the night progresses. Four to five REM sleep periods occur a night, and approximately 20% of total sleep is spent in REM. Experimental sleep studies have indicated that completion of an entire cycle is necessary to benefit from sleep. Sleep deprivation is considered to be cumulative, and studies have indicated that an individual can "make up" for sleep deprivation through a period of recovery sleep.

Non-REM sleep is the anabolic phase, in which RNA and proteins are synthesized, especially in the CNS. This stage is prolonged by increased body tiredness. Deprivation of non-REM sleep produces lethargy and depression. REM sleep is characterized by dreaming and the process of memory storage. This stage assists with the maintenance of op-

---

*Hay, D., and Oken, D.: The psychological stresses of intensive care unit nursing. In McConnell, E.A.: Burnout in the nursing profession: coping strategies, causes, and costs, St. Louis, 1982, The C.V. Mosby Co., p. 254.

timistic mood, attention, and self-confidence. REM sleep also seems to facilitate emotional adaptation to the physical and psychological environment, and is needed in large quantities after stress and worry.

The characteristic course of ICU syndrome commonly begins on the second to the fifth day after admission to the ICU. The patient usually experiences a perceptual distortion of a visual, tactile, proprioceptive, or, less frequently, auditory type. The distortion is often associated with anxiety, motor restlessness, inability to concentrate, and mild confusion. It may progress into a paranoid delusional state, gross disorientation, illusions, or even hallucinations.

The nurse, as an integral part of the health team, can be instrumental in minimizing the risks of ICU psychosis. Vigilant assessments must be made to reduce the noxious stimuli that result from an ICU environment. Care plans should be implemented that reduce and/or eliminate predisposing environmental factors and that allow for adequate individualized preoperative preparation (in surgery patients), and establishment of a trusting relationship. Routine orientation checks with frequent reorientation as indicated should be performed. Visiting hours should be reevaluated and individualized as indicated. Frequent family visitation should also be stressed. The nursing history should ascertain the patient's characteristic sleep pattern. It is important that care be organized, planned, and performed to prevent sleep deprivation and allow for periods of uninterrupted sleep. Pain should be controlled as much as possible with analgesia. Nursing care should be planned to preserve as much of a normal day/night cycle as possible to reduce the intensity of any delirium. Explanation and reexplanation of equipment, machines, and procedures is a necessity. The patient should be encouraged to verbalize as well as to ventilate feelings and perceptions of perceptual illusions, if present. Reinforcement of reality and the self-limiting character of perceptual illusions and the associated disorientation is also of prime importance.

Medical interventions have been directed toward the use of chemotherapeutic agents and the use of a psychiatric liaison. Drug therapy, if used, is usually introduced after the emergence of the delirium. Haloperidol (Haldol) has been used as treatment, because it reduces confusion and agitation without overly sedating patients. For sleep medication, hypnotics that do not suppress REM sleep should be prescribed. It is important to note that correction of factors that predispose to altered mental status, e.g., metabolic disturbances, acidosis, digoxin toxicity, electrolyte imbalances, and any pulmonary insufficiency should be corrected before drug treatment.

ASSESSMENT

1. History—medical, surgical, psychosocial
2. Presence and nature of the following signs and symptoms
   a. Behavioral
      (1) Progressive disorientation (generally first to time, then to place, finally to person)
      (2) Cognitive impairment
      (3) Inability to concentrate and mild confusion; may accompany delusions, hallucinations
      (4) Delusions
      (5) Hallucinations
      (6) Motor restlessness
   b. Somatic
      (1) Altered BP
      (2) Evidence of decreased peripheral perfusion
      (3) Tachycardia
      (4) Hyperventilation
      (5) Anorexia
3. Patient/family's perception of and reaction to diagnosis, progression of disease, and treatment modalities
4. Coping mechanisms of patient/family; key relationships and support systems
5. Wound for evidence of infection, e.g.
   a. Erythema
   b. Inflammation
   c. Drainage

GOALS

1. Reduction of patient/family anxiety with provision of information and explanations about ICU syndrome and its self-limiting nature
2. Decreased associated problems (e.g., infection, self-injury, arrythmias)
3. Decrease in the development/intensity of ICU syndrome
4. Patient uses available support systems (e.g., family/significant others)
5. Shortened stay in the ICU with associated decreased costs

POTENTIAL PROBLEMS	EXPECTED OUTCOMES	NURSING ACTIVITIES

■ Patient/family's anxiety related to ICU syndrome	■ Reduction in anxiety with provision of information, explanations, and reinforcement	■ Prevention
		  Ongoing assessment of patient/family's level of anxiety
		  Reinforcement of self-limiting character of ICU syndrome
		  Encouragement of verbalization of feelings and illusions experienced by patient
		  Explanation in lay terms of possibility of "perceptual illusions" while in ICU
		Monitor for
		  Patient/family's verbalization of anxiety or "nervousness"
		  Patient restlessness or inability to sleep
		  Tense body posture
		  Anxious facial expression
		  Anorexia
		If problem occurs
		  Provide information as needed
		  Encourage verbalization by patient/family
		  Sedate, as ordered, prn
		  Reinforce self-limiting character of ICU syndrome

■ Wound/cannula site infection secondary to confusion and agitation	■ Infection-free state	■ Prevent by
		  Employing strict aseptic technique with dressing changes
		  Changing dressings q24 hr and prn
		  Explaining to patient importance of keeping dressings intact until suture line is healed and/or cannulas are removed
		Monitor for
		  Local signs and symptoms of wound/cannula site infection
		  Elevated body temperature
		  Elevated WBC count
		Notify physician of aforementioned abnormalities
		If problem occurs
		  Administer antibiotics, as ordered
		  Administer local wound/cannula care, as ordered

■ Confusion and agitation (ICU syndrome)	■ Patient's mentation and orientation will remain "normal"	■ Prevention
		  Normalize environmental stimuli as much as possible
		  Establish trusting relationship with patient/family
		  Adequate, individualized preoperative teaching for surgery patients
		  Continuously orient patient to ICU milieu
		  Encourage verbalization of feelings by patient
		  Control pain as much as possible with analgesia, as ordered
		  Plan nursing care to preserve as much of patient's normal day/night cycle as possible
		  Individualize visiting hours if and when possible
		  Explain and reexplain equipment, machines, and procedures, as necessary
		  Reinforce reality and self-limiting character of perceptual illusions and disorientation
		Monitor for
		  Inappropriate conversing
		  Combative behavior
		  Obvious confusion
		  Increased activity level and/or motor restlessness
		  Inability to concentrate
		Notify physician of aforementioned abnormalities
		If problem occurs
		  Institute environmental normalization if possible (lowering lights, increasing privacy, decreasing noise, etc.)
		  Extend sleep/rest periods when physical stability allows
		  Administer any chemotherapeutic agents, as ordered
		  Reassess and reemphasize preventive nursing activities, as needed

POTENTIAL PROBLEMS	EXPECTED OUTCOMES	NURSING ACTIVITIES

■ Self-injury by patient	■ Minimal self-injury sustained by patient	■ Prevention
		  Continuously assess patient's orientation
		  Sedate patient, as ordered, prn
		  Restrain patient, as ordered, prn, to prevent self-injury
		  Reduce confusion by implementing nursing activities outlined in Problem, Confusion and agitation
		Monitor for
		  Combative behavior
		  Unexplained ecchymoses, cuts, and/or abrasions
		Notify physician for abnormalities in aforementioned
		If problem occurs
		  Sedate patient, as ordered, prn
		  Restrain patient, as ordered, prn
		  See Problem, Confusion and agitation

INFECTION CONTROL IN THE CRITICAL CARE UNIT

Medical technology has developed to the extent that critically ill patients who previously would have succumbed to their underlying illness are surviving in greater numbers. This survival is often threatened by the spectre of infection—patients who survive their illness may experience increased morbidity and mortality secondary to infection. Critical care nurses have a responsibility to be aware of infection control problems so that they can take steps to prevent these complications. This standard will attempt to explore common infection control problems and discuss nursing activities useful in overcoming them.

Very few things in the world are sterile or remain sterile after contact with the environment. Normal flora are microorganisms that reside in many areas of the body without causing infections. These organisms vary from one body area to another and also from one host to the next based on individual factors such as age, presence of chronic disease, temperature, and acidity.[3] Microorganisms that cause infection in a healthy person are called pathogens. Organisms that are part of a person's normal flora but can cause infection when the host's defenses break down are called opportunistic pathogens.

Infection entails the replication of organisms in the tissues of a host; if this results in overt clinical manifestations, then an infection is said to exist.[1] Infections are also classified as endogenous, in which microorganisms are transmitted from one area of the body to another producing infection, or exogenous, in which the source of the offending microorganism is the external environment. Colonization implies the populating of a body area (e.g., skin, mucous membranes) by microorganisms with no tissue invasion or production of disease.[7]

Infection results from the interaction between an infectious agent and a susceptible host. This interaction—called transmission—occurs by means of contact between the agent and the host. Three interrelated factors—the agent, the host, and some means of transmission—represent the chain of infection. For an infection to occur, a significant number of pathogenic organisms must be present, an individual must be susceptible to the infection, and a means for the agent to have appropriate contact with the susceptible host must occur.

Certain physiological factors increase the risk of infection, such as very young or old age, chronic diseases, uremia, lymphomas, leukemias, neoplasms, treatment with steroids or other immunosuppressive agents, radiation therapy, antibiotics, shock, or trauma.[1]

The methods of transmission have been divided into four categories, which are as follows:

1. Contact transmission, which includes
   a. Direct contact, in which the infectious agent is transported from the infected host to another susceptible host
   b. Indirect contact, which occurs when the microorganism is transmitted via contaminated inanimate objects (commonly called fomites)
   c. Droplet spread, which occurs when infectious particles are suspended in the air as a result of talking, coughing, or sneezing (requires close contact [less than 3 feet])
2. Airborne transmission, which occurs when droplet nuclei or dust particles containing the infectious agent are suspended in the air (transmitted over greater distances)
3. Vehicle transmission, which occurs when mediums that harbor infectious agents contact a susceptible host (e.g., food, water, blood)
4. Vector-borne transmission, which occurs when microorganisms are moved via insects, mosquitoes, fleas, or ticks, causing disease.

Breaking the chain of infection involves interrupting one or more events in the series. This can be done through control of sources of bacteria; through control of transmission by using isolation or single-dose, single-use equipment; and by maximizing host immunity, e.g., through immunizations, increasing nutritional status, medications, etc.

Hospitals are conducive to the development and spread of infection. Major reservoirs of pathogens include the patient's own community-acquired flora, microorganisms introduced in the hospital environment through medical personnel or inanimate patient care equipment, intrinsically contaminated commercial products, or other colonized or infected patients.[14]

A nosocomial or hospital-acquired infection is one that

was neither present nor incubating at the time of admission. An infection that becomes apparent after discharge from the hospital but was clearly developing during the hospitalization is also considered nosocomial. It has been estimated that on a nationwide basis approximately 5.5% of all hospital patients will develop a nosocomial infection,[5] which may lengthen their stay by up to 15 days, and in the case of bacteremias, increases mortality. It has been estimated that as many as one half of all reported nosocomial infections are preventable.[1]

Bacterial infections account for the majority (90%) of recognized infections,[5] although this may reflect the difficulties of confirming fungal, viral, and parasitic infections. Table 61-1 outlines bacteria and fungi and Table 61-2 lists viruses of importance in the hospital setting. There are currently more than 400 different viruses classified, and this number is growing. The role of viruses as normal flora is undetermined.[3,9]

The longer survival of critically ill patients and the increasing resistance of bacteria to antibiotics are resulting in reports of nosocomial infections by organisms previously thought to be nonpathogenic and of increased microbial resistance in laboratory isolates. It is generally acknowledged that our antibiotic arsenal seldom remains more than a few drugs ahead of the resistant bacteria that colonize and infect patients.

Significant factors that lead to the endemic occurrence of multidrug-resistant bacteria in hospitals include (1) admission or readmission of patients with preexisting GI, genitourinary, respiratory, or wound colonization or infections with resistant strains of bacteria; (2) in-hospital spread of bacteria from person to person, usually via transient hand carriage (this may result in a few infected but many colonized patients); (3) indirect spread of resistant organisms between patients caused by environmental contamination; and (4) the effects of antibiotic pressure, which encourages the suppression of sensitive flora with subsequent colonization by more resistant bacteria.[26]

Along with the benefits to patient care that have resulted from the development of specialized units to care for seriously ill patients there have also been certain hazards, notably that of producing a concentration of highly susceptible patients at greater risk of nosocomial infection. After 3 days in a critical care unit, a patient runs a 50% risk of colonization with exogenous bacteria and a 23% chance of hospital-acquired infection,[14] with the risk increasing as the stay is prolonged. After 10 days the risk of colonization is over 90% and the risk of infection is 75%.[14]

Among the several risk factors responsible for the high rate of colonization/infection of critical care unit patients are (1) compromised host resistance secondary to underlying illness; (2) changes in the patient's flora that accompany serious illness; (3) antibiotics used to treat life-threatening disease that change host flora, thus predisposing to colo-

nization with multidrug-resistant bacteria; (4) the variety of invasive procedures done for therapeutic and monitoring purposes; (5) life-saving procedures done on an emergency basis with compromised aseptic technique; (6) therapeutic immunosuppression; and (7) close proximity to other patients who are predisposed to similar infections.[1]

Prevention of cross-infection among critical care unit patients depends on medical and nursing personnel maintaining a high level of awareness of the susceptibility of such patients to nosocomial infection. Studies confirm that the prime vectors in the transmission of microbes in a critical care unit are the personnel who work in the unit and that the main route of contamination is direct contact. The sources of infection can be traced to other patients in the unit, to personnel, and to equipment. Although airborne spread represents a definite threat, it occurs less commonly than contact by direct or fomite routes.[13]

In addition to the animate environment, the inanimate environment in a medical institution provides possible sources of infecting organisms. Generally, objects that have the closest contact with a possible host, especially invasive devices such as IV or Foley catheters, are considered the most significant sources of infecting organisms.[3] Thus environmental contamination may serve as a source for transmission of nosocomial infection whenever contaminated patient care equipment, instruments, or medicines introduce pathogenic microorganisms through any body orifice or directly into a wound.

General objectives for infection control in critical care units include the following:

1. To minimize the risk of infection to the critically ill patient by
   a. Meticulous hand washing and personal hygiene
   b. Appropriate sterilization, cleaning, and monitoring of equipment that comes into contact with the patient
   c. Institution, maintenance, and monitoring of housekeeping procedures
2. To prevent patient-to-patient spread of organisms by means of personnel, fomites, direct contact, or airborne transmission
3. To segregate patients potentially hazardous to others by
   a. Establishing and maintaining isolation policies for the unit
   b. Practicing satisfactory containment techniques
4. To be aware of the scope of infection and familiar with the guidelines for the prevention of infection

The primary goal in specimen collection is to obtain material representative of the suspected infectious pathogen (uncontaminated by other microorganisms) to facilitate a laboratory diagnosis. In general, all culture specimens should be collected and transported in sterile containers that are properly labeled with the patient's name, the site from

TABLE 61-1. Common agents that cause nosocomial infections

ORGANISM	NORMAL LOCATION	ORGANISM AS PATHOGEN
Gram-positive bacteria		
Staphylococcus aureus	Skin, hair, naso-oropharynx	Boils, pneumonia, food poisoning, wound infections
Staphylococcus epidermidis	Skin, hair, naso-oropharynx	Bacterial endocarditis, wound infections, stitch abscesses
Streptococcus group A	Oropharynx, perianal area, anus	Erysipelas, impetigo, pharyngitis, scarlet fever
Streptococcus group B	Genitalia, adult vagina, colon	Endometritis, wound infections, infant septicemia or meningitis
Streptococcus group D	Colon	Urinary tract infections, wound infections, subacute endocarditis
Streptococcus pneumoniae	Anterior nares, oropharynx	Pneumonia, meningitis, endocarditis
Streptococcus viridans	Oropharynx, skin, respiratory tract	Subacute bacterial endocarditis, meningitis
Corynebacterium	Skin, eye conjunctiva, nasooropharynx	*Corynebacterium diphtheriae* is causative agent of diphtheria
Gram-negative bacteria		
Escherichia coli	Colon, perineum	Urinary tract infections, enteritis
Klebsiella pneumonia	Colon, perineum, naso-oropharynx	Pneumonias, wound infections, urinary tract infections
Proteus mirabilis	Colon, perineum	Urinary tract infections, pneumonia, gastroenteritis
Serratia marcescens	Ubiquitous in nature, not common as flora	Urinary tract infections, septicemia, wound infections
Haemophilus influenzae	Nasooropharynx	Meningitis, pneumonia, conjunctivitis, subacute bacterial endocarditis
Neisseria meningitidis	10% to 15% of population are asymptomatic carriers in naso-oropharynx	Meningitis, pneumonia
Neisseria gonorrhoeae	Not normal flora	Gonorrhea, pelvic inflammatory disease, arthritis, septicemia, ophthalmia of newborn
Pseudomonas aeruginosa	Colon	Urinary tract infection, pneumonia, wound infections, septicemia; may infect burn wounds or decubitus ulcers
Bacteroides fragilis	Oropharynx, colon, vagina	Peritonitis, endometritis, septicemia, wound infections
Salmonella	Not normal flora—some asymptomatic carriers exist	Gastroenteritis, diarrhea, typhoid fever *(Salmonella typhi)*
Shigella	Not normal flora	Diarrhea, dysentery
Other opportunistic pathogens		
Candida albicans	Ubiquitous in environment; disease is usually caused by factors that compromise host	Superficial infections (vaginitis, oral thrush); disseminated disease in compromised host
Nocardia asteroides	May be normal flora of skin or naso-oropharynx	Opportunistic pathogen in compromised host—may cause pneumonia or septicemia
Cryptococcus neoformans	Found in soil—opportunistic pathogen	May be introduced into skin and cause local lesions or be inhaled and produce pulmonary disease in compromised host
Histoplasma capsulatum	Found in soil—opportunistic pathogen	May cause skin lesions, pulmonary disease
Aspergillus	Ordinarily found in nature—opportunistic pathogen	May cause pulmonary disease, skin lesions, myocarditis, disseminated disease in compromised host

Modified from Mikat, D.M., and Mikat, K.W.: A clinician's dictionary guide to bacteria and fungi, ed. 4, Indianapolis, Eli Lily & Co.

TABLE 61-2. Viral infectious agents

Viruses causing respiratory disease

Influenzavirus
Adenovirus
Enterovirus
Respiratory syncytial virus
Parainfluenza virus
Myxovirus

Viruses causing GI disease

Hepatitis A virus
Hepatitis B virus

Viruses causing CNS disease

Poliovirus
ECHO virus
Coxsackievirus
Herpes simplex virus

Viruses causing skin lesions/rashes

Smallpox virus
Varicella-zoster virus
Measles virus
Herpesvirus

Modified from Castle, M.: Hospital infection control, principles and practice, New York, 1980, John Wiley & Sons, Inc., and Hargiss, C.O., and Larson, E.: Am. J. Nurs. **83**:2165-2186, 1981.

which the specimen was obtained, the type of specimen, the date, time, and manner in which the specimen was obtained, and a request for the specific test desired. The specimen should be delivered to the lab as soon as possible.

Lab results must always be interpreted with consideration of the patient's clinical condition. Human errors such as mislabeling can and do occur, the culture specimen can be contaminated at any point, and lab testing is not always exact. When there is doubt as to the significance of results, repeat culturing may be appropriate.

Table 61-3 discusses common types of specimens obtained, the proper techniques for obtaining and handling these specimens, and clinically significant findings.

NOSOCOMIAL URINARY TRACT INFECTIONS

The urinary tract is the most common site of nosocomial infection, accounting for approximately 40% of the total number of infections reported by acute care hospitals and affecting an estimated 600,000 patients per year.[28] Most nosocomial urinary tract infections are related to urinary tract manipulation or instrumentation, most commonly indwelling Foley catheters. The indwelling Foley catheter is a familiar, common part of nursing care today, but unfortunately it is too often taken for granted. Many physicians and nurses do not fully appreciate the serious risks of catheterization, and in fact some consider bacteriuria and infection to be an inevitable consequence of the procedure.

While it is true that most patients with catheter-associated bacteriuria either recover spontaneously when the catheter is removed or respond without complication to appropriate antibiotic therapy, some infections can lead to pyelonephritis, septicemia, and other serious sequelae.[4]

A single catheterization incurs a 1% to 2% risk of significant bacteriuria and infection in general.[24] This risk may increase to 10% to 20% in pregnant women, elderly patients, diabetic patients, or patients who have a structural or neurological abnormality causing urinary retention.[2] Catheter-associated bacteriuria cannot be eliminated by current methods; however, its incidence may be reduced to acceptable levels with the use of careful aseptic technique at the time of insertion, the use of intermittent catheterization, and the use and careful maintenance of closed drainage systems.

A nosocomial urinary tract infection is considered to be present when colony counts in urine of more than 100,000 organisms per ml of urine or pyuria of 10 WBCs is found in a patient with prior negative urine analysis and/or culture or if a previously infected patient has new organisms cultured with a clinical continuation or deterioration of symptoms.[10]

Normal bowel flora organisms are commonly associated with nosocomial urinary tract infections. *Escherichia coli* is the most common organism, but others include *Enterobacter, Proteus, Klebsiella, Pseudomonas, Staphylococcus,* and group D streptococci. As stated previously, many of the microorganisms are part of the patient's endogenous bowel flora, but they can also be acquired by cross-contamination from other patients or hospital personnel or by exposure to contaminated solutions or nonsterile equipment. Other pathogens that can cause infections in the patient who has undergone catheterization are *Serratia marcescens* and *Pseudomonas cepacia*—these are of clinical significance because they do not commonly reside in the GI tract. Their isolation from patients suggests exogenous contamination.[28]

Infecting microorganisms gain access to the urinary tract by several routes. Microorganisms can be introduced into the bladder through the use of contaminated equipment, aseptic solutions, or poor aseptic technique and if the periurethral area is not cleansed adequately before the insertion of the catheter and routinely thereafter. Contamination may also occur by interrupting the closed sterile drainage system at the catheter-tubing junction or by allowing reflux of urine into the bladder from contaminated collection bags and tubing. Finally, passive transmission by unwashed, contaminated hands remains a major cause of cross-infection of catheters.[2]

NOSOCOMIAL POSTOPERATIVE WOUND INFECTIONS

The skin itself has active functions, namely protection, excretion, and sensory functions. Disruption of the continuity of the skin, tissue integrity, or the physiologic function

TABLE 61-3. General guidelines for microbiologic specimens and interpretation

CULTURE TYPE	COLLECTION TECHNIQUE	CLINICAL SIGNIFICANCE
Swabs		
Nares	Use sterile swab in transport media approved for culture use	Culture positive with clinically relevant organism
Throat		
Endocervix	Firmly swab, but do not rub area	
Vagina		
Urethra		
Urine		
Clean catch (midstream)	Cleanse perineal area to reduce skin flora contamination	> 100,000 organisms/ml of urine
	Collect 7 to 10 ml of midstream flow in sterile container	
	Send to lab within 60 to 90 minutes or refrigerate immediately and send within 24 hours	
Straight catheterized	Cleanse perineal area as for clean catch; use aseptic technique when inserting catheter	10,000 to 100,000 organisms/ml of urine
	Place specimen in sterile container—transport to lab within 60 minutes	2 to 4 positive polymorphonuclear leukocytes
Foley catheter	Prepare sampling port with disinfectant	Same as straight catheterized specimen
	Aspirate urine with sterile syringe and needle	
	Remove needle to inject urine into sterile container	
	Transport as for straight catheterized specimen	
Wound swab	Superficial debris should be removed by gently wiping area with cotton soaked in sterile water or saline	Organisms seen on gram stain
	Swab active site, not skin area	Polymorphonuclear leukocytes present
	Send to lab within 60 minutes, or refrigerate and send within 24 hours	
	No bacteriostatic solution should be used to clean wound before culture	
Feces	Obtain fresh stool in clean container	Ova, parasites, bacterial pathogen isolated
	Do *not* refrigerate	
	Send to lab within 30 to 60 minutes	
Sputum		
Expectorated or induced	First morning specimen is best	Purulent material
	Collect material coughed up, not saliva	Organism seen on gram stain and <2 epithelial cells on gram stain (indicates less chance of contamination by mouth flora)
	Place in appropriate sterile container (depending on test being done)	
	Send to lab within 60 minutes	
Tracheal aspiration	Use sterile suction catheter and aseptic technique	Same as expectorated or induced
	Send to lab within 60 minutes	
IV catheter tip	Use aseptic technique, prepare site before removal of catheter	>15 colonies of organism
	Cut with sterile scissors	Positive culture in broth medium
	Place in sterile container	NOTE: Not reliable indication of patient condition—complicating factors include differentiating contaminants from organism responsible for infection
	Send to lab within 2 hours	
Blood	Use aseptic technique—prepare site and probing finger with iodine	Any positive cultures
	Avoid using uncovered stopcocks or in-use lines for specimen collection	Complicating factor—it is often hard to distinguish contaminants from real bacteremias; may need to do serial cultures for confirmation
	Collect in specified sterile container—disinfect tube top before injecting specimen	
	Send to lab within 60 minutes	
CSF	Use sterile gloves, aseptic technique	Positive gram stain for organisms
	Prepare site with iodine	Any positive cultures
	Place CSF in sterile tube	
	Send to lab within 30 minutes	

Modified from Hargis, C.O., and Larson, E.: Infection control: putting principles into practice, Am. J. Nurs. **83:**2165-2186, 1981; and Presswood, G.M.: Collection, transport, and interpretation of microbiologic specimens, Crit. Care Q. **3:**11-26, March 1983.

of any other anatomic structure is classified as a wound. Wounds may result from mechanical, thermal, chemical, or radiation trauma. Wound healing involves a series of processes that attempt to restore the tissue to its normal functioning.

The first phase of the repair process after an injury is hemostasis, which begins when platelets adhere to the exposed collagen in the walls of the severed vessels, followed by inflammation, which functions primarily by clearing away cellular debris and combating any microbes present through the action of lymphocytes and macrophages.[6]

The second phase of healing begins with the migration and proliferation of epithelial cells and invasion by fibroblasts at the site of the wound. This helps to seal the wound and protect it from contamination. Collagen secreted by the fibroblasts that adhere to the wound margins also contributes to wound contraction and adds strength to the wound site.

The final phase of healing is cell differentiation, which begins once the entire wound surface is covered with a thin layer of epithelial cells. During this phase the final repairs are made, with realignment and organization of cellular material, resulting in a healed wound.[6]

Surgery involves the violation of the body's primary defense against the entry of bacteria—the skin. Surgical wounds can be classified according to the likelihood and degree of wound contamination at the time of operation, as shown in Table 61-4.

Surgical wound infections are the second most common nosocomial infection and are an important cause of increased costs, morbidity, and mortality in patients. In general, a wound infection can be assumed if purulent material drains from the wound, even if a culture is negative or not taken.[25]

This definition is accepted primarily because (1) a positive culture does not necessarily indicate infection, since many wounds, infected or uninfected, are colonized by bacteria, and (2) infected wounds may not yield pathogens by culture because the patient has been previously treated with antibiotics or because of inadequate culture techniques.[25]

The risk of developing a surgical wound infection is largely determined by three factors: (1) the amount and type of microbial contamination of the wound, (2) the condition of the wound at the end of the operation (largely determined by surgical technique and the disease processes encountered during the operation), and (3) host susceptibility, i.e., the patient's intrinsic ability to deal with microbial contamination.[25]

The frequency and severity of each complication depends on the infecting pathogen and the site of infection (e.g., any infection involving an implanted foreign body or substantial necrotic tissue is likely to have serious sequelae).[25]

Surgical wound infections are usually localized to the wound and with appropriate treatment do not result in major complications. However, infections can result in several kinds of severe local and systemic complications, including destruction of tissue and separation of the wound, metastatic infection, bacteremia, and shock.[25]

Significant areas of preoperative concern include the general health of the patient and the presence of underlying diseases or conditions such as obesity, malnutrition, diabetes, or older age. A coexistent remote infection is associated with an increased risk of infection. Whether operative wound infection results from hematogenous seeding of the wound by the remote source or from a general depressant effect on host resistance caused by the remote infection is unknown. However, patients with remote infection should not undergo any elective surgery until the preexisting infection has been eradicated.[21]

Most surgical wound infections probably result from organisms that gain access to the wound at the time of operation.[1] Adequate physical facilities and adherence to standard operating room procedures are important in reducing the risks of intraoperative contamination of wounds. Contamination from the surgical team may result from direct contact with the hands or shedding from the skin or mucous membranes. The likelihood of this is reduced by hand scrubbing with an antibacterial soap to remove or reduce the number of bacteria present and using sterile gowns and gloves as an additional barrier. Other intraoperative mea-

---

TABLE 61-4. Classification of surgical wounds

Clean wound

Uninfected operative wounds with no inflammation encountered
No operative entry into respiratory, GI, genitourinary, or oropharyngeal cavity
No break in surgical technique
Infection rate 1.8%[1,25]

Clean contaminated wounds

Operative entry into GI, respiratory, or genitourinary tract
Absence of infected contents
Includes operations involving biliary tract, appendix, vagina, oropharynx
Infection rate 8.9%[1,25]

Contaminated wounds

Includes open, fresh, accidental wounds
Operations complicated by major breaks in surgical technique or gross spillage from GI tract or infected body fluids
Incisions in which acute inflammation is encountered
Infection rate 21.6%[1,25]

Dirty and infected wounds

Suggests that organism causing postoperative infection was in operative field before operation
Contaminated or traumatic wound with foreign body or necrotic tissue
Obvious infection, inflammation noted during surgery
Perforated viscus
Infection rate 38.4%[1,25]

sures that reduce the likelihood of wound infection include scrupulous aseptic technique and the exclusion of medical personnel with any evidence of infection (e.g., upper respiratory, skin infection), according to the policy developed by the infection control committee in the hospital.

Exogenous sources of contamination include the operating room air, poor operative technique or wound management, type of suture used, and the surgical instruments themselves if they are not adequately sterilized.

The prevention of infection in the immediate postoperative period involves preventing direct contamination of the wound. One may also reduce the risk of wound infection by ensuring adequate drainage of the wound. If not allowed to drain freely, blood, pus, body fluids, and necrotic material may collect and provide a growth medium for microorganisms. A dressing will provide protection and immobilization of the wound as well as collect wound drainage. Dressings should be changed as frequently as necessary to avoid saturation and the creation of a moist, warm environment, which facilitates bacterial growth.

NOSOCOMIAL PNEUMONIAS

Lower respiratory tract infections constitute the third most common type of nosocomial infection in the United States, accounting for about 15% to 20% of all nosocomial infections among hospitalized patients. Nosocomial infections of the lower respiratory tract are particularly dangerous, because they tend to complicate and extend hospitalization and produce a mortality of up to 50%.[24]

The primary functions of the respiratory tract are to clean, warm, and humidify ventilated air and to maintain adequate gas exchange. Humans possess an intricate system of pulmonary defense mechanisms that includes the nasal hairs, the sneeze and cough reflexes, ciliary transport, and antibodies on the surface of the mucous membranes that line the upper respiratory tract. These result in a practically sterile lung parenchyma. Heredity, age, nutritional status, environment, and the individual's resistance to disease can modify the pulmonary protective mechanisms. Bed rest, dehydration, hypoxia, anesthesia, alcoholic intoxication, and coma also affect the proper functioning of the respiratory tract defenses.[19]

The oropharynx of a healthy person is normally populated with organisms such as *Staphylococcus epidermidis, Staphylococcus aureus,* and *Streptococcus pneumoniae* but ordinarily does not provide a suitable growth environment for gram-negative bacilli. However, acutely or chronically ill patients are more susceptible to both colonization and infection with gram-negative bacteria, because they are frequently underhydrated and poorly nourished and have greatly compromised defense mechanisms. The incidence of gram-negative colonization for patients admitted to a critical care setting is reported to be 22% within the first 24 hours of admission![19]

Patients whose pulmonary defense mechanisms are compromised by associated conditions such as respiratory tract disease, tracheal intubation, coma, acidosis, or antimicrobial therapy are most likely to be colonized. Patients colonized with gram-negative bacteria are more likely to develop pneumonia than patients not colonized.[13] Pneumonia results from an inability of the lungs' defense mechanisms to clear or kill an aspirated challenge.

Bacteria are believed to invade the lower respiratory tract by three routes: (1) aspiration of oropharyngeal organisms, (2) inhalation of aerosols containing bacteria, as may occur through exposure to contaminated respiratory therapy equipment; and (3) hematogenous spread from a distant site of infection.[24]

Although many types of microorganisms, including bacteria, fungi, viruses, and parasites cause nosocomial pneumonia most cases are caused by bacteria. Approximately 51% of nosocomial pneumonias are caused by gram-negative bacteria such as *Klebsiella, Enterobacter,* and *Pseudomonas aeruginosa.*[19] Other causes of nosocomial pneumonia are gram-positive bacteria such as *Staphylococcus aureus* and *Streptococcus.* Endogenous sources of gram-negative bacteria include the GI tract, which may be seen when patients aspirate vomitus and subsequently develop a pneumonia. Exogenous sources can include contaminated respiratory therapy equipment.

A cough productive of purulent secretions, fever, and elevated WBC and radiographic evidence of new or increasing infiltrates of the lungs all contribute to the diagnosis of nosocomial pneumonia.[20]

Patients most likely to develop nosocomial bacterial pneumonia are those who (1) have had a recent surgical operation; (2) have conditions that make aspiration likely; (3) are exposed to contaminated respiratory therapy equipment, receive improper respiratory care, or have instrumentation of the respiratory tract; (4) are colonized in the oropharynx with aerobic gram-negative bacteria; or (5) have impaired immunological function.[24]

The use of respiratory therapy equipment routinely bypasses some of the pulmonary defense mechanisms, thus increasing the patient's chance of acquiring a nosocomial pneumonia. Endotracheal tubes prevent effective coughing, and they traumatize the mucociliary complex, causing increased mucous production and decreased clearance. Assisted ventilation for patients having respiratory failure or other critically ill patients can be a source of infecting microorganisms. Up until 5 to 10 years ago, the risk of introducing nosocomial pathogens through respiratory therapy equipment was greatly underestimated. The current use of disposable respiratory therapy equipment has done much to minimize the risk of respiratory infections. Most respiratory therapy departments are aware of their responsibilities in preventing nosocomial pneumonia and to that end have set up policies and procedures for decontamination and sterilization of equipment.

NOSOCOMIAL BACTEREMIA

IV therapy is a fundamental part of modern patient care and is given to approximately 30% to 50% of hospital patients,[23] many of whom are critical care unit patients. IV therapy allows for direct access to a patient's vascular system to administer fluid, electrolytes, and medication and also allows for hemodynamic monitoring. The benefits of IV therapy are clear, but unfortunately the IV system also provides a potential route for microorganisms to enter the vascular system, bypassing normal skin defense mechanisms. Infections related to IV therapy include phlebitis, suppurative thrombophlebitis, and bacteremia.[26]

One of the more serious infections—bacteremia—may occur in any one of three clinical settings: (1) localized infection that can no longer be contained, overtax host defenses, and allow for hematogenous seeding (e.g., peritonitis); (2) bacteremia that originates from a local infection (e.g., cellulitis) or occurs in the absence of any identifiable local infection; and (3) microorganisms that are introduced directly into the bloodstream through an invasive vascular device.[15]

Each year nosocomial bacteremias develop in approximately 194,000 patients in US hospitals. Up to one half of the patients in whom bacteremia develops die.[15] Bacteremias can be classified as primary (specifically related to contaminated IV catheters, infusates, or intravascular monitoring devices) or secondary (as a complication of an infection of another site). Most nosocomial bacteremias occur endemically and are secondary to postoperative wound or intraabdominal infection, urinary tract infection, or pneumonia.[15] The emphasis here will be on primary bacteremias associated with contaminated IV therapy or intravascular devices, monitoring equipment, or infusates, as these infections are highly preventable with conscientious adherence to infection control measures.

A nosocomial bacteremia is defined as the isolation of any organism from a properly obtained blood culture specimen in a patient who was admitted without signs and symptoms of infection or the isolation of a new organism from a subsequent culture in a previously culture-positive patient.[10]

Some factors that influence a patient's risk of acquiring an IV catheter–related infection include[12] (1) patient susceptibility, e.g., burn, chronically ill, or immunocompromised patients are at increased risk; (2) type of catheter used, e.g., plastic catheters are associated with increased infection rates; (3) method of insertion, e.g., cutdown insertions have a higher risk of infection than percutaneous insertions; (4) duration of IV therapy—the rate of positive catheter cultures and associated bacteremia increases after 2 to 3 days; and (5) presence of monitoring devices within the infusion system.

The use of intraarterial infusions for hemodynamic monitoring has increased in recent years. Over 80,000 patients are monitored each year in US hospitals.[17] There are multiple sites for extrinsic contamination of these monitoring systems, including transducer domes,[12] stopcocks,[12] infusate,[17] and inadequately sterilized transducers.[12]

Factors that may contribute to recurrent contamination of pressure monitoring systems and the continuing risk of infection in patients include (1) ignorance of infectious hazards posed by the system; (2) inadequate knowledge about recommended techniques for assembling, inserting, and maintaining the systems in patients and cleaning and sterilizing components after use; (3) reuse of disposable equipment; and (4) high demand for monitoring equipment leading to inadequate time for cleaning.[1]

ASSESSMENT

1. Patient status
   a. Extremes of age
   b. Level of orientation: comatose, status after stroke
   c. Length of hospitalization
   d. Level of mobility
2. Presence of chronic disease
   a. Diabetes
   b. Cardiovascular disease
   c. Chronic obstructive pulmonary disease
   d. Renal failure
   e. Anemia
3. Skin integrity
   a. Surgical or traumatic wound
   b. Burns
   c. Bony prominences
4. Immunosuppressed states
   a. Presence of neoplasms
   b. Presence of leukemias, lymphomas
   c. Previous treatment with immunosuppressive agents such as steroids, chemotherapy, radiation therapy
   d. Congenital or acquired immunodeficiency
5. Medical instrumentation/therapeutic factors
   a. Surgery
   b. Assisted ventilation or presence of tracheostomy
   c. Urinary tract manipulation: intermittent catheterization, indwelling Foley catheter, cystoscopy
   d. Intravascular devices: IV catheter, arterial lines, CVP lines
   e. Dialysis: hemodialysis or peritoneal
6. Medications
   a. Antibiotics
   b. Transfusions
7. Laboratory and diagnostic data
   a. CBC: elevated or decreased WBC
   b. Presence of lymphocytes
   c. Culture results
   d. Hypothermia or hyperthermia
   e. Symptomatology: positive chest x-ray film, dysuria, bacteriuria, pyuria, purulent drainage from wound, productive cough, etc.

8. Communicable infection or disease
   a. Type of infectious agent
   b. Route or method of transmission
   c. Potential for cross-contamination
   d. Need for isolation
   e. Need for decontamination/disinfection of equipment
   f. Medical treatment or equipment placing patient at risk for infection

GOALS

1. Minimization of risk of infection to the critically ill patient
2. Recognition of risk factors for hospital-acquired infections as they apply to each patient
3. Support of patient's defense mechanisms against infection
4. Recognition of signs of infection and interpretation of culture results according to the patient's status
5. Prevention of patient-to-patient spread of infection
6. Segregation of patients potentially hazardous to others
7. Absence of or quick resolution to hospital-acquired infections

POTENTIAL PROBLEMS	EXPECTED OUTCOMES	NURSING ACTIVITIES

Catheter-associated urinary tract infection[2,4,28]

■ Urinary tract infection secondary to catheterization	■ Absence or resolution of catheter-associated urinary tract infection	■ Be aware of appropriate indication for catheterization
		  Postoperative catheterization, which may be required if patient is unable to void 8 to 12 hours after surgery
		  Cord-injury patients with varying degrees of bladder dysfunction who require intermittent or indwelling catheter drainage
		  To facilitate surgery on urethra or associated structures
		  To observe output measurements in comatose or shock patients
		  In cases of obstruction
		Insert catheter, as ordered, according to the following guidelines
		  Insert smallest size catheter, using strict aseptic, atraumatic technique
		  Tape catheter securely to avoid urethral irritation
		  Leave urinary catheters in place only for as long as necessary
		  For selected patients, other methods of urinary drainage may be useful alternatives (e.g., condom catheterization, intermittent catheterization, suprapubic catheterization)
		Wash hands immediately before and after any manipulation of catheter site and apparatus; this is critical determinant in limiting spread of infection
		Maintain closed sterile drainage system; do not disengage catheter and drainage tube unless catheter must be irrigated
		Avoid irrigation unless obstruction is anticipated (e.g., as might occur with bleeding after prostatic or bladder surgery)
		  Use large-volume sterile syringe and sterile irrigant for each irrigation procedure
		  If frequent irrigations are required, use sterile three-way continuous irrigation system
		Specimen collection—if volume of fresh urine is needed for examination, cleanse distal end of catheter, or preferably sampling port, with disinfectant; then aspirate urine with sterile needle and syringe
		  Empty urine bag carefully to avoid contamination of emptying spout
		  Measuring graduates should be individualized to each patient and maintained as clean
		Urinary flow—maintain unobstructed flow
		  Position and arrange tubing and bag to ensure free, downhill, continuous flow of urine
		  Keep bag below level of bladder
		  Avoid clamping catheter
		    Overdistension of bladder causes ischemia of vessels of bladder wall and is probably important factor in development of subsequent cystitis
		To minimize chance of cross-infection, avoid placing infected and uninfected patients in same room

POTENTIAL PROBLEMS	EXPECTED OUTCOMES	NURSING ACTIVITIES
Nosocomial wound infection		
■ Wound infection secondary to surgical procedure	■ Absence of surgical wound infection	■ *Preoperative factors* 　Encourage short preoperative stay for all elective surgery to decrease chance of nosocomial colonization 　Optimize patient's nutritional balance, as both malnutrition/obesity increase patient's chance of developing wound infection; monitor dietary intake and nutritional status—administer TPN if necessary 　Correct chronic diseases to extent possible 　　Diabetes—monitor blood, sugar, urine glucose; administer insulin and glucose if needed, as ordered 　　Anemia—monitor blood values and administer replacement blood if needed, as ordered 　　COPD—monitor PaO_2 levels, administer O_2 supplementation, as ordered; include preoperative teaching of deep breathing and coughing 　Administer antibiotics to eradicate remote infection before elective surgery if needed, as ordered 　Administer prophylactic antibiotics in selected patients who are at high risk for developing nosocomial wound infection 　Shave skin just before surgery 　Perform preoperative surgical preparation with antiseptic solution *Intraoperative factors* 　Preoperative scrub by surgical team with antiseptic solution 　Use masks, gowns, gloves, caps, and shoe covers 　Observe aseptic technique 　Remove foreign bodies, necrotic or contaminated tissues during surgery *Postoperative factors* 　Careful hemostasis and gentle handling of wound 　Observe wound closely and accurately document condition, describing 　　Nature of drainage, including amount, color, consistency, odor 　　Condition of suture line (open/closed) and skin around wound (swollen, excoriated) 　　Signs of infection (erythema, warmth, pain) at site 　Change dressings as frequently as needed to avoid saturation and subsequent bacterial proliferation 　Use aseptic technique during dressing changes 　Culture any purulent drainage and document any changes in appearance of wound; notify physician of any changes in appearance of wound
Nosocomial pneumonia[19,20,24]		
■ Nosocomial pneumonia related to 　Compromised ventilatory status 　Respiratory therapy 　Tracheostomy	■ Absence of nosocomial pneumonia 　Maximal respiratory status	■ Assess respiratory status including skin color, rate of respirations, breath sounds, characteristics of cough 　Prevent nosocomial pneumonia by 　　Changing position frequently for immobilized patients to prevent pooling of lung secretions 　　Teaching and encouraging deep breathing and coughing with use of incentive spirometer, unless contraindicated by patient's status 　Administer analgesics for pain that interferes with effective coughing and deep breathing; allow for proper wound support during coughing and deep breathing 　Administer fluids, as ordered, to provide for adequate hydration, which allows patient to mobilize secretions 　Mouth care should be done frequently to decrease chance of nosocomial colonization 　Assist with removal of secretions by administering clapping, vibrating, postural drainage, and suctioning, if necessary; administer airway humidification if needed, as ordered

POTENTIAL PROBLEMS	EXPECTED OUTCOMES	NURSING ACTIVITIES
		Wash hands after contact with respiratory secretions whether or not gloves are worn
		Ensure use of sterile fluids in nebulizers or ventilator reservoirs, which should be dispensed aseptically (i.e. lip or rim of bottle should not touch equipment)
		Unused fluid should be discarded after 24 hours
		Water that has condensed in reservoir tubing should be discarded and not allowed to drain back into reservoir
		Suction patient using "no-touch" technique or gloves on both hands and sterile suction catheter for each series of suctioning
		Use unit dose or small multiple-dose medication vials if possible; if multiple-dose vials must be employed, aseptic technique should be used in drawing up medication and unused portions be discarded within 24 hours
Nosocomial bacteremia[12,23,26]		

■ Sepsis/bacteremia secondary to
  Bacterial seeding from concurrent infection
  Contaminated intravascular catheter, infusate, or intravascular device
	■ Absence or resolution of nosocomial infection of urinary tract, lower respiratory tract, or wound infection, which may cause bacterial seeding of circulatory system
	Absence of contaminated IV catheter, infusates, or devices
	Absence of phlebitis, cellulitis at IV site
		■ Prevent lower respiratory tract, urinary tract, and wound infections (see specific problem)
		Use IV therapy only for definite therapeutic and diagnostic indications and discontinue as soon as possible
		Employ aseptic technique for insertion of any IV catheter
		  Scrub IV site with antiseptic before insertion
		  Secure IV catheter at insertion site and cover with sterile dressing; mark with date of catheter insertion
		  Change peripheral IV sites q48-72 hr
		Inspect IV site daily for color and condition of skin, warmth, erythema, cellulitis, purulent drainage, tenderness, or pain
		  Document observations—discontinue IV if local infection/infiltration is suspected
		Aseptically prepare IV solutions; change routinely q24 hr and discontinue at once if contamination is suspected
		  If IV solution is suspected to be contaminated, record fluid lot number and send sample of fluid for culture
		  Inspect IV bottle for visible turbidity, leaks, cracks, particulate matter, and manufacturer's expiration date before using
		Change IV administration tubing routinely q48 hr
		Employ invasive pressure monitoring only in clinical situations in which information gathered by this technique can clearly influence decisions in patient management
		Wash hands before inserting or manipulating pressure monitoring system
		  Wear sterile gloves for insertion of intravascular catheter for pressure monitoring and use aseptic technique
		  Maintain pressure monitoring systems as closed systems; keep manipulation for blood specimens/samples at minimum
		Do not reuse disposable components of pressure monitoring systems
		Use normal saline or bacteriostatic H_2O for flush solutions and solutions used in transducer domes; glucose-containing solutions are known to support growth of microorganisms
		  Change flush solutions q24 hr
		During calibration of pressure monitoring system, avoid contact between sterile fluid column in cannula and tubing and nonsterile solution or equipment
		Replace chamber dome and administration tubing q48 hr
		After use, clean/disinfect or sterilize transducers according to manufacturer's recommendations; store so as to prevent recontamination before use on another patient
		Change central (e.g., pulmonary artery) catheter line q3-4 days

ISOLATION TECHNIQUES

Patients in critical care units may need isolation at certain times. Accomplishing this in the most economical, efficient, and safe way for both patients and personnel is often a point of controversy. The way a specific illness or disease is transmitted should determine the means of isolation employed, the protective attire used, and whether articles from the room require special handling.

To that end, the Centers for Disease Control have recommended categories of isolation; groups of diseases with similar isolation requirements are placed into corresponding categories.[11] Over 90% of US hospitals have adopted this approach according to a national survey done in 1976.[8]

Rooms needed for isolation can vary from regular multibed rooms to single-bed private rooms. A private room is indicated for infections transmitted by the airborne route or for patients who might expose roommates unnecessarily in a multibed room.

Gowns are indicated if the infectious agent can be transmitted on clothing. The gowns should be worn once and discarded.

Masks are needed if the infectious agent can be transmitted by aerosols or droplets. They should be used only once, changed if they become wet, and discarded after use.

Gloves are worn if the infectious agent can be spread by direct patient contact or indirect contact with articles contaminated by the patient's secretions/excretions. Gloves should be used once and then discarded. This should always be followed by hand washing.

Hand washing is the most important means of preventing the spread of infection. Hands should be washed before and after patient contact, even when gloves are used. The purpose of hand washing is primarily the removal of dirt by sudsing, friction, and rinsing with running water. Antibacterial soaps are recommended for personnel engaging in patient care activities.

Linens that are contaminated by the patient's secretions/excretions should be handled aseptically. Double-bagging of linens from patients in isolation is recommended. The linens should be labeled as contaminated so laundry personnel may take the necessary precautions to protect themselves.

Patient care articles and reusable supplies should be sterilized, disinfected, or discarded after use. If articles are to be sterilized, they should be placed in a plastic bag and marked contaminated, so that central sterile supply personnel may take proper precautions in handling them.

Table 61-5 is a brief outline of the different types of isolation and the nursing activities associated with them. Each nurse needs to become familiar with the types of isolation used in his/her hospital as outlined by the Infection Control Committee. The Centers for Disease Control have issued a comprehensive guide for isolation practices as of August, 1983 for review by hospital personnel.

■ ■ ■

Because health care personnel appreciate the importance of infection control in patient care today, patient care can hopefully be maximized. As illustrated throughout this standard, nosocomial infections are highly preventable with increased attention to detail and scrupulous adherence to established infection control procedures.

TABLE 61-5. Isolation techniques

Strict/unusual isolation

Highly communicable diseases or diseases transmitted by more than one route

Includes anthrax, diptheria, rabies, Lassa fever

Traditional or full isolation needed

Private room—door closed

Gowns, gloves, masks for all entering room

Hand washing before entering and leaving room and as indicated during patient care

Patient care articles and equipment in room should be kept to a minimum and be preferably disposable; disposables should be double-bagged before discarding; reusable equipment should be sent to central sterile supply in autoclavable bag.

Linens should be double-bagged and marked as contaminated

Disposable dishes/trays

Lab specimens should be placed in appropriate container with lid securely fastened, then double-bagged

Chart should not be brought into patient's room

If patient is transported, receiving service and escort should be notified; wheelchair/stretcher should be draped with clean sheet; patient should be masked and gowned

Cleaning personnel should be notified of proper precautions

Respiratory isolation

Infections passed by airborne route

Includes common childhood diseases (i.e., chickenpox, rubella, measles, mumps), Staphylococcal pneumonia, meningococcal meningitis (until after 24 hours of IV antibiotics)

Precautionary measures include

Private room—door closed

Masks for all who enter patient's room

Gowns not required, unless uniform is likely to become contaminated with respiratory secretions

Gloves not necessary

Articles contaminated by respiratory secretions should be double-bagged before being discarded or disinfected before reuse

Hand washing before entering and leaving room and as indicated during patient care activities

If patient is transported, receiving area/escort should be notified; wheelchair/stretcher should be draped with clean sheet; patient should be masked

Patient should be instructed to cough/sneeze into tissues and dispose of them properly

Terminal disinfection includes airing out of the room—time varies according to number of air exchanges per hour in room or presence of exhaust fan

Special respiratory isolation

Used for pulmonary tuberculosis—a disease passed by airborne route and of lesser infectivity than diseases requiring respiratory isolation

Precautionary measures include

Private room with good ventilation (i.e., door open, exhaust fan, window open); object is to increase air currents

Masks are not required unless patient cannot be taught to cough/sneeze into tissues or if patient is intubated

Gowns not required

Gloves not required

Soiled tissues should be double-bagged before being discarded

Blood precautions

Indicated for diseases transmissible by contact with blood or items contaminated by blood

Includes malaria, hepatitis B, hepatitis non-A, non-B, AIDS

Precautionary measures include

Private room not necessary

Masks not required

Gowns not required

Careful hand washing before entering and leaving room and as indicated during patient care activities

Gloves for handling blood specimens/articles contaminated by blood

Articles contaminated by blood should be discarded or sent to central sterile supply for sterilization

Blood specimens sent to lab should be marked to alert lab personnel of need for proper handling

Needles should be handled carefully—not replaced into sheath after use (often a cause of inadvertant needle sticks) but clipped and placed in puncture-resistant container

Modified from Infection control at the New York Hospital–Cornell Medical Center, ed. 5, New York, 1982, The Committee on Infections of the New York Hospital; and Isolation techniques for use in hospitals, Atlanta, 1970, U.S. Department of Health, Education, and Welfare, Public Health Service, Centers for Disease Control.

TABLE 61-5. Isolation techniques—cont'd

Enteric precautions

Intended for diseases passed by direct contact with infected feces or articles heavily contaminated with excretions; transmission depends on oral ingestion of offending microorganism

Includes *Salmonella, Shigella,* Hepatitis A, campylobacter, cholera

Precautionary measures include

    Private room for children; adults do not require private room unless incontinent or diarrhea is of such severity that patient hygiene is affected

    Scrupulous hand washing before entering and leaving room and as indicated during patient care activities

    Gloves should be worn for handling feces or potentially contaminated items

    Gowns for all personnel having direct patient contact

    Urine and feces should be flushed directly into toilet or discarded in dirty utility room; bed pans should be disinfected after use

    Masks not required

    Patient care articles contaminated by excreta should be discarded or sent to central sterile supply for disinfection/sterilization

    Linens should be double-bagged and marked as contaminated; they should be changed as soon as possible if they become soiled

    Disposable dishes/trays should be used

Precautions for multidrug-resistant organsisms

Intended for patients who are infected with resistant organisms—to prevent chance of cross-contamination among patients

Precautionary measures include

    Private room desirable but not required—depending on site of infection (i.e., patient with urinary tract infection with resistant organism should not be roomed with patients with indwelling Foley catheters)

    Scrupulous hand washing before entering and leaving patient's room and as indicated during patient care activities

    Gloves for handling patient's secretions/excretions or potentially contaminated articles

    Gowns for direct patient contact

    No patient care articles for common usage—patient should have individualized items (i.e., urine measuring graduate, water pitcher, etc.)

Wound and skin precautions

These precautions are used for diseases that are transmitted through direct contact with wounds or indirect contact with articles heavily contaminated with wound secretions or drainage

Includes staphylococcal and streptococcal wound or skin infections or any wound infection with extensive drainage not confined to a dressing

Precautionary measures include:

    Private room desirable, but not required; preferable that patient not be roomed with patients who have recently had surgery

    Gowns for all personnel having direct contact with infected wounds or skin area

    Careful hand washing before entering and leaving room and as indicated during patient care activities

    Gloves when having direct contact with infected area or handling articles contaminated by wound drainage.

    Soiled dressings should be double-bagged; articles used for dressing care should not be shared with other patients but left at bedside, discarded on discharge or sent to central sterile supply if reuseable

    Linens should be double-bagged and marked as contaminated

REFERENCES

1. Bennett, J.V., and Brachman, P.S., eds.: Hospital infections, Boston, 1979, Little, Brown and Co.
2. Bielski, M.: Preventing infection in the catheterized patient, Nurs. Clin. North Am. **15:**703-713, 1980.
3. Castle, M.: Hospital infection control: principles and practice, New York, 1980, John Wiley & Sons, Inc.
4. Cunka, B.A.: Nosocomial urinary tract infections, Heart & Lung **11:**545-551, 1982.
5. Dixon, R.E.: Effects of infections on hospital care, Ann. Intern. Med., **89:**749-753, 1978.
6. Flynn, M.E., and Rovee, D.T.: Wound healing mechanism, Am. J. Nurs. **82:**1544-1558, 1982.
7. Fuchs, P.C.: Epidemiology of hospital associated infections, Chicago, 1979, Educational Products Division, American Society of Clinical Pathologists.
8. Garner, J.S.: Isolation techniques in critical care units, Crit. Care Q. **3:**29-41, March 1980.
9. Hargiss, C.O., and Larson, E.: Infection control: putting principles into practice, Am. J. Nurs. **83:**2165-2186, 1981.
10. Infection control at the New York Hospital–Cornell Medical Center, ed. 5., New York, 1982, The Committee on Infections of the New York Hospital.
11. Isolation techniques for use in hospitals, Atlanta, 1970, U.S. Department of Health, Education and Welfare, Public Health Service, Centers for Disease Control.
12. Kaye, W.: Catheter and infusion related sepsis: the nature of the problem and its prevention, Heart Lung **11:**221-227, 1982.
13. LaForce, F.M.: Hospital acquired gram-negative rod pneumonias: an overview. In Dixon, R.E., ed.: Nosocomial infections, 1981, Yorke Medical Books.
14. Laufman, H.: Surgical intensive care and nosocomial infection, Infect. Surg. 23-30, Oct. 1982.
15. Maki, D.G.: Nosocomial bacteremias: an epidemiological overview, Am. J. Med. **70:**719-732, 1981.
16. Maki, D.G.: Control of colonization and transmission of pathogenic bacteria in the hospital, Ann. Intern. Med., **89** (part 2 suppl.):777-780, 1978.
17. Maki, D.G., and Hassemer, C.A.: Endemic rate of fluid contamination and related septicemia in arterial pressure monitoring, Am. J. Med. **70:**733-738, 1981.
18. Mikat, D.M., and Mikat, K.W.: A clinician's dictionary guide to bacteria and fungi, ed. 4, Indianapolis, 1981, Eli Lilly & Co.
19. Oakes, C.A.: Lower respiratory infections, Crit. Care Q. **3:**57-62, March, 1980.
20. Podjasek, J.H.: Respiratory infection in the mechanically ventilated patient: an overview, Heart Lung **12:**5-9, 1983.
21. Polk, H.C., and Finn, M.: Prevention of surgical wound infections QRB, 18-22, March, 1979.
22. Presswood, G.M.: Collection, transport, and interpretation of microbiologic specimens, Crit. Care Q. **3:**11-26, March 1983.
23. Simmons, B.P.: Guidelines for the prevention of intravascular infections, Atlanta, 1981, Department of Health and Human Services, U.S. Department of Public Health Services, Centers for Disease Control.
24. Simmons, B.P.: Guidelines for prevention of nosocomial pneumonia, Atlanta, 1981, Department of Health and Human Services, U.S. Department of Public Health Service, Centers for Disease Control.
25. Simmons, B.P.: Guidelines for the prevention of surgical wound infections, Atlanta, 1981, Health and Human Services, U.S. Department of Public Health Service, Centers for Disease Control.
26. Stamm, W.E.: Infections related to medical devices, Ann. Intern. Med. **89** (part 2 suppl.):764-769, 1978.
27. Weinstein, R.A., and Kabins, S.A.: Strategies for the prevention and control of multi-drug resistant nosocomial infections, Am. J. Med., **70:**449-454, 1981.
28. Wong, E.S.: Guidelines for the prevention of catheter associated urinary tract infections, Am. J. Inf. Control **11:**28-33, 1982.

ACQUIRED IMMUNE DEFICIENCY SYNDROME

Acquired immune deficiency syndrome (AIDS) is a severe sustained immune defect of unknown cause that predisposes the individual to multiple disease states. The more commonly encountered diseases that are secondary to the immune defect are a disseminated form of Kaposi sarcoma, pneumocystis carinii pneumonia, and life-threatening opportunistic infections. Autoimmune phenomena and other types of malignancies are also associated with AIDS.

AIDS is predominantly identified in homosexual men; however, it has also been identified among Haitians of recent immigration, IV drug abusers, and individuals suspected to have contracted the illness through contaminated blood products (e.g., hemophiliacs, patients receiving large volumes of blood).

The immune deficiency effects a subset of lymphocytes, T-lymphocytes, which function in cell-mediated immunity and immune surveillance. Immune surveillance describes the ability to recognize and destroy potentially malignant cells; a deficiency of T-lymphocytes predisposes the individual to neoplasms. Defects in cell-mediated immunity, that part of the immune system that is active against slowly developing bacterial infections, intracellular organisms, and many viral and fungal infections, will predispose to opportunistic infections. Hyperfunction of the humoral immune system is also suspected of leading to autoimmune phenomena in some individuals.

The cause of the immune defect is unknown; however, a viral agent, from a group of viruses known at retroviruses, is suspected of being a causative factor. Transmission of this agent appears to follow a pattern similar to that of hepatitis B, (i.e., having enteric, parenteral, and sexual routes of transmission). Thus precautions against contact with blood and body fluids are employed when a patient is hospitalized with a diagnosis of AIDS.

The patient with AIDS typically gives a history that may include weight loss, fevers, night sweats, lymphadenopathy, diarrhea, and a nonproductive cough that may have persisted for 6 to 18 months. Individuals with Kaposi sarcoma may also have multiple purplish nodules on the skin and mucous membranes and involvement of the GI and respiratory tracts.

The critical care nurse more often encounters patients with AIDS when they develop life-threatening opportunistic infections. The most prevalent of the opportunistic infections is pneumocystis carinii pneumonia, an interstitial pneumonia of insidious onset accompanied by dyspnea, tachypnea, cyanosis, nonproductive cough, and initial respiratory alkalosis. Initially, symptoms of respiratory compromise are often far more severe than diagnostic studies such as chest radiographs and arterial blood gas values would appear to indicate. Pneumocystis carinii pneumonia may be treated with IV trimethoprim and sulfamethoxazole (Bactrim, Septra) or with Pentamidine, an experimental agent obtained from the Centers for Disease Control. Despite treatment, profoundly compromised alveolar ventilation is often progressive, requiring mechanical ventilation.

Additional serious opportunistic infections associated with AIDS commonly manifest as pneumonia, meningitis, or encephalitis secondary to aspergillosis, candidiasis, cryptococcosis, cytomegalovirus, toxoplasmosis, atypical mycobacterium, nocardiosis, and strongyloidosis. Esophagitis may be caused by candidiasis, cytomegalovirus or herpes simplex. Enterocolitis secondary to cryptosporidiosis and extensive mucocutaneous herpes is also included among the opportunistic infections of AIDS. While patients with AIDS may develop single infections, they more often exhibit multiple concomitant infections.

Management of the opportunistic infections is aimed at support of the involved system(s). When available, pharmacologic agents specific for the identified organism are employed. Experimental agents are often employed in the treatment of uncommon organisms. Most of the aforementioned organisms are ubiquitous to the environment and do not cause disease in healthy individuals. However, in the acute care setting, additional isolation precautions may need to be employed to prevent health care workers from serving as vectors to other immunocompromised patients.

The prognosis for a patient with AIDS is related to the degree of immunocompromise and the nature of the secondary disease that develops. Kaposi sarcoma without accompanying opportunistic infection may be treated with chemotherapy and has the most favorable prognosis. Individuals who develop multiple opportunistic infections tend to be more profoundly immunosuppressed and have a poor prognosis for survival beyond 1 year. Despite successful treatment of initial infections, patients commonly succumb to recurrent or additional infections.

Trials with immune response modifiers such as interferon are being conducted in an attempt to restore immune function; however, no consistently successful curative treatment has yet been found.

ASSESSMENT

1. History to include
   a. Nature, onset, and duration of prodromal symptoms, including
      (1) Weight loss
      (2) Anorexia
      (3) Diarrhea
      (4) Fevers
      (5) Night sweats
      (6) Nonproductive cough
      (7) Dyspnea
      (8) Lymph node enlargement
   b. Past history of
      (1) Hepatitis
      (2) Sexually transmitted diseases
      (3) Amebiasis
      (4) Viral illnesses
      (5) Other infectious diseases
      (6) Exposure to needles
   c. Social history to include
      (1) Recreational drug use
      (2) Ethnic background
      (3) Sexual preference
2. Physical assessment to include baseline parameters of all systems, with special attention to
   a. Respiratory
   b. Neurological
   c. Skin and mucous membranes—description, location, and drainage of lesions
   d. Lymph node enlargement
3. Results of lab and diagnostic tests

   a. CBC, WBC, lymphocyte count (lymphopenia seen in most patients)
   b. Anergy panel (cutaneous anergy is a common indicator of depressed cell-mediated immunity)
   c. Serum electrolytes
   d. Antibody titers (indicating exposure to infectious agent)
   e. Culture reports for identification of opportunistic infection
   f. Radiography, bronchoscopy reports for presence of interstitial infiltrates and confirmation of pneumocystis carinii pneumonia
   g. Endoscopic procedures for presence of Kaposi sarcoma in GI tract
   h. CSF analysis
   i. Lymphocyte function studies (if available)
      (1) Inversion of T-helper/suppressor ratio (normal 0.9 to 3.5); patients with AIDS may have values as low as 0.1
      (2) Lymphokine assays to demonstrate activity of cellular immune system
      (3) Lymphoproliferative response studies

GOALS

1. Absence, control, or resolution of opportunistic infections, nosocomial infections, or sepsis
2. Optimal respiratory function
   a. Adequate alveolar ventilation—arterial blood gas levels within normal limits
   b. Absence of respiratory distress
3. Intact neurological function and absence of symptoms
4. Absence of fever
5. Fluid and electrolyte levels within normal limits
6. Adequate nutritional state with weight gain or maintenance within normal limits
7. Patient/significant others are able to develop support systems and coping strategies to deal with illness
8. Before discharge patient is able to
   a. Define environmental and life-style risk factors affecting prognosis
   b. Describe measures to control transmission of AIDS

POTENTIAL PROBLEMS	EXPECTED OUTCOMES	NURSING ACTIVITIES
■ Severe opportunistic infections related to profound immune compromise manifested by Pneumonia Encephalitis Meningitis Enterocolitis Esophagitis Extensive mucocutaneous herpes	■ Resolution of current infection Support of involved system and associated signs and symptoms Absence of other opportunistic infection	■ Prevent by Protecting patient from cross-contact with other patients with opportunistic infections Adherence to standard infection control practices (see Standard 61, Infection control in the critical care unit Instructing patient/family regarding life-style practices and environments that may predispose to opportunistic infections Administering prophylactic agents (e.g., Bactrim), as ordered Monitor for Presence of fever, noting febrile pattern WBC including differential ESR Infectious agents identified on culture reports Signs and symptoms of infection in most commonly involved systems Dyspnea, tachypnea, cyanosis, nonproductive cough Change in mentation, behavior; headache, nuchal rigidity, photophobia Profuse diarrhea, abdominal cramping Development of lesions on skin and mucous membranes If problem occurs Institute specific supportive measures based on involved system and infectious agent See Standard 42, *Meningitis/encephalitis*; Standard 2, *Acute respiratory failure* Prepare patient for administration of pharmacotherapy, ensuring patient is knowledgeable regarding side effects of experimental agents Instruct patient/family concerning need for additional isolation precautions Administer antibiotic, antiviral, or antifungal agents specific for opportunistic infection, as ordered Monitor patient's response to support measures and pharmacotherapy
■ Inadequate nutritional state related to Increased metabolic demands associated with fevers Nausea and vomiting associated with chemotherapy GI involvement of Kaposi sarcoma Profound diarrhea from opportunistic infection	■ Weight gain or weight maintained within normal limits Positive nitrogen balance	■ Assess baseline nutritional status, including Current weight and degree of recent weight loss Skin turgor Muscle mass; note muscle wasting Monitor for Nausea and vomiting and relationship to medication therapy Anorexia Dysphagia Daily weight Frequency, volume, and consistency of stools Calorie consumption Consult with nutritionist to plan diet with adequate protein and calories for metabolic requirements Administer antiemetics before meals, chemotherapy, or other pharmacotherapy, as appropriate Administer antidiarrheals and specific agents for opportunistic infection causing diarrhea Decrease metabolic caloric demand Administer antipyretics or hypothermia, as ordered Plan care to conserve patient's energy If significant malnutrition exists Administer hyperalimentation and intralipids (see Standard 57, *Total parenteral nutrition*)

POTENTIAL PROBLEMS	EXPECTED OUTCOMES	NURSING ACTIVITIES
■ Inadequate support systems Social isolation related to Imposed isolation precautions Attitudes encountered concerning life-style Patient's desire not to share information concerning life-style with family or business associates Friend's/health care workers' fear of exposure	■ Patient describes available support system and satisfaction with adequacy of same Patient/family verbalizes understanding of isolation precautions	■ Assess adequacy of support systems Presence of significant others Attitudes of significant others toward illness Coping abilities and mechanisms of patient, significant others Assist patient/significant others to identify and obtain additional emotional support Organized community groups* Social service referrals Family support Spiritual support Instruct patient, significant others, and health care personnel regarding extent and rationale for isolation precautions Blood and body fluid precautions to prevent transmission of suspected "AIDS agent" Respiratory isolation to prevent health care personnel from acting as vectors for pneumocystis carinii pneumonia to other immunocompromised patients Strict isolation for extensive mucocutaneous herpes Reassure patient, visitors, and health care personnel that majority of opportunistic agents do not cause disease in those who are not immune deficient Provide social contact and communicate positive, accepting attitude to patient through frequent visits and employing nonverbal techniques such as touch Recognize own attitudes toward patient's life-style and how this may be verbally or nonverbally communicated Provide environmental stimulation with radio, clock, reading materials, if appropriate
■ Acute respiratory insufficiency Hypoxia Respiratory alkalosis/acidosis Inadequate alveolar ventilation Related to Interstitial pneumonia associated with opportunistic infection Respiratory involvement of malignancy	■ Absence of signs and symptoms of respiratory distress Dyspnea, tachypnea Increased respiratory effort Arterial blood gas levels within normal limits	■ Prevent by Protecting patient from other individuals with opportunistic infections Administering prophylactic Bactrim and Septra Monitor for Rate and depth of respirations and breath sounds Signs and symptoms of compromised respiratory function, seen initially in these patients as Tachypnea, nonproductive cough, dyspnea Increased respiratory effort, cyanosis, and increased anxiety Change in mentation Increase in temperature Abnormalities in arterial blood gas levels Initial compensatory respiratory alkalosis End stage respiratory acidosis Increased alveolar-arterial oxygen difference (A-a gradient); measures gas transfer from alveolar spaces into blood; infections in lung occlude air spaces in these patients and do not always show up initially but can be detected by A-a gradient Normal A-a gradient in 30- to 40-year-old individual is 11 to 16 mm Hg Formula for determination of A-a gradient on room air where A = alveolar and a = arterial $$P_{AO_2} = P_{IO_2} - \frac{Pa_{CO_2}}{0.8} \ (P_{IO_2} = 713 \times F_{IO_2})$$ $$P_{AO_2} - Pa_{O_2} = \text{A-a gradient}$$ Monitor trend of A-a gradient; note increase indicating worsening lung condition

*Information about these groups may be obtained by contacting the National Gay Task Force, (800)221-7044.

POTENTIAL PROBLEMS	EXPECTED OUTCOMES	NURSING ACTIVITIES
		Monitor radiograph for evidence of increased infiltrates (although this is not diagnostic of severity of respiratory insufficiency); if problem develops, see Standard 2, *Acute respiratory failure;* Standard 6, *Mechanical ventilation*

■ Sepsis
  Hypotension
  Inadequate tissue perfusion
  Metabolic acidosis
Related to
  Multiple opportunistic/nosocomial infections secondary to immune deficiency
	■ Absence of hypothermia/hyperthermia
	BP within normal limits for patient
	Arterial blood gas levels, serum CO_2 within normal limits
	Adequate tissue perfusion
		■ Prevent by administering prophylactic antibiotics, if indicated
		Monitor for
		  Hypotension
		  Temperature for hypothermia/hyperthermia and change in pattern of fever
		  Tachycardia
		  WBC with differential for granulocytopenia and increase in bands
		  ESR
		  C and S reports
		  Mentation changes
		  Urine output q1 hr
		  Circulation to periphery
		  Arterial blood gas levels for metabolic acidosis
		  Serum CO_2 and K^+
		  Radiograph
		If problems occur
		  Septic shock
		    Maintain cardiac output and tissue perfusion with prescribed
		      Pharmacological agents
		      Volume replacement
		  Institute hypothermia/hyperthermia, as ordered, to maintain temperature within normal limits
		  Administer prescribed antibiotics based on C and S reports
		  Administer sodium bicarbonate to correct metabolic acidosis, as ordered
		
		See STANDARD 65 *Disseminated intravascular coagulation*
		STANDARD 17 *Shock*

■ Fluid and electrolyte imbalances related to
Profound diarrhea from opportunistic infections
Increased metabolic requirements of fever and sepsis
	■ Electrolyte levels within normal limits
	Moist mucous membranes
	Urinary output in excess of 30 ml/hour
		■ Prevent by
		  Maintaining fluid intake at minimum of 2000/ml/day unless contraindicated, as ordered
		  Consulting with nutritionist to provide diet that will promote normal bowel function
		  Maintaining body temperature within normal limits
		Monitor
		  Vital signs and T q4 hr
		  Accurate intake and output
		  CVP
		  Signs and symptoms of dehydration
		    Decreased skin turgor
		    Dry mucous membranes
		  Serum electrolytes
		  BUN and creatinine
		  Urine for electrolytes
		  Fluid loss associated with diarrhea
		  Weight loss
		  Arrhythmias
		  Signs and symptoms of electrolyte imbalance
		    Lassitude, irritability, weakness, nausea, vomiting, neuromuscular abnormalities, twitching
		If problem occurs administer the following, as ordered
		  Electrolyte replacement

POTENTIAL PROBLEMS	EXPECTED OUTCOMES	NURSING ACTIVITIES

		Nutritional support
		  Total parenteral nutrition
		  Intralipids
		  Tube feeding
		Antipyretic medication to maintain metabolic requirements
		Antidiarrheal medications
		Specific agents against opportunistic infections

■ Alterations in mentation, neurological status, related to
  CNS involvement of opportunistic infection
  Pharmacological side effects
  Psychological effects of illness
	■ Baseline neurological status intact or improved	■ Monitor for signs and symptoms associated with meningitis and encephalitis, including
		  Headache
		  Nuchal rigidity
		  Photophobia
		  Change in mentation
		  LOC
		  Vomiting
		  Fevers
		Observe for changes in patient behavior and note possible precipitating or related factors, including environmental stressors or recent psychologically stressful events
		Monitor for anticipated CNS side effects of medication therapy, particularly experimental agents
		Explain to patient/family about CNS/behavioral changes associated with drug therapy, expected duration of change, and any anticipated alteration in medications
		Maintain safe environment and protect patient from injury
		Minimize environmental stimuli when appropriate
		Provide emotional support and assist patient/family to maximize coping mechanisms appropriate to stressful event
		Administer psychotherapeutic drugs, as ordered
		If problem occurs, see Standard 42, *Meningitis/encephalitis*

■ Patient/family's fear and anxiety related to
  Unknown outcomes of illness
  Possible terminal event
	■ Patient/significant others able to express fears and describe measures that will assist them	■ Assess patient/family's expectations regarding outcomes of illness
		Consult with physician to provide accurate and consistent information regarding prognosis
		Observe for behavior patterns that indicate fear or anxiety
		  Fear of being alone
		  Insomnia
		  Agitation
		Encourage verbalization of patient/family's feelings about prognosis; accept expressions of anger, denial, etc.
		Recognize and support level at which patient/family are in grieving process
		Assist patient to obtain support concerning feelings of guilt about life-style or perceiving this disease as ''punishment'' for sexual preference

■ Insufficient knowledge to comply with discharge regimen	■ Patient/family verbalize
	  Discharge plan and intent to comply
	  Life-style and environmental risk factors for development of opportunistic infections
	  Life-style alterations to limit transmission of AIDS
		■ Discharge teaching to include recommendations to
		  Avoid unnecessary exposure, particularly intimate contact with individuals with known infections or viral illnesses
		  Avoid exposure to old, dusty environments and environments containing bird droppings
		  Limit number of sexual partners and avoid sexual practices involving direct oral or rectal contact; employ condom for ejaculation
		  Avoid travel to areas in which infections are endemic
		  Maintain caloric requirements and balanced diet
		  Refrain from blood donation

MULTIPLE TRAUMA

Multiple trauma refers to injury of two or more systems of the body. When an accident involves significant force, the body may sustain multiple injuries. Assessment is based on the principle of *triage*. Assessment for detection of life-threatening injuries should be employed first, followed by administration of appropriate life-sustaining therapy.

A triage system for evaluation of the trauma patient has been developed* with life-threatening injuries given first priority in the following order:

1. Life-threatening injuries
   a. Cardiovascular
      (1) Cardiac arrest
      (2) Cardiopericardial injuries
      (3) Hypovolemia (e.g., hemorrhage or severe burn)
   b. Respiratory
      (1) Obstructed airway
      (2) Injured chest wall—flail chest
      (3) Decreased thoracic air space
         (a) Pneumothorax
         (b) Hemothorax
         (c) Diaphragmatic rupture
   c. CNS
      (1) Coma—closed head injury
      (2) Spinal cord injury
2. Urgent injuries
   a. Visceral
      (1) Spleen and liver—intraperitoneal bleeding
      (2) Bowel and pancreas
         (a) Bowel and pancreas— intraperitoneal bleeding
         (b) Bowel—bacterial contamination
         (c) Pancreas—liberation of pancreatic enzymes
      (3) Kidney and bladder
         (a) Kidney trauma
         (b) Ruptured bladder, urethra
   b. Cardiovascular
      (1) Traumatic aortic injury—impending rupture
      (2) Continued bleeding from intraabdominal and vascular injuries
      (3) Laceration of arterial or venous supply to an extremity—viabili of extremity threatened
3. Delayed injuries
   a. Fractures of extremities
   b. Soft tissue injury
   c. Spine and pelvic trauma, fractures
   d. Maxillofacial injury

Immediate management of the trauma patient includes provision of a patent airway with adequate oxygenation, blood volume replacement as needed, control of hemorrhage, and emergency relief measures (e.g., pericardiocentesis, chest tube, intubation) for life-threatening injuries.

These intitial resuscitation activities continue while efforts for repair of specific injuries are begun, with priority attention given to the most life-threatening cardiac and respiratory injuries.

Trauma patients that are most likely to be cared for in the critical care unit include those with the following:
1. Multisystem injury
2. Blunt thoracic trauma with cardiac and/or pulmonary injury
3. Pulmonary aspiration of gastric contents
4. Posttraumatic pulmonary insufficiency
5. Multiple transfusions
6. Prolonged hypotension
7. Sepsis and/or grossly contaminated wounds
8. Preexisting cardiovascular, respiratory, or renal disease
9. Sustained head injury

Hemodynamic monitoring in the critical care unit usually includes measurement of arterial pressure, CVP, PAP, cardiac output, and other hemodynamic parameters. Pulmonary artery catheters are particularly useful in assessing the response of an impaired left ventricle to fluids and blood products. PAP and PCWP can also assist in differentiating pulmonary and cardiac abnormalities.

*Civetta, J.M.: Assessment of the patient following multisystemic trauma, Summary proceedings, Seventeenth Annual Symposium on Critical Care Medicine, Las Vegas, Nev., 1979, University of Southern California School of Medicine, Postgraduate Division, and Institute of Critical Care Medicine.

ASSESSMENT

1. History and nature of trauma sustained, including time, events, and weapons, if any
   a. Known foreign objects that remain in wound
   b. Wound, contusions, or abrasions to any body parts
   c. Apparent bleeding sites
   d. Suspected presence of abdominal crisis
   e. Neurological abnormalities; progression/regression of LOC from preadmission status
2. Stabilization treatment in progress
   a. Means to establish and maintain a patent airway, oxygenation
   b. Means for control of hemorrhage (e.g., pressure dressings, volume replacement)
   c. Treatment for hypotension, shock
   d. Treatment for fractures, (e.g., splints, backboards)
   e. Prophylactic antibiotic therapy to clear bacteria from circulation
   f. Means to maintain adequate urinary output (e.g., fluids, cardiotonic medications)
3. Hemodynamic stability; adequacy of cardiac output and tissue perfusion
   a. Signs and symtpoms indicating specific cardiac abnormalities
      (1) Pericardial friction rub
      (2) Evidence of progressing tamponade
      (3) Radiographic evidence of enlarged heart; widened mediastinum indicative of aortic injury
      (4) ECG evidence of myocardial injury
      (5) Sinus tachycardia with small, diminishing pulse pressure
      (6) Recurrent arrhythmias
      (7) New conduction defects
      (8) Distention of neck veins
   b. Results of lab studies, including
      (1) Chest radiograph
      (2) ECG
      (3) Ultrasound study
      (4) IV contrast study
      (5) Pericardiocentesis
      (6) Cardiac enzymes
      (7) Radioisotope scanning
      (8) Cardiac catheterization
      (9) Aortography
4. Adequacy of respiratory function
   a. Patent airway
   b. Respiratory rate and quality
   c. Respiratory distress—note presence of dyspnea, gasping, stridorous breathing, wheezing, retractions, cyanosis
   d. Subcutaneous emphysema
   e. Chest movements—note presence of asymmetrical movements

   f. Diaphragmatic movements
   g. Chest wall integrity for intactness
   h. Position of trachea for midline
   i. Breath sounds—note decreased, distant, and/or dull breath sounds; adventitious sounds (e.g. rales, rhonchi)
   j. Hyperresonant chest on percussion
   k. Signs/symptoms of pulmonary edema
   l. Signs/symptoms of hypoxia including agitation, tachypnea, dyspnea, and labored respirations
   m. Signs and symptoms revealed by radiographic studies consistent with
      (1) Pneumothorax
      (2) Hemothorax
      (3) Intrapulmonary hematoma
      (4) Pulmonary contusion
      (5) Foreign object (e.g., bullet) within pulmonary parenchyma
      (6) Mediastinal widening
      (7) Pneumomediastinum
      (8) Apical or another area of increased density (may suggest injury of a major vessel or contusion of the lung)
      (9) Laceration of the lung
5. Adequacy of CNS function
   a. Peripheral motor activity—note presence of purposeful movements or spontaneous responses
   b. LOC—note presence of confused, disoriented, lethargic, stuporous, or even unresponsive behavior and dulled mentation; if stuporous or unresponsive, assess reaction to verbal, noxious stimuli
   c. Vision
      (1) Pupils—assess size and response to light; note inequality
      (2) Visual disturbances—note concurrent vertigo, dizziness, headache
   d. Signs and symptoms of increased ICP
   e. Presence and nature of drainage from ears, nose, mouth, and head; test for presence of glucose
   f. Presence of seizure activity
      (1) Note body source and progression
      (2) Duration
      (3) Type of tremor/seizure
   g. Results of lumbar tap
      (1) Increased ICP
      (2) Bloody or cloudy CSF
   h. Signs and symptoms of fractures
      (1) Skull radiograph results indicating a large separation of fractured bone fragments
      (2) Depression of any area on the scalp
      (3) Leakage of CSF from nose or ear
      (4) Severe ecchymosis of eyelids or over mastoid process

i. Result of CT scan
6. Signs and symptoms of injury or rupture of an intraabdominal organ
    a. Localized or generalized peritonitis
       (1) Increasing abdominal discomfort/pain distention
       (2) Tenderness, rebound tenderness
       (3) Muscle rigidity, spasm
       (4) Decreased bowel sounds
       (5) Tachycardia, fever
       (6) Shoulder pain (may be from diaphragmatic irritation)
    b. Injury of solid viscera (liver, spleen, pancreas) including hemorrhage, enlargement of organ, abdominal distention, reflex ileus, rectal bleeding
    c. Results of lab and diagnostic tests
       (1) Radiographs—note presence of pneumoperitoneum: retroperitoneal air, elevation of diaphragm with air under diaphragm
       (2) Abdominal tap
       (3) Intraluminal studies and selective celiac and superior mesenteric angiography
       (4) CBC; note presence of leukocytosis
       (5) Elevated serum and urine amylase levels
7. Signs and symptoms of genitourinary system injury
    a. Tenderness in the suprapubic area, perineum, scrotum, and pubic rami on pelvic compression
    b. Expanding masses or masses in the flank and suprapubic area, perineum, and scrotom
    c. Laceration, contusions, avulsion, or amputation of the penis
    d. Hemorrhage
    e. Hematuria
    f. Pelvic examination revealing pelvic hematoma, lesions of the urethra, and blood at urethral meatus
    g. Results of abdominal radiographs indicating lower rib fracture, presence of foreign body near the genitourinary system
8. Musculoskeletal system for injuries, function
    a. Sensation, motor function of extremities
    b. Pain—location, nature
    c. Bruises, lacerations
    d. Swelling, deformity
    e. Pulses, pallor
9. Results of lab and diagnostic tests, including
    a. CBC
    b. Coagulation studies: PT, APTT
    c. ECG
    d. Pertinent radiographs—chest, abdomen, or fracture site(s)
    e. Serum electrolyte levels
    f. Liver function tests
    g. Cardiac enzymes

h. Indices of renal function
i. Urinalysis
j. Arterial blood gas levels
k. Specific scans, echograms, angiograms, endoscopies (depending on the injury sustained)
10. Assess nutritional status
11. Assess level of patient/family's anxiety regarding the traumatic injury sustained, immobility and disabilities, diagnostic procedures, and therapeutic regimen

GOALS

1. Respiratory
    a. Respiratory function sufficient for adequate oxygenation and ventilation
    b. Patent airway
    c. Full lung expansion
2. Cardiovascular
    a. Hemodynamic stability
    b. Adequate cardiac output
3. Neurological
    a. Patient alert and oriented to time, place, and persons
    b. Sensations and spontaneous movements of extremities and torso within normal limits
    c. Absence or resolution of head injury; stabilization of spinal cord injury
4. GI/Genitourinary
    a. Function of abdominal organs within normal limits
    b. Absence and/or resolution of signs of abdominal trauma, catastrophe, including injury to
       (1) Liver
       (2) Spleen
       (3) Pancreas
       (4) Kidney, bladder, urethra
       (5) Bowel, peritoneum
5. With fractures
    a. Stabilization of fractures present
    b. No apparent bleeding from fracture site
6. With infection
    a. Infection free
    b. Absence of atelectasis
    c. Absence of infection associated with open traumatic injuries
7. Resolution and/or prevention of complications, including renal insufficiency, stress ulcer, embolic phenomena, coagulopathy
8. Absence and/or minimal deformity or contractures
9. Restoration to optimal physical and psychological functioning
10. Absence of malnutrition
11. Reduction in patient/family's anxiety with provision of information, explanations, and comfort
12. Before discharge, patient/family is able to
    a. Verbalize knowledge of

(1) Activity progression and precautions

(2) Dietary management and modifications

(3) Medications—identification, dosage, schedules for administration, possible adverse effects, and precautionary measures

(4) Untoward signs and symptoms requiring medical follow-up

b. Perform specific therapeutic measures such as dressing changes

c. Describe plan for follow-up care

POTENTIAL PROBLEMS	EXPECTED OUTCOMES	NURSING ACTIVITIES
▪ Respiratory insufficiency related to *obstructed airway,* which may result from Mandibular fracture(s) Massive bleeding from intraoral injuries Altered sensorium Aspiration of blood, gastric contents Edema of larynx (common in auto crash trauma)	▪ Respiratory sufficiency with patent, unobstructed airway Absence of respiratory distress Alveolar ventilation adequate with Paco₂ within patient's normal limits	▪ Monitor for Rate and quality of respirations Respiratory distress—note presence of deep, gasping, rapid, shallow, labored, dyspneic, or stridorous breathing; wheezing Adequacy of ventilation Hold hand above patient's nose and mouth and feel force of expired air Observe chest movements Monitor Paco₂ levels Occlusion of airway by tongue, secretions, or blood Arterial blood gas results for hypoxemia, hypercapnia If partial/total obstructed airway is apparent Hyperextend head (except in patients with suspected cervical or spinal cord injury) If airway obstruction is still present, remove clotted blood, loose teeth, dentures, vomitus, foreign objects from patient's mouth with fingers Apply humidified O₂ mask as ordered Prepare patient for and assist with intubation for mechanical ventilation, which is often required for patients with Fractures of several ribs Severe mandibular fractures Massive oropharyngeal tissue injury Obtundation from head injury *See* STANDARD 6 *Mechanical ventilation*
▪ Respiratory insufficiency related to *flail chest,* which may result from Fracture of four or more ribs Fracture of sternum at junction of ribs (separation of costochondral cartilages producing free-floating sternum)	▪ Flail chest stabilized with adequate alveolar ventilation, without undue splinting, and without further lung contusion caused by fractured ribs Cardiac output and arterial O₂ saturation, Pao₂ within normal limits	▪ Monitor for Splinting Swelling and/or crepitation over rib cage Light palpation revealing fractured rib Paradoxical movement of chest with breathing Arterial blood gas results for decrease in arterial O₂ saturation, Pao₂ Pain Chest radiograph results indicating fracture Notify physician of these abnormalities If flail chest occurs Administer analgesics, as ordered Assist physician with local infiltration of anesthetic, if necessary Maintain sandbag traction, light hand pressure, or pillow splint for stabilization if intubation is not immediately possible or necessary Prepare patient for and assist with intubation; see Standard 6, *Mechanical ventilation*
▪ Respiratory insufficiency related to *pulmonary vessel injury* with *hemothorax,* which may be associated with bleeding from the following arteries Pulmonary Main hilar Pleurocutaneous	▪ Hemodynamic stability with adequate cardiac output, normovolemia Pulmonary vessels intact	▪ Monitor for evidence of Shock, hypovolemia, blood loss Hypoxemia, hypercapnia Signs and symptoms of pulmonary contusion Atelectasis Decreased breath sounds Bloody secretions Hazy chest radiograph in area of suspected contusion

POTENTIAL PROBLEMS	EXPECTED OUTCOMES	NURSING ACTIVITIES

		Chest radiograph results revealing
		  Pneumothorax
		  Hemothorax
		Prepare patient for and assist with chest tube insertion if procedure is necessary
		  Monitor chest tube drainage; note amount, nature of drainage
		    If dark and pulsatile, pulmonary artery tear may be the source
		    If bright red and pulsatile, pulmonary vein or surrounding artery may be torn
		If chest entrance wound is present, monitor for tear of aorta and other major arterial vessels and for cardiac tamponade; see Problem, Hemodynamic instability, if chest entrance wound is present
		If pulmonary vessel injury occurs, assist with needle aspiration or tube thoracotomy, as needed
		Prepare patient for surgery, if planned (often required for major, ongoing blood losses, large retained clot after chest tube insertion, major bronchial tear)

■ Respiratory insufficiency related to *sucking wound*
Destroys pressure gradient between atmosphere and pleural space
Leads to atelectasis, pneumothorax, mediastinal shift, impaired venous return to heart
	■ Adequate alveolar ventilation
	Absence or resolution of sucking chest wound
	Absence of air leak
		■ Monitor for
		  Sound of sucking wound of chest; note open wound
		  Signs/symptoms of pneumothorax, mediastinal shift, impaired venous return to heart, atelectasis
		If sucking wound occurs
		  Maintain airtight dressing (gauze with petroleum jelly coating); should be applied at end of expiration when diaphragm has expelled residual air and fluid from pleural space through wound opening
		Prepare for and assist with insertion of chest tube
		Maintain patient in semi-Fowler position

■ Respiratory insufficiency related to *pulmonary contusion* with hemorrhage and edema
Signs of pulmonary contusion become more obvious hours after trauma because of natural inflammatory process and because low pressure pulmonary system is prone to accumulation of fluid used during resuscitation
	■ Absence or resolution of pulmonary contusion	■ Monitor for
		  Dropping PaO_2 levels
		  Requirements for greater inspired O_2 concentrations to achieve adequate oxygenation (PaO_2)
		  Higher inspiratory pressures required for delivery of desired tidal volume (decreased compliance)
		  Chest radiograph results revealing diffusely hazy picture throughout lung fields consistent with pulmonary interstitial edema; localized or diffuse pattern of haziness and atelectasis consistent with pulmonary contusion
		Notify physician of these abnormalities
		If pulmonary contusion occurs
		  Administer respiratory support if needed, as ordered
		  Supplemental humidified O_2
		  Intubation and mechanical ventilation, if needed
		  See Standard 6, *Mechanical ventilation*
		Administer fluids cautiously
		  Accurate intake and output
		  Administer diuretics as ordered
		  Weigh daily; note weight gain, which is to be avoided
		Place patient on Roto-Rest bed to help promote constant pulmonary drainage

■ Posttraumatic respiratory insufficiency; adult respiratory distress syndrome related to
Sepsis (systemic and/or pulmonary)
Long bone fracture (fat emboli)
Direct pulmonary injury
Massive transfusion of whole blood
	■ Adequate oxygenation and ventilation
	Arterial blood gas levels within normal limits
	Clear lungs as evidenced by chest radiograph and auscultation
		■ Monitor for syndrome, particularly in patients at high risk, including
		  Hypoxemia
		  Decreased pulmonary compliance
		  Measurements of lung volumes reveal fall in resting volume or functional residual capacity (FRC)
		  Diffuse infiltrates, which may progress to consolidation, indicating worsening of syndrome
		If posttraumatic respiratory insufficiency occurs, administer therapy, as ordered, directed at recruiting collapsed and partially occluded alveoli, which will directly increase FRC of lung and improve oxygenation/ventilation

POTENTIAL PROBLEMS	EXPECTED OUTCOMES	NURSING ACTIVITIES
Aspiration of gastric contents Fluid overload Ischemic pulmonary injury (i.e., hemorrhagic shock)		If artificial mechanical ventilation is instituted, see Standard 6, *Mechanical ventilation* If mechanical ventilation with PEEP is instituted, see Standard 7, *Positive end-expiratory pressure* Administer fluids carefully to avoid hypervolemia and pulmonary interstitial edema (which is directly associated with fluid overload) Administer diuretics as ordered—monitor patient's response carefully Monitor weight daily; improvement in respiratory function is often associated with loss of some of extra body fluid used for resuscitation

■ Respiratory insufficiency related to reduced air space that results from Pneumothorax Bronchial tear Hemothorax Diaphragmatic tear Phrenic nerve injury and diaphragmatic paralysis	■ Adequate alveolar ventilation with full lung expansion Absence of respiratory distress	■ Monitor for signs and symptoms of pneumothorax and/or hemothorax
		  Tachypnea
		  Respiratory distress, dyspnea
		  Asymmetrical chest movements
		  Altered LOC caused by hypoxia; anxiety
		  Diaphoresis
		  Tachycardia with weak pulse
		  Pallor
		  Hypotension
		Additional signs that are indicative of pneumothorax
		  Sudden, sharp chest pain; pleural pain
		  Distant breath sounds on affected side
		  Hyperresonance on percussion
		  Chest radiograph indicating collection of air in pleural space
		  Shift of trachea to unaffected side
		  Distended neck veins
		  Swelling and palpable crepitations around neck (particularly injuries to apex of lung)
		Additional signs that are indicative of hemothorax
		  Chest pain
		  Dullness with percussion
		  Chest radiograph results revealing fluid level in pleural space area
		  Drop in Hct if blood loss is significant
		  Sudden drop in BP, CVP, and cardiac output; oliguria
		If pneumothorax and/or hemothorax occur, monitor vital signs q15-30 min and serial Hct levels
		Prepare for and assist with
		  Thoracentesis
		  Chest tube insertion
		If hemothorax occurs (in addition)
		  Administer fluids, blood, and blood products as ordered; closely monitor patient's response
		Monitor for signs of bronchial tear
		  Signs/symptoms of pneumothorax
		  Massive air leak into mediastinum, pleural space
		  Persistent atelectasis
		  Inability to sufficiently expand injured lung
		Monitor for signs of diaphragmatic tear, particularly in patient's with history of blunt chest and abdominal trauma
		  Elevated diaphragm by radiograph and clinical examination
		  Persistent lower lobe atelectasis
		Assist with upright chest radiograph, fluoroscopy, and other tests to rule out injury to phrenic nerve and paralysis of diaphragm, revealed in part of reduced diaphragmatic movement

POTENTIAL PROBLEMS	EXPECTED OUTCOMES	NURSING ACTIVITIES

■ Hemodynamic instability related to *hemorrhage* resulting from
Torn or ruptured aorta
Tear of subclavian or innominate artery
Tear of coronary artery
Cardiac rupture
	■ Hemodynamic stability
	Adequate cardiac output, blood volume
	Hemodynamic parameters/vital signs within patient's normal limits
	Urine output 0.5 ml/kg/hour in adults; 1 to 2 ml/kg/hour in children/infants
		■ Monitor
		  Vital signs q¼-1 hr until stable
		  For presence of signs/symptoms of shock
		    Marked hypotension, tachycardia
		    Weak, thready pulses
		    Peripheral vasoconstriction (coolness, clamminess)
		    Pallor
		    Restlessness
		  For external blood loss (through wounds, body orifices, tubes inserted for drainage)
		  For presence of expanding chest wall hematoma
		  Results of serial Hct and Hgb (q6-12 hr and prn until stable)
		  Fluid intake and output, scrupulously
		  For signs/symptoms of cardiac tamponade caused by accumulation of blood in pericardium, mediastinum
		  For presence of injuries that may be associated with (internal/external) hemorrhage: chest or upper abdominal wound
		  For chest radiograph results revealing widened mediastinum; contused myocardium; hematoma at apex of heart; foreign body (e.g., bullet) near major vessels; rib fractures; flail chest and/or fractured sternum; hemothorax; and for injury to major artery
		Note diminished or absent pulses on affected upper extremity; monitor for
		  Neurological deficits associated with ischemia, thrombosis; cerebral embolism; ischemic brachial plexus injury, which is revealed by neurological deficits of arm
		  Presence of bruit over major vessel (may indicate traumatic arteriovenous fistula formation)
		  Substernal pain
		Notify physician of any abnormality
		If hemorrhage occurs
		  Administer fluids, blood, and blood products, as ordered; if arterial venous tear suspected, administer into catheterized vessel proximal to suspected arterial/venous tear
		  Carefully monitor patient's hemodynamic response
		  Keep patient supine until resuscitation effort improves hemodynamic/circulatory parameters; avoid Trendelenburg position if head, neck, and chest injuries are suspected
		  Prepare patient for arteriography and/or surgery as planned
		  Assist with insertion of central venous, pulmonary artery lines
		  Monitor CVP and PAP q½-1 hr and prn during resuscitation efforts
		  Measure circumference of all body systems parts that may be bleeding, particularly abdomen and lower extremities

■ Hemodynamic instability related to *myocardial contusion*	■ Hemodynamic stability
	Resolution of signs/symptoms of myocardial contusion
		■ Monitor for
		  ECG evidence of myocardial ischemia, injury
		  New conduction defect
		  Recurrent arrhythmias, particularly sinus tachycardia, atrial arrhythmias, bundle branch block, and ventricular arrhythmias
		  Elevated cardiac enzyme levels
		  Concurrent hemodynamic compromise—low cardiac output not produced by obvious valvular or septal rupture
		  Signs of heart failure, e.g.
		    Fatigue; tachycardia
		    Diaphoresis
		    Tachypnea, dyspnea, orthopnea
		    Rales, rhonchi
		    Restlessness
		    Edema
		    Increased venous pressure, distended neck veins
		    Decreased urine output
		    Gallop rhythm
		    Pulsus alternans

POTENTIAL PROBLEMS	EXPECTED OUTCOMES	NURSING ACTIVITIES
		Pericardial rub, other signs of pericarditis
		Cardiac tamponade (e.g., tear of coronary artery, etc.)
		Exsanguinating intrathoracic hemorrhage (e.g., in pericardial laceration or myocardial rupture
		Ventricular aneurysm
		Notify physician of any of these abnormalities
		If myocardial contusion occurs
		Administer supportive therapy, as ordered
		Mild inotropic agents
		Beta–adrenergic-blocking agents
		Diuretics
		Fluids
		O_2
		See standards appropriate for problems associated with myocardial contusion: Standard 21, *Arrhythmias;* Standard 15, *Heart failure (low cardiac output);* Standard 12, *Acute myocardial infarction*
		Prepare patient for diagnostic studies, as planned, which may include
		Ultrasound study
		Radioisotope scan
		IV contrast study of right heart
■ Hemodynamic instability related to *cardiac tamponade*	■ Absence or resolution of cardiac tamponade Hemodynamic stability: BP, P within patient's normal limits	■ Monitor for signs/symptoms of cardiac tamponade, including
		Rapidly advancing signs of shock—hypotension, decreasing pulse pressure, rising venous pressure, tachycardia, cold clammy skin
		Progressive venous distention in neck and arms
		Kussmaul sign (neck veins paradoxically expand with inhalation)
		Pulsus paradoxus (pulse stronger with exhalation, weaker with inhalation)
		Distant heart sounds
		Decreasing voltage of QRS complex on ECG
		Characteristic pericardial friction rub and ECG S-T segment and T wave abnormalities
		Widening mediastinum, cardiac silhouette as evidenced by chest radiograph results
		Notify physician of these abnormalities
		If cardiac tamponade occurs
		Prepare patient for pericardial aspiration, if planned, and assist with procedure; after procedure, monitor for recurrent cardiac tamponade, which may indicate bleeding artery and need for pericardial window
		Administer IV fluid, blood products as ordered; carefully monitor patient's response
		Administer cardiotonic, diuretic agents as ordered for cardiac failure and pulmonary edema
		See Standard 18, *Pericarditis* for nursing activities regarding pericardial effusion/cardiac tamponade
■ Hemodynamic instability related to traumatic *pericardial rupture,* resulting from Herniation of heart Torsion of great vessels Rupture of heart itself	■ Resolution of traumatic pericardial rupture	■ Monitor for signs of traumatic pericardial rupture, primarily signs of cardiac decompensation and low cardiac output Notify physician of signs of cardiac decompensation Prepare patient for emergency surgery, if planned
■ Hemodynamic instability related to *valvular injuries* Mitral regurgitation resulting from Laceration of leaflet	■ Valvular function adequate for sufficient forward blood flows Hemodynamic stability: BP, P within patient's normal limits	■ Monitor for Acute mitral regurgitation Evidence of acute increase in left atrial pressure, PCWP (25 to 30 mm Hg or more), which produces characteristic symptoms, including dyspnea, orthopnea, paroxysmal nocturnal dyspnea Early systolic murmur

POTENTIAL PROBLEMS	EXPECTED OUTCOMES	NURSING ACTIVITIES

Rupture of chordae tendineae
Hemorrhage into and avulsion of papillary muscle (necrosis, then rupture)
Aortic regurgitation associated with
Tear of aortic leaflet
Avulsion of commissural attachment
Aortic intimal tear with prolapse of leaflet into ventricular outflow tract
Tricuspid regurgitation
	Absence and/or resolution of valvular injuries	Holosystolic murmur, heard best at apex of axilla in left lateral decubitus position and not transmitted to neck—S_1 soft; S_3 present
		Chest radiograph results revealing enlarged left atrium
		  Pulmonary congestion, edema; Kerley B lines
		ECG revealing left axis deviation
		Cardiac catheterization revealing
		  Diminished or decreased pressure gradient at mitral valve
		  Mitral regurgitation on cineangiography
		  Elevated left atrial pressure—big V waves
		Echocardiographic results indicating mitral valve regurgitation
		If acute mitral regurgitation is sustained, evidence of chronic mitral regurgitation develops; ECG may reveal
		  Left ventricular hypertrophy
		  Left atrial hypertrophy
		  Atrial fibrillation
		Notify physician of any of these abnormalities
		Monitor for aortic regurgitation
		  Primary picture is of left ventricular failure
		  Auscultation revealing
		    Soft S_1, loud S_2
		    Basal decrescendo diastolic murmur
		    Low rumbling middiastolic or presystolic apical murmur (Austin-Flint murmur)
		    Midsystolic murmur at apex
		  Wide pulse pressure
		  Hypertension in lower extremities (BP in lower extremities may be 60 to 100 mm Hg higher than in arms)
		  Quick-rising pulses (water-hammer)
		  Chest radiograph results revealing
		    Dilatated aorta
		    Enlarged left ventricle
		    Signs of left ventricular failure (e.g., pulmonary interstitial edema, vascular redistribution)
		  ECG revealing signs of left ventricular hypertrophy
		    High-voltage R and S waves
		    S-T segment and T wave changes
		  Cardiac catheterization results revealing
		    Little or no pressure gradient at aortic valve (aortic pressure falls to 40 mm Hg or less and left ventricular end diastolic pressure markedly increases associated with regurgitation of blood from the aorta to left ventricle)
		    Increase in aortic systolic pressure may occur
		    Aortic regurgitation with cineangiocardiography
		  Echocardiogram
		    Dilatated, hyperdynamic ventricle
		    High-frequency vibrations of anterior mitral valve leaflet
		    Early closure of mitral valve
		    Coarse fluttering of AV during diastole when flail AV present
		Notify physician of any abnormality
		Monitor for tricuspid regurgitation
		  Holosystolic murmur—maximal point near sternum; increased with inspiration; not transmitted to axilla
		  V waves in jugular venous hypertension and CHF
		  Pulsating liver
		  Chest radiograph revealing enlarged right atrium, vena cava
		  ECG revealing right axis deviation
		  Cardiac catheterization revealing
		    Elevated right atrial pressure
		    Dilatated right atrial and right ventricular cavities
		    Regurgitation of contrast material from right ventricle to right atrium during systole; prominent V wave develops
		    V waves in and proximal to right atrium

POTENTIAL PROBLEMS	EXPECTED OUTCOMES	NURSING ACTIVITIES
		Echocardiographic and radionuclide studies reveal enlarged right ventricle
		If tricuspid regurgitation is sustained, signs of right ventricular failure develop, which may include
		Right ventricular impulse along left sternal border
		Elevated systemic venous pressure
		Peripheral edema
		Anorexia, nausea
		Hepatomegaly, hepatic systolic pulsation
		Evidence of low cardiac output
		Fatigue
		Tachycardia
		Reduced peripheral perfusion
		Notify physician of aforementioned abnormalities
		If valvular insufficiency occurs, administer therapy to support cardiac function as ordered, which may include
		Cautious fluid administration so as not to overload the heart
		Diuretics
		Inotropic agents
		If signs of heart failure occur, see Standard 15, *Heart failure (low cardiac output)*
		Prepare patient for cardiac catheterization, if planned
		Prepare patient for surgery, if planned

■ Hemodynamic instability related to *rupture of cardiac septa, chamber walls,* which may include
Ventricular wall rupture
Interatrial septal defect
Ventricular septal defect
Left ventricular–right atrial communication
Aortic–right ventricular communication
Process may include acute laceration or less acute contusion and hemorrhage, followed by necrosis, sloughing, and perforation
	■ Hemodynamic stability
	Cardiac chambers, septum intact
		■ Monitor for signs of septal, chamber rupture (in patients with history of chest compression)
		Cardiovascular collapse
		Low cardiac output
		Profound heart failure
		Pulmonary congestion, interstitial edema
		Notify physician of these abnormalities
		If rupture occurs
		    Administer fluid, blood, blood products, as ordered
		    Monitor patient's vital signs continuously via bedside monitor; note q5 min
		    Prepare patient for surgery according to plan of care

■ Altered LOC related to
Closed head injury
Concussion
Contusion
Skull fracture
Exacerbation/onset of acute medical problem (e.g., diabetes)
Cerebrovascular accident
Drug overdose, poisoning
Hysteria
	■ Patient oriented to persons, place, and time
	Neurological examination within normal limits
	Absence or resolution of increased ICP
		■ Assess LOC and note in particular
		Decreased alertness, orientation to surroundings
		Restlessness, confusion, stupor
		Monitor for
		Hemodynamic changes associated with increased ICP
		    Widening pulse pressure
		    Slow bounding pulse, bradycardia
		Slowed, slurred speech
		Neck stiffness
		Abnormal respiratory pattern
		Inequality of pupil size and reaction to light
		Mild fever
		Nausea and/or vomiting
		Changes in ICP measurements
		Fluid intake and output imbalance; particularly note polyuria associated with increased intracranial pressure
		Patient's movement and sensation of all extremities; note differences and notify physician
		Presence of ecchymoses around eyes, chin, and/or ears

POTENTIAL PROBLEMS	EXPECTED OUTCOMES	NURSING ACTIVITIES

		If these signs and symptoms are present
		  Evaluate for skull fracture (frontal and basal), and gently palpate skull for depressions, protrusions, lacerations
		  Check for drainage from ears, nose, and mouth
		  Test ear and nose drainage for presence of glucose, indicating spinal fluid
		  Examine ears, nose, and hair for foreign objects
		Notify physician of these abnormalities
		If signs/symptoms of head injury are present, prepare patient for tests as ordered, which may include
		  CT scan
		  Arteriography
		  EEG
		
		See STANDARD 33 *Head trauma*
		
		If cerebral swelling is suspected and patient is conscious, instruct patient to avoid further increases in ICP by bearing down during elimination or blowing nose
		Reevaluate patient's neurological status, including LOC, motor and sensory functions, and pupillary reactions q½-1 hr and prn
		Keep patient's head elevated 30 degrees

■ Skeletal injuries: spinal cord injury, which most commonly occurs at C5, C6, and/or C7; and T12, L1	■ Stabilization of fracture
	Degree of sensation and movement of extremities remains stable or improves
	GI function within normal limits
	Hemodynamic stability, adequate cardiac output
		■ Monitor for signs of spinal trauma
		  Sensation and movement of extremities
		  Sensation of torso
		  Reflexes to extremities, torso
		If spinal cord injury is suspected, particularly if lesion is high in cord, monitor for signs of decreased sympathetic tone including hypotension, bradycardia, hypothermia
		Notify physician of any of these abnormalities
		If spinal cord injury occurs
		  Closely monitor vital signs q¼-1 hr until stable
		  Administer fluids, vasopressor medication as ordered
		  Perform ongoing neurological evaluation, including
		    LOC
		    Pupillary size, equality, and reaction
		    Sensation, movement of extremities
		    Sensation of torso
		    Reflexes in upper and lower extremities
		    Evaluation for presence of Babinski reflex
		  Maintain patient in straight alignment; support extremities and back (e.g., with pillows)
		  Ensure straight alignment of body and head when turning patient (if allowed to turn)
		Prepare patient for placement of tongs if procedure is necessary
		Maintain tongs and traction, as ordered, once applied
		Place patient on Roto-Rest bed* if indicated

■ Skeletal injuries: fracture of extremity	■ Fracture heals with proper alignment of bone
	Sensation and movement of extremity within normal limits
		■ Monitor for
		  Deformity, swelling, or open wounds on admission
		  Pain—location, nature, and severity
		  Reduced movement and ROM; marked pain with movement
		  Reduced sensitivity to extremity; note paresis, followed by paresthesia
		  Reduced circulation to any extremity
		  Note pallor, coolness, thready pulses

*A new device, the Roto-Rest bed, has been used in critically ill patients to effect lateral-to-lateral position changes and continuous rotation to influence distribution of pulmonary blood flow. Selection of extreme lateral position can be made, particularly in cases of respiratory failure with primarily unilateral involvement. Dependent positioning of the uninvolved lung to match ventilation and perfusion can be accomplished simply. Rapid resolution of a large pulmonary contusion serves to illustrate the clinical use of the apparatus.

POTENTIAL PROBLEMS	EXPECTED OUTCOMES	NURSING ACTIVITIES

		Notify physician of any of these abnormalities
		Assist with maintaining immobilization of fractures
		If casts are applied, monitor circulation to extremities (pulses, warmth, color) and patient's ability to move extremities
		Maintain sterile dressings on open fracture (nonadherent dressings soaked in saline solution or povidone-iodine may be ordered)
		Monitor for signs of bleeding associated with fracture
		    Increasing circumference of extremity, pelvis (lower abdomen)
		    Dropping Hct
		    Signs of developing shock, i.e., hypotension, tachycardia, etc.
		If spinal fracture is suspected, keep patient flat and spine in straight, immobile alignment
		For spinal fracture, see Problem, Skeletal injuries: spinal cord injury
		For rib fractures where flail chest is suspected, see Problem, Respiratory insufficiency related to flail chest
		For skull fractures, see Problem, Altered LOC

■ Skeletal injuries with associated fatty microemboli and reactive edema of lungs, brain, and kidneys (resulting from fracture of long bones and ribs)	■ Absence or resolution of fatty microemboli
	Pulmonary, cerebral, and kidney function within normal limits
		■ Monitor for signs and symptoms of
		    Pulmonary interstitial edema and hypoxia
		    Delirium
		    Hematuria and fatty droplets in urine
		    Petechiae, which may appear on chest, in axillary folds, in sclera, and under eyelids
		Notify physician of these abnormalities
		If fatty microemboli occur, see Standard 31, *Embolic phenomena*

■ Trauma to internal organ systems: peritonitis	■ Absence or resolution of peritonitis	■ Monitor for signs and symptoms of peritonitis, particularly in the patient with history of blunt trauma to abdomen
		    Increasing abdominal pain
		    Tenderness, rebound tenderness, and/or rigidity
		    Abdominal muscle spasm
		    Abdominal guarding
		    Decreased bowel sounds
		    Abdominal distention
		    Tachycardia, fever, leukocytosis
		    Signs and symptoms of hypovolemia, shock
		Observe for signs and symptoms of rupture of GI tract or other abdominal organs
		Radiograph may reveal pneumoperitoneum if associated rupture of any portion of GI tract occurs
		If peritonitis occurs, see Standard 45, *Peritonitis*

■ Esophageal injury; evaluate for in patients with upper to middle chest injury(ies) with trauma; may be associated with injuries to aorta, trachea, left main stem bronchus	■ Intact esophagus
	Normal esophageal function
		■ Monitor for
		    Pneumomediastinum on radiograph (occurs in small percentage)
		    Complaints of substernal pain, neck and epigastric discomfort
		If problem is suspected, more certain diagnosis can be made by carefully inserting tube into upper esophagus through which water-soluble opaque material can be passed and visualized by radiograph; assist physician with this procedure, as needed
		If problem is detected, prepare patient for surgery, as ordered
		Assist with insertion of chest tube to drain mediastinum, if needed

■ Injury, rupture of urinary drainage system	■ Intact bladder
	Urine output within patient's normal limits
		■ Monitor for
		    Urine output through bladder catheter q2 hr; note presence of gross hematuria and urine in small volumes
		    Suprapubic pain with rebound tenderness
		    Shock from bleeding
		    Presence of large suprapubic mass; suprapubic swelling
		    Large boggy mass above prostate on rectal examination (usually done by physician)

POTENTIAL PROBLEMS	EXPECTED OUTCOMES	NURSING ACTIVITIES
		Monitor lab study results, including
		Urinalysis for presence of red blood cells
		Kidney, ureter, and bladder (KUB) radiograph for pelvic fracture; increased darkness in vesicular area may indicate extravasation
		Excretory urograms for injury to kidney and leakage
		Retrograde cystogram, which is reliable for demonstrating frank extravasation
		IV pyelogram
		Notify physician of any pertinent findings
		Prepare patient for and assist with pertinent diagnostic studies, as ordered
		If bladder injury occurs
		Administer therapy as ordered to treat shock, hemorrhage; closely monitor patient's hemodynamic response
		Prepare patient for surgery, which may include
		Drainage of injured site
		Closure of tear
		Placement of cystostomy tube (in addition to indwelling urethral catheter)
■ Trauma to kidney(s) (suspect if trauma to abdomen)	■ Kidney function within normal limits, including urine output, urine and serum creatinine, electrolyte levels; BUN; specific gravity; urine and serum osmolality	■ Determine presence of ecchymosis, bruise, contusion, or laceration in midlower abdomen
		Monitor for hematuria, flank pain, hypotension, and dropping Hct, which may indicate ongoing bleeding; abdominal mass in flank area may be hematoma associated with trauma to kidneys
		Monitor lab studies for indices of renal function
		Urine output, specific gravity
		BUN
		Serum creatinine levels and urinary clearance
		Serum and urine electrolyte levels
		Serum and urine osmolality
		Uric acid
		Notify physician of notable abnormalities
		Administer therapy aimed at maintaining adequate renal blood flow, maintaining fluid and electrolyte balance, and preventing further renal damage (e.g., avoiding nephrotoxic antibiotics)
		Prepare patient for and assist with certain diagnostic procedures, which may include
		KUB radiograph
		Urogram (after treatment for shock)
		Renal angiography
		Prepare patient for surgery, if planned, particularly in presence of persistent bleeding, if laceration can be sutured; if injury is severe, nephrectomy may be needed
		Monitor for signs and symptoms of perinephric infection; observe for evidence of perinephric abscess
		Flank pain with radiation to upper abdomen, back, or shoulder
		Tenderness and spasm of flank and upper abdominal muscles; discomfort often relieved with thigh in flexed position
		Nausea, vomiting
		Fever
		Malaise
		Leukocytosis
		Palpable mass
		Evidence of concurrent pyelonephritis
		If present, notify physician and administer therapy as ordered, e.g., antibiotics or surgical drainage

POTENTIAL PROBLEMS	EXPECTED OUTCOMES	NURSING ACTIVITIES
■ Injuries to membranous urethra, which often occur in association with fracture of pubic bone	■ Kidney-bladder function within normal limits, including normal urinary output	■ Monitor for Gross hematuria; hemorrhage Inability to void Lower abdominal or perineal pain Tender suprapubic mass (containing blood and urine) Results of cystourethrogram Notify physician of any of these abnormalities If problem occurs Administer therapy, as ordered, including fluids and blood products to maintain blood volume and maintenance of bladder catheter, which may have small amount of traction applied Closely monitor intake and output, specific gravity of urine, and indices of kidney function, and continue aforementioned monitoring activities
■ Rupture of diaphragm	■ Diaphragm intact Diaphragmatic function within normal limits Absence of respiratory distress Alveolar ventilation within patient's normal limits	■ Monitor for respiratory distress Presence of tachypnea, dyspnea Serial blood gas results indicating hypoventilation (hypercapnia) Difficulty in delivery of inspiratory volume during mechanical ventilation, e.g., high inspiratory pressures on volume ventilators or low volume delivered on pressure-limited ventilators Monitor chest radiograph results for Mediastinal shift Elevated diaphragm and upper abdominal organs Occasionally, protrusion of abdominal organs through diaphragm into chest Persistent lower lobe lung atelectasis Notify physician of these abnormalities Administer supportive care as ordered, which may include artificial ventilation If intubation is necessary, see Standard 6, *Mechanical ventilation* Prepare patient for surgery, if planned
■ Rupture of spleen, which occurs frequently in association with Fractures of lower ribs Childhood trauma (with or without rib fractures) Presence of diseases that make spleen very friable (malaria, typhoid, sarcoidosis, infectious mononucleosis)	■ Splenic function within normal limits; absence of signs of internal bleeding	■ Monitor for ruptured spleen, particularly in patients with history of blunt abdominal trauma, with fractures of lower left ribs Monitor for Left flank pain Pain and tenderness in left upper quadrant of abdomen Left shoulder pain (occurs in about 75% of patients with ruptured spleen and is associated with diaphragmatic irritation; also called *Kehr sign*) Developing signs of peritoneal irritation Evidence of blood loss and falling Hct Moderate leukocytosis and temperature elevation (usually does not occur) Radiograph results revealing displacement of gastric air bubble and loss of splenic outline Assist with diagnostic abdominal tap, which is positive for blood in about 75% of patients with ruptured spleen Notify physician of aforementioned abnormalities Prepare patient for surgery as planned and ordered
■ Trauma to or rupture of liver Occurs less commonly than rupture of spleen (more force is required) Bleeding may occur and cease spontaneously	■ Liver function within normal limits; absence of signs of internal bleeding	■ Monitor for signs of rupture of the liver, including Right upper quadrant pain with muscle rigidity and tenderness Right shoulder pain (from diaphragmatic irritation) Swelling in right upper quadrant Note presence of concurrent signs of peritonitis indicating possible ongoing hemorrhage Monitor hemodynamic status closely; note hypotension, tachycardia Notify physician of presence of any of these abnormalities

POTENTIAL PROBLEMS	EXPECTED OUTCOMES	NURSING ACTIVITIES
Is suspected in presence of blunt abdominal trauma or fractures of lower right ribs or when concurrent laceration of right kidney is present		If trauma to liver is suspected 　Monitor vital signs closely (q15-30 min) until stable 　Note signs of shock, i.e., hypotension, tachycardia, oliguria, peripheral vasocons friction 　Monitor results of serial Hct determinations; note abnormal values 　Measure abdominal girth serially (q1-2 hr) 　Note increasing size, tenseness of abdomen If liver trauma or rupture occurs 　Administer fluids, blood, and blood products, as ordered 　Closely monitor patient's response as before 　Monitor serial liver function tests; particularly note coagulation studies, protein levels, transaminase levels, etc.
■ Infection related to 　Local factors 　　Ischemia and devitalization of tissue 　　Reduced blood flow to injured tissue, with deficient delivery of immunoproteins and leukocytes to combat bacterial contamination 　　Hematoma formation 　　Penetration of contaminated foreign object 　　Puncture of bowel with massive fecal soilage of peritoneum 　Systemic factors 　　Systemic hypoxia 　　Hemorrhagic shock 　　Severe tissue injury (depletes body of proteins that prepare bacteria for phagocytosis by polymorphonuclear leukocytes) 　　History of recent alcohol intake (depresses phagocytic leukocyte function)	■ Absence or resolution of infection Afebrile Wounds, fracture heal without undue necrosis or devitalization of tissue	■ Prevention 　Administer humidified O_2, as ordered 　Administer adequate nutrients to meet calculated metabolic requirements to aid in healing and support of immunological activity against infection 　Apply sterile dressings to open wounds, as ordered 　Adhere to appropriate aseptic technique in handling endotracheal tube, tracheostomy, bladder catheter, and arterial and IV lines; remove these lines according to hospital protocol and as soon as patient's status allows, as ordered 　Administer antibiotics, if ordered 　Administer topical antibiotics, as ordered 　Assist with debridement of wounds, if needed 　Prepare patient for surgery for evacuation of hematoma or fluid collections (these can be media for infection) 　Provide for vigorous chest physiotherapy tailored to fit patient's needs 　See Standard 8, *Chest physiotherapy* 　Assist patient with ambulation as soon as feasible, according to plan of care Monitor 　Temperature q1-2 hr; note fever 　For signs of wound infection—discomfort, erythema, swelling, purulent drainage 　CBC results indicating leukocytosis; elevated ESR 　For chest radiograph results compatible with atelectasis, subdiaphragmatic abscess; abdominal radiograph results indicating fluid collection 　Abdominal ultrasound results 　C and S results of wound, sputum, blood, and other appropriate sites If infection occurs 　Administer antibiotics, as ordered 　Continue preventive measures identified before 　Prepare patient for drainage of infected collections and/or debridement of necrotic foci if either procedure is necessary
■ Acid-base imbalance	■ Parameters of acid-base balance within normal limits, including Arterial pH O_2 CO_2 Bicarbonate Electrolyte levels, particularly 　K^+ 　Na^+ 　Cl^- 　CO_2	■ Prevent by 　Administering electrolyte solutions based on patient's calculated requirements and serum levels 　Administering O_2 and supportive ventilation according to patient's needs, as ordered Monitor 　Signs and symptoms of hypoxia 　Results of arterial blood gas determinations 　Serum lactate levels, if determined 　Serum electrolyte levels Notify physician of abnormalities

POTENTIAL PROBLEMS	EXPECTED OUTCOMES	NURSING ACTIVITIES

		Administer therapy as ordered to correct acid-base problem, which may include
		  Correction of electrolyte imbalance, if present
		  Metabolic acidosis
		    Sodium bicarbonate
		    Improvement of blood flows with fluids, blood products
		    Cardiac support with inotropic and/or vasodilating agent
		  Respiratory acidosis
		    Vigorous chest physiotherapy; if necessary, mechanical ventilation may be instituted
		  Respiratory alkalosis
		    Sedation
		    Adjustment of ventilator settings for intubated patient
		    Decrease in tidal volume, respiratory rate
		  Metabolic alkalosis
		    If pronounced, ammonium chloride may be administered

■ Renal failure, which may result from prolonged low blood flows and ischemia	■ Indices of renal function within normal limits, including
	  Urine volume
	  Specific gravity
	  Urine electrolytes
	  Urine osmolality
	  Urine-plasma electrolyte, urea, creatinine, and osmolality ratios
	  Free H$_2$O clearance
	  Serum BUN
		■ Prevent with early resuscitation by administering fluids and blood products, as ordered
		Carefully monitor patient's hemodynamic status and daily weights
		Carefully monitor urine output; good indicator of adequate renal blood flow
		Monitor other indices of renal function, including
		  Urine specific gravity
		  Urine electrolyte levels
		  Creatinine clearance*
		  Urine-plasma urea ratio
		  Urine-plasma creatinine ratio
		  Urine-plasma osmolality ratio
		  Free H$_2$O clearance (falls in patients with acute renal failure)
		  Serum BUN
		If problem occurs, see Standard 52, *Acute renal failure*

■ Stress ulceration, with upper GI bleeding
Patients at greatest risk include those with
  Multisystem trauma
  Major intracranial injury or surgery
  Shock
  Burns
  Infection/sepsis
  Renal dysfunction
  Respiratory insufficiency
  Corticosteroid therapy
  Coagulopathy, GI disorder
	■ Absence or resolution of stress ulceration	■ Prevent stress ulceration with therapy as ordered, which may include
		  H$_2$ antagonist (e.g., cimetidine)
		  NG tube
		  Antacids titrated to gastric pH
		  Anticholinergics (particularly for patients with intracranial trauma and for patients who are to undergo surgery)
		  Provision for adequate nutritional intake
		  Prevention with therapy for precipitating causes, including
		    Shock
		    Burns
		    Infection
		    Renal dysfunction
		    Respiratory insufficiency
		Monitor for
		  Bloody NG drainage
		  Complaints of nausea, epigastric distress
		  Dropping Hct
		  Increasing abdominal girth
		  Melenic, heme-positive stools
		If stress ulceration occurs, see Standard 49, *Acute upper gastrointestinal bleeding*

■ Alterations in nutritional status caused by trauma	■ Restoration of previous nutritional status	■ Assess nutritional status; see Standard 2, *Acute respiratory failure,* Problem, Decreased appetite If GI tract is functioning, begin enteral feeding; see Standard 2, *Acute respiratory failure,* Problem, Decreased appetite

---

*Soft tissue and muscle damage results in an increased load of creatinine for kidney clearance. Therefore consider both urine and plasma creatinine levels.

POTENTIAL PROBLEMS	EXPECTED OUTCOMES	NURSING ACTIVITIES
		If GI tract is not functioning and/or caloric requirements are too high, begin parenteral nutrition; see Standard 57, *Total parenteral nutrition*
■ Anxiety, which may be associated with Nature of traumatic injuries sustained Inability to move some body parts Loss of sensation Diagnostic tests Therapeutic regimen	■ Reduction in patient/family's anxiety with provision of information, explanations, and encouragement	■ Ongoing assessment of anxiety Assess patient/family's knowledge of disease process including abnormalities in sensation and movement, need for critical care; diagnostic tests, and therapeutic regimen Explain in simple terms relationship of traumatic injury to rationale for various therapeutic interventions Prepare patient for and, if appropriate, assist with diagnostic tests Provide opportunity for and encourage patient/family's questions, verbalization of fears and anxieties Provide for and encourage patient/family's participation in care Encourage patient/family with acknowledgement of daily and weekly gains/improvements Provide comfort measures Provide emotional support; administer care in unhurried manner Assess reduction in level of patient/family's anxiety
■ Insufficient knowledge for compliance with discharge regimen*	■ Before discharge patient/family verbalizes knowledge of discharge regimen, including activity progression	■ Assess patient/family's preliminary knowledge and understanding of discharge regimen Collaborate with physician, physiotherapist, and other members of health team in development of discharge regimen Instruct patient/family as needed in activity progression; tailor information to injury and/or surgery patient has experienced Chest surgery with sternotomy and major abdominal surgery Avoid lifting heavy objects (over 5 pounds) for several weeks Avoid lifting objects over 15 pounds for several months, as directed Patient should consult physician before resuming more vigorous activities such as playing golf or active sports Encourage patient that chest movements or use of abdominal muscles with such activities as coughing, doing housework, driving may cause some discomfort for several weeks In first few weeks at home, mild analgesic may be ordered for use, as needed Caution patient to seek medical attention for undue/unusual discomfort Fractures In conjunction with physician and physiotherapist, instruct patient in extremity movement, muscle-strengthening exercises, weight bearing according to nature of fracture and extent of healing
	Patient/family verbalizes knowledge of dietary modifications	Instruct patient in necessary dietary modifications and practices such as Chew and swallow slowly For patients with diabetes after severe pancreatitis, see Standard 56, *Diabetic ketoacidosis* If renal failure/dysfunction is present, see Standard 52, *Acute renal failure* See other appropriate standards according to patient's problems and dietary modifications required
	Patient/family is able to perform specific therapeutic measures, such as dressing changes, use of splints, devices, and others	Instruct patient/family in specific therapeutic measures, such as dressings, as appropriate and as ordered Provide opportunity for return demonstration Provide for availability of dressings, splints, etc.

*If responsibility of critical care nurse includes this type of follow-up care.

POTENTIAL PROBLEMS	EXPECTED OUTCOMES	NURSING ACTIVITIES
	Patient/family verbalizes knowledge of medications	Instruct patient in discharge medications, including Purpose and importance Identification Dosage/number of pills Frequency and timing Possible adverse effects Precautionary measures Avoidance of other medications without physician's consent
	Patient/family identifies untoward signs and symptoms requiring medical follow-up	Review untoward signs and symptoms that require medical follow-up; describe possible residual effects that may persist for 3 to 4 months after specific trauma sustained See other appropriate standards according to patient's priority problems and residual dysfunction Cardiac abnormalities Respiratory abnormalities Renal abnormalities Neurological abnormalities
	Patient/family's behavior indicates acceptance of any body image change or limitations	Discuss with patient/family importance of and support them in successful emotional adjustment to any body image change or limitations in function Encourage verbalization of questions, fears, and anxiety regarding any body image change or limitations Provide referrals to agencies, if appropriate
	Patient/family is able to describe plan for follow-up care	Describe plan for follow-up care, including purpose for, when and where to go, who to see, and what specimens to bring Provide opportunity for and encourage patient/family's questions Assess patient's potential compliance with discharge regimen

BURNS

The skin is the largest organ of the body, covering its entire surface. It has two distinct layers, called the *epidermis* and the *derma*. The epidermis, the outer thin avascular layer of stratified squamous epithelial cells, functions as a barrier against environmental hazards. The thicker derma consists of a closely interwoven layer of dense areolar connective tissue, blood vessels, and nerve endings; hair follicles; and sweat and sebaceous glands.

The skin functions as a barrier between the body's internal and external environment and plays an active role in the prevention of infection and trauma. It also protects the body from excessive fluid loss, yet permits elimination of excess water and other waste products. It helps to regulate body temperature, prevents the damaging effects of sunlight (ultraviolet light), secretes oil to soften and lubricate, produces vitamin D with exposure to ultraviolet light, and is an important sense organ with receptor endings for pain, temperature, and touch.

Injury to the skin as in burns will either decrease or eliminate these functions, depending on the amount of skin lost (see Figs. 5 and 6) and the depth of damage (see Table 64-1).

The three most common etiologies of burns are flame (thermal), electrical, and chemical. Additional etiological classification includes burns with and without inhalation injury.

Burns can potentially result in multisystem failure throughout the period of management. Loss of skin integrity leads to increased capillary permeability and thrombosis, cellular necrosis, massive fluid shifts with increased evap-

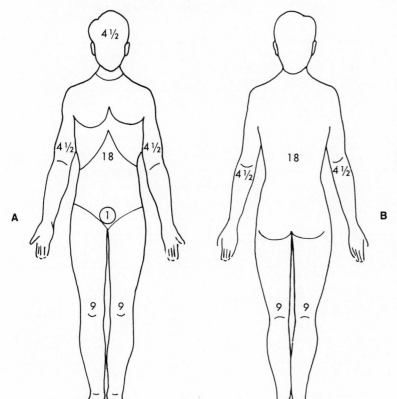

FIG. 5. Estimation of size of burn (percentage of body surface involved) by rule of nine. **A,** Anterior; **B,** posterior. Nines are assigned to specific areas (anterior and posterior) and may be summed as follows:

Head	9
Right upper extremity	9
Left upper extremity	9
Torso	36
Perineum	1
Right lower extremity	18
Left lower extremity	18
TOTAL	100

It is advisable to color code depth of burns for estimating size to give a better picture of the injury to the patient.

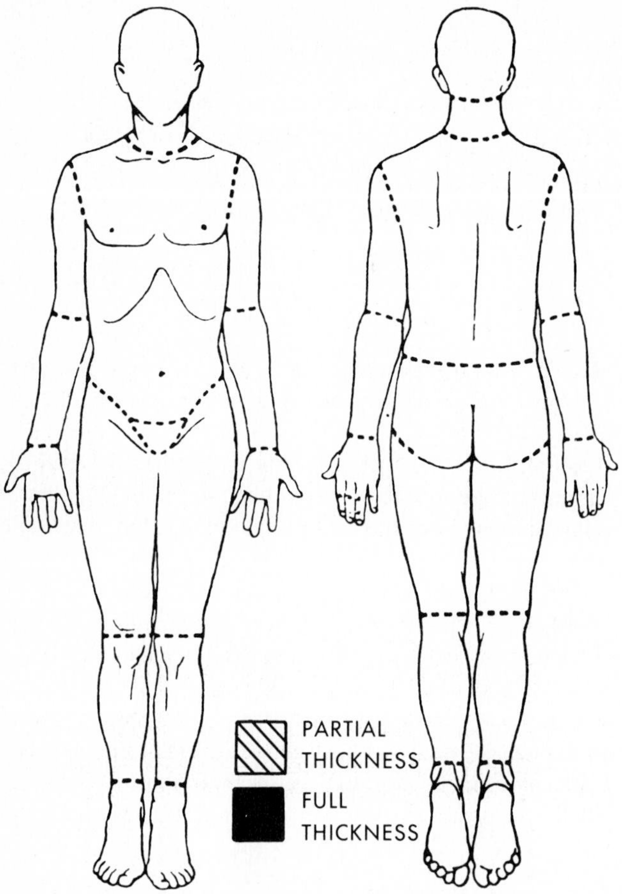

PARTIAL THICKNESS

FULL THICKNESS

Date:_____

Height:_____ Weight:_____

2°_____+3°_____=_____%

Resuscitation Requirements

1st 24 hours:

2nd 24 hours (D5W):

Calorie Requirements

A. Feeding Chosen:_____

B. # cc's required to achieve C.C.R.:_____

Percent Surface Area Burned
(Berkow Formula)

AREA	0-1 YEAR	1-4 YEARS	5-9 YEARS	10-14 YEARS	15 YEARS	ADULT	2°	3°
Head	19	17	13	11	9	7		
Neck	2	2	2	2	2	2		
Ant. Trunk	13	13	13	13	13	13		
Post. Trunk	13	13	13	13	13	13		
R. Buttock	2½	2½	2½	2½	2½	2½		
L. Buttock	2½	2½	2½	2½	2½	2½		
Genitalia	1	1	1	1	1	1		
R. U. Arm	4	4	4	4	4	4		
L. U. Arm	4	4	4	4	4	4		
R. L. Arm	3	3	3	3	3	3		
L. L. Arm	3	3	3	3	3	3		
R. Hand	2½	2½	2½	2½	2½	2½		
L. Hand	2½	2½	2½	2½	2½	2½		
R. Thigh	5½	6½	8	8½	9	9½		
L. Thigh	5½	6½	8	8½	9	9½		
R. Leg	5	5	5½	6	6½	7		
L. Leg	5	5	5½	6	6½	7		
R. Foot	3½	3½	3½	3½	3½	3½		
L. Foot	3½	3½	3½	3½	3½	3½		
TOTAL								

FIG. 6. Estimation of size of burn by percentage of body surface.

TABLE 64-1. Depth of burns

BURN DEPTH	SKIN INVOLVEMENT	SENSATION	APPEARANCE	COURSE
First degree	Epidermis	Normal pain Tingling	Erythema Slight edema Blanching on compression	Regeneration within 1 week Peeling
Second degree	Varying depth of epidermis (partial thickness)	Increased sensitivity to pain and temperature; may not be sensitive to contact	Dry or blistered Erythema Edema Moist wound Cherry red or dull shite	May spontaneously generate within 2 weeks if infection is prevented Depigmentation and scarring
Third degree	All skin layers (full thickness)	Anesthesia Painless	Wet or dry leathery surface Cherry red to white or black Wet or dry	No chance of regenera- tion; requires grafting Scarring Decreased function Alteration of appearance

TABLE 64-2. Fluid replacement formulas*

Baxter formula

First 24 hours — Ringer lactate 4 ml/kg body weight/percentage of body surface burn + 2000 ml D5W
NOTE: One half of calculated requirement of first 24 hours after burn should be administered within 8 hours after injury; remainder should be administered in next 16 hours

Second 24 hours
  40% to 50% burn — 2000 ml D5W + 500 ml colloids
  50% to 70% burn — 2000 ml D5W + 800 ml colloids
  Greater than 70% burn — 2000 ml D5W + 1200 ml colloids

Brooke Army formula

First 24 hours — Ringer lactate 1.5 ml/kg body weight/percentage of body surface burn + colloids 0.5 ml/kg body weight/percentage of body surface burn
Colloids include blood, dextran, or plasma
NOTE: Calculate replacement from time of injury
Give one half of calculated fluid during first 8 hours, one third in second 8 hours, and one fourth in third 8 hours

Second 24 hours — 2000 ml D5W + colloids
NOTE: Give one half amount in first 24 hours

*For other formulas, see Pruitt, B.A.: Fluid and electrolyte replacement in the burned patient, Surg. Clin. North Am. **38**:1291, 1978.

orative losses of heat and water, increased metabolic expenditures of energy (calories), constant threat of invasive sepsis, and altered defense mechanisms with generalized immunosuppression. Therefore a burn injury presents a clinical profile that demands a thorough understanding of fluid and electrolyte balance, cardiopulmonary physiology, renal function, GI integrity, metabolic alterations, sepsis, and neurological/psychological management.

The pathophysiology and management of burns can be classified into three periods: emergent period (shock phase), acute period (phase of eschar separation/healing), and rehabilitation period (phase of reconstruction and reentry).

The emergent period is characterized by increased capillary permeability and fluid shifts, which cause inadequate tissue and organ perfusion. Management during this period primarily consists of fluid resuscitation (see Tables 64-2 and 64-3) and pulmonary, cardiovascular, and renal support. This period, which may last anywhere from 48 hours to several days, ends with the mobilization of fluid and the establishment of cardiopulmonary and renal stability.

The acute period is the phase of eschar separation. This period lasts until the wound, if partial thickness, heals spontaneously, or if full thickness, is covered with autografts. A primary concern during this period is the prevention of

TABLE 64-3. Formulas for intravenous resuscitation

| NAME | TYPE AND VOLUME OF FLUID | | SPECIAL MONITORING RECOMMENDATIONS |
	FIRST 24 HOURS	SECOND 24 HOURS	
Burn budget (Moore)	Colloid—5% of body weight first 12 hr 2.5% of body weight second 12 hr 0.45 saline—according to renal output; approximately 1200 ml Ringer's lactate—1000-4000 ml depending on burn depth D5W 1500 to 5000 ml depending on estimated surface loss	Colloid—2.5% of body weight—other fluids as on day 1	Adjust according to urine output and clinical status
Evans	Colloid—1 ml/kg/% burn Normal saline—1 ml/kg/1% D5W 2000 ml (less in children)	One half of first 24 hr	Urine putout Vital signs
Old Brooke	Colloid—0.5 ml/kg/% Ringer's lactate—1.5 ml/kg/% D5W 2000 ml One half in first 8 hr—one half in next 16 hr	One half of first day's colloids plus crystalloids	Urine output 30 to 50 ml/hr
MGH	Plasma—125 ml/% burn Normal saline—15 ml/% burn	One half of first day plus 2000 ml D5W	Urine output Vital signs
Parkland	Ringer's lactate—4 ml/kg/% burn One half in first 8 hr One half in next 16 hr	Colloid—0.5 ml/kg/% D5W 2000 One half of first day's Ringer's lactate	Urine output 30 to 50 ml (adults) 1 ml/kg/hr (children < 3 yrs) 15 to 25 ml/hr (children > 3 yrs)
Hypertonic resuscitation	Na⁺ 250 mEq/liter Cl⁻ 150 mEq/liter Lactate 100 mEq/liter Average rate 300 ml/hr	D5W	Adjust formula to urine output 30 to 40 ml/hr (adults), mental state, peripheral capillary filling, vital signs
New Brooke	Ringer's lactate—2 to 3/kg/% One half first 8 hr One half next 16 hr	D5W one half of first 24 hr total plus colloid 0.3 to 0.5 ml/kg/%	Urine output 30 to 50 ml/hr
Hypertonic albuminated (Jelenko)	1000 ml 5% D5W and 120 mEq NaCl 120 mEq Na lactate 12.5 g albumin	Most patients complete resuscitation 24 hr No recommendations for second 24 hr	Infuse so that mean arterial BP is 60 to 110 mmHg, urine output 30 to 50 ml/hr

From Munster, A.M.: Burn care for the house officer, Baltimore, 1980, The Williams & Wilkins Co., pp. 18-19.

complications. The primary complications are infection leading to septicemia, inability to provide adequate caloric support, contractures, scarring, and systemic failure, especially cardiopulmonary and renal failure.

The rehabilitation period actually begins when the patient is admitted. This period is concerned with the functional physical restoration and psychosocial reentry of the patient into society. Vigorous rehabilitation including physiotherapy and occupational therapy helps to prevent contractures and hypertrophic scarring and helps achieve maximal function of affected body parts.

The patient should be encouraged to assume gradual responsibility for ADL in preparation for discharge and cosmetic reconstruction. Ongoing psychological support and encouragement are needed from the day of admission to assist the patient in coping with the tremendous physiological and psychological trauma associated with a burn injury.

ASSESSMENT

1. History
   a. Burn history
      (1) Time of burn (when)
      (2) Open or closed space (where)
      (3) How long since injury
      (4) What type of injury (thermal, electrical, chemical, radiation)
   b. Previous history
      (1) Presence of underlying conditions

(2) Allergies

(3) Medications

(4) Family history

(5) Social history

(6) Review of systems

c. Presence of concomitant trauma injury

2. Physical examination

  a. Burn assessment

    (1) Extent of burn wound size (percentage)

    (2) Depth of burn wounds (degrees)

    (3) Evaluation of smoke inhalation: history of closed-space injury; face, neck, thorax burns; singed nasal and facial hairs; carbonaceous sputum; arterial blood gas levels and carboxyhemoglobin measurements; chest radiograph results; signs and symptoms of respiratory distress; laryngoscopy and/or bronchoscopy results

    (4) Presence of circumferential full-thickness burns; escharotomy evaluation (chest and extremities) through frequent pulse and circulation checks

  b. Systems assessment

    (1) Respiratory status: airway patency, lung assessment and integrity; evaluation of oxygenation and ventilation

    (2) Cardiac status: vital signs; cardiac and hemodynamic parameters; circulation and pulse evaluation

    (3) Renal status: hourly urine output (30 ml/hour or more for adults and 1 ml/kg/hour for children); hemoglobinuria/myoglobinuria; trauma to genitourinary tract

    (4) GI status: bowel sounds; abdominal and organ assessment; admission weight; stomach decompression

    (5) Neurological/psychological status: sensorium; head/spinal cord trauma; serum chemical levels (alcohol, drugs, etc.)

3. Lab and diagnostic data, including

  a. CBC for decreased Hct, RBC count, and leukocytosis

  b. Electrolytes and admission blood profile, coagulation studies, etc.; note abnormalities

  c. Urine work-up: urinalysis, C and S, electrolytes, myoglobin, etc.; note abnormalities

  d. Head, chest, and abdominal radiograph results for fracture, etc.

  e. ECG for arrhythmias

  f. Results of spinal fluid examination indicating presence of blood/RBCs (this test optional)

  g. Arterial blood gas and carbon monoxide levels

  h. Serum/urine screens for alcohol, drugs; VDRL; hepatitis, pregnancy, etc.

4. Patient/family's level of anxiety about disease process, diagnostic procedures, and therapy planned

5. Patient/family's understanding of purpose of debridement and surgery, expected prognosis, and psychological reactions

6. Patient's level of anxiety regarding pain, disfigurement, finances, effect on personal life and vocation

GOALS

1. Reduction in patient/family's level of anxiety with provision of information, explanations, and encouragement

2. Respiratory sufficiency

  a. PaO_2 and $PaCO_2$ within patient's normal limits

  b. Absence of rales, wheezes, and stridor

3. Normovolemia

4. Electrolyte and CBC levels within normal limits

5. Hemodynamic stability: absence of arrhythmias; BP, P, and urine output within normal limits

6. Infection free; absence of wound infection

7. Adequate intake of nutrients and vitamins to meet calculated daily requirements; weight stabilization or weight gain; positive nitrogen balance with adequate wound healing

8. Absence or resolution of complications including renal failure, pulmonary edema or emboli, anemia, malnutrition

9. Resolution of burn wound with granulation or skin grafting

10. Restoration to optimal physical, emotional, and psychological functioning

11. Absence of or minimal disability and disfigurement

12. Acceptance of alteration of body appearance

13. Before discharge patient/family is able to

  a. Describe specific wound care, with return demonstration as appropriate

  b. Describe the rehabilitation program and demonstrate activities (e.g., exercises) accurately

  c. Describe dietary and medication regimen

  d. Ask questions regarding self-care

  e. State necessary information regarding follow-up visits to physician and/or clinic

POTENTIAL PROBLEMS	EXPECTED OUTCOMES	NURSING ACTIVITIES
■ Patient/family's anxiety related to limited understanding of disease process, diagnostic tests, surgical procedures, and expected outcome	■ Patient/family demonstrates decreased level of anxiety with provision of information, explanations, and encouragement	■ Ongoing assessment of level of anxiety and understanding Describe burn process, signs and symptoms patient is experiencing, and therapy employed Explain rationales for various diagnostic and therapeutic procedures as they relate to present condition Provide time for and encourage questions and verbalization, stimulate discussion of feelings and fears Explain diagnostic and therapeutic procedures; assist as necessary Solicit patient's cooperation and participation in care Explain precautionary techniques to prevent infection, including Wearing sterile gown, mask, and gloves according to patient's condition and hospital policy Encourage family to participate in care of patient Keep patient/family informed of patient's progress Provide for psychiatric consult to assist patient/family in coping with feelings and situation, if needed

■ Patient/family's anxiety related to alteration in body image with associated
Disfigurement
Interruption in life-style
Unavoidable dependency
Grief and hostility
Pain
	■ Resolution and/or adaptation to present body appearance
	Verbalization of fears, grief, and acceptance of body image
		■ Assess patient's
		  Family interaction
		  Religious, ethnic, and cultural background
		  Perception of illness
		  Values, ideals, and aspirations in life
		  Past experiences with stress, illness; coping mechanisms
		  Level of comprehension
		Address patient by name and explain all procedures; elicit his/her cooperation and assistance
		Allow family visits at frequent intervals
		Relate awareness of patient's feelings and encourage verbalization and discussion of fears and anxieties
		Provide care in gentle, unhurried manner
		Allow use of telephone, outgoing cards, letters, etc.
		Approach and administer care in consistent positive manner with attitude and desire to help
		Express warmth and sincerity in praising patient for accomplishment of goals
		Show respect for patient's integrity and self-worth
		Support and encourage patient with self-care; readjust environment so that patient is able to reach things
		Provide for physical comfort and emotional support
		Provide psychiatric consult if needed, as ordered
		Administer sedatives and analgesics, as ordered and particularly before treatments
		  Provide diversional activities
		Encourage patient to talk about plans for future
		Refer patient to appropriate resources for aid in finances, education, and family problems, as needed

■ Acute respiratory failure related to
Airway obstruction
Pulmonary edema
Atelectasis
Pneumonia
Pulmonary emboli
Carbon monoxide inhalation
Pneumothorax
Eschar formation on chest and neck that restricts respiration
Adult respiratory distress syndrome
Inhalation injury
	■ Patent airway with adequate ventilation and oxygenation
	Arterial blood gas results within patient's normal limits
	Resolution of respiratory failure
	Absence of signs and symptoms of hypoxia
		■ Determine history of smoke, fume, or flame inhalation, including injury occurring in confined space
		Monitor for
		  Moist respirations
		  Respiratory distress: tachypnea, dyspnea, rales, wheezing, stridorous, harsh or diminished breath sounds, and adventitious sounds
		  Bloody or black-tinged sputum
		  Frank burns of tongue
		  Red pharynx
		  Cherry red lips
		  Hoarseness or voice change
		  Burns of head, face, and neck
		  Pallor, cyanosis of skin and mucous membranes
		  Arterial blood gas results indicating acidosis, hypoxemia

POTENTIAL PROBLEMS	EXPECTED OUTCOMES	NURSING ACTIVITIES

		Monitor for severe burns of the neck and chest that result in eschar formation, prepare for escharotomy
		   Prepare scalpel and suture material
		   Assist in procedure
		Administer antibiotics and steroid therapy, if ordered
		Notify physician of any abnormality and prepare for therapy
		If problem occurs, see Standard 2, *Acute respiratory failure*
		If intubation and mechanical ventilation are necessary, see Standard 6, *Mechanical ventilation*
		Provide respiratory treatments, i.e., chest physiotherapy, ROM exercises, O_2 therapy
		Administer respiratory medications, if ordered, and antibiotics according to culture results, as ordered

■ Hypovolemia related to
   Fluid loss from burned areas or vascular depletion caused by third spacing
   Hemorrhage from burned area and/or stress ulcers
   Hypervolemia related to vigorous fluid administration
   Increased total body water related to lack of fluid mobilization or vascular depletion caused by third-space losses
	■ Normovolemia
	  Weight and circulating blood volume within patient's normal limits
	  Hemodynamic stability
		■ Monitor for signs and symptoms of hypovolemia, including
		   Hypotension, orthostatic hypotension
		   Tachycardia
		   Decreased CVP, cardiac output, PAP, and PCWP if available
		   Decreased urine output
		   Increased Hct
		   Poor skin turgor
		   Dry mucous membranes
		   Extreme thirst
		   Gross bleeding or fluid loss from wound, NG tube, or other drainage tube
		   Signs of internal bleeding
		   Results of guaiac tests on all drainage
		   Restlessness and disorientation
		Notify physician of abnormalities
		Prepare and administer fluid, including
		   Crystalloid solutions and electrolytes
		   Blood and blood products
		Use formulas as basis for administering fluid resuscitation, as ordered (see Tables 64-2 and 64-3)
		Titrate fluid replacement with hourly urine output and other hemodynamic parameters, as ordered
		Start oral fluids in frequent small amounts, as ordered, with gradual increase as tolerated
		Monitor for signs of hypervolemia associated with vigorous fluid administration
		   Increase in BP, tachycardia
		   Increased CVP, PAP, cardiac output, and PCWP
		   Increased urine output
		   Marked weight gain
		   Dyspnea, wheezes, moist rales
		   Chest radiograph results revealing interstitial edema
		   Distended neck veins
		   Disorientation
		   Nausea
		Notify physician of any of these abnormalities
		Monitor for signs and symptoms of inadequate fluid replacement and continued hypovolemia
		Monitor for signs and symptoms of vascular depletion caused by increased third-space loss
		Monitor for signs and symptoms of renal failure; if renal failure occurs, see Standard 52, *Acute renal failure*
		Monitor serum and urine chemistries

■ Sepsis secondary to wound infection	■ Absence or resolution of infection	■ Use mask, sterile gown, and gloves when caring for patient Employ strict sterile technique when caring for wound

POTENTIAL PROBLEMS	EXPECTED OUTCOMES	NURSING ACTIVITIES

	Absence of clinical manifestation of infection	Administer agents to support immune mechanism according to hospital policy, (e.g., tetanus toxoid, tetanus immune globulin [Hyper-Tet], gamma globulin, convalescent plasma, pseudomonas vaccine, and hyperimmune serum, if ordered)
		Encourage personnel or visitors with upper respiratory, GI, or skin infections to avoid visiting while infected
		Keep patient utilities separate; employ disinfectant and sterilization technique for equipment or materials used for patient's care
		Debride or assist with debridement, as ordered
		Administer topical agents and wound and/or graft dressings aseptically, as ordered
		Culture all wounds, if ordered
		Shave body hair as appropriate and as ordered
		Administer prescribed dietary regimen to support defenses against infection and promote wound healing
		Monitor for signs and symptoms of infection, including
		    Leukocytosis; note CBC results daily
		    Complaint of headache, chills, malaise; decreased sensorium
		    Anorexia, nausea, vomiting
		    Increased respiratory, pulse rate
		    Decreased BP; hemodynamic instability
		    Decreased urinary output; monitor accurate intake and output q1 hr
		    Hypothermia/hyperthermia
		    Cyanosis and/or facial flushing; decreased peripheral circulation
		    Petechiae on skin; sites of bleeding
		    Decrease in bowel sounds and ileus
		    Positive culture results from wound, sputum, blood, stool, and/or urine
		Notify physician of any abnormality
		Administer therapy, as ordered
		Monitor for signs and symptoms of DIC

■ Malnutrition related to
  Inadequate intake of nutrients
  Increased metabolic requirements associated with burn injury
  Bowel dysfunction
  Hepatic/pancreatic dysfunction
	■ Absence and/or resolution of malnutrition
	  Positive nitrogen balance
	  Consumes most of recommended caloric requirements
	  Weight gain if appropriate
	  Wound healing well
		■ Assess cultural and social dietary habits, food preferences, nutritional status, and food allergies and set nutritional requirement accordingly (usually high in protein and high in calories) in collaboration with dietitian and physician
		Gradually progress to desired nutritional intake based on caloric needs and requirements, as ordered
		Administer antacid, as ordered
		Administer supplementary vitamin therapy, as ordered
		Ensure required caloric and fluid intake
		    List foods taken daily
		    Have dietitian plan meals and substitutes with patient
		    Allow home-cooked foods within set limits
		    Provide supplementary nourishment with snacks
		    Accurate intake and output
		    Daily weights
		Provide conditions conducive to eating
		    Frequent oral hygiene
		    Provide for cleaning dentures, as needed
		    Assist with eating or feed patient, if needed
		    Position for comfort, ease in reaching food
		    If tube feeding is needed
		        Ensure patency and proper location of tube
		        Place patient in semi-Fowler position
		        Aspirate feeding tube before each feeding or periodically during continuous infusion
		        Notify physician for abnormally large aspirate and heme positive test on aspirate and low pH
		        Check feedings for any change of consistency or odor
		        Warm feedings to room temperature before administering
		        Start with small amount of feeding, given as continuous drip or intermittent drip/bolus method

POTENTIAL PROBLEMS	EXPECTED OUTCOMES	NURSING ACTIVITIES
		Monitor for adverse effects: abdominal cramping, diarrhea, nausea, vomiting, gastric distention
		Notify physician if occurs; alter nutritional program, as ordered
		Slowly increase amount of feeding, as ordered
		Auscultate for bowel sounds q4-8 hr
		If hyperalimentation is required, see Standard 57, *Total parenteral nutrition*
		Ongoing assessment of nutritional status and therapy
		Weight loss and gain; state of muscle mass
		General appearance; note presence of
		Dry, flaky, and cracked skin
		Dry and discolored tongue
		Sunken eyeballs
		Loss of appetite
		Lethargy
		Poor skin turgor, flaccidity
		Delayed wound healing
		Decreased muscle control, tremors, and twitching
		Monitor GI function chemistries
■ Contractures/deformities	■ Absence and/or resolution of contractures/deformities Adherence to rehabilitation program Restoration of optimal physical function	■ Assess for areas prone to develop contractures and deformities
		Collaborate with physician and therapist regarding activities to prevent contractures and deformities
		Explain rationales for all activities
		Application of splints, traction or functional devices to fingers, limbs; evaluate for properly applied devices
		Maintain burned area in position of physiological function
		Passive and active ROM exercises q2-4 hr
		If necessary place patient in a clinically therapeutic bed (e.g., Stryker, CircOlectric) and explain rationale
		While patient is in bed, prevent contractures of burn areas as follows
		Head and anterior aspect of neck—no pillows; small foam pad may be placed under head
		Posterior aspect of neck—pillow under upper chest
		Upper chest, axilla, and arms—arms abducted at 90 degrees and slightly above shoulder level
		Ankles and feet—feet at 90 degrees; dorsiflexion at ankles using footboard
		Encourage patient to assist in care, i.e., eating
		Ambulate, as ordered
		Gradually increase patient's self-care, graded activities, and social activities as condition permits
		Use bed cradle to keep sheets off burned areas
		Maintain heat and humidity in room at comfort level
		Monitor for any increase of alkaline phosphatase and decrease in serum Ca^{++} levels, which may be associated with Ca^{++} deposition near joints and tendons
		Prepare patient for corrective/reconstructive surgery, as ordered
		Ensure intake of prescribed amount of nutrients to ensure healing
		Observe measures to prevent infection
■ Insufficient knowledge for compliance with discharge regimen*	■ Sufficient information to comply with discharge regimen Patient/family's behavior indicates successful emotional adjustment to situation	■ Assess patient/family's level of understanding, ability to comprehend, and any physical limitations regarding follow-up plan of care and discharge regimen
		Discuss patient's role in success of rehabilitation program, including patient's emotional adjustment, with patient/family and health team
		Encourage verbalization of questions, doubts, and fears

*If responsibility of critical care nurse includes such follow-up care.

POTENTIAL PROBLEMS	EXPECTED OUTCOMES	NURSING ACTIVITIES

	Patient/family correctly performs procedures, use of special equipment devices, splints, exercises, and ADL
	
	Patient/family identifies signs and symptoms of wound infection and when to notify physician
	
	Patient/family describes dietary, medication, and activity regimens
	
	Patient/family describes plan for follow-up care
		Explain thoroughly burn care with return demonstration
		  Normal bathing
		  Application of lubricating cream to burn site and grafts (e.g., lanolin-based cream)
		  Application of any antibiotics and/or dressings, as ordered
		Procure supplies, equipment, and splint for patient's use after discharge
		Demonstrate with return demonstration ROM exercises, application and use of equipment and devices
		Describe signs and symptoms of wound infection, including
		  Redness
		  Swelling
		  Tenderness, pain, and warmth to touch
		  Any sudden bleeding or drainage
		Explain and discuss
		  Need for gradual resumption of activities
		  Importance of well-balanced diet, particularly high-calorie, high-protein diet if wound is not completely healed; stress importance of maintaining appropriate weight
		  Need for medications prescribed and then identification, route, dosage, action, side effects
		Explain importance of ongoing and follow-up care, including
		  Keeping appointment for physiotherapy, if applicable
		  Purpose for visits, when and where to go, who to see, and what specimens to bring
		Provide opportunity for and encourage questions and verbalization of anxiety regarding discharge regimen and any residual disability
		Stress importance of safety measures in preventing burns
		Assess patient/family's potential compliance with discharge regimen

DISSEMINATED INTRAVASCULAR COAGULATION

Disseminated intravascular coagulation (DIC) syndrome, also known as the *defibrination syndrome, consumption coagulopathy, intravascular coagulation syndrome,* and *diffuse intravascular clotting,* is one of the most serious of the acquired coagulation disorders. It is difficult to diagnose and treat. DIC syndrome involves an abnormal activation of the clotting process, resulting in generalized consumption of platelets and clotting factors. This precipitates the formation of thrombi and emboli. Consequently, there is a widespread deposition of platelets and fibrin in the microvasculature. This precipitates the formation of thrombi and emboli. The fibrinolytic process is then activated to dissolve the fibrin clots. Fibrin-split products are one of the end products of the process of lysing the clot and have an anticoagulant effect. The overall result of a massive stimulation of the coagulation process and the activation of the fibrinolytic process results in a severe hemorrhagic diathesis. In addition to bleeding, ischemia of major organs and tissue by emboli occluding the microvasculature, and anemia caused by hemorrhage, are major clinical problems.

Normally, there is a balance between the coagulation process and the fibrinolytic process. This balance of the two processes checks the occurrence of widespread clotting or hemorrhage. The coagulation process is activated intrinsically or extrinsically. The intrinsic pathway is activated in response to endothelial damage, whereas the extrinsic pathway is activated in response to tissue injury. Despite the pathway stimulated, the end result is the same: prothrombin is converted to thrombin and fibrinogen is converted to fibrin, resulting in clot formation. The fibrinolytic process is then activated for clot dissolution.

DIC is not usually seen as a primary disorder but results as a secondary complication of another disease. It is postulated that the primary disease may damage the cells that stimulate the coagulation process. The coagulation process can be activated by means of the intrinsic or extrinsic pathway, depending on whether the damage occurred to endothelial cells or other tissue.

DIC has been associated with conditions including overwhelming viral or bacterial sepsis and shock, especially gram-negative septicemia and acute severe hemolysis; abruptio placentae; carcinoma, particularly if metastases are present; coagulopathies associated with liver failure; and a variety of other circumstances in which thromboplastic materials may enter the circulation or in which diffuse endothelial damage is present.

Generally accepted clinical criteria for the diagnosis of DIC include depletion of coagulation Factors V and VIII and fibrinogen (less than 100 mg/100 ml); thrombocytopenia (less than 100,000/mm^3); production of excessive amounts of circulating fibrin-split products; and increased fibrinolytic activity of the blood. Prolonged PT and APTT time are also possible clinical indicators of DIC.

In acute DIC, hemorrhagic manifestations generally predominate as seen in petechiae and GI bleeding. Other signs and symptoms may include severe abdominal, back, and muscle pain; nausea and vomiting; dyspnea and acrocyanosis (generalized diaphoresis with mottled, cold fingers and toes); convulsion, coma, and shock.

The major goal—to stop the hemorrhage—is accomplished by terminating the accelerated coagulation process. Heparin is the agent of choice. The ultimate cure, however, depends on accurate diagnosis and proper treatment of the primary disease that precipitated the DIC syndrome.

Although heparin is the usual agent of choice, it should be administered early in the course of treatment to be most effective.

Once heparin therapy has been initiated, replacement therapy (use of blood, platelets, fresh frozen plasma, and cryoprecipitate) may be required for severe depletion of platelets and coagulation factors. Packed RBCs provide RBC replacement with less volume than whole blood, because the plasma has been extracted. Fresh frozen plasma is an excellent source of several clotting factors and fibrinogen. Fresh frozen plasma is kept frozen until its use. It should not be stored after thawing, because the factors are degraded in the prolonged thawed state. Platelets, which should not be refrigerated, are prepared from whole blood and are indicated for thrombocytopenia. Cryoprecipitate is a concentrated source of clotting factors and fibrinogen. Any replacement therapy should follow initiation of heparin; otherwise the blood and blood products will also be rapidly consumed in the accelerated coagulation process.

The overall therapy for DIC can be very complex and is associated with considerable risk.

ASSESSMENT

1. History, presence, and nature of
   a. Sudden onset of hemorrhage associated with profound circulatory collapse
   b. Underlying conditions precipitating DIC, i.e., infections, carcinomas, leukemias, immune complex diseases, obstetrical conditions, etc.
   c. Thromboembolic diathesis as manifested by angina, confusion, convulsions, coma, fever, and azotemia
   d. Coagulation disorders, i.e., vitamin K deficiency and deficiency of Factors VIII and IX
   e. Intake of medications that alter the coagulation mechanism, e.g., aspirin, coumadin
   f. Hepatic abnormalities with or without hepatomegaly
   g. Hemarthrosis, i.e., blood in joint space
   h. Diffuse bleeding from body orifices, venipuncture and incisional sites, respiratory, renal, or upper GI tract
   i. Ecchymosis, hematomas, hematuria, and menorrhagia
   j. Arterial hypotension often associated with shock
2. Lab and diagnostic data, including
   a. Platelet counts indicate thrombocytopenia
   b. Clotting factors depleted in plasma, i.e., reduced fibrinogen with increased fibrinogen degradation products and decreased Factors V and VIII
   c. Other coagulation tests: results of PT or APTT tests are usually prolonged
   d. Presence of fragmented RBCs in peripheral blood
   e. Arterial blood gas results indicating acidosis
   f. ECG for any arrhythmias
   g. Chest radiograph for presence of reactive interstitial edema associated with diffuse deposition of microemboli in the lungs
   h. Results of throat, blood, sputum, urine, and stool cultures
3. Patient/family's knowledge and understanding of disease process, diagnostic procedures, and therapy planned
4. Patient/family's level of anxiety related to disease process, therapy employed, and anticipated prognosis

GOALS

1. Reduction of patient/family's anxiety with provision of information and explanations
2. Hemodynamic stability—adequate perfusion of central and peripheral organ systems
3. Respiratory function sufficient to maintain adequate oxygenation and ventilation; absence of respiratory distress syndrome
4. Rapid resolution or control of impaired coagulation
5. Resolution of the underlying conditions associated with DIC
6. Prevention of complications associated with generalized bleeding diathesis and thrombosis
7. Adequate intake of nutrients, vitamins to meet calculated daily requirements, to maintain weight or to achieve weight gain
8. Sufficient information for compliance with discharge regimen; patient/family is able to
   a. Accurately describe activity, dietary, and medication regimen
   b. Identify signs and symptoms requiring medical attention
   c. Describe plan for follow-up care

POTENTIAL PROBLEMS	EXPECTED OUTCOMES	NURSING ACTIVITIES
■ Patient/family's anxiety related to Insufficient knowledge of disease process, diagnostic procedures, and therapy employed	■ Patient/family's behavior demonstrates decreased level of anxiety with provision of information and explanations	■ Ongoing assessment of level of patient/family's anxiety
	Patient/family verbalizes understanding of disease process and its relation to diagnostic procedures and therapy employed	Assess patient/family's knowledge and understanding of disease process, anticipated diagnostic procedures, and therapy employed
		Describe the nature of disease syndrome, reasons for signs and symptoms patient is experiencing, and rationales for various diagnostic and therapeutic interventions to be employed
	Patient/family verbalizes questions, fears, and any anxieties related to aforementioned	Explain and assist in preparing patient for anticipated diagnostic procedures
		Encourage patient/family's questions, verbalization of fears and anxieties
	Patient/family participates actively in planning and implementing care	Involve patient/family in planning and assessing care
		Provide reassurance
		Evaluate for decrease in level of anxiety with provision of information and explanations
		Provide appropriate consultation for patient/family with clergy and social service

POTENTIAL PROBLEMS	EXPECTED OUTCOMES	NURSING ACTIVITIES
Pain	Relief of pain Reduction in nonverbal evidence of pain	Assess behavioral response to pain, intensity, location, and associated LOC Offer and/or administer pain medications, as ordered; if IM or subcutaneous route is used, use small-bore needles Position for utmost comfort with proper body alignment Encourage patient to verbalize fears and anxieties related to pain and course of disease process Apply warm and cold compresses on joints, as ordered; if needed, use bed cradle and immobilized affected joint Plan nursing activities to allow uninterrupted rest periods Support patient/family Evaluate for reduction of pain
■ Impaired coagulation as evidenced by Thrombosis formation with consumption of platelets and coagulation factors Hemorrhage Hypotension Acidosis	■ Early resolution of impaired coagulation Hemodynamic stability Normotensive Arterial blood gas levels within normal limits	■ Prevent by administering immediate therapy for presence of etiological factors, including sepsis, cancer, leukemias, immunological abnormalities, obstetrical complications Monitor for Any bleeding including occult, internal, hemorrhaging from orifices, mild oozing from injection sites; petechiae and ecchymosis Hematest results on all urine, stool, and emesis Signs and symptoms that may indicate DIC without bleeding include fatigue, malaise, weakness, myalgia, peripheral thrombosis, sudden vision changes, hypotension, acrocyanosis (generalized sweating with mottled, cold toes and fingers), nausea and vomiting, severe muscle, back, abdominal, bone, and joint pain; dyspnea and cyanosis, oliguria; convulsions, coma, and shock Lab test results for prolonged APTT and PT; thrombocytopenia; low fibrinogen levels; elevated fibrin-split products, strongly positive protamine sulfate test; reduced factor assay levels, particularly II, V, and VII; CBC for decreased Hct, Hgb, and leukocytosis; electrolytes for hyperkalemia; and arterial blood gas levels for decreased bicarbonate levels and acidosis Hypotension and hyperthermia/hypothermia, vital signs including temperature q2 hr and prn Quality of peripheral pulses Changes in mental status, i.e., headaches, vertigo, irritability, and confusion Chest radiograph results for infiltrate or pleurisy Notify physician of any abnormalities If problem occurs Administer blood products as ordered; observe necessary precautions, which include Monitoring vital signs and temperature before, during, and after transfusion, and monitoring for any untoward reaction, i.e., skin reactions Double-checking patient's name and product on label before administration Using ultrafilter in transfusing blood and packed cells Administer heparin if ordered and monitor lab results, i.e., APTT accordingly Estimate blood loss Daily weights Serial Hgb and Hct results q12-24 hr and prn Measure intake and all drainage, i.e., NG drainage, melena, urine output Administer adequate nutritional intake, as ordered, in small frequent feedings Prevent further bleeding Mouth care Use soft toothbrush or cotton swabs with mild mouthwash

POTENTIAL PROBLEMS	EXPECTED OUTCOMES	NURSING ACTIVITIES
		May use carbonated drinks to break crust in mouth without bleeding
		Apply liquid lubricant on lips
		Medications
		Given preferably by oral, rectal, and IV routes
		Use smallest gauge needle, rotate sites, and apply steady pressure for 3 to 5 minutes whenever injections are given
		Use electric shaver to reduce any incidence of abrasions
		Administer stool softeners as ordered, if needed
		Handle patient gently at all times to protect skin and prevent mucosal trauma
		Elevate head if patient is dyspneic, and administer O_2 if ordered
		Apply cold and/or hot compresses as appropriate for joint and bone pain; use bed cradle and immobilize affected area
		Refer to monitoring activities to detect further signs and symptoms of bleeding
		Notify physician of any abnormalities
■ Insufficient knowledge to comply with discharge regimen*	■ Patient/family has sufficient information to comply with discharge regimen	■ Assess patient/family's level of understanding and ability to comprehend follow-up plan of care and discharge regimen
	Patient/family accurately describes medication, dietary, and activity regimens	Explain relationship of disease process to prescribed therapy
	Patient/family identifies signs and symptoms requiring medical attention	Provide required information so that before discharge patient/family is able to
	Patient/family accurately describes plans for follow-up care	Describe medication regimen
		Names of drugs and purpose
		Specific dosage schedule
		Expected adverse side effects, how to deal with them, and when to notify physician
		Describe activity regimen
		Describe dietary regimen, i.e., therapeutic diet, if ordered
		If recurrence of underlying condition is possible, describe signs and symptoms
		Describe follow-up visits including purpose for, when and where to go, who to see, and what specimens to bring
		Provide opportunity for and encourage patient/family's questions and verbalization
		Assess patient/family's potential compliance with discharge regimen

*If responsibility of critical care nurse includes such follow-up care.

DRUG OVERDOSE

Drug overdose is commonly seen in the emergency facility. Prescription drugs as well as over-the-counter agents supply the adult with a variety of avenues for self-inflicted harm. Attempted suicide accounts for most drug-induced emergencies, often related to a traumatic life event surrounding the incident of drug ingestion. Bereavement is one of the most common crises implicated in drug overdose. Sometimes the anticipation of an event precipitates the drug ingestion. The commonly seen drugs in the overdose situation are barbiturates, narcotics, sedatives, aspirin, acetaminophen, and tranquilizers. Less often, overdose includes the abuse of amphetamines, anticholinergics, and opiates.

Diagnosis of drug overdose is confirmed by history, signs and symptoms, and lab values. The history must include time and amount of ingestion, substance used, recent significant life events, and prior psychiatric support. Often, histories are conflicting or absent, and diagnosis is contingent on symptomatology and lab data.

Signs and symptoms of drug overdose vary with the drug ingested. CNS involvement, ranging from lethargy and coma to confusion and convulsions, is a common presenting deficit. Respiratory depression or stimulation and cardiac arrhythmias leading to cardiopulmonary collapse often follow. Fluid and electrolyte imbalance, aspiration pneumonia, and disturbances in acid-base balance may complicate the clinical picture.

Lab data is essential in the diagnosis and treatment of drug overdose. Toxicology screens of blood, urine, and gastric contents are important values in early management. Liver function tests, CBC, electrolyte levels, and arterial blood gas measurements are observed throughout the clinical course to assess complications of drug ingestion.

Treatment is initially aimed at identification and removal of the ingested substance. The induction of emesis in the conscious patient is begun only after ingestion of a strong acid or base is ruled out. The comatose patient or the patient having a seizure is lavaged through a large-bore gastric tube. Charcoal administration after gastric lavage or emesis binds toxic metabolites, and ionic cathartics facilitate removal of drug byproducts. Forced alkaline diuresis may be instituted early in overdose management. If the drug that was used is known, prompt administration of drug-specific antidotes other than charcoal, if available, reverses toxic effects or prevent further absorption.

Supportive care of the overdose victim is determined by the body systems compromised and the drug ingested. CNS manifestations are controlled through management of agitation, convulsions, or depression. Respiratory hyperactivity is managed with prevention of metabolic disturbance, and respiratory depression is supported mechanically. Maintenance of fluid and electrolyte balance prevents shock and renal damage.

The variety and combination of drug-induced emergencies demand constant assessment (see Table 17). Frequently, organ compromise is delayed or prolonged because of drug interaction, concurrent alcohol intake, or prior system failure. Drug overdose patients require critical care assessment and monitoring for the prevention and treatment of life-threatening system disturbance.

Nursing management also includes patient and family support as well as continual assessment of lingering suicidal tendencies. Protection of the patient from further self-inflicted harm is first in nursing prevention. Nursing awareness of fluctuating neurological states, ranging from combativeness to coma, allows for anticipation of secondary life-threatening events. Throughout the hospital stay, the patient's need for nonjudgmental support is important to successful verbalization and staff management of the crisis. The family and/or significant others are recognized as support systems and are addressed educationally and emotionally about the overdose event. Follow-up counselling for the patient and family is stressed when the diagnosis of overdose is confirmed.

Table 66-1 illustrates the manifestations of the major drug overdose emergencies.

ASSESSMENT

1. Detailed history of incident
   a. Identification of drug ingested
   b. Estimation of amount of drug ingested
   c. Combination of drugs ingested
   d. Combination of alcohol and drug
   e. Estimation of time of incident

TABLE 66-1. Clinical manifestations of drug overdose

DRUG	NEUROLOGICAL	RESPIRATORY	CARDIOVASCULAR	METABOLIC
Aspirin	Hyperthermia Stimulation	Hyperpnea Respiratory alkalosis	Hypertension	GI hemmorrhage Metabolic acidosis
Acetaminophen	Hypothermia Depression	Normal	Normal	Hepatocellular ne- crosis GI irritability
Anticholinergics	Hyperthermia Stimulation Dilatated pupils Seizures Hyperreflexia	Compromise caused by cardiovascular col- lapse Decreased rate	Tachycardia Hypotension Ventricular arrhythmias	Low serum K+ Urinary retention Ileus
Tricyclic antide- pressants	Hyperthermia Stimulation Dilatated pupils Seizures Hyperreflexia	Compromise caused by cardiovascular col- lapse Decreased rate	Tachycardia Hypotension Ventricular arrhythmia	Low serum K+ Urinary retention Ileus
Barbiturates Slow-acting	Hypothermia Early CNS depression Nystagmus Abnormal deep tendon reflexes	Depression Respiratory arrest Pneumonia Pulmonary edema	Hypotension Dilatation of circulatory tree because of di- minished autonomic nervous system in- nervation	Hypoglycemia Skin blisters
Long-acting	Hypothermia CNS depression hours after ingestion	Depression Respiratory arrest Pulmonary edema Pneumonia	Hypotension Dilatation of circulatory tree	Hypoglycemia
Narcotics	Hypothermia Pinpoint pupils, unless hypoxic Stupor Spinal cord stimulation Spasticity Hyperreflexia	Depression	Hypotension caused by decreased sympa- thetic tone Dilatated periphery	Dry mouth
Benzodiazepines	Hypothermia Dilatated pupils Slow pupil response Depressed Coma	Depression	Irritable myocardium Hypotension	Vomiting Dry mouth
Amphetamines	Hyperthermia Nervous Dilatated pupils Convulsions Muscle spasm	Stimulation	Tachycardia Hypertension Arrhythmias	Nausea Vomiting
Cholinergics	Normothermia Tremors Headache Convulsions Coma	Dyspnea Pulmonary edema	Bradycardia Complete heart block	Anorexia Diarrhea Cramping
Sedative/hyp- notics	Hypothermia Lethargy Coma Hyporeflexia	Depression Cyanosis	Collapse Hypotension	Vomiting

LAVAGE	ANTIDOTE	NURSING MANAGEMENT	TREATMENT
Lavage with saline up to several hours after ingestion	Aluminum hydroxide	Transfuse prn Vitamin K for abnormal clotting factors	Sodium bicarbonate Fluid diuresis K$^+$ supplement
Ipecac, 30 ml, with several glasses H$_2$O Gastric lavage if comatose	Acetylsysteine, up to 72 hours after ingestion	Avoid steroids, antihistamines, phenobarbital, which increase toxicity of metabolite	Treat for hepatic encephalopathy
Lavage with normal saline	Charcoal, 50 to 100 g, initially Physostigmine, 2 mg, over 2 to 3 min; repeat q15 min	Lidocaine, procainamide, quinidine are contraindicated because they depress myocardium, enhance toxicity	Sodium bicarbonate Hyperventilate if on ventilator Propranolol for tachycardia
Lavage with normal saline	Charcoal, 50 to 100 g initially Physostigmine, 2 mg, over 2 to 3 min; repeat q15 min	Lidocaine, procainamide, quinidine are contraindicated because they depress myocardium, enhance toxicity	Sodium bicarbonate Hyperventilate if on ventilator Propranolol for tachycardia
Lavage; use Ewald tube	Charcoal, 50 to 100 g initially; repeat q12 h, with 20 to 60 g	Fluid replacement for hypotension No pressors One ampule dextrose 50%	Osmotic alkaline diuresis
Lavage with normal saline	Charcoal, as above	Monitor for pulmonary edema	Forced alkaline diuresis Hemodialysis Hemoperfusion
Lavage with normal saline	Naloxone, 0.4 mg IV; repeat q5 min until 3.2 mg total is given; this may induce vomiting	Maintain airway Check for pulmonary edema, noncardiac	Observe for cardiac or respiratory arrest
Lavage with normal saline	Charcoal, as above	Respiratory support, airway	Hydration
Forced emesis or lavage if comatose	Sedation, as ordered	Observe for arrhythmias, seizures	Phentolamine, propranolol, as adrenergic blockers
Lavage with normal saline	Atropine, 0.4 mg IV	Observe for seizures, arrest	Atropine, as ordered
Lavage with normal saline	Charcoal, as above	Be aware that excretion route is kidneys Support compromised systems	Hydration

f. Explanation of precipitating life crisis
g. Identification of support systems
2. Physical signs and symptoms
   a. Neurological
      (1) Depression
      (2) Agitation
      (3) Mental status changes
      (4) Headache
      (5) Pupil reaction, size
      (6) Visual changes
      (7) Convulsions
      (8) Hallucinations
      (9) Hyperreflexia
      (10) Absent reflexes
      (11) Gag reflex
      (12) Vertigo
      (13) Slurred speech
      (14) Spasticity
   b. Respiratory
      (1) Respiratory depression, apnea
      (2) Hyperventilation
      (3) Rales
      (4) Wheezes
      (5) Salivation changes
   c. Cardiovascular
      (1) Arrhythmia
      (2) Hypotension
      (3) Hypertension
      (4) Alteration in heart rate
      (5) Peripheral pulses
   d. Renal
      (1) Anuria
      (2) Oliguria
      (3) Alteration in urine pH
      (4) Alteration in urine concentration
   e. Temperature
      (1) Hypothermia
      (2) Hyperthermia
   f. Fluid and electrolyte levels
      (1) Skin turgor
      (2) Mucous membrane turgor
      (3) ECG changes
      (4) Muscle cramping
   g. GI
      (1) Nausea
      (2) Vomiting
      (3) Diarrhea
      (4) Abnormal vomitus, stool
      (5) Abdominal cramping
      (6) Bleeding
3. Monitor lab values for
   a. Toxicology screen
   b. Arterial blood gas levels
   c. CBC
   d. Electrolytes
   e. BUN
   f. Creatinine
   g. Glucose
   h. Urinalysis
   i. Urine chemistry screen
   j. Liver function tests
4. Psychosocial aspect of incident
   a. Significant others
   b. Precipitating stressor
   c. History of prior attempts
   d. Effect of incident on patient, significant others (shame, depression)

GOALS

1. Return to baseline CNS status
2. Respiratory sufficiency; adequate oxygenation and ventilation, with arterial blood gas levels within patient's normal limits
3. Hemodynamic stability; adequate cardiac output, peripheral perfusion, normovolemia, absence of arrhythmia
4. Parameters of renal function within normal limits
5. Normothermia
6. Fluid and electrolyte balance
7. Absence of GI irritability
8. Infection-free state
9. Absence of overdose recurrence
10. Understanding of hospital routine
11. Before discharge the patient/family:
    a. Demonstrates comprehension of the effects of drug intake
    b. Identifies specific factors that encourage drug ingestion
    c. Identifies symptoms requiring medical attention and appropriate actions to take to obtain it
    d. Asks pertinent questions regarding self-care

POTENTIAL PROBLEMS	EXPECTED OUTCOMES	NURSING ACTIVITIES

■ Altered LOC	■ LOC within normal limits
	Patient oriented to time,
	place, person
		■ Administer the following, as ordered
		  Specific antidote
		  Saline lavage
		  Charcoal
		  Diuresis
		Assess patient's response
		Monitor for
		  CNS depression
		    Stupor
		    Lethargy
		    Coma
		  CNS stimulation
		    Hyperactivity
		    Seizures
		    Confusion
		Notify physician of any abnormality
		If CNS depression occurs
		  Stimulate CNS
		    Attempt to arouse patient through verbal stimulation
		    Allow family to talk to patient
		    Turn frequently to encourage movement
		    If no response occurs, assess the following carefully
		      Pain response
		      Response to sternal or fingernail pressure
		  Observe neurological parameters, e.g.
		    Pupil size, reaction
		    LOC
		    Reflexes
		    Pain response
		    Orientation
		    Vital signs
		    Extremity strength
		If CNS stimulation occurs
		  Sedate cautiously, as ordered
		If seizures occur
		  Protect from harm
		  Observe seizure for
		    Length
		    Extremities affected
		    Progression
		    Muscles involved
		    Eye, tongue deviation
		  Maintain patent airway
		    Insert oral airway
		    Turn to side
		    Suction
		    Administer O_2, as ordered
		    Prevent aspiration
		  Administer anticonvulsants, as ordered
		  Observe LOC before, during, and after seizure

■ Alterations in respiratory
state; depression or
stimulation of respiratory center by drug
	■ Absence or resolution of
	signs and symptoms of
	respiratory depression or
	stimulation
	Adequate oxygenation and
	ventilation with arterial
	blood gas levels within
	normal limits
		■ Monitor for alterations in respiratory status
		  Changes in rate
		  Changes in depth
		  Dyspnea
		  Skin color changes
		  Changes in quality, patterns of respirations
		  Changes in arterial blood gas levels
		Promote adequate respiratory function
		  Turn and position q2 h
		  Administer chest physiotherapy q4 h

POTENTIAL PROBLEMS	EXPECTED OUTCOMES	NURSING ACTIVITIES
		If altered respiratory status occurs, administer the following, as ordered O₂ therapy Mechanical ventilation

■ Cardiovascular collapse related to drug ingestion	■ Adequate cardiac output
	Hemodynamic stability
	BP and peripheral perfusion within normal limits
		■ Monitor circulatory parameters, especially for the following alterations
		Hypotension
		Hypertension
		Changes in heart rate
		Arrhythmias
		Change in mental status
		Pallor
		Poor peripheral pulses
		Rapid respirations
		Change in skin temperature
		Thirst
		Poor skin turgor
		Decreased CVP, PCWP
		If cardiovascular collapse occurs, monitor the following
		Cardiac rhythm, rate
		Vital signs
		Peripheral perfusion
		  Pulses
		  LOC
		  Urine output
		  Color
		CVP, PCWP
		Intake/output q1 h
		Arterial blood gas
		Administer the following, as ordered
		Fluid challenge
		Transfusions
		O₂, ventilatory support
		Medications

■ Renal dysfunction related to drug metabolites, hypoperfusion	■ Indices of renal function within normal limits
	Hemodynamic stability
	Cardiac output, BP, P within normal limits
		■ Monitor renal function through observation of
		Lab data
		  Creatinine
		  BUN
		  Urinalysis
		  Specific gravity
		  Serum electrolytes
		  Urine electrolytes
		Change in urine output
		  Oliguria
		  Anuria
		Change in fluid state
		  Edema
		Change in mental state
		  Confusion
		  Drowsiness
		Cardiac arrhythmias
		  Electrolyte imbalance
		Change in weight
		Change in BP
		If hypotension or renal dysfunction occur, administer the following therapy, as ordered
		Manage hypovolemic shock with fluid replacement
		Record intake/output q1 h

POTENTIAL PROBLEMS	EXPECTED OUTCOMES	NURSING ACTIVITIES
		Monitor and manage metabolic acidosis by arterial blood gas analysis
		Replenish electrolyte loss
		Administer medications such as sodium bicarbonate, mannitol, as ordered
		Prepare for dialysis, if indicated; see Standard 52, *Renal Failure;* Standard 53, *Peritoneal Dialysis;* Standard 54, *Hemodialysis*
■ Temperature changes related to drug effect on basal metabolic rate	■ Restoration of normal body temperature	■ Monitor body temperature q2 h, specifically observing for Hyperthermia Hypothermia If hypothermia occurs, administer the following, as indicated Blankets Warming mattress If hyperthermia occurs, administer the following, as ordered Cooling blanket Sponge bath

■ Fluid and electrolyte imbalance caused by drug metabolism	■ Electrolyte balance within normal limit
	Normovolemia
	BP, P, CVP, PCWP, and urine output within normal limits
	Baseline weight maintained
		■ Monitor for alteration in fluid and electrolyte balance
		Weight
		Fluid balance
		Hydration status
		  Edema
		  Rales
		  Specific gravity
		  Abnormal skin turgor
		  Mucous membranes
		  Thirst
		  BP
		  Pulse (thready, bounding)
		  Intake/output ratio
		  Lab data
		    Serum osmolality
		    Urine osmolality
		    Serum electrolytes
		    Urine electrolytes
		    Hct
		If fluid and/or electrolyte imbalance occur
		Monitor the following
		  Vital signs q1 h
		  Cardiac rhythm
		  Daily weights
		  Lab data
		  Intake/output q1 h
		Administer the following, as ordered
		  Fluid replacement, diuresis
		  Electrolyte replacement

■ GI irritability caused by drug ingestion	■ GI function within normal limits Absence of signs and symptoms of GI distress	■ Monitor for Nausea Vomiting Diarrhea Abdominal cramping Distention Bleeding If GI irritability occurs Observe symptoms Treat pain, as ordered Measure fluid loss and replace, as ordered Monitor electrolyte and blood loss and replace, as ordered

POTENTIAL PROBLEMS	EXPECTED OUTCOMES	NURSING ACTIVITIES
■ Superinfection, related to aspiration pneumonia, increased susceptibility	■ Absence or resolution of infection	■ Prevention Provide for 　Adequate nutritional intake, as ordered 　Place patient in low to semi-Fowler position to prevent aspiration 　Inflate tracheal tube cuff, if patient is intubated Monitor for the following 　Change in temperature 　Alterations in WBC count 　Changes in urine, blood, or sputum cultures 　Changes on radiograph 　Adventitious breath sounds 　　Rales 　　Rhonchi 　　Diminished breath sounds 　Sputum color, consistency 　Urine color, odor If superinfection occurs 　Administer antibiotics, as ordered 　Check temperature q2 h; note hyperthermia 　Administer sponge bath, if needed 　Apply cooling blanket, as ordered 　Administer fluids for adequate hydration, as ordered
■ Recurrence of overdose related to inadequate resolution of crisis, insufficient education	■ Patient/family demonstrates 　Acceptance of limitations 　Knowledge of stressors 　Awareness of new coping mechanisms	■ Inform patient and family about drug and its effects Discuss impact of stress Assist patient in identifying support systems Encourage participation in support group Encourage verbalization of fears Provide for psychiatric support and follow-up on unit, mobilizing other resources, as indicated (i.e., psychiatrist)
■ Emotional trauma secondary to hospitalization	■ Understanding of hospital suicide precautions Understanding and acceptance of psychiatric evaluation	■ Explain hospital routine Impart nonjudgmental, caring attitude Reinforce integrity Allow verbalization about incident Encourage family and significant others to participate in rehabilitation
■ Poor compliance with psychiatric follow-up, poor understanding of overdose implications	■ Patient/family indicates compliance with discharge regimen as evidenced by Comprehension of drug effects Comprehension of overdose hazards Understanding of need for support, medical and familial Identifies symptoms of drug ingestion Family awareness of drug effects, implications, need for follow-up	■ Encourage family support of patient Assess understanding of problem Plan time for interaction Monitor patient's ability to verbalize with/without family Assess patient/family coping mechanisms Monitor ability to deal with anger, depression Explore constructive release mechanisms Support psychiatric follow-up Explore patient's feelings about psychiatrist Monitor patient's interest in care through asking questions

POISONING

Poisoning is one of the most common pediatric medical emergencies among young children. Boys are more frequently involved than girls, and the physically active, mobile, and curious child under 5 years of age is most vulnerable. The younger child has a tendency to ingest common household items, the older child, medicines. Almost one half of all poisonings occur in the kitchen, and one fifth occur in the bathroom. The more common causes of poisoning in children under 5 years old are aspirin, soaps, detergents, cleansers, bleaches, vitamins, minerals, insecticides, plants, polishes and waxes, hormones, tranquilizers and other analgesics, and antipyretics; as acetaminophen use increases.

The diagnosis of poisoning is made by history, presenting signs and symptoms, and lab data. The signs and symptoms of poisoning are also common to many conditions of childhood, making diagnosis difficult without a positive history. The possibility of poisoning should always be considered in children who present with signs and symptoms of questionable etiology.

Signs and symptoms of poisoning by ingestion, inhalation, or skin absorption may include GI disturbances with anorexia, vomiting, diarrhea, and abdominal pain. Symptoms of CNS involvement may occur and are usually of either depression or stimulation. Depression of the CNS can result in lethargy, stupor, and coma. Stimulation can result in convulsions, restlessness, and confusion. Further symptoms of poisoning may include shock, cardiac arrhythmias, and cardiac failure. There may be notable gray cyanosis that develops as a result of the conversion of hemoglobin to methemoglobin when specific drugs and chemical poisons are present. The patient may become oxygen depleted and have respiratory symptomatology. Other symptoms may develop as a result of the poisoning.

The lab tests used for diagnosis are those specific for identification of the toxic substance. Specimens from the stomach, blood, and urine are analyzed.

The general method of treatment of acute poisoning is identification and removal of the substance, prevention of further absorption, facilitation of elimination, administration of an antidote, and supportive therapy of the various organ systems related to symptomatology.

In the emergency room, treatment is directed toward identification and removal of the poison. If the substance is not caustic or is not a hydrocarbon, removal by emesis or lavage will be instituted. Vomiting is never induced if the child is comatose or having seizures. The goal is to remove the substance before absorption. To facilitate the removal of the poison, fluid diuresis and, in a few specific instances, dialysis may be used.

Additional measures to prevent further absorption of the substance are often necessary, because all gastric contents are not removed by these techniques.

Antidotes may be administered to inactivate the ingested substance. Activated charcoal is a common local antidote. There are some specific antidotes for particular substances ingested; however, these are relatively few. If the ingested substance is caustic, attempts will be made to neutralize it and to prevent its absorption.

Once emergency treatment has been rendered, general supportive therapy becomes the priority. This type of therapy is greatly dependent on the substance involved and its actions on body systems.

The CNS may be affected and control of seizures and treatment of agitation or depression may be required. Respiratory support for adequate respiratory exchange may be necessary. Treatment of shock with fluids and replacement of electrolyte losses as well as prevention of renal failure may also be part of supportive therapy. Other vital functions may be seriously affected. It is for these reasons that children in an acute poisoning episode are at risk and have need for critical care.

ASSESSMENT

1. Careful history surrounding poisoning incident
   a. Identification of ingested substance
   b. Estimation of how much was ingested
   c. When ingestion occurred
2. Physical signs and symptoms
   a. Neurological
      (1) Agitation
      (2) Depression
      (3) Convulsions
      (4) Delirium

(5) Headache
(6) Mental changes
(7) Disturbances of equilibrium
(8) Pupil response
(9) Visual disturbance

b. Cardiac
(1) Alteration in heart rate
(2) Arrhythmia
(3) Hypotension

c. Renal
(1) Anuria
(2) Hematuria
(3) Oliguria
(4) Color of urine

d. Respiratory
(1) Hyperventilation
(2) Respiratory depression
(3) Coughs
(4) Wheezes
(5) Rales
(6) Abnormal odor on breath
(7) Alteration in salivation

e. GI
(1) Nausea
(2) Vomiting
(3) Diarrhea
(4) Abnormal color of vomitus and stool

f. Temperature
(1) Hypothermia
(2) Hyperthermia

g. Skin
(1) Burns
(2) Interruption of skin integrity
(3) Edema
(4) Cyanosis
(5) Skin staining or discoloration
(6) Hair loss

(7) Absence or presence of perspiration
(8) Abnormal color of tissues

3. Monitor lab data for results of
   a. CBC
   b. Serum electrolytes
   c. Blood glucose
   d. Blood levels of specific ingested substance
   e. Blood gas levels
   f. BUN
   g. Creatinine
   h. Urinalysis
   i. Urine chemistry

4. Developmental level of the child
   a. Effect of incident on child (guilt, punishment)
   b. Effect of hospitalization on child
   c. Developmental tasks according to age

5. Response of parents to child's illness and hospitalization
   a. Level of anxiety
   b. Guilt
   c. Degree of understanding on incident and therapeutic management

GOALS

1. Restoration of normal CNS functioning
2. Normal cardiac function and circulatory perfusion
3. Normal renal function
4. Normal respiratory function
5. Normal fluid and electrolyte function
6. Resolution of GI irritation
7. Restoration of normal body temperature–regulating system
8. Absence of infection
9. Supportive therapy for child and family during crisis period
10. Effective parental coping mechanisms
11. Hospitalization as positive developmental experience
12. Discharge planning related to prevention

POTENTIAL PROBLEMS	EXPECTED OUTCOMES	NURSING ACTIVITIES
■ Alteration of CNS related to toxic action of poison involved	■ Detection of alteration Supportive therapy Return to optimal level of functioning	■ Prevent by Administration of specific antidote for ingested substance Early detection of further CNS changes Monitor for Stimulation Confusion Restlessness Delirium Convulsions Depression Lethargy Stupor Coma NOTE: CNS depression is ominous complication of poisoning

POTENTIAL PROBLEMS	EXPECTED OUTCOMES	NURSING ACTIVITIES
		Intervention if problem occurs
		Stimulation
		Cautious administration of sedatives
		Convulsions
		Protect patient from injury
		Observe seizure
		Activity and progression
		Muscular involvement
		Body parts involved
		Tongue deviation
		Duration of seizure
		Determine LOC before, during, and after seizure
		Administer anticonvulsants, as ordered by physician
		Maintain adequate ventilation and airway
		Insert airway if possible (only when jaw is relaxed)
		Side-lying position
		Suction
		O_2
		See Standard 41, *Seizures*
		Depression
		Stimulation of CNS
		Serial observation of the following
		Vital signs
		LOC
		Orientation
		Pupil size and reaction to light
		Muscle strength of extremities
		Reflexes
		Response to pain
▪ Peripheral circulatory collapse related to toxic action of poison	▪ Restore and maintain adequate circulatory blood volume and tissue perfusion	▪ Prevent by
		Continuous monitoring of indices of circulatory perfusion
		Monitor for
		Change in skin temperature
		Pallor
		Declining BP
		Rapid shallow respirations
		Rapid, thready pulse
		Thirst
		Restlessness, nervousness, apprehension
		Change in LOC
		Change in temperature
		Declining CVP
		GI disturbances
		Intervention if problem occurs
		Serial monitoring of vital signs
		Serial measurement of CVP
		Volume expansion through IV administration, as indicated and as ordered
		Intake and output q1 hr
		Administration of medication, as ordered
		Body positioning
		Blood gas analysis
		Administration of O_2
		Respiratory support
		Cardiac monitoring
▪ Renal damage related to toxic action of poison involved or renal ischemia produced by shock	▪ Indices of renal function within normal limits	▪ Prevent by
		Continuous monitoring of parameters of circulatory perfusion and renal function

POTENTIAL PROBLEMS	EXPECTED OUTCOMES	NURSING ACTIVITIES
		Monitor for
		Change in lab data
		BUN
		Creatinine
		Urinalysis
		Specific gravity
		Urine electrolytes
		Serum electrolytes
		ECG
		Change in urine output
		Decreased volume
		Presence of edema
		Change in mentation
		Drowsiness
		Disorientation
		Change in cardiac rhythm
		Arrhythmia related to electrolyte imbalance
		Change in weight
		Change in BP
		Intervention if problem occurs
		Management of shock, as ordered
		Management of metabolic acidosis, as ordered
		IV fluid and electrolyte replacement
		IV fluid and electrolyte maintenance
		Accurate measurement and recording of intake and output
		Administration of medications, as ordered
		Mannitol
		Furosemide
		Dialysis
		Peritoneal (see Standard 53, *Peritoneal dialysis*)
		Hemodialysis (see Standard 54, *Hemodialysis*)
■ Alteration of respiratory function related to respiratory depression and/or obstruction	■ Respiratory function normal as indicated by arterial blood gas levels	■ Prevent by
		Continuous monitoring of respiratory status
		Implementation of medical and nursing regimen to provide and maintain adequate respiratory function
		Monitor for
		Change in arterial blood gas levels
		Change in respiratory status
		Rate
		Depth
		Quality
		Degree of difficulty
		Color
		Intervention if problem occurs
		Respiratory support
		O_2 therapy
		Intubation
		Mechanical ventilation (see Standard 6, *Mechanical ventilation*)
■ Fluid and/or electrolyte imbalance related to poisoning episode	■ Weight within normal limits	■ Prevent by
	Electrolytes within normal parameters	Parenteral maintenance
		Fluid replacement
		Electrolyte replacement according to serum levels and maintenance requirements
		Monitor for
		Change in fluid and nutritional intake
		Change in weight
		Change in state of hydration
		Mucous membranes
		Skin turgor
		Thirst
		Tears

POTENTIAL PROBLEMS	EXPECTED OUTCOMES	NURSING ACTIVITIES
		Behavior
		Urine specific gravity
		Change in indices of intravascular volume
		BP
		P
		CVP
		Urine output and specific gravity
		Changes in lab data
		Serum electrolytes
		Hct
		Intervention if problem occurs
		Frequent assessment of vital signs
		Accurate measurement and recording of intake and output
		Daily weight
		Accurate parenteral administration of fluids and electrolytes
		Monitor IV q1 hr for rate of flow and amount infused (use infusion pump if available)
		Observe IV site q1 hr
		Monitor lab data
■ GI irritation related to specific action of ingested poison	■ GI system intact and functioning normally	■ Monitor for
		Nausea
		Vomiting
		Diarrhea
		Bleeding
		Distention
		Pain
		Intervention if problem occurs
		Documentation of symptoms
		Symptomatic treatment
		Documentation of patient's response to treatment
■ Alteration in body temperature regulation related to toxic action of poison involved	■ Maintenance of normal body temperature	■ Prevent by
		Measuring body temperature q1-2 hr
		Monitor for
		Change in body temperature
		Hypothermia
		Hyperthermia
		Intervention if problem occurs
		Hyperthermia
		Cooling mattress
		Tepid sponge
		Hypothermia
		Heating mattress
		Blankets
■ Bacterial superinfection related to increased susceptibility	■ Absence of infection	■ Prevent by
		Serial monitoring of blood and urine cultures
		Administration of antibiotics, as ordered
		NOTE: Antibiotic therapy is not instituted routinely as prophylactic treatment
		Monitor for
		Temperature elevation greater than 101° F (38.3° C)
		Change in lab values
		WBC and differential
		Cultures of blood and urine
		Chest radiograph
		Intervention if problem occurs
		Temperature elevation
		Check temperature q2-4 hr or as indicated
		Tepid sponge
		Cooling mattress
		Encourage fluid intake (per appropriate route)
		Institute mode of therapy as per physician's order
		Antibiotics

POTENTIAL PROBLEMS	EXPECTED OUTCOMES	NURSING ACTIVITIES
■ Family crisis related to Poisoning episode Need for hospitalization Guilt Anxiety	■ Facilitate coping mechanisms within the family	■ Assess degree of stress and ability to cope Determine level of understanding of child's condition, treatment, and need for hospitalization Offer factual information Clarify misconceptions Encourage parenteral expression of feelings about incident and hospitalization Establish relationship Plan time for interaction Reassure parents Support parents Determine with parents their degree of involvement in care of their child Maintain parental sense of adequacy to care for their child Periodically evaluate effect of interventions on parents' behavior
■ Emotional stress related to trauma of hospitalization	■ Reduced emotional trauma	■ Prevent by Minimal separation of parents and child Continuity of care Monitor for Presence of separation anxiety Phase of separation anxiety (if present) Protest Despair Denial Presence of fears of Bodily harm Mutilation Loss of body integrity Strangers Unfamiliar surroundings Presence of feelings of Guilt Wrongdoing Loss of love Anger Intervention if problem occurs Separation anxiety Presence of parents Parent participation Presence of security object Fears Orientation to surroundings Consistent nursing personnel Correct misconceptions Provide accurate information Feelings Verbalization Play Drawing
■ Recurrence of poisoning episode related to Insufficient education Environmental conditions Developmental age of child	■ Change in attitude through increased knowledge of developmental influences on poisoning incidence and poisoning prevention	■ Assessment and translation of findings into educational program, which may include Accident prevention Risk factors that most often result in injury Significant areas in household that cause problems relevant to age of child Protective measures helpful in accident avoidance Human development Gross motor and fine motor coordination for age Importance of exploration, investigation for children

Neonatal-Pediatric

THE UNSTABLE PREMATURE INFANT

The term *premature* refers to an infant born before the completion of 37 weeks of gestation. The problems associated with prematurity are primarily related to the relative immaturity of the organ systems. The immature infant is not sufficiently developed, physically or physiologically, to meet basic needs in extrauterine life. Maturity is determined by actual gestational age.

The premature infant, though small, may be an appropriate size for his/her gestational age. (Approximately three fourths of newborns who weigh less than 2500 g are born prematurely.) However, poor intrauterine growth may be an additional handicap, further complicating the postnatal course. Anomalies, if present, are further hazards to survival. Moreover, the handicap of immaturity limits the infant's ability to cope with any stresses, including illness.

Other factors related to premature delivery frequently cause mechanical disadvantages that can complicate the infant's postnatal outcome, for example, breech presentation, multiple birth, prolapsed cord, abruptio placentae and related abnormalities, premature rupture of membranes, and greater uterine tone and/or contractility.

About 8% of live births in the United States are premature. Less than 1% of live births are premature infants weighing less than 1000 g.

Etiological factors associated with prematurity include chronic hypertension, limited prenatal care, malnutrition, smoking, and drug use (including alcohol and caffeine). Often these factors overlap and are associated with poor socioeconomic conditions. There is increased likelihood for premature delivery when there is a history of premature delivery(ies). Recent experience indicates a higher incidence of prematurity when there is a history of induced abortion.

Assessment of gestational age is important. As indicated before, the infant's relative immaturity is an index of risk for potential problems. It also presents clues as to what can/should be expected, and it is the basis for specific nursing assessment and interventions. For example, an infant of 34 to 36 weeks gestation may be able to suck at the mother's breast. An infant of less than 32 weeks gestation will probably require tube feedings. An infant of 28 weeks gestation may rely on parenteral feedings for several weeks.

Immaturity is manifested by differences in activity and neurological responses. The more immature infant is less active with a weaker cry and less muscle tone and resistance. Movements are irregular and jerky, because the immature muscles cannot sustain contraction. The CNS, lungs, liver, and other organs have not completely developed.

Prematurity accounts for more than one half of newborn deaths, though the mortality for premature infants is about 30%. Mortality is closely correlated with gestational age and birth weight. Infants that are both immature and small for gestational age have a poorer outlook. Respiratory distress syndrome (RDS) is the most common cause of death. Intraventricular hemorrhage also remains a leading cause of death, with an incidence of about 30% premature patients and a mortality that is estimated to be over 60%.

In some centers, survival is as high as 95% for premature infants between 1500 and 2500 grams. It should be noted that the highest survival rates for sick newborns are in level III nurseries, not level II, leading to the conclusions that (1) there must be careful screening to assure appropriate transfers to higher level units and (2) emphasis should be on prenatal maternal transfers so that infants can be stabilized and not be subjected to the rigors of transport.

About 25% of very low birth weight infants (less than 1000 g) and about 10% of infants over 1000 g are born with less than 26 weeks of gestation. These very premature infants have less than a 25% survival rate.

Morbidity is also considerably higher, as much as 10 times greater for premature infants than for full-term infants. As indicated before, immaturity is not only in itself a handicap but also limits an infant's ability to cope with problems that may evolve. Clinical signs of problems may be less easily identified because of overlapping signs of immaturity.

Certain problems occur with greater frequency in the premature infant. RDS is the major pulmonary problem. Another common problem is necrotizing enterocolitis (NEC), which is a most serious complication considering its insidious onset, rapid course, and high mortality. NEC is the most common reason for neonatal surgery. Additionally, even slight elevations of serum bilirubin levels are cause for concern, because the immature liver is slow to conjugate and excrete bilirubin, thus increasing the risk of kernicterus.

Another problem occurring with greater frequency in the premature infant is patent ductus arteriosus (PDA), often associated with and complicating a variety of neonatal problems. The premature infant is also predisposed to pulmonary edema. More than one third of infants born weighing less than 1500 g or at less than 35 weeks gestation suffer periventricular-intraventricular hemorrhage. The incidence is highest among those born at less than 32 weeks gestation.

The outlook for later growth and development of surviving premature infants is not yet fully known. In general, current prognoses are optimistic. Overall, the incidence of severe handicaps may be as high as 15%, but 85% of infants born under 1200 grams are assessed to be neurologically normal at 1 year. It seems that those who develop neurological symptoms in the neonatal period are most at risk for subsequent neurological problems. There does seem to be a greater incidence of sudden infant death syndrome (SIDS), peaking at 1 to 3 months of age, especially among infants under 1500 g at birth. Later lower respiratory tract problems seem to be related to the occurrence of bronchopulmonary dysplasia, not RDS. BPD results from immaturity of the airways and cardiovascular system as well as from therapy (e.g., positive pressure ventilation and oxygen). Another complication of oxygen therapy is retrolental fibroplastic sequelae, which retain an incidence of 2% (one half of which is blindness) in infants 1000 to 1500 g and 17% (less than one third of which is blindness) in infants 1000 g and under.

To assess subsequent somatic growth and psychosocial development of premature infants, one must subtract the number of weeks preterm at birth from the infant's age at time of assessment (e.g., a 2-month-old infant born at 32 weeks gestation should be compared to a 3-week-old term infant). Thus, adjusted for prematurity, normal height and weight is generally achieved by 1 year. The small infant does not remain a small child. Subsequent growth determinants are related to genetic predisposition and environmental factors.

Later developmental lags are probably associated with factors other than prematurity, for example, CNS injuries, nutritional deficiencies in the perinatal period, intrauterine growth retardation, and hypoxia. Regarding these latter, the long-range impact of critical neonatal care has not been fully evaluated.

A significant sequela to both the immediate separation of infant and mother and the prolonged hospitalization of the high-risk infant who requires critical care can be subsequent child neglect and abuse as well as other parenting problems, including marital discord. Research indicates that structured interventions can prevent these problems from occurring and promote faster weight gain and other signs of infant growth and development.

Parental responses and coping patterns are variable. Guilt often interplays with other emotions. Sometimes there is a denial stage. Often, the response of parents is unrelated to the severity of the infant's problems. In addition, each parent may be at different stages of accepting and different levels of coping at any given time. This is often caused by one supporting the other and then "breaking down" when the other is available for support. Or, parental difficulties may be caused by nurturance or communication deficits in the relationship. Assessing and promoting effective coping must be an integral goal in the plan of care if parents are to assume their care-taking responsibilities adequately.

The parents' stress is often related to the sudden end of their prenatal planning and the fact that their expectations of a normal, healthy baby have been shattered. In addition, their daily life is totally disrupted. The routine of visiting the hospital, often for short, fractured visits spaced at sometimes irregular intervals, is exhausting and made more so by the stressfulness of the situation with its accompanying fear and anxiety. The fatigue disrupts sleep-rest patterns and biorhythms. Couples often report a cessation of sexual relations. If a referral center is used, the inconvenience and expense of travel may add to the burden. For families with other children the impact of the disorganization of routine, especially when prolonged, can be deleterious, leaving little reserve for coping with repeated setbacks, a final negative outcome, or any special care needs following the baby's discharge. If the infant's condition is critical, i.e., if the baby is sick as well as premature, there are often unavoidable limitations on parent-infant contact, which may be detrimental to the attachment process and/or increase worry and anxiety. The qualitative differences in types of parent-infant, especially maternal-infant, contact have been found to be significant in the early development of premature infants and also the adequacy of later parenting.

ASSESSMENT

1. Gestation
   a. Gestation is estimated in weeks beginning with mother's first day of last menstrual period; before birth,

uterine size, ultrasonography, and amniocentesis may be used
  b. Neurological examination
  c. Physical examination
2. Appropriate intrauterine growth (compare infant with standard charts; infants who fall in the ninetieth percentile are considered small or large for gestational age)
  a. Weight (about 50% of low birth weight infants are premature)
  b. Length (length is more closely related to maturity than weight)
  c. Head circumference (head circumference should be determined at weekly intervals in low birth weight infants to assess aberrations from expected growth)
3. Maternal obstetrical history of previous premature delivery
4. History of complications during gestation
  a. Maternal age under 16
  b. Toxemia
  c. Multiple gestation
  d. Infection
  e. Third trimester bleeding
  f. Hemoglobinopathy
5. History of complications during and immediately after delivery

  a. Fetal distress
  b. Low Apgar score at either 1 minute or 5 minutes
    (1) Below 4 at 1 minute
    (2) Below 8 at 5 minutes
  c. Postnatal resuscitation (stimulation, suctioning, oxygenation, intubation, positive pressure ventilation—either manual or mechanical)
6. Results of serial lab tests
  a. Arterial blood gas levels
  b. Serum glucose, bilirubin, electrolytes

GOALS

1. Premature infant grows and thrives
2. Family is able to cope with the unanticipated crises of the birth experience and remain an intact, mutually nurturing dyad or group
3. Successful parent-infant bonding
4. Infant develops normally, considering gestational age
5. Adequate but not excessive oxygenation
6. Adequate nourishment with weight gain
7. Neutral thermal environment maintained
8. Normal psychosocial and psychomotor growth
9. Parents develop and have confidence in their parenting skills

POTENTIAL PROBLEMS	EXPECTED OUTCOMES	NURSING ACTIVITIES

■ Apnea (respiratory pause greater than 20 seconds) related to
Prematurity
Intracranial bleeding
PDA
RDS
Pneumonia
Maternal oversedation
CNS immaturity
Cold stress
Electrolyte imbalance
Hypoglycemia
Apnea may be presenting sign of variety of neonatal problems
	■ Adequate respiratory function maintained
	Absence of apnea, hypoxemia
		■ Attach infant with identified risk factors to respiratory monitor, setting alarms to detect respiratory pauses greater than 15 seconds
		Attach all infants under 1800 g to respiratory rate monitor, as above
		Observe for
		  Cyanosis
		  Seizures
		  Prominent bounding pulses
		  Heart murmur
		Note tachycardia, irritability, hematemesis, albuminuria
		Monitor arterial blood gas levels and acid-base balance
		Monitor transcutaneous Po_2
		Maintain core temperature in lower neutral range
		Provide tactile and auditory stimulation, including periodic rocking and nonnutritive sucking
		Position infant in prone position
		Administer O_2, as ordered (usually 20% to 30%), for cyanosis and/or hypoxemia
		Administer naloxone, as ordered, if maternal oversedation is identified
		Administer theophylline, as ordered, to increase alveolar ventilation through central stimulation (usually po after initial IV dose)
		  Monitor serum theophylline q1-2 day to prevent toxicity
		Provide descriptive documentation of apneic episodes
		  Note duration
		  Note presence or absence of
		    Bradycardia
		    Cyanosis
		    Abdominal distention
		  Note activity and position of infant before, during, and after episode, e.g., feeding, sleeping, prone, supine
		  Note temperature of infant and Isolette

POTENTIAL PROBLEMS	EXPECTED OUTCOMES	NURSING ACTIVITIES

		Note resumption of respirations
		  Whether spontaneous
		  Whether stimulation is required
		  Note type and amount of stimulation required
		Stimulate infant during apneic period
		  Stroke feet, hands, face, back
		  Then move to extremities and trunk
		  Start with gentle stimulation and continue more vigorously, as required

■ Hypothermia related to
  Hypoglycemia
  Hypoxia
  Sepsis
  Insufficient environmental temperature
Hypothermia may be presenting sign of infection
Cold stress increases metabolism; if hypoglycemia ensues, anaerobic metabolism leads to metabolic acidosis
	■ Body heat conserved
	Alleviation/resolution of underlying causes of fluctuant temperature
		■ Dry infant immediately at birth and place under radiant heat source
		  Do not allow infant to touch metal or other conductive surface
		  Do not place infant in drafts
		Wrap infant in warmed blanket (remember that radiant heater does not prevent heat loss by convection)
		Transport infant in Isolette to maintain neutral thermal environment
		  Warmers and/or incubators in both delivery room and nursery should be preheated
		  Use warmed linen
		  NOTE: Neutral thermal environment is one in which O_2 requirement (i.e., consumption) is lowest for maintaining body temperature
		Use servocontrolled unit (radiant warmer or Isolette)
		  Position skin probe over liver
		  Use heat-reflecting adhesive to prevent probe sensing environmental heat
		  Set heater output between 98.6° and 99.5° F (37° and 37.5° C)
		  Maintain abdominal skin temperatures between 96° and 97.7° F (35.8° and 36.5° C)
		  Use warmed blankets when holding infant outside Isolette or warmer
		  NOTE: Servocontrol mechanism limits gradient between skin and environmental air temperature; when infant's temperature goes above or below desired temperature, mechanism automatically turns off or on accordingly; overheating (abdominal temperatures over 97.7° F [36.5° C]) and/or rapid rewarming may cause apnea; basis for this heat-induced apnea mechanism is not known
		Monitor
		  Axillary temperature q30 min until stable, then q2 hr
		  Signs and symptoms of cold stress
		    Reduced activity
		    Flaccid movements
		    Pallor
		    Cyanosis
		    Cold to touch
		    Pupils dilatate
		    Slow, shallow, irregular breathing
		    Bradycardia
		Investigate changes in infant's temperature; assess infant's thermal response to hypoxic episodes (oxyhemoglobin may fail to dissociate)
		  Note postural flexion into fetal position
		Warm blood and other infusions to body temperature
		Warm O_2 to ambient temperature
		  Monitor O_2 temperature
		  Maintain Oxyhood temperature at 87.8° to 93.2° F (31° to 34° C)
		Increase infant's temperature gradually; after first week, larger and/or more stable premature infant should have servocontrol discontinued
		Clothe and wrap infant, allowing face to be exposed to cooler temperatures (84.2° to 86° F [29° to 30° C])
		Assess stability of core temperature; as infant grows and becomes stable, temperature is maintained without supplementary heat input and infant may be transferred to bassinet
		Ambient nursery temperature should be about 77° F (25° C)

POTENTIAL PROBLEMS	EXPECTED OUTCOMES	NURSING ACTIVITIES
■ Hyperthermia related to Overheating Sepsis	■ Normal temperature	■ Monitor environmental temperature Maintain thermoneutral environment as described in Problem, Hypothermia Note signs and symptoms of hyperthermia Flushing Tachycardia Labored respirations Skin moisture Seizure activity Apneic episodes Notify physician if these occur If hyperthermia occurs, administer therapy as ordered and monitor patient's response
■ Delayed parent-infant bonding and/or inhibited attachment related to Separation from infant Prolonged hospitalization of infant Grieving over loss of healthy, normal newborn Poor outlook for positive outcome and/or unpreparedness because of early arrival	■ Parents demonstrate nurturant responses to infant Parents communicate their feelings about infant Successful patient-infant bonding	■ As soon as infant has been stabilized in high-risk nursery, allow parents to visit (this may be just father at first; in this instance, introduction and orientation will have to be repeated for mother) This visit should include parents touching and examining baby; parents may need help to initiate contact, relaxation techniques and therapeutic touch may assist parents at this time Minimize environmental potentiation of crisis Prepare parents for equipment and setting before they enter nursery Explain purpose of equipment, particularly tubes and wires attached to infant; explain that amount of equipment is not index to how sick infant is (remember technology appears even more overwhelming in comparison to infant's small size) At end of visit, clarify parents' perceptions of situation; help them set realistic goals Recognize grief and withdrawal caused by perceived condition Encourage verbalization of feelings of shock, failure, guilt, anger Recognize defense mechanisms, e.g., denial, anger, rejection Recognize negative comments as expression of need for support Visiting times should be flexible; encourage parents to visit frequently; identify staff members by name; relationship with primary nurse is optimal, but parents should be acquainted with other staff members also If visits decrease or become sporadic or irregular, follow up with phone call Point out signs of progress and growth; help parents anticipate nonlinear course so they are not needlessly overwhelmed by apparent setbacks, e.g., if infant is moved back to radiant warmer from Isolette or if IV therapy is restarted Model nurturant behavior; provide opportunities for parents to care for infant; reinforce nurturant behaviors; describe to parents their special value to infant Support and reinforce parent-infant attachment (it is important when someone other than parents, e.g., grandparent, will be primary caregiver that this person is included in attachment process from soon after birth) Set realistic prognostic expectations for survival; do not hesitate to be optimistic in early period; focus on immediate and day-to-day goals and progress Clarify misconceptions with factual information (nurse should be present at conferences with physicians to be better prepared to provide explanation) Encourage breast-feeding Teach advantages Nutrient Immunological Psychological/interactive Teach methods of expression (supply is directly related to amount and frequency of breast stimulation) Stimulation of let-down reflex

POTENTIAL PROBLEMS	EXPECTED OUTCOMES	NURSING ACTIVITIES
		Hot moist towels for 10 minutes or warm shower
		Relaxation and centering techniques
		Breast massage
		Manual
		Electric or hand pump
		Care of pump
		Frequency: q3 hr during day
		Assist mother to breast-feed
		Breast-feeding should be initiated as soon as possible
		Reassure mother as she initiates breast-feeding
		Explain infant's learning needs, weak suck, etc.
		Maximize privacy
		In-between feedings should not be with nipple; use dropper technique
		Position baby for maternal comfort and to allow adequate grasp of nipple; premature infant should be positioned on side on pillows so that mother can support head while keeping arms and shoulders relaxed
		Support and reassure mother
		Show interest in how *she* is feeling
		Convey importance of *her* milk for *her* baby
		Discuss methods of support with husband; explain that support is for mother, not for breast-feeding itself
		Importance of massaging interscapular area
		Importance of mother's nutritional and fluid intake
		Relaxation techniques
		Instruct parents regarding storage of breast milk
		Label with name, date, and time
		Refrigerate for 2 to 3 days and then discard (milk may be frozen and kept for 6 months; when removed from freezer, it should be used within 48 hours); refrigeration is preferable to freezing because leukocytes are destroyed in freezing
		Use plastic containers, because leukocytes stick to glass
■ Hypoxia secondary to apnea, RDS, cardiac insufficiency, anemia, shock	■ Adequate oxygenation	■ Assess respiratory status
		Attach infant to cardiorespiratory monitor and turn on alarm; observe infant's breathing pattern
		Note and record apneic episodes
		Monitor and record
		Respiratory rate
		Breathing pattern; note
		Retractions
		Flaring nostrils
		Grunting
		Skin color
		F_{IO_2} (q2 hr)
		Airway pressures
		Assist with intubation, if necessary

See STANDARD 6   *Mechanical ventilation*
      STANDARD 70   *Neonatal respiratory distress*

Suction tracheobronchial tree, as needed
Administer chest physiotherapy frequently in compromised infant
  Gentle percussion may be applied by hand or with fingers (nipples or small masks may be substitute of more convenient size to adequately rotate over various lung segments)
  Posturing is important
  Vibration for small premature infant is controversial
  Either manual or electric vibration can be used
Administer aminophylline po or IV for intractable frequent apnea if needed, as ordered

See STANDARD 70   *Neonatal respiratory distress*

POTENTIAL PROBLEMS	EXPECTED OUTCOMES	NURSING ACTIVITIES

		Support infant's respiratory efforts
		  Avoid restraining infant (restraints reduce sensory stimulation)
		  Change infant's position regularly; prone positions enhance ventilation/perfusion ratios and reduce asynchronous chest wall motion
		  Nonnutritive sucking has been found to enhance oxygenation
		    Allow infant to suck on soft nipple
		  During apneic spells, stimulate infant gently at first
		    Stroke feet, hands, face, back
		    Then move to extremities and trunk
		    More vigorous stimulation may be required
		  CPAP may be prescribed
		    Administer good skin care around nares when prongs are used; topical steroids may be prescribed
		    Monitor for
		      Gastric distention and aspirate prn
		      Signs of pneumothorax or pneumomediastinum
		  Minimize conditions that increase O₂ consumption
		    Hyperthermia
		    Cold stress

■ Peripheral cyanosis
  Related to vasoconstriction and decreased oxygen extraction at tissue level with subsequent peripheral acidosis
  Resulting from
    Autonomic vasomotor instability
    Immaturity
    Hypothermia
    Local venous or arterial obstruction (thrombi, spasm)
    Sepsis
    Metabolic acidosis
    Medications
  Most peripheral cyanosis is physiological
	■ Adequate tissue perfusion
	  Adequate oxygenation
		■ Monitor
		  Color of extremities and nail beds
		  Capillary filling; note delayed filling
		  Acid-base balance
		  Breathing pattern
		    Weak, irregular respirations imply CNS involvement
		    Tachypneic or labored respirations may be caused by pulmonary or cardiac problems
		  Axillary temperature; see Problem, Hypothermia
		    Assess gradient between skin and environmental temperatures
		Observe for signs of sepsis, including lethargy, change in feeding pattern; see Problem, Sepsis
		Notify physician of abnormalities in aforementioned
		If cyanosis occurs
		  Administer therapy to correct underlying etiological problems, as ordered
		  Administer O₂, as ordered

■ Hypoglycemia (less than or equal to 25 mg/dl) related to
  Delayed feedings
  Low liver glycogen stores
  Cold stress
  Continuous low blood sugar may result in increased risk of cerebral damage; untreated hypoglycemia may be fatal
  Immaturity limits adrenal medullary response to low glucose
	■ Serum glucose within normal limits
	  Absence or resolution of adverse side effects of low blood sugar
	  Maintenance of fluid and electrolyte balance
		■ Assure adequate glucose intake
		  Early feeding is important; monitor intake
		  If infant is not taking oral feedings, parenteral glucose must be given (10% dextrose in water [D10W], 75 ml/kg body weight/day) as prescribed by physician
		Beware of increased metabolic demands of cold stress, hypoxia, etc.
		Monitor blood sugar by manual blood glucose monitoring strip (e.g., Dextrostix) at 12 hours of age, then q4-8 hr for 48 hours
		Be alert to signs and symptoms of hypoglycemia
		  Lethargy, either as isolated finding or with irritability and tremulousness (may be one of first signs)
		  Jittery movements or muscle twitching
		  Apnea
		  Cyanosis or pallor
		  Convulsions
		  Irritability
		  Hypotonia
		  Hypothermia
		  Diaphoresis
		If blood glucose is below 45%, notify physician and administer therapy as prescribed
		  IV therapy may be increased to 15% dextrose in water (D15W)
		  Steroids may also be prescribed

POTENTIAL PROBLEMS	EXPECTED OUTCOMES	NURSING ACTIVITIES

■ Ineffective individual coping by either mother or father or both, ineffective family coping by parental dyad or significant household group of mother related to Psychophysical exhaustion
Excessive stress
Excess anger or guilt
Financial stress
Fear
	■ Parents are able to provide mutual support for each other
	Each parent is able to devise effective strategies for coping
		■ Recognize and assess impact of events on mother
		Assess coping style and effectiveness of coping strategies
		Identify supports and assess adequacy and effectiveness
		Identify additional stressors
		  Separation from other children
		  Travel distance/time to hospital
		Assess coping style of father and ability to provide support
		Identify additional stressors
		  Travel back and forth between neonatal center, hospital in which mother is, and home, and perhaps even another location where other children are
		  Work schedule
		  Loss of work time and income
		  Frustration from noncomplementary visiting hours or phone privileges
		  Financial pressures
		Identify anticipatory grieving
		  Expressed feelings of sadness
		  Loss of appetite
		  Inability to sleep
		  Irritability
		  Guilt
		  Preoccupation thinking about baby, especially in relation to one's own involvement or effect on events and outcomes
		  Crying
		  Withdrawal
		  Depression
		  Thinking baby might die
		  Recognize that further away neonatal center is, more intensified may be parental fear of survival
		Note infrequent visiting pattern
		Identify intentional maternal-paternal separation as factor of perception of severity of illness
		Refer to social workers and counselors, as appropriate
		Recognize that absence of grief may be an ominous sign of impending family disorganization and conflict
		  Refer to organized family support programs, including self-support groups

■ Sensory deprivation and/or bombardment	■ Infant receives appropriate stimulation from environment
	Infant develops socially responsive behavior
	Infant learns behaviors that influence subsequent stimuli
	  Parents and staff respond appropriately to infant's cues
	Infant associates feeding with pleasant social stimuli
		■ Provide verbal stimulation
		  Soft talk and gentle tactile stimuli should precede other care giving
		  Hold face within 9 inches of infant and in his/her line of vision
		Avoid repeated and sudden noise or jerky handling of infant
		Control noise level in unit
		Provide bright and moving visual stimuli
		Provide tactile stimulation
		  Rock and stroke infant gently and rhythmically
		  Avoid touching infant with cold objects, e.g., stethoscope
		Play music at intervals
		  Continuous playing of music or radio talk should be avoided
		Lower lights during night hours
		Provide social stimulation
		  Provide continuity of care by primary nurse and same caregiver each shift as much as possible
		  Talk to infant whenever he/she is being handled
		  Talk to infant whenever near him/her
		    Initiate talk in en face position
		  Provide stroking and cuddling even when infant cannot be taken from Isolette or warmer
		Assess infant's social responsiveness
		  Alertness
		  Visual responsiveness
		    Inanimate stimuli
		    People

POTENTIAL PROBLEMS	EXPECTED OUTCOMES	NURSING ACTIVITIES
		Ability to be consoled
		Muscle tone
		Self-quieting behavior
		Smiling behavior
		Note responses of pleasure, dissatisfaction, or inattention to various interactions
		Signs of attention include
		Head turning
		Staring
		Slowed heart rate and respiratory rate
		Change in motor activity, visual function
		Continuous, repetitious stimuli do not arouse interactive behaviors
		Avoid stimulating infant when he/she is irritable; assure parents that infant can hear and see them; help parents recognize infant's response to various stimuli and when infant is able to receive stimuli
		Support parents' interaction with infant
		Make baby as attractive as possible
		Allow parents to bring in clothes and toys
		Encourage parents to see and touch infant frequently
		Infant should be fully awake when offered feedings
		Stimulate infant, change diaper, etc., before offering feeding
		Provide nonnutritive sucking at regularly scheduled intervals if/when infant is NPO; during these periods, infant should be held for at least 20 minutes
		Stimulates rooting reflex
		Develops proprioception of sucking activity
		If dropper or gavage feedings are necessary, infant should be offered nipple so that sucking becomes associated with food intake and relief of hunger
■ Abdominal distention Stomach may become distended from positive airway pressure—either CPAP or mechanical/manual ventilatory assistance	■ Diaphragm movement not inhibited Absence of abdominal distention	■ Measure abdominal circumference just above umbilicus at time of admission; thereafter take this measurement daily (at same time each day and before feeding)
		Note distention in relation to feeding pattern
		Whether abdomen usually becomes distended with feedings; whether this distention is gross or limited to gastric area
		Length of time that distention persists
		If distention persists until subsequent feeding time, aspirate via gastric tube
		Note quantity of air aspirated as well as other stomach contents; discard air and mucus and replace partially digested formula
		Note changes in pattern of distention in relation to feeding
		Institute more frequent measurements of abdominal girth
		Report increasing abdominal girth and other abnormal changes to physician
		Remove air from stomach q½-2 hr or prn when infant is receiving ventilatory assistance
		Observe for signs of respiratory distress
		Adjust infant's feeding schedule as tolerated
		Smaller, more frequent feedings may be better tolerated
		Experiment with varied infant positions
		Leave NG tube open and in place to decompress stomach
		Position infant in prone or right lateral position after feeding (efficacy of this posturing in reducing residual volume is variable and physiological basis for it is debatable)
■ Dehydration and electrolyte imbalance related to Third spacing associated with NEC, peritonitis, early postnatal period, etc.	■ Fluid and electrolyte balance Adequate but not excessive fluid intake	■ Monitor hourly intake and output strictly; record
		Include medications given and blood specimens taken
		Weigh diapers if stools are loose
		Monitor hydration status
		Weigh daily at same time and before feeding and record (more frequent weights may be indicated)

POTENTIAL PROBLEMS	EXPECTED OUTCOMES	NURSING ACTIVITIES

Increased insensible fluid loss (as much as 190%) associated with phototherapy, radiant warmer, endotracheal intubation
Increased fluid needs associated with fever, stress, increased caloric expenditures/demands
Shock associated with perinatal asphyxia, reduced cardiac output, hemorrhage, neurogenic factors, coagulation disorder, sepsis
Resulting in cardiac arrhythmias related to
Hypokalemia associated with increased aldosterone secretion
Hemodynamic changes
Hypoxia
Healthy premature infant is also prone to high frequency of arrhythmias because of immature autonomic nervous system and immature cardiac conduction tissue
		Skin turgor
		Eyes
		Anterior fontanelles
		Mucus membranes
		Urine output
		Lab data
		  Hct (should be maintained at 40%; this index may be falsely elevated because of fluid restriction)
		  Serum Na$^+$ and glucose
		  BUN, serum osmolality; these values will be altered not only by hydration, but also by therapeutic administration of urea and osmotic diuretics
		  Urine specific gravity and osmolality
		  Urine output
		  Serum creatinine
		Monitor and record
		  Peripheral pulses
		  Skin temperature of hands and feet; note temperature gradient
		  Skin color
		  CVP, BP, and P (CVP should be maintained at 3 to 8 cm H$_2$O or as ordered); note pulse pressure
		  Cardiac rate and rhythm continuously by oscilloscope
		  Hematest results of stools and gastric drainage
		Notify physician of abnormalities and initiate appropriate intervention, according to unit protocol or as ordered; this may include administration of
		  Fluids
		  Cardiotonic, vasopressor, antiarrhythmic medications
		  Diuretics
		  Blood products
		Administer IV infusions, as prescribed*; record hourly (infusion pumps should be used)
		Note signs of overload: CHF, pulmonary edema, PDA, weight increase
		Replace NG drainage according to physician's orders

■ Intraventricular hemorrhage related to
Prematurity
Cerebral hypoxic insults
Fluctuant arterial BP
Perinatal asphyxia
Increased venous pressure secondary to
RDS, pneumothorax, or positive pressure ventilation
Increased cerebral blood flow secondary to fluid or vasopressor therapies
Occurs in more than 50% of infants who weigh less than 1500 g at birth
	■ Minimization of cerebral insult
	Absence of encephalopathy
	Absence of other CNS sequelae
		■ Observe for changes in LOC and other CNS activity, including
		  Unreactive pupils; generalized tonic seizures; temperature instability; flaccid quadripesis
		  Hypotonia, decrease in spontaneous and elicited movements; vertical drift of eyes (usually downward)
		Monitor
		  Head circumference and note rate of growth; note increase in anterior fontanelles; note bulging
		  Temperature
		  Heart rate
		  BP
		  Hct; note hct that does not increase following transfusions
		  Arterial blood gas levels
		  Blood glucose; note glucose and water disequilibrium
		Monitor ICP if available (note that with marginal arterial BP, even relatively slight increase in ICP may seriously compromise cerebral perfusion)
		Assist with serial lumbar punctures

---

*The daily maintenance water requirement for the low birth weight infant includes: insensible water loss, 32%; urinary output, 56%; and stool loss, 6%. Additionally, there are water needs for tissue synthesis of 0.85 ml/g of weight gain. Low volumes are usually infused during the first days of life because of lower metabolic rates and decreased activity, and to allow for the expected physiologic contraction of extracellular fluid volume. (Excessive fluid administration has been associated with PDA.) Care must be taken to keep infusion rates constant because variable blood flow volume has been associated with the occurrence of intraventricular bleeding.

POTENTIAL PROBLEMS	EXPECTED OUTCOMES	NURSING ACTIVITIES
		Administer drugs to reduce CSF, as ordered
		Osmotic agents
		Carbonic anhydrase inhibitors
		ATPase inhibitors
		Administer steroids (dexamethasone) to reduce cerebral edema, as ordered
		Administer phenytoin (Dilantin) and/or phenobarbital, as ordered, to prevent cerebral hypoxia and control seizures
■ Impaired skin integrity related to thin, fragile skin of small premature infant further compromised by poor tissue perfusion and interstitial edema or dehydration At younger gestational age, infants have less subcutaneous fat stores	■ Intact integument	■ Note dry, scaling skin
		Provide skin care around nares when prongs are used
		Administer topical steroids if prescribed
		Administer topical tocopherol (vitamin E) in accord with unit protocols or as ordered
		Monitor IV infusions carefully to prevent infiltration
		Note pressure points, turn child, and provide support appropriately
		Change position frequently
■ Sepsis	■ Absence of infection	■ Prevent exposure to nosocomial infection by the following activities
		Practice strict aseptic technique with all procedures (mask and gloves only when indicated, e.g., umbilical catheterizations)
		Limit visitors
		Allow only parents to handle infant
		(Parents or staff with upper respiratory infection, open wounds, diarrhea, etc., are not permitted in nursery)
		Teach parents proper hand-washing technique
		Parents wear long-sleeved gowns over clothing when entering nursery
		Allow parents to touch only their own infant
		Instruct parents not to handle other infants' supplies or to move things from one Isolette or crib to another
		Use special precautions with invasive life-support procedures
		Respiratory therapy equipment should be changed daily
		Humidifiers should be changed daily; fill with sterile H_2O (q8 hr)
		Do not allow condensation in tubing to drain back to humidifier
		Change IV tubing q48 hr, solutions q24 hr; cover stopcocks at all times
		Change continuous NG feeding apparatus q8 hr
		Restart feedings (whether formula or breast milk) q4 hr
		Date multidose vials when first opened (because of very small doses used with these patients, they are not consumed quickly)
		Culture multidose vials according to unit policy routines
		Take cultures of formulas weekly
		Monitor for signs of infection (these may involve any organ system)
		Cultures should be taken at admission as per protocol of unit
		Few signs and symptoms are unique to sepsis; any infant who is regressing should be evaluated for sepsis (repeat cultures)
		Apnea
		Tachypnea
		Bradycardia or tachycardia
		Hypotension
		Lethargy or poor feeding
		Irritability
		Abdominal distention
		Hepatosplenomegaly
		Cyanosis or mottling
		Jaundice
		Petechiae or bleeding
		Hypothermia or hyperthermia
		Acidosis

POTENTIAL PROBLEMS	EXPECTED OUTCOMES	NURSING ACTIVITIES
		Note local signs of infection related to therapies, e.g., eyes of infant who has been in humidifid Oxyhood, heel stick sites, sites of IVs, umbilical cord stump
		Report abnormal observations to physician
		Take repeat cultures if symptoms suggesting sepsis appear
		Obtain laboratory evaluation, as ordered
		Assist with lumbar puncture
		Gram stain and culture—both bacterial and viral
		Protein and glucose
		Cell count and differential
		CBC with differential and platelet count
		Chest radiograph
		Urinalysis
		Monitor culture results (while definitive diagnosis of infection/sepsis is made with positive cultures, antibiotic therapy must be started immediately if clinical assessment indicates there is an infection; regimen may be altered when sensitivity results are available
		Administer IV antibiotics, as prescribed (dosage schedules for neonates differ from those of older children and adults because of slower renal clearance)

■ Malnutrition related to
  Inadequate caloric intake caused by small gastric capacity (3 to 5 ml) and poor absorption of fats and vitamins
  Prolonged or frequent periods without enteral feedings
  Increased caloric requirements related to
    Hypothermia
    Respiratory distress
    Infection
  Loss of calories through diarrhea
  Normally higher metabolic rate of small for gestational age infants
	■ Adequate caloric intake
	  Infant growth
	  Appropriate weight gain
		■ Monitor intake and output q1 hr
		  Oral intake record should include type and caloric content of feedings
		  Administer TPN, as ordered (TPN solutions should be prepared by pharmacist under ultraviolet hood)
		  Monitor
		    Weights daily
		    Head circumference weekly
		    Urine Clinitest q4 hr if stabilized (q½-1 hr until stable)
		    When TPN is discontinued, monitor Dextrostix q1 hr for 6 to 8 hours
		  Administer Intralipid as ordered; this may be infused simultaneously with TPN through Y connector or intermittently
		  Administer intermittent or continuous gavage feedings (gavage feeding may be indicated also when premature infant is too immature to suck and swallow)
		  NG or orogastric feedings
		    Insert No. 5 French feeding tube through nose or mouth, down esophagus, and into stomach
		    Confirm placement
		      Aspirate stomach contents
		      Auscultate 2 to 5 cc injection of air into stomach via tube; this may be visualized by gastric distention (remove air immediately)
		    Position infant on right side with head and thorax elevated slightly
		    Allow measured amount of formula to flow by gravity
		    Keep infant on right side with head and thorax elevated or position on abdomen for at least 1 hour
		    Note and record emesis (emesis of 1 to 2 ml is normal in premature infant)
		  Nasojejunal feedings*†
		    This method is indicated when gastric gavage is contraindicated, e.g., recurrent aspiration, persistent respiratory distress, and mechanical ventilation make gastric feedings unsafe
		    Tube is usually inserted by physician

*Passage of gastric tube may stimulate vagal response, resulting in serious bradycardia and/or apnea. Gastric distention during and following feeding may also stimulate this reflex.

†Oral medications should be administered through a gastric tube when jejunal or duodenal feedings are used.

POTENTIAL PROBLEMS	EXPECTED OUTCOMES	NURSING ACTIVITIES
		Correct placement is verified by radiograph before feedings are initiated
		Note radiograph results
		Restrain upper extremities prn
		Feeding should be warmed to body temperature
		Use infusion pump; initial rate is usually 2 to 3 ml/kg body weight/hour and may be increased 1 ml/hour q6-8 hr as tolerated
		Change infusion catheters q8 hr
		Do not allow formula or breast milk to remain at room temperature for more than 4 hours
		Agitate Volutrol at least once q1 hr to mix H₂O and soluble components of breast milk
		Aspirate residual in jejunum q2-4 hr; it should be less than 1 ml; notify physician if residual increases
		Measure gastric residual if ordered when jejunal/duodenal tube is in place; this is not considered routinely necessary by some
		Monitor and record stool consistency and guaiac
		Initial feeding is 3 to 5 ml
		Feeding quantity is gradually increased
		Monitor for complications
		Perforation
		Intussusception
		Catheter blockages
		Changes in intestinal flora
		Diarrhea
		Nasoduodenal feedings*
		Some neonatal clinicians have found this method more advantageous than jejunal route
		Exact nutrient absorption from duodenum and jejunum is not certain
		During continuous drip feedings (which are indicated whenever amount tolerated by bolus is insufficient for nutrition)
		Check catheter position q2 hr
		Note emesis
		Test for guaiac
		Bile may indicate reflux or misplacement of tube
		Notify physician if abnormalities are observed
		Holding infant is not precluded by either intermittent or continuous tube feedings
		Oral nipple feedings may be used for infant mature enough to suck and swallow
		Feedings should begin with 3 to 5 ml volume
		Guidelines for increasing or withholding feedings may be specified by physician
		Note gastric residuals (residuals may not indicate intolerance of feeding; residual of as much as 5 ml may persist even when feeding is reduced; meanwhile, it may not increase with increased feedings)
		Rock infant in nurse's or parent's lap for 5- to 20-minute periods at prescribed intervals (at least twice each shift)†
		When infant is 5 days old, temperature stability should be adequate; larger babies may be able to tolerate this sooner (during first few days, smaller premature infant can be rocked in nurse's hands or arms under heat source or in Isolette)
		Administer therapeutic touch several times a day for 5 to 20 minutes‡

---

*Oral medications should be administered through a gastric tube when jejunal or duodenal feedings are used.
†Rocking has been found to stimulate newborn growth. The effects of rocking may be enhanced by interpersonal contact.
‡The exact mechanism of its effect in this situation is not fully understood. It may enhance energy and/or O₂ consumption, thus increasing reserves. The infant's need for proprioceptive stimulation may be involved.

POTENTIAL PROBLEMS	EXPECTED OUTCOMES	NURSING ACTIVITIES
■ PDA related to Immaturity Increased pulmonary vascular resistance	■ Absence of apnea Adequate oxygenation	■ Monitor for Characteristic "machinery murmur" throughout systole and diastole (usually maximal at upper left sternal border) Characteristic bounding radial pulses (radial pulses usually difficult to palpate in absence of PDA) Signs of pulmonary edema Signs of CHF: hepatomegaly, weight gain, elevated CVP, periorbital edema in recumbent position, cool and/or cyanotic extremities Notify physician of abnormalities in aforementioned Administer the following, if ordered Indomethacin to promote ductus closure Digoxin to improve myocardial function Take heart rate before giving drug; hold dose and notify physician if rate is less than 120 Diuretics to reduce fluid congestion Theophylline to prevent apnea
■ NEC	■ Absence of NEC	■ Monitor for Changes in feeding pattern Poor absorption of feedings Emesis Presence of bilious material in gastric aspirate Hematest positive stools or emesis Increasing abdominal distention Note history of hypoxic or hypotensive episodes, including fetal distress Withhold enteral feedings according to unit protocols following occurrence of above symptoms or hypoxic episodes (usually for 1 week to 10 days) *See* STANDARD 71 *Neonatal necrotizing enterocolitis* Encourage and support breast-feeding
■ Hyperbilirubinemia related to immaturity, delayed initiation of feedings Vitamin K excess Acidosis Hypoalbuminemia Sepsis Hemolysis Hypothermia Hypoxia	■ Absence or resolution of hyperbilirubinemia Absence of kernicterus* and bilirubin encephalopathy†	■ Observe for jaundice; document and report observations Spectral reflectance, a noninvasive quantitative method, may be used for greater accuracy and to determine need for further laboratory testing Monitor Total bilirubin levels, including direct and indirect, daily on all premature, low birth weight, and sick infants for first 7 days of life (jaundice appears with higher levels of bilirubin in these infants and thus hyperbilirubinemia may not be recognized if visible jaundice is used as sole criterion) Serum acid-base balance Provide early feeding (within first 12 hours of life) according to unit protocols, unless contraindicated (5% or 10% glucose in water, formula, or breast milk) Administer phototherapy‡ as ordered Phototherapy for unstable premature infants is usually started at 8 mg bilirubin/dl

*Kernicterus is the presence of unconjugated bilirubin in the basal ganglia and is associated with a syndrome of high-pitched cry, hypertonicity, and opisthotonos followed by athetosis, asymmetrical spasticity, hearing loss, and dental anomalies. The exact pathogenesis is not yet known.

†Bilirubin encephalopathy refers to a broad spectrum of neurological damage associated with hyperbilirubinemia including dyslexia, hyperactivity, poor motor coordination, and intellectual impairment. The exact correlation of these symptoms with kernicterus is not clearly understood, and neither is the process by which bilirubin damages CNS nuclei.

‡Phototherapy reduces serum bilirubin levels. Whether it also reduces the development of kernicterus is not known. (Kernicterus has been reported in both full-term and premature infants who received phototherapy but also had multiple complications, as listed, that potentiate kernicterus development.) Phototherapy degrades bilirubin compounds to water-soluble, readily excreted compounds and also increases the excretion of unconjugated bilirubin and bilirubin metabolites into the bile and urine. This occurs in the outer 2 mm of the skin and is most effective when a large surface is exposed. The most effective light is narrow-spectrum blue light, although broad-spectrum daylight is also used. Staff should be shielded from the blue light to prevent nausea and dizziness. Clinical studies have contradicted animal studies regarding the long-term effects of phototherapy. No measurable long-term effects have yet been identified.

POTENTIAL PROBLEMS	EXPECTED OUTCOMES	NURSING ACTIVITIES
		Apply eye shields to closed eyes (check eyes for signs of conjunctivitis); change shield daily
		Uncover infant for maximum exposure
		Change position q2 hr
		Verify regular maintenance checks of phototherapy lights to assure proper wavelength
		Cover ultraviolet light with plastic shield to protect infant from ultraviolet radiation
		Monitor temperature; prevent overheating
		Replace insensible H_2O loss
		Monitor and record urine specific gravity; notify physician of increase
		Give supplemental glucose H_2O between feedings if infant is taking po feedings (this will vary with size and gastric capacity of infant)
		Turn lights off when drawing blood specimens
		Observe for side effects of phototherapy
		Cutaneous erythema
		Increased skin pigmentation
		Increased intestinal transit time
		Abdominal distention
		Loose green stool
		Hyperthermia
		Increased skin blood flow
		Decreased growth (there is subsequent catching up)
		Hypocalcemia
		Apnea (related to eye shields)
		Alterations in behavior
		Recognize increased insensible fluid loss (usually twofold to threefold increase) and monitor intake-output balance accordingly
		Assist with exchange transfusion* if needed (clinical criteria—or most effective time—for intervening with exchange transfusion in premature infants is not known; generally, transfusion in these infants is done at lower bilirubin levels because associated hypoxia, acidosis, hypoglycemia, or infection may make them more susceptible to neurotoxicity; however, interrelationships of these various factors or stresses are not known)
		Administer albumin before transfusion, if ordered (reportedly, this increases efficiency of exchange transfusion, theoretically as a result of volume expansion)
		Preferred route is umbilical artery and vein (withdrawing from artery and infusing into vein)
		Place infant under radiant warmer and attach to cardiorespiratory monitor
		Exchanged blood should be less than 1 day old
		Warm exchanged blood to 95° to 98.6° F (35° to 37° C)
		Before and after transfusion, monitor the following parameters
		Hct and Hgb
		Platelets
		Arterial blood gas levels and pH
		Heart rate, respiratory rate, BP, and T q10-15 min; record after every 100 ml transfused
		Serum electrolytes, including Ca^{++}
		Total serum protein
		Total and direct serum bilirubin
		Reticulocytes
		Manual blood glucose strips (e.g., Dextrostix) and serum glucose

*Exchange transfusion remains the most efficient method of decreasing serum bilirubin. There is a 5% mortality associated with this procedure related to the infant's clinical status before the transfusion. An estimated 1% mortality exists during or within the first 6 hours after the procedure.

POTENTIAL PROBLEMS	EXPECTED OUTCOMES	NURSING ACTIVITIES

		During transfusion observe for signs of
		    Hypotension
		    Hypoglycemia
		    Hypocalcemia
		    Hyperkalemia
		    Hyponatremia
		    Bradycardia
		    Acidosis
		    Hypoxia
		    Hypovolemia
		    Thrombocytopenia
		    Volume overload
		    Acidosis/alkalosis
		Ca^{++} may be prescribed per unit volume of blood infused, especially if pretransfusion level is low (less than 7.5 mg/100 ml)
		After exchange, monitor manual blood glucose strips (e.g., Dextrostix) q15-20 min for 2 hours (hypoglycemia is common after effect)
		Observe for signs of complications of exchange transfusion
		    Alterations in ICP
		    NEC
		    Arrhythmias (related to myocardial hypoperfusion)
		    Thrombi or emboli
		    Sepsis
		Notify physician of abnormalities in aforementioned, and alter therapy as ordered
		    Exchange transfusion may have to be repeated
		Monitor for kernicterus (rare with therapeutic lowering of bilirubin levels)
		    High-pitched cry
		    Hypertonicity
		    Opisthotonos
		    As condition progresses
		        Athetosis
		        Asymmetrical spasticity
		        Hearing loss
		        Dental anomalies
		Notify physician of aforementioned abnormalities
		Administer therapy, as ordered, and monitor patient's response

■ Retrolental fibroplasia (retinopathy of prematurity) caused by hyperoxia	■ Absence of effects of retinotoxic O_2 levels	■ Maintain minimal level of inspired O_2 (FIO_2) that is sufficient to maintain PaO_2 at 50 to 70 mm Hg ($FIO_2 \leq 0.4$ is usually adequate) Monitor FIO_2 and record concentration q1-2 hr FIO_2 should be prescribed based on arterial blood gas levels Infants who receive O_2 for any period should have optic fundi examined by ophthalmologist during and after O_2 therapy, at discharge, and at 5 months of age or 3 months after discharge Arrange for consultation as per hospital routine Instruct parents regarding discharge follow-up; arrange clinic appointment Administer tocopherol (vitamin E), as prescribed

POTENTIAL PROBLEMS	EXPECTED OUTCOMES	NURSING ACTIVITIES
■ Parents lack confidence in their skills to care for infant at home—related to perceived ''special needs,'' dependency on staff, anxiety	■ Infant will thrive and receive appropriate physical and psychological nurturing Parents demonstrate readiness to assume infant's care and enthusiasm for homecoming Appropriate parent-infant attachment	■ Prepare parents for assuming care of baby at home Help parents plan for infant's homecoming Recognize that parents probably were not prepared for early delivery Allow parents to discuss this experience and their feelings; while primary attention is directed to newborn, mother may feel neglected, inadequate, or guilty Instruct parents in care of baby; fathers should be included in active care participation in nursery Feeding techniques Infant should be awake and alert Methods to stimulate sucking, e.g., moving nipple in baby's mouth, pressure on chin, stroking chin Bathing Normal and individual sleep/wake patterns and other behaviors, e.g., crying Special needs Signs and symptoms of and immediate intervention for aspiration As discharge time nears, assess preparation of home situation Refer to public health nurse or Visiting Nurse Association Discuss specific preparations Assess parents' readiness to assume responsibility for infant's care

GROWTH RETARDATION

In the past, newborns whose birth weight was 2500 g or less were termed *premature*. However, it is now known that not all newborns weighing less than 2500 g are premature (meaning born before 38 weeks gestation). The term *low birth weight* is used to designate infants weighing less than 2500 g, regardless of cause and without regard to length of gestation. When infants of low birth weight are properly classified according to gestational age, approximately one third are small for their gestational age.

The term *intrauterine growth retardation* is applied to infants whose birth weight is below that which is expected according to gestational age. Terms such as *small for dates, small for gestational age (SGA),* and *dysmature* have been used to refer to fetal underdevelopment. Infants whose birth weight is in the 10th percentile or less for their gestational age on the intrauterine growth curve are considered growth retarded.

In early fetal life, growth results from an increase in cell number. Insults during this vulnerable period of fetal growth result in organs with fewer cells than normal but with cells of normal size. The infant at birth does not appear wasted, but all growth parameters are below normal. During the later part of fetal development, increases in cell size become dominant. Insults during this period of cell hypertrophy result in cells of normal number but smaller size. The infant appears wasted. Weight may be the only abnormally low growth parameter (less than expected). The skin is dry with loose skin folds. Hair may be thin and sparse. The infant is alert and appears to be hungry. Meconium staining may be evident.

There are two major factors that determine fetal growth: the adequacy of the "supply line" (mother and placenta) and the inherent growth potential of the fetus. Intrauterine growth retardation may be caused by maternal, placental, and fetal factors. Maternal factors include malnutrition, hypertension, preeclampsia, alcohol and/or drug abuse, cigarette smoking, advanced diabetes, heart disease, and chronic renal disease. Placental factors include premature separation, single umbilical artery, placental infarction, and the twin transfusion syndrome. Fetal factors include chronic intrauterine infection, congenital malforma-

tions, multiple gestation, and chromosomal abnormalities.

The diagnosis of intrauterine growth retardation is confirmed by characteristic physical and neurological signs and symptoms at birth. The assessment of gestational age for all newborns should be part of the nursery admission procedure. Using a system such as the one described by Dubowitz,* the nurse can determine the infant's gestational age and plot this on the Denver intrauterine growth curve to determine if the infant is at or below the 10th percentile. Treatment begins by anticipating the birth of a growth-retarded infant and/or identifying the infant as growth retarded at birth. Adequate provisions for warmth and resuscitation must be available in the delivery room. Growth-retarded infants do not readily tolerate the stress of labor, thus asphyxia should be anticipated and resuscitative measures instituted if necessary.

Hypoglycemia may be present at birth and should be anticipated during the first 48 to 72 hours, because the infant's already-low glycogen stores are exhausted. Close monitoring of the blood sugar by a blood glucose monitoring strip (e.g., Chemstrips, Dextrostix) is part of nursing care. If low glucose is detected, precise serum glucose determinations should then be made.

Oral formula or breast milk feedings are begun as soon as possible, but not later than 4 hours of age. Treatment by IV infusion of glucose is necessary when laboratory serum glucose determinations indicate a blood glucose level below 20 to 25 mg/dl in low birth weight infants and 30 to 35 mg/dl in term infants less than 3 days old. The Hct is followed closely to detect polycythemia, which may be asymptomatic.

Prognosis for the growth-retarded infant depends on a number of factors, including the cause, severity and duration of the insult and the recognition and management of neonatal disorders. Research is ongoing related to long-term outcomes. Parents must understand the importance of close follow-up.

---

*Dubowitz, L., Dubowitz, V., and Goldberg, C.: Clinical assessment of gestational age in the newborn infant, J. Pediatr. **77:**1-10, 1970.

ASSESSMENT

1. Maternal history of
   a. Infection
   b. Hypertension
   c. Preeclampsia
   d. Alcohol/drug abuse
   e. Smoking
   f. Advanced diabetes
   g. Renal disease
   h. Malnutrition
   i. Multiple gestation
2. Determination of infant's gestational age, using criteria developed by Dubowitz
3. Infant's weight below 10th percentile for gestational age according to Denver intrauterine growth curve
4. Monitor lab data
   a. Hct
   b. Blood sugar
   c. Immune globulin type M (IgM)
   d. Electrolytes
   e. TORCH screen
5. Signs and symptoms of complications
   a. Seizures
   b. Respiratory distress
   c. Hyperbilirubinemia
   d. Meconium aspiration
   e. Hypothermia
   f. Hypoglycemia

GOALS

1. Blood glucose within normal limits
2. Adequate nutrition for weight gain
3. Thermal stability
4. Parent-infant attachment
5. Before discharge, parents
   a. Verbalize understanding of infant's condition
   b. Demonstrate ability to bathe, feed, and care for infant
   c. State plans for follow-up visits

POTENTIAL PROBLEMS	EXPECTED OUTCOMES	NURSING ACTIVITIES
■ Perinatal asphyxia caused by chronic hypoxia and/ or hypoxic stress during labor	■ Asphyxiated state recognized and appropriate treatment instituted at birth	■ Anticipate growth-retarded infant from maternal history Monitor fetal heart during labor Suction airway immediately at birth Provide O_2 as indicated by infant's condition Observe for meconium-stained fluid, skin, and nails

■ Hypoglycemia as result of reduced glycogen stores	■ Blood sugar maintained between 45 to 120 mg/dl	■ Monitor blood glucose by Dextrostix at birth and q3-4 hr; notify physician if below 45 mg/dl
		Observe infant carefully for signs of hypoglycemia
		   Jittery movements
		   Apnea
		   Lethargy
		   Seizures
		   Color change
		   Poor suck reflex
		Begin feedings as soon as possible after birth and no later than 4 hours of age

■ Hypothermia as result of limited subcutaneous insulation	■ Axillary temperature maintained in neutral thermal zone (97° to 98° F [36° to 36.5° C])	■ Monitor axillary temperature at least q2-3 hr; if infant is in Isolette, check Isolette temperature and adjust as necessary
		Observe for symptoms of thermal instability
		   Cold skin temperature
		   Lethargy
		   Grunting respirations
		   Poor feeding
		Avoid placing infant on cold surfaces or in drafty locations
		Institute warming measures
		   Dry off infant
		   Add additional blanket
		   Place infant in Isolette and attach servocontrol mechanism
		   Warm infant slowly (1°/hour) to avoid hyperthermia

■ Polycythemia
   Etiology is unclear, but may be result of placental insufficiency
	■ Hct maintained below 65%	■ Monitor Hct at birth and follow as necessary
		Observe for signs of increased blood viscosity
		   Respiratory distress
		   Cyanosis
		   Seizures
		If indicated, assist physician with partial exchange transfusion; monitor vital signs; keep accurate records of withdrawn blood and infused plasma

POTENTIAL PROBLEMS	EXPECTED OUTCOMES	NURSING ACTIVITIES
■ Congenital anomalies	■ Abnormalities recognized and appropriate management instituted	■ Thorough physical assessment at birth or on admission to nursery Notify physician of abnormalities Administer supportive care according to abnormality present, as ordered

■ Hyperbilirubinemia as result of hemolysis	■ Indirect bilirubin maintained below level acceptable for weight and gestational age	■ Observe and record infant's color q4 hr
		Monitor indirect bilirubin at least q8 hr beginning 48 hours after delivery
		If phototherapy is indicated
		  Keep infant warm by placing in Isolette and recording temperature q4 hr; remove infant only for feedings
		  Apply eye patches over closed lids
		  Remove eye patches for eye care and feeding q4 hr and replace
		  Offer H_2O between feedings to prevent dehydration and to promote excretion of bilirubin via intestinal route

■ Late anemia as result of rapid weight gain and low iron stores	■ Hct maintained within normal limits for age	■ Administer iron supplement, as ordered Instruct parents in proper administration of iron supplement
■ Delayed parent-infant attachment	■ Parent-infant interaction and attachment occur	■ Encourage early and frequent visitation Encourage parents to touch, cuddle and hold infant Allow parents to verbalize concerns Provide parents with explanations of treatment and equipment

■ Parents have insufficient knowledge and/or skills to comply with discharge regimen	■ Parents verbalize understanding of cause(s) and effects of infant's growth retardation
	Parents demonstrate ability to care for infant
	Parents state provision for follow-up care
		■ Assess parents' knowledge and understanding of infant's condition
		Teaching program* that includes
		  Cause and effect of underlying problem (should be done by physician and reinforced by nurse)
		  Newborn care—bathing, feeding, diaper care, etc.
		  Follow-up—necessity of timing and where and by whom to be provided

*If responsibility of critical care nurse includes such follow-up care.

NEONATAL RESPIRATORY DISTRESS

Respiratory distress in the newborn may be caused by conditions of pulmonary and nonpulmonary origin. The most common pulmonary causes are *hyaline membrane disease (HMD), meconium aspiration syndrome,* and *transient tachypnea of the newborn.* The failure of the newborn to establish respirations at birth is also considered respiratory distress. Congenital heart disease, CNS disorders, and metabolic and hematological disturbances are nonpulmonary causes of respiratory distress.

HMD is a disease of prematurity. Respiratory distress occurs as a result of an inadequate amount of surfactant, a substance that lines the alveoli and prevents alveolar collapse. Insufficient surfactant levels result in atelectasis and increased pulmonary resistance. This, in turn, results in hypoxia and hypercapnia. Infants with HMD exhibit mixed acidosis. Respiratory acidosis results from difficulties in gas exchange. Metabolic acidosis is a result of hypoxia and anaerobic metabolism. A chest radiograph reveals the typical "ground glass" appearance of the lungs.

There is no definitive treatment for HMD. Treatment is aimed at supporting the infant until surfactant is produced in sufficient quantity. This is accomplished by providing or assisting ventilation; correcting acid-base disturbances; providing nutritional support; and maintaining BP and Hct levels.

Meconium aspiration syndrome usually occurs in term infants and is the neonatal consequence of fetal asphyxia. In addition to obstruction of the airway, chemical pneumonitis may result from an inflammatory response to meconium. At delivery, it is important to visualize the vocal cords and to carefully suction the meconium before the infant takes a breath and before resuscitative measures are instituted.

Treatment in the nursery is again supportive. Vigorous pulmonary therapy followed by suctioning is repeated as indicated. Oxygen and/or mechanical ventilation may be necessary. Nutritional support, maintenance of acid-base balance and BP are important priorities. One complication of meconium aspiration syndrome is pneumothorax, which should be suspected if the infant's clinical status deteriorates suddenly. The lungs, in time, are capable of removing the meconium, and marked recovery is usually noted after 48 hours.

Transient tachypnea of the newborn usually follows an uneventful term pregnancy. It is characterized by tachypnea in the absence of significant retractions or rales. The infant may be cyanotic on room air. Delayed resorption of fetal lung fluid following birth is believed to be the cause.

Respiratory distress is manifest at or shortly after birth. This respiratory distress is self-limited and the majority of these infants recover in 5 to 10 days without sequelae. Management is supportive and is directed towards maintaining oxygenation and adequate nutrition.

Surgical conditions such as tracheoesophageal fistula and diaphragmatic hernia are nonpulmonary causes of respiratory distress. Other nonpulmonary causes are congenital heart disease, hypoglycemia, hypothermia, loss of blood, and CNS disturbances.

A variety of symptoms may be present in infants with respiratory distress (see Assessment). They may be present at birth or they may be delayed for several hours. An expiratory grunt, as the infant attempts to keep alveoli from collapsing by increasing "back pressure" in the respiratory system, is characteristic of HMD.

Management of respiratory distress is aimed at identifying the cause, maximizing pulmonary function, and minimizing oxygen consumption. Respiratory assistance can be provided by the use of supplemental oxygen and by CPAP. The monitoring of blood gas levels is essential, as is attention to electrolytes, nutrition, and cardiovascular status. Thermoregulation is imperative to minimize oxygen consumption.

The prognosis for these infants is dependent on a number of factors, including the cause of the respiratory distress and the recognition and management of neonatal disorders. Hypoxia may have an effect on the infant's subsequent development. Careful monitoring of arterial blood gas levels and appropriate adjustment of oxygen levels has reduced the incidence of retrolental fibroplasia. All infants who have received oxygen should have an ophthalmoscopic examination before discharge. Chronic pulmonary disease is becoming more common as a result of intensive respiratory therapy and the use of ventilators and positive pressure therapy. Long-term data is only now becoming available on the consequences of intense respiratory therapy. Infants receiving such treatment will require close follow-up after discharge.

ASSESSMENT

1. Maternal history of
   a. Premature delivery
   b. Bleeding
   c. Meconium-stained amniotic fluid
2. Pulmonary causes leading to respiratory distress
   a. Transient tachypnea of the newborn
   b. HMD
   c. Aspiration syndrome(s)
   d. Airway obstruction
   e. Pneumothorax
   f. Pneumonia
   g. Pulmonary hemorrhage
3. Nonpulmonary causes leading to respiratory distress
   a. Congenital heart disease
   b. Metabolic factors
      (1) Hypoglycemia
      (2) Hypothermia
      (3) Hyperthermia
   c. CNS factors
      (1) Drug effect
      (2) Cerebral hemorrhage
      (3) Meningitis
   d. Hematological factors
      (1) Polycythemia
      (2) Anemia
      (3) Acute blood loss
   e. Sepsis
   f. Persistent fetal circulation
4. Continuous monitoring of PO_2 via transcutaneous sensor
5. Continuous monitoring of heart rate, temperature, and respirations
6. Signs and symptoms of respiratory distress
   a. Suprasternal, substernal, and intercostal retractions
   b. Nasal flaring
   c. Expiratory grunt
   d. Cyanosis in room air
   e. Tachypnea/apnea
   f. Tachycardia/bradycardia
   g. Decreased breath sounds on auscultation
7. Results of lab data
   a. Arterial blood gas levels
   b. Blood glucose
   c. Hct
   d. Electrolytes
   e. Blood culture
8. Chest radiograph findings
9. Signs and symptoms indicating need for assisted ventilation, with guidelines for the following modes of assisted ventilation

   a. Oxygen via Oxyhood
      (1) Absent or mild retractions
      (2) Blood gas analysis within normal limits in less than 40% oxygen
   b. CPAP
      (1) Spontaneous respirations, grunting, tachypnea
      (2) Recurrent apnea
      (3) Mild to moderate retractions
      (4) Requires 40% to 60% oxygen to maintain blood gases within normal limits
      (5) Rising Pa_{CO_2}
   c. Mechanical ventilation
      (1) Severe retractions
      (2) Apnea
      (3) Requires greater than 60% oxygen to maintain blood gases within normal limits
      (4) Pa_{CO_2} greater than 70 mm Hg
10. Complications of assisted ventilatory therapy
    a. Bronchopulmonary dysplasia
    b. Pneumothorax
    c. Intracranial hemorrhage
    d. Retrolental fibroplasia
11. Parental response to neonatal illness
    a. Understanding of cause of respiratory distress
    b. Understanding of rationale for and effects of treatment
    c. Guilt associated with failure to produce a "normal" baby
    d. Coping mechanisms and support system

GOALS

1. Absence and/or resolution of respiratory distress
2. Maximum pulmonary function
3. Minimum metabolic requirement and oxygen consumption
4. Nutritional intake supportive for growth
5. Successful weaning from oxygen and/or assisted ventilatory therapy
6. Absence of complications resulting from oxygen and/or assisted ventilatory therapy
7. Absence of infection
8. Successful parent-infant attachment
9. Before discharge, parents
   a. Verbalize understanding of cause, therapeutic management, and prognosis
   b. Demonstrate ability to bathe, feed, and care for infant
   c. State plans for follow-up care by pediatrician and, if indicated, specialists

POTENTIAL PROBLEMS	EXPECTED OUTCOMES	NURSING ACTIVITIES

■ Hypoxia and respiratory insufficiency related to inadequate ventilation, airway obstruction	■ Maximal pulmonary function
	Absence of respiratory distress
		■ Position infant for maximal lung expansion
		  Extend infant's head by placing small blanket roll under shoulders; *do not hyperextend*
		  Elevate head of bed slightly
		  Keep infant's hands off chest
		  Change position from sides to back at least q2 hr
		Observe and auscultate for bilateral air entry at least q1 hr; possible causes of decreased or unequal air entry
		  Kinked endotracheal tube or ventilator tubing
		  Endotracheal tube displaced into nasopharynx
		  Endotracheal tube displaced into right main stem bronchus
		  Airway clogged with secretions
		  Pneumothorax
		Monitor transcutaneous Po_2 continuously
		  Calibrate machine according to manufacturer's directions
		  Keep high and low alarms in ON position
		  Rotate position of sensor q3-4 hr
		  Be aware of possible causes of abnormal reading
		    Endotracheal tube or ventilator tubing kinked
		    Airway clogged with secretions
		    Endotracheal tube displaced
		    Pneumothorax
		    Other
		Maintain patency of airway
		  Suction at least q2 hr and prn for removal of secretions
		    Oxyhood—suction nasopharynx and oropharynx
		    CPAP—suction nasopharynx and oropharynx
		    Endotracheal tube
		      Instill 0.33 to 0.5 ml sterile saline solution to loosen secretions
		      Reattach ventilator and ventilate 30 seconds
		      Turn head to one side
		      Using gloved hand and sterile catheter, quickly suction
		      Replace on ventilator for 30 seconds, then repeat steps 3 and 4 on other side
		Chest physiotherapy for infants with poor air exchange and positive radiological findings of atelectasis
		Monitor Hct at least daily; record amount of blood withdrawn for lab analysis

■ Increased metabolism related to increased tissue O_2 consumption	■ Minimum metabolic requirement and adequate tissue oxygenation	■ Avoid excessive stimulation
		Maintain neutral thermal environment
		  Provide care within Isolette or under radiant heater
		  Monitor and record axillary temperature q2-3 hr (thermoneutral zone is 97° to 98° F [36° to 36.5° C])
		  If warming measures are necessary, warm infant slowly (1°/hour) to avoid hyperthermia
		Administer O_2 via heated humidified nebulizer with temperature at same level as ambient air
		Administer gavage feedings to minimize energy expenditure
		  Have formula or breast milk at room temperature
		  Administer slowly, maximum 2 ml/minute

■ Acid-base disturbance	■ Acid-base balance	■ Monitor arterial blood gas levels q2-4 hr according to patient's condition
		Notify physician of any abnormal results
		Keep flow sheet for recording blood gas results and interventions as ordered
		  Respiratory acidosis—correct by reducing CO_2 levels by use of controlled ventilation
		  Metabolic acidosis—correct by slowly infusing prescribed amount of sodium bicarbonate diluted in a one-to-one ratio with sterile H_2O
		  Respiratory alkalosis—correct by reducing breathing rate

POTENTIAL PROBLEMS	EXPECTED OUTCOMES	NURSING ACTIVITIES

■ Nutritional imbalance
Fluid and electrolyte im-
balance
	■ Fluid and electrolyte bal-
	ance
	Nutritional intake support-
	ive for growth
		■ Monitor results of serial serum Na^+, K^+, and Cl^- determinations
		Keep bedside flow sheet for recording all intake/output
		Intake
		  Gavage feedings
		    Insert NG or orogastric feeding tube
		    Verify tube placement in following three ways
		      Absence of bubbles when tip placed under H_2O
		      Aspiration of gastric contents
		      Auscultate while injecting 0.5 to 1 cc of air through feeding
		        tube; listen below xiphoid process for air entry into stom-
		        ach; remove air
		    Elevate head of bed slightly
		    Administer breast milk or formula at room temperature
		    Administer feeding slowly, maximum 2 ml/minute, to minimize
		      metabolic activity and to reduce pressure on diaphragm
		    Observe for
		      Cyanosis
		      Tachypnea
		      Apnea
		      Bradycardia
		      Abdominal distention
		      Emesis
		    After feeding, place infant on side
		    Record type and amount of feeding as well as infant's response
		  IV infusions
		    Use infusion pump to maintain constant flow rate
		    Keep IV at rate ordered
		    Protect IV site
		    Inspect IV site q1 hr for infiltration or leakage
		    Record q1 hr
		      Type of solution
		      Amount infused
		      Running balance in relation to rate ordered
		  Hyperalimentation (see Standard 57, *Total parenteral nutrition*)
		Output
		  Daily weights on same scale
		  Weigh diapers to determine urine output
		  Test urine q4 hr for specific gravity, pH, and presence of sugar,
		    protein, and blood
		  Record number, color, and consistency of stools; test stool for
		    guaiac
		  Record amount of blood withdrawn for lab analysis
		Monitor for signs and symptoms of dehydration
		  Elevated Hct
		  Elevated total protein level
		  Poor skin turgor
		  Loss of 5% total body weight within 24 hours
		  Elevated Serum Na^+
		  Elevated urine specific gravity
		  Decreased urine output
		Notify physician of aforementioned abnormalities, and alter thera-
		  peutic regimen as ordered

■ O_2 toxicity	■ Absence or minimization of O_2 toxicity	■ Measure and record FIO_2 q1 hr Administer prescribed amount of O_2 Verify all changes in FIO_2 with an O_2 analyzer Calibrate O_2 analyzer at least once each shift Humidify and warm all O_2

POTENTIAL PROBLEMS	EXPECTED OUTCOMES	NURSING ACTIVITIES

■ Infection	■ Prevention or absence of infection	■ Meticulous handwashing
		Change Isolette weekly; change Isolette sleeves every 2 to 3 days
		Suction with gloved hand and sterile catheter
		Care of ventilatory equipment
		    Change tubing and/or Oxyhood and humidifier q24 hr
		    Refill humidification source with sterile H_2O each shift
		    Check tubing for condensation and drain into basin; do not drain back into humidifier
		Change indwelling feeding tube daily
		Care of IV infusion
		    Change IV bottle, tubing, and stopcocks q24 hr
		    Cleanse umbilical catheter insertion site daily according to unit protocol
		    Observe insertion site for inflammation, discharge, etc.
		Monitor for signs and symptoms of infection
		    Thermal instability
		    Inflammation of umbilical stump
		    Lethargy
		    Apnea
		Assist physician in drawing of blood cultures, spinal taps, etc.
		Administer antibiotics, as ordered

■ Respiratory insufficiency related to use and function of Oxyhood and assisted ventilatory equipment	■ Maximal therapeutic effects of assisted ventilatory equipment	■ Oxyhood
		Use hood of appropriate size*
		    Small: less than 2½ pounds (1134 g)
		    Medium: 2½ to 8 pounds (1135 to 3629 g)
		    Large: over 8 pounds (3630 g)
		Do not plug holes; they allow for removal of CO_2
		Do not seal space between hood and infant's neck
		CPAP
		    Use nasal prongs of size appropriate for nares
		    Keep nasal prongs securely in nares; remove q4 hr to give care
		        Stimulate skin under nares
		        Cleanse and dry nostril openings and skin thoroughly
		        Check for redness due to pressure
		        Replace and anchor securely
		    Connections of tubes and gauges must be tight with no air leakage
		    Administer prescribed amount of CPAP
		    Monitor and record amount of CPAP q1 hr
		Mechanical ventilation
		    Monitor pulse and respiration during intubation
		    Use endotracheal tube of appropriate size†
		        2.5 inside diameter: under 1000 g
		        3.0 inside diameter: 1000 to 1500 g
		        3.5 inside diameter: 1500 to 2200 g
		        4.0 inside diameter: over 2200 g
		    Secure endotracheal tube in proper position; obtain radiographic confirmation of tube position
		    Keep an extra tube of appropriate size at bedside
		    Set alarms at reasonable limits and keep in ON position
		    Maintain bedside flow sheet for q1 hr recording of
		        All settings (pressures, rate, CPAP, PEEP, FIO_2, etc.)
		        Changes made and by whom
		    Check tubes for kinking, which can result in blocked airway
		    Keep tubing free of accumulated moisture
		    Place manual resuscitator bag with appropriate size mask at bedside and within reach in case of ventilator failure or extubation

*Williams, T.J., and Hill, J.W., eds.: Handbook of neonatal respiratory care, Riverside, Calif., Bourns, Inc., p. 55.
†Avery, G.B.; Neonatology, Philadelphia, 1975, J.B. Lippincott Co., p. 268.

POTENTIAL PROBLEMS	EXPECTED OUTCOMES	NURSING ACTIVITIES
■ Inability to wean from O_2 due to Anemia Sepsis Hypoglycemia Inadequate nutritional state Pneumothorax Severe asphyxia or CNS disturbance Bronchopulmonary dysplasia	■ Successful weaning from O_2	■ Monitor infant for signs and symptoms of Anemia Sepsis Hypoglycemia Poor nutritional state Pneumothorax Severe asphyxia or CNS disturbance To lower F_{IO_2} Repeat Pa_{O_2} before each decrease and/or use transcutaneous P_{O_2} as guide Reduce environmental O_2 in 5% decrements per hour; when below 30%, reduce in 2% decrements Observe infant for Cyanosis Pallor Tachypnea Hypothermia Record all changes and infant's response Notify physician of any difficulty in weaning, and administer corrective therapy, as ordered
■ Difficulties in parent-infant bonding caused by separation, guilt, and anxiety	■ Resolution of parental guilt feelings and beginning of parent-infant attachment process	■ Encourage parents to verbalize feelings regarding illness of their child; reassure parents as to ''normalcy'' of guilt feelings Encourage parents to communicate with each other and with other parents Promote parent-infant involvement during hospitalization Refer to the infant by his/her name Encourage early and frequent visitation and phone contact Involve parents in infant's care, i.e., feeding, bathing, diapering Encourage parents to touch and hold infant as much as feasible Ask parents to bring in ''something'' for infant—clothes, family picture to hang at cribside, new small stuffed animal, music box, etc.
■ Insufficient parental knowledge and/or skills to successfully care for infant after discharge	■ Parents Verbalize cause of respiratory distress, rationale and effects of treatment, and prognosis Demonstrate ability to care for infant at home State provisions for follow-up care by pediatrician and other specialists	■ Ongoing assessment of parents' knowledge and understanding of condition and treatment Explain and clarify when indicated Reassure parents of their ability to care for infant after discharge Referral to local visiting nurse agency Involve parents in infant's care throughout hospitalization Teaching plan* to include Etiology, management, and prognosis (should be done initially by physician and nurse and reinforced by nurse) Demonstration of newborn care—bathing, feeding, diapering, etc.; return demonstration by parents Explanation and demonstration of special procedures and/or medication administration; return demonstration by parents Importance and necessity of follow-up care

*If responsibility of critical care nurse includes such follow-up care.

HEMOLYTIC DISEASE CAUSED BY Rh/ABO INCOMPATIBILITY

Hemolytic disease of the newborn is most commonly caused by Rh or ABO incompatibility. Hemolysis is the result of an antigen-antibody reaction in the fetus or newborn. Incompatible RBCs leak into the maternal circulation where antibodies are produced and pass back into the fetal circulation, causing hemolysis.

The most serious form of the disease occurs in Rh incompatibility when the mother is Rh negative and the fetus is Rh positive. Sensitization occurs at the time of placental separation. The first pregnancy is usually not affected. During subsequent pregnancies, the transfer of maternal antibodies into the fetal circulation causes the hemolytic process. This disease begins in utero. Its severity can be gauged by maternal antibody titers and by repeated amniocentesis. Because bilirubin is excreted via the placenta, the main risk to the fetus is anemia. The fetus responds to this anemia by attempting to increase erythropoiesis, which is responsible for the hepatosplenomegaly seen in affected infants. The most severe form of the disease is hydrops fetalis. Progressive anemia leads to hypoxia, heart failure, and generalized edema.

After birth, jaundice usually becomes evident within the first few hours of life. The degree of anemia reflects the severity of the disease. Immediate exchange transfusion at birth is indicated in the presence of hydrops fetalis or CHF. The diagnosis can be confirmed by the direct Coombs test, which demonstrates the presence of maternal antibodies on the infant's red blood cells.

The most effective treatment for Rh disease is prevention. Since the early 1960s it has been possible to prevent maternal sensitization through the administration of a vaccine that destroys fetal antigens before they stimulate the production of antibodies. This vaccine must be administered to the mother within 72 hours after delivery and repeated after each pregnancy.

Hemolytic disease from ABO incompatibility is usually of a much milder form. Most often, the mother is type O and the fetus type A or B. First pregnancies may be affected, since anti-A or anti-B antibodies are already present in maternal blood. Severe forms of the disease are rare. The diagnosis is made in the newborn based on clinical and hematological findings. Jaundice is common, as is mild anemia. Peripheral blood smears reveal the presence of spherocytes. A direct Coombs test may be weakly positive or negative, but maternal serum analysis reveals the presence of anti-A or anti-B titers. Exchange transfusions are generally not indicated in cases of ABO incompatibility.

When immediate transfusion is not indicated at birth, the infant's bilirubin and Hct levels should be closely followed every 4 to 6 hours. The danger to the infant is that of kernicterus (bilirubin toxicity), which results in CNS damage. Several factors influence this risk, including the concentration of serum bilirubin, albumin-binding capacity, gestational age, acid-base balance, and the use of drugs that may interfere with the ability of albumin to bind bilirubin.

Exchange transfusion is indicated to treat hyperbilirubinemia or severe anemia (see Assessment). A double volume exchange of 170 ml/kg body weight replaces 85% of the infant's blood. Fresh Rh negative blood is preferred. The use of old blood may cause hyperkalemia. Blood preserved with acid citrate dextrose (ACD) predisposes the infant to hypocalcemia, rebound hypoglycemia, and acidosis. The exchange is done through the umbilical vein, alternately removing and infusing 5 to 20 ml of blood, and usually takes about 1 hour. Several exchange transfusions may be necessary as bilirubin rebounds and hemolysis continue to occur. In some institutions, an exchange transfusion may be preceded by the administration of albumin to increase availability of binding sites.

Phototherapy is of value in mild to moderate cases of hemolytic disease and is usually the only treatment necessary for ABO incompatibility. It should not be used in place of an exchange transfusion when bilirubin levels are rising rapidly, but it may be used following an exchange transfusion. Once phototherapy has begun, skin color is no longer an adequate indicator of bilirubin concentration, since photodecomposition of bilirubin occurs in the capillaries of the skin.

If kernicterus can be prevented, the prognosis for these infants is excellent. Anemia may occur in the second week as remaining antibodies continue to hemolyze the newborn's red blood cells. It is important to explain this to parents, because these infants may require blood transfusions after discharge. This form of anemia does not respond to iron therapy.

ASSESSMENT

1. Family history
   a. Rh incompatibility
      (1) Rh negative mother
      (2) Rh positive father
      (3) Rising titer of anti-D antibodies in maternal serum
   b. ABO incompatibility
      (1) Mother's blood type O
      (2) Previous child with ABO disease
2. Results of prenatal amniotic fluid testing
   a. Intrauterine diagnosis of fetal hemolytic disease
   b. Fetal lung maturity
3. Results of lab studies (neonate)
   a. Indirect bilirubin
   b. Hgb and Hct
   c. Peripheral blood smear
   d. Direct and indirect Coombs test
   e. Blood and Rh type
   f. Reticulocyte count
   g. Platelet count
4. Signs and symptoms of hydrops fetalis
   a. Prematurity
   b. Severe pallor
   c. Subcutaneous edema
   d. Hepatosplenomegaly
   e. CHF
   f. Ascites
5. Signs and symptoms of anemia in infant without hydrops fetalis
   a. Mild edema
   b. Pallor
   c. Hepatosplenomegaly
   d. Hypoglycemia
6. Indications for exchange transfusion
   a. At birth
      (1) Hydrops fetalis
      (2) CHF
   b. Cord Hgb less than 14 mg in premature infant or 11 mg in full-term infant
   c. Term infant
      (1) Bilirubin greater than 6 mg/dl in first 6 hours
      (2) Bilirubin greater than 10 mg/dl in first 12 hours
      (3) Bilirubin 20 mg/100 ml at any time

   d. Premature infant*

Birth weight (grams)	Maximum bilirubin
less than 1250	10 mg/dl
1250 to 1499	13 mg/dl
1500 to 1999	15 mg/dl
2000 to 2499	17 mg/dl
2500 and up	18 mg/dl

   e. Rate of rise of bilirubin 0.5 mg/dl/hour
7. Complications of exchange transfusion
   a. Vascular
      (1) Embolization
      (2) Thrombosis of portal vein
      (3) Perforation of vessel
   b. Cardiac
      (1) Volume overload
      (2) Arrhythmias
      (3) Arrest
   c. Metabolic
      (1) Hypoglycemia
      (2) Hyperkalemia
      (3) Hypernatremia
      (4) Hypocalcemia
      (5) Acidosis
   d. Clotting
      (1) Thrombocytopenia
      (2) Overheparinization
   e. Infections
      (1) Hepatitis
      (2) Bacteremia
   f. Other
      (1) Perforated intestine
      (2) Mechanical injury to donor cells
      (3) NEC
      (4) Hypothermia
8. Parental response to neonatal illness
   a. Understanding of hemolytic process
   b. Understanding of the course of treatment
   c. Guilt related to birth of "abnormal" infant
   d. Coping mechanism and support system

GOALS

1. Absence of kernicterus
2. Absence of anemia
3. Maximum therapeutic effect of phototherapy and/or exchange transfusion
4. Absence or resolution of complications of exchange transfusion
5. Successful parent-infant attachment

*Korones, S.B., and Lancaster, J.: High-risk newborn infants: the basis for intensive nursing care, ed. 3, St. Louis, 1981, The C.V. Mosby Co.

6. Before discharge, parents
   a. Verbalize understanding of etiology and management of infant's hemolytic disease
   b. Demonstrate ability to bathe, feed, and care for infant
   c. Understand need for close monitoring of Hct after discharge
   d. State plans for follow-up care

POTENTIAL PROBLEMS	EXPECTED OUTCOMES	NURSING ACTIVITIES

■ Competition for albumin-binding sites
Cold stress
Hypoxia
Drugs
Hypoglycemia
	■ Maximum availability of bilirubin-binding sites	■ Monitor temperature q4 hr
		Observe for respiratory distress (see Standard 70, *Neonatal respiratory distress*)
		Read literature regarding each drug infant receives; request alternate drug when indicated
		Monitor Dextrostix q4 hr
		Observe for signs and symptoms of hypoglycemia
		  Jittery movements
		  Apnea
		  Lethargy
		  Seizures
		  Color change
		Notify physician if any of aforementioned occurs and alter therapy, as ordered

■ Hypoglycemia caused by islet cell hyperplasia in Rh disease	■ Normoglycemia (45 to 120 mg/dl)	■ Keep IV at rate ordered
		Monitor Dextrostix q4 hr
		Observe for signs and symptoms of hypoglycemia
		  Jittery movements
		  Apnea
		  Lethargy
		  Seizures
		  Color change
		Notify physician if any of aforementioned occurs and alter therapy, as ordered

■ Kernicterus (bilirubin toxicity)	■ Absence of kernicterus	■ Monitor serum bilirubin q4 hr
		Observe for signs and symptoms of kernicterus
		  Decreased sucking ability
		  Reduced muscle tone
		  High pitched cry
		  Opisthotonos
		  Muscle regidity
		  Inform physician immediately if any of aforementioned are present
		Prepare for immediate exchange transfusion

■ Hyperbilirubinemia; delayed resolution of hyperbilirubinemia related to use and function of phototherapy equipment	■ Maximum therapeutic effect of phototherapy
	Bilirubin level within normal limits
		■ Keep infant nude (can wear diaper)
		Keep infant's eyes covered while under lights
		  Apply eye patches over closed lids
		  Do not apply too tightly
		  Remove q4 hr for eye care, and inspect for conjunctivitis
		Use plastic shield to separate lights from infant
		Assess energy output of lights each shift
		  Measure energy output by spectroradiometer
		  Record number of hours bulbs used
		  Change bulbs according to manufacturer's directions
		Monitor bilirubin and Hct q4 hr
		  Turn lights *off* when drawing blood
		  Skin color is not indicative of serum bilirubin once phototherapy begins

POTENTIAL PROBLEMS	EXPECTED OUTCOMES	NURSING ACTIVITIES

■ Side effects of phototherapy
  Hyperthermia
  Increased H_2O loss
  Increase in rate of metabolism
  Loose stools
  Maculopapular rash
	■ Absence/resolution of side effects and maintenance of fluid balance	■ Weigh infant daily
		  Keep infant in Isolette
		  Record temperature q4 hr
		  Record intake and output
		    Offer H_2O between feedings
		    If IV is present, maintain at rate ordered
		    Measure urine specific gravity
		    Record color, consistency, and number of stools
		  Observe skin for
		    Presence of rash
		    Skin color q4 hr (turn off lights to observe)
		  Keep diaper area clean and dry
		  Notify physician if any side effects occur
		  Remove eye patches q4 hr and observe for conjunctivitis

■ Complications of exchange transfusion
 	
  Air embolus
 	
  Cardiac arrhythmias
 	
  Metabolic imbalance
 	
  Sepsis
  Aspiration
  Perforated intestine
 	
  Thrombocytopenia
	■ Absence or resolution of complications	■ Monitor and record infant's response to procedure
		  Check blood slip with blood received to assure correct blood
		  Observe for and anticipate complications during and after procedure
		    Use stopcock to prevent air from entering umbilical line
		    Flush umbilical catheter before insertion
		    Attach infant to cardiac monitor
		    Have O_2 and suction in working order
		    Monitor and record
		      T, P, R, and BP q10 min during procedure, then q15 min four times, q30 min six times
		      Amount of blood infused and withdrawn
		      Presence of arrhythmias
		    Do procedure under radiant warmer
		    Obtain baseline electrolytes
		    Administer fresh blood, as ordered
		    Administer blood at room temperature
		    Observe for signs and symptoms of hypocalcemia
		      Irritability
		      Tachycardia
		      Twitching
		      Prolonged Q-T interval
		    Administer calcium, as ordered
		      Infuse slowly
		      Observe for bradycardia
		    Hypoglycemia (see aforementioned signs and symptoms)
		  Maintain strict sterile technique
		  Aspirate stomach before procedure
		  Keep NPO after procedure
		  Observe for signs and symptoms of perforation
		    Abdominal distention
		    Bloody stools
		    Bilious vomiting
		    Hypotension
		    Pallor
		  Monitor platelet count
		  Observe all puncture sites for bleeding
		  No venipuncture or IM injections should be given until platelet count is known (unless absolutely necessary)
		After transfusion, notify physician of any symptoms of complications, and administer corrective therapy, as ordered

POTENTIAL PROBLEMS	EXPECTED OUTCOMES	NURSING ACTIVITIES
■ Bilirubin rebound following exchange transfusion (caused by binding of extravascular tissue bilirubin to fresh albumin)	■ Bilirubin level remains stable and within normal limits	■ Monitor serum bilirubin immediately after exchange transfusion and q4 hr Prepare for repeat exchange transfusion
■ Anemia Vulnerable RBCs remain in circulation with phototherapy In second week after exchange transfusion as remaining antibodies destroy more cells	■ Hct level is within normal limits	■ Monitor Hct at birth and q4 hr during first 24 hours, then at least q8 hr Assist physician with blood transfusion, if indicated Administer blood at room temperature Administer at ordered rate Monitor vital signs q15 min during administration Instruct parents Explain physiology Stress need for follow-up Tell parents of possible need for transfusion after discharge
■ Difficulties in parent-infant bonding caused by separation, guilt, and anxiety	■ Resolution of guilt feelings and beginning of parent-infant attachment process	■ Provide parents with explanations of treatment regimen and equipment Promote parental involvement during hospitalization Encourage early and frequent visitation and phone contact Allow parents to verbalize feelings; reassure them that guilt feelings are normal If baby is receiving phototherapy, remove eye patches and allow parents to feed while out from lights
■ Parents have insufficient knowledge and/or skills to comply with discharge regimen	■ Parents are able to Describe mechanism of hemolytic disease Explain rationale and effects of treatment Discuss need for close observation and follow-up for anemia, and recognize possibility of need for future transfusion Demonstrate ability to care for infant State provisions for follow-up care	■ Assessment of parents' knowledge of hemolytic disease and treatments used Involve parents in infant's care Referral to local visiting nurse agency Teaching program,* including Physiology of hemolytic disease Rationale for and effects of treatment Demonstration of newborn care; return demonstration by parents Potential for anemia and possible transfusion after discharge Importance of follow-up care

*If responsibility of critical care nurse includes such follow-up care.

NEONATAL NECROTIZING ENTEROCOLITIS

The most common neonatal preoperative diagnosis is necrotizing enterocolitis (NEC), an idiopathic, potentially lethal septic necrosis of the intestines occurring primarily in very immature newborn infants. The incidence of this problem has been increasing, perhaps reflecting the enlarged susceptible population resulting from improved survival rates of premature and low birth weight infants. Of all cases of NEC diagnosed, 80% to 90% occur in infants weighing less than 2500 g and more than 50% occur among those weighing under 1500 g; three fourths of these weigh less than 1000 g. Term infants are also susceptible (approximately 10% to 20% of cases). In term infants, NEC seems to be associated with polycythemia, diarrhea, low birth weight, or small size for gestational age. It also occurs in older infants, children, adolescents, and adults associated with chronic respiratory disease, chronic bowel disease, severe diarrhea, obstructive intestinal lesions, and immunological compromise.

The cause remains uncertain and has been presumed to be miltifactorial, largely because it is difficult to decipher among the many involved factors that may be truly causal and those that are merely associated by virtue of the population at risk and related therapies. Many factors previously suggested as predisposing to NEC pathogenesis have since been found to be equally common among infants of matching weight. The greatest predisposing risk factor is currently considered to be prematurity, with increasing incidence associated with lower birth weights. It is also accepted that intestinal bacteria are necessary for development of NEC. Hence it invariably occurs after the infant has begun feeding, usually by 96 hours of age and less than 72 hours after the first feeding. The onset is often sudden and rapidly progressive with a downhill clinical course as rapid as 4 to 48 hours until the infant succumbs. On the other hand, symptoms may appear slowly with variable intensity and disappear if feedings are discontinued only to recur when feeding resumes.

Pathogenesis is attributed to the immature infant's overshooting the reflexive circulatory redistribution response to hypoxemia, hypothermia, or shock states. In this normal physiological reflex, blood is shunted from organs that tolerate ischemia comparatively well to those that would suffer irreversible damage if deprived of oxygen. This selective ischemia decreases mesenteric circulation. Ischemia may also result from local vasospasm and thromboembolic phenomena, hypovolemia, or reduced cardiac output related to heart failure, MI, or arrhythmias. (In older patients, volume may also be depleted with third spacing following severe burns and extensive surgery or with dehydration secondary to gastroenteritis.)

Bowel ischemia may augment the slower peristalsis of immaturity and result in functional intestinal obstruction, which may then be further exacerbated by ischemic mucosal injury. If the ischemia is extreme or prolonged, mucus secretion is reduced, which eventually progresses to proteolysis and autodigestion. The mucosal ischemia provides an ideal situation for bacterial growth. The organisms involved are essentially normal bowel flora: *Escherichia coli*, enterococci, alpha streptococci, enterobacteria, and *Proteus*. Intestinal colonization may be altered by variations in the nursery's microflora, which may influence the incidence and severity of apparent cluster outbreaks of NEC identified in some units. Anaerobic bacteria, *Clostridium*, and *Bacteroides fragilis* have also been isolated from the stool of NEC patients. The gas-forming bacteria invade areas damaged by proteolysis and autodigestion, resulting in pneumatosis. Bacterial toxins pass readily into the portal circulation through the damaged mucosa, and can potentially cause hepatic toxicity or septic shock.

The type of feeding and the volume of intake combine with intestinal integrity and maturity to affect bacterial activity. The immature colon cannot handle the glucose, fat, or electrolyte load, causing intravascular fluid to rush into the gut to promote isoosmolarity. The large amount of fluid cannot be absorbed by the lower colon and is lost through diarrhea, resulting in hypovolemia. For this reason, hyperosmolar formulas are no longer used in small infant's feedings. However, there may be further carbohydrate malabsorption related to hypoxia. Slow absorption with or without stasis provides an environment for excess bacterial growth, to which the vulnerability of the mucosa has been previously described. Meanwhile, increased gas production increases intestinal distention, further disrupting peristalsis and thus contributing to a pathological cycle.

Thrombocytopenia and DIC have been documented to

varying degrees and with varying incidences among NEC patients. Their pathogenesis, role in the disease process, and contribution to mortality remain open to hypothesis and investigation. Thrombocytopenia has been identified without other hematological findings associated with DIC. It is variably associated with varyingly severe bleeding manifestations (oozing venipuncture and incision sites; intraventricular, pulmonary, and abdominal hemorrhage; hemopericardium). Despite normal bone marrow, this form of DIC does not respond immediately to platelet transfusion, perhaps because of microthrombosis or platelet consumption in the gut. DIC has been considered a complication of the disease, caused by the release of thromboplastin by the damaged bowel. DIC has also been suggested as a triggering factor in NEC pathogenesis. Localized platelet microthrombosis caused by intestinal ischemia could promote the necrotic process in the bowel, perhaps without even evoking generalized consumption coagulopathy. Diffuse coagulopathy occurring as a later sequela is usually irreversible without bowel resection. Rapid clinical deterioration occurs within hours. Peritonitis occurs if the gas dissecting under the mucosa perforates the bowel wall.

Treatment of NEC is aimed at resting the injured bowel, providing nutritional support, and managing complications such as sepsis, coagulopathy, or shock syndromes. Usually, medical intervention is sufficient, and surgery is not required. Therapy is initiated when suspicion is aroused by early suggestive signs. To prevent further damage, this is done without waiting for other symptoms, radiographic evidence, or other lab data. Oral feedings are discontinued and gastric contents are removed via NG tube. The NG tube is left in place so that gastric decompression may be maintained by either continuous intermittent suction or frequent manual aspiration. Systemic gentamicin or kanamycin is usually used, perhaps in addition to topical administration of these drugs via NG tube. Cultures of stool, blood, and gastric aspirate should be done to validate sensitivity. Sensitivity studies of the species of *Klebsiella* prevalent in the particular nursery at the time should also be considered in determining initial therapy, because *Klebsiella* is the most commonly associated organism. Fluid resuscitation is an important part of therapy because of the third spacing associated with bowel necrosis. Hydrocortisone may be given to counteract the endotoxemic vasodilation that leads to shock. Circulatory support may also require isoproterenol (Isuprel) and plasma. Exchange transfusion is sometimes used to increase humoral immunology (deficient in the newborn) or to retard DIC. Provision for adequate nutrition using TPN fulfills requirements for growth and healing and enables the bowel to rest completely for at least 2 weeks after symptoms have subsided. Enteral feeding must be restarted cautiously, monitoring residuals so that overfeeding or compromised GI motility can be identified. Parenteral nutrition should be continued and tapered accordingly as adequate enteral nutrition is attained, a process that may take as long as a month (more commonly 2 or 3 weeks).

In the past, surgery was considered necessary only with signs of bowel perforation or peritonitis. Currently, surgery is advocated before perforation, when there is continued physiological deterioration beyond 72 hours of supportive therapy and bowel rest. If the platelet count drops below 100,000/mm^3 or persists at reduced levels above 100,000/mm^3, gangrene is suspected and surgery is indicated. Waiting increases the risk of hemorrhage and DIC. Hyponatremia or metabolic acidosis that does not improve within 4 hours of therapy is another indication. Surgery involves bowel resection and creation of a temporary ileostomy or colostomy. All necrotic and acutely inflamed bowel is removed. Primary anastomosis is contraindicated because of potential further ischemia and persistent peritonitis. There may be multiple stomas, because necrosis is often patchy. Minimal dissection of bowel is preferred.

Postoperative care includes continued gastric decompression for 7 to 10 days, antibiotic therapy according to peritoneal culture reports for at least 10 days after evidence of sepsis subsides, and continued parenteral nutrition. A high proximal stoma (above the midjejunum) will be closed first, usually after about 3 weeks, to resume GI function and enteral alimentation. Then, if there are multiple stomas, those distal to the functional stoma are usually closed first, leaving the final reanastomosis until after bowel integrity has been verified by barium study. Mechanical and functional abnormalities may occur subsequently. These include stricture and short-gut syndrome, the diagnosis of which may be made as long as 3 months postoperatively. Ischemic strictures at the involved site are also a complication that follows medical therapy. In about one third of the cases, ischemic strictures are multiple, although they may become symptomatic at different times. In many cases, these are asymptomatic and discovered only by routine barium follow-up examination. If there is severe restriction, abdominal distention and vomiting (with or without bile) will occur.

With early recognition, survival from NEC is better than 80%. Its insidious onset, the subtle nature of early symptoms, and its rapid pathological course make astute nursing observation critical in recognition and timely intervention. Survival following surgery has also improved with the increased use of laboratory studies instead of radiographic clinical signs, which often lag behind histopathological severity. Survival has increased for both small and large babies. Septicemia, DIC, peritonitis, and multiple organ failure are responsible for the mortality. The incidence of strictures is reportedly unchanged despite other outcome changes. Long-term prognosis is excellent: physical development and GI function are both unimpaired. In older patients, the clinical course is similar. Mortality in this group is higher because of delayed diagnosis, failure to recognize the syndrome, and delayed treatment.

ASSESSMENT

1. History of perinatal stress (recognizing that NEC may occur when none of these is evident)
   a. Prematurity (especially less than 34 weeks)
   b. Birth asphyxia
   c. Neonatal shock
   d. Respiratory distress
   e. Premature rupture of membranes
   f. Placenta previa or abruptio placentae
   g. Maternal sepsis
   h. Toxemia of pregnancy
   i. Breech or cesarean delivery
2. Abdominal girth measurement on admission and serially before feedings
3. Symptoms of infection, stress, hypoxia, and immunological abnormalities
4. Other nonspecific early symptoms
   a. Thermal instability
   b. Lethargy
   c. Metabolic acidosis
   d. Jaundice
   e. Apnea
   f. Vomiting
5. Poor absorption of feedings (it should be remembered that a majority of premature infants do not absorb their feedings initially)
6. GI symptoms (usually appear 12 to 24 hours after increasing gastric residuals are noted)
   a. Abdominal distention
   b. Vomiting (bilious emesis)
   c. Localized erythema and induration of abdominal wall
   d. Occult blood in stools
   e. Decreased bowel movements

7. Diagnostic radiographic results confirming NEC, including
   a. Nonspecific intestinal dilatation appearing as multiple separate dilatated loops with air-fluid levels in upright position
   b. Intraperitoneal air
   c. Pneumatosis cystoides intestinalis (linear strip or bubbles of gas alongside gas-filled loop; the bubbles may appear like cysts)
   d. Portal venous gas
8. Lab data results
   a. C and S reports
   b. CBC with differential, PT and APTT, platelet count
   c. Serum electrolytes
   d. Serum glucose
   e. Blood gas levels
   f. Blood in stools, emesis, NG drainage
9. Advanced symptoms, including
   a. Hyperglycemia
   b. Frank intestinal bleeding
   c. Peritonitis (reddening or shininess of abdominal wall)
   d. Progressive DIC
   e. Metabolic acidosis

GOALS

1. Integrity of bowel
2. Adequate nutrition
3. Parents verbalize understanding of disease and therapeutic regimen
4. Parents demonstrate interest and desire to participate in care of patient
5. Infant thrives
6. Family unit remains functional

POTENTIAL PROBLEMS	EXPECTED OUTCOMES	NURSING ACTIVITIES

■ Poor absorption of feedings (retained gastric contents are usually undigested formula; this progresses from clear formula at first to bile-tinged material)	■ Absorption of po intake adequate for growth	■ Successful therapy relies on early recognition
		Aspirate gastric contents before each feeding, noting quality and quantity
		Report increasing residuals or bile-stained material immediately
		Encourage and support breast-feeding (breast milk is more easily absorbed by newborn, especially premature infant)
		Parenteral alimentation as ordered by physician and prepared by pharmacist
		Monitor and record
		  Daily weight
		  Hourly intake and output
		  Clinitest q2 hr (less frequently when glucose tolerance has stabilized, usually after 2 days)
		  Serum electrolyte and osmolality per medical routine (usually daily for first week) for any imbalances

Dehydration and electrolyte imbalance resulting from poor absorption	Fluid and electrolyte balance	Monitor serum electrolytes and osmolality; urine output, specific gravity, and osmolality Notify physician of abnormalities and alter therapy, as ordered

POTENTIAL PROBLEMS	EXPECTED OUTCOMES	NURSING ACTIVITIES

■ DIC* secondary to
  Tissue necrosis
  Bleeding
  Sepsis
  In newborn, infections of
  bacterial and viral origin
  are most common stim-
  uli activating clotting
  process
	■ Absence or resolution of
	  coagulopathy
	  Adequate blood volume
	  (Euvolemia)
		■ Administer therapy as ordered to ameliorate underlying or associated
		    problems, e.g., sepsis, hypoxia, shock
		    Be alert to early suggestive signs, e.g., lethargy
		  Observe for evidence of progressive bleeding
		  Monitor for
		    Persistent oozing from puncture sites
		    Petechiae
		    Ecchymoses
		    Hematuria
		    Hematemesis
		    Bloody stools
		    Skin pallor
		  Monitor and record blood loss, including small amounts for laboratory
		    specimens
		  Monitor serial lab tests for infants at risk (do not use heparinized
		    syringe or catheter to obtain specimens)
		    PT
		    APTT
		    Platelets
		    Thrombin time
		    Fibrinogen
		    Fibrin degradation products
		    Factor V
		    Hemoglobin
		  Hematest stools, gastric secretions, and emesis
		  Administer vitamin K, as ordered
		  Maintain aseptic technique
		  Maintain neutral thermal environment
		  Administer IV antibiotics, as ordered
		  Administer IV heparin, as ordered, to maintain whole blood clotting
		    time at 20 to 30 minutes and APTT at 60 to 70 seconds.
		  Assist with exchange transfusion (this is controversial therapy)
		  Apply pressure over bleeding sites (pressure dressings should be
		    avoided because area needs to be observed for adequate circulation,
		    which may be easily impaired in premature or low birth weight
		    infant)
		  Avoid IM injections
		    Be attentive to venipunctures and capillary heel sticks for prolonged
		      bleeding
		    Notify physician of abnormalities
		  Administer transfusions as ordered, which may be necessary as in-
		    dicated by coagulation studies; sometimes exchange transfusions
		    are done; heparin has been found to be less effective in newborns
		    than in adults
		  See Standard 65, *Disseminated intravascular coagulation*

■ Sepsis	■ Maximal protective re-
	  sources maintained; ab-
	  sence or resolution of
	  sepsis
	  Minimal exposure to noso-
	  comial infection
		■ Encourage and support breast-feeding
		    Explain importance of breast milk in supplying protective immu-
		      nological activity of secretory IgA (IgA is principal immuno-
		      globulin in intestinal secretions and is lacking for several days
		      in newborns)
		    In addition, colostric leukocytes provide passive immunity against
		      enteric pathogens
		    Teach manual and pump expression techniques so that breast milk
		      may be given if infant cannot suck at breast, requires tube feed-
		      ings, small feedings, or NPO periods; keep breast milk in plastic
		      (not glass) containers, because leukocytes adhere to glass

*DIC in the neonatal period has a higher than 60% mortality. Two thirds of infants who die with NEC have developed DIC; approximately one sixth of NEC survivors have had DIC symptoms. Correction of coagulopathy before hemorrhage is considered key to survival.

POTENTIAL PROBLEMS	EXPECTED OUTCOMES	NURSING ACTIVITIES

		Use appropriate aseptic technique
		  Particularly in relation to feeding and invasive procedures
		  Change tubing q48 hr on all IVs and q8 hr on continuous feedings
		  Remove NG tubes between intermittent feedings if residuals are not large
		    Catheter is not only potential reservoir for bacteria, but foreign body that can cause irritability and inflammation in tissue; such irritated or inflamed tissue may be susceptible to further damage (see description of pathology)
		  NG tube should not be left in place for intermittent feedings if infant demonstrates discomfort
		  NG tube may be left in place if there is no apparent irritation and if infant does not pull at it, since frequent reinsertion can be traumatic and may injure tissue
		  Nasojejunal tubes should be changed q72 hr
		  Discard opened formula that has been kept at room temperature for more than 4 hours; no more than 4-hour supply of formula or breast milk should be assembled for continuous drip feedings; unfrozen breast milk should not be used after 72 hours in refrigerator
		Be alert to signs of sepsis in neonate to assure early treatment
		Monitor for
		  Change in feeding pattern (usually first sign)
		  Lethargy
		  Irritability
		  Temperature elevation in stable thermal environment
		  Notify physician of any signs of infection
		  Monitor potential infection sources, including culture results

■ Parental anxiety, apprehension and misunderstanding
  Anxiety and apprehension do not follow continuum of progress; parents' perceptions and feelings may be labile
  Often both parents will not exhibit same feelings at same time
	■ Parents' behavior demonstrates
	  Reduced level of anxiety
	  Ability to discuss concerns and fears, ask questions, and verbalize realistic expectations of potential outcomes
		■ Assess parents' level of anxiety, perceptions, and depth of understanding
		  Recognize denial and disbelief
		  Appreciate and accept
		  Encourage and strengthen parents' ability to complement and support each other
		  Allow parents to express feelings of remorse, helplessness, anger, guilt, and pain; encourage validation of feelings
		  Assure parents that such feelings are normal
		  Provide atmosphere that allows convenient and comfortable interaction with staff
		  Provide continuity in assigning nurses to care for patient
		Provide ongoing explanations of all treatments and routine care, appropriate to parents' level of understanding
		  Encourage questions
		  Provide realistic information and reassurance
		Prepare parents in advance for potential complications as well as likely outcomes; this helps to ameliorate uncertainty and establish trust
		Allow parents to participate in infant's care as much as possible
		  During most critical periods, encourage visits
		  Explain rationale for minimal handling, and encourage contact such as stroking forehead or fingers

■ Compromised parent-infant attachment	■ Parents visit, call, and express concern	■ Assess parents' interactions with infant
		Share nuances of infant's behavior with parents; encourage verbal interactions with baby
		Reinforce appropriate patterns of behavior
		Talk to infant in front of and with parents
		Be aware of surrogate attachment patterns nurses may develop with infant patients (especially those requiring critical care) and avoid unconscious exclusion of parents
		  Encourage frequent parental visits
		  Encourage phone calls between visits

POTENTIAL PROBLEMS	EXPECTED OUTCOMES	NURSING ACTIVITIES

■ Respiratory insufficiency related to abdominal distention	■ Adequate oxygenation
	Diaphragm movement is not inhibited
		■ Note subtle changes in breathing pattern; intervene with assistance to minimize work of breathing and assure adequate ventilation; tilt warmer and position infant to minimize abdominal pressure on diaphragm
		Monitor
		   Arterial blood gas values for any abnormalities
		   Abdominal girth
		Note distention in relation to feeding
		Remove air from stomach q30 min and prn
		   Note amount

■ Exacerbation of symptoms following treatment, or recurrence of symptoms	■ Resumption of feeding regimen with adequate absorpiton Bowel integrity	■ Maintain NPO for 7 to 10 days to rest injured bowel Resume feedings slowly in small amounts Do not continue feedings if significant residuals persist Avoid formula feedings Substrates in formula contribute to production of hydrogen gas, which would augment pathogenic activity of gas-forming bacteria Measure serial abdominal girth measurements before feedings; note sudden or continuing increase

■ Progressive inflammation and damage to mucosal wall of intestine	■ Integrity of bowel
	Absence or resolution of enterocolitis
		■ Umbilical catheter should be removed if NEC is suspected
		Prevent injury of gut wall
		   Avoid excessive handling
		   Do not palpate abdomen unnecessarily
		   Avoid diapering
		   Take axillary temperature
		Allow bowel to rest by withholding feedings, as ordered; be attentive to infant's tolerance for po intake; monitor absorption of feedings; monitor for signs of perforation
		   Apnea
		   Shock
		   Sudden drop in temperature
		   Bradycardia
		   Sudden listlessness
		   Rag doll limpness
		   Involuntary rigidity of abdomen
		   Radiograph (usually taken q4-6 hr)
		Notify physician of any abnormalities
		   Administer medications and treatments, as ordered

■ Perforation and/or peritonitis	■ Absence or resolution of peritonitis	■ Note increasing reddening or shininess of abdominal wall Monitor abdominal girth; note increase Notify physician of any changes Peritonitis is indication for immediate surgery See following postoperative care
Postoperative ■ Sepsis and/or wound infection	■ Wound intact, well healed, infection free	■ Keep suture line clean; this may be challenge because of proximity of stoma on small abdomen of premature infant; avoid dressings (may serve as reservoirs for infection) Monitor surgical site and temperature for any abnormalities and notify physician if abnormalities occur If sepsis occurs, administer antibiotics, as ordered If wound infection occurs, administer antibiotics and local wound care, as ordered
■ Respiratory insufficiency	■ Adequate oxygenation	■ Turn patient q1-2 hr Administer chest physiotherapy prn Administer assisted ventilation, as indicated *See* STANDARD 6 *Mechanical ventilation* Monitor arterial blood gas levels; breathing pattern

POTENTIAL PROBLEMS	EXPECTED OUTCOMES	NURSING ACTIVITIES

■ Skin breakdown from enzymes in ileal drainage Immature infant's skin is less resistant to excoriation than others	■ Skin remains clean, dry, and intact	■ Improvise appropriate stoma bags
		  Infant urine collection bags may be cut and shaped for this purpose
		  Plastic medicine cups can be adapted by cutting stoma-size hole in bottom of cup; then aspirate cup contents prn
		  Karaya powder is helpful
		Monitor skin condition

■ Wound disruption caused by catabolism	■ Wound heals
	Weight gain
	Closure of colostomy or ileostomy
		■ Assure adequate nutrition; administer TPN, as prescribed
		Resume feedings via NG tube, as ordered
		Employ good skin care
		Maintain aseptic technique
		Monitor
		  Daily weights
		  Caloric intake

■ Electrolyte imbalance	■ Fluid and electrolyte balance within normal limits	■ Accurately record intake and output including all drainage q1 hr Administer replacement for bowel secretions to augment IV intake, as ordered
■ Dehydration from ileostomy diarrhea, especially if more than 50% of small intestine was removed	■ Adequate hydration Adequate absorption of nutrients	■ Monitor accurate intake and output to assess fluid balance and determine replacement needs Administer appropriate IV therapy, as ordered, including TPN NPO until ileostomy is closed, if indicated
■ Short-gut syndrome, which may be protracted; this may be caused by size of intestinal portion that remains or by disease process	■ Parents verbalize signs and symptoms of short-gut syndrome and bowel stricture	■ Review evidence of short-gut syndrome with parents and encourage them to report these, e.g., changes in feeding patterns, bowel patterns, abdominal distention, weight loss, vomiting, diarrhea

■ Parental anxiety and/or apprehension	■ Parents demonstrate confidence in their own child care abilities relative to their infant's special needs
	Parents verbalize or demonstrate understanding of discharge management of feeding difficulties
		■ Enable parents to continue participating in infant's care after immediate postoperative period, including ostomy care; colostomy is closed after weight gain improves and before discharge
		Help parents become familiar with infant's individuality
		Give parents appropriate phone numbers, etc.
		  Assure them their calls are welcome any time and that you are interested
		  Suggest some specific times to encourage them to call even if there are no identified problems
		Arrange appropriate follow-up care
		Prepare parents for homecoming
		  Explain to parents that it may take several weeks or even months for remaining bowel fo function adequately
		  Multiple formula changes may be necessary
		  Inform parents that rehospitalization may be necessary for appropriate IV therapy, including hyperalimentation
		  Repeat these explanations often, as necessary; parents will need encouragement

CROUP SYNDROME

The term *croup* is commonly applied to a group of infectious conditions of the larynx and trachea seen in infants and young children. The condition is characterized by a brassy cough and inspiratory stridor. Stridor is usually indicative of a high respiratory obstruction. Substernal inspiratory retractions may be present and also may be indicative of upper airway obstruction. Hoarseness or aphonia are variable symptomatic findings.

These infections are of great significance because of the small size of the airway in children. An inflammatory process such as croup can render the airway even smaller and place the infant or child at risk of obstruction.

There are a large number of infectious agents that can cause croup. Viral agents have now been identified as the cause of croup in a high percentage of patients. Parainfluenza virus is probably the most common agent. Other viral agents include adenoviruses, respiratory syncytial virus, and influenza viruses. Croup caused by a virus usually has a gradual onset and course, although an influenza virus may cause an abrupt onset and severe course.

Bacterial agents that cause croup are *Haemophilus influenzae* type B, *Corynebacterium diphtheriae*, pneumococci, and group A streptococci. *H. influenzae* croup is usually an extreme emergency. It is usually characterized by supraglottic obstruction with a red, swollen epiglottis and has a rapid course.

Viral croup is seen more commonly in the younger child from age 3 months to 3 years. Bacterial croup is seen more commonly in children from 3 years to 7 years. Males have a higher incidence of croup than females. There is no known reason for this. Croup seems to occur more frequently in cold weather.

Allergic laryngeal edema can be severe and dangerous. Inhaled irritants may produce laryngeal spasm in some children. Croup syndrome may be produced by foreign body aspiration and subsequent subglottic obstruction. Croup is a classical example of a respiratory infection in which the main problem is upper airway obstruction. Laryngeal edema and spasm are the major causes of this obstruction. The significant physiological problem that results from this is hypoxemia. Low arterial PO_2 is frequently seen, whereas PCO_2 retention is unusual. The PCO_2 is low because of the hyperventilation stimulated by the hypoxemia. There are several clinical forms of croup. *Laryngotracheobronchitis*, also known as *viral* or *subglottic croup*, is the most common form. As the name suggests, the infection involves the subglottic area of the larynx, trachea, and bronchi. The onset is gradual with a history of upper respiratory infection before the appearance of the croupy cough and stridor. The temperature is not usually elevated. Symptoms of respiratory distress appear as the laryngeal obstruction progresses. Stridor becomes associated with sternal, subcostal, and abdominal retractions. The expiratory phase of respiration is prolonged and may be associated with wheezing. Breath sounds are decreased with rhonchi and scattered rales. Cyanosis is a late sign and is indicative of severe obstruction.

The management of viral croup includes the use of mist to reduce laryngeal edema. Racemic epinephrine is effective but must be used with caution because of the rebound effect. Corticosteroids have been used effectively in children with spasmodic croup, but their use remains controversial in infectious croup. If these measures are not successful in reducing the degree of respiratory distress, an artificial airway must be considered.

The majority of children with laryngotracheobronchitis usually do not progress beyond the cough, stridor, and mild distress stage. The condition runs its course within 3 to 7 days with complete recovery. Of all the children with laryngotracheobronchitis, only a small percentage will need to be cared for in a critical care unit.

The most severe form is *acute epiglottitis*, also referred to as *bacterial* or *supraglottic croup*. As previously mentioned, it is most commonly caused by *H. influenzae* type B. It has a rapid, progressive, and fulminant course. The onset is abrupt. The younger child usually has high fever and respiratory distress. The older child complains of a severe sore throat and difficulty in swallowing. Pooling of secretions in the pharynx and drooling are common signs because of the dysphagia. This child usually assumes a sitting position with chin thrust forward, mouth open and tongue slightly protruding. The voice may be absent, hoarse, or muffled. Temperature is elevated. Within hours after onset, the child may be in marked respiratory distress with stridor, retractions, and nasal flaring. The diagnosis is made

627

by visualizing the large, edematous, cherry red epiglottis. This should *only* be done in a controlled setting with a team ready to perform an immediate intubation or tracheostomy. Stimulation of the epiglottis while attempting to visualize it has produced complete obstruction and death. Lateral radiographs of the larynx may be of value in confirming the enlarged epiglottis without resorting to direct visualization. Leukocytosis of more than $15,000/mm^3$ is usually present. Blood cultures will identify *H. influenzae* type B (or other causative organisms).

When the diagnosis of epiglottitis is suspected, the approach should be to provide an artificial airway. Medical management of the child without an artificial airway should not be attempted. If an airway is not provided promptly, the mortality may be quite high. Preparation should be for controlled intubation or tracheostomy. Corticosteroids have not proven to be of significant value over airway instrumentation. Parenteral antibiotics are indicated. Ampicillin and chloramphenicol are the drugs of choice.

The child with epiglottitis usually responds rapidly to antibiotics and may be extubated or decannulated in 48 to 72 hours.

The nurse in the critical care area will most certainly be involved in the care of all children with acute epiglottitis.

ASSESSMENT

1. Recent history of minor upper respiratory infection
2. Physical signs and symptoms
   a. Laryngotracheobronchitis
      (1) Characteristic brassy cough
      (2) Inspiratory stridor (crowing noise)
      (3) Retraction
      (4) Prolongation of exhalation with wheezing
      (5) Diminished breath sounds
      (6) Rhonchi and scattered rales
      (7) Hypoxemia
   b. Acute epiglottitis
      (1) High fever
      (2) Brassy cough
      (3) Inspiratory stridor
      (4) Dysphagia
      (5) Retractions
      (6) Nasal flaring
      (7) Irritability
      (8) Restlessness
      (9) Tripod position—sitting up, arms in front, chin thrust forward, mouth open and drooling
      (10) Hypoxemia
3. Monitor lab data for results of
   a. Lateral neck and chest radiographs
   b. WBC and differential
   c. Throat culture
   d. Blood culture
   e. Serum *H. influenzae* antigen
   f. Arterial blood gas levels
4. Developmental level of the child
   a. Effect of illness on child (guilt, punishment)
   b. Effect of hospitalization on child
      (1) Fear of strangers
      (2) Fear of bodily harm
      (3) Fear of separation and abandonment
   c. Developmental tasks according to age
5. Response of parents to child's illness and hospitalization
   a. Level of anxiety
   b. Degree of understanding of illness and therapeutic management
   c. Guilt

GOALS

1. Resolution of acute respiratory distress
2. Relief of upper airway obstruction
3. Absence of infection
4. Normal cardiac function
5. Normal fluid and electrolyte balance
6. Normal sleep/wake pattern
7. Child's and parent's behavior indicates a reduction in anxiety
8. Hospitalization as a positive developmental experience for the child
9. Parent's behavior demonstrates effective coping mechanisms

POTENTIAL PROBLEMS	EXPECTED OUTCOMES	NURSING ACTIVITIES
■ Acute respiratory failure related to laryngeal obstruction	■ Respiratory function normal as indicated by arterial blood gas levels	■ Prevent by Continuous monitoring of respiratory status Implementation of medical and nursing regimen to provide and maintain adequate respiratory function Monitor for Change in arterial blood gas levels Change in degree of respiratory distress Tachypnea Tachycardia Retractions Nasal flaring Color Stridor

POTENTIAL PROBLEMS	EXPECTED OUTCOMES	NURSING ACTIVITIES
		Breath sounds
		Posture
		Mentation
		NOTE: Decrease in stridor, increase in heart rate, and decrease in respiratory rate are indicative of emergency situation
		Intervention if problem occurs
		Pediatric emergency procedure
		Intubation
		Tracheostomy
		Mechanical ventilation (see Standard 6, *Mechanical ventilation*)
		NOTE: Epiglottitis of acute onset represents one of the few true pediatric emergencies
■ Fluid and/or electrolyte imbalance related to degree of respiratory distress	■ Weight within normal limits Electrolytes within normal parameters	■ Prevent by
		Parenteral maintenance
		Fluid replacement
		Electrolyte replacement according to serum levels and maintenance requirements
		Monitor for
		Change in fluid and nutritional intake
		Change in weight
		Change in state of hydration
		Mucous membranes
		Skin turgor
		Thirst
		Tears
		Behavior
		Urine specific gravity
		Change in indices of intravascular volume
		BP
		P
		CVP
		Urine output and specific gravity
		Changes in lab data
		Serum electrolytes
		Hct
		Intervention if problem occurs
		Frequent assessment of vital signs
		Accurate measurement and recording of intake and output
		Daily weights
		Accurate parenteral administration of fluids and electrolytes
		Monitor IV q1 hr for rate of flow and amount infused (use infusion pump if available)
		Observe IV site q1 hr
		Monitor lab data
■ Infection related to presence of parainfluenza virus, *H. influenzae,* group A streptococcus, or pneumococci	■ Infection free Complication free	■ Prevent by
		Proper hand-washing techniques
		Administration of antibiotics, as ordered
		Monitor for
		Temperature elevation greater than 101° F (38.2° C)
		Extension of infectious process to other regions of respiratory tract such as middle ear and lungs
		Lab values
		WBC count and differential
		Cultures—throat and blood
		Chest radiograph
		Intervention if problem occurs
		Temperature elevation
		Check temperature q2-4 hr or as indicated
		Administer antipyretics, as ordered
		Tepid sponge
		Cooling mattress
		Encourage fluids (as per appropriate route)

POTENTIAL PROBLEMS	EXPECTED OUTCOMES	NURSING ACTIVITIES

		Extension of infectious process
		    Assess respiratory status, as indicated
		    Institute mode of therapy, as per physician's orders
		        Antibiotics
		        Mist tent
		        Chest physiotherapy

■ CHF related to degree of respiratory failure	■ Cardiac function within normal limits	■ Prevent by
		    Following medical and nursing regimen in management of respiratory distress and failure (see Problem, Acute respiratory failure)
		Monitor for
		    Tachycardia
		    Tachypnea
		    Dyspnea—grunting, nasal flaring, coughing
		    Weight increase
		    Urinary output decrease
		    Feeding difficulty
		Intervention if problem occurs
		    Frequent assessment of vital signs
		    Fluid restriction as ordered
		    Daily weights
		    Accurate measurement and recording of intake and output
		    Sitting position
		    Careful feeding to avoid aspiration
		    Administration of (as ordered by physician)
		        Digoxin
		        Furosemide
		        O_2
		        Chest physiotherapy

■ Sleep deprivation related to respiratory distress	■ Sleep/wake pattern restored to preillness state	■ Prevent by
		    Decreased amount of sensory stimulation
		    Minimal disturbance of patient by nursing and other health team members
		    Proper body positioning to ease work of breathing and provide for maximum comfort
		    Decreased amount of emotional stress; allow parents to remain with child
		Monitor for
		    Change in LOC
		        Difficult to arouse
		        Responds to verbal stimuli
		        Responds to painful stimuli
		    Change in level of mentation
		        Confusion
		        Disorientation
		    Change in mood
		        Passive
		        Aggressive
		        Crying
		        Irritable
		    Change in work of breathing
		        Degree of difficulty
		        Degree of comfort
		NOTE: Changes in any or all of aforementioned may indicate hypoxemia
		Intervention if problem occurs
		    Plan sleep/wake pattern by
		        Decreasing amount of stimuli (noise) and limiting time when nursing and medical team activities take place
		        Using sleep-promoting activities (stroking, rubbing, gentle soft voices)

POTENTIAL PROBLEMS	EXPECTED OUTCOMES	NURSING ACTIVITIES
		Providing for maximal comfort by adjusting body position to ease the work of breathing (head elevated)
		Sedatives are contraindicated
■ Emotional stress related to trauma of hospitalization	■ Reduced emotional trauma	■ Prevent by
		Minimal separation of parents and child
		Continuity of care
		Monitor for
		Presence of separation anxiety
		Phase of separation anxiety (if present)
		Protest
		Despair
		Denial
		Presence of fears
		Bodily harm
		Mutilation
		Loss of body integrity
		Strangers
		Unfamiliar surroundings
		Presence of feelings of
		Guilt
		Wrongdoing
		Loss of love
		Anger
		Intervention if problem occurs
		Separation anxiety
		Presence of parents
		Parent participation
		Presence of security object
		Fears
		Orientation to surroundings
		Consistent nursing personnel
		Correct misconceptions
		Provide accurate information
		Feelings
		Verbalization
		Play
		Drawing
■ Family crisis related to	■ Facilitate coping mecha-	■ Assess degree of stress and ability to cope
Illness of child	nisms within the family	Determine level of understanding of child's condition, treatment, and need for hospitalization
Need for hospitalization		Offer factual information
Lack of knowledge about condition		Clarify misconceptions
Guilt		Encourage parental expression of feelings about illness and hospitalization
Anxiety		Establish relationship
		Plan time for interaction
		Reassure parents
		Support parents
		Determine, with parents, their degree of involvement in care of their child
		Maintain parental sense of adequacy to care for their child
		Periodically evaluate effect of the interventions on parents' behavior

ASTHMA/STATUS ASTHMATICUS

Asthma is a reversible, episodic, obstructive condition affecting the lower respiratory tract. It is characterized by wheezing and various degrees of dyspnea. The wheezing is caused as airway flow is restricted by bronchospasm, edema, and increased mucus production.

The onset of asthma is usually in early childhood, between the ages of 3 and 8 years. Boys are affected more than girls in the early years. During adolescence and thereafter, both are affected equally. Asthma may be controlled but not cured.

All children with asthma have a hypersensitivity of the smooth muscle of the airways to a variety of factors. Bronchospasm may occur in response to inhalants such as dust, molds, animal hair, and airborne pollens. Cold air and rapid changes of temperature may provoke an asthmatic attack. Foods, as a source of allergy, also may precipitate an attack. Such foods include egg white, cow's milk, fish, chocolate, and nuts.

It is well documented that asthma is a complex disorder with biochemical, infectious, immunological, endocrine, and psychological factors playing roles of varying degrees of importance.

Episodes of asthma may be insidious or abrupt in onset. Those associated with infections are commonly insidious and prolonged, whereas those associated with specific allergens are abrupt and brief once the allergen is removed.

The asthmatic episode is characterized by increasing dyspnea, coughing, wheezing, and a prolongation of the expiratory phase of respiration. Coarse and fine rales are present. The episode is progressive, and as pulmonary ventilation becomes more limited, the heart and respiratory rates increase along with retractions, nasal flaring, and cyanosis. The skin may be flushed and moist with prominent sweating. The child becomes restless and fatigued. Abdominal pain may be present if coughing is severe. Very often the child will vomit, and this will somewhat relieve the symptoms. This effect is only temporary, however.

Diagnosis is made by family history of atopic disease, child's history of episodes of coughing and wheezing, clinical signs and symptoms, lab data, and response to previous therapy.

The conventional mode of therapy during an asthmatic episode is primarily pharmacological. The medications used are those specific for bronchodilation, relief of mucosal edema, liquefaction, and expectoration of mucus. These medications include epinephrine, phenylephrine, ephedrine, aminophylline, and theophylline. Beta agonists such as terbutaline, metaproterenol, isoproterinol, and albuterol (salbutamol) are also used. Other therapy, in conjunction with medication, includes moisturized oxygen and IV fluid administration.

If the child fails to respond clinically to the administration of the aforementioned medications, the diagnosis of *status asthmaticus* is generally made. There is no precise definition for status asthmaticus. It is said to exist when the asthmatic episode is severe and unresponsive to conventional therapy.

Status asthmaticus is a pediatric medical emergency. Therapy is directed toward maintaining adequate ventilation. Arterial blood gas levels are monitored closely. Moisturized oxygen is administered, because these children are usually hypoxemic. The usual pharmacological agents are administered, and, in addition, corticosteroids. IV fluid replacement and maintenance are important to ensure adequate hydration. Measures are taken to correct the associated metabolic acidosis by the administration of sodium bicarbonate, and respiratory assistance.

If respiratory failure is imminent, isoproterenol by continuous infusion may be given. If this is not successful and respiratory failure ensues, assisted ventilation by a mechanical ventilator may be required.

The nurse in the critical care area will be involved in the care of children with a severe episode of asthma and, of course, of those with status asthmaticus.

ASSESSMENT

1. Family history of allergy
2. History of eczema or food intolerance
3. History of episodes of coughing and wheezing
4. Recent history of infection
5. Physical signs and symptoms
   a. Dyspnea
   b. Wheezing
   c. Productive cough

d. Prolonged expiratory phase of respiration
e. Coarse and fine rales
f. Tachypnea
g. Retractions
h. Nasal flaring
i. Tachycardia
j. Cyanosis
k. Perspiration
l. Apprehension
m. Restlessness
n. Fatigue
6. Response to conventional pharmacological therapy
a. Sympathomimetics
b. Theophyllines
c. Beta agonists
7. Monitor lab data for results of
a. Arterial blood gas levels

b. Throat and sputum smear and culture (eosinophilia is common)
c. Chest radiograph
d. WBC count
e. Pulmonary function studies

GOALS

1. Resolution of acute respiratory distress
   a. Relief of bronchospasm
   b. Relief of mucosal edema
   c. Removal of secretions
2. Normal fluid and electrolyte balance
3. Absence of infection
4. Normal sleep/wake pattern
5. Supportive therapy for child and parents during asthmatic crisis
6. Discharge planning for the control of chronic asthma

POTENTIAL PROBLEMS	EXPECTED OUTCOMES	NURSING ACTIVITIES

■ Acute respiratory failure related to
Bronchospasm
Mucosal edema
Mucus production
	■ Respiratory function within normal limits	■ Prevent by
		Continuous monitoring of child's respiratory status
		Implementation of medical regimen
		  Bronchodilating adrenergic drugs
		  Vasoconstrictive adrenergic drugs
		  Corticosteroids
		  Moisturized O_2
		  Hydration
		Implementation of nursing regimen
		  Percussion and vibration
		  Postural drainage
		  Suctioning
		  Body positioning to enhance respiratory effort and facilitate removal of secretions
		Monitor for
		  Change in arterial blood gas levels
		  Change in response to pharmacological agents
		  Change in degree of the following parameters
		    Respiratory rate and quality
		    Heart rate
		    Wheeze
		    Cough
		    Breath sounds
		    Color
		    Mentation
		NOTE: Significant decrease in or absence of inspiratory breath sounds, severe retractions during inspiration, use of accessory muscles, diminished LOC, and cyanosis despite administration of O_2 are signs of acute respiratory failure and are considered medical emergency
		Intervention if problem occurs
		  Intubation
		  Mechanical ventilation (see Standard 6, *Mechanical ventilation*)

■ Acidosis related to respiratory insufficiency	■ Serum pH within normal limits	■ Prevent by Continuous monitoring of respiratory status Monitoring of serial arterial blood gas levels Respiratory support Monitor for Change in arterial blood gas levels

POTENTIAL PROBLEMS	EXPECTED OUTCOMES	NURSING ACTIVITIES
		Intervention if problem occurs Respiratory support Drug therapy NOTE: Acidosis must be corrected for pharmacological agents to be effective
▪ Fluid and/or electrolyte imbalance related to degree of respiratory distress	▪ Weight within normal limits Electrolytes within normal parameters	▪ Prevent by Parenteral maintenance Fluid replacement Electrolyte replacement according to serum levels and maintenance requirements, as ordered Monitor for Change in fluid and nutritional intake Change in weight Change in state of hydration Mucous membranes Skin turgor Thirst Tears Behavior Urine specific gravity Change in indices of intravascular volume BP P CVP Urine output and specific gravity Changes in lab data Serum electrolytes Hct Intervention if problem occurs Frequent assessment of vital signs Accurate measurement and recording of intake and output Daily weights Accurate parenteral administration of fluids and electrolytes Monitor IV q1 hr for rate of flow and amount infused (use infusion pump if available) Observe IV site q1 hr Monitor lab data
▪ Respiratory infection related to asthmatic episode	▪ Infection free Complication free	▪ Prevent by Administration of antibiotics and sulfonamides to which invading organisms are sensitive, as ordered by physician NOTE: Penicillin and related semisynthetic derivatives (i.e., ampicillin and oxacillin) are used cautiously because of known possible serious reactions when used with asthmatics Monitor for Temperature elevation greater than 101° F (38.2° C) Change in color of sputum Extension of infectious process to further areas of respiratory tract Lab values WBC count and differential Cultures—throat, sputum, blood Chest radiograph Intervention if problem occurs Temperature elevation Check temperature q2-4 hr or as indicated Administer antipyretics, as ordered Tepid sponge Cooling mattress Encourage fluid intake (as per appropriate route)

POTENTIAL PROBLEMS	EXPECTED OUTCOMES	NURSING ACTIVITIES

		Extension of infectious process
		  Assess respiratory status, as indicated
		  Institute mode of therapy, as per physician's orders
		    Antibiotics, sulfonamides
		    Humidified O_2
		    Chest physiotherapy

■ Sleep deprivation related to respiratory distress	■ Sleep/wake pattern restored to preillness state	■ Prevent by
		  Decreased amount of sensory stimulation
		  Minimal disturbance of patient by nurse and other health team members
		  Proper body positioning to ease work of breathing and to provide for maximal comfort
		  Decreased emotional stress; allow parents to remain with child
		Monitor for
		  Change in LOC
		    Difficult to arouse
		    Responds to verbal stimuli
		    Responds to painful stimuli
		  Change in level of mentation
		    Confusion
		    Disorientation
		  Change in mood
		    Passive
		    Aggressive
		    Crying
		    Irritable
		  Change in work of breathing
		    Degree of difficulty
		    Degree of comfort
		NOTE: Changes in any or all of aforementioned may indicate hypoxemia
		Intervention if problem occurs
		  Plan sleep/wake pattern by
		    Decreasing amount of stimuli (noise) and limiting time in which nursing and medical team activities take place
		    Using sleep-promoting activities (stroking, rubbing, gentle soft voices)
		    Providing for maximal comfort by adjusting body position to ease the work of breathing (head elevated)
		    Sedative contraindicated

■ Increased anxiety level of child and parents related to severity of asthmatic episode	■ Reduced anxiety level as demonstrated by behavior of child and parents	■ Prevent by
		  Therapeutic intervention to relieve symptoms
		  Accurate information as to physical status
		  Establish trusting relationship; provide reassurance
		Monitor for
		  Change in facial expression
		  Change in body posture
		  Change in mood
		  Change in behavior
		Intervention if problem occurs
		  Establish trusting relationship
		  Encourage verbalization related to asthma and asthmatic episodes
		  Convey accurate information
		  Reassure child and parents as to positive outcome
		  Do not leave child or parents alone during crisis
		  Evaluate effectiveness of nursing interventions as demonstrated by level of anxiety of child and parents

POTENTIAL PROBLEMS	EXPECTED OUTCOMES	NURSING ACTIVITIES
▪ Family crisis related to 　Illness of child 　Need for hospitalization 　Lack of knowledge 　　about condition 　Guilt 　Anxiety	▪ Coping mechanisms within 　family facilitated	▪ Assess degree of stress and ability to cope 　Determine level of understanding of child's condition, treatment, and 　　need for hospitalization 　Offer factual information 　Clarify misconceptions 　Encourage parental expression of feelings about illness and hospi- 　　talization 　　Establish relationship 　　Plan time for interaction 　　Reassure parents 　　Support parents 　Determine with parents their degree of involvement in care of their 　　child 　Maintain parental sense of adequacy to care for their child 　Periodically evaluate effect of interventions on parents' behavior
▪ Insufficient control of asth- ma related to increasing frequency of episodes	▪ Control of chronic asthma	▪ Assess level of understanding of disease process and implications on 　child and family 　Establish teaching plan to include 　　Explanation of disease 　　Signs and symptoms of impending asthmatic attack 　　Factors influencing asthma 　　　Allergens 　　　Respiratory irritants 　　　Upper respiratory infection 　　　Exercise 　　　Emotional upset 　　Home management 　　　Medication (purpose, dosage, and time taken) 　　　Medical follow-up 　　　Breathing exercises 　　　Supportive therapy 　Evaluate parents' and child's knowledge of home health routine by 　　having them verbalize information

REYE SYNDROME

Reye syndrome is an acute toxic encephalopathy and fatty degeneration of viscera affecting mainly the liver, brain, and kidney. The encephalopathy consists of cerebral swelling without evidence of inflammation. It was first described in 1963. Since then more than 2000 cases have been reported to the Centers for Disease Control. Its cause and pathogenesis remain unknown. The pathology is multisystemic, affecting the respiratory, central nervous, renal, metabolic, and cardiovascular systems. Therapy consists of empirically based, supportive regimens. Most symptoms seem to be reversible if there is no hypoxic brain damage. Mortality has declined to less than 30%; with diagnosis and therapy in the earliest stage, there is almost 100% survival. (Previously there was less than 20% survival.) Death is usually attributed to increasing ICP secondary to cerebral edema.

Reye syndrome occurs in children from infancy through adolescence as a sequela to an uncomplicated, acute, or mild febrile infection, usually a viral one in the upper respiratory tract accompanied by anorexia. The prodromal illness is commonly chickenpox or influenza B. Occasionally it is a diarrhea. The average age is 7 years; there have been few adult cases. Males and females are equally affected. Incidence is greater among whites than blacks. The geographical distribution remains unexplained. Lower incidence rates are found in Pacific states and higher rates in the north-central and mountain states. There is also an identifiable rural/suburban/urban pattern. It is assumed that incidence is higher than recognized because of the likelihood that noncomatose patients remain undiagnosed.

The prodromal illness may last from 1 day to 2 weeks. As the child begins to demonstrate spontaneous recovery, severe sudden vomiting occurs and persists with or without a low-grade fever. This vomiting characterizes the recognizable onset of Reye syndrome.

The progression of sensorial changes is variable. When vomiting begins, the patient may be irritable and lethargic but well oriented. In some patients, lethargy persists with no progression to unconsciousness. Some will experience disorientation, confusion, and agitated delirium with episodes of screaming. Deterioration with fever, hyperventilation, hypertonia, convulsions, and coma may be rapid.

Although it is now recognized that the majority of patients recover uneventfully without becoming comatose, progression to deeper coma with decorticate/decerebrate movement and respiratory arrest may ensue if there is no intervention. This disease course has been classified into five stages (see Assessment). What controls the rate of progression is unknown. In victims under 1 year of age, neurological changes are often less distinct, and the vomiting history may not be easily demarcated. Meanwhile, hypoglycemia and coma may be more marked in these patients than in older children.

The duration of the entire course may be less than 24 hours, or it may last 1 week or more. Typically, the encephalopathy persists for 24 to 96 hours with gradual neurological improvement. The outcome is usually apparent within 3 to 4 days. Prognosis seems to be related to the rate of progress through the disease stages and the stage at which supportive therapy is initiated. Neurological impairment is not an uncommon sequela and is usually associated with delayed return of consciousness, perhaps as long as several weeks. With supportive intervention, most noncomatose patients will not progress to deeper coma and will experience an improved appetite with cessation of vomiting within 24 hours. Usually these patients can be discharged within 2 to 3 days after admission.

Some hypotheses regarding the cause of Reye syndrome have suggested that susceptibility is related to exposure to viruses or toxins, whereas others suggest that these factors precipitate the syndrome in already susceptible individuals. There may be an interaction between a virus and a toxin, or the biochemical response to such an interaction may be caused by an enzymatic deficiency or a Krebs cycle defect. The syndrome may actually represent the similar clinical and pathological manifestations of a variety of etiologically unrelated conditions. An association with relatively high salicylate levels has been identified, but no causal relationship can be demonstrated. It has been hypothesized that the salicylate role may be as a synergistic cofactor with the as yet unidentified host factors in combination with the antecedent illness. Meanwhile, some patients have developed the disease without having used salicylate. Also, no correlation has been found between serum salicylate levels and neurological grade of disease development.

Treatment is focused on maintaining homeostatic function through the acute phase and preserving neurological integrity. Emphasis is on maintaining MAP and preventing increased ICP. ICP monitoring is crucial. IV 10% glucose solutions are started if liver function tests are abnormal. If there are occasional rises above 20 mm Hg in ICP during the period of elevated serum ammonia, more aggressive therapy may be initiated. This includes intubation and controlled ventilation with paralyzation of the patient. Hypothermia may also be employed. Rewarming is not started until ammonia levels return to normal and EEG returns to type 2. Paralyzation is accomplished to prevent shivering and should be continued until core temperature reaches 95° F (35° C). Fluid intake is restricted. Osmotic diuresis is indicated if ICP increases. Sedation with thiopental or barbiturates is used when ICP elevations persist or when patient movements result in mild elevations.

Outcome is greatly improved with early recognition and intervention, especially before the development of neurological signs. It is felt that the protracted and dangerous rises in ICP are precipitated by temporary increases, normally insignificant in the well individual. Hence early initiation of measures that inhibit the movements and responses that alter ICP are key to recovery. Recovery from stage 3 or 4 (see Assessment) may take many months, and these survivors manifest a variety of residual neurological deficits, ranging from subtle perceptual deficits to psychomotor retardation and other overt symptoms. For patients less than 1 year old, prognosis is somewhat poorer in terms of both survival and neuropsychological integrity.

ASSESSMENT

1. History of prodromal upper respiratory infection and/or viral syndrome within previous week
2. Early signs and symptoms are indication for SGOT/ SGPT determination: severe and persistent vomiting
   a. With or without high fever (101° F [38.3° C])
   b. With or without diarrhea
3. Symptoms and signs suggesting CNS dysfunction (usually acute onset)
   a. Tachypnea with respiratory alkalosis and marked dyspnea
   b. Confusion/delirium/agitation
   c. Hypertonia
   d. Confulsions
   e. Coma (deterioration may be rapid)
4. Elevated SGPT/SGOT levels are indications for other laboratory studies and diagnostic procedures, including
   a. Serum glucose, electrolytes, and urea
   b. Serum ammonia
   c. CBC with differential
   d. Acid-base status
   e. PT

   f. Total serum bilirubin
   g. Serum salicylate levels
   h. Serum and urine toxic screen
   i. Serological studies to rule out hepatitis A or B virus, cytomegalovirus, and Epstein-Barr virus
   j. Arterial blood gas levels
   k. Liver biopsy, which may be done for nondiagnostic investigational purposes (e.g., epidemiological or pathological studies; Microvesicular fat droplets may be noted
   l. Lumbar puncture
      (1) CSF chemistry (note low glucose level)
      (2) CSF culture and sensitivity
   m. EEG; a typical pattern may be observed, but this is not in itself diagnostic
5. Presence of specific disease stage
   a. Stage 1
      (1) Vomiting, lethargy, sleepiness
      (2) Abnormal liver function tests
      (3) Type 1 EEG
   b. Stage 2
      (1) Disorientation, delirium, combativeness, hyperventilation hyperactive reflexes
      (2) Type 2 EEG
   c. Stage 3
      (1) Hyperventilation, decorticate rigidity, and obtunded state
      (2) Type 2 EEG
   d. Stage 4
      (1) Deepening coma, decerebrate rigidity, loss of oculocephalic reflexes, fixed pupils with hippus, dysconjugate eye movements
      (2) Improved liver function
      (3) Type 3 or 4 EEG
   e. Stage 5
      (1) Seizures, loss of deep tendon reflexes, respiratory arrest, flaccidity
      (2) Liver function may be normal
      (3) Type 4 EEG
6. Patient/family's level of anxiety related to disease condition, signs and symptoms, and therapeutic interventions

GOALS

1. Reduction of parents' anxiety and feelings of inadequacy in coping with sudden acute life-threatening situation
2. Adequate oxygenation and tissue perfusion
3. Adequate hydration and electrolyte balance
4. ICP readings within normal limits
5. Cardiac, renal, hepatic, and respiratory function within normal limits
6. Absence of neurological deficit or mental impairment
7. Resumption of preillness activity level

POTENTIAL PROBLEMS	EXPECTED OUTCOMES	NURSING ACTIVITIES
■ Respiratory distress Alkalosis secondary to hyperventilation	■ Absence/resolution of respiratory distress Acid-base balance	■ Administer chest physiotherapy q1 hr, and reposition patient unless contraindicated; administer O_2 therapy with humidification if ordered (monitor arterial blood gas results) Observe respirations and assess breath sounds Notify physician of abnormalities, and alter therapy as ordered Assist in intubation and mechanical ventilation if needed, as ordered Hyperventilation is used to maintain Pco_2 at 20 to 25 mm Hg See Standard 6, *Mechanical ventilation*

■ Rapidly progressive neurological deficit caused by cerebral edema
Cerebral perfusion is decreased because of increased ICP; resulting hypoxia may be exacerbated by hypoxemic condition
	■ Neurological function within normal limits
	Cerebral perfusion pressure at or greater than 50 mm Hg
	Resolution of cerebral edema
		■ Assess neurological status q1 hr
		Check reflexes: Babinski, deep tendon, doll's eye, pupillary
		Note posturing
		Assess LOC
		NOTE: If pancuronium bromide is being used to paralyze patient for mechanical ventilation, only pupils can be checked; posturing may be noted as dose wears off
		Note seizure activity; record
		  Type
		  Foci
		  Frequency
		  Duration
		Position patient with head elevated 30 degrees
		Avoid sudden position changes
		Take seizure precautions, including restraints and padded siderails; see Standard 41, *Seizures*
		Monitor and record q1 hr
		  BP
		  Arterial blood gas levels and pH
		  Intake and output
		    Fluid intake is restricted to one half to two thirds daily maintenance needs
		Monitor ICP continuously
		Direct measurement of ICP is indicated in patients with stage 2 signs and symptoms (see Assessment)
		Calculate and record cerebral perfusion pressure q1-2 hr, depending on fluctuation*
		ICP monitoring is discontinued when recovery is apparent (after 3 to 4 days), and extubation is achieved *or* there is no recovery and pressure remains stable for about 1 week (4 to 6 days)
		Sequence for discontinuing ICP monitoring, as ordered (this process will take 36 to 72 hours; there should be 6- 12-hour equilibration between each step)
		  Decrease mechanical ventilation slowly so Pco_2 rises gradually (5 mm Hg q4-8 hr)
		  Discontinue muscle relaxants
		  Taper drug therapy
		  Discontinue mechanical ventilation
		  Discontinue sedation
		  Discontinue ICP monitoring
		Administer O_2 therapy, as ordered
		Keep Pco_2 at 20 to 25 mm Hg by hyperventilation (to maintain decreased cerebral blood flow)
		Modify respiratory therapy to avoid increases in ICP
		Observe ICP fluctuation related to respiratory therapy
		  Administer physiotherapy gently
		  Hyperventilate for 1 minute before suctioning (frequent suctioning may require sedation)
		  Administer minimal PEEP to prevent increased intrathoracic pressure
		  PEEP should be less than or equal to 2 cm H_2O

*Cerebral perfusion pressure = MAP − ICP.

POTENTIAL PROBLEMS	EXPECTED OUTCOMES	NURSING ACTIVITIES
		Temperature monitoring is important concomitant of ICP monitoring Administer osmotic diuretic, as prescribed Hypothermia may be ordered to reduce cerebral blood flow through decreased cerebral metabolism

■ Inappropriate secretion of antidiuretic hormone	■ Fluid and electrolyte balance	■ Monitor
		  Urine osmolality
		  Urine specific gravity
		  Urine Na$^+$
		  Serum electrolytes and osmolality
		  Intake and output; restrict fluids, as ordered
		  Signs and symptoms of H_2O intoxication—confusion, stupor, coma, seizures
		    May be masked because they are consistent with Reye syndrome
		Notify physician of abnormalities and administer therapy, as ordered

■ Diabetes insipidus	■ Normal circulatory volume	■ Monitor BP, intake and output, and urine specific gravity q15-30 min Replace urinary output q30 min or q1 hr, as ordered, until specific gravity is greater than or equal to 1.010 Administer vasopressor infusion, as ordered Maintain NPO

■ Hyperammonemia related to renal failure	■ Reduction of serum levels of ammonia	■ Administer neomycin, as ordered
		Administer peritoneal dialysis, if ordered; see Standard 53, *Peritoneal dialysis* (this mode of therapy in Reye syndrome is controversial)
		Assist with exchange transfusions, if prescribed
		  Monitor
		    Heart rate and rhythm
		    BP
		    Respiratory rate
		    Temperature
		    Glucose using manual blood glucose monitoring strip (e.g., Dextrostix)
		    Arterial blood gas levels and pH
		    Electrolytes, including Ca^{++}
		    Serum ammonia
		    Hct
		    Hgb
		  Administer calcium gluconate before and during procedure, as ordered
		Continue monitoring aforementioned parameters after transfusion
		  Hypoglycemia and hypotension are risks during immediate post-transfusion period

■ Hepatic failure	■ Absence of hepatic decompensation	■ Monitor
		  PT and APTT q12 hr
		  Ammonia, SGOT, SGPT, total serum protein, bilirubin, alkaline phosphatase, and amylase
		  Blood glucose using manual blood glucose monitoring strip (e.g., Dextrostix) q4 hr
		  Serum glucose q1 day
		Administer fresh frozen plasma before liver biopsy, as ordered; assist with liver biopsy

■ Infection	■ Absence of infection	■ Maintain asepsis with all invasive monitoring procedures, IVs, etc. Culture all catheter tips when removed Monitor for signs of local infection and sepsis Monitor temperature q1-2 hr and prn Notify physician if these abnormalities occur, and alter therapy as ordered

POTENTIAL PROBLEMS	EXPECTED OUTCOMES	NURSING ACTIVITIES
■ Hyperpyrexia	■ Afebrile	■ Monitor temperature q1 hr or more frequently if unstable Administer tepid sponge baths Apply hypothermia, as ordered Use servocontrol mechanism or monitor temperature q15 min when patient is on hypothermia blanket Antipyretics are contraindicated

■ Impending death	■ Family prepared for impending death	■ Reassure parents that they are not to blame for death
		  Review medical facts
		  Allow parents to review history of illness, their response to symptoms, and events before and during hospitalization
		  Assure parents that they did all that they should have done and that their actions were appropriate
		Encourage parents to verbalize their feelings
		  Recognize steps in grieving process
		  Accept expressions of anger, denial, etc.
		Include siblings' needs when discussing situation with parents
		  Help parents understand children's age-related perceptions of death so that they may give appropriate explanations and consolation

■ Fear and anxiety related to separation from family, sensory bombardment of critical care unit environment, etc. Waking child who was obtunded on admission is not familiar with all procedures he/she has been experiencing	■ Reduction of anxiety Behavior appropriate to prehospitalization level of psychosocial development	■ Explain all procedures to child Include those events he/she may observe occurring with other patients Describe environment to child to reduce fear and to answer questions about machinery Orient child to time, place, and multiple people who come and go in unit Provide social stimulation by talking to the patient; do not approach patient, manipulate tubing, etc. without conversing with him/her; allow choices when possible Encourage and promote the parents' participation in care Allow child to verbalize feelings about hospital experiences

■ Parents' anxiety related to disease condition and therapy; they may feel confused, frightened, and guilty	■ Reduction of parents' anxiety and feelings of guilt and inadequacy
	Parents are able to describe events in course of child's disease without assigning inappropriate correlations
		■ Provide support to parents
		  Reassure parents that they gave appropriate care, took correct action, and sought help in timely manner
		  Describe what is known about Reye syndrome
		  Explain procedures
		  Explain child's status and anticipated course
		  Assure parents that it is not common for siblings to contract same disease
		  Allow parents to express their feelings
		  Time and attention must be given to help parents cope with suddenness of situation (and possibly rapid deterioration) and sense of helplessness in face of problem that has incomplete medical answers
		  Allow parents to be at patient's bedside and to touch and stroke child
		  Note visiting patterns
		    Frequency
		    Regularity
		    Whether parents come together
		  Assess parent-infant interactions
		    Stimulate and reinforce social interaction/dialogue (premature infants take less initiative and give less feedback than full-term infants)
		    Point out individual attractive features; assure parents that apparent unattractiveness is typical of premature infants and their baby will grow to look normal
		    Note whether parents make positive comments about infant, infant behavior, and impact of infant on them

POTENTIAL PROBLEMS	EXPECTED OUTCOMES	NURSING ACTIVITIES
		Note evidence of parents' self-esteem, emotional exhaustion, support for each other
		Note whether parents demonstrate nurturant behavior
		Note whether parents are attentive to infant's behavior
		Gradually decrease parents' dependence on staff
		Parents should be able to spend time with infant without interference from staff
		Infant's supplies should be at crib so that parents do not have to continually ask questions or seek assistance from staff
		Allow parents to improvise and do things in comfortable manner; allow them to arrange infant's things
		Infant's schedule (bath, etc.) should be geared to parents' visiting
		Offer approval and reinforce proper techniques
		"Nesting" or live-in arrangements for parents to provide all care before discharge of infant has been investigated with significant results
		Arrange for follow-up care and support
		Clinic appointments
		Visiting nurse or public health nurse referrals
		Social service referrals (social services should be actively involved from soon after birth so that social problems can be assessed and appropriate intervention initiated)
		Follow-up phone calls by primary nurse and nursery staff to offer support and identify problems
		Encourage phone calls to ask questions, refer problems, or seek encouragement

DIAPHRAGMATIC HERNIA

Diaphragmatic hernia in the newborn consists of incomplete embryonic formation of the diaphragm, which allows displacement of abdominal viscera into the thorax, displacing the lungs and heart and causing severe respiratory distress. Occasionally, the viscera move freely through the defect so they are sometimes in the thorax and sometimes in the abdomen. Position usually affects migration in these instances, so that when the infant is horizontal, organs move back and forth into the thorax.

This defect occurs in about 1 in 5000 births. The left side is involved in over 80% of cases. The herniation may occur in the posterolateral segment, in the anterior portion directly beneath the sternum (foramen of Morgagni), or at the esophageal hiatus.

The most common diaphragmatic hernia (and the most serious) is posterolateral, known as *Bochdalek hernia*. It results when the triangular pleuroperitoneal canal fails to close. In the majority of cases, a sac covers the abdominal contents. If the abdominal viscera migrate into the thorax early in gestation, left lung development is affected, resulting in hypoplasia. The heart is displaced to the right, and the right lung is smaller than normal. If the migration of abdominal organs occurs later, there is less hypoplasia of the left lung. When the left side is involved, the intestine, stomach, and spleen compress the lung and displace the mediastinum to the right; when the lesion is on the right side, the liver and/or intestine are involved. Right side involvement is less severe, because the liver limits the degree of herniation into the chest cavity.

The less common *Morgagni hernia* usually results from incomplete muscularization of the diaphragm and most commonly occurs on the right side. Symptoms are usually less severe, and the patient may be asymptomatic.

The severity of symptoms is related to the amount of lung compressed and the relative hypoplasia of lung tissue, which varies. With a moderate degree of herniation, the lung may be histologically normal although smaller. Hypoplasia reflects retarded growth and maturation of the lungs resulting in decreased lung volume, diminished branching of the bronchial tree, and failure of alveoli to multiply. Sometimes there are fewer bronchial branchings with each leading to a normal number of alveoli. Growth in the contralateral lung will also be compromised, though to a lesser extent. The lungs are stiff and noncompliant, requiring high distending pressure. Hypoplastic lungs are associated with small pulmonary vascular beds, a decreased number of pulmonary resistance vessels per unit of lung tissue, and increased pulmonary vascular smooth muscle. These effects increase pulmonary vascular resistance and pressures. Pulmonary vascular resistance is also increased by hypoxemia and hypercapnia. Abnormally high PAP may produce right ventricular hypertrophy. A right to left shunting through the ductus arteriosus results and persists after surgical repair.

The presenting sign is severe respiratory distress, usually immediately at birth. This quickly worsens. The serial Apgar scores may deteriorate. Immediate surgical intervention is indicated. Surgical repair may be via thorax or abdomen. The latter is usually preferred because of the difficulty in finding appropriate space and correctly placing all the organs in the abdomen. Frequently, a temporary ventral hernia must be left to accommodate the viscera. Often, other intraabdominal anomalies are found. A chest tube is placed postoperatively, regardless of the approach used. To stabilize the mediastinum, air will be injected or withdrawn until radiograph shows its position is satisfactory.

Management of these patients focuses on maintenance of adequate oxygenation and ventilation. Preoperatively, this must be accomplished without distending the intestines or overdistending the hypoplastic lungs. The infant is positioned on the affected side with the head of bed elevated to maximize ventilation of the contralateral, healthier lung. The patient may be intubated and oxygen supplied. Positive pressure is avoided, if possible. An NG tube is inserted to decompress the intestines via continuous aspiration. Postoperatively, respiratory support and scrupulous management of fluid, electrolyte, and acid-base balance are essential. The lungs are gradually expanded with low pressure ventilation, as needed. Higher distending pressures may be required to expand the alveoli. Nutritional support with TPN is indicated to enhance oxygenation and promote healing and growth. Tolazoline, chlorpromazine, and acetylcholine may be prescribed to counteract pulmonary vasoconstriction. The extracorporeal membrane oxygenator has been used in some centers.

The high mortality of patients with this problem (over 50%) is related to the severity of the pulmonary hypoplasia, which prevents adequate gas exchange. There does not seem to be any relationship between survival and gestational age or birth weight. The earlier the symptoms appear, the greater the severity and thus the poorer the prognosis. Thus the highest mortality is associated with patients who have difficulty initiating postnatal respirations. Mortality is also higher when there are accompanying cardiovascular anomalies.

Ventilatory function usually is regained in a few weeks despite early postoperative stiffness. Pneumothorax and midgut volvulus are potential postoperative complications. Pneumothorax on the contralateral side is a fairly common cause of death. Persistent PDA is another common complication, a result of disturbed lung growth that involves increased pulmonary artery smooth muscle (which increases pulmonary vascular resistance and thus promotes right to left shunting).

Survivors generally have persistent lower airway obstructive disease and compensatory overdistention of alveoli. This results in normal static lung volumes but reduced forced expiratory volumes. Pulmonary vasculature remains reduced on the affected side.

ASSESSMENT

1. Presence of signs and symptoms of diaphragmatic hernia, including
   a. Birth asphyxia
   b. Progressive respiratory distress and increasing cyanosis following clamping of umbilical cord
   c. Scaphoid (concave) abdomen (indicates displacement of a considerable amount of intestine)
   d. Vomiting
   e. Barrel chest
2. Auscultation
   a. Displacement of cardiac impulse to one side of chest (heart sounds heard on right)
   b. Diminished breath sounds in the involved hemithorax
   c. Bowel sounds in thorax
   d. NG injection of air is heard as "whooshing" sound throughout chest
3. Diagnostic radiograph results confirming diaphragmatic hernia (a chest radiograph is always indicated as soon as possible in the presence of respiratory distress)
   a. Absence of diaphragmatic margin on affected side
   b. Presence of inappropriate thoracic structures
   c. Mediastinal displacement
4. Results of lab tests,* including
   a. Arterial blood gas levels
   b. Serum electrolytes
   c. Radiograph
5. History of polyhydramnios

GOALS

1. Adequate oxygenation
2. Adequate nourishment with weight gain
3. Successful parent-infant bonding
4. Normal psychosocial and psychomotor growth
5. Family will be able to cope with crisis and remain an intact, mutually nurturing dyad or group
6. Parents will develop and have confidence in their parenting skills

*Usually there is marked acidosis with accompanying hyperkalemia.

POTENTIAL PROBLEMS	EXPECTED OUTCOMES	NURSING ACTIVITIES
Preoperative		
■ Respiratory insufficiency	■ Adequate oxygenation	■ Assess respiratory status; note 　Respiratory rate, breathing pattern, color 　Notify physician of abnormalities Insert large NG tube to decompress air-filled intestines 　Apply suction Position infant so that lung on unaffected side is allowed to fully expand Assist with intubation and mechanical ventilation as ordered to maintain P_{O_2} at 50 to 60 mm Hg 　Rapid, shallow respirations are preferred because too much positive pressure may rupture lungs Administer O_2 immediately if cyanosis of mucous membranes is present Resuscitator bag is contraindicated to prevent overinflation of unaffected lung *See* STANDARD 6　*Mechanical ventilation*

POTENTIAL PROBLEMS	EXPECTED OUTCOMES	NURSING ACTIVITIES

■ Acidosis related to anaerobic metabolism	■ Acid-base parameters within normal limits, including Pao_2, $Paco_2$, bicarbonate, base excess, lactate	■ Maintain rapid respiratory rate 50 to 60/minute
		Administer curare or pancuronium if needed to maintain pH over 7.2, as ordered
		Administer sodium bicarbonate infusion, as ordered
		Monitor
		    Arterial blood gas levels q1 hr
		    Respiratory status
		    Heart rate and rhythm
		    Level of activity
		Notify physician of changes, and alter therapy as ordered

■ Delayed bonding because mother does not see baby at delivery and/or baby is rushed away for emergency treatment
This initial separation during immediate postnatal period can be exacerbated by prolonged hospitalization and parental grief because newborn is sick and/or dying
	■ Parents interact with infant as soon as possible
	Successful parent-infant bonding
	Parents communicate their feelings about infant
		■ Explain disease process and need for therapy prescribed
		Explain procedures, their purpose, etc. to parents
		    Allow repetitive questions
		Allow and encourage frequent visits
		    Give parents telephone number of unit and name of primary nurse; encourage them to call to check on baby, ask questions, etc.
		Encourage parents to touch and stroke infant; encourage parents to participate in infant's care to whatever extent possible
		Assess parent-infant interactions
		    Stimulate and reinforce social interaction/dialogue
		Encourage verbalization of both positive and negative feelings
		Assure parents that feelings of failure, guilt, frustration, bitterness, anger, sorrow, and disappointment are normal, i.e., shared by others in similar circumstances
		Reassure parents that they are not to blame for problem
		    Allow them to review history of pregnancy, labor, and delivery
		    Review medical facts
		Point out infant's responsive behaviors
		Point out infant's individual characteristics
		Educate parents regarding infant's special needs and problems
		Encourage questions
		Prepare parents for prolonged hospitalization and follow-up
		    Tell them what to expect
		    Assure them that they will be able to see and handle infant to greater extent after initial acute period
		If/when situation appears grave, give honest explanations to parents
		Recognize denial, anger, and withdrawal as steps in grieving process and mechanisms of defense
		    Encourage parents to observe infant and repeat explanations; this will help parents to formulate and accept "real" situation
		    Allow parents to verbalize feelings
		Discuss siblings at home so that parents may verbalize impact of situation on family interaction
		Recognize parents as individuals

Postoperative
■ Respiratory insufficiency related to
Pneumothorax
	■ Absence or resolution of respiratory insufficiency
	Full lung expansion
	Intact contralateral lung
		■ Prevention
		
		Use low peak-inspiratory and end-expiratory pressure, as ordered
		Maintain patency of chest tubing
		    Milk q1-2 hr, as necessary
		    Monitor drainage q1-2 hr (chest tubes are connected to straight drainage without suction)

Mediastinal shift	Absence or resolution of mediastinal shift	Monitor
		    Chest radiograph q2-4 hr
		    Breath sounds q½-1 hr
		    Breathing pattern

POTENTIAL PROBLEMS	EXPECTED OUTCOMES	NURSING ACTIVITIES
Hypoxia caused by reduced lung expansion*	Adequate oxygenation and ventilation	Administer mechanical ventilation via endotracheal tube, as ordered Maintain inspiratory pressure at less than or equal to 20 cm H$_2$O Monitor arterial blood gas levels Notify physician of any changes in respiratory status and alter therapy, as prescribed

■ Hypotension	■ Adequate tissue perfusion maintained through hemodynamic stability
	BP within normal limits for newborn
		■ Monitor
		  BP, P
		  Urine output, including specific gravity (minimal output should be 1 ml/kg/hour)
		  Color
		  Temperature
		  Level of activity
		Notify physician of abnormalities in aforementioned, and alter therapy as ordered

■ Malrotation of abdominal organs This is usually assessed and corrected at time of surgery	■ Intake of nutrients sufficient to achieve weight gain	■ Accurately measure and record intake and output Observe for distention and poor absorption following feeding Weigh infant daily Administer feedings, as ordered Gastrostomy tube is in place postoperatively

■ Infection	■ Absence of infection	■ Use appropriate aseptic techniques
		  Change respiratory therapy tubing daily or according to hospital protocol
		  Place fresh sterile H$_2$O in humidifiers q8 hr
		  Change IV tubing, IV solutions q24 hr
		  Refrigerate breast milk or formula after it has been opened; discard after 4 hours at room temperature
		  Thawed breast milk may be kept in refrigerator for 24 hours
		Teach parents proper hand-washing technique
		Monitor for signs of infection
		  Apnea
		  Lethargy
		  Change in absorption of feeding
		  Acidosis
		  Hypotension
		  Hypothermia
		Monitor culture results
		Report any abnormal observations to physician and alter therapy, as ordered

■ Retrolental fibroplasia (retinopathy of prematurity) caused by hyperoxia	■ Absence of effects of retinotoxic O$_2$ levels	■ Maintain inspired O$_2$ concentrations at minimal level necessary to achieve adequate oxygenation
		  Monitor FIO$_2$ and record concentration q1-2 hr
		    FIO$_2$ should be prescribed based on arterial blood gas levels
		  Monitor PaO$_2$
		    q4 hr if FIO$_2$ is less than 40%
		    q2 hr if FIO$_2$ is greater than 40%
		    q1 hr using transcutaneous PO$_2$ monitoring
		Administer vitamin E, as ordered
		Arrange for consultation by ophthalmologist as per hospital routine†
		Instruct parents regarding discharge follow-up; arrange clinic appointment

*Improvement of respiratory status postoperatively depends on the degree of hypoplasia.
†Infants who receive O$_2$ for any period should have optic fundi examined by ophthalmologist during and following O$_2$ therapy, at discharge, and at 5 months of age or 3 months after discharge.

POTENTIAL PROBLEMS	EXPECTED OUTCOMES	NURSING ACTIVITIES
■ Delayed wound healing, infection	■ Wound intact and heals without infection	■ Monitor incision site for Drainage Erythema Edema Notify physician of any abnormalities Keep area dry and clean Dressing is not necessary
■ Parental anxiety related to lack of confidence in their parenting skills, their perception of infant's special needs, etc.	■ Reduction of anxiety Infant receives appropriate physical and psychological nurturing Parents demonstrate readiness to assume care of infant	■ Prepare parents for assuming care at home Allow parents to discuss their experiences and feelings Instruct parents in care of baby (include father) Feeding techniques Bathing Signs and symptoms of and intervention for respiratory distress Arrange public health nurse or Visiting Nurse Association referral Assess parent-infant interactions See Standard 68, *The unstable premature infant*, Problem, Lack of confidence in parenting skills

TRACHEOESOPHAGEAL FISTULA

Tracheoesophageal fistula (TEF) is an abnormal congenital or acquired communication between the trachea and esophagus.

In most cases of congenital TEF, there is also an associated esophageal interruption, or atresia (Fig. 7, *A*). If this is the case, swallowed fluid enters the proximal esophageal pouch, then is aspirated into the trachea, causing a chemical pneumonia (most often the right upper lobe). Gastric contents are regurgitated through the distal esophagus and fistula into the lungs, and air travels from the lungs into the stomach (causing gastric distention). TEF should be suspected in an infant with excessive drooling, respiratory distress (particularly choking or cyanosis during feeding), frequent pneumonia, and excessive gastric air.

Occasionally, the infant may have congenital TEF without esophageal atresia (Fig. 7, *B* and *C*). In these cases, the infant may not demonstrate excessive drooling or gastric air but will have frequent aspiration pneumonia, coughing spells, and cyanosis.

Acquired TEF may occur after trauma, penetrating wounds, or prolonged tracheal and esophageal intubation and with carcinoma.

The diagnosis of congenital TEF with esophageal atresia should be suspected in the infant with excessive gastric air

on the chest radiograph and is confirmed by the inability to pass a catheter from the esophagus into the stomach. To detect congenital or acquired TEF without esophageal atresia, contrast studies with esophagogram or bronchoscopy may be performed. Contrast radiography is *extremely* hazardous in newborns, however, since aspiration of even small amounts of contrast medium causes severe chemical pneumonitis. Therefore these studies are avoided in the small infant if the diagnosis can be made another way. Any patient should be monitored for signs of aspiration during contrast radiography, and emergency suction and intubation equipment should be readily available.

Once the diagnosis is established, catheterization of the blind esophageal pouch (with associated esophageal atresia) or stomach (with simple fistula) and gastrostomy are performed to prevent further aspiration and gastric reflux. Surgical intervention is necessary once the patient's respiratory status is acceptable.

If associated esophageal atresia is present, the surgeon will attempt primary anastomosis of proximal and distal esophageal segments with closure of the TEF. If esophageal segments are too short to join directly, the fistula is closed using a retropleural approach, and an esophagostomy (for emptying of the blind pouch) and gastrostomy (for feeding)

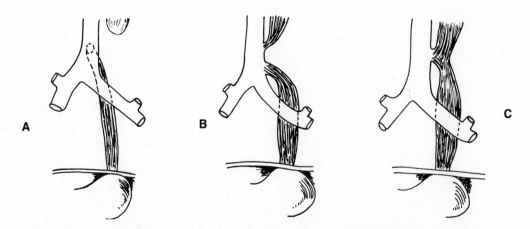

FIG. 7. A, Most common form of congenital TEF with esophageal atresia. **B** and **C,** TEF without esophageal atresia.

are created. Several months later, esophageal reanastomosis or reconstruction is then performed. If an uncomplicated TEF is present, it is closed through a cervical or thoracotomy incision. Local resection of lung tissue is performed as needed.

Following surgery, the patient is kept NPO with gastrostomy or parenteral nutrition for 3 to 14 days. The most common postoperative complications include leakage from the esophageal anastomosis, esophageal stricture, continued respiratory infection, recurrent fistulas, and dysphagia.

Children with congenital TEF have increased incidence of associated congenital heart disease, renal anomalies, GI anomalies (especially imperforate anus), skeletal and neurological problems, and thrombocytopenia.

ASSESSMENT

1. Gestational history (gestational age, perinatal distress, cyanosis at birth or during feeding, excessive drooling)
2. Congenital fistula
   a. Respiratory distress: cyanosis, tachypnea, nasal flaring, copious secretions, retractions, decreased lung aeration, evidence of pneumonia or pneumonitis by radiograph or clinical examination
   b. Cardiovascular status: evidence of cyanotic heart disease or heart failure (see introduction to Standard 28, *Cardiac surgery: pediatric*)
   c. Level of hydration: fontanelle in infants less than 18 months old, mucous membranes, skin turgor, tearing in patients over 3 months old
   d. Nutritional status: amount of subcutaneous fat, recent daily caloric intake, wound healing, and serum glucose in infants
   e. Temperature: presence of fever or hypothermia (in infants)
   f. Hematological status: leukocytosis or thrombocytopenia
   g. Associated anomalies: imperforate anus or other GI anomalies; skeletal, renal, or neurological disorders
3. Acquired fistula
   a. Cause of fistula (wound, trauma, prolonged intubation, carcinoma)
   b. Respiratory status: evidence of pneumonia or pneumonitis by radiograph or clinical examination, excessive sputum production, cyanosis, dyspnea, tachypnea, nasal flaring, retractions, orthopnea
   c. Evidence of infection: leukocytosis, fever, sputum production, wound inflammation
   d. Presence of other complications of penetrating tracheoesophageal injury
   e. Presence of complications of carcinoma and necessary therapy
4. Patient/family's anxiety about and comprehension of disorder and therapy

GOALS

1. Adequate respiratory status, including absence of further aspiration and resolution of current pneumonia
2. Adequate nutritional status and fluid and electrolyte balance
3. Absence of respiratory or wound infection
4. Patient/family's comprehension of disease, treatment plan, and prognosis, with manageable stress levels
5. Patient/family's comprehension of necessary home health care and medical follow-up
6. Patient/family's demonstration of appropriate skills in performing home health care

POTENTIAL PROBLEMS	EXPECTED OUTCOMES	NURSING ACTIVITIES
■ Respiratory distress related to aspiration pneumonia, gastric reflux, chemical pneumonitis, and postoperative atelectasis, pneumothorax, or anastomosis dehiscence	■ Stable respiratory status as measured by Normal respiratory rate Minimal respiratory effort (no use of accessory muscles) Absence of pulmonary infection on radiograph and clinical examination Absence of further aspiration pneumonia and resolution of existing pneumonia	■ Monitor respiratory rate and lung aeration, and notify physician if increased distress is present Normal adult's respiratory rate: 10 to 18/minute Normal newborn's respiratory rate: 30 to 50/minute Normal 6- to 18-month-old child's respiratory rate: 20 to 30/minute Normal 2- to 10-year-old child's respiratory rate: 18 to 30/minute Normal adolescent's respiratory rate: 12 to 20/minute NOTE: Consider patient's individual normal range Monitor for signs of increased respiratory effort, and notify physician if present Adults and children: use of accessory muscles, nasal flaring, cyanosis, diaphoresis, increased pulmonary congestion on radiograph and/or clinical examination Infants will demonstrate aforementioned with more severe retractions, head bobbing (up to age of 4 months), grunting, and mottling or pallor instead of (or in addition to) cyanosis *Maintain NPO as soon as diagnosis is suspected* and for 3 to 14 days postoperatively, as ordered Have suction equipment, O₂, and resuscitator bag at bedside

POTENTIAL PROBLEMS	EXPECTED OUTCOMES	NURSING ACTIVITIES
		Suction oropharynx frequently to prevent aspiration of secretions (after surgery, do not allow suction catheter to extend to area of tracheal or esophageal suture lines; it may be necessary to use marked catheter for comparison when suctioning)
		If patient is intubated and mechanically ventilated following surgery, see Standard 6, *Mechanical ventilation*
		Insert Raplogle tube into proximal pouch of esophagus (if esophageal atresia is present) to provide continuous removal of secretions
		Record tube output as part of patient's daily output
		Irrigate and aspirate tube to ensure patency, using small amounts of sterile saline solution or air (0.5 to 1 cc) q1-2 hr
		Elevate head of bed 20 to 30 degrees, and keep patient on side or prone as much as possible before surgical repair (to prevent aspiration and to reduce gastric reflux)
		If patient has pharyngostomy or esophagostomy, patient should be turned to side of "ostomy" to facilitate drainage
		If gastric tube or gastrostomy is inserted to remove gastric contents (to prevent gastric reflux), check its placement and function by irrigating with small amounts of normal saline solution or air (1 to 5 cc) q2 hr (reaspirate irrigation material after each check)
		Prepare patient for and monitor patient during any diagnostic radiographic studies (bring emergency equipment—resuscitator bag, endotracheal tube, etc.—to radiology, and do not leave patient unattended at any time during studies)
		If parenteral alimentation is begun, see Standard 57, *Total parenteral nutrition*
		NOTE: These neonates are especially prone to development of NEC; monitor for evidence of Hematest positive stools and abdominal distention; see Standard 72, *Neonatal necrotizing enterocolitis*
		Provide gastrostomy and esophagostomy stomal care; monitor for peristomal excoriation, and notify physician of any stomal breakdown
		Turn patient frequently; keep skin warm and dry; massage any bony prominences to stimulate circulation
		Monitor Hgb and Hct; notify physician of significant changes
		Weigh patient daily, and notify physician of any significant weight gain or loss (greater than 1 kg/24 hours in adults, greater than 200 g/24 hours in children, and greater than 50 g/24 hours in neonates)
		Monitor fluid intake and output; calculate patient's daily fluid requirements, and discuss with physician if patient is not receiving them
		Monitor level of hydration
		Palpate fontanelle in infants under 18 months—will be sunken if dehydration is present
		Mucous membranes should be moist, and tearing should be present in infant beyond age of 3 months
		Skin should not "tent" when pinched
		Urine output should be adequate (1 to 2 ml/kg/hour) with normal specific gravity (1.005 to 1.020)
		Notify physician if there is evidence of dehydration
		Once oral feedings are resumed, monitor closely for dysphagia and/or aspiration; notify physician immediately if either occurs, and be prepared to institute emergency measures if respiratory distress develops
		May wish to add food coloring to initial fluid intake and stop feedings if color appears in respiratory secretions
■ Patient/family's anxiety regarding diagnosis, surgery, prognosis, hospitalization, and change in appearance (caused by scarring or stoma)	■ Patient/family (as appropriate) demonstrates comprehension of diagnosis, surgical and medical plan of care, and prognosis	■ Prepare patient/family for any diagnostic or surgical procedures (for children, play or art may be used to provide information in a less threatening manner); focus on what patient will see, feel, or hear
		Orient patient/family to the nursing care unit, staff, and policies

POTENTIAL PROBLEMS	EXPECTED OUTCOMES	NURSING ACTIVITIES
	Patient/family's stress levels do not interfere with their ability to support one another and function appropriately	Provide patient/family with sufficient opportunity to discuss fears, concerns, and questions (if gastrostomy or esophagostomy is necessary, patient/family will need assistance in coping with patient's change in appearance) Frequently orient patient to time and place after any surgical intervention or sedation Frequently explain care regimen to patient/family; include description of and explanation for tubes and NPO Provide child with frequent reassurances that he or she is a "good boy" or "good girl," and be able to tell patient when parents or other significant family members will return Assist parents of newborn in mourning for the loss of healthy, perfect child and adjustment to fact that their child has congenital defect; parents will need reassurances that they could not have prevented their child's congenital lesion Make sure that patient/family is given consistent explanations
■ Infection related to aspiration pneumonia, surgical anastomosis dehiscence, and poor nutritional status NOTE: If acquired fistula has been caused by penetrating injury, infection can result	■ Absence of infection with no evidence of pneumonia on radiograph or clinical examination, wound infection, (erythema, heat, drainage), leukocytosis, fever (or hypothermia in infants), or sepsis	■ Monitor temperature: notify physician and obtain blood cultures if fever occurs (greater than 100.4° F [38° C]); because infant can become hypothermic with infection, monitor also for temperature instability Auscultate lungs and report any evidence of congestion NOTE: Empyema may occur with dehiscence of esophageal anastomosis if retropleural approach was not used for surgical correction Monitor blood counts for evidence of infection Note wound appearance; report any heat, erythema, or drainage, and obtain culture of wound if these occur Administer any ordered antibiotics—check patient's dosage and allergies before administration If patient is receiving steroids or chemotherapy, observe closely for evidence of infection and be particularly cautious with assignments of patient's roommates (to prevent introduction of other sources of infection or contamination) Provide care of any existing stoma and prevent peristomal excoriation
■ Patient/family may have inadequate information to comply with home health care regimen and health maintenance*	■ Patient/family demonstrates comprehension of and ability to perform home health care Patient/family demonstrates knowledge of planned physician follow-up and future surgical and medical intervention	■ Provide adequate time for teaching and return demonstration of home health care regimen; include medications, "ostomy" or wound care, return checkup visits, and signs of emergency requiring immediate medical intervention Provide patient/family with list of appropriate physicians and why, how, and where to contact them Parents of infant will require information on timing of immunizations—usually immunizations should be delayed until several weeks after child has recovered from surgery Provide reinforcement of home health care teaching by all members of health team (all should use same terminology when communicating with patient/family) If needed, provide ongoing therapy with family to help them deal with patient's altered appearance and health care needs Initiate appropriate community health referrals Collect sputum specimen for C and S and Gram stain studies if patient demonstrates any evidence of respiratory infection Administer appropriate antibiotics, as ordered; check dosage and patient allergies before administration Administer steroids, as ordered; check dosage and monitor wound healing (and observe for evidence of GI bleeding) during course of administration

*If responsibility of critical care nurse includes such follow-up care.

POTENTIAL PROBLEMS	EXPECTED OUTCOMES	NURSING ACTIVITIES

		During gastrostomy feedings and once oral feedings are resumed, put small amount of food coloring into food and monitor for any evidence of aspiration; be prepared to discontinue feedings and institute emergency measures quickly (have suction equipment close at hand)
		Provide chest physiotherapy
		  Do not place patient in Trendelenburg position for drainage as it may promote gastric reflux
		  Use rib-springing exercises and innovative games with children to promote deep breathing
		Provide care of thoracotomy pleural drainage tubes (with water seal drainage) following surgical repair, as needed
		  Maintain water seal
		  Monitor for evidence of pneumothorax (decreased breath sounds, tachypnea, increased respiratory effort, and hyperresonance to percussion) or hemothorax (decreased breath sounds and dullness to percussion, tachypnea, increased respiratory effort, increased chest tube drainage of 100 ml/hour in adults or greater than 3 ml/kg/hour in children); notify physician if these occur

■ Poor nutrition related to inability to maintain oral feedings, severe illness, and stress	■ Adequate nutritional status as measured by
	Appropriate weight gain
	Adequate subcutaneous tissue
	Moist mucous membranes
	Good skin turgor
	Adequate wound healing
		■ Calculate patient's daily caloric requirements; ensure adequate caloric intake via parenteral alimentation or gastrostomy feedings
		Monitor infant's serum glucose or Dextrostix as needed; notify physician of any evidence of hypoglycemia (glycogen storage in infants is minimal)
		If gastrostomy feedings are ordered
		  Secure tube carefully once appropriate placement is determined
		  Begin gastrostomy feedings with small, dilute amounts and advance volume and osmolarity slowly, as patient's tolerance permits
		  Before each feeding, aspirate tube and measure any residual formula; do not advance feedings if residual is greater than 5 ml in infant and 20 ml in adult (or as hospital policy dictates)
		  Monitor for abdominal distention (measure abdominal girth q2 hr) and diarrhea when feedings are increased in volume or osmolarity; if either occur, notify physician and reduce feeding
		  Gastrostomy feedings *should be accomplished through gravity drainage only and never through pressure* (gastric perforation can occur)
		  Provide oral stimulation with pacifier for infant during feeding
		  Follow feedings with 5 to 10 ml normal saline solution or sterile H₂O to flush tubing; then leave tube unclamped but elevated (so air and regurgitant matter can reflux up tubing instead of into esophagus) for several minutes (30 to 40) after each feeding

Bibliography

RESPIRATORY

Abels, L.F.: Acute respiratory failure, Crit. Care Q. **1:**1-82, 1979.

Abels, L.F.: Mosby's manual of critical care, St. Louis, 1979, The C.V. Mosby Co.

Adams, N.R.: The nurse's role in systematic weaning from a ventilator, Nurs. '79 **9:**34-41, Aug. 1979.

Berk, J.L., et al., eds.: Handbook of critical care, ed. 2, Boston, 1982, Little, Brown & Co.

Brannia, P.K.: Physical assessment of acute respiratory failure, Crit. Care Q. **1:**27-41, March 1979.

Brooks, C.G.: Artificial mechanical ventilation of the adult. Part I. Getting it started, Crit. Care Nurse **1:**15-17, May-June 1981.

Brooks, C.G.: Artificial mechanical ventilation of the adult. Part II. Fine tuning, Crit. Care Nurse **1:**8-14, July-Aug. 1981.

Broughton, J.O.: Understanding blood gases, Madison, Wis., 1979, Ohio Medical Products.

Brunner, L., and Suddarth, D.: Textbook of medical surgical nursing, ed. 4, Philadelphia, 1980, J.B. Lippincott Co.

Burrell, Z.L., and Burrell, L.O.: Critical care, ed. 4, St. Louis, 1982, The C.V. Mosby Co.

Bushnell, S.S.: Respiratory intensive care nursing, Boston, 1979, Little, Brown & Co.

Cameron, M.I.: What patients need most before and after thoracotomy, Nurs. '78 **8:**28-36, May 1978.

Cline, B.A., and Fisher, M.L.: A.R.D.S. means emergency, Nurs. '82 **12:**62-67, Feb. 1982.

Clutario, B.C., and Holzman, B.H.: Uncommon diseases, extrapulmonary diseases, systemic diseases, and toxins. In Scarpelli, E.M., et al., eds.: Pulmonary disease of the fetus, newborn and child, Philadelphia, 1978, Lea & Febiger.

Conn, A.W., Edmonds, J.F., and Barker, G.A.: Cerebral resuscitation in near-drowning, Pediatr. Clin. North Am. **26:**691-701, 1979.

Cunningham, J.H., et al.: Interstitial pulmonary edema, Heart Lung **6:**617-623, 1977.

Dammert, W., and Mast, C.P.: Tracheostomy. In Levin, D.L., Morriss, F.C., and Moore, G.C., eds.: A practical guide to pediatric intensive care, St. Louis, 1979, The C.V. Mosby Co.

Divertie, M.B.: Adult respiratory distress syndrome, Mayo Clin. Proc. **57:**371-378, 1982.

Dossey, B., and Passons, J.M.: Pulmonary embolism: preventing it, treating it, Nurs. '81 **11:**26-32, March 1981.

Eisenbach, D.: The pathophysiology of adult respiratory distress syndrome, Nurs. '80 **10:**54, May 1980.

Elpern, E.H.: Asthma update: pathophysiology and treatment, Heart Lung **9:**665-670, 1980.

Flenley, D.C.: Blood gas and acid base interpretation, Resp. Care, **27:**311-317, 1982.

Fish, J.E., and Summer, W.R.: Acute lower airway obstruction: asthma. In Moser, K.M., and Spragg, R.G., eds.: Respiratory emergencies, ed. 2, St. Louis, 1982, The C.V. Mosby Co., pp. 144-165.

Fuchs, P.: Oxygen delivery systems, Nurs. '80 **10:**34-43, Dec. 1980.

Fuchs, P.: Continuous mechanical ventilation, Nurs. '79 **9:**26-33, Dec. 1979.

Gallagher, T.J., et al.: Terminology update: optimal PEEP, Crit. Care Med. **6:**323-336, 1978.

Hopewell, P.C.: Adult respiratory distress syndrome, Basics Resp. Dis. **7:**1-6, March 1979.

Hudgel, D., and Madsen, L.: Acute and chronic asthma: a guide to intervention, Am. J. Nurs. **80:**1791-1795, 1980.

Kirilloff, L.H., and Tibbals, S.C.: Drugs for asthma: a complete guide, Am. J. Nurs. **83:**55-61, 1983.

Lanford, A.: Name that acid-base, Crit. Care Nurse **1:**10-12, March-April 1981.

Mancini, M.R., et al.: Status asthmaticus, Nurs. '82, 58-63, March 1982.

Martz, K.V., Joiner, J., and Shepherd, R.M.: Management of the patient-ventilator system: a team approach. St. Louis, 1979, The C.V. Mosby Co.

Mathewson, H.S.: Respiratory therapy in critical care, St. Louis, 1976, The C.V. Mosby Co.

Michaelson, E.D.: Oxygen therapy and delivery in obstructive pulmonary disease, Heart Lung **7:**627-632, 1978.

Mitchell, R.S., and Petty, T.L., eds.: Synopsis of clinical pulmonary disease, ed. 3, St. Louis, 1982, The C.V. Mosby Co.

Modell, J.H., et al.: Clinical course of 91 consecutive near-drowning victims, Chest **70:**231-238, 1976.

Moser, K.M., and Spragg, R.G., eds.: Respiratory emergencies, ed. 2, St. Louis, 1982, The C.V. Mosby Co.

Murphy, P.A., and Schare, B.L.: Timely techniques in caring for the patient with an endotracheal tube, Nurs. '81 **11:**70-73, Sept. 1981.

Nielsen, L.: Assessing patients' respiratory problems, Am. J. Nurs. **80:**2192-2196, 1980.

Nielsen, L.: Ventilators and how they work, Nurs. **80:**2202-2205, 1980.

Nielsen, L.: Potential problems of mechanical ventilation, Am. J. Nurs. **80:**2206-2213, 1980.

Nielsen, L.: Weaning patients from mechanical ventilation, Am. J. Nurs. **80:**2214-2217, 1980.

Peterson, B.: Morbidity of childhood near-drowning, Pediatrics **59:**364-370, 1977.

Promistoff, R.A.: Administering oxygen safely: when, why, how, Nurs. '80 **10:**54-56, Oct. 1980.

Rachow, E., and Fein, I.A.: Fulminant noncardiogenic pulmonary edema in the critically ill, Crit. Care Med. **6:**360-363, 1978.

Rhodes, M.L.: Acute respiratory failure in chronic obstructive lung disease, Crit. Care Q. **1:**1-11, March 1979.

Scarpelli, E.M., et al., eds.: Pulmonary disease of the fetus, newborn and child, Philadelphia, 1978, Lea & Febiger.

Shapiro, B.A., et al.: Clinical application of respiratory care, ed. 2, Chicago, 1979, Year Book Medical Publishers, Inc.

Shafer, T.: Nursing care of the patient with ARDS, Crit. Care Nurse **1:**34-42, March-April 1981.

Shrake, K.: The ABC's of ABG's, Nurs. '79 **9:**26-33, Sept. 1979.

Spearman, C., and Sheldon, R.: Egan's fundamentals of respiratory therapy, ed. 4, St. Louis, 1982, The C.V. Mosby Co.

Stevens, P.M.: Positive end expiratory pressure breathing, Basics Resp. Dis. **5:**1-6, Jan. 1977.

Sweetwood, H.: Acute respiratory insufficiency, Nurs. '77 **7:**24-31, 1977.

Tecklin, J.S.: Positioning, percussing and vibrating patients for effective bronchial drainage, Nurs. '79 **9:**64-71, 1979.

Vaughan, P.: Acute respiratory failure in the patient with chronic obstructive lung disease, Crit. Care Nurse **1:**44-46, Sept.-Oct. 1981.

Wade, J.: Comprehensive respiratory care: physiology and technique, ed. 3, St. Louis, 1982, The C.V. Mosby Co.

Waldron, M.W.: Oxygen transport, Am. J. Nurs. **79:**272-275, 1979.

Whitcomb, M.E.: The lung: normal and diseased, St. Louis, 1982, The C.V. Mosby Co.

Pleural compromise

Bricker, P.L.: Chest tubes: the crucial points you mustn't forget, RN **43:**21-26, Nov. 1980.

Cohen, S.: How to work with chest tubes, Am. J. Nurs. **80:**685-705, 1980.

Culpepper, J., et al.: Malpositioned nasogastric tube causing pneumothorax and bronchopleural fistula, Chest **81:**389, 1982.

Erickson, R.: "Chest tubes: they're really not that complicated." Nurs. '81 **11:**34-42, May 1981.

Farber, D.L., et al.: Hemoptysis and pneumothorax after removal of a persistently wedged pulmonary artery catheter, Crit. Care. Med. **9:**494-495, 1980.

Gillespie: Thoracic trauma, Emerg. Med. (Nov. 1980) 69-88.

Hinson, J., et al.: Catamenial pneumothorax in sisters, Chest **80:**634-635, 1981.

Hollimon, P., et al.: Pneumothorax attributable to nasogastric tube, Arch. Surg. **116:**970, 1981.

McSwain: A stab at pneumothorax, Emerg. Med. 109-110, 1981.

Netter, F.: The CIBA collection of medical illustrations, vol. 5, The heart, New York, 1969, The CIBA Co.

Ofoegbu, R., et al.: Pleurodesis for spontaneous pneumothorax, Am. J. Surg. **140:**679-681, 1980.

Macoviak, J., et al.: Tetracycline pleurodesis during active pulmonary-pleural air leak for prevention of recurrent pneumothorax, Chest **81:**78-81, 1981.

Perdue, P.: Urgent priorities in severe trauma: life-threatening respiratory injuries, RN **44:**27-33, 1981.

Pierce, J., et al.: More on familial spontaneous pneumothorax, Chest **78:**263, 1980.

Rhea, J., et al.: Tension pneumothorax, Am. Fam. Physician **25:**149, 1982.

Slay, R., et al.: Transient ST elevation associated with tension pneumothorax, J.A.C.E.P. **8:**16-18, 1979.

West, J.: Pulmonary pathophysiology, ed. 2, Baltimore, Williams & Wilkins Co., 1982.

Chest tubes

Bates, B.: A guide to physical examination, Philadelphia, 1983, J.B. Lippincott Co.

Brew, C., and Dracup, K.: Helping the spouse of critically ill patients, Am. J. Nurs. **78:**50-53, 1978.

Bricker, P.L.: Chest tubes: the crucial points you mustn't forget, RN **43:**22-27, Nov. 1980.

Butler-Maher, A.: A systems approach to nursing the patient with multiple systems failure, Heart Lung **10:**871, 1981.

Duncan, C., and Erickson, R.: Pressures associated with chest tube stripping, Heart Lung **11:**166-171, 1982.

Dziurbijko, M.M., and Larkin, J.C.: Including the family in preoperative teaching, Am. J. Nurs. **78:**1892-1893, 1978.

Erickson, R.: Consultation: stripping chest tubes, Nurs. '83 **13:**96, March 1983.

Erickson, R.: Solving chest tube problems, Nurs. '81 **11:**62-68, June 1981.

Erickson, R.: Chest tubes: they're really not that complicated, Nurs. '81 **11:**34-43, May 1981.

Molter, N.C.: Needs of relatives of critically ill patients: a descriptive study, Heart Lung **8:**332-339, 1979.

Programmed instruction: how to work with chest tubes, Am. J. Nurs. **80:**685-712, 1980.

Rich, W., and Reichenberger, M.: Managing flail chest: a matter of maintaining breath . . . and life, Nurs. '81 **11:**30-31, Dec. 1981.

Schwartz, L.P., and Brenner, Z.P.: Critical care transfer: reducing patient stress through nursing intervention, Heart Lung **8:**540-546, 1979.

CARDIOVASCULAR

Abels, L.F.: Mosby's manual of critical care, St. Louis, 1979, The C.V. Mosby Co.

Adams, N.: Reducing the perils of intra-cardiac monitoring, Nursing '76 **6:**66-74, 1976.

Adams, N.: Hemodynamic monitoring, Crit. Care Q. **2:**1-86, 1979.

Andreoli, K., et al.: Comprehensive cardiac care, ed. 5, St. Louis, 1983, The C.V. Mosby Co.

Bailen, M.T.: Intra-aortic balloon pumping. Lectures presented at the Cardiovascular Laboratory, College of Physicians and Surgeons, Columbia Presbyterian Medical Center, New York, 1976-1979.

Barash, P.G., et al.: Intra-operative use of Swan-Ganz catheter data, New Haven, Conn., 1978, Yale School of Medicine, Department of Anesthesia.

Berk, J.L., et al., eds.: Handbook of critical care, Boston, 1982, Little, Brown & Co.

Bolton, E.: Procedural guidelines for the use of balloon-tipped, flow directed catheters, Crit. Care Nurse **1**:33-40, Feb. 1981.

Bregman, D.: Mechanical support of the failing heart, Curr. Probl. Surg. **13**:1-84, Dec. 1976.

Brunner, L., and Suddarth, D.: The Lippincott manual of nursing practice, ed. 3, Philadelphia 1982, J.B. Lippincott Co.

Brunner, L., and Suddarth, D.: Textbook of medical surgical nursing, ed. 4, Philadelphia, 1980, J.B. Lippincott Co.

Burrell, Z.L., and Burrell, L.O.: Critical care, ed. 4, St. Louis, 1982, The C.V. Mosby Co.

Caprini, J.A., et al.: Heparin therapy. I, Cardiovasc. Nurs. **13**:13-16, 1977.

Caprini, J.A., et al.: Heparin therapy. II, Cardiovasc. Nurs. **13**:17-20, 1977.

Chung, E.: Quick reference to cardio-vascular diseases, ed. 2, Philadelphia, 1983, J.B. Lippincott Co.

Cohen, S., Nursing care of patients in shock: pharmcotherapy. Part I, Am. J. Nurs. **82**:943-964, 1982.

Cromwell, R., et al.: Acute myocardial infarction: reaction and recovery, St. Louis, 1977, The C.V. Mosby Co.

Cudkowicz, L., and Sherry, S.: Current status of thrombolytic therapy, Heart Lung **7**:97-100, 1978.

Daily, E.K., and Schroeder, J.S.: Techniques in bedside hemodynamic monitoring, ed. 2, St. Louis, 1980, The C.V. Mosby Co.

Davidson, S.V.S., et al.: Nursing care evaluation: concurrent and retrospective review criteria, St. Louis, 1977, The C.V. Mosby Co.

Edwards Laboratories: Understanding hemodynamic measurements made with the Swan Ganz catheter, Santa Ana, Calif., 1977, Edwards Laboratories.

Fitzmaurice, J.B.: Venous thromboembolic disease: current thoughts, Cardiovasc. Nurs. **14**:1-4, 1978.

Foxworth, G.D.: Rehabilitation for hospitalized adults after open-heart procedures: the team approach, Heart Lung **7**:834-839, 1978.

Gildae, J.H., et al.: Congenital cardiac defects, Am. J. Nurs. **78**:255-278, 1978.

Goldman, M.J.: Principles of clinical electrocardiography, ed. 9, Los Altos, Calif., 1976, Lange Medical Publications.

Guide to physiological pressure monitoring, Waltham, Mass., 1977, Hewlett-Packard Co.

Harrington, D.: Disparities between direct and indirect arterial systolic blood pressure measurements, CVP **6**:40-44, Aug.-Sept. 1978.

Hart, L.K., and Frantz, R.A.: Characteristics of postoperative patient-education programs for open-heart surgery patients in the United States, Heart Lung **6**:137-142, 1977.

Hazinski, M.G.: The cardiovascular system. In Armstrong, M.E., et al., eds.: McGraw-Hill handbook of clinical nursing, New York, 1979, McGraw-Hill Book Co.

Hazinski, M.G.: Congenital heart lesions, Chicago, 1978, Bio-Services Corp.

Hurst, J.W., et al.: The heart, ed. 4, New York, 1978, McGraw-Hill Book Co.

Johansen, K.: Aneurysms, Sci. Am. **247**:110-111, July 1982.

Lalli, S.: The complete Swan-Ganz, RN **41**:65-77, 1978.

Leech, J.E.: Psychosocial and physiologic needs of patients with arterial occlusive disease during the preoperative phase of hospitalization, Heart Lung **11**:442-449, 1982.

Long, G.D.: Managing the patient with abdominal aortic aneurysm, Nurs. '78 **8**:20-27, 1978.

Marriott, H.J.L., and Conover, M.H.B.: Advanced concepts in arrhythmias, St. Louis, 1983, The C.V. Mosby Co.

Meltzer, L., et al., eds.: Concepts and practices of intensive care for nurse specialists, Bowie, Md., 1976, Charles Press Publications, Inc.

Miller, S.P., and Shada, E.A.: Preoperative information and recovery of open heart surgery patients, Heart Lung **7**:486-493, 1978.

Monson, D.O., et al.: Management of the pediatric cardiac surgical patient. In Golden, M.D., ed.: Intensive care of the surgical patient, ed. 2, Chicago, 1980, Year Book Medical Publishers, Inc.

Moss, A.J., et al.: Heart disease in infants, children and adolescents, ed. 2, Baltimore, 1977, The Williams & Wilkins Co.

Neu, H.: Early treatment of infection of unknown origin, Indianapolis, 1976, Eli Lilly & Co.

Petty, T.L.: Respiratory failure and the heart revisited, 1982, Heart Lung **11**:29-32, 1982.

Prakash, O., et al.: Cardiorespiratory and metabolic effects of profound hypothermia, Crit. Care Med. **6**:165-171, 1978.

Prakash, O., et al.: Erratum: cardiorespiratory and metabolic effects of profound hypothermia, Crit. Care Med. **6**:339-346, 1978.

Rakoczy, M.: The thoughts and feelings of patients in the waiting period prior to cardiac surgery: a descriptive study, Heart Lung **6**:280-287, 1977.

Robbins, S.L.: Pathologic basis of disease, ed. 2, Philadelphia, 1979, W.B. Saunders Co.

Rodman, M.: Drugs for treating shock, RN **39**:77-86, 1976.

Sadler, P.D.: Nursing assessment of postcardiotomy delirium, Heart Lung **8**:745-750, 1979.

Schwartz, S.I., et al., eds.: Principles of surgery, ed. 3, New York, 1979, McGraw-Hill Book Co.

Sedlock, S.: Interpretation of hemodynamic pressures and recognition of complications, Crit. Care Nurse **1**:39-44, Nov.-Dec. 1980.

Sedlock, S.: Cardiac output: physiologic valuables and therapeutic intervention, Crit. Care Nurse **1**:14-22, Feb. 1981.

Shearer, J.K., and Caldwell, M.: Use of sodium nitroprusside and dopamine hydrochloride in the postoperative cardiac patient, Heart Lung **8**:302-307, 1979.

Sokolow, M., and McIlroy, M.B.: Clinical cardiology, Los Altos, Calif., 1977, Lange Medical Publications.

Sorensen, M.B., et al.: Cardiac output measurement by thermal dilution, Ann. Surg. **183**:67-72, 1976.

Thompson, W.L.: The patient in shock. In The proceedings of a symposium on recent research developments and current clinical practice in shock, Kalamazoo, Mich., 1976, Upjohn Co.

Tucker, S.M., et al.: Patient care standards, ed. 3, St. Louis, 1984, The C.V. Mosby Co.

Vinsant, M., and Spense, M.: Commonsense approach to coronary care: a program, ed. 3, St. Louis, 1981, The C.V. Mosby Co.

Wells, S., Stokes, S., and Mahoney, K.: Manual of cardio-vascular assessment, Reston, Va., 1983, Reston Publishing Co., Inc.

Wenger, N.K., Hurst, J.W., and McIntyre, M.C.: Cardiology for Nurses, New York, 1980, McGraw-Hill Book Co.

Woods, S.: Monitoring pulmonary artery pressures, Am. J. Nurs. **76:**1765-1771, 1976.

Zschoche, D.A.: Mosby's comprehensive review of critical care, ed. 2, St. Louis, 1981, The C.V. Mosby Co.

Transluminal coronary angioplasty

Bell, W., and Meck, A.: Guidelines for the use of thrombolytic agents, N. Engl. J. Med. **301:**1266-1270, 1979.

Block, P.: Coronary angioplasty: current status, Surg. Rounds, 62-69, May 1982.

Bullas, J.: Fibrinolytic therapy: nursing implications, Crit. Care Nurse **1:**43-46, 1981.

Cowley, M., et al.: Efficacy of PTCA: technique, patient selection salutary results, limitations, and complications, Am. Heart J. **101:**272-280, 1981.

Gruntzig, A., et al.: Nonoperative dilatation of coronary artery stenosis, N. Engl. J. Med. **301:**61-67, 1979.

Mason, D.: International experience with PTC recanalization by streptokinasethrombolysis reperfusion in acute myocardial infarction: new, safe, landmark approach to salvaging ischemic muscle and improving ventricular function, Am. Heart J. **102:**1126-1133, 1981.

Ott, B.B.: Percutaneous transluminal coronary angroplasty and nursing implications, Heart Lung **11:**294-298, 1982.

Purcell, J. and Griffin, P.: PTCA, Am. J. Nurs. **81:**1620-1626, 1981.

Slack, J.D., Slack, L.A., and Orr, C.: Recurrent severe reaction to iodinated contrast media during cardiac catheterization, Heart Lung **11:**348-352, 1982.

Stertzer, S., et al.: Transluminal coronary artery dilatation, Pract. Cardiol. **5:**25-32, 1979.

Vliestra, R., et al.: PTCA: initial Mayo Clinic experience, Mayo Clin. Proc. **56:**287-293, 1981.

Cardiomyopathies

Breu, C.S., Lindenmuth, J.E., and Tillisch, J.H.: Treatment of patients with congestive cardiomyopathy during hospitalization: a case study, Heart Lung **11:**229-236, 1982.

Dracup, K.: Unraveling the mysteries of cardiomyopathy, Nurs. '79 **9:**84-87, May 1979.

Dossey, B., Guzzetta, C., and Kenner, C.: Critical care nursing, Boston, 1981, Little, Brown & Co.

Egoville, B.B.: IHSS: what to teach the patient who has it, Nurs. '80 **10:**50-55, April 1980.

Haughey-Weidman, C.: Alcoholic cardiomyopathy: when abstinence makes the heart grow stronger, Nurs. '80 **10:**54-58, Sept. 1980.

Love, M., and Oertel, T.: Mitral valve prolapse and idiopathic hypertrophic subaortic sterosis: two sources of chest pain in young adults, J.E.N. **9:**21-6, Jan.-Feb. 1983.

Trobaugh, G.: Cardiomyopathies. In Happenny, J., et al., eds.: Cardiac nursing, Philadelphia, 1982, J.B. Lippincott Co., pp. 651-655.

Hypertensive crisis

Anderson, R.J., et al.: Oral clonidine loading in hypertensive urgencies, JAMA **246:**848-850, 1981.

Borhani, N.O.: Epidemiology of hypertension as a guide to treatment and control, Heart Lung **10:**245-254, 1981.

Finnerty, F., Jr.: Treatment of hypertensive emergencies, Heart Lung **10:**275-281, 1981.

Freier, D.T., Eckhauser, F.E., and Harrison, T.S.: Pheochromocytoma, Arch. Surg. **115:**388-391, 1980.

Ginkus-O'Connor, N.: Intravenous drugs used in treating hypertensive emergencies, Heart Lung **10:**848-855, 1981.

Hill, M., and Fink, J.: In hypertensive emergencies, act quickly, Nurs. '83 **13:**34-41, Feb. 1983.

Hill, M., and McCombs, N., eds.: Symposium on hypertension, Nurs. Clin. North Am. **16:**299-376, 1981.

Hypertension, Am. J. Nurs. **80:**925-950, 1980.

Krakoff, L., and Laragh, J.: The renin system in the diagnosis of hypertension, Somerville, N.J., 1977, Hoechst-Roussel Pharmaceutical, Inc.

Krupp, M., and Chatton, M.: Hypertensive cardiovascular disease, Curr. Med. Diagn. Treatment **1:**183-193, 1982.

Langford, H.G.: Electrolyte intake, electrolyte excretion and hypertension, Heart Lung **10:**269-274, 1981.

Messerilli, F., and Ventura, H.: Ca antagonists and hypertension, Drug Ther. **7:**39-44, Nov. 1982.

Patient behavior for blood pressure control, JAMA **241:**2534-2537, 1979.

The role of clinical electrophysiological testing in the treatment of ventricular tachycardia

Altman, G.: Alcoholic cardiomyopathy, Cardiovasc. Nurs. **17:**25-30, 1981.

Fisher, P., et al.: Role of implantable pacemakers in control of recurrent ventricular tachycardia, Am. J. Cardiol. **49:**194-204, 1982.

Gilbert, C., and Akhtor, M.: Right heart catheterization for intracardiac electrophysiologic studies: implications for the primary care nurse, Heart Lung **9:**85-91, 1980.

Horowitz, L., Josephson, M., and Kastor, J.: Intracardiac electrophysiologic studies as a method for the optimization of drug therapy in chronic ventricular arrhythmia. Prog. Cardiovasc. Dis. **23:**81-97, 1980.

Josephson, M., and Serdis, S.: Recurrent ventricular tachycardia. In Clinical cardiac electrophysiology: techniques and interpretations, Philadelphia, 1979, Lea & Febiger.

Livelli, F., et al.: Response to programmed ventricular stimulation: sensitivity, specificity and relationship to heart disease, Am. J. Cardiol. **50:**452-458, 1982.

Mason, J., and Winkle, R.: Accuracy of the ventricular tachycardia–induction study for predicting long term efficacy and inefficacy of antiarrhythmic drugs, N. Engl. J. Med. **303:**1073-1077, 1980.

Moss, J., and Schwartz, P.: Delayed repolarization (OT or OTV prolongation) and malignant ventricular arrhythmias, Mod. Concepts Cardiovasc. Dis. **50:**85-90, 1980.

Rusken, J., DiMarco, J., and Hasan, G.: Out of hospital cardiac arrest: electrophysiologic observations and section of long term antiarrhythmic therapy, New Engl. J. Med. **303:**607-613, 1980.

Vascular disease: medical and surgical management

Abramson, D.I.: Medical and surgical management of chronic occlusive arterial diseases, Pract. Cardiol. **6:**136-152, 1980.

Bernstein, E.F.: Noninvasive diagnostic techniques in vascular disease, ed. 2, St. Louis, 1982, The C.V. Mosby Co.

Cranley, J.J., and Hyland, L.J.: Diagnoses in peripheral vascular diseases, Contemp. Surg. **14:**45-80, April 1979.

Haimovici, H.: Vascular emergencies, New York, 1982, Appleton-Century-Crofts.

Juergens, J.L., Spittell, J.A., and Fairbairn, J.F.: Peripheral vascular diseases. Philadelphia, 1980, W.B. Saunders Co.

Najarian, J.S., and Delaney, J.P.: Vascular surgery, Miami, 1978, Symposia Specialists, Inc.

Perry, M.O., and Silane, M.F.: Occlusive disease of peripheral arteries. In Goldsmith, H.S.: Practice of surgery, Philadelphia, 1981, Harper & Row, Publishers, Inc.

Spittell, J.A.: Peripheral arterial disease: evaluation, Pract. Cardiol. **5**(6):25-32, 1979.

Spittell, J.A.: Peripheral arterial disease: management, Pract. Cardiol. **5**(7):37-41, 1979.

Thompson, J.E., and Garrett, W.V.: Peripheral arterial surgery, N. Engl. J. Med. **302:**491-501, 1980.

NEUROLOGICAL

Adams, R.D., and Victor, M.: Principles of neurology, New York, 1981, McGraw-Hill Book Co.

Chusid, J.C.: Correlative neuroanatomy and functional neurology, Los Altos, Calif., 1975, Lange Medical Publications.

Chaplin, J., and Demers, A.: Primer of neurology and neurophysiology, New York, 1978, John Wiley & Sons, Inc.

Ciba Pharmaceutical Co.: Clinical symposia of nervous system, vols. 15, 18, 19, 26, and 29, Summit, N.J., 1963, 1966, 1967, 1974, 1977, Ciba-Geigy Corp.

Forster, F.M.: Clinical neurology, ed. 4, St. Louis, 1978, The C.V. Mosby Co.

Green, B., Marshall, L., and Gallagher, T., eds.: Intensive care for neurological trauma and disease, New York, 1982, Academic Press, Inc.

Howe, J.R.: Patient care in neurology, Boston, 1977, Little, Brown & Co.

Lewis, A.J.: Mechanisms of neurological disease, Boston, 1976, Little, Brown & Co.

Noback, C., and Demarest, R.: The human nervous system, ed. 2, New York, 1975, McGraw Hill Book Co.

Nursing Skillbook: Coping with neurological problems proficiently, Pennsylvania, 1980, Nursing '80 Books.

Peele, T.L.: The neuroanatomic basis for clinical neurology. ed. 3, New York, 1977, McGraw-Hill Book Co.

Plum, F., and Posner, J.B.: Diagnosis of stupor and coma, Philadelphia, 1980, F.A. Davis Co.

Rapper, A., Kennedy, S., and Zervas, N., eds.: Neurological and neurosurgical intensive care, Baltimore, 1983, University Park Press.

Taylor, J.W., and Ballenger, S.: Neurological dysfunctions and nursing intervention, New York, 1980, McGraw-Hill Book Co.

Wehrmaker, S., and Wintermute, J.: Case studies in neurological nursing, Boston, 1978, Little, Brown & Co.

GASTROINTESTINAL

Alden, J.: Gastric and jejunoileal bypass: a comparison in the treatment of morbid obesity, Arch. Surg. **112:**799-806, 1977.

Boyer, C.A., and Oehlberg, S.M., eds.: Symposium of diseases of the liver, Nurs. Clin. North Am. **12:**257-356, 1977.

Brunner, L., and Suddarth, D.: The Lippincott manual of nursing practice, ed. 2, Philadelphia, 1981, J.B. Lippincott Co.

Brunner, L., and Suddarth, D.: Textbook of medical surgical nursing, ed. 4, Philadelphia, 1980, J.B. Lippincott Co.

Buckwalter, J., and Herbst, C.: Complications of gastric bypass for morbid obesity, Am. J. Surg. **139:**55-60, 1980.

Burrell, Z.L., and Burrell, L.O.: Critical care, ed. 4, St. Louis, 1981, The C.V. Mosby Co.

Callan, J.P.: Surgical treatment of morbid obesity, JAMA **241:**1271, 1979.

Cimetidine-warfarin interaction may cause hemorrhage, Nurses' Drug Alert **3:**9-16, 1979.

Condon, R., and Nyhus, L., eds.: Manual of surgical therapeutics, ed. 4, Boston, 1978, Little, Brown & Co.

Croushore, T.M.: Postoperative assessment: the key to avoiding most common nursing mistakes, Nurs. '79 **9:**47-51, 1979.

Ellis, P.D.: Portal hypertension and bleeding esophageal and gastric varices: a surgical approach to treatment, Heart Lung **6:**791-798, 1977.

Griffin, W., et al.: A prospective comparison of gastric and jejunoileal bypass procedures for morbid obesity, Ann. Surg. **186:**500-509, 1977.

Halverson, J.: Obesity surgery in perspective, Surgery **87:**119-127, 1980.

Hocking, M., et al.: Jejunoileal bypass for morbid obesity, N. Engl. J. Med. **308:**995-999, 1983.

Kinney, J.M., et al., eds.: Manual of surgical intensive care, Philadelphia, 1977, W.B. Saunders Co.

Kratzer, J.B., and Rauschenberger, D.S.: What to teach your patient about his duodenal ulcer, Nurs. '78 **8:**54-56, 1978.

Long, G.D.: G.I. bleeding: what to do and when, Nurs. '78 **8:**54-56, 1978.

Miller, B.: Jejunoileal bypass: a drastic weight control measure, Am. J. Nurs. **81:**564-568, 1981.

Mozzisik, C. and Martin, E.W., eds.: Gastric partitioning: the latest surgical means to control morbid obesity, Am. J. Nurs. **81:**569-572, 1981.

McConnell, E.A.: After surgery: how you can avert the obvious hazards and the not so obvious ones, too, Nurs. '77 **7:**32-39, 1977.

Malkiewicz, J.: For a really thorough abdominal examination: the fine art of giving a physical, RN **45:**58-63, Oct. 1982.

Nasrallah, S.M.: The management of acute pancreatitis, Crit. Care Q. **5:**15-20, Sept. 1982.

Printen, K., et al.: Stomal ulcers after gastric bypass, Arch. Surg. **115:**525-527, 1980.

Slota, M.: Abdominal assessment, Crit. Care Nurse **2:**78-81, March-April 1982.

Schimmel, L., et al., eds.: A new mechanical method to influence pulmonary perfusion in critically ill patients, Crit. Care Med. **5:**277-279, 1977.

Steinheber, F.: Bleeding from the upper gastrointestinal tract, Hosp. Med. **15:**47-64, 1979.

Schlag, M.K.: Pre and postoperative fluids and electrolytes: nursing assessment and intervention, OR Nurse **4:**10-15, Sept. 1982.

Tucker, S.M., et al.: Patient care standards, ed. 2, St. Louis, 1980, The C.V. Mosby Co.

Wapnick, S., et al.: La Veen continuous peritoneal-jugular shunt, JAMA **237:**131-133, 1977.

RENAL

Berk, J.L., et al., eds.: Handbook of critical care, Boston, 1976, Little, Brown & Co.

Brundage, D.J.: Nursing management of renal problems, ed. 2, St. Louis, 1980, The C.V. Mosby Co.

Burrell, Z.L., and Burrell, L.O.: Critical care, ed. 4, St. Louis, 1981, The C.V. Mosby Co.

Davidson, S.V., et al.: Nursing care evaluation: concurrent and retrospective review criteria, St. Louis, 1977, The C.V. Mosby Co.

Dary, J.M.: Care of the critically ill acute renal failure patient, Crit. Care Nurse **1:**47-52, Nov.-Dec. 1981.

Flamenbaum, W., and Leslie, B.R.: Diagnosis and management of renal failure in surgical patients, Orthop. Clin. North Am. **9:**845-857, 1978.

Gutch, C.F., and Stoner, M.H.: Review of hemodialysis for nurses and dialysis personnel, ed. 4, St. Louis, 1983, The C.V. Mosby Co.

Juliani, L., and Reamer, B.: Kidney transplant: your role in aftercare, Nurs. '77 **7:**46-53, 1977.

Nursing Update: Diuretics, Nurs. '83 **13:**64-65, Aug. 1983.

Stark, J.L.: How to succeed against acute renal failure, Nurs. '82, **12:**26-33, July 1982.

Stark, J.L., and Hunt, V.: Helping your patient with chronic renal failure, Nurs. '83 **13:**56-64, Sept. 1983.

Simon, N.M., et al.: Chronic renal failure. I. Pathophysiology and medical management, Cardiovasc. Nurs. **12:**7-16, 1976.

Smith, E.C., and Freedman, P.: Dialysis: current status and future trends, Heart Lung **4:**879-883, 1975.

Tichy, A.M.: Renal failure, Crit. Care Update **9:**7-21, Aug. 1982.

Tucker, S.M., et al.: Patient care standards, ed. 2, St. Louis, 1980, The C.V. Mosby Co.

Van Meter, M.: Anatomy self-test: the kidneys, RN **46:**55-56, July 1983.

Zschoche, D.A.: Mosby's comprehensive review of critical care, ed. 2, St. Louis, 1981, The C.V. Mosby Co.

METABOLIC

Abels, L.F.: Mosby's manual of critical care: practices and procedures, St. Louis, 1979, The C.V. Mosby Co.

Aberman, A.: An update on diabetic ketoacidosis, Emerg. Med. **14:**143-144, 1982.

Anderson, M.A., Aker, A.N., and Hickman R.O.: The double-lumen Hickman catheter, Am. J. Nurs. **82:**272-273, 1982.

Bjeletich, J.: Repairing the Hickman catheter, Am. J. Nurs. **82:**274, 1982.

Bjeletich, J., and Hickman, R.O.: The Hickman indwelling catheter, Am. J. Nurs. **80:**62-65, 1980.

Broviac, J.W., Cole, J., and Scribner, B.H.: A silicone rubber atrial catheter for prolonged parenteral alimentation, Surg. Gynecol. Obstet. **136:**602-606, 1973.

Brunner, L., and Suddarth, D.,: Textbook of medical surgical nursing, ed. 4, Philadelphia, 1980, J.B. Lippincott Co.

Brunner, L., and Suddarth, D.: The Lippincott manual of nursing practice, ed. 3, Philadelphia, 1980, J.B. Lippincott Co.

Campbell, C.: Nursing diagnosis and intervention in nursing practice, New York, 1978, John Wiley & Sons, Inc.

Cataland, C.: Hypoglycemia: a spectrum of problems, Heart Lung **7:**455-462, 1978.

Chambers, J.: Save your diabetic patient from early kidney damage Nurs. '83 **13:**58-64, May 1983.

Colley, R., and Wilson, J.: Meeting patients' nutritional needs with hyperalimentation: how to begin hyperalimentation therapy, Nurs. '79 **9:**76-83, May 1979.

Colley, R., and Wilson, J.: Meeting patients' nutritional needs with hyperalimentation: managing the patient on hyperalimentation, Nurs. '79 **9:**57-61, June 1979.

Colley, R., and Wilson, J: Meeting patients' nutritional needs with hyperalimentation: providing hyperalimentation for infants and children, Nurs. '79 **9:**50-63, July 1979.

Connors, J.F.: Diabetic ketoacidosis: a case for self-discipline, Nurs. Mirror **153:**50-52, Nov. 1981.

Crowley, M., and Baker: Preparing nurses for Hickman catheter care: a self-learning module. Oncol. Nurs. Forum **7:**17-19, 1980.

Dreffler, R.J., et al.: Home-care of the Hickman/Broviac Catheter, Oncol. Nurs. Forum, **9:**59-63, 1982.

Fitzgerald, B.P.: TPN: the only road home, Nurs. '82, **12:**44-49, Sept. 1982.

Fleming, R., Witzke, D., and Beart, R.: Catheter-related complications in patients receiving home parenteral nutrition, Ann. Surg. 2: 580-584, 1980.

Fonkalsrud, E.W., et al.: Occlusion of the vena cava in infants receiving central venous hyperalimentation, Surg. Gynecol. Obstet. **154:**189-192, 1982.

Heimbach, D.M., and Ivy, T.D.: Technique for placement of a permanent home hyperalimentation catheter, Surg. Gynecol. Obstet. **143:**634-636, 1980.

Hickman, R.O., et al.: A modified right atrial catheter for access to the venous system in marrow transplant recipients, Surg. Gynecol. Obstet. **148:**871-875, 1979.

Isselbacher, K.J., et al., eds.: Harrison's principles of internal medicine, ed. 9, New York, 1980, McGraw-Hill Book Co.

Johnstone, J.D.: Infrequent infections associated with Hickman catheters, Cancer Nurs. **5:**125-129, April 1982.

Lumb, P.D., et al.: Aggressive approach to intravenous feeding of the critically ill patient, Heart Lung **8:**71-80, 1979.

Manfredi, C., et al.: Developing a teaching program for diabetic patients, Cont. Ed. Nurs. **8:**46-52, 1977.

Massar, E., et al.: Peripheral vein complications in patients receiving amino acid/dextrose solutions, JPEN **7:**159-162, 1982.

Mayers, M., et al.: Quality assurance for patient care, New York, 1977, Appleton-Century-Crofts.

Nemchik, R.: Diabetes today: the new insulin pumps, RN **46:**52-59, May 1983.

Nemchik, R.: Diabetes today: current therapy for retinopathy, RN **46:**34-40, June 1983.

Nurses' Drug Alert **2:**145-160, Dec. 1978.

Skillman, T.G.: Diabetic ketoacidosis, Heart Lung **7:**594-602, 1978.

Stock-Barkman, P.: Confusing concepts: is it diabetic shock or diabetic coma? Nurs. '83 **13**:32-41, June 1983.

Tucker, S., et al.: Patient care standards, ed. 2, St. Louis, 1980, The C.V. Mosby Co.

Walters, J., and Feeman, J.: Parenteral nutrition by peripheral vein. In Mullen, J., Crosby, L., and Rombeau, J., eds.: The surgical clinics of north america, symposium on surgical nutrition, Philadelphia, 1981, W.B. Saunders Co.

Weil, M.H., and Henning, R.J.: Handbook of critical care medicine, Miami, 1978, Symposia Specialists, Inc.

White, N.: Glycohemoglobin: a new text to help the diabetic stay in control. Nurs. '83 **13**:55-58, Aug. 1983.

Williams, S.R.: Essentials of nutrition and diet therapy, ed. 3, St. Louis, 1982, The C.V. Mosby Co.

Wilson, J., and Colley, R.: Meeting patients' nutritional needs with hyperalimentation: administering peripheral and enteral feedings, Nurs. '79 **9**:62-69, Sept. 1979.

GENERAL
Emotional and spiritual care of the critically ill

Adams, M., et al.: Psychological responses in critical care units, Am. J. Nurs. **78**:1504-1512, 1978.

Blackwell, B., and Carlson, C. E.: Behavioral concepts and nursing intervention, ed. 2, Philadelphia, 1978, J.B. Lippincott Co.

Bliss, J.: Sharing another's death, Nurs. '76, **6**:30, April 1976.

Borg, N., et al.: Core curriculum for critical care nursing, ed. 2, Philadelphia, 1981, W.B. Saunders Co.

Budd, S., and Brown, W.: Effect of a reorientation technique on postcardiotomy delirium, Nurs. Res. **23**:341-348, 1974.

Burton, G.: Interpersonal relations: a guide for nurses, ed. 4, New York, 1977, Springer Publishing Co., Inc.

Davidhizar, R.: Recognizing and caring for the delirious patient, J. Psychiatr. Nurs.**16**:38-41, May 1978.

Dickinson, C.: Search for spiritual meaning, Am. J. Nurs. **75**:1789-1794, 1975.

Donnelly, G.F., and Sutterley, D.C.: Coping with stress: a nursing perspective, Rockville, Md., 1981, Aspen Systems Corp.

Fish, S., and Shell, J.: Spiritual care: the nurse's role, Downers Grove, Ill., 1978, Inter-Varsity Press.

Gaffnett, C.: Your patient's dying: now what? Nurs. '79, **9**:27-33, Nov. 1979.

Helton, M.C., Gordon, S.F., and Nunnery, S.L. the correlation between sleep deprivation and the intensive-care unit syndrome, Heart Lung **9**:464-468, 1980.

Kinney, M., et al.: AACN's clinical reference for critical care nursing, New York, 1981, McGraw-Hill Book Co.

Krieger, D.: Foundations for holistic health nursing practices: the renaissance nurse, Philadelphia, 1981, J.B. Lippincott Co.

Kushner, H.: Renewal, Ladies' Home Journal, pp. 48-51, May 1983.

Lasater, K.L., and Grisanti, D.J.: Postcardiotomy psychosis: indications and interventions, Heart Lung **4**:724-729, 1975.

Lynch, J.: The simple act of touching, Nurs. '78 **8**:31-36, June 1978.

Massura, E.R.: The view from both sides of intensive care, Focus AACN **9**:3-5, Aug.-Sept. 1982.

Obayuwana, A.: Hope: a panacea unrecognized, J. Natl. Med. Assoc. **72**:67-69, 1980.

Piepgras, R.: The other dimension: spiritual help, Am. J. Nurs. **68**:2610-2613, 1968.

Pranulis, M.: Loss: a factor affecting the welfare of the coronary patient, Nurs. Clin. North Am. **7**:445-455, 1972.

Pumphret, J.: Recognizing your patient's spiritual needs, Nurs. '77 **7**:64-70, Dec. 1977.

Ramlow, M.: Hope, Focus AACN **9**:10, Aug.-Sept. 1982.

Sadler, P.D.: Incidence, degree and duration of postcardiotomy delirium, Heart Lung **10**:1084-1092, 1981.

Sadler, P.D.: Nursing assessment of postcardiotomy delirium, Heart Lung **8**:745-750, 1979.

Self, P., and Viau, J.: 4 steps for helping a patient alleviate anger,'' Nurs. '80, **10**:66, Dec. 1980.

Shelly, J.: Spiritual care . . . planting the seeds of hope, Crit. Care Update **9**:7-15, Dec. 1982.

Walsleben, J.: Sleep disorders, Am. J. Nurs. **82**:936-940, 1982.

Williams, J.: Understanding the feelings of the dying, Nurs. '76 **6**:50-56, March 1976.

Acquired immune deficiency syndrome

Allen, J., and Mellin, G.: The new epidemic: immune deficiency, opportunistic infections, and kaposi's sarcoma, Am. J. Nurs. **88**:1718-1722, 1982.

Gold, J.: Pneumocystis carinii: a pneumonia on the rise, Your Patient and Cancer, 30-38, Sept. 1981.

Henig. R.: AIDS: a new disease's deadly odyssey, Time Magazine, 28-44 Jan. 1983.

Katz, A., Lenth, J., and Nysather, J.: The immune system: it's development and functions, Am. J. Nurs. **76**:1614-1617, 1976.

Marx, J.: Spread of AIDS sparks new health concern, Science **219**:42-43, Jan. 1983.

West, S.: One step behind a killer, Science **219**:36-45, March 1983.

Multiple trauma

Berk, J.L., et al., eds.: Handbook of critical care, Boston, 1976, Little, Brown & Co.

Civetta, J.M.: Assessment of the patient following multisystemic trauma. Lecture presented at the Seventeenth Annual Symposium on Critical Care Medicine, Las Vegas, 1979, University of Southern California School of Medicine, Postgraduate Division, and Institute of Critical Care Medicine.

Clutter, P.: Abdominal trauma and hypovolemic shock, Crit. Care Update **9**:5-9, Feb. 1982.

Flint, L.M.: Intraperitoneal injuries, Heart Lung **7**:273-277, 1978.

Lance, E., and Sweetwood, H.: Chest trauma, Nurs. '78 **8**:28-33, 1978.

Molyneux-Luick, M.: The ABC's of multiple trauma, Nurs. '77 **7**:30-36, 1977.

Richardson, J.D.: Management of non-cardiac thoracic trauma, Heart Lung **7**:286-292, 1978.

Burns

Brunner, L., and Suddarth, D.: Textbook of medical surgical nursing, ed. 4, Philadelphia, 1980, J.B. Lippincott Co.

Brunner, L., and Suddarth, D.: The Lippincott manual of nursing practice, ed. 3, Philadelphia, 1980, J.B. Lippincott Co.

Burrell, Z.L., and Burrell, L.O.: Critical care, ed. 4, St. Louis, 1981, The C.V. Mosby Co.

Hayter, J.: Emergency nursing care of the burned patient, Nurs. Clin. North Am. **13**:223-234, 1978.

Mathewson, H.S.: Respiratory therapy in critical care, St. Louis, 1976, The C.V. Mosby Co.

McCrady, V.: Burn management, Crit. Care Q. **1**:1-111, 1978.

Meltzer, L., et al., eds.: Concepts and practices of intensive care for nurse specialists, Bowie, Md., 1976, Charles Press Publications, Inc.

Pruitt, B.A., Jr.: Fluid and electrolyte replacement in the burned patient, Surg. Clin. North Am. **58**:1291-1312, 1978.

Tucker, S., et al.: Patient Care standards, ed. 2, St. Louis 1980, The C.V. Mosby Co.

Wooldridge-King, M.: Nursing consideration of the burned patient during the emergent period, Heart Lung **11**:353-361, 1982.

Disseminated intravascular coagulation

Burrell, A.L., and Burrell, L.O.: Critical care, ed. 4, St. Louis, 1981, The C.V. Mosby Co.

Condon, R., and Nyhus, L., eds.: Manual of surgical therapeutics, ed. 4, Boston, 1978, Little, Brown & Co.

Hall, M.: Another link in the chain: disseminated intravascular coagulation, Nurs. Mirror **154**:53-54, 1982.

Hudak, C., et al.: Critical care nursing, ed. 2, Philadelphia, 1977, J.B. Lippincott Co.

Isselbacher, K.J., et al., eds.: Harrison's principles of internal medicine, ed. 9, New York, 1980, McGraw-Hill Book Co.

Jennings, B.: Improving your management of DIC, Nurs. '79 **9**:60-67, 1979.

McGillick K.: DIC: the deadly paradox, RN **45**:41-43, Aug. 1982.

Vogelpohl, R.A.: Disseminated intravascular coagulation: a review of the diagnostic tests and the medical and nursing intervention, Crit. Care Nurse **1**:38-43, May-June 1981.

Zschoche, D.A.: Mosby's comprehensive review of critical care, ed. 2, St. Louis, 1981. The C.V. Mosby Co.

Drug overdose

Arena, J.M.: Clinical symposia, The treatment of poisoning, vol. 30, no. 2, Summit, New Jersey, 1978, CIBA Pharmaceutical Company.

Elenbaas, Robert M., ed: Critical care quarterly, vol. 4, no. 4. Poisonings and overdose, Rockville, Md., 1982, Aspen Systems Corporation.

Goldfrank, L., et al.: General management of the poisoned and overdosed patient, Hosp. Physician **17**:61-74, Aug. 1981.

Greenland, P., and Howe, T.A.: Cardiac monitoring in tricyclic antidepressant overdose, Heart Lung **10**:856-859, 1981.

Levy, G.: Gastrointestinal clearance of drugs with activated charcoal, N. Engl. J. Med. **307**:676-678, 1982.

Kaufman, B.S.: Attempted Suicide with overdoses of barbiturates, tranquilizers and narcotics: diagnoses and management. From Summary Proceedings: Annual Symposium on Critical Care Medicine, University of Southern California School of Medicine, March, 1983.

Thompson, W.L.: Poisoning: the twentieth-century black death, Critical Care State of the Art, vol. 1, The Society of Critical Care Medicine, New York, 1980.

Poisoning

Arena, J.M.: Clinical symposia. The Treatment of poisoning, vol. 30, no. 2, Summit, N.J., 1978, CIBA Pharmaceutical Co.

Dreisbach, R.H.: Handbook of poisoning-diagnosis and treatment, ed. 9, Los Altos, Calif., 1977, Lange Medical Publications.

Elenbaas, Robert M., ed.: Critical Care Quarterly, vol. 4, no. 4, Poisonings and overdose, Rockville, Md., 1982, Aspen Systems Corp.

Goldfrank, L., et al.: General management of the poisoned and overdosed patient, Hosp. Physician **17**:61-74, Aug. 1981.

Greenland, P., and Howe, T.A.: Cardiac monitoring in tricyclic antidepressant overdose, Heart Lung, **10**:856-859, 1981.

Kaufman, B.S.: Attempted suicide with Overdoses of Barbiturates, Tranquilizers and Narcotics: Diagnoses and Management. From Summary Proceedings: Annual Symposium on Critical Care Medicine, University of Southern California School of Medicine, March, 1983.

Kempe, H.C., Silver, H.K. and O'Brien, D.: Current pediatric diagnosis and treatment, ed. 4, Los Altos, Calif., 1976, Lange Medical Publications.

Thompson, W.L.: Poisoning: the twentieth-century black death, Critical Care State of the Art, vol. 1, The Society of Critical Care Medicine, New York, 1980.

Vaughan, V.C., et al.: Nelson textbook of pediatrics, ed. 11, Philadelphia, 1979, W.B. Saunders Co.

NEONATAL-PEDIATRIC

Aladjem, S., and Brown, A.K., eds: Perinatal intensive care, St. Louis, 1977, The C.V. Mosby Co.

Alfonso: Newborn's potential for interaction, JOGN Nurs. **7**:9, 1978.

Baumgart, S.: Radiant energy and insensible water loss in the premature newborn infant nursed under a radiant warmer, Clin. Perinatol. **9**:483, 1982.

Blumenthal, I., et al.: Effect of posture on the pattern of stomach emptying in the newborn, Pediatrics **63**:532, 1979.

Boutros, A., et al.: Management of Reye's syndrome: a rational approach to a complex problem, Crit. Care Med. **5**:234, 1977.

Boutros, A., et al. Reye's syndrome: a predictably curable disease, Ped. Clin. North Am. **27**:539, 1980.

Brown, E.G., and Sweet, A.Y., eds.: Neonatal necrotizing enterocolitis, New York, 1980, Grune and Stratton, Inc.

Brunner, R.L., et al.: Neuropsychological consequences of Reye's syndrome, J. Pediatr. **96**:706, 1979.

Burrington, J.D.: Necrotizing enterocolitis in the newborn infant, Clin. Perinatol. **5**:29, 1978.

Chinn, P.L.: Issues in lowering infant mortality: a call for ethical action, Adv. Nurs. Sci. **1**:63-78, 1979.

Clark, L.J.H., and Godfrey, S.: Asthma, Philadelphia, 1977, W.B. Saunders Co.

Collins, D.L., et al.: A new approach to congenital posterolateral diaphragmatic hernia, J. Pediatr. Surg. **12**:149, 1977.

Coran, A.G., et al.: Esophageal atresia. In Surgery of the neonate, Boston, 1978, Little, Brown & Co.

Cornell, E.H., and Gottfried, A.W.: Intervention with premature human infants, Child Dev. **47**:32, 1976.

Curran, C.L., and Kachoyeanos, M.K.: The effects on neonates of two methods of chest physical therapy, MCN **4:**309-313, 1979.

Dibbins, A.W. Congenital diaphragmatic hernia: hypoplastic lung and pulmonary vasoconstriction. Clin. Perinatol. **5:**93, 1978.

Dreisbach, R.H.: Handbook of poisoning: diagnosis and treatment, ed. 9, Los Altos, Calif., 1977, Lange Medical Publications.

Dubowitz, L.M., et al. Visual function in the preterm and fullterm newborn infant, Dev. Med. Child Neurol. **22:**465-475, 1980.

Dweck, H.S.: Feeding the prematurely born infant, Clin. Perinatol. **2:**183, 1975.

Edwards, M.: Nursing case study: Reye's syndrome, Nurs. Times **93:**1039-1040, 1977.

Evans, H.E., and Glass, L.: Perinatal medicine, Hagerstown, Md., 1976, Harper & Row, Publishers, Inc.

Fomon, S.J.: Human milk in premature feeding, Am. J. Public Health **67:**361-363, 1977.

Friedman, S., and Sigman, M.: Preterm birth and psychological development, New York, 1981, Academic Press.

Greenwood, R.D., and Rosenthal, A.: Cardiovascular malformations associated with tracheoesophageal fistula and esophageal atresia, Pediatrics **57:**87-91, 1976.

Hamosh, M., et al. Fat digestion in the stomach of premature infants, J. Pediatr. **93:**674, 1978.

Hazinski, M.F.: Pediatric critical care: a nursing perspective, St. Louis, 1984, The C.V. Mosby Co.

Heird, W.C., and Anderson, T.L.: Nutritional requirements and methods of feeding low birth weight infants, Curr. Prob. Pediatr. **7:**, 1977.

Hendren, W.H., and Kim, S.H.: Pediatric thoracic surgery. In Scarpelli, E.M., et al., eds: Pulmonary disease of the fetus, newborn and child, Philadelphia, 1978, Lea & Febiger.

Johnson, S.H.: High risk parenting: nursing assessment and strategies for the family at risk, New York, 1979, J.B. Lippincott Co.

Jonson, B., et al.: Continuous positive airway pressure: modes of action in relation to clinical applications, Pediatr. Clin. North Am. **27:**687, 1980.

Kattan, M.: Long-term sequelae of respiratory illness in infancy and childhood, Pediatr. Clin. North Am. **26:**525-535, 1979.

Kempe, H.C., Silver, H.K., and O'Brien, D.: Current pediatric diagnosis and treatment, ed. 4, Los Altos, Calif., 1976, Lange Medical Publications.

Kinsey, V.E., et al.: Pao$_2$ levels and retrolental fibroplasia: a report of the cooperative study, Pediatrics **60:**655-668, 1977.

Klaus, D., ed.: Parent to infant attachment: special issue, Birth Fam. J. **5:**183-253, 1978.

Klaus, M.H., and Kennell, J.H.: Interventions in the premature nursery: impact on development, Pediatr. Clin. North Am. **29:**1203, 1982.

Klaus, M.H., and Kennell, J.H.: Parent-infant bonding, ed. 2, St. Louis, 1982, The C.V. Mosby Co.

Knights, C.E.: Practical aspects of transcutaneous gas monitoring, Perinatol.-Neonatol. **7:**39, 1983.

Korones, S.B., and Lancaster, J.: High-risk newborn infants: the basis for intensive nursing care, ed. 3, St. Louis, 1981, The C.V. Mosby Co.

Landau, L.I., et al. Respiratory function after repair of diaphragmatic hernia. Arch. Dis. Child. **52:**282, 1977.

La Salle, A.J., et al.: Congenital tracheoesophageal fistula without esophageal atresia, J. Thorac. Cardiovasc. Surg. **78:**583-588, 1979.

Leib, S.A., et al.: Effects of early intervention and stimulation on the preterm infant, Pediatrics **66:**83, 1980.

Lemons, J.A., et al.: Differences in the composition of preterm and term human milk during early lactation, Pediatr. Res. **16:**266, 1982.

Levin, D.L.: Morphologic analysis of the pulmonary vascular bed in congenital left sided diaphragmatic hernia, J. Pediatr. **92:**805, 1978.

Lovejoy, F.H., et al.: Clinical staging in reye syndrome, Am. J. Dis. Child. **128:**179, 1974.

Marshall, L.F., et al.: Pentobarbital therapy for intracranial hypertension in metabolic coma. Reye's syndrome, Crit. Care Med. **6:**1-5, Jan.-Feb. 1978.

Marwood, R.P., and Davison, O.W.: Antenatal diagnosis of diaphragmatic hernia, Br. J. Obstet. Gynecol. **88:**71, 1981.

Measel, C.P., and Anderson, S.: Non-nutritive sucking during tube feedings: effect on clinical course in premature infants, JOGN Nurs. **8:**265-272, 1979.

Mickell, J.J., et al.: Intracranial pressure monitoring in Reye-Johnson syndrome, Crit. Care Med. **4:**1-7, Jan.-Feb. 1976.

Miner, H.: Problems and prognosis for the small-for-gestational-age and the premature infant, MCN **3:**221-226, 1978.

Miranda, S.B. Visual abilities and pattern preferences of premature infants and fullterm neonates, J. Exp. Child Psychol. **10:**189, 1970.

Moss, T.J., and Adler, R.: Necrotizing enterocolitis in older infants, children, and adolescents, J. Pediatr. **100:**764, 1982.

Naplepka, C.D.: Understanding thermoregulation in newborns, JOGN Nurs. **5:**17-19, 1976.

Neifert, M.R.: Medical management of breastfeeding, Keep. Abreast J. Hum. Nurt. **3:**274-282, 1978.

Newman, S.L., et al.: Reye's syndrome: success of supportive care, N. Engl. J. Med. **299:**1079, 1978.

Oh, W.: Fluid and electrolyte therapy in low birth weight infants receiving parenteral nutrition, Clin. Perinatol. **9:**637, 1982.

O'Neill, J.A.: Necrotizing enterocolitis in the newborn: operative indications, Ann. Surg. **182:**274, 1979.

Patton, B., ed: Symposium on neonatal care, Nurs. Clin. North Am. **13:**1-84, 1978.

Priestley, B.L.: Low birth weight: born too early or too small, Nurs. Mirror **148:**38-40, 1979.

Problems in neonatal intensive care, Briefs **43:**25-27, Feb. 1979.

Purohit, D.M., et al.: Effect of tolazoline on persistent hypoxemia in neonatal respiratory distress, Crit. Care Med. **6:**14, 1978.

Rausch, C.B.: Effects of tactile and kinesthetic stimulation on premature infants, JOGN Nurs. **10:**34, 1981.

Rigatto, H.: Apnea, Ped. Clin. North Am. **29:**1105, 1982.

Ross, G.S.: Parental responses to infants in intensive care: the separation issue reevaluated, Clin. Perinatol. **7:**47, 1980.

Roberts, F.B.: Perinatal nursing, New York, 1977, McGraw-Hill Book Co.

Rothfeder, B.: Feeding the low birthweight neonate, Nurs. '77 **7:**58-59, 1977.

Sarasohn, C.: Care of the very small premature infant, Ped. Clin. North Am. **24:**619, 1977.

Schanler, R.J., and Oh, W.: Composition of breast milk obtained from mothers of premature infants as compared to breast milk obtained from donors, J. Pediatr. **96:**679, 1980.

Schechner, S.: For the 1980s: how small is too small? Clin. Perinatol. **7:**135, 1980.

Schullinger, J.N., et al.: Neonatal necrotizing enterocolitis: survival, management and complications—a 25-year study, Am. J. Dis. Child. **135:**612, 1981.

Slade, C.L.: Working with parents of high risk newborns, JOGN Nurs. **6:**21-26, 1977.

Slota, M.C.: Pediatric problems: diaphragmatic hernia, Crit. Care Nurse **2:**32, 1982.

Solkoff, N., and Matuszak, D.: Tactile stimulation and behavioral development among low birthweight infants, Child Psychiatry Hum. Dev. **6:**33, 1975.

Starko, K.M., et al.: Reye's syndrome and salicylate use, Pediatrics **66:**859, 1980.

Stoll, B.J., et al.: Epidemiology of necrotizing enterocolitis: a case control study, J. Pediatr. **96:**447, 1980.

Sugar, M.: Consistent caretakers in the premature nursery, Child Psychiatry Hum. Dev. **8:**32, 1978.

Vaughan, V.C., et al.: Nelson textbook of pediatrics, ed. 11, Philadelphia, 1979, W.B. Saunders Co.

Waldman, R.J., et al.: Aspirin as a risk factor in Reye's syndrome, JAMA **247:**3089, 1982.

Wohl, M.E.B., et al.: The lung following repair of congenital diaphragmatic hernia, J. Pediatr. **90:**405, 1977.

Weeks, H. L.: What every ICU nurse should know about Reye's Syndrome, J. Mat. Child Nurs. **1:**231-238, 1976.

Williams, J.K., et al.: Thermoregulation of the newborn, MCN **1:**355-360, 1976.

Williams, T.J., and Hill, J.W., eds.: Handbook of neonatal respiratory care, Riverside, Calif., Bourns, Inc., 1979.

Yu, V.Y.H.: Effect of body position on gastric emptying in the neonate, Arch. Dis. Child. **50:**500, 1975.

Zamansky, H.A., et al.: Care of the critically ill newborn in an infant care center, Am. J. Nurs. **76:**566-581, 1976.

Appendixes

ABBREVIATIONS

A-a gradient alveolar-arterial oxygen difference
ABO blood types A, B, and O
ADH antidiuretic hormone
ADL activities of daily living
AIDS acquired immune deficiency syndrome
AMI acute myocardial infarction
APTT activated partial thromboplastin time
ASD atrial septal defect
AV atrioventricular (cardiovascular); arteriovenous (renal)
BP blood pressure
BUN blood urea nitrogen
°C degree(s) Celsius
C and S culture and sensitivity
CA^{++} calcium ion
CABG coronary artery bypass grafting
CBC complete blood count (including hematocrit, hemoglobin, white blood cell count)
cc cubic centimeter
CHF congestive heart failure
Cl$^-$ chloride anion
CNS central nervous system
CO$_2$ carbon dioxide
COPD chronic obstructive pulmonary disease
CPAP continuous positive airway pressure
CPB cardiopulmonary bypass
CPR cardiopulmonary resuscitation
CSF cerebrospinal fluid
CT computed tomography
CVA cerebrovascular accident
CVP central venous pressure
DIC disseminated intravascular coagulation
dl deciliter (100 ml)
ECG electrocardiogram
EEG electroencephalogram

ESR erythrocyte sedimentation rate
°F degree(s) Fahrenheit
FEV$_1$ fraction of air (volume) expired in 1 minute
FEV (FEVC) forced expiratory volume (capacity)
FIO$_2$ fraction of inspired oxygen
FRC functional residual capacity
g gram
GI gastrointestinal
Hct hematocrit
Hgb hemoglobin
HMD hyalin membrane disease
hr hour
ICP intracranial pressure
ICU intensive care unit
IgA immune globulin type A
IgM immune globulin type M
IHSS idiopathic hypertrophic subaortic stenosis
IM intramuscular
IPPB intermittent positive pressure breathing
IV intravenous
K$^+$ potassium ion
KUB kidney, ureter, and bladder
LAP left arterial pressure
LOC level of consciousness
LUQ left upper quadrant
LV left ventricular
MAO monoamine oxidase
MAP mean arterial pressure
mg milligram
MI myocardial infarction
min minute(s)
mm Hg millimeters of mercury
Na$^+$ sodium ion
NaHCO$_3$ sodium bicarbonate

NEC necrotizing entercolitis (neonatal)
NG nasogastric
NMR nuclear magnetic resonance
NPO nothing per os (nothing by mouth)
O₂ oxygen
P pulse
Pao₂ partial arterial pressure of oxygen
Paco₂ partial arterial pressure of carbon dioxide
PAP pulmonary artery pressure
PAD pulmonary artery diastolic
PAS pulmonary artery systolic
PCWP pulmonary capillary wedge pressure
PDA patent ductus arteriosus
PEEP positive end expiratory pressure
% percent
pH symbol for the logarithm of the reciprocal of the hydrogen ion concentration, thus reflecting hydrogen ion concentrations. High hydrogen ion concentration is reflected by low pH level; low hydrogen ion concentration is reflected by high pH level.
po per os (by mouth)
Po₂ partial pressure of oxygen
PP perfusion pressure
PPN peripheral parenteral nutrition
prn as needed
PT prothrombin time
q every

R respiration
REM rapid eye movement (sleep)
RBC red blood cell
RDS respiratory distress syndrome
Rh the Rh antigen in the blood (coined when human blood tested with blood of Rhesus monkeys and the Rh antigen found)
ROM range of motion
SAH subarachnoid hemorrhage
SB Sengstaken-Blakemore (tube)
SIDS sudden infant death syndrome
SGA small for gestational age
SGOT serum glutamic oxaloacetic transaminase
SGPT serum glutamic pyruvic transaminase
stat immediately
TCA transluminal coronary angioplasty
TEF tracheoesophageal fistula
TGV transposition of great vessels
TIA transient ischemic attack
TLC total lung capacity
TPN total parenteral nutrition
VC vital capacity
VDRL venereal disease research laboratories test
VSD ventricular septal defect
V_T tidal volume
WBC white blood cell

SURGICAL PROCEDURES: ASSESSMENT

1. Patient/family's knowledge and level of understanding regarding operative therapy
   a. What they have been told
   b. Expectations
   c. Fears regarding surgery and outcome
   d. Previous surgical experiences
2. Significant intraoperative data
   a. Type of anesthesia; amount and reversal given
   b. Type, time, and amount of narcotic agents and muscle relaxants; amount and reversal given
   c. Medications administered during procedure; amount, time, frequency
   d. Any problems encountered during procedure: type, time, treatment, duration, effects, and side effects
   e. Any elective special techniques used such as hypotension, hypothermia
      (1) Medication used for control: amount, length of time, effects and side effects; level systolic blood pressure reduced to
      (2) If hypothermia: period and length of time induced, temperature reading, effects and side effects, rewarming regimen
   f. Blood loss and replacement
   g. Intake and output during procedure
   h. Blood determinations including serum electrolytes, hemoglobin, hematocrit, arterial blood gas levels (monitored intraoperatively)
   i. Diuretics administered during procedure (e.g., furosemide, mannitol, or urea)
   j. Length of surgery
3. Significant operative procedure data
   a. Procedure performed
      (1) Thoracic
         (a) Biopsy
         (b) Nature and extent of tissue excised
         (c) Nature of repair
      (2) Cardiac
         (a) Number, type, and location of coronary artery bypass grafts
         (b) Site of valvular replacement and type of valve used
         (c) Defect repaired; type of graft material used

         (d) Length of surgery and time on cardiopulmonary bypass
      (3) Vascular: aneurysms; decompressive portovenous shunting procedures
         (a) Location, type, and extent of vessel repair
         (b) Presence and type of graft
      (4) Neurological
         (a) Biopsy
         (b) Partial or total tumor removal
         (c) Aneurysm wrapping or clipping
         (d) Clot evacuation
         (e) Type of shunt insertion; pressure valve placed
      (5) Gastrointestinal (including bypass surgeries)
         (a) Nature of gastrointestinal tract repair (e.g., plication of ulcer, amount of tissue resected)
         (b) Type of anastomosis
      (6) Renal transplantation
         (a) Type of transplant (e.g., cadaver, living related donor)
         (b) Placement of transplanted kidney and type of anastomosis
   b. Pathology apparent at surgery
      (1) Thoracic
         (a) Appearance of abnormal tissue (e.g., traumatized tissue; fibrotic, emphysematous changes; degree of tracheal stenosis)
         (b) Extent of tumors, cysts, abscesses, etc.
         (c) Extent of tissue resected
      (2) Cardiac
         (a) Location and extent of coronary artery disease, including distal arterial blood flows and myocardial dysfunction (as revealed by preoperative and intraoperative assessment)
         (b) Graft blood flows
         (c) Location and extent of valvular stenosis and/or insufficiency; vegetations present
         (d) Presence and extent of ventricular aneurysm; estimated proportion of ventricle involved; and amount of ventricle resected
         (e) Presence and extent of septal defect; the type and size of patch used
      (3) Vascular: aneurysms

(a) Size, type, and location of aneurysm

(b) Visible areas of ischemia, necrosis

(c) Vessel "clamp" time (absence of blood flow through artery while repair is being accomplished)

(4) Neurological

(a) Benign versus malignant tumor

(b) Tumor type and extent

(c) Degree of carotid artery stenosis if carotid endarterectomy performed

(d) Nature of malfunction requiring shunt revision

(e) Other significant operative findings such as increased intracranial pressure, cerebral edema, fluid accumulation, cranial nerve involvement

(5) Gastrointestinal

(a) Decompressive portovenous shunting procedures

(i) Type of vessel anastomosis

(ii) Portal pressures before and after anastomosis is made

(b) Pancreatic and gastrointestinal surgery—presence and extent of (as appropriate)

(i)   Tumor

(ii) Ulcer

(iii) Ulcerative colitis

(iv)   Adhesions

(v)   Obstruction—partial or total

(vi)   Ischemic bowel

(vii) Necrotic debris

(viii) Cyst, abscess(es)

(ix)   Peritonitis

(x)   Fluid inside or outside peritoneum

(6) Renal transplantation—appearance of patient's diseased kidneys (e.g., atrophy, polycystic biopsy)

c. Presence of drains: number, type, and location; suction or gravity

d. Presence of any operative factors requiring special precautions

(1) Maintenance of blood pressure in prescribed range

(2) Positioning

(3) Observation for dysfunction of certain organs such as occurs after prolonged clamping of a major vessel, with organ dysfunction related to disease process, or associated with operative trauma

e. Any complications of surgical procedure: treatment, effects, side effects, anticipated course/prognosis

f. Information and detail surgeon has provided patient/family regarding operative therapy and pathology

NEONATAL-PEDIATRIC DATA

Normal blood pressures (systolic)

Newborn: 60 to 90 mm Hg
1 to 12 months: 74 to 100 mm Hg
1 to 2 years: 80 to 110 mm Hg
2 to 6 years: 82 to 112 mm Hg
6 to 8 years: 84 to 116 mm Hg
8 to 10 years: 88 to 120 mm Hg
10 to 12 years: 94 to 130 mm Hg
12 to 14 years: 100 to 134 mm Hg
14 to 16 years: 104 to 140 mm Hg
16 to 18 years: 108 to 142 mm Hg

Normal heart rates*

Infant: 110 to 160/minute
Toddler: 90 to 130/minute
Preschooler: 90 to 120/minute
School-age child: 80 to 110/minute
Adolescent: 60 to 90/minute

Normal respiratory rates*

Newborn: 30 to 50/minute
6 to 18 months: 20 to 30/minute
2 to 10 years: 18 to 30/minute
Adolescent: 12 to 20/minute

*Increased heart and respiratory rates are expected in the distressed child.

Calculation of maintenance fluids

Weight	Formula
0 to 10 kg	100 ml/kg (neonates may tolerate up to 150 ml/kg if renal and cardiac functions are adequate)
11 to 20 kg	1000 ml for the first 10 kg + 50 ml/kg for each kilogram over 10 kg
21 to 30 kg	1500 ml for the first 20 kg + 25 ml/kg for each kilogram over 20 kg

Average daily caloric requirements

High-risk neonate: 120 to 150 calories/kg
Normal neonate: 100 to 120 calories/kg
1 to 2 years: 90 to 100 calories/kg
2 to 6 years: 80 to 90 calories/kg
7 to 9 years: 70 to 80 calories/kg
10 to 12 years: 50 to 60 calories/kg

APPENDIX D

PEDIATRIC MEDICATION DOSAGES

DRUG NAME (TRADE NAME)	GENERAL TYPE	DOSAGE*†	CAUTIONS*	METABOLISM/ EXCRETION
Acetaminophen (Tylenol)	Antipyretic	Oral: 60 mg/yr of age *or* 5-10 mg/kg/dose q4-6 hr Maximum oral dose: 650 mg Rectal: (over 1 yr); 100 mg/yr of age *or* 5-10 mg/kg/dose q4-6 hr Maximum rectal dose: 1200 mg	Overdose may produce hepatotoxicity; skin rash or fever may also develop	Hepatic metabolism with urinary excretion of metabolites
Acetazolamide (Diamox)	Carbonic anhydrase inhibitor (diuretic and anticonvulsant)	Diuretic: 5 mg/kg/day as single dose IV or IM Anticonvulsant: 10-15 mg/kg/day in single dose or 2-3 doses orally	May produce increased urine potassium losses; can result in paresthesias	Renal excretion: eliminated unchanged in urine
Amikacin (Amikin)	Antibiotic	Neonates: 15/mg/kg/day given in divided doses q12 hr IM or IV Infants or children: 15-22.8 mg/kg/day given in divided doses q8 hr IM or IV *or* 420 mg/m² body surface area/day given q12 hr IV or IM Therapeutic serum levels: Peak—20-30 mg/liter Trough—4-8 mg/liter Toxic—35 mg/liter	Give IV dose *slowly;* may produce ototoxicity, nephrotoxicity, eosinophilia, or rash	Renal excretion
Aminophylline (Aminodur, Cardophyllin, Diophyllin, Methophyllin, Somophyllin)	Bronchodilator	For status asthmaticus: 4-7 mg/kg IV over 15-20 min, then 1.0 mg/kg/hr as continuous infusion For bronchodilation: Oral maintenance: 5-7 mg/kg/dose given q6 hr Rectal dose: 5 mg/kg given q6 hr Maximum dose for bronchodilation: 20 mg/kg/day	Potentiates epinephrine; incompatible with ACTH, potassium, penicillin, chloramphenicol, methicillin, erythromycin, tetracycline, meperidine, pressor amines, and phenytoin	Primarily hepatic metabolism with 10% excreted unchanged in urine

From Hazinski, M.F.: Nursing care of the critically ill child, St. Louis, 1984, The C.V. Mosby Co.
*These drug dosages and cautions have been verified whenever possible with the following sources: Biller, J.A., and Yaeger, A.M., eds.: The Harriet Lane handbook, ed. 9, Chicago, 1981, Year Book Medical Publishers, Inc.; Gilman, A.G., Goodman, L.S., and Gilman, A., eds.: Goodman and Gilman's The pharmacological basis of therapeutics, ed. 6, New York, 1982, Macmillan Publishing Co.; Waring, W.W., and Jeansonne, L.O., eds.: Practical manual of pediatrics, ed. 2, St. Louis, 1982, The C.V. Mosby Co.
†Please note that the dosages listed in this table represent approximate dosages used for children. These dosages must always be modified according to patient condition and response to therapy.

DRUG NAME (TRADE NAME)	GENERAL TYPE	DOSAGE	CAUTIONS	METABOLISM/ EXCRETION
		For prevention of apnea: 1-2 mg/kg/oral dose, given q6-8 hr Therapeutic serum levels (theophylline levels are assayed): For bronchodilation: 10-20 mg/liter For apnea: 5-12 mg/liter		
Amoxicillin—see penicillins				
Ampicillin—see penicillins				
Atropine	Anticholinergic	0.01-0.02 mg/kg/IV dose (this dose may also be given subcutaneously) Maximum dose: 0.4 mg	May produce tachycardia, or AV dissociation; hyperpyrexia may also occur	Distributed throughout body, then excreted through urine
Benzathine penicillin—see penicillins				
Calcium chloride (27% calcium, usually administered as 10% solution containing 1 g/10 ml)	Electrolyte replacement	IV supplement: 20-50 mg/kg/ dose (this dose may also be given orally) Maximum dose: 1 g	May produce bradycardia if infused rapidly; administer at a rate *no faster* than 100 mg/min; may produce vascular irritation so monitor infusion site	Used throughout the body
Calcium gluconate (9.4% calcium, usually administered as 10% solution containing 1g/10 ml)	Electrolyte replacement	IV supplement: 100-200 mg/ kg/dose (this dose may also be given orally) Maximum dose: 2 g	Monitor for bradycardia during infusion; maximum infusion rate: 100 mg/min	Used throughout the body
Carbenicillin—see penicillins				
Cephalexin (Keflex)	Antibiotic	25-100 mg/kg/day given in divided doses q4-6 hr orally Maximum dose: 4 g/day	Patients with penicillin sensitivity may have cross-sensitivity reaction; risk of nephrotoxicity may be enhanced if administered concurrently with aminoglycoside antibiotic	Renal excretion
Cephalothin (Keflin)	Antibiotic	50-100 mg/kg/day given in divided doses q4-6 hr IV or deep IM Maximum dose: 12 g/day	May produce vascular irritation (see also Cephalexin)	Renal excretion
Chloral hydrate (Noctec)	Sedative and hypnotic	1-30 mg/kg/dose, orally or rectally Maximum dose: 2 g/dose or 50 mg/kg/day	Administer with caution if hepatic disease is present	Hepatic metabolism

DRUG NAME (TRADE NAME)	GENERAL TYPE	DOSAGE	CAUTIONS	METABOLISM/ EXCRETION
Chloramphenicol (Chloromycetin)	Antibiotic	Loading dose for severe infections: 20 mg/kg IV or po Maintenance dose: Neonates—25-50 mg/kg/ day, given in divided doses q6 hr IV or po Infants and children—50-100 mg/kg/day given in divided doses q6 hr IV or po Therapeutic serum levels: Peak—20 mg/liter Range—10-20 mg/liter Toxic level—>25 mg/liter	Monitoring of blood levels is *essential;* bone marrow suppression can occur; administer with caution if hepatic or renal dysfunction is present	Hepatic inactivation with urinary excretion of metabolites
Chlorothiazide (Diuril)	Diuretic	20-40 mg/kg/day orally (given in 1 or 2 doses)	May cause hyperbilirubinemia, hypokalemia, hyperglycemia, or metabolic alkalosis	Renal excretion
Cimetidine (Tagamet)	Antacid	20-40 mg/kg/day, given in divided doses q6-8 hr IV or po Maximum dose: 2400 mg/day	May produce diarrhea, rash, neutropenia, myalgia, or gynecomastia	Renal excretion
Clindamycin (Cleocin)	Antibiotic	Oral: 8-25 mg/kg/day given in divided doses q6-8 hr Parenteral: 15-40 mg/kg/day IV or IM given in divided doses q6-8 hr Maximum dose: 4.8 g/day	Use with caution if hepatic or renal disease is present	Hepatic metabolism
Cloxacillin—see Penicillins				
Codeine	Analgesic	0.5-1.0 mg/kg/dose, given po or subcutaneously q4-6 hr Maximum dose: 3 mg/kg/day	May produce cardiorespiratory depression (but less depression than occurs with morphine or meperidine)	Hepatic metabolism with inactive forms excreted in the urine
d-Tubocurarine—see Tubocurarine				
Dexamethasone (Decadron)	Adrenocortical steroid	For increased intracranial pressure: 0.5-1.0 mg/kg IV or IM for loading dose then 0.25-0.5 mg/kg/day For treatment of asthma or upper airway obstruction: 0.25-0.5 mg/kg/day given in divided doses q6 hr	If chronic therapy is discontinued, dose must be tapered before discontinuation to prevent adrenal insufficiency; this drug may interfere with the action of phenytoin sodium (Dilantin); steroid therapy may produce gastrointestinal bleeding, delayed wound healing, or increased susceptibility to infection	Renal excretion
Diazepam (Valium)	Anticonvulsant, muscle relaxant	For status epilepticus: 0.1-0.5 mg/kg/IV dose Maximum dose: 10 mg Relaxant: 0.1-0.8 mg/kg/day given orally in divided doses *or* 0.1-0.3 mg/kg/dose IV or IM	May produce hypotension or respiratory depression	Hepatic metabolism

DRUG NAME (TRADE NAME)	GENERAL TYPE	DOSAGE	CAUTIONS	METABOLISM/ EXCRETION
Dicloxacillin—see Penicillins				
Digoxin (Lanoxin)	Cardiac glycoside	Oral digitalizing dose (given in divided doses over 18-24 hr): Preterm neonate—0.025-0.050 mg/kg Term neonate—0.04-0.08 mg/kg 2 wk-2 yr—0.06-0.08 mg/kg 2 yr-10 yr—0.5-1.0 mg Intravenous digitalizing dose: calculated at two-thirds oral dose Maintenance dose: calculated at one-eighth digitalizing dose given q12 hr Therapeutic serum level: <1 yr up to 3.0-3.5 ng/ml >1 yr 0.6-2.5 ng/ml	May produce arrhythmias	Renal excretion (60% to 75%)
Diphenylhydantoin—see Phenytoin				
Dobutamine (Inotrex)	Beta-adrenergic agonist	For treatment of low cardiac output as continuous infusion: 2-10 mcg/kg/min; dosages and effects in neonates may be different	May produce tachyarrhythmias, hypotension	Rapidly inactivated in the body
Dopamine (Intropin)	Beta-adrenergic agonist	For the treatment of low cardiac output as continuous infusion: 1-5 mcg/kg/min produces "dopaminergic" effects (especially increased renal blood flow and glomerular filtration rate) 5-10 mcg/kg/min produces primarily beta₁ effects, especially increased cardiac contractility and cardiac output Dosages >10 mcg/kg/min produce primarily alpha-adrenergic effects (especially peripheral vasoconstriction) Dosages and effects in neonates may be different	May result in increased pulmonary artery pressure; renal blood flow is probably reduced once the dosage exceeds approximately 10 mcg/kg/min; may produce tachyarrhythmias	Rapidly inactivated in the body
Doxycycline (Vibramycin)	Antibiotic	Initial dose: <45 kg: 4.4-5 mg/kg/day, given in divided doses q12 hr IV or po >45 kg: 200 mg/day given in divided doses q12 hr IV or po Maintenance dose: <45 kg: 2.2-2.5 mg/kg/day, given in divided doses q12 hr IV or po >45 kg: 100 mg/day as single dose or 2 doses divided q12 hr IV or po	Can produce vasculitis and subcutaneous burn so monitor infusion site; give with caution if renal or hepatic disease is present	Renal excretion (20%-60%) and fecal excretion NOTE: There is greater elimination of this drug in the feces than other tetracyclines, making this one of the safest tetracyclines to administer to the patient with renal failure

DRUG NAME (TRADE NAME)	GENERAL TYPE	DOSAGE	CAUTIONS	METABOLISM/ EXCRETION
Epinephrine (Adrenalin)—see also Racemic epinephrine	Alpha- and beta-adrenergic agonist	Aerosol: 1:100 solution nebulized for 1 min; *not to be confused with 1:1000 solution* For status asthmaticus: 0.01 ml/kg/dose subcutaneously (of 1:1000 aqueous solution) Maximum dose: 0.5 ml As a vasopressor: 0.01 ml/kg/dose (of 1:1000 solution) *or* 0.05-1.0 mcg/kg/min as continuous infusion	May produce tachyarrhythmias, nausea, vomiting, headaches, or hypertension; this drug increases myocardial oxygen consumption, often increases systemic vascular resistance or pulmonary artery pressure, and may reduce renal blood flow	Hepatic metabolism with urinary excretion of metabolites
Erythromycin (Erythrocin, Pediamycin, Ilosone, E-Mycin)	Antibiotic	Oral dose: 30-100 mg/kg/day given in divided doses q6-8 hr IV dose: 10-30 mg/kg/day given in divided doses q4-6 hr	Do not give IM; use with caution in patients with liver disease; gastrointestinal side effects are common	Concentrated and/or inactivated in the liver with biliary excretion; renal excretion (10%-15%) may be present
Ethacrynic acid (Edecrin)	Diuretic	1.0 mg/kg/IV dose *or* 2-3 mg/kg/oral dose	Causes increased potassium loss in the urine	Renal excretion (66%) and hepatic metabolism (33%)
Furosemide (Lasix)	Diuretic	For treatment of congestive heart failure: 1.0-2.0 mg/kg/dose IV, IM, or orally; up to 4 mg/kg/dose may be administered orally For treatment of renal failure: 2.0-6.0 mg/kg/dose IV (may be repeated)	Produces potassium and chloride loss in the urine; may produce a hypochloremic metabolic alkalosis; ototoxicity has been reported	Renal excretion (and a small amount is excreted in feces)
Gentamicin (Garamycin)	Antibiotic	3.0-7.5 mg/kg/day, IV or IM given in divided doses q8 hr Therapeutic serum level: Peak—6-8 mg/liter (or mcg/ml) Trough—1-2 mg/liter	Has been reported to cause renal and ototoxicity, especially when peak concentrations exceed 10 mg/liter or trough concentrations exceed 2 mg/liter; infuse over a minimum of 15-30 min	Primarily renal excretion
Glucose solutions	Electrolyte replacement	D_{25}: 1-2 ml/kg/dose D_{50}: 0.5-1.0 ml/kg/dose Should be diluted before administration in peripheral IV	May produce vascular irritation or burn	Used throughout the body; may also be excreted in the urine
Glucose and insulin	For treatment of hyperkalemia	Acute treatment of hyperkalemia: 0.5-1.0 ml D_{50}/kg *plus* 0.1 unit regular insulin/8-12 g dextrose infused *or* 0.5-1.0 ml D_{50}/kg *plus* 0.02-0.04 units regular insulin/kg	Give lower range of insulin dose for premature infants	Used throughout the body; may also be excreted in the urine
Glycerin (Glyrol)	Osmotic diuretic	0.5-1.5 g/kg/day orally (titrated to control increased intracranial pressure)	May produce increased serum osmolality resulting in rebound cerebral edema and increased intracranial pressure; may also produce hyperglycemia and glycosuria	Used in the body and excreted in the urine
Hydrochlorothiazide + spironolactone (Aldactazide)	Diuretic	1.65-3.3 mg/kg/day given orally	See cautions of spironolactone	Renal excretion

DRUG NAME (TRADE NAME)	GENERAL TYPE	DOSAGE	CAUTIONS	METABOLISM/ EXCRETION
Hydrocortisone (Cortef, Hydrocortisone, Solu-Cortef)	Adrenocortical steroid	Gram-negative shock: 50 mg/kg IV then 50-70 mg/kg/day given in divided doses Status asthmaticus: 10 mg/kg/day IV given in divided doses q6 hr Physiologic replacement: 12.5-15 mg/m^2/day IV or IM in one dose or 25.0 mg/m^2/day po in 3 doses	May produce Cushing's syndrome (including hypertension, weight gain, muscle atrophy, fluid retention, psychiatric disturbances, or osteoporosis), impaired immunologic status and/or wound healing, steroid dependence, nausea, vomiting, hyperglycemia, or gastrointestinal ulceration; if patient has received chronic therapy, dosage should be tapered before discontinuation, to prevent adrenal insufficiency	Renal excretion (cortisol metabolites are excreted as 17-hydroxycorticosteroid)
Isoetharine hydrochloride (Bronkosol)	Beta$_2$ adrenergic agonist (bronchodilator inhalant)	0.25-0.5 ml is usually diluted with 3 ml normal saline and given in an oxygen aerosol; 3-7 inhalations are usually administered q4 hr	May produce tachycardia, headache, or hypertension	Hepatic metabolism
Isoproterenol (Isuprel, Aludrine)	Beta-adrenergic agonist	For bradycardia: 0.05-0.1 mcg/kg/min IV continuous infusion For hypotension: 0.05-0.5 mcg/kg/min For bronchodilation: 1-2 inhalations q4-6 hr (1:500 mesometer)	May produce tachyarrhythmias at even low doses; patient may feel anxious, nauseated, or dizzy, or the patient may complain of headache; inhalation overdose may produce ventricular arrhythmias	Hepatic metabolism
Lidocaine (Xylocaine)	Antiarrhythmic	1 mg/kg/IV bolus dose Maximum dose: 5 mg/kg Continuous infusion: 10-20 mcg/kg/min	May produce seizures in toxic doses	Hepatic metabolism and renal excretion
Mannitol 10%-20% (Osmitrol)	Osmotic diuretic	Increased intracranial pressure: 0.15-0.3 g/kg/q1-2 hr or continuous infusion of 0.05-0.15 g/kg/hr; may be titrated to maintain serum osmolality of 310 mOsm/liter If necessary, up to 0.25-2.0 g/kg/day may be administered to control increased intracranial pressure	May produce increased serum osmolality resulting in rebound cerebral edema and increased intracranial pressure; monitor serum and urine osmolality and serum electrolyte concentrations	Renal excretion
Meperidine (Demerol)	Analgesic narcotic	1 mg/kg/dose IV Maximum dose: 100 mg	May produce respiratory depression, or decreased gastrointestinal motility; may produce excitation, hyperpyrexia, or delirium in patients receiving monamine oxidase (MAO) inhibitors	Hepatic metabolism
Metaproterenol sulfate (Alupent, Metaprel)	Beta$_2$ adrenergic agonist	Inhalant: (0.65 mg or approximately 0.2 ml in 3 ml saline) 2-3 inhalations Syrup or tablet: 1.3-2.6 mg/kg/day given in 3 doses	Adverse reactions include tachycardia, hypertension, palpitations, nervousness, nausea, and vomiting	Renal excretion

DRUG NAME (TRADE NAME)	GENERAL TYPE	DOSAGE	CAUTIONS	METABOLISM/ EXCRETION
Morphine sulfate	Analgesic narcotic	For analgesia: 0.1 mg/kg/dose IV or subcutaneously For hypercyanotic spells ("Tet" spells): 0.1-0.2 mg/kg/dose IV or subcutaneously Continuous IV infusion: 100 mcg/kg/hr Maximum dose: 15 mg	May produce respiratory depression; chronic administration can produce addiction; also may produce decreased gastrointestinal motility or nausea; administer naloxone for reversal of morphine (see naloxone)	Conjugated throughout the body, then excreted in the urine; free morphine may accumulate in kidneys, lungs, liver, and spleen for hours after administration
Moxalactam	Antibiotic	50-75 mg/kg/day, given in divided doses q8 hr For treatment of meningitis or other severe infections: 100 mg/kg/day, given in divided doses q8 hr	See cephalothin	Renal excretion
Nafcillin—see Penicillins				
Naloxone (Narcan)	Opioid antagonist	0.005-0.010 mg/kg/dose IV or IM	May stimulate respirations and may enhance pain perception	Hepatic metabolism
Nitroglycerin	Vasodilator	Continuous infusion IV dose: 1-25 mcg/kg/min (NOTE: maximal dose reserved for patients with severe pulmonary hypertension) Topical ointment (2%): 0.5-1.5 cm reapplied q½-6 hr, or long-acting disks changed q12 hr	Produces hypotension in the hypovolemic patient; may require simultaneous volume infusion; may also produce severe headache; since IV nitroglycerine is adsorbed by polyvinyl chloride tubing and buretrols, special IV administration equipment is necessary	Hepatic metabolism
Nitroprusside—see Sodium nitroprusside				
Oxacillin—see Penicillins				
Pancuronium (Pavulon)	Paralyzing (nondepolarizing) agent	Intermittent IV dose: Neonates: 0.02 mg/kg Older infants and children: 0.1-0.15 mg/kg for loading dose, then 0.1 mg/kg/ q30-60 min Continuous infusion: 0.1 mg/ kg/hr IV	Drug effect can be accentuated by hypothermia, acidosis, some anesthetics, decreased renal function, and aminoglycoside antibiotics; may produce tachycardia and venous pooling	Hepatic metabolism and renal excretion
Paraldehyde	Anticonvulsant	For status epilepticus: 0.15 mg/kg IV (may be repeated) or 0.3 ml/kg rectally	Intravenous dose must be administered using a glass syringe and special tubing	Depolymerized in the liver and ultimately excreted in the urine or exhaled

DRUG NAME (TRADE NAME)	GENERAL TYPE	DOSAGE	CAUTIONS	METABOLISM/ EXCRETION
The penicillins				
Penicillin G (Pentids, Pfizerpen G)	Antibiotic	Newborn <7 days: 50,000-100,000 units/kg/day, given in 2 doses IV or IM Newborns >7 days: 100,000-200,000 units/kg/day, given in divided doses IV or IM q6-8 hr Child: 25,000-300,000 units/kg/day, given in divided doses IV, IM, or po q4-6 hr	Monitor for sensitivity reaction or rash NOTE: Potassium penicillin contains 1.68 mEq potassium ion per 1 million units; sodium penicillin contains 1.68 mEq sodium ions per 1 million units	Primarily renal excretion (60%-90%) with small amount excreted in bile
Amoxicillin (Amoxil, Larotic, Polymox)	Antibiotic	Under 20 kg: 20-40 mg/kg/day orally, given in divided doses q8 hr Greater than 20 kg: 200-500 mg/kg/day orally, given in divided doses q8 hr	May produce diarrhea (although this occurs less frequently than with ampicillin); monitor for sensitivity reaction or rash; may be taken with meals	Primarily renal excretion (70%) within 6 hr
Ampicillin (Amcill, Omnipen, Polycillin)	Antibiotic	Neonate <7 days: 50-100 mg/kg/day, given in divided doses q8 hr IV or po Beyond the first week: 100-200 mg/kg/day, given in divided doses q8 hr IV or po Severe infections (IV or IM): <40 kg: 200-400 mg/kg/day given in divided doses IV or IM q4-6 hr; >40 kg: 8-12 g/day, given in divided doses IV or IM q4-6 hr Maximum dose: 12 g/day	May produce diarrhea; monitor for sensitivity reaction or rash; less complete absorption occurs if oral dose taken with meals	Primarily renal excretion (70%) within 6 hr
Benzathine penicillin (Bicillin, Permapen)	Antibiotic	0.3-1.2 million units/single (deep) IM dose	Monitor for sensitivity reaction or rash	Primarily renal excretion (70%)
Carbenicillin (Geopen, Pyopen)	Antibiotic	50-200 mg/kg/day, given in divided IV doses q6-8 hr NOTE: Oral administration not recommended since the drug is poorly absorbed in the gastrointestinal tract Severe infections: 400-600 mg/kg/day, given in divided doses, q4-6 hr Maximum dose: 40 g/day	May produce thrombocytopenia or anaphylaxis; may interact with gentamicin; this drug produces large urinary potassium losses; contains large amounts of sodium ion (4.7 mEq sodium/g); give with caution if renal impairment is present	Hepatic metabolism and renal excretion
Cloxacillin (Cloxapen, Tegopen)	Antibiotic	Under 20 kg: 50-100 mg/kg/day, given orally in divided doses q6 hr Greater than 20 kg: 1-2 g/day, given orally in divided doses q6 hr Maximum dose: 4 g/day	Monitor for sensitivity reaction or rash	Primarily renal excretion with significant hepatic metabolism

DRUG NAME (TRADE NAME)	GENERAL TYPE	DOSAGE	CAUTIONS	METABOLISM/ EXCRETION
The penicillins—cont'd				
Dicloxacillin (Dycill, Dynapen, Veracillin)	Antibiotic	Under 40 kg: 12.5-25 mg/kg/day, given orally in divided doses q6 hr Greater than 40 kg: 0.5-1.0 g/day, given orally in divided doses q6 hr	Administer 1-2 hr before meals to maximize absorption; monitor for sensitivity reaction or rash	Primarily renal excretion with significant hepatic elimination
Nafcillin (Unipen)	Antibiotic	Newborn: <7 days—40 mg/kg/day, given in 2 doses; >7 days—60 mg/kg/day, given in divided doses q6-8 hr Older infants and children: 50-100 mg/kg/day, given orally or 100-200 mg/kg/day given IM (in 2 doses) or IV (in divided doses q4-6 hr) NOTE: Oral administration is not recommended since the drug is poorly absorbed in the gastrointestinal tract	May produce sensitivity reaction or rash	Primarily hepatic metabolism with small amount (10%) excreted unchanged in the urine
Oxacillin (Bactocill, Prostaphlin)	Antibiotic	50-100 mg/kg/day, given in divided doses q4-6 hr	May produce hematuria or nephritis; monitor for sensitivity reaction or rash	Primarily renal excretion with significant hepatic elimination
Procaine penicillin (Bicillin, Crysticillin, Duracillin, Wycillin)	Antibiotic	0.3-1.2 million units as single IM injection NOTE: The procaine provides a slight anesthetic effect—each 300,000 units contains approximately 120 mg procaine	Monitor for sensitivity reaction or rash	Primarily renal excretion (60%-70%) with small amount excreted in bile
Pentobarbitol (Nembutol)	Barbiturate Sedative	For sedation: 2-3 mg/kg/dose orally For barbiturate coma: loading dose: 2-5 mg/kg IV; then additional doses provided as needed to maintain serum pentobarbitol level of 20-40 mcg/ml (or 2.0-4.0 mg/dl)—usually 0.5-3.0 mg/kg/hr are required	May produce hypotension or arrhythmias	Hepatic and renal excretion
Phenobarbitol	Barbiturate Anticonvulsant	For status epilepticus: 5 mg/kg/IV dose—may give as many as 3 doses For chronic anticonvulsant: 4-6 mg/kg/day, given orally in 2 doses Therapeutic serum level: 15-40 mcg/ml	May produce drowsiness and respiratory depression	Hepatic metabolism with renal excretion (25%)

DRUG NAME (TRADE NAME)	GENERAL TYPE	DOSAGE	CAUTIONS	METABOLISM/ EXCRETION
Phenytoin (Dilantin)	Anticonvulsant antiarrhythmic	For status epilepticus: 10-15 mg/kg/IV dose Maximum dose: 1250 mg Maintenance anticonvulsant: 5-8 mg/kg/day Antiarrhythmic: 2-4 mg/kg/IV dose *or* 2-8 mg/kg/day given orally Therapeutic serum level: 10-25 mcg/ml	May produce bradycardia, decreased myocardial contractility, hypotension, or ventricular fibrillation; may produce central nervous system depression	Primarily hepatic metabolism
Potassium chloride	Electrolyte replacement	IV supplement: 0.5-1 mEq/kg/ dose, given over 1-2 hr; concentration of KCl in peripheral IV should not exceed equivalent of 40 mEq/ liter, to prevent vascular irritation Oral supplement: 2-4 mEq/kg/ day	IV infusion tubing should be labeled carefully to prevent inadvertent bolus infusion; rapid infusions can produce arrhythmias or cardiac arrest; administer with caution if renal failure is present	Used throughout the body, and excreted by the kidneys
Prednisone	Adrenocortical steroid	1.5-2.0 mg/kg/day, given orally, in a single or several divided doses	Chronic therapy can produce growth retardation; chronic therapy dose should be tapered before drug is discontinued to prevent adrenal insufficiency; steroid therapy can cause gastrointestinal bleeding, delayed wound healing, or increased susceptibility to infection	Renal excretion
Procainamide (Pronestyl)	Antiarrhythmic	IV bolus: 3-10 mg/kg/dose, given over 5 min Maximum bolus dose: 500 mg Continuous infusion: 20-50 mcg/kg/min Oral dose: 15-50 mg/kg/day Therapeutic serum level: 4-8 mg/liter	May depress cardiac contractility or produce thrombocytopenia; toxic effects include AV dissociation	Hepatic metabolism
Propranolol (Inderal)	Antiarrhythmic, beta-adrenergic blocker	For treatment of arrhythmias: 0.01-0.1 mg/kg, given IV over 10 min For treatment of hypercyanotic ("Tet") spells: 0.15-0.25 mg/ kg, given slowly IV For treatment of hypertension: 0.5-1 mg/kg/day, given in divided IV doses Oral dose: 0.2-8 mg/kg/day, given in divided doses	May produce severe bradycardia, AV conduction disturbances, and decreased cardiac contractility; also known to cause hypotension, nausea, and vomiting	Hepatic metabolism

DRUG NAME (TRADE NAME)	GENERAL TYPE	DOSAGE	CAUTIONS	METABOLISM/ EXCRETION
Quinidine	Antiarrhythmic	Oral dose: 15-60 mg/kg/day, given in divided doses	May depress myocardial contractility; may also produce a rise in serum digoxin levels if these drugs are given concurrently	Hepatic metabolism
Racemic epinephrine (Vaponefrin, Micronefrin)	Bronchodilator	0.125-0.25 ml of 2.25% solution diluted to 3 ml with normal saline and administered by nebulizer; occasionally, a dose of 0.05 ml/kg/dose is calculated and diluted to 3 ml with normal saline and administered by nebulizer	If administered in conjunction with a beta-adrenergic blocker, the racemic epinephrine can potentiate existing bronchospasm; may also produce tachyarrhythmias, headache, nausea, or palpitations	Hepatic metabolism
Sodium bicarbonate	Electrolyte replacement	1-2 (or 1-4 if acidosis severe) mEq/kg/dose *or* kg wt $\times$ base excess $\times$ 0.3 = _____ mEq NaHCO$_3$ needed to correct the calculated base deficit Maximum dose: 8 mEq/kg/24 hr	Metabolism of bicarbonate produces carbon dioxide so that ventilation must be adequate to prevent the development of hypercapnia; may produce vascular irritation if administered through a peripheral IV	Used throughout the body
Sodium nitroprusside (Nipride)	Vasodilator	0.1-8 mcg/kg/min, given as continuous infusion Toxic thiocyanate levels: >10 mg/dl	Will produce hypotension in hypovolemic patients; may require simultaneous volume infusion; may produce headaches NOTE: Metabolism of this drug results in the formation of *cyanide* and *thiocyanate*, so levels of thiocyanate should be checked if therapy continues for 48 hr (check sooner if hepatic dysfunction is present)	Hepatic metabolism
Spironolactone (Aldactone)	Diuretic	1.5-3.3 mg/kg/day orally	Since this drug enhances renal potassium reabsorption, hyperkalemia can result; this drug is often administered in conjunction with a "potassium wasting" diuretic such as furosemide; may potentiate ganglionic blocking agents	Hepatic metabolism with renal excretion of metabolites
Streptomycin	Antibiotic	Infants: 15-40 mg/kg/day, in divided doses IM q12 hr Children: 40 mg/kg/day, given in divided doses IM q12 hr Maximum dose: 2 g/day	May produce central nervous system depression or ototoxicity; reduce dosage in the presence of renal insufficiency	Primarily renal excretion
Succinylcholine (Anectine)	Paralyzing (neuromuscular blocking) agent	1-2 mg/kg/IV dose	Effects may last 10 min; must be able to intubate immediately to prevent respiratory insufficiency; side effects include bradycardia, hypotension, and arrhythmias	Hydrolyzed by pseudocholinesterase in the liver and plasma

DRUG NAME (TRADE NAME)	GENERAL TYPE	DOSAGE	CAUTIONS	METABOLISM/ EXCRETION
Terbutaline (Brethine)	Beta₂ adrenergic agonist (bronchodilator)	For treatment of status asthmaticus: 7-10 mcg/kg/dose given subcutaneously Oral dose: 75 mcg/kg/dose (usually, 10 times the effective subcutaneous dose is given orally)	Side effects include tachycardia, palpitations, headaches, nervousness, tremors, drowsiness, nausea, vomiting, and sweating	Renal excretion (60%), and hepatic metabolism (40% conjugated in the liver), with some (3%) biliary excretion
Tetracycline (Achromycil)	Antibiotic	Older infants and children: Oral: 25-50 mg/kg/day, given in divided doses q6 hr IV: 10-15 mg/kg/day, given in divided doses q12 hr IM: 10-25 mg/kg/day, given in divided doses q8-12 hr Children >40 kg: Oral: 1-2 mg/day, given in divided doses q6 hr Parenteral: 10-20 mg/kg/day, given IM or IV in divided doses	Recommended for use in children *only when other antibiotics are not suitable;* may produce increased intracranial pressure, tooth staining, and decreased bone growth; oral dose should be taken 1 hr before meals, and should never be taken in conjunction with oral calcium supplements	Primarily excreted in the urine and feces
Theophylline (Accurbron, Aerolate, Aqualin supprettes, Bronkodyl, Elixophyllin, Lanophyllin, Oralphyllin, Theo-II, and Theolair)	Bronchodilator	5-8 mg/kg/dose, given orally or IV q6 hr (rectal administration also possible) For treatment of apnea: 1-2 mg/kg/oral dose, given q6 hr Therapeutic serum levels: Bronchodilation—10-20 mg/liter For treatment of apnea—5-12 mg/liter Toxic levels—>20 mg/liter	May produce palpitations, tachyarrhythmias, anorexia, nausea, vomiting, anxiety, irritability, insomnia, dizziness, hypokalemia, alkalosis, or seizures NOTE: This drug antagonizes propranolol; concurrent administration of phenothiazides will antagonize the chronotropic effect of the theophylline; erythromycin administration will inhibit the clearance of theophylline	Primarily hepatic metabolism, a small amount (10%) is recovered unchanged in the urine
Tobramycin (Nebcin)	Antibiotic	5-7.5 mg/kg/day, given in divided doses q8-12 hr Therapeutic serum levels: Peak—6-8 mg/liter Trough—1-2 mg/liter	May produce nephrotoxicity or ototoxicity	Primarily renal excretion
Tocainide	Antiarrhythmic	Adult dosages range from 1200-2400 mg/day Pediatric dosages not yet determined	Monitor heart rate, rhythm, and systemic perfusion Toxic effects include nausea and neuropathies	Hepatic metabolism and renal excretion
Trimethoprim (TMP) or sulfamethoxazole (SMZ) (Bactrim, Septra)	Antibiotic	Minor infections: 8-10 mg/kg/day TMP *or* 40-50 mg/kg/day SMZ given in divided doses q12 hr For treatment of pneumocystis carinii pneumonia: 20 mg/kg/day TMP *or* 100 mg/kg/day SMZ given in divided doses q6 hr	Reduce dosage if renal failure is present; may produce bone marrow depression	Primarily renal excretion

DRUG NAME (TRADE NAME)	GENERAL TYPE	DOSAGE	CAUTIONS	METABOLISM/ EXCRETION
d-Tubocurarine (Curare)	Paralyzing (neuromuscular blocking) agent	Neonates: 0.3 mg/kg initially, then 0.15 mg/kg/dose Infants and children: 0.2-0.4 mg/kg initially, then 0.04-0.2 mg/kg/dose	Drug effects are enhanced if gentamicin or related antibiotics are administered simultaneously; this drug may produce heart rate and blood pressure lability; *patient ventilatory support must be adequate*	Primarily renal excretion (33%-75%) with some biliary excretion (11%)
Urea	Osmotic diuretic	1gm/kg, given q4-6 hr, titrated to control intracranial hypertension	May produce increased serum osmolality and rebound cerebral edema and further increase in intracranial pressure; monitor serum and urine osmolality and serum electrolyte concentrations	Renal excretion
Vancomycin (Vancocin)	Antibiotic	Neonates: 30-45 mg/kg/day, given in divided doses q8-12 hr Infants and children: 40 mg/kg/day, given IV q6 hr	May produce nephrotoxicity or phlebitis	Primarily renal excretion
Vasopressin (Pitressin)	Antidiuretic hormone	Aqueous: 1-3 ml/day, given subcutaneously in 3 divided doses Tannate in oil: 0.2 ml/dose IM q1-3 days Nose drops: 1-2 drops in each nostril q4-6 hr prn	May produce arrhythmias when given IV	Rapidly inactivated by body enzymes
Verapamil (Cordilox)	Antiarrhythmic	IV: 0.15-0.25 mg/kg/dose Oral: 20-80 mg/dose q6-8 hr	May produce decreased cardiac contractility resulting in hypotension; can also produce decreased renal clearance of digoxin (if these drugs are given concurrently) causing digoxin levels to rise	Hepatic metabolism (80%)

PEDIATRIC CONTINUOUS INFUSION DOSAGE CHARTS ("DRIP CHARTS")*

NOTE: The following charts enable determination of the exact mcg/kg/minute given by continuous infusion of drugs concentrated as 1, 50, or 100 mg/100 ml. If standard drug concentrations are not used, a formula may be used to make a medication concentration that will allow administration of *1 mcg/kg/minute* for *each ml/hour* administered of the drug (e.g., if 3 ml/hour of the drug are administered, the patient is receiving 3 mcg/kg/minute). This formula would require a drug concentration that varies with the weight of the child as follows:

Patient's weight (kg) × 6 = mg of medication/100 ml

*From Hazinski, M.F.: Nursing care of the critically ill child, St. Louis, 1984, The C.V. Mosby Co.

For example, a 7 kg child receiving dopamine would have a dopamine concentration of 7 × 6 or 42 mg/100 ml. Then, if the infusion rate is 5 ml/hour, that child receives 5 mcg/kg/minute of dopamine. If the infusion rate is changed to 10 ml/hour, the child receives 10 mcg/kg/minute of dopamine. This calculation is also useful for continuous infusion of drugs such as dobutamine, nitroprusside, and nitroglycerine.

If isoproterenol will be administered, it may be desirable to prepare a medication concentration that will allow administration of *0.1 mcg/kg/minute* for each *ml/hour* of the drug that is administered. In this case the drug concentration will vary with the weight of the child as follows:

Patient's weight (kg) × 0.6 = mg of medication/100 ml

PEDIATRIC CONTINUOUS INFUSION RATES (for 1 mg/100 ml concentration)*

	WEIGHT in kg																							
	2	3	4	5	6	7	8	9	10	11	12	13	14	15	16	17	18	19	20	21	22	23	24	25
1 ml/hr	.08	.055	.042	.033	.028	.024	.021	.019	.017	.015	.014	.013	.012	.011	.01	.009	.009	.009	.008	.008	.008	.007	.007	.007
2 ml/hr	.16	.11	.084	.066	.056	.05	.042	.04	.034	.03	.028	.026	.024	.02	.02	.018	.018	.017	.017	.016	.015	.015	.014	.013
3 ml/hr	.24	.165	.126	.1	.08	.07	.06	.057	.051	.045	.042	.083	.036	.03	.03	.029	.028	.026	.025	.023	.023	.022	.02	.019
4 ml/hr	.32	.22	.17	.13	.11	.1	.08	.076	.068	.06	.056	.052	.05	.04	.04	.039	.037	.035	.033	.032	.032	.03	.028	.027
5 ml/hr	.40	.275	.21	.165	.14	.12	.11	.10	.09	.08	.07	.065	.06	.055	.05	.049	.04	.044	.042	.040	.038	.036	.035	.033
6 ml/hr	.48	.33	.25	.2	.17	.14	.13	.11	.10	.09	.08	.078	.07	.066	.06	.058	.055	.053	.05	.048	.046	.044	.042	.04
7 ml/hr	.56	.385	.29	.23	.19	.17	.15	.13	.12	.11	.10	.09	.083	.077	.07	.068	.064	.06	.058	.056	.053	.051	.049	.047
8 ml/hr	.64	.44	.34	.26	.22	.19	.17	.15	.136	.12	.11	.10	.096	.09	.08	.078	.074	.07	.067	.064	.06	.058	.056	.053
9 ml/hr	.72	.495	.38	.297	.25	.22	.19	.17	.15	.135	.126	.12	.11	.1	.09	.088	.083	.08	.075	.07	.068	.065	.063	.06
10 ml/hr	.8	.55	.42	.33	.28	.24	.21	.19	.17	.15	.14	.13	.12	.11	.1	.098	.092	.09	.084	.08	.076	.073	.07	.067
11 ml/hr	.88	.6	.46	.36	.31	.26	.23	.21	.187	.165	.15	.14	.13	.12	.11	.107	.10	.097	.09	.087	.084	.08	.077	.073
12 ml/hr	.96	.66	.5	.4	.33	.29	.25	.23	.2	.18	.17	.16	.14	.13	.12	.118	.11	.106	.10	.095	.09	.08	.08	.08
13 ml/hr	1.04	.715	.55	.43	.36	.31	.27	.25	.22	.195	.18	.17	.16	.14	.13	.127	.12	.11	.11	.10	.1	.087	.09	.087
14 ml/hr	1.12	.77	.59	.46	.39	.34	.29	.27	.24	.21	.2	.18	.17	.15	.14	.137	.13	.12	.12	.11	.106	.10	.097	.094
15 ml/hr	1.2	.825	.63	.495	.42	.36	.315	.29	.26	.22	.21	.195	.18	.165	.15	.147	.14	.132	.125	.12	.114	.11	.104	.1

*Values expressed represent mcg/kg/min.

PEDIATRIC CONTINUOUS INFUSION RATES (for **50 mg/100** ml concentration)*

										WEIGHT in kg														
	2	3	4	5	6	7	8	9	10	11	12	13	14	15	16	17	18	19	20	21	22	23	24	25
1 ml/hr	4.2	2.8	2.0	1.7	1.4	1.2	1.0	.93	.83	.76	.69	.64	.6	.56	.52	.49	.46	.44	.42	.40	.38	.36	.35	.33
2 ml/hr	8.3	5.6	4.2	3.3	2.8	2.4	2.1	1.85	1.7	1.5	1.4	1.3	1.2	1.1	1.0	.98	.93	.88	.83	.79	.76	.72	.69	.67
3 ml/hr	12.5	8.3	6.2	5.0	4.2	3.6	3.1	2.8	2.5	2.3	2.0	1.9	1.8	1.7	1.6	1.5	1.4	1.3	1.25	1.2	1.1	1.09	1.04	1.0
4 ml/hr	16.7	11.0	8.3	6.7	5.6	4.8	4.2	3.7	3.3	3.0	2.8	2.6	2.4	2.2	2.1	2.0	1.9	1.8	1.7	1.6	1.5	1.4	1.38	1.3
5 ml/hr	20.8	13.9	10.4	8.3	6.9	6.0	5.2	4.6	4.2	3.8	3.5	3.2	3.0	2.8	2.6	2.5	2.3	2.2	2.1	2.0	1.9	1.8	1.7	1.67
6 ml/hr	25.0	16.7	12.5	10.0	8.3	7.0	6.3	5.6	5.0	4.5	4.2	3.8	3.6	3.3	3.1	2.9	2.8	2.6	2.5	2.4	2.3	2.2	2.1	2.0
7 ml/hr	29.0	19.4	14.6	11.7	9.7	8.3	7.3	6.5	5.8	5.3	4.9	4.5	4.2	3.9	3.6	3.4	3.2	3.1	2.9	2.8	2.7	2.5	2.4	2.3
8 ml/hr	33.0	22.0	16.7	13.3	11.0	9.5	8.3	7.4	6.7	6.0	5.6	5.1	4.8	4.4	4.2	3.9	3.7	3.5	3.3	3.2	3.0	2.9	2.8	2.7
9 ml/hr	37.5	25.0	18.7	15.0	12.5	10.7	9.4	8.3	7.5	6.8	6.2	5.8	5.4	5.0	4.7	4.4	4.2	3.9	3.8	3.6	3.4	3.3	3.1	3.0
10 ml/hr	41.7	27.8	20.8	16.7	13.9	11.9	10.4	9.3	8.3	7.6	6.9	6.4	6.0	5.6	5.2	4.9	4.6	4.4	4.2	4.0	3.8	3.6	3.5	3.3
11 ml/hr	45.8	30.6	22.9	18.3	15.3	13.1	11.5	10.2	9.2	8.3	7.6	7.0	6.5	6.1	5.7	5.4	5.1	4.8	4.6	4.4	4.2	4.0	3.8	3.7
12 ml/hr	50.0	33.3	25.0	20.0	16.7	14.3	12.5	11.0	10.0	9.0	8.3	7.7	7.1	6.7	6.2	5.9	5.6	5.3	5.0	4.8	4.5	4.3	4.2	4.0
13 ml/hr	54.0	36.0	27.0	21.7	18.0	15.5	13.5	12.0	10.8	9.8	9.0	8.3	7.7	7.2	6.8	6.4	6.0	5.7	5.4	5.2	4.9	4.7	4.5	4.3
14 ml/hr	58.3	38.9	29.0	23.3	19.4	16.7	14.6	13.0	11.7	10.6	9.7	9.0	8.3	7.8	7.3	6.7	6.5	6.1	5.8	5.6	5.3	5.0	4.9	4.7
15 ml/hr	62.5	41.7	31.0	25.0	20.8	17.9	15.6	13.9	12.5	13.4	10.4	9.6	8.9	8.3	7.8	7.3	7.0	6.6	6.3	6.0	5.7	5.4	5.2	5.0

*Values expressed represent mcg/kg/min.

PEDIATRIC CONTINUOUS INFUSION RATES (for 100 mg/100 ml concentration)*

	WEIGHT in kg																							
	2	3	4	5	6	7	8	9	10	11	12	13	14	15	16	17	18	19	20	21	22	23	24	25
1 ml/hr	8.33	5.56	4.17	3.33	2.8	2.4	2.1	1.85	1.67	1.5	1.39	1.3	1.2	1.1	1.0	.98	.93	.88	.83	.79	.76	.72	.69	.67
2 ml/hr	16.67	11.1	8.30	6.67	5.56	4.8	4.2	3.7	3.3	3.0	2.8	2.6	2.4	2.3	2.1	1.96	1.85	1.75	1.7	1.6	1.5	1.4	1.39	1.33
3 ml/hr	24.9	16.7	12.5	10.0	8.3	7.1	6.2	5.6	5.0	4.5	4.2	3.8	3.6	3.3	3.1	2.9	2.8	2.6	2.5	2.4	2.3	2.2	2.1	2.0
4 ml/hr	33.3	22.2	16.7	13.3	11.1	9.5	8.3	7.4	6.7	6.0	5.6	5.1	4.8	4.4	4.2	3.9	3.7	3.5	3.3	3.2	3.0	2.9	2.8	2.7
5 ml/hr	41.7	27.8	20.9	16.7	13.9	11.9	10.4	9.3	8.3	7.6	6.9	6.4	6.0	5.5	5.2	4.9	4.6	4.4	4.2	4.0	3.8	3.6	3.5	3.3
6 ml/hr	50.0	33.3	25.0	20.0	16.7	14.3	12.5	11.0	10.0	9.0	8.3	7.7	7.0	6.6	6.3	5.9	5.5	5.3	5.0	4.8	4.5	4.3	4.2	4.0
7 ml/hr	58.3	38.9	29.0	23.3	19.4	16.7	14.6	13.0	11.7	10.6	9.7	9.0	8.3	7.7	7.3	6.9	6.5	6.1	5.8	5.6	5.3	5.1	4.9	4.7
8 ml/hr	66.6	44.4	33.3	26.7	22.2	19.0	16.7	14.8	13.3	12.0	11.1	10.3	9.5	8.8	8.3	7.8	7.4	7.0	6.7	6.4	6.1	5.8	5.6	5.3
9 ml/hr	75.0	50.0	37.5	30.0	25.0	21.0	18.7	16.7	15.0	13.6	12.5	11.5	10.7	9.9	9.4	8.8	8.3	7.9	7.5	7.0	6.8	6.5	6.2	6.0
10 ml/hr	83.3	55.6	41.7	33.3	27.8	23.8	20.8	18.5	16.7	15.0	13.9	12.8	11.9	11.1	10.4	9.8	9.3	8.8	8.3	7.9	7.6	7.2	6.9	6.7
11 ml/hr	91.6	61.0	45.9	36.7	30.6	26.2	22.9	20.4	18.3	16.7	15.3	14.0	13.0	12.2	11.5	10.8	10.2	9.6	9.2	8.7	8.3	8.0	7.6	7.3
12 ml/hr	100.0	66.7	50.0	40.0	33.3	28.6	25.0	22.0	20.0	18.2	16.7	15.4	14.3	13.3	12.5	11.8	11.0	10.5	10.0	9.5	9.1	8.7	8.3	8.0
13 ml/hr	108.0	72.0	54.0	43.0	36.0	31.0	27.0	24.0	21.7	19.7	18.0	16.7	15.5	14.4	13.5	12.7	12.0	11.4	10.8	10.3	9.9	9.4	9.0	8.7
14 ml/hr	116.6	77.8	58.4	46.7	38.9	33.3	29.0	25.9	23.3	21.0	19.4	17.9	16.7	15.6	14.6	13.7	13.0	12.3	11.7	11.0	10.6	10.0	9.7	9.3
15 ml/hr	125.0	83.4	62.5	50.0	41.7	35.7	31.0	27.8	25.0	22.7	20.8	19.2	17.9	16.7	15.6	14.7	13.9	13.2	12.5	12.0	11.4	10.9	10.4	10.0

*Values expressed represent mcg/kg/min.

ADULT MEDICATION DOSAGES

DRUG	INDICATION	DOSAGE*	CAUTIONS
Calcium chloride	Electrolyte replacement in cardiac arrest, hypocalcemia, tetany, hypoparathyroidism	500 mg IV initially, with further dose dependent on serum Ca^{++} levels Arrest: 0.5 to 1.0 g IV, not to exceed 1 ml/min† (or 0.7 to 1.4 mEq/min) or 200 to 800 mg into ventricular cavity	Venous irritation with IV use Bradycardia Arrhythmias, arrest Constipation Syncope, tingling sensation May cause severe arrhythmias in digitalized patient
Calcium gluconate	Electrolyte replacement	500 mg to 1 g IV initially;‡ repeat according to serum Ca^{++} levels	Venous irritation with IV use Bradycardia Arrhythmias, arrest Constipation Syncope, tingling sensation Severe arrhythmias in digitalized patient
Dextrose	Replacement therapy for hypoglycemia Reduction of cerebral edema	Dextrose 50%: 25 to 50 g slowly over 1 to 2 min. Maximal 0.5 g/kg/hr Dextrose 25% 1 to 2 ml/kg/dose	Venous irritation at IV site, may cause tissue sloughing with extravasation May cause rapid fluid shifts and circulatory overload
Digitalis			
Digitoxin	Cardiotonic glycoside, which reduces heart rate, increases contraction strength, and works as antiarrhythmic, specifically in treatment of CHF, paroxysmal atrial tachycardia, atrial fibrillation, and atrial flutter	Loading dose: 0.5 to 1.6 mg IV or po in divided doses over 24 hours Maintenance dose: 0.1 mg q1 day (range .05 to 0.3 mg q1 day IV or po)	May cause arrhythmias (heart blocks, premature ventricular contractions, bradycardia), which can precipitate hypotension and CHF Nausea/vomiting Yellow-green halos, blurred vision Agitation, weakness
Digoxin	Cardiotonic glycoside, which reduces heart rate, increases contraction strength, and works as antiarrhythmic, specifically in the treatment of CHF, paroxysmal atrial tachycardia, atrial fibrillation, and atrial flutter	Loading dose: 0.5 to 1.5 mg IV or po in divided doses over 24 hours Maintenance dose: 0.125 to 0.5 mg IV or po daily	May cause heart block, conduction disturbances, and arrhythmias, which can precipitate hypotension and CHF Fatigue Hallucinations Visual disturbances such as yellow-green halos, blurring Nausea/vomiting Do not give calcium salts to digitalized patient, as life-threatening arrhythmias may result

*The drug dosages listed in this table may change according to the patient's system performance, e.g., shock or renal failure. Drug administration and effective ranges are judged by individual clinical response.
†1 g calcium chloride = 13.5 mEq or 270 mg calcium.
‡1 g calcium gluconate = 4.5 mEq or 90 mg calcium.

DRUG	INDICATION	DOSAGE	CAUTIONS
Dobutamine	Adrenergic agent used in refractory heart failure to increase cardiac output and contractility	2.5 to 10.0 mcg/kg/min IV infusion; maximum infusion, 40 mcg/kg/min	May cause tachycardia, hypertension, increased anginal episodes, and premature ventricular ectopy Contraindicated in IHSS Incompatible with alkaline solutions Effect reduced in presence of beta-blocking agents
Dopamine	Adrenergic agent used in treatment of shock, to increase cardiac output and contractility, BP, or blood flow to vital organs	1 to 4 mcg/kg/min* "Dopaminergic" effects, renal dilatation, increased urine output 4 to 8 mcg/kg/min Primary beta-1 adrenergic effects, increased heart rate, increased cardiac contractility; "dopaminergic" effects may persist at this dose ≥8 to 10 mcg/kg/min Alpha-adrenergic effects, peripheral vasoconstriction, marked vasoconstriction at >15 mcg/kg/min	May cause tachycardia, increased ventricular ectopy, hypertension Extravasation may cause sloughing and necrosis of local tissue Incompatible with alkaline solutions Doses exceeding 50 mcg/kg/min may cause oliguria in normotensive patients Hypovolemia should be treated before initiation of dopamine infusion for shock
Isoproterenol	Beta-adrenergic stimulant, which increases heart rate, causes vasodilation, and increases conduction velocity; useful in treating heart blocks and arrhythmias; causes bronchial dilatation	0.02 to 0.06 mg IV, then 0.01 to 0.2 mg IV or .5 to 5.0 mcg/min IV infusion IM: 0.2 mg initially, followed by 0.02 to 1.0 mg prn	May induce headache, palpitations, flushing, nausea and vomiting Bronchial irritation, occasionally edema may result May induce angina Contraindicated if tachycardia is present May expect reduced effect if beta blockers have been used
Norepinephrine	Alpha-adrenergic agent, which elevates BP, increases cardiac output and contractility, and slows sinus rate	8 to 16 mcg/min, with increases of 2 to 4 mcg q15 min until desired BP is reached	Causes necrosis of tissue if extravasation occurs; phentolamine, 5 to 10 mg, infused in area may alleviate sloughing Decreased urine output may result Angina, palpitations, arrhythmias, and hypertension may result from high doses
Sodium polystyrene sulfonate	Resin that removes potassium from GI tract; used in hyperkalemia	15 g daily to four times/day in H_2O or sorbitol 3 to 4 ml/g resin, po 30 to 50 g/dl sorbitol q6 hr per rectum	May cause constipation or diarrhea, nausea and vomiting Sodium retention and/or hypokalemia may result
Potassium chloride	Replacement therapy for hypokalemia	Loading dose: orally, 40 to 100 mEq in divided doses daily for marked depletion of K^+ Maintenance dose: 20 mEq po q1 day 10 to 20 mEq/hr IV (Maximum rate of administration is 30 to 40 mEq/hr) Generally use concentrations of 40 to 60 mEq/L or less, total daily dose not to exceed 150 mEq	Hyperkalemia may result from rapid infusion; flaccid limbs, muscle weakness, nausea/vomiting, arrhythmias, and heart blocks may indicate hyperkalemia Contraindicated in patients with renal failure Never administer by IV push or IM

*These effects and dosages are approximate and the individual response of the patient should always be considered when titrating the dose.

DRUG	INDICATION	DOSAGE	CAUTIONS
Nitroglycerin	Relaxes vascular smooth muscle and dilatates arterial and venous beds; used in control of hypertension, CHF associated with infarction, and angina pectoris	5 mcg/min initially by IV infusion; increase q3-5 min until desired response is obtained	Titrate infusion to PCWP and/or BP Contraindicated in patients with hypotension, hypovolemia, increased ICP, constrictive pericarditis or cardiac tamponade Nitroglycerin adheres to usual IV tubing; special nonabsorbent tubing or dosage adjustment is required
Sodium bicarbonate	Alkaline agent used to correct acidosis induced by altered metabolic states	Acidosis: 2 to 5 mEq/kg IV, infused over 4 to 8 hr periods Cardiac arrest: 1 mEq/kg IV initially; may repeat in doses of 0.5 to 1.0 mEq/kg after 10 minutes If assessment of arterial blood gases is not available, give 0.5 mEq/kg q10 min until circulation is restored	May increase failure in CHF patients, increase BP in hypertension, as well as increase edema Not for use in renal failure Precipitates calcium salts, inactivates catecholamines, i.e., epinephrine
Sodium nitroprusside	Relaxes vascular smooth muscle and dilatates blood vessels, reducing BP Increases cardiac output in CHF	0.5 to 10.0 mcg/kg/min; average dosage 3 mcg/kg/min	Extravasation may cause tissue sloughing Headache, dizziness, nausea, and vomiting may result Hypotension may indicate need for reduction in dose Acidosis may result, especially in patients with renal failure Agent is light sensitive and must be protected with foil; after dilution in IV, must be reconstituted q4-24 hr according to manufacturer's guidelines

Index